GOOD PRACTICE

A Guide to Real General Practice

CHRIS HEATH FRCP MRCGP

Published by Paragon Publishing, Rothersthorpe
First published 2017

ISBN 978-1-78222-482-2

Book design, layout and production management by Into Print
www.intoprint.net
+44 (0) 1604 832149

Printed and bound in UK and USA by Lightning Source

Order additional copies from your favourite bookseller by using the ISBN above or, in case of difficulty, copies are available from
Heathgoodpractice@gmail.com
at £65 each including p and p to UK mainland. (PayPal)
Please contact for shipping costs elsewhere.

This Notebook belongs to:
Dr:

GMC No:
Passport No:
Smear No:
Prescriber No:
Useful Phone Numbers:

Partners: Home: Mobile: E Mail:

Ambulance:
Emergency:
Routine:
District Nurses:
Community Midwife:
Health Visitor:
CMHT

Hospitals/Labs/Physio/X Ray/A and Es etc:
1)
2)
3)
4)
5)

Consultants/specialities: (Good, bad, indifferent and why. Interests/personality/ comments etc) **Contact details: Notes:**

Note: Admissions: Blood P.R.: Fresh: Surgical.
                       Melaena: Medical.
                       Upper G.I. bleeding usually under endoscopists
                       (Physicians)
                       Gallstones: Usually Surgical if acute
                       Renal stones: Urological until it becomes obstructed
                       then Surgical.

Local peculiarities:

Duty PSW OOH:
Sharps Hotline:
OOH service:

OOH Child Protection:
Nursing Homes:

Undertakers:

Pharmacies:

Police:

CONTENTS

1   Politics, Who we are, The CQC etc 8
2   Administration, Training, The Consultation and Teaching. 128
3   Basic Biology 260
4   Acute Medicine in General Practice. 270
5   Alcohol. 303
6   Allergy 307
7   Analgesics. 315
8   Anticoagulants, Clotting, Thrombolysis, Blood etc. 320
9   The Breast. 332
10 Cancer and Terminal Care 337
11 Cardiology 396
12 Some Useful Clinical Signs, Eponymous diseases 448
13 Dermatology 461
14 Diabetes, Metabolism. 474
15 Diet, Diets, Vitamins and Nutrition. 504
16 Driving. 543
17 Odd drugs 549
18 Ear, Nose and Throat 574
19 Gastroenterology 584
20 Geriatrics 604
21 Haematology 607
22 Hormones. 610
23 Immunisations and Vaccinations 624
24 Infections, Antibiotics, Microbiota. 642
25 Legal Issues 695
26 Liver 720
27 Miscellaneous. 726
28 Musculoskeletal, Orthopaedics, Sports, NSAIDs. 740
29 Neurology. 798
30 Ophthalmology 846
31 Paediatrics 858
32 Pathology 954
33 Pregnancy, Obstetrics and Gynaecology, Contraception 1002
34 Psychiatry and Controlled Drugs 1053
35 Respiratory. 1097
36 Sex and Sexually Transmitted Infections 1122
37 Sleep 1130
38 Travel 1145
39 Urology. 1150
40 Work 1180
    References 1190

Good Practice

Good Practice:
The Polemic

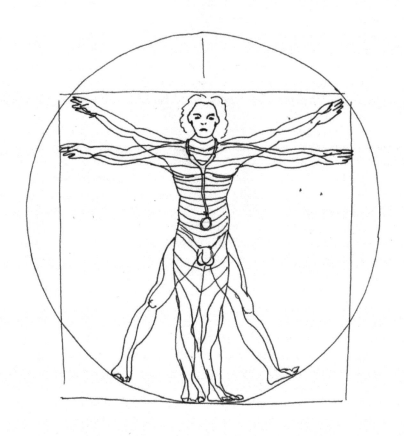

PART ONE

1: Politics, Who we are, The CQC etc

Good Practice, Patient Centred but non P C Family Medicine.

This book is the product of forty years at the front end of NHS medicine and a third to a half a million consultations. There probably aren't any doctors qualifying today who will work half the hours or see half this number of patients in their careers thanks to their restricted working weeks. It has taken five years to write and correct and although some of the information will always remain relevant, some factual details will change quite quickly. This has been particularly true of such things as medical politics, immunisation recommendations, treatments, medical scandals, enquiries and so on. It has been hard to keep up with some of these and I just had to draw the line at an arbitrary date because some lessons, like heart hospitals not talking to relatives just never seemed to sink in. Please write to me if you have suggestions, revisions or corrections or better ways of managing the conditions covered in the text. I will be happy to include them in future updates and credit you appropriately. If you disagree with my views on how poorly some modern doctors, medical schools, Royal Colleges, The GMC, politicians or managers behave then it probably isn't worth contacting me.

I have done my best to be accurate and up to date with all advice, doses and treatments but suggest all physicians check their own doses and medications and satisfy themselves that the advice I am offering is safe, appropriate and satisfactory before using it. I take no responsibility for any harm that you may inadvertently cause.

I have been in NHS practice for forty years. I have worked in a mixture of specialities, Medicine and Surgery, Obstetrics and Gynaecology, Anaesthetics, Intensive Care and Psychiatry. I was a career Paediatrician for over 5 years, eventually lecturing Child Medicine at a teaching hospital before having Damascene change of heart. This led me to leave hospital medicine and do thirty years as what in America is called a Primary Care Physician in three different General Practices. I have been a GP Trainer and an Appraiser ever since appraisal for GP s began in 2002. I took a few months sabbatical away from appraisal to complete this book and was refused permission to continue appraising. Perhaps when you have read the book you will see why.

As far as my hospital life was concerned, I went to medical school, – no one from my family or my secondary school had ever done so before, in September 1970. I qualified in 1975, having done preclinical training and a locum or two on the wards as a student. Then I did gruelling house jobs, a long apprenticeship of SHO and registrar jobs and I finally lectured my chosen speciality of Paediatrics at a grand teaching hospital. These were "one in two" and "one in three" rotas. In other words, working weeks of 130-140 hours each. There was teaching "by humiliation", (although this was rare in my experience), my registrar, the next person on call with me in my first house job of trauma and general surgery lived twenty miles away at night and weekends. He was often reluctant to come in and help. You saw a procedure, then copied it, then taught it in quick succession in a "see one, do one, teach one" sequence. You often felt quite alone. I was doing central venous cannulation as an junior SHO in 1976, something I heard on the radio that a senior registrar was unable to do while volunteering in Sierra Leone in 2014. She would have been five years or so older than me but less technically experienced in this one respect at least. The senior nurses on the wards were generally antagonistic and unhelpful to me and to the other house staff throughout my junior medical grades until my tenure in any job had lasted a year or so and by then they might have got to know the new doctors and softened a little. I remember a programme on television called "Cardiac Arrest" about a junior doctor fighting exhaustion, antagonistic nurses and unreasonable relatives while trying to treat seriously ill patients and learn his trade simultaneously. Few believed that hospitals could be as unfriendly as that. They **were** then, but are far less so, for a variety of reasons now. They were hard and sometimes challenging working conditions but they produced a technically able, experienced, confident and a usually more proficient, safer work force than exists today and one which offered the patient continuity, familiarity and consistency.

In the last few months of 2014 the GMC became alarmed at the emotional sensitivity and seeming suicide proneness of many modern doctors, especially those being complained against. It told medical schools to start teaching "emotional resilience". The subtext for doctors of my generation was that the overwhelmingly female and intellectualised medical profession of today was oversensitive, -"soft". Undoubtedly part of the problem is the alienation, slowness and naivety of the GMC complaints structure, procedure and staff. There are almost no doctors with experience of General Practice (GP is 90% of the work of the NHS) at the GMC. (Stop Press: Throughout the writing of this book there were no GPs on the GMC Council. But by 2017, one had appeared, Professor Anthony Harnden with 26 years GP experience. You could say that the twelve members on average had two years each.) But there is also a current increasingly female and Working Time Directive protected medical workforce. They are far less naturally "resilient" than my generation. By 2015 it was announced that the suicide risk of GMC investigated doctors was 13 x the general population. 28 doctors had probably killed themselves while under investigation between 2005 and 2013. Speakers at the 2015 LMC's conference said that the GMC investigation process ignored basic human rights and forced many doctors to endure investigations lasting as much as five years. The presumption was "guilty until proven innocent", the current situation is "unfair, unkind and unacceptable" said one speaker. Responding to a similar LMC debate in Scotland the conference demanded reforms to speed up processes, reduce the stress of investigations and better support doctors who had their fitness to practise called into question.

The Medical Protection Society conducted a survey of doctors under GMC investigation in 2015 and 47% did not believe that they had received enough support during the process, a quarter considering actually leaving the profession because of the investigation itself. All doctors who comment on the process speak about being considered guilty until proven innocent, the glacial slowness, the isolation they felt and the distance from reality of the GMC organisation itself.

On the other hand perhaps doctors today are hypersensitive, a bit over susceptible to depression compared with a few decades ago. Is that possible? Are we becoming too soft, too emotional? Have the medical schools gone too far in unseating the white male Dr Finlay? It might well be imagined that a career of working with sick, depressed, demanding, unreasonable, suffering and dying patients might seem a wholly negative and therefore emotionally depressing environment. So why shouldn't its practitioners become depressed? That would be natural surely. On the other hand I can only remember ONE seriously depressed student or doctor in my first thirty years and there was only one consultant I worked with in my entire early medical life who committed suicide. He was a lovely committed, caring consultant Paediatric Oncologist. So I don't believe depression has to come with the job:

I believe a sea change, described extensively elsewhere, in the sort of people selected for medical school has happened during my medical career. Today, doctors seem unprepared for the long hours necessary to become proficient at their craft, the sacrifices they have to make to learn the techniques, knowledge and skills. They are unwilling to adapt to the servitude and availability, to the patients often needing to come before family and self and so we have a poorly committed, resentful, floundering and chronically depressed young medical profession. The job hasn't changed, the character and personality of people allowed to do it have. Too few army officers and rugby players, too many young mums and female part timers. A major new (2016) review of 200 studies in nearly 50 countries (!) confirmed high rates of depression and suicidal ideation amongst medical students. (Rotenstein JAMA Dec 2016 17324): The prevalence of depressive symptoms or depression in medical students was 27%, 11% reporting suicidal ideation at medical school. Only 16% sought treatment. The authors relate the high levels of depression found in residents (29%) and the high levels in students (27%). I just wonder why nearly all the harrowing stories of suicide and misery I have heard in junior doctors recently seem to be about very high functioning, high achieving females. Given the majority of psychiatric illness in doctors does seem to be in female doctors, given that women in medicine have more time off sick than their male colleagues and the majority of medical students are now female, why do we continue to dominate an emotionally demanding and unforgiving profession with the gender that seems to have this particular vulnerability? Surely this is unfair on the female student/doctor, her colleagues, her patients and the tax payer.

Despite all the above, the training is certainly far less arduous today than it was even a couple of decades ago, the hours of duty a fraction of what they were, and as I constantly say, the profession has been emasculated over the last 20 years. Doctors feel entitled to and receive less criticism and more support from colleagues today so they don't need the thick skins of their forbears. It did come as a slight surprise however that 14% of General Practitioners of today had suicidal thoughts (Mind, 2016) with their protected and supported training, their day off a week and their home by 7pm working life. I couldn't help thinking what had they got to be depressed about? No, seriously, try adding an evening and night on call every third night, a few out of bed night visits plus a weekend surgery, Saturday and Sunday every third week.........

The latest results:

Having contacted every medical school in the UK and asked them myself while preparing this book, it turns out that doctors seem to be selected now almost solely on academic performance so this new personal sensitivity isn't surprising. How DO you assess at the age of 18, a candidate's subsequent maturity, common sense, trustworthiness, fortitude, confidence, groundedness, friendliness, determination, generosity of spirit and backbone – all the characteristics that good doctors have and aren't necessarily selected by our present minimum 3 A stars at A Level? What we select for now is academic prowess, skill at exams, lack of life experience, high pressure coaching, determined family and professional support and we get a highly sexually and racially biased group of emotionally naive medical students. With a disproportionately small number of white male candidates. (White males 26% medical students, 43% of the population. Dr Theodore Dalrymple, Telegraph). Mainly female highly academic 3 A-star students are not the sort of people whose life experience or personality would naturally have acquired them the determination, self worth, confidence, self reliance and thick skin of the GMC's "emotional resilience". Multiple studies have shown these academic female doctors' higher rates of sickness, both physical and emotional, as well as increased suicide rates. Indeed, It might be that the profession is being specifically selected to be **unable to develop those tough characteristics**. I have trained and appraised many young doctors who were entirely unprepared for the emotional demands that medicine makes. Face to face interviews and assessments of candidate's actual personalities are rare. It begs the question however, whether a thick skin and self confidence are things you can select for at interview or subsequently teach. In the past these characteristics were an inevitable consequence of doing the job. It was a tough, relentless apprenticeship. But we were, by and large, more self reliant, less emotionally vulnerable. We had to be. We were respected by patients for this commitment, dedication and vocation and it did make us far more self reliant than today's generation of doctors. Apparently. When I listened to striking doctors (2015-2016) being interviewed, one sixth of whom were, it was clear, taking their £500,000 – £850,000 medical education and going to Australia or New Zealand for "fewer hours and better pay", I realise what a cultural shift in doctors' attitude has taken place. Australia already had 7,500 of our doctors in 2016, so how long are we going to be supporting their health service when ours is the one that clearly needs more well trained doctors?

There was talk after the 2016 doctors' strike of a reduction in applications for medical school places, of a perception, after all the strike associated moaning by juniors that the job might be a bit more challenging than most teenagers would be happy with. This, of course was not the case: There were a total in 2015 of 82,034 applications for 7,424 places. (One place for eleven applicants). The numbers, of course hide multiple applications to different medical schools by the same applicant. The number of individual applicants was 20,100. Success at getting in depended on country of origin:

40% for UK applicants
10% for EU applicants
20% for non EU applicants.

I did several years in hospital, mainly as a Paediatrician but I then realised that the life of a GP rather than a consultant would offer greater control over the quality of care I could give and allow me the *personal* independence to do the job properly. For doctors, life then was much, much harder than it is now. For patients, the care was generally much better. I estimate I have seen about a third to half a million patients in all over the forty years since I started clinical practice and because of the hours we worked before statutory working time restrictions, at any given stage in my career, I had seen about twice as many patients as my equivalent doctor today. I was twice as experienced at the same age.

Like everyone, I assumed the NHS and the healthcare it gave would get better and better as time went on. But any patient who went into hospital or who saw their GP regularly in the 70's or 80's will tell you that apart from the technology and some clinical outcomes, the overall quality of the Health Service is noticeably worse now than it was then. The basic quality of medical and nursing care, the personal attitudes of respect and politeness, professional relationships, language skills, standards of behaviour, even dress codes, – things we all thought were sacrosanct, have changed for the worse for reasons undebated, unexplained and with general public regret. You only have to look at the health related headlines of the last twenty years to see how badly wrong things have gone.

Pip in Great Expectations smells Jaggers' soap scented hands and at first wonders if he could be a doctor. Then **"But No I thought, he couldn't be a doctor, or he would have a quieter and more persuasive manner"**. Is that how people regard doctors now?

Look at how Josephine Tey, famous writer of detective novels gets a bed ridden 1950's Scotland Yard detective to describe the nurse who enters his room:

"She stood there slender and remote, as elegant in her way as Marta was; her white cuffed hands clasped loosely in front of her narrow waist; her white veil spreading itself in imperishable dignity; her only ornament the small silver badge of her diploma. Grant (The detective) wondered if there was anywhere in this world a more unshakable poise than that achieved by the matron of a great hospital". Few of us regard doctors or nurses with such unqualified admiration today.

This is a handbook of facts, the sort of thing that I always wished that I could have had ready access to during my 30 plus years as a GP and the ten years of hospital medicine that preceded it. But it is also a critique of many aspects of a service that has let huge numbers of patients down for purely political reasons and often refuses to recognise or address its own short comings. There are some personal opinions thrown in based on four decades of experience at the sharp end of the NHS. It is obvious to everyone who has seen the progress of the NHS over the last few decades that many things are dysfunctional from top to bottom in what was once our nation's pride and joy. It is quite clear to patients and many doctors why the scandals and disasters happen. The only puzzle is why politicians, administrators, regulators, trainers and Royal Colleges didn't see them coming and why many refuse to address them now. From the point of view of experienced doctors, we see that training has deteriorated, in hospitals and General Practice. The abilities of GPs and hospital staff, their clinical skills up to and (according to the RCP) Consultant level, but also their ability simply to communicate with their patients, their dedication and vocation, standards of dress, behaviour and commitment have all worsened over probably the last two to three decades. Even the quality of caring – perhaps the most puzzling, damaging and important loss for patients and relatives has deteriorated markedly in many diverse units and departments all over the country. Perhaps this is not universal: Examples of excellent practice abound in hospitals and G.P. but the national soul searching has applied to ward and management nursing staff, academic departments of nursing, CQC inspectors and administrators, senior and junior managers as well as doctors of various grades and seems an entirely new phenomenon in our National Health Service. I have had decades of professional and personal experience and feedback from patients and colleagues, hospital doctors and nurses as well as fellow trainers, appraisers and G P s. Many friends and family members have visited their GPs as patients and been to hospital as in and out patients in recent years all over the country. They have recounted their experiences to me and about a quarter of their interactions over the last twenty or so years seem have been clearly unsatisfactory in one way or another. Most patients who look back twenty or more years say that standards and attitudes were better then. So why are they now worse, who is supposed to police and improve these "standards" and who is to blame for the slow and progressive loss of something that we used once to take for granted and value so highly ? It is also obvious that almost every attempt by politicians and academics to change the way the service is run, funded and organised has resulted in a worse experience for the patient.

Now we are told there will be a legal sanction of "Wilful Neglect" (2014), that nurses will have to be taught to "Care" and we have needed a lawyer, – a QC, Robert Francis, to tell us to put the patient's interests at the heart of our activities. I never thought that day would come. When I qualified in the mid seventies it was a different medical world, – but clearly in many ways a much better one from the point of view of the patient.

I firmly believe there are simple but almost certainly politically unacceptable answers to all the disasters of the last few decades – Including Harold Shipman himself. In his case, it was the political and subsequent administrative response that has caused most of the harm not just Shipman himself. He was one psychopath amongst a quarter of a million UK doctors but his legacy of harm continues through the misunderstanding by political legislators of an infrequent but essential role of GPs. In particular of the need to have ready access to strong pain control in primary care at all times. How has the political response damaged patient care? Let me explain. It is through the constantly recurring:

The Unforeseen Consequences Rule of NHS Change:

Because Shipman used Diamorphine to murder his innocent victims, our politicians have reacted by deciding to make the legal requirements of obtaining, auditing and disposing of Controlled Drugs almost impractically complicated for busy doctors to undertake. As a consequence almost no GPs carry proper pain killers now because the regulations on controlled drug management are so complicated and impractical that most doctors (90% of GPs in fact) have, shockingly, left acute pain relief to someone else. The whole ethos of primary care being a Boy Scout service ready to help in any emergency, anywhere, has now disappeared. The patient experience of sudden acute pain is currently often a miserable one of ambulances that are delayed, out of hours doctors who don't have access to strong pain killers, (these are now stored in central, inaccessible locations) or in some cases notoriously administer drugs that are now unfamiliar and give overdoses that kill the patient. When they get to A and E the doctors can be overwhelmed by trivial cases, or at weekends the over 50% of cases that can be alcohol related (Emerg. Med J online Dec21 2015), or understaffing and frequently leave the patient suffering on trolleys in corridors for hours. One of my patients who dislocated his hip had to wait several hours before he was given any effective pain relief at all. He was horrified by the inhumanity of the experience. I was angry, upset and frustrated by the depressing familiarity of it.

Every single disaster in this scene of woe is a direct result of soft contemporary politics denuding the certainties of traditional medicine: The over 2/3 feminisation of medical schools and the emasculation of medicine generally, combined with the Working Time Directive means fewer full time doctors and fewer doctors (generally male), willing to do the arduous rotas of A and E. The doctors there are undertrained. Equality and Diversity legislation, the over education of nurses, misdirected human rights legislation, the endless and progressive attempt to knock doctors off their pedestals of authority and control, particularly white male doctors, means that doctors no longer control the clear provision of a consistent quality of care. A destructuring of organisational hierarchies within the NHS, – the inevitable unforeseen consequences of misguided politicians and lawyers who have never treated a sick patient. All of these have had some influence in this catalogue of disasters. If you think I am exaggerating, try and find alternative rational explanations for the daily failures we read about in our newspapers.

You may have noticed that doctors don't wear white coats anymore, or ties or have long sleeves – unless they are the Swiss surgeons on TV caring for injured Formula one drivers, or American doctors on websites or private British doctors, Physicians, GPs or Surgeons in adverts and in real life private hospitals. Here is what GPs look like and how they dress when patients: 1) Choose them rather than being allocated to them and 2) Pay good money to see them on top of their direct taxation. You have to admit this doctor looks like a doctor. This is not what most NHS doctors go onto the wards looking like. See Census of Consultant Physicians Cover (on page 33).

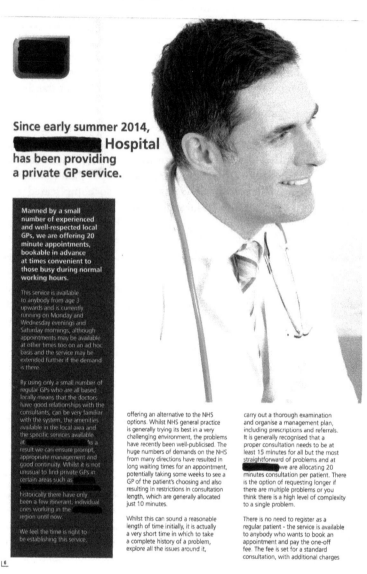

Since early summer 2014, ▮▮▮▮▮▮▮▮ Hospital has been providing a private GP service.

Manned by a small number of experienced and well-respected local GPs, we are offering 20 minute appointments, bookable in advance at times convenient to those busy during normal working hours.

This service is available to anybody from age 3 upwards and is currently running on Monday and Wednesday evenings and Saturday mornings, although appointments may be available at other times too on an ad hoc basis and the service may be extended further if the demand is there.

By using only a small number of regular GPs who are all based locally means that the doctors have good relationships with the consultants, can be very familiar with the system, the amenities available in the local area and the specific services available at ▮▮▮▮▮▮▮▮. As a result we can ensure prompt, appropriate management and good continuity. Whilst it is not unusual to find private GPs in certain areas such as ▮▮▮▮▮▮▮▮

historically there have only been a few itinerant, individual ones working in the ▮▮▮▮▮▮▮▮ region until now.

We feel the time is right to be establishing this service,

offering an alternative to the NHS options. Whilst NHS general practice is generally trying its best in a very challenging environment, the problems have recently been well-publicised. The huge numbers of demands on the NHS from many directions have resulted in long waiting times for an appointment, potentially taking some weeks to see a GP of the patient's choosing and also resulting in restrictions in consultation length, which are generally allocated just 10 minutes.

Whilst this can sound a reasonable length of time initially, it is actually a very short time in which to take a complete history of a problem, explore all the issues around it,

carry out a thorough examination and organise a management plan, including prescriptions and referrals. It is generally recognised that a proper consultation needs to be at least 15 minutes for all but the most straightforward of problems and at ▮▮▮▮▮▮▮▮ we are allocating 20 minutes consultation per patient. There is the option of requesting longer if there are multiple problems or you think there is a high level of complexity to a single problem.

There is no need to register as a regular patient - the service is available to anybody who wants to book an appointment and pay the one-off fee. The fee is set for a standard consultation, with additional charges

6

You may have been an inpatient and seen that our doctors don't seem to dress smartly any more at all. Your initial thoughts that standards and attitudes are deteriorating may have been assuaged by the thought that there was a good reason for this. The rolled up sleeves and lack of ties are supposed to cut down infection. Actually they don't. Private hospitals and European hospitals where male doctors do still tend to wear ties and long sleeves have far lower infection rates than NHS hospitals where they wander around like night club drop outs. No one has ever proven that ties (tucked in to shirts or otherwise) and long sleeves contribute to cross infection. Even Alan Johnson the Health Secretary who introduced the "bare below the elbows" recommendation admitted that there was "Little scientific evidence to support the move". Ironically all staff wear identity badges now and these as much as neckties, lanyards and watches (and now, so the evidence shows, stethoscopes), can become colonised with transferable bacteria. So to be consistent about the bare below the elbows we doctors and nurses should really all be bare above the waist and scrub all exposed skin between seeing each patient. But then there is increasing evidence that hand scrubs, gels and disinfectants, medicated soaps and talcs are, of course, creating multi treatment resistant superbugs against which we will have no active agent, topical or systemic. So all those disinfectants are helping to cause the killer infections we fear the most.

Like so many changes affecting what used to be called "standards" the unforeseen consequence of this new slovenliness is a diminution in status, authority, of perceived structure, even security and respect (sorry to use those old fashioned terms but most patients over 40 will relate to the concepts) within the doctor/patient relationship. And the indirect effect is that of knocking the doctor, particularly the consultant, off his pedestal. But then maybe that **was** the idea.

I was pleased to see an article from the previously silent BMJ on doctors' dress code: "Scrubs or jeans – what should doctors wear to work?" by Kathy Oxtoby in July 2015 which highlighted some of these issues. Although this review did say that doctors currently look a mess and were the worst dressed group of professionals in hospitals, hard to identify and seriously deprofessionalised, the solution she gave was a uniform. Not a return to respectable formal "professional" clothing. Not a morning inspection by the consultant or registrar.

The author made no mention of the effect on patients of the doctors' dishevelled appearance, the dishonest reasons for ending long sleeves, white coats and ties, the fact that they do not cause infection and in hospitals where they are worn, infection rates are often at their lowest. She did say that hospital doctors today look a mess and implied that patients found it harder to trust and respect someone who looked like they were still students on their gap year or returning from an all night party. Isn't that all obvious?

This is one soft political ideology and its consequence: Make the doctor less authoritarian, and instead of them becoming more human the result is that you make the doctor less of an authority and give them less of an air of authority. The result: the patient then has no one trustworthy to trust. Familiarity breeds contempt. One thing every doctor needs to learn early in their career is that inspiring trust and confidence especially by a professional approach, appearance and attitude makes your job easier and helps patients get better quicker.

Another about which I give the facts later is: Make the doctor less likely to be male and you make the profession warmer and more caring: Well the actual result has been the exact opposite. 70% of medical students and new doctors are now female. You would suppose this would make a more empathetic medical profession. The actual result for the patient is that, despite there being more doctors overall, you are less likely to see **any** doctor these days. This is because female doctors are more likely to be part – time, assistants or job sharers so they do far fewer hours in their careers and continuity of care everywhere is reduced. Also women doctors like doing Paediatrics but they do not as a rule choose careers in Surgery, Casualty, Orthopaedics or full time GP partnerships – these are generally considered to be less family friendly. This is nationally acknowledged as a major cause of the crisis in A and E and other specialities.

The latest figures show (2016) 18% of consultants are part time (all or nearly all female), across the UK. 40% of consultant posts remain unfilled, in some areas 60% are unfilled, perhaps because despite the record numbers of doctors coming through training, so many are opting for part time careers. In the 2016 State of the Nation Report, covered by all national newspapers, the shocking statistic that only 10% of medical graduates intended to work full time was disclosed. Ironically the failure of female doctors to do Emergency Medicine has caused closures of casualty units but the popularity of Paediatrics amongst women has done the same. In 2015 it was disclosed in a number of daily papers that Paediatric units across the country were in crisis because they could not afford expensive agency locum staff. The reason? 70% of their full time staff were female and so many of them were off on maximum maternity leave then returning to work only part time. Too many women in a speciality cripples Paediatric units, just like too few women closes casualty units. By 2016 the Sunday Times was predicting a virtual end to adequate staffing levels in Paediatric units across the country (14/8/16) and a severe curtailment of normal services. This was because (Nigel Edwards, Nuffield Trust Chief Executive) "There had not been enough training of Paediatric junior staff due to the exacting standards we expect and PART TIME WORKING". Well only one of those two factors is new and easily explicable.

It all comes down to a simple fact: Social medicine can't work if too many of its practitioners put family above patients and are significantly less than full time.

I also believe that the most empathetic and understanding doctors I have worked with, bar none, have all been male. Many (not all) female doctors, despite now being the majority, still over compensate for a subjective sense of competitive disadvantage in their professional abilities. Some feel they have to replace confidence with intransigence, flexibility with distance, fairness with hardness. Also male and female doctors don't **work** the same way:

Female doctors refer more patients for investigations and second opinions. Most research suggests 30% more – and so secondary care, hospital departments and casualty units are now busier, presumably with larger numbers of relatively healthy patients. Female doctors make fewer intuitive guesses, have fewer gut feelings, rely more on objective (and expensive) evidence, a mindset that makes them intrinsically less suited to areas such as Primary Care and Emergency Medicine. Any professional area which depends upon diagnostic intuition and risk taking.

The **Working Time Directive** sounds like a good idea to avoid tired staff by limiting the working week to 48 hours but the consequence is that we have a poorly experienced and less competent medical work force than at any time since the start of the NHS. We also have one of the youngest medical work forces (due to some new medical school building) in the Western world. Young, inexperienced, unwilling to work longer and working half to a third of the hours of their predecessors of a couple of decades ago. Reassuring isn't it?

If you have been an in-patient over a weekend you will also know there is no consistency or continuity between on call teams in hospitals at weekends and a higher death rate at weekends too. Staff don't seem to stay around to hand over – apart from nurses and they spend hours in the office away from the ward at each shift change, "handing over". For doctors this is in no small part due to shorter rotas and lack of experience due to the WTD. As I have said elsewhere, my career has seen junior doctors' working weeks **reduced to a third (This is the Working Time Directive averaged limit). The 2016 contract reduced single week hours from a maximum of 91 to 72 hours and the number of nights from seven to four, the maximum number of consecutive days from 7 to 5.** Today there is an averaged 48 hours maximum – down from my 1970's one in two rota of 136 hours. So juniors today have a third of the experience, a third of the knowledge, confidence, safety, competence and ability of their forbears at all stages in their careers up to and including consultant. As far as junior obstetricians are concerned, when surveyed, four fifths (82%) of trainees believed that the Directive had reduced training opportunities and half (52%) observed that job satisfaction had been reduced. Just over half of trainees believed that their work-life balance had improved. A survey by the Association of Surgeons in Training showed that of 1510 surgical trainees responding, 67% did clinical work while off duty to "protect their training, " 75% were not happy to be working an EWTD compliant rota and 84% had seen no improvement in work-life balance. In the 2016 Royal College of Physicians annual census (13,003 consultants) "There had been a gradual fall over the last five years in perceptions of how well Certificate of Completion of Training holders (applicants for consultant posts) feel trained in their speciality". I am not surprised – All as a result of the" good idea" of reducing working hours. Outcome: Disaster for patients. Insecurity and inexperience for doctors.

As if to emphasise how wrong this whole policy has been, a new study (BMJ 2016 352.i719, 5 Feb) objectively demonstrated that longer continuous working shifts (over 28 hours continuously for hospital doctors), do not cause harm to patients. This is something many older, more experienced doctors have long suspected. – mine were up to 80 hour weekends in the 70's and 80's. No one is suggesting today's juniors should work as hard as we did then *(or could work those hours)*. But the demand by the current feminised working time directed workforce to keep their sessions and working weeks *so* short and family friendly seems more and more to do with self interest than altruism and is destined to prevent them from ever reaching their predecessors' standard of competence.

So to summarise: In the last couple of decades of my career, the working week for doctors has reduced from 136 hours (on a 1 in 2 rota) to a third of that, 48 hours. Meanwhile, sickness absence has increased 300%, all other forms of illness, from depression to physical and emotional causes and of course suicide, have gone up. Female doctors, also are less likely to report their emotional and mental illnesses (Gen Hosp Psychiatry 2016 2016 Andrew *et Al). In the same time the percentage of female doctors has more than trebled. "Women physicians complete suicide at the same rate as male physicians whereas in the general population women complete suicide far less often than their male counterparts" Dr Andrew*

Well, there it is: an NHS where soft politics and decisions made by governments, Medical School Selection Committees, Royal Colleges, The D o H and no one knows who, have unforeseen consequences, often negative, on the patient. Someone somewhere may have wanted those pompous male consultants brought down a peg or two and misused infection control and feminism to do it but in the long run they changed all our lives for the worse. Part time doctors with open necked shirts, rolled up sleeves, party hair and short frocks, slippers and dangly earrings. How can you take a junior doctor seriously who looks too young (like I did for the first 20 years after I qualified) but who also wears none of the cultural badges of seriousness and responsibility and doesn't EVEN look like he or she is trying to be taken seriously?

"Doctoring is an art, not a science: and any layman interested in science sufficiently to follow the literature knows more about it than those doctors, probably the large majority, who practice only to earn their bread". "A life spent making mistakes is not only more honourable but more useful than one spent doing nothing "

So said George Bernard Shaw in The Doctor's Dilemma.

Patients may have faith in doctors: "Belief has nothing to do with medicine-I am into knowledge not belief". Dr Michael Cunningham, Consultant Gastroenterologist, Geneva.

The best way to be an effective doctor is to persuade your patients that you actually like them.

Everyone has an opinion on how a good doctor should practice and what makes a good doctor in the first place. These opinions will vary but we all know when we have been treated by an inadequate one. Today most people not only have an opinion on how doctors should conduct themselves but on how their own illness should be treated. "Expert patients" can be well read and informed or widely misread, deluded and misinformed. All doctors should strive to be expert in their field but to know the limits of their expertise. This especially applies to a speciality where you have to know something about everything like General Practice.

These days data is far more readily available than a hundred years ago. A tidal wave of facts on the Internet, totally unedited and unqualified and anyone with an iPhone can try matching their information against your knowledge as their GP. What you have, hopefully, if you are a good doctor, as well as power, is knowledge, experience, wisdom and a degree of authority. The latter takes familiarity, time, contact and trust to acquire and to exercise but authority, some seriousness and demeanour are just as important as accessibility and friendliness. Probably more important. It is a difficult balancing act. Demeanour means taking time to consider how you are being perceived by the patient, not naively believing that appearances don't matter. They most assuredly do.

While writing this I read a Sunday Times editorial where the relatives of a British traveller killed abroad were distressed and horrified to be dealt with by a consular staff member in shorts and a T shirt. This is how many bereaved and frightened patients feel when dealt with by doctors who are similarly inappropriately, disrespectfully, informally dressed. Not all medicine is fun, entertaining and making friends and although we don't have to dress like undertakers it is inappropriate that most junior doctors, both male and female now dress even less smartly than assistants at mobile phone stores.

This is not meant to be a complete guide to General Practice. If it were it would be thousands of pages long and be about everything in medicine. I assume you will know where to access travel prophylaxis advice, updated immunisation information, new drug data, differential diagnoses, detailed haematology, physiological data and so on. I assume you will have access to MIMS, Palliative Care Guidance, BNF, Clinical Evidence, NICE and other Guidelines etc. It is more a collection of my own opinions reflecting those of most real patients and personal desk top lecture notes that I have found useful. There is a lot that I haven't included so feel free to stick extra pages in wherever you like.

GPs do most of the medicine and see by far the most patients in the NHS- that is why it is so wrong for GPs to be underrepresented on the GMC and GP to be under represented in medical school training. The GMC at last acquired its one member with GP experience onto its Governing Council during the writing of this book. (One of the twelve Council members had been a GP and he was the first I had seen, in 2017). Name a non surgical subject (except radiology) and GP s do the majority of it. Psychiatry? Our local unit has been so inaccessible unreliable, uncaring and inconsistent that to all intents and purposes, it has barely existed at all for the last 25 years and the local GPs have had to take uncomfortable treatment initiation and management decision risks daily. The same went for adolescent psychiatry and a number of other specialist departments. This is not the picture of the thriving, dedicated, integrated, caring, treasured NHS that Westminster politicians always portray when they talk about it. But it is the result of politicians and soft politics, not doctors, managing our health care for decades. It remains to be seen whether Local Commissioning Groups will improve this and have the honesty and courage to put patients before politics and self interest. First signs are not promising. CCGs began in 2012. By 2016 GPs were "Tiring of CCGs" according to GP magazines and given the slowness of clinical improvements and the speed of some family members' business involvements it is not hard to see CCGs as Fund Holding Mark 2. The Kings Fund and Nuffield Trust report of July 2016 found that only 1 in 5 GPs felt they could influence CCGs (surely the whole point of them?) Two years earlier 35% felt they were able to influence CCGs.

The book is in two parts: Polemic – a discussion and opinions on how the NHS works, including training, organisation, what is going wrong and a limited foray into politics and part 2, Lecture Notes under system headings.

Basically as I have already said, getting the NHS fit again comes down to more personal responsibility, for patients and staff, less politics and probably fewer better staffed services. Certainly more beds. About 25% more permanent beds, especially acute and mental health beds.

Since 1987 the number of NHS beds has approximately halved. Every year 80,000 people (this excludes Scotland which doesn't keep its own figures) have long planned operations cancelled due to a shortfall built into the system. My own mother was admitted to my DGH on three occasions for her much needed hip replacement, cancelling the milk and being wished good luck by her friends each time. Each time she was told after waiting all day on the orthopaedic day unit there was no bed and she had to go home. She found the get well soon cards on her mat three separate times from the same friends. Eventually she decided to pay for the operation to be done privately.

This is more than just a text book, it is a personal guidebook based on 40 years of hard work and seeing things frequently going wrong. My own ancient London medical school, The Middlesex Hospital, one of the best in the country, was closed and demolished twenty years ago in an epically stunning, stupid and destructive act of vandalism. According to "Migrating Doctors" (Clinical Medicine 2017 Vol. 17 No 1) 36% of our doctors obtained their primary medical qualification abroad, a greater proportion than any other European country. How is it (the article questions) that the fifth richest economy in the world is so dependent on doctors from countries whose health needs exceed ours? They have contributed £15Bn to the exchequer in saved medical school fees but as you will see, do not necessarily always come with an equivalent medical school set of skills or from the GMC's statistics, appear equally able from the patient's point of view. The situation is doubly ironic when you consider a fifth of our home trained doctors plan to emigrate to Australia or New Zealand. This country imports thousands of foreign doctors each year who pass the GMC entrance exams in Medicine and English, a huge percentage of whom subsequently fail British assessments of competence. About a quarter cannot speak English acceptably by any objective standard. They are now allowed to fail the MRCGP exam five times before finally considered below a British standard. Why only five? The BAPIO representing doctors who qualified in India took The RCGP to court saying the exam was culturally biased. Of course it is. It is meant to assess the candidate's readiness to work, speak, communicate with, integrate and diagnose British patients. General practice demands that the GP understands more about the patient than what disease causes what symptoms. The best GPs are part of their community, trusted, relied on and integrated into it. Wherever they came from. Cultural attitudes and language are the foundations of that relationship. But we do need, urgently, to build four or five British medical schools if we are going to stop being dependent on foreign doctors forever. We also need a proper understanding with our junior doctors regarding their half of the contract. They get the most expensive state education and one of the highest income careers available. In return they should agree to work in the UK, mostly full time and not go on strike over (what to my generation of doctors seems) unreasonable demands. It seems that every significant political interference or reorganisation for decades has resulted in direct harm to the way staff work with patients, to have resulted in diminished kindness and empathic care. These two things are unauditable and unquantifiable but more important to the patient than anything else the NHS can offer. I think that good humane medical and nursing care are basically a part personal, part emotional and part professional response to the doctor's and nurse's first contact with any sick patient. A humane RE – Action. Some of what has gone wrong is that managers and politicians who have never doctored or nursed have tried to make doctors and nurses quicker and more efficient. They have applied management and political thought processes to jobs that are difficult to organise, regiment and catalogue in that way without dehumanising them. A managed approach might work if the job were standardised and predictable, if you were selling cans of beans or teddy bears but generally speaking, greater efficiency, speedier processing, higher bed occupancy, process focussed and protocol driven working completely ruins the patient experience AND that of the staff. And puts lives and health at risk.

I believe that doctors and nurses if left to their own devices and without targets, protocols, pathways of "care" would never have become as alienated from their patients as we all seem to have done in the last twenty years. We are not selling a product but in a real sense we are selling ourselves. Instead, how we work is now taken out of our hands, the process becomes the sole reason you go onto the ward or book appointments in surgery, the needs of the organisation are paramount, not the patient. So nurses don't wander the ward nursing, offering drinks, conversation and friendship. Going where they are needed. They give five minutes to each bed occupant in succession, checking temperature, blood pressure, confirming tablets have been dispensed, the DNAR form has been signed and that their own work sheet is filled in. They become inflexible. They spend hours of their day on form filling and record keeping or "handing over" when very little of this record keeping should actually be necessary. The shift hand over used to take ten minutes. Now the ward is deserted for ages.

Oh and I also believe that doctors should doctor and nurses should nurse. That means that an experienced doctor should always override the clinical decisions of a nurse. Whatever her protocol or priorities dictate. You cannot have different perspectives at conflict over the management on one patient.

In this book I will include blank pages in each of the chapters so that you can add your own lecture notes, updates, advances, selected improvements, guidelines, favourite drugs and changes that you find useful and then keep it as a living guide throughout your career.

Many current official guidelines are subsequently found to be wrong even by their authors and you will have to develop a system that works for you and your patients and never blindly apply protocols, check lists and official guidelines just because they happen to exist. Quite often they are harmful and your gut feeling and experience are far more reliable guides of what to do.

There are of course some basic things that never change, the importance of appearing confident, professional, smiling and being open and friendly, BUT NOT OVER FRIENDLY, of looking and listening and always, at every consultation: the laying on of hands. We avoid touching the patient at our peril.

Many aspects of new General Practice, for instance the awful tendency to ask the patient what they think is wrong and what they would like us to do: Exemplified by Saurabh Jha in Medscape Nov 2016 "He's a patient and he's come for your opinion not his." The bizarre reticence new doctors have for the act of touching patients, caused by sexual assault paranoia and the assumption that they will always need a chaperone for intimate examinations are quite simply wrong. Self destructively wrong.

Your eyes, hands and common sense are your most effective tools but you do need to use them all without fear or favour.

"Deduction and diagnosis are a simple matter of getting to the nature of things and the nature of things is what great endeavours like medicine, science, writing and poetry aspire towards".

(from "Just looking-How the revolution in medical education influenced the works of Arthur Conan Doyle and William Carlos Williams" by Will Entrekin)

But basically we must always remember that we are paid to help the patient get better, nothing else. If we forget that we are doing the wrong job.

The Politics:

God and the doctor we alike adore, but only when in danger not before;
The danger o'er, both are alike requited, God is forgotten, and the doctor slighted.
John Owen 1563-1622

The NHS has become intertwined with the national life and politics of Britain in a way that was inconceivable at its outset. It takes 18% of public spending, about £110Bn per year (2013) compared with 12% on education and 5% on defence.£5.7Bn of this is lost in fraud due to the inevitable poor oversight of a huge state run monopoly. £350m to dishonest claiming by my colleagues in GP but there is a whopping £1Bn in "procurement fraud". We know that if every Trust and Health Authority bought its laundry services or latex gloves or sterilisation services from one supplier there would be huge reductions in cost but this £1Bn is sheer fraud, dishonesty.(This report from the former anti fraud Tsar Jim Gee in Sept 2015) One Birmingham dentist alone dishonestly claimed £1.4m for dead patients before she was jailed. It is the biggest employer in Europe, with 1.7

million employees, the fifth biggest employer in the world, still (2016) in this digital age, the biggest purchaser of faxes in the world, one of the most inefficient organisations, with some parts overworked and at constant over capacity and some intrinsically inefficient, seemingly as part of its design. In 2014 it employed 147,000 doctors and 372,000 nurses. (Official figures) About 35,000 are GPs and we do 90% of the patient interactions in the NHS so what ARE the other 112,000 doctors doing? Despite this huge budget, when Monitor compared the NHS in 2015 with healthcare in Australia, Canada, France, Germany, the Netherlands, Sweden and the US, they found that no other system offered consistently higher healthcare at a lower cost. England had the cheapest service of the eight countries in fact at $3659 (£2333, E2962) per person per year compared with an average of $6087 in the other seven countries. Health is expensive everywhere.

But the NHS pretends to be all things to all people and remains untouched by both wings of politics. To the political left it is a sacred cow because the NHS is the most direct and accessible way that the weak and vulnerable are cared for in our society and to the political right because any real interference would be seen as the strong bullying the vulnerable weak. Until recently doctors were hated by both sides of the political spectrum. The socialists disliked the middle class overpaid medical professionals that controlled how medical care was provided and the conservatives resented the state paying the high salaries of the self employed and internally disciplined medical profession. We couldn't win, but at least the patients used to like us.

The result has been that the service keeps on growing, is constantly expected to do more and more and the medical profession has only recently come under any serious kind of state supervision or control. I use the terms "serious" and "supervision" advisedly. The care it provides is often of poor quality – partly because it is all freely available at the point of demand, for everyone and partly because no *real* assessment of the day to day abilities of NHS doctors is ever carried out once they are in post. The relatively new Appraisal system, imposed after the Harold Shipman scandal, simply encourages doctors to self educate in a relatively standard way but the appraiser is not permitted to sit in with the doctor or read his or her notes or to assess their consultation skills and knowledge at all. Not quite what the politicians promised or the patients had hoped for. Two thirds of doctors (August 2017) thought Appraisal was pointless and certainly had no positive effect on their practice. In fact only 16% thought it was in any way beneficial. Given how far the appraisal apple has fallen from the original tree, that is hardly surprising.

All politicians therefore try to manage the juggernaut and all fail abysmally. I hope to explain why.

Just look at the headlines, news paper and broadcast talking points in just a few months of months of 2013/14:

1) £13 Billion written off because Blaire and Brown wasted the money on NHS computerisation that didn't work. This could have applied to several NHS computer systems, all characterised by "poor oversight and management" and lack of "joined up thinking" and perhaps over ambition to supervise and control a service that costs a lot and tries to do too much. This headline referred to computerised patient records. I discuss computerised medical records more fully a little later. This is another example of what sounds like a good idea but is misplaced and harmful outside interference with the medical process. It was really introduced to enable auditing, control, supervision and payment of the activities of employed doctors, particularly in

General Practice but has led to a computer centred focus in the consultation and a distraction of the doctor's concentration away from the patient. The only advantage of Electronic Medical Records from the individual patient's perspective is the Summary Care Record, held at an accessible site with limited health data, accessible to approved medical personnel (with a smart card) and which all patients have been opted into. The somewhat more honest American primary care physician internet chatter is far more direct and democratic in its distaste for the computerisation of medical records than ours. In their case it seems to be at the behest of Medicair and Medicaid to streamline payment but has resulted in the same screen directed consultation. The doctor now spends far more time studying the screen and the keyboard than the patient. Across the Atlantic it is much the same but they publically and vocally object to it more than we do. Computerisation targets for EMRs-Electronic Medical Records, had been introduced, *imposed*, on American primary care physicians over 2014. They were so unpopular that over 50% of the profession had missed their Medicair and Medicaid targets by 2015 and were supposed to be fined. Only a national outcry and rushed legislation saved the day for common sense and suspended the fines. Computers and consulting, – even the basic personality traits that allow you to relate to computers on the one hand or to human beings on the other, are clearly chalk and cheese. I have found this to be as true of partners as of patients.

2) £40m to be cut from the NHS budget in the next 3 years. The NHS budget in 2012 was £104Bn. So that is 0.04 of the budget (like a 4p cut from a budget of £100). Was this even worth mentioning?

3) There are only 5 A and E consultants on call in the whole of the UK on many average nights in our advanced first world country. This level of cover would have been unheard of twenty years ago. So why can't casualty departments now find doctors who want to work in the challenging and difficult environment of busy A and E departments, doing unsociable hours, weekends and family unfriendly work/life unbalanced jobs? The answer is simple: But no one discusses it out loud:

2/3 of medical graduates are now female – nearly all of whom get pregnant within five years of qualifying and all of whom work no more than 2/3 the career hours of the few new male graduates. Women generally speaking avoid careers that require a high out of hours commitment in training, long and physically demanding working conditions and have unsociable hours once they achieve consultant status. They are disproportionately represented in part time, job share and non surgical specialities. The figures are given elsewhere but the highest number of women in any surgical speciality is in Paediatric surgery where they make up only 25% of the total. So if women don't want to work in casualty and two thirds of graduates are women then this MAY have something to do with there being no medical staff in A and E departments. The majority of weekend casualty consultations are alcohol related. – That is code for traumatic/violent. No wonder our very young, predominately female medical profession prefers part time Paediatrics and General Practice. Indeed the representative of the College of Emergency Medicine quoted the **"feminisation of medicine"** as the primary cause of the shortage when interviewed on Radio 4 in January 2014. It may be worth mentioning here that every General Practice I know which has lost a full time male partner over the last few years has found only part time female applicants interested and available to interview and has had to replace one full time male with two female part time partners.

It is this new feminine demographic change which now effectively prevents a 7day NHS, a 24 hour General Practice, a properly staffed A and E and Secondary Care and was summarised by an article in the medical press in May 2015:

Thus "Fewer GPs are opting to become partners since the 2004 contract was introduced. The number of salaried GPs has rocketed by 206% in the last 10 years as the latest workforce figures from the Health and Social Care Centre show. The number of GP partners has dropped by 9% in the same time"

"Partnership can be seen as a restrictive career choice"-said Dr Vicky Weeks, Chairwomen GPC Sessional Sub Committee. "Gone are the days when you put your feet under the desk for 9 sessions a week".

The BMA's largest ever poll of GPs recently found that sessional GPs often choose their role because of the flexibility it brings, with 72% of locums and 52% of salaried GPs saying their post offered a better work life balance. By mid 2015, despite BMA polling finding "overwhelming support for independent contractor status", it also found 75% of salaried and locum GPs under 30 years old did not plan to become partners. It didn't say if they were all female.

The patients now hate the loss of continuity and access which they had grown used to with the previously male dominated full time work force. They see the different characteristics of the ways the sexes work, -female doctors as well as being the part timers, refer more for second opinions and take clinical fewer risks. They take longer over each consultation even though they keep better notes. A study published in the BMJ in 2017 showed that patients who saw "The same General Practitioner a greater proportion of the time" experienced fewer admissions. You get to know your patient if you have seen them often and they know if they can rely on you. Conversely you know if and when they are genuinely ill. But only if you are available enough when they are ill. Most new female GPs are part time and most part timers are female. It's not rocket science, its General Practice or how it used to be. The bed starved NHS needs can't-be-too-careful admissions like an Ebola Epidemic. Data from 230,000 records for patients in England aged 62-82 between 2011 and 2013 showed that those with a "High continuity of care" had over 12% fewer admissions for ambulatory care sensitive conditions than those with low continuity of care. Part time doctors make work for the rest of us.

Hospital doctors are the same: The latest Royal College of Physicians Census shows a year on year progression in part time consultants with the highest percentage in the history of the NHS. Virtually everyone a woman.

This, of course, is the time scale when the medical schools have feminised the medical profession and this whole agenda is due to women. The war against the white male is being won. Medical women, once settled in a career generally no longer **do full a time commitment, they demand a life/work balance, they don't do half the medical careers on offer or half the (tougher) rotas, they don't do partnerships and they would say their posts offer a better work life balance. But what do their patients say? What has this organisational chaos done to the service the NHS now offers?** Many patients would argue that many female part timers and port folio doctors have lost any sense of commitment, continuity or vocation at all.

By November 2015 the invasion and occupation was well underway: GMC data showed women represented 63% of GPs under 40, 56% of GPs 40-49 and 37% over 50 years old. Clearly a feminist mind set had taken control of medical school selection committees sometime in the last 20 years. Female GP trainees outnumber males 2 to 1 and account for over half of the UK profession overall – although I expect this is considerably less than half the hours worked by the profession. The same report commented that female medical students outnumber male but that male hospital surgeons were 72% and male ophthalmologists 56% of their professional work forces. BME GPs by this time had risen by a quarter since 2010.

The 2014/5 Consultant Census showed an increased need for the Generalist Physician and Geriatric Consultant in hospitals as 65% of hospital admissions are over 65 years of age and these patients have many complex medical problems all at once affecting multiple systems. Not something that a Urologist, Rheumatologist, Cardiologist, Ophthalmologist, Gastroenterologist, Respiratory Physician etc one after the other can be roped in to sort out. It was just in these groups of generalists that (outside London anyway) there were the greatest increase in jobs advertised and not filled. Physician numbers had increased by 3.2% over the preceding year, to a total of 13,003 in all, but **a fifth were now part time**. 40% of advertised posts remained unfilled – Now I wonder whether the part time commitment of the female consultants explains current lack the of total applicants. Don't forget that if a medical school and a training scheme are training a female who is going to work half time then she is elbowing out a male applicant who would be full time and twice as productive for the same educational cost in money and hours. He will also take less time off sick and obviously have less maternity leave. She comes off the conveyor belt and does half the hours – but hey, there isn't a male doctor around to apply for the full time post because she and her female colleagues filled the only places at medical school and the training grades so there are no full time applicants because there are only women in the pool.

Female GPs refer in to hospitals 30% more patients than male doctors for second opinions. I do not know whether the research that disclosed this troubling difference made allowance for the part-timism of most female GPs and therefore their relative lack of experience compared with similarly aged male doctors. Or whether it factored in the age or stage of career of the over referring female GPs, the fact that they aren't full time and therefore can't "get the patient back soon to check on them", or whether it is just that women are less confident and more risk averse throughout their careers. Is it simply a gender risk taking issue? The fact is however that no primary care system can function without the primary carers taking a significant degree of responsibility. And for responsibility read risk. That is what General Practice **IS**. So here are three reasons why casualties are much busier and they are all due to the recent feminisation of General Practice:

Patients have less continuity and a poorer relationship with the huge number of part time female GPs in practice now and would just as readily establish contact with their local casualty department, somewhere they can at least get an appointment easily with a full time doctor.

Women doctors don't want to work careers in casualty departments because of their life/work and family priorities and because of the female dominant out-put of medical schools there are fewer and fewer male doctors around to staff A and E departments.

There are more patients in casualty because female GPs refer 30% more patients to secondary care for a second opinion.

To add to the chaos caused by women avoiding the harder disciplines of A and E (and no doubt an evolving Orthopaedics and General Surgery manpower crisis) there was, by August 2015 the flip side of that demographic causing problems. Too many female doctors going into a speciality – in this case, Paediatrics, immediately taking time off to have families and often never going back to full time working. The Daily Telegraph of August 27th ran the headline "Doctor shortage could force children's units to shut". Stating that "So many female doctors work part time or go on maternity leave, one in four neonatal posts is empty with the service heavily reliant on expensive locums". The Royal College of Paediatrics and Child Health carried out the survey and blamed the 75% of new Paediatricians who are female and start families early for leaving units short staffed. 78% of clinical directors felt their units would be at risk within six months."A high proportion of doctors are choosing to work less than full time once they have children" said Dr Simon Clark from the RCPCH. The college was hoping nurses or GPs might fill the gaps.

By 2014/2015 locums were keeping the "undermanned" NHS afloat in many specialities, not just Paediatrics and Casualty. In 2014 £1bn was spent on locum fees, one doctor earning a ridiculous £500,000. The headlines of several national newspapers regularly decried the cost of temporary medical staff and the seeming paradox that there were now constant holes in the staffing structure of the NHS. – This despite the government constantly defending itself by saying there were record numbers of doctors. What is the explanation? This was and is of course, that more doctors are now part time, off on maternity leave and anywhere but treating patients. Everyone in the profession knows this but no one in government or the media has the honesty say it out loud. Women.

No one knows who has made the highly irrational, unaffordable, self destructive, inexplicable and sexist policy decision to overwhelm the medical profession with women. There is no possible rational explanation unless you believe in some sort of tacit political conspiracy to dismantle the once male dominated profession by feminist medical school selection committees.

Academic doctors have been shown by numerous pieces of research to be unrepresentatively left wing compared with front line physicians, GPs and surgeons. Perhaps it is happening by accident. Perhaps no one in the NHS is tasked with thinking about the future consequences of decisions made today. It certainly seems like that when we hear almost daily of a "man power" crisis, a casualty melt down, the cost of locums and problems with foreign trained doctors hastily brought in to fill the gaps. Perhaps central policy makers and democratic decision making have no control over the selection policies of independent medical schools. If that is the case then it is a bit like letting each independent ship yard decide what ships it wants to build for the Navy and the country finding itself with 500 mine sweepers. Certainly it hasn't been the result of a democratic, service responsive, long term, gap filling, cost effective or open consultation. Or any forward thinking or central planning. No one in their right mind could say medicine, from the perspective of the patient's experience, has improved because of the influx of mainly female doctors. My friends on selection committees of medical schools say the obvious, that girls interview better at 17 years old and often do better at the A Level subjects required. If this is the case, then a report published in February 2015 and broadcast on the Today Program which said that "deprived areas" of the country do not even offer the academic subjects necessary for medicine means that the target demographic is getting smaller and smaller. So if you are a state educated white northern male teenager who wants to be a doctor in the 21st century, forget it. We are getting a medical profession that does not reflect the British public in geography, sex or race and from the feedback I get every day, the public does not want this or like it. We are sleepwalking to the edge of staffing and demographic disaster that soft politics from soft headed authority is guilty of time and time again in the NHS.

In this case the decision makers are the blinkered selection committees of medical schools. These selection committees are racist, against white applicants, sexist against males and southern biased-at least if you believe the medical profession should reflect the society it serves.

Remind me to mention unforeseen consequences again later.

Just to end on, the same feminisation is taking place in the same specialities in the USA. In August 2015 a national report of a 2012 assessment was published which showed: The percentage of female trainees was lowest in orthopaedics at 13.8%, the highest for Obstetrics/Gynae 82.4%, and women were represented at over 50% in

Dermatology 64%

Internal medicine/Paediatrics 58%

Family Medicine 55%

Pathology 55%

Psychiatry 55%

they didn't say, but I am willing to bet the figures are well UNDER 50% for General Surgery, ER, and most specialised surgery.

If you cannot see that the 15% to 65% female transition during my career has had no demonstrable advantage and multiple severe disadvantages for the patients, you clearly work for a medical school selection committee.

4) 37,000 patients die of unrecognised sepsis every year. Infection, particularly in children is hard to recognise early. It takes acumen, familiarity, extensive previous contact, practical knowledge and in short – experience. At every level of British medicine the lack of experience and reduction in clinical skills is becoming more of an issue in hospitals and GP practices. This is primarily due to the halving of the hours worked by junior doctors in training due to the E.U. Working Time Directive. Juniors would work more than a 100 hours a week in 1975 when I qualified. This was restricted to 56 hours in 2003 and no more than 48 hours since 2009. How can they now be as competent or as experienced as the generations that preceded them if they are seeing so many fewer patients- **probably half,** in their period of training? I illustrate this elsewhere but the poor training and relative lack of practical skills of senior training grade doctors compared with their predecessors was highlighted in "Commentary", The Royal College of Physicians Journal in an article recently. This applied to hospital doctors but trainers of GPs also bemoan the lack of case experience and clinical confidence of fully qualified GP s compared with previous generations.

5) The elderly now know their casualty staff better than their GPs thanks to the "disastrous" change in working practices that followed the last contract negotiations.(-The Secretary of State)

The BMA "ran rings" around the Department of Health negotiators under the last labour government and undoubtedly permitted an unexpected salary windfall for GPs over the subsequent several years as well as the effective ending of quality out of hours cover. The substitute GP out of hours service is now completely inadequate. It isn't really an out of hours General Practice Service at all. Run by private companies (the defunct GP Cooperatives were probably the best compromise), the services cover large areas with small numbers of doctors, many of whom have no knowledge or contact with the local practices or communities. They often over use casualty and the ambulance service. Casualty Departments are therefore the first port of call for many patients and some individuals can visit them upwards of 200 times a year, knowing their casualty doctor better than their GP (according to The Secretary of State, 2013). This shows the failure of Social Services and Community Psychiatric Services to be funded and to work properly, the failure of many G Ps to take proper responsibility for all their patients, especially the socially and psychiatrically dysfunctional, or to be available for house calls right up to the 6.30pm hand over deadline, the failure of real "Care in the Community" and the fallacy of "Free to all at the point of demand".

Counter intuitively The College of Emergency Medicine reviewed A and E attendance and published its results in May 2014. They said that of 3000 patients attending casualty in a 24 hour period the preceding March, only 15% could have been treated in the community. Last year NHS England suggested 25% could be and they replied to the 15% figure by saying that previous assessments of the number of A and E attendees who could be dealt with by GPs varied from 10 to 45%. Given that the problem is that most of these cases are ones that have an acute onset, the **"issue seems to be a GP failure to accommodate the acute presentation of illness".**

I suppose this in its turn all depends on whether GPs are genuinely available at short notice (as we all should be), what illnesses an individual GP is prepared to treat at home, whether he or she is willing to review the patient four hours later, whether a trusted colleague will be covering the patient and can be handed over to. This will be related to how well the GP knows and trusts the parents/relatives/patients to call for help, how available and accessible that GP and his or her practice is to the patient in the first place. If you are in the ideal position of being a full time partner, 9 sessions a week, in a practice of no more than six or seven (full time) partners, a personal list system, responsible cross cover, good communication and therefore offering CONTINUITY, then the patient need not always be dumped on secondary care. On the other hand, if you are a sessional GP, in a practice with twelve or more mostly part time or sessional partners, frequent locums, lots of external commitments, no named list system so you are unfamiliar with the patient and their family, if you have to get home to pick up your kids from school and you have several phone calls or visits to do first and you are only supposed to be on 'til one o'clock and you don't know the duty afternoon doctor very well because you are part time, then sending that mild asthmatic in through casualty sounds very tempting. The latter scenario is, of course, partly a function of how many part time female partners a practice has.

6) The consultant contract is only **now** to be renegotiated so that they are properly available out of hours and at weekends. Some consultants are currently able to claim £150,000 in overtime a year.

Stop Press: Overtime pay had continued to increase, up by a third by 2016 with one Lancashire consultant claiming the obscene sum of £350,000 in one year. No progress has been made there in several years, so good luck with that, Secretary of State. One obvious issue, one elephant in the front room is that Britain is just not educating enough doctors and certainly not enough male (full time) doctors. Therefore consultants in some specialities use their scarcity as a bargaining tool and charge a premium to work extra hours, do extra clinics, waiting list initiatives etc.

What did the Government think would happen when their negotiators ended the GP 60 to 100 hour standard working week? The NHS only ever worked properly when doctors at all levels worked truly unhealthy and unsociable hours because we felt it was our vocation, part of the job. We got respect and status in return, occasionally slightly preferential treatment by our colleagues but our health, marriages and relationships suffered. We were at work when our children were growing up (most of us were men because women tend to prioritise families over patients, not the other way round) and we were so tired we all fell asleep at meetings, social gatherings and parties. In my case I felt that it was a fair exchange. I had been given the most expensive post graduate education available and a career with a good income and greater choice than almost any other. Currently medical education costs between £500,000 and £850,000 but 2/3 of doctors receiving it are family friendly women. They do not want full time jobs, jobs in challenging working environments or partnerships in General Practice. An increasing number of (mainly) female consultants retire early. Listen to the GMC feedback chat from junior doctors on their working conditions and you have to conclude that they have less of a vocation, a greater work life self interest and no idea of what medicine was like even twenty years ago, let alone before that. The Working Time Directive Generation. Consultants are not readily going to exchange their half of their new contract and do more hours and weekends – any more than GP s are going to volunteer to take on out of hours cover as well as (in the case of full time GP s) their 60 hour working week.

7) The Frances report has 290 recommendations to put the patient back at the heart of all NHS decision making – So where had the patient been allowed to get to, why and by whom?

I believe, as I have said, that it has been interference by politicians pure and simple and the imposition of constant soft political agendas which have caused most of the NHS disasters of the last decade. So instead of being led by their own clear professional and ethical standards, frequent alterations in work priorities and goals and altered management schedules have distanced nurses particularly but also doctors from their primary caring role. As so often is the case, politicians, managers and sometimes lawyers have messed about with various aspects of what was previously a functioning health system and each time made it worse from the patient's perspective because they simply don't know how health care works. They look at it (note that Sir Stuart Rose of Marks and Spencer was being seconded to advise NHS managers of failing Trusts in 2014) simply from business and managerial perspectives. No wonder CARE came lower than turnover in the list of priorities.

Nursing is a time consuming and inefficient way of allocating expensive staff. It is hard to define what good nurses do that makes them better than bad nurses or what makes good nurses care more than others. What they do doesn't seem very complicated and you can have the same number of nurses, the same number of patients in the same number of beds on different wards with very different outcomes. So from a manager's and a cost cutting politician's point of view why not reduce their numbers, reduce some of that wasteful talking to the patients, sitting on bedsides, holding hands and refine their job down to a list of essential roles to be done in a defined time frame?

Health and efficiency!

So that would be the thought process and the people responsible. Politicians, accountants, managers, some fresh out of business school or university, making decisions on staffing and work priorities. Occasionally it would be a committee of academic nurses or doctors. Few of them would probably be old enough to have been hospital patients themselves for any length of time and to know that good nursing takes time and space. Few would be medics, by definition or if they were they would be at least one step removed from day to day active patient contact: Teachers or academics.

A policy decision would be made and these changes would then be introduced into the working priorities of every doctor and nurse. Something like the Liverpool Pathway. Changes brought about by politicians (there are many frustrated politicians who are trained as nurses and doctors) implemented by managers and carried out by doctors and nurses. Instead of responding to each individual patient's needs and being independently free to care according to our own assessments of each patient's contemporary needs, we (doctors and nurses) were forced to lose that independence and purpose and swap it for a predetermined shopping list of tasks. And now, of course we find ourselves alone in the dock for complying with our new contracts.

Most real nursing – the stuff that patients value, is reactive, not proactive and consists of being **available** and performing several roles at once. But this requires nurses to be on the ward in sufficient numbers, accessible, responsive, suitably skilled but not over skilled (no ward nursing role really requires a degree level education does it?) willing to undertake any and all nursing care as the need arises. It is the same in nursing as in medicine: the cleverer and higher qualified the doctor or nurse, the less able and willing they are to deal with messy mundane day to day bread and butter problems.

How many nurses are reasonable?

Combine all this interference with a reduction in numbers and disasters are bound to happen.

Tentatively, NICE mooted one nurse to eight patients as a reasonable general ward ratio in May 2014. NICE also suggested one nurse to four patients in casualty cubicles as well as two nurses per patient with a life threatening illnesses in A and E – in January 2015. Those seem reasonable figures for both general wards and casualty departments to me.

So we would all agree with that – Yes? Political interference with basic old fashioned health care always makes the patient experience worse. Agreed?

So in that case lets really take all politics out of health care:

Stop over educating nurses to degree standard and thereby often putting two hands on the rudder. A colleague of mine of 35 year's experience was recently refused permission to admit a patient with chest pain over the phone by a "cardiovascular" nurse because she didn't believe the doctor's analysis and diagnosis. I cannot tell you how angry this sort of thing makes me at the lack of trust, the reliance on (no doubt) rigid protocols rather than experience and first hand observation. Also the danger **to the patient** of this sort of harmful paradox. The patient was indeed in the process of having an acute infarct-that is the point of the story. He had to be admitted via casualty. Nurses are trained NOT to be diagnosticians, they only focus straight ahead. My neighbour, a practice nurse of thirty years standing came to me a few months ago, distraught because her sick father was refused a doctor's appointment by his busy practice receptionist and seen by their nurse practitioner instead. His symptoms; painless jaundice, abdominal swelling, dehydration and anorexia. The nurse practitioner arranged bloods and gave him a three week appointment until my neighbour and I discussed what every medical student knows about painless jaundice. She phoned the GP and her father got his 2 week referral. Painless jaundice = cancer until proven otherwise – every medical student knows this. Shortly after this, he deteriorated and his family took him to casualty as the only way of getting him seen quickly. This is a typical scenario in the 21st century NHS. Of course he had pancreatic cancer. Two weeks later he died. This combination of power and inflexibility in many nurse practitioners that

I have come across is extremely dangerous to ill patients who never come as a standard package. Departments and GPs who rely on them are often short changing patients, often expecting far too much of the nurse. Doctors are supposed to think laterally, trained to ask why, what if and what else? In the same week I heard this story there was a programme on National Radio ("Case Notes") publicising the importance of a doctor's "Gut Feelings" in detecting occult and atypical illness. In fact the reliability of doctors' suspicions, based on past experience and "felt" rather than rationalised thought processes has been well recognised for years

(BMJ Sept 25 2012 08.11./BMC Family Practice 2013 14 (1)) etc.

No nurse with a degree, a position of power, an admission algorithm and no real diagnostic experience should ever trump a doctor with years of experience and a sick patient in front of them. This is back to front and can never be in the long term interest of any patient. The evidence against such doctor substitutes continues to accumulate whenever it is objectively measured.

In a competition of diagnostic accuracy between humans and "machines", published in 2016, physicians "handily beat" algorithms designed to diagnose conditions based on vignettes of patient history. Specifically, physicians accurately identified the diagnosis in clinical vignettes of patient health histories about twice as often as computer based symptom checkers did. – According to a research letter published online Oct 2016 in JAMA Int Medicine.

Women again: Stop medical schools preferentially training doctors who are poor value for money: Those doctors who will work no more than 2/3 of their potential career hours, take half of their first five years off, then pick and choose their careers, avoiding A and E, avoiding the tougher surgical specialities, avoiding full time careers and partnerships in General Practice and thus adversely affecting their continuity and quality of care, harming their long term therapeutic and professional relationships by a job share or part time career and so on – in other words, cut down the number of women students. Certainly, stop medical schools giving more than two thirds of places to women as they do now. From a tax payer's perspective can we afford any more than 25% of our medical work force to be women?

End the compulsory six monthly Equality and Diversity training for GP trainers and appraisers. This has the tacit but unavoidable implication that any foreign doctor, however under trained or with irrelevant training or with certain difficult cultural attitudes or with poor English skills is uncriticisable or must be handled preferentially. This may not have been the original intention but it has certainly been the result.

Like it or not there is a climate – if not of fear, within medicine regarding criticising foreign graduates about language and cultural issues, then at least of resigned, reluctant resentment. You criticise their abilities at your own peril.

Doctors from a number of foreign countries, including those that supply most of our foreign graduates, India, Pakistan, Egypt and Nigeria are many times more likely to defer and fail appraisals, to fail membership exams, to be complained about, be referred to the GMC and be struck off. This does not apply to doctors from ethnic minorities trained or born in Britain and of course there are many doctors from these countries who are excellent and out-perform the average British trained doctor. But only 20% of doctors trained abroad are at the British mean level of knowledge according to data published in 2014. So what we need are more British medical schools not more foreign graduates, surely? Jeremy Hunt announced in September 2016 that medical schools would start to address this with 1,500 extra places a year in 2018. This is in an attempt to become self sufficient in doctors almost 70 years after the birth of the NHS. I really hope that they are value for money in terms of potential career hours and as well as the obligation to work in the UK for 4 years after qualifying, there is a full time obligation too.

Ban medical NHS staff with full face veils (burqas) and the associated cultural attitudes, who cannot communicate emotions to the patient or touch male patients – and about whom British patients would be bemused and distressed in equal measure. This may be a rare situation as yet but it was one experienced by a disabled patient of mine who was told by a female radiographer with her face covered that she could not help him out of his wheel chair or touch him if he collapsed. What happens if I have one of my "turns" he said. Let's hope you don't she replied.

The Legal Situation:

The GMC recommends that an employer can insist on the removal of any garment that inhibits communication-such as those that cover the face. A tribunal upheld the right of a local authority to require the removal of a face veil by a teacher as non discriminatory. Given the importance of communication and the consistent application of such a policy.

The current GMC advice, based on relevant case law applied to teaching but at least as relevant in medicine is that "any garment that might inhibit communication, such as a face veil should be removed. This is non discriminatory and the action was supported on appeal."

Stop doctors identifying themselves by their first names – yet another erosion of the authority of the medical profession seemingly embraced without question by all doctors under thirty. Let's try and restore some authority and dignity into medicine. Patients, generally, have had enough informality and chaos. They long for some authority, seriousness, professionalism again.

End the fallacious dumbing down via casual work clothing which really has nothing to do with infection control as it was initially promoted and restore the authority of senior ward nurses and consultants to enforce and embrace a smart dress code. You only have to look at American and European medical websites or interviews with their real doctors on television or publicity literature or some of our own elite hospitals to see that their doctors still wear white coats and smart clothes, ties included. Do you think they don't care about infection? See the following diagrams and tell me first impressions aren't important when you are feeling ill, vulnerable and anxious.

Here are various pictures of doctors: The front cover of the RCP Consultant census designed no doubt to be inclusive:(60% female and probably 40% BEM, most of them pretty untidy but the most scruffy in the ward round is the one I assume to be the consultant. Generally speaking this is a patient's heart sink on call team.

The other two pictures are from The Royal Marsden Hospital information booklet, showing one of their consultants and the other diagram is from an NHS brachytherapy information booklet for patients. Try and ignore the severely rheumatoid fingers of the doctor's right hand. Both show the sort of doctor that patients **hope** to have looking after them – dressed seriously, soberly, long sleeves, tie, even, dare I mention it, a WHITE COAT, – and someone who looks like he made an effort today, a professional. Every patient over 25 remembers when all doctors looked professional, respectable in the true meaning of that word. Britain now has the youngest medical profession in the western world and it shows.

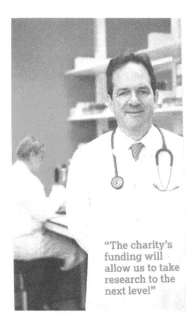

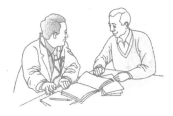

Urologist, so that a full range of tests can be carried out and an assessment of the prostate made.

How is prostate cancer diagnosed?
The doctor will initially ask the patient questions to check their general medical health and see if they are experiencing any symptoms associated with prostate cancer (although, as has been mentioned, such symptoms are not specific to prostate cancer).

Physical examination
Having made a general examination, the doctor will then need to perform a rectal examination to feel the gland. A gloved, lubricated finger is inserted into the back passage (rectum) to check the size and shape of the prostate gland.

 A Patient's Guide to Prostate Cancer

"The charity's funding will allow us to take research to the next level"

Royal College of Physicians | **Royal College of Physicians of Edinburgh** | ROYAL COLLEGE OF PHYSICIANS AND SURGEONS OF GLASGOW

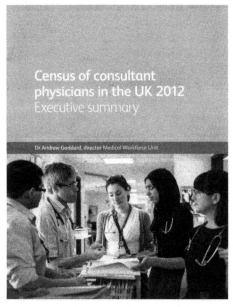

Census of consultant physicians in the UK 2012
Executive summary

Dr Andrew Goddard, director Medical Workforce Unit

When I qualified my working week was up to 136 hours (on a 1 in 2 with the weekend on call) The Working Time Directive currently specifies a maximum of 48 hours a week averaged over 26 weeks for trainee doctors. So my generation of doctor worked up to three times harder than today's doctor, was better trained, gave a better service, was SAFER and ironically had less time off sick (this is discussed later).

There was an ongoing campaign to garner sympathy on the GMC website about how hard life as a doctor on the ward was, predating the strike call in 2015. The changes to consultant and GP contracts and a dramatic change in what I would call the ethos of service amongst doctors seem to undermine this claim in my view and that of many of my generation. Life for GPs and hospital doctors is infinitely less stressful now than 20 or 30 years ago but the quality of care, continuity and survivability for patients, especially out of hours have all deteriorated over the same time. How could we (particularly the government who freed the slaves) have thought it would be otherwise? The NHS was built on long hours, dedication and vocation and the patients appreciated the doctors and nurses for what they all regarded as doing more than just a job. The NHS hasn't doubled equivalent medical staff numbers to compensate for their reduction in hours. It hasn't doubled the length of medical training so that doctors will have the equivalent experience and be as competent as their trainers. In return for the longest hours worked by any profession, patients tended (though there were exceptions) not to abuse or take the doctors or the service for granted. Few would have visited casualty 200 times in one year then or phoned the out of hours service every night forty years ago. I am afraid patients perceive a different medical profession today, one less deserving of sympathy and respect.

There are many other differences in the NHS now compared with when it started on 5th July 1948.

As well as doctors working fewer hours, there are never any empty beds today either. The number of NHS beds has inexplicably been halved to 150,000 in the 30 years since 1987 – you would think that illness was rarer and easier to treat. Bed occupancy can be over 100% with patients waiting in trolleys for a discharge or a death. The crisis in A and E is multifactorial but what is the point of seeing and managing a patient in casualty, deciding that they need admitting, if the bed occupancy is always 100% and all the beds are full? We need more beds and more staff. We need **less efficiency**, more flexibility in the system all year round and all wards having some empty beds. We must increase the number of beds, especially on acute wards by 10-25%. No hospital should ever be on "divert" (as our local DGH is constantly) simply because it failed to predict a car crash or the annual Norovirus epidemics.

End the Working Time Directive and tell all junior medical staff that their working week could be up to 100 hours for the first 5 years after qualifying. It was for me. This is what medicine was like for everyone when I qualified. This in itself leads to emotional resilience as well as clinical confidence.

Since one sixth to one seventh of fully trained GPs (after an investment by the taxpayer of at least £500,000 each) are planning to take their skills and settle abroad (2014, mainly Australia and New Zealand, not Sierra Leone or The Central African Republic) shouldn't all medical students also sign a contract to work for the NHS for at least 5 years after qualifying or reimburse their educational costs? Too draconian? Think about it. Given the comparative failure rate of foreign trained doctors taking MRCGP, appraisals and other professional exams, the competition to get in to UK medical schools and their high entrance requirements, a British training is expensive, highly prized and second to none. It guarantees a high income, a good quality doctor and personal career flexibility. I think the Tax payer who funds it has the right to expect a reasonable return for his investment. Now (2015) moves are afoot to allow foreign trained doctors to sit the standard British Membership exam a fifth time. Most British graduates pass first time or if very unlucky, second.

So do you still think we should remove all politics from medicine?

8) The weekend death rate is 40% higher almost certainly due to non availability of medical staff and the lack of what during the week are considered routine investigations. In November 2015 a UCH paper was published showing the death rate amongst newborn was 7% higher at weekends. That amounts to 770 extra deaths of babies per year. This paper came out between the overwhelming vote in favour of striking by NHS Junior doctors and the actual strikes taking place. During this period much of the invective from junior staff in the GP press was how medical staff already worked weekends, there was no public demand for it anyway, if there were it wouldn't make much difference and if it could be provided it would be unaffordable. Another study (September 2015) showed that patients admitted for care at weekends had a higher risk of death within 30 days than those admitted during the week. This general mortality difference is undoubtedly due to the Working Time Directive, the way the NHS is organised to avoid paying overtime to ancillary staff, the consultants' new contract, the new life/work balance expected by junior doctors these days and the much easier working conditions of doctors over the last 20 years. This is despite their feedback to The GMC website about how hard life on the wards is today! These changes in working conditions for junior doctors have led to an inevitable reduction in patient contact time and practical experience (competence) but there are also changes to commitment in new consultant contracts and a dramatic change in what I would call the ethos of service amongst younger doctors. What used to be called vocation. So there are many causes for this weekend increase in mortality risk for patients.

The Department of Health accepts that there are 12,000 "Avoidable Deaths" each year within the NHS – that's over 30 each day. I wonder how many of these are due to the changes in lifestyle of junior and senior doctors in hospital (and in General Practice) that have slipped into place over the last twenty years.

In an editorial in the RCP monthly house magazine "Clinical Medicine" in December 2015, the point was made that the weekend mortality excess (they said of 6000 patients) of patients admitted at weekends was common to many health care systems. They quote "The Doctor Foster Unit" as finding an increase in mortality of emergency and elective weekend admissions and said "reduced staffing across all grades is a highly likely contributor", as is reduced diagnostics, rota changes and unnecessary waits for patients requiring emergency treatment. They also say that weekend patients are sicker overall (Freemantle) – which possibly suggests that we might need more staff on duty at weekends than Monday to Friday surely? There is also the conundrum that patients already in hospital on a Sunday have a lower mortality on that day than compared with weekdays. Presumably this is because no one is carrying out procedures, operations or investigations because there are no doctors or ancillary staff around to do them. The editorial continues saying "It is a poor defence of UK medical services to say that foreign services are as bad as us". Quite. The actual numbers are difficult to clarify and constantly seized on by the striking BMA. The Government was sticking to 6-11,000 extra deaths in the February 2015 Prime Minister's question time about the junior doctors' strike and their attempt to improve services at weekends.

Life for GPs and hospital doctors is infinitely less hard work now than 20 or 30 years ago even though sickness and absence due to stress and minor illness is ironically several orders (actually three times) higher. Indeed, the GMC now wants medical schools to teach "emotional resilience" and given all the above it is not before time. Add all this up and you might be forgiven for thinking we have a generation of doctors who work less hard, who are mainly female and part time, are less dedicated, less committed, get ill easier, who are thinner skinned emotionally, are less experienced, less capable and as a direct consequence the quality of care, continuity and survivability for patients out of hours have all deteriorated. This is probably true "in hours" too, given the doctors' relative lack of experience and confidence (the diminishing ability to perform practical procedures even at new consultant level is frequently referred to in "Clinical Medicine" the journal of the Royal College of Physicians). How could we have thought that it would be otherwise?

The seven day NHS used to exist. Blair and Brown with the GP contract and the end of 24 hour cover ended it in General Practice. The shameful commercialisation of out of hours cover and the withdrawal of contracts from cooperatives was the Coup de Grace. In hospitals, the consultant contract, the working time directive of 48 hours for junior staff, the feminisation of the medical schools and the profession has led to a family friendly, patient unfriendly working ethos.

The Government, perhaps encouraged by such campaigns as that of the Sunday Times regarding the risks of getting ill out of hours is (2015) is attempting to address the issue of **poor out of hours cover** "despite more NHS doctors than ever before" by changing doctors' contracts (2015). An official study (The High Intensity Specialist Led Acute Care Project) revealed in July 2015 that some hospitals have 10 times as many consultants covering emergencies on a weekday as on a weekend. It showed there are huge variations between hospitals too. ("which explained the 4,400 extra deaths attributable to substandard care at weekends"-Sunday Times). The study of 14,500 consultants in 115 Trusts showed an average of 3.6 as many senior doctors around in hospitals on Wednesdays compared with Sundays. The worst showed a 10:1 ratio, the best a 2:1 ratio. Six out of 10 trusts admitted front line gaps in cover on acute wards because of consultant shortages. **Junior doctors were found to be no more likely to be on call at weekends than consultants**. This is the fact that is most surprising to me. Only 3.6% of junior doctor's total hours worked were on the Sunday shift 7am – 7pm. These figures show the BMA's claim (and the torrent of E Mail self justification on medical websites supporting it from hospital doctors) that they work a 7 day week to be false. One female junior doctor self righteously E Mailed a GP on line magazine to say that she had done extra hours every day of her 5 day week and her consultant "never grumbled when he was called". I qualified in 1975, did a 1 in 3 rota for about 15 years and so did 33% of all available Sunday 7am-7pm sessions, not 3.6% like today's junior doctors. Today we have a predominantly female GP workforce, >50% for the first time in NHS history and a rapidly increasing consultant and GP work force of female part timers. (ref: RCP Census and feedback from every GP friend whose vacancy has been advertised).

There are other working differences these days: The GP work force is younger: 31% of the workforce is under 40 yrs, 30% 40-50 yrs, 28% 50-60 yrs and only 12% over 60 years. Older doctors are not equally distributed, Yorkshire and The Humber having the largest proportion of doctors younger than 40 yrs old, (38%) but they make up only 26% in the East of England.

	In London (2015)	In the South West:	In Scotland:	Wales:
Under 40yrs	30%	28%	31%	28%
40-50 yrs	27%	31%	30%	29%
50-60yrs	24%	32%	31%	31%
Over 60 yrs	18%	9%	9%	12%

I am willing to bet that many of the doctors taking their four decades of experience and wisdom to retire early are put off returning by the cost of GMC registration, the ease with which patients can make and pursue trivial complaints, the exorbitant cost of medical indemnity insurance and the complex, nit picking, detailed requirements of appraisal and revalidation. This latter has spawned an overblown industry of educators and IT specialists which simply had no role and did not exist twenty years ago. As well as doctors working fewer hours, offering less continuity and less experience, the beds they cover these days are never empty. Bed occupancy can be over 100% in the UK with patients waiting on trolleys for a discharge or a death. **We need more beds and more staff.** We need less efficiency, more flexibility in the system all year round and wards with some empty beds.

PS: In April 2014 The OECD produced a report agreeing with this point of view: It said more than 50,000 NHS beds had been lost since 2001 and we had the second lowest number of beds in Europe. The Daily Mail had on its front page in February 2017 that we were still continuing removing bed capacity even now. 15,000 beds gone in the last 6 years, -this is 10% or 24 hospitals' worth. France has twice the number, admittedly not a good comparison since the French Health Service is generally used as an example of an indulgent and bloated one but ours is now cachectic and pared beyond the bone. The UK spends 8.4% of GDP on health compared with and OECD average of 8.8%. We will spend less in 2020 as a proportion of GDP than in 2005. Most other countries have a smaller percentage state contribution however, making up the difference with part of the cost of their health care directly FROM THE PATIENTS. It is only in the UK that the "Free at the point of demand" mantra keeps being chanted in the corridors of healthcare.

France spends more as a percentage of GDP, the UK has lower public expenditure on healthcare than France (but where 77% of the total amount spent on health is by the state the rest by the patient, UK 83.2%), but France has more doctors (3.3/1000 population, UK 2.8) more MRI scanners, (7.5/million population, UK 5.9) a shorter wait for elective surgery, (7% wait more than 4 months UK 21%), better life expectancy, (81.5, UK 80.6) and lower infant mortality (3.5/1000 live births, UK 4.2) (Civitas The Health of the Nation 2016 P 41).You surely cannot attribute all this, including infant mortality, to the Mediterranean effect?

We have 2.95 beds per 1000 population compared with 6.4 in France, 7.65 in Austria and 8.27 in Germany! Clearly our cost cutting has gone beyond safe or sensible limits.

We spend $3,405/patient/year, tie bottom (of the major nations) according to the "Clinical Medicine" editorial of Dec 2015 with New Zealand in the advanced nation international chart of health expenditure. The USA is top at $8,502/patient/year, Germany spends $5002, the Netherlands $5217, Norway $6177 and France $4124.

9) "Successful Trusts" to loan their managers to "Failing Trusts" to share "Best Practice". Will they also lend beds and experienced doctors who are available at nights and weekends and in casualty departments at busy times and nurses who are willing to nurse?

10) Should nurses be allowed to wear veils? (See above) There is a strongly held view amongst patients and a growing number of medical staff that the human rights agenda that now pervades every policy and publication with an NHS, GMC, Department of Health, Royal College, Deanery, RGN or associated organisation's badge on it is directly harming patient care. This discussion is emblematic of the issue. By which I mean the human rights of staff and some patients are adversely affecting the medical care and "rights" of the majority of patients. The unwillingness of staff to pursue health tourists, the tolerance and understanding granted to medically unjustified procedures such as male and female circumcision. There are at least 60,000 FGM patients in this country (one source said twice this number) and to date (2015) not one prosecution has been made against the parents, procurer or surgeon. What about the NHS Surgeons who top up their income doing male circumcisions, a procedure with absolutely no benefit and many genuine disadvantages in a country that does not have a desert climate? Risk of infection in a dry climate can be the only rational reason circumcision was adopted by two of the three Abrahamic religions. So how **can** a nurse behind a burqa care, communicate or connect if she is shielded and inaccessible and therefore hiding from the patient? Surely this issue should not even need debating in the UK in the 21st century? The GMC has now clarified its stance on the issue as one related to interference with communication. If that can be said to be happening, you can ask for the veil to be removed and no equality or human right has been infringed.

11) GPs and consultants should be compelled to go back to providing 7 day a week care. This became a touchstone of the Cameron Government in 2015 given the high mortality rates at weekends, the overuse of casualty departments, the general disengagement of many GP practices from the community in which we used to be so embedded. The volcanic anger this patient centred proposal supposedly caused in the profession gives bemused entertainment to all doctors qualified more than 15 years ago. Nearly all the self justifying pleading in the medical press against weekend and night time cover ignores the facts that junior doctors are under trained and under experienced today due to the rotas they currently work and that there are up to ten times as many doctors covering emergencies in hospitals during the week as at weekends. There are at least 4,400 deaths attributable to poor care at weekends according to the Sunday Times. The loudest protesters are, of course, junior doctors and most of those are now women. They are on call not for 33% of daytime Sundays as I was on my 1 in 3 rotas or 50% on my 1 in 2 rotas but for 3.6% of daytime Sundays. No wonder they don't want to alter their Life/work balance.

So this attempt at making medicine a vocation again with the needs of the patient at its heart and more on call is doomed to failure if the feminisation of medical schools and graduates, with their 60-65% careers, the needs of their growing families, the part-timism of General Practitioners, the growth of non-partners, portfolio careers and life/work balance, the working time directive and so on are to continue.

Continuity of care in General Practice was not an issue when I entered practice. You did an average 80 or 90 hour week (I remember the wry smiles my colleagues and I gave when the teachers were striking to reduce their 40 hour week and their working year to even fewer weeks) but I was half asleep when I wasn't at work. Also although I was saturated with patients, experience and pathology I do feel I missed out on seeing most of my children growing up. There was, however, a sense of my paying the country back for the privilege of a medical education. Does that not exist now?

12) GPs should make a point of contacting all their older patients every so often because the new contract has allowed many of them to quietly drop pastoral visits and much old style routine care. Good GPs should know who is on their list and know their patient's extended family as well. If patients are house bound, suffer a long term illness or take any regular medication, real family doctors will have a routine visiting schedule organised for each patient. If a GP's list is below 2000 there is no excuse for not keeping tabs on them all. If their list is around 1800, as many are, all housebound patients should be on a regular visiting rota. My list was between 2,200 and 2,300 for 30 years and all housebound patients were seen regularly.

13) The GMC suggested it adopt new powers from 2014 to assess the English language ability of all doctors working in the UK. **About time.** Yet again, patients rights and safety have been subservient to politics for years – as in fact they still are in many spheres, despite The Frances report. Under E.U. law, no German, (eg Daniel Ubani), Croatian, Bulgarian, Greek, Lithuanian, Romanian, Slovenian etc needed to prove that they could speak English at all in early 2014 although this was finally being addressed by the end of 2014. NHS employers have been hopelessly weak at assessing the REAL language skills of doctors and nurses for decades. The GMC website set up for comments on this proposal was 100% in favour of this change but why has politics put patients at such an obvious risk for so long? It might also like to review the standards it sets on the **comprehensibility** of those who it passes as fit to communicate – accent and vocabulary are as important as basic language skills within most consultations and in all specialities – especially for older patients, those who are hard of hearing or a little confused. There are 26,000 doctors from the EU on the medical register and far more from further afield.

I frequently go to lectures by doctors who are Senior Registrars, Deans, Lecturers or even Consultants, some in post for many years and who are virtually incomprehensible. This is either through heavy accent, pronunciation, poor diction or vocabulary. The audience gets the gist of the lecture from the hand out, the overheads, from the E Mail summary afterwards or from the whispered "What did he just say?" to a neighbour.

Patients come back from outpatients virtually every day with the depressing "She was very nice but I couldn't understand a word she said".

We are a first world country. Why do we need to rob developing countries of their doctors or take people who cannot speak the world's foremost language of scientific papers, navigation, Shakespeare, rock music, The Beatles, Hollywood, the BBC and air traffic control? Why can't we properly assess them before employing them? This obviously applies to their medical as well as language skills.

Our current system sometimes gives us a second class health service with, I estimate an incomprehensible – up to 20-25% of foreign trained doctors from various parts of the world. Even worse, many doctors are taken from countries where, as I have said elsewhere, training standards and curricula are inadequate or partly irrelevant for the British NHS. Sometimes (as with some Indian medical schools in 2015) corrupt. No wonder some do badly at professional examinations and assessments and need the unfair leg up of regular Equality and Diversity teaching given to appraisers and trainers to blur standards. A foreign doctors' pressure group, the BAPIO, sued the RCGP in 2014 claiming a cultural bias in the college's examinations and although they lost the case, claimed a "moral victory". They promised to try the legal action again. I can only hope that the Royal College has the courage of its patients' and most of its members' convictions. The College has now mooted that foreign graduates can take the AKT part of MRCGP as many as 5 times and fail it four times – and then still be considered competent to be MRCGP and a British GP. Would you want your family treated by someone who either didn't know the medicine or the English and so failed this part of the exam four times? What is a membership qualification worth? Is MRCGP supposed to hold its head up in the same company as other memberships and Fellowships which for the most part ARE tests of excellence and quality markers?

I thought I was alone in expressing this concern about a relatively small number of foreign trained doctors until I started asking various colleagues. Then I found many consultants and GPs, not all of whom trained in the UK agreed with me. Certainly the Royal Colleges and the GMC do if you judge by their decisions. It became front page news in several papers in April 2014 with the publication of "the most rigorous assessment of foreign trained doctors to date". Half of the 1300 foreign trained doctors allowed to work in the UK every year would fall short if they had to pass standard UK assessments said the Times front page article – especially those trained outside the EU. Patient groups said that this skills gap would damage trust in doctors (which in my experience is already highly selective) and they warned NHS "Chiefs" not to fill staffing gaps with foreign doctors.-What do you think they have been doing since 1948 and what are they planning to do for the huge looming GP deficit now?? The RCGP has called for General Practice to be designated a "Shortage Occupation" to make it even easier for overseas doctors to work here. Some casualty gaps are filled by Indian doctors interviewed by skype. Currently (2015) 22% of practitioners were trained overseas – an increase from 19% in 2004. In Barking and Dagenham 71% of GPs were trained overseas. Dr Kailash Chand, Deputy Chairman of the BMA in April 2015 said: "The important things are to make sure their clinical knowledge, communication skills and understanding of British culture are up to scratch." Good point.

Some of these figures come from a BMJ article in which academics from Cambridge and UCL showed 80% of foreign trained doctors do worse than British doctors in Membership exams. (Roughly 60% of British trained doctors pass MRCP first time but only 35% of those trained outside the EU). Researchers said this was to do with **medical knowledge** rather than other factors. This is despite them having passed a GMC exam designed to make sure they can function at the same level as British trained doctors. How worrying is that? How easy is the GMC exam anyway? **"Only 20% of international medical graduates are at the level of a median British graduate".** And "You look at the questions and think: I wouldn't want a physician who doesn't know the answer to that" said the leader of the study.

16% of all new doctors are foreign and another worrying paper, this time from Durham University, found that foreign trained doctors were 60% more likely to fail annual reviews of competence.

India supplies the most foreign doctors to Britain and in my experience Indian doctors are amongst the best but also the worst foreign doctors, likewise the next country, Pakistan. I have had the pleasure of working with some superb doctors from both countries but also had to try to understand the garbled English and fill in the basic knowledge of others. The rest of the list is, in order of numbers, Nigeria, Egypt, Ireland and so on. Add to these knowledge and language gaps, the occasional cultural difficulties and attitudes of some doctors from some countries and the picture yet again is one where politics in the form of political diversity, equality and correctness dogma has been triumphant over patient safety and quality of care. For instance:

Why **do** GP appraisers and trainers have to undergo Equality and Diversity training twice a year anyway? How does this improve clinical and communication standards amongst those being trained and appraised? How does it relate to or improve the quality of care received by the patient? Surely it simply implies that cultural, language and professional variations must be tolerated rather than brought up to a "British standard" and if you as an appraiser or trainer find fault in a foreign trained graduate because they have a poor grasp of English, or British attitudes, relationships or culture then there is clearly something wrong with your own politics and **your** attitude – and by the way, that of your patients.

The UCL paper suggested pass marks for foreign doctors to gain UK entry should be higher. The GMC in the article was quoted as saying: 1300 doctors a year from abroad passed the exams but subsequent performance suggested "Half of them should not have qualified." The same article described the extent to which the NHS has come to depend upon these foreign doctors ("Half of whom should not have qualified"). In the five years to 2012, 670 doctors were struck off, 420 (almost 2/3) were from abroad. This must be considered to be one of the very few truly unbiased reports on foreign doctors in the UK. The whole area is now wrapped up in so much political and racial static that it has become almost impossible to even raise the subject in official forums. Patients on the other hand, given permission, will talk about their experiences with far less constraint. Virtually every public statement and report is typified by the attitude and bias expressed by the GP Magazine headline of 21st July 2016 "BME doctors face unconscious bias and remain less likely to pass exams". (See figures below*)

The truth is however that there is a cultural *disbelief regarding the failures* of imported doctors amongst the medical managers, educators, academics and commentators not shared by patients and front line medics. Look at the **Front Page** of middle England's mouth piece, The Daily Mail, Sept 24th 2016: "Patients at risk from E.U. doctors". This may not be an academic journal but it accurately reflected the experience of many patients. This was an article quoting Niall Dickson, Head of The GMC talking about the loophole of EU membership that allows European doctors to work in the UK without professional competence checks. (Via the Free movement of labour). This is a "real weakness when it comes to protecting the public" "Some European doctors struggle when they come to practise here, medicine is very culturally specific" (See the discussion about the failure rate of foreign doctors and MRCGP and the RCGP being taken to court by the Indian doctors association). "It is only 2 years since the British authorities managed to assess whether European doctors were able to speak English". Said the Head of the GMC. There are 30,500 EU doctors practising in the UK and 3,500 more arrive each year. The GMC's own figures show that EU doctors are twice as likely to be suspended, struck off or given a warning than UK qualified doctors. It is clear that for whatever reason foreign trained doctors whether from developing countries or the EU are not offering the same quality of care that British trained doctors are.

There are 95,000 foreign trained doctors in the NHS – a quarter of the total at the time of the academic papers above.

In 2015 it was reported that 22% of GPs were trained overseas in an article about UK trained doctors shunning General Practice (Doctors.net). As we all know, in some parts of the UK there are almost no foreign trained doctors and in other parts almost no home grown GPs. In Barking and Dagenham 71% of GPs were trained overseas by 2015. Does this happen in other countries to the same extent?

It is not only patients, – even the medical establishment is beginning to realise this is a real problem at last with Dr Richard Vautrey GPC Deputy Chairman saying (April 2015) "We simply don't train enough within the UK to meet the needs of a growing population" – So: we either need more medical schools or a determined effort to stop the population growing. Perhaps the announcement at the Conservative Party Conference 2016 that the NHS would train up to 1500 more doctors a year and end the 6000 a year student number cap will achieve this. It would take 10 years and the joint announcement demanding repayment of education costs if graduates leave the country in less than 4 years would be essential. I can't help thinking some restriction on sex bias of medical schools or fertility of the recently qualified should have been included if the Government were really serious about cost effectiveness though.

The latest GMC figures (2015) are slightly different but reflect the overall medical population:

PMQ World Region	No. of doctors	%	No. of GPs	%	No. of Specialists	%
EEA (excluding UK)	29,269	11.0%	4,072	6.3%	13,916	16.7%
International	68,871	25.8%	10,871	16.7%	20,368	24.5%
UK	169,006	63.3%	50,165	77.0%	48,828	58.7%
Total	267,146	100.00%	65,108	100.00%	83,112	100.00%

PMQ is primary medical qualification and may not be the nationality of the doctor.

In the latest report *on doctors and ethnicity (July 2016), The GMC said the pass rate for

white UK graduates was   76%,
BME UK graduates   63%,
and PMQ outside EEA   41%.

14) Paediatric training should be a compulsory part of all GP training schemes because of the frequent failure of GPs to recognise seriously ill children. I was a Paediatric Lecturer before going into General Practice and only changed my mind about my career as an afterthought. Of course Paediatrics should be an absolute training requirement since in many practices anything up to half the consultations can be with children and at some times of year most of them are febrile. GPs are missing sepsis and so are casualty officers but the average DGH Paediatric unit cannot cope with its current workload let alone every "off colour" hot child that a playing safe GP sends in for a second opinion. I once heard a GP registrar who hadn't done a Paediatric job say she was just going to send every sick child into hospital. Hospitals are dangerous and risky places for children – if you send a well child in then you are just as likely to get a sick one out.

15) Compensation paid out by the NHS has risen by 20% in one year, with 16,000

people lodging claims in 2012/13. This amounts to £15.7Bn (this is a staggering 1/7 of the NHS budget) and bizarrely is based upon the cost of totally private care for the injured party. A lifetime of private care if a baby is brain damaged at birth. – **This is as if the NHS did not actually exist** and the care would not **actually** be provided by GPs, district nurses and NHS consultants. These are rules that were laid down when the NHS was started and have never been updated, something that clearly takes 1/7 of the care away from sick and dying patients. The system puts the money into the pockets of lawyers (Look at some compensation websites if you really want to see how lawyers generate their income) and often into the current accounts of patients who are actually getting their care free.

In 2015 the Conservative Government proposed a cap of £100,000 on excessive legal fees in compensation cases. This is not a cap in compensation pay-outs to the client but in excessive fees charged by their lawyers. These often exceed the compensation payment to the patient itself. We surely need rational but limited compensation sums awarded to the litigants too, sums estimated assuming that the NHS will do most of the care free or even, dare I say it, a compensation free NHS. This is not so difficult to justify: We are not an expensive private profit based health business system like the US. We have a tax payer funded free at the point of demand, pared down, run on a shoe string, provides everything state system. The innocent tax payer is penalised by the court for the hospital or doctor's error or bad luck. No system has ever shown that litigation improves clinical care and in the UK compensation comes out of funding for patient care. Because of constant premium increases, there were (August 2015) calls for Crown Indemnity to cover GP's medical Insurance. Why don't we just say that complaints will be heard, mistakes corrected, apologies issued, miscreants dealt with by professional bodies and victims looked after by the NHS but no compensation paid?

In an interview in October 2016 The Health Secretary, Jeremy Hunt proposed a faster way of dealing with obstetric disasters without the blame and secrecy culture that costs so much and causes such delay. He quoted £1.5 Bn per year in maternity pay outs and an average of 11.5 years to settle obstetric brain damage claims. Clearly the current system benefits only lawyers and causes harm to everyone else involved.

An article in the Sunday Times in April 2017 mentioning a patient who steadfastly refused to claim compensation, quoted NHS Resolution (The former NHS Litigation Authority) saying £56Bn could be needed to deal with all the cases arising from mistakes and failures up to march 2016. (This is half a year of running costs for the NHS, ps: there is only £70Bn circulating at any time in the British economy). They added that they received 11,000 new clinical negligence claims in 2015-16. They resolved 5,000 without payment of damages.

16) 1700 mental health beds have closed since 2011 and the Head of South London and Maudsley NHS Trust describes NHS mental health services as "In Crisis". 9% of the beds available in 2011/12 had been closed and there were no beds in London for several weekends in 2013/14. One London mental health patient had to be found a bed in Somerset. Nick Clegg announced that mental health was going to be a priority in January 2014 and almost immediately the dire state of Children and Adolescent's mental health emergency services was disclosed.

Well you need to increase local mental health bed numbers by 20% and fund locally trained medical staff as a matter of urgency to begin to address the pitiful state of UK mental health services. You also need to fund new regional adolescent units almost everywhere. – And you need to staff them with the right doctors. If any doctor needed to speak English competently, colloquially, to have a knowledge of the patients' background, their cultural and historical environment, even their national sense of humour and irony, it is the psychiatrist. Much of their therapy is a talking cure; they live and die by communication. Cues, intonations, inferences, humour – inappropriate or not, misplaced cultural references can all be part of the coded communication. How can anyone do that properly without excellent language and cultural knowledge? You could ask: How can anyone do that if their first language isn't English?

17) Three quarters of GP practices provide no service on either Saturday or Sunday ever. So David Cameron's promise to restore weekend Primary Care cover is going to prove either impossible or hopelessly expensive. With the part-timism of female GPs – and women are the majority of the profession, the now famous unwillingness of many female doctors to work nights and weekends (see the A and E crisis), the unwillingness of slaves once set free to re-enter servitude, I think it will take a major contract show down or withdrawal of most of the funding for everything else GPs do to coax real doctors back into doing first-on out of hours cover again.

18) A coalition of foreign doctors is taking the Royal College of General Practitioners to court because foreign trained doctors are 4 times more likely to fail the Membership Examination (2014). The College denies a racist bias. (-the actual failure rate sometimes quoted is 69% for some foreign applicants 9% for UK trained doctors in "GP Exams" – and this is after three years of UK GP training (Mail Online Oct 19 2013 – mainly Indian, Pakistani and Nigerian applicants). My experience of the training of registrars, the political indoctrination of trainers and appraisers, the MRCGP examination, the constant Equality and Diversity Indoctrination and the lack of factual candour of the Membership examination is that the College falls over itself to be antiracist in all its dealings. To the detriment of patient care sometimes. I am surprised the College faced down the British Association of Physicians of Indian Origin long enough to win the case. It is liberal to the point of paranoia. The long term outcome will be one of two things: No 1) The College has been racist – but that will be impossible to prove because all evidence for at least 20 years has shown exactly the opposite or 2) The obvious alternative. – and this seems to be confirmed by the public level of complaints, recent objective research published in various journals, the GMC's level of removals from the register as well as the exam data – that some foreign trained doctors just really aren't up to UK standards and shouldn't have passed GMC or RCGP exams. In mid 2015 serious proposals were being made that 5 attempts be allowed at the AKT part of MRCGP solely because foreign graduates were finding it hard to pass.

Certainly it is hard to see how some foreign doctors are up to British trained standards and no amount of Equality and Diversity indoctrination of Trainers and Appraisers will change that.

This latter conclusion, that many foreign doctors are sub standard seems supported by a number of front page headlines drawing attention to GMC decisions in 2013 and 2014: The Times April 2014: "Doctors from India are 4X more likely to be struck off than those trained in the UK. – The disclosures triggered concern about the scrutiny of foreign trained doctors after a recent decision to relax government rules on recruitment from overseas. GMC statistics show that in the last 5 years, 117 Indian and Pakistani trained doctors have been struck off against 142 British trained doctors. That is 1 in a 1000 UK trained doctors, 1 in 250 Indian trained doctors and 1 in 350 Pakistani trained doctors. In all, 75% of struck off doctors came here from abroad (up from 61% in 2009). Overseas doctors now make up one in three UK doctors, "Half of foreign doctors are below UK standards" and A and E vacancies are being filled by Indian doctors who have been interviewed on Skype. The country with the largest number of struck off doctors is India, followed by Pakistan, Egypt and Nigeria." etc

I have worked with some superb doctors from India and Pakistan. In fact one of the best three GPs and two of the best three surgeons I know are either Indian or Pakistani.

But

1) when compulsory Equality and Diversity Training is imposed on Trainers and Appraisers

(which surely implies that a certain loosening of language and clinical standards is only fair?) and

2) There is a disproportionate number of upheld complaints and strikings off against doctors from a relatively small number of foreign countries and

3) The failure rates of "Routine Appraisal Tests" and Membership Exams is so much higher in overseas doctors than for UK trained doctors

4) Foreign trained doctors are far more likely to defer and fail re accreditation compared with UK trained doctors

5) Two papers published in 2014 (BMJ and the Lancet) showed that only 20% of foreign trained doctors "were at the median British level" of exam competence

6) There was a national enquiry in India in mid 2015 about extensive corruption in the testing, reliability and awarding of medical degrees in a number of their most famous medical schools which had involved the deaths of some whistle blowers,

surely a reasonable conclusion is that the quality of medicine of many foreign trained doctors is poorer than British trained doctors and that we are putting British patients at risk by admitting so many and not testing their abilities properly?

19) The NHS has been writing off £500m annually in treatment given to foreign nationals and not chased up after they had left the country. I simply don't believe this was all for life threatening emergencies. It was for the severe pain of my mother's hip who is visiting and she can't cope anymore, or my sister happens to be visiting and is now in labour with her twins, both situations I have seen. Just think how many services, staff, new equipment this "theft" from the British tax payer could pay for. This is typical of the result of decades of grey politics stemming from "free at the point of demand", no restrictions, the no obligations, just rights "wet care" that the NHS has evolved to give. Doctors are indoctrinated not to challenge patients from day 1 in medical school. This global largess was not in the original plan and certainly not what the public wants when asked and when they think about it, so why do we allow it? We cave in to sympathetic foreign news coverage, human rights spokespeople and the completely unrepresentative politicians of the liberal left as if we were a world power with infinite resources and largess and had a population who wanted its money spent on the curing sick of the rest of the world. It begins with Great Ormond St separating third world Siamese twins or treating the war injured of the Middle East and African conflicts and this humanity becomes conflated with treating everyone from everywhere on demand.

20) More British children die every day than in Sweden because of poor care. Rickets is on the rise in the UK, because of the increasing number of brown skins, paranoia about

melanoma amongst those with pink skins and our inside, computer focused lives these days. Only 16% of our diabetic adolescents are well controlled compared with double that number in Germany and our adolescent mental health services are poor and being cut. The only surprise there is that Germany **only** manages to control a third of **its** adolescent diabetics.

21) Up to a quarter of all NHS Trusts are failing to provide "satisfactory" care to their patients, even after the Mid Staffs and Francis enquiry. The government replies by saying that its new inspection regime will sort that out. That would be inspection by the CQC: – the whistle blower persecuting, incompetent amateur inspector using, newly revamped, run by ex managers of dysfunctional and abusive Health Authorities/Trusts and now refocussing on "real care...." CQC ?

22) The BMA is "Now supporting a 7 day a week NHS" which will save at least 4,400 lives if the Monday to Friday death rate is extended to the weekend too. It says there are resource implications and does not want routine medical conditions and operations etc dealt with 7 days a week but does want to be part of ensuring acutely ill patients get better care at weekends. Little does it know the outcry from the feminised medical profession this clearly life saving and patient centred proposal will cause. The BMA will change its stance somewhat by 2015 when it sees the overwhelming difficulty of reminding a less dedicated, less vocational, less self sacrificial, more domesticated and less masculine profession that the patient used to come first.

23) The NHS is "Dismissive" when claims of poor care for seriously ill and dying patients are made against it by relatives. This is according to a review carried out by Ann Clwyd whose husband died in hospital in Cardiff a year or two ago. The nurses caring for him at the end "Showed coldness, indifference, even contempt" according to the emotional and articulate description of his MP wife. I have never worked on a unit where the dying were not given water or kept warm or the dignity of having their nakedness covered or sufficient pain relief. I found her description as shocking as it was inexcusable. Were the nurses so over worked they had no time to give basic humane care to fellow human beings? Were they given other priorities and forgot what they were really there to do, to look after patients?, Were there too few of them or too many beds? Were they so protocol driven or all degree status nurses so that they felt above basic nursing? I just don't know. But clearly whoever were the senior nurses on the ward failed to reorder the work and care priorities and attitudes of their team day after day. Surely they cannot just be allowed to get away with this?

Part of the problem is that all complaints procedures take too long. Positions and feelings polarise and compromise becomes impossible and, of course, people forget what actually happened within weeks. Only lawyers and "judges" fail to realise this reality. When one couple of patients complained about my refusing the husband a sick certificate, (he said he was unable to work because of anxiety but I knew he had a cash window cleaning business on the side and hadn't the time to "work") the process involved three interviews, several written submissions, hours of work and a file an inch or more thick after eighteen months. The case was dismissed and you will have to take my word that the complainants' testimony was complete nonsense.

24) In November 2013 it emerged that Colchester cancer unit staff were bullied into falsifying appointment and treatment times so that they seemed to meet national targets. Staff members had blown the whistle, an inadequate internal review had not addressed the

problem, the Chief Executive failed to resign and Bernard Jenkin the North Essex MP said "It is a terrible indictment of the culture of the Health Service that we have replaced values with targets" and a sense of resigned disappointment was felt all round. The unit was put in "Special Measures".

It is ironic that politicians, the very people who are primarily responsible for the target led, clip board culture, command and control, top down attitudes that have caused virtually all these scandals and the suffering and deaths in their wake are the first to divest themselves of all blame. Of course it is politicians and managers who are responsible for setting and enforcing the impossible targets in the first place and pretending that every ward, every department and every unit is capable of providing the same level of service and care along with all their other administrative priorities. They can't. There are good units in the NHS and there are bad units. Targets per se don't make a blind bit of difference.

25) A fifth of the maternity budget pays for the less than 1:1000 deliveries that go wrong and result in multimillion compensation claims, 1/5 of the whole budget to cover the pay outs which are still calculated assuming there is no free healthcare in the UK. The Secretary of State and the Public Accounts Committee agree that this is an unjust and unjustifiable, unsustainable situation. Several of their predecessors have said the same thing. Unfortunately the lawyers are in charge, not the people or their nominal representatives and they always get rich and most parliaments are full of them. Well, all they have to do is cap or end compensation claims against the NHS. Make a law that says no one can sue the NHS or a doctor for more than, say, £50,000. At the moment, thousands of innocent victims are harmed by having millions of pounds of funding diverted from clinical care. In return for capping this, every serious incident should be investigated within a limited time span, say 6 months, by an independent tribunal quickly and honestly and their recommendations for changes to clinical practices and staffing levels implemented compulsorily. The "victim" is given "priority care" thereafter. No prosecution of a doctor for a medical mistake or negligence has ever been shown to improve standards or reduce further mistakes. What does is persuading the relevant department to review its procedures, start regular unit clinical review meetings, adequate cover arrangements or rotas.

(Complications, Atul Gawande)

26) Four million over 75 year olds to be registered with a named GP who knows their medical history and who (to quote the Health Secretary) "doesn't have to ask about 65 questions about their history every time they phone up". Ambulances will be able to phone GPs directly. Why not have a named GP for every patient? That was the original idea of the NHS after all.

Some of us never stopped doing this because we always felt the backbone of good Family Medicine is a personal relationship with your doctor. The last coalition Health Secretary blamed the 2004 Labour contract for ending registration with GPs and introducing the (ludicrous, unpopular, doomed to fail, hated by all patients) registration with the practice structure, which all good practices actually ignored. Andy Burnham, the labour health spokesman said it was the "Coalition's fault" that It was harder to get any appointment with **anyone** in your practice under the government". The Health Secretary at the time replied that GPs will soon have to be responsible for care 24 hours a day 7 days a week, and 40% of ticking boxes had been cut out by the coalition.!! What he actually meant was GPs would supervise others providing nocturnal and weekend care.

27) The new charge of Wilful neglect will now be a stick to threaten uncaring staff

with although nowhere in the world has the prosecution of medical staff after the event been shown to improve standards of care for patients. As I said above, the nursing and medical professions didn't suddenly stop caring nationally over the last decade by magic. For nurses it was partly due to a reduction in numbers, partly what they did with their time spent on the ward (too much record keeping, reporting and administration) and partly altered working practices (management directed and audited, task focussed schedules and lists instead of patient responsive and independent working). So give the nurses their professional freedom and independence back and you won't need to threaten them with anything.

28) Ambulances are now waiting not for the recommended 15 minutes to off load sick patients at casualty but for up to 5 hours – An A and E consultant was interviewed on the radio and blamed the ridiculously high occupancy rates and the consequent lack of beds in all hospitals, the absence of general Consultants to discharge patients at weekends and the inability to discharge patients into social care in the community.

How did they manage to find a casualty Consultant to interview?

29) Poor care at Lanarkshire to be investigated due to the increase in death rate compared with similar units. If this is the HSMR, the Dr Foster Organisation's Hospital Standardised Mortality Ratio, then it may not be quite as reliable as you think and it may be losing some of its currency.

Some hospitals, for instance, have higher recorded death ratios because of their atypical catchment areas, their inpatient specialities or their patient intake may be different. Although the Mid Staffs failures in care were first highlighted by their high HSMR, other hospitals have found their ratios were improved by the opening of a local hospice which took all the dying patients out of their figures or other factors outside their control. (Deadly Hospitals. File on Four: Feb 14, 2014)

30) Consultants to be forced to be on call at weekends and see all emergency admissions within 14 hours. Consultants can earn huge amounts in overtime in some specialities but actually do more on call than many average junior doctors by some assessments. For instance: Juniors do Sunday day times on call as only 3.6% of their total work rota according to the Sunday Times (July 2015) And Isn't medicine supposed to be an apprenticeship?

31) The head of the CQC says NHS staff are out of control and that a target culture and micromanagement by politicians as well as a collective fear by staff of criticising the system are all to blame. Given the history of the last year, most NHS staff would say precisely this about the CQC.

32) The main hospital in Northern Ireland, the Royal Victoria Hospital put out a major incident call on a Wednesday of a normal week because the hospital and casualty unit were both full and there was a "Lack of A and E staff" to deal with the influx. This left 42 patients on trolleys in the department. The main issue seemed to be too few doctors applying to work in casualty departments leaving them chronically understaffed. No doubt the dangerous over 100% bed occupancy that is the norm in the NHS also had something to do with it as well. This lack of casualty doctors is a new phenomenon. Two thirds of medical graduates are now female and A and E is an arduous, confrontational, stressful, high pressure and often unpleasant working environment. It necessitates hard rotas, both in training and working. Female doctors value their families and their life/work balance it seems, more than their male colleagues and now there is the Working Time Directive

protecting both sexes from the long hours of their predecessors that were the norm a few decades ago. Could these facts be linked? Women do not "do casualty" according to the spokesman of the College of Emergency Medicine on the Today Programme in 2014 and by that year A and E units were spending £120m/year on locums. Three trusts used locums 50% of the time.-This is just to **normally** staff A and E departments.

Clearly the NHS has been the laboratory in which every government and political or economic theory has had free reign over six decades with the result that patients have been the least important stake holder and what happens to them only a peripheral issue. It has to cope with society's problems and politics – TB, Hepatitis B, and a lot of the Rickets and HIV is due to immigration policy, sexual health, abortion and many obstetric problems are due to social, welfare and tax policy, go to a casualty unit on Friday or Saturday and see the cost that alcohol excise duty pouring into the Treasury part of government exacts on another part. Our political system and compensation culture is run by lawyers, accountants and human rights activists and it shows. The patient, directly or indirectly pays the bill. Nobody in their right mind could think that the NHS works well anymore. Certainly not with the idea that patient is at its centre.

The Sun launched a **"Major Investigation"** into the "NHS in crisis" in the Summer of 2014: It cited record numbers using GP services, record numbers being turned away and swamping A and E units because patients cannot get appointments with GPs.

Other facts it mentioned were 10.6m Britons having surgery the previous year, drug prescriptions up 60% since 2004 and GPs conducting 40m more consultations than in 2009. The worst performing areas quoted were Bradford, Slough, Redbridge, Newham where 20% of people were unable to get an appointment with their GP. Even in the best performing areas – Bath and North East Somerset 5% couldn't get appointments. A third of people felt (YouGov poll) that NHS services had got worse in the last year and the paper, with its typical frankness, blames obesity, lax immigration policy and people living longer. They comment that funding access to GPs is the key and that (this time from the Times) 40m people will be turned down for an appointment (original source RCGP). Subsequent research suggested that it would be 50m for the year.

A RCGP spokeswoman blamed lack of investment and an elderly population. Obviously no spokeswoman from the unfailingly unworldly and P.C. RCGP would blame sloth, greed, immigration, over dependency, feminisation and part-timism of the medical profession or anything else as non PC as these. They suggested another 8000 GPs to cope with the workload. Let us hope some of them will be male, trained in the UK or at least to UK standards and full time. GPs conduct 90% of the consultations of the NHS and have seen a drop from 10.75% (2005) to 8.4% (2012) of the budget of the NHS. The RCGP now want this to be raised to 11%. Why not more?

So it is hard to get an appointment with a GP now – which is as much to do with your GP being at home with her kids half the time and changing GP demography as it is lower thresholds for consulting amongst patients. The doctor's appointment was some-thing when I was a boy that was an occasion of formality, worth and value. The question of overuse, consulting with trivia or taking the "service" for granted didn't arise when I was a child. Indeed my parents, despite paying to set the NHS up, never saw it as a familiar "service". It was something to be respected and valued. The doctor was not "serving" us and providing a service like a plumber or a prostitute, we were "consulting" him like a trusted, respected, expert advisor and friend. How different the situation by 2015 when 80% of London GPs were so angered by regular non attendees that they demanded fines for DNAs. A 2015 study by LMCs in Leicester, Leicestershire and Rutland showed 68,000 appointments, 5% of the total were missed by patients – 16 million across England annually. (GP 10/11/15) In another study published in June 2015 it transpired that a million booked consultations went unattended. Nationally the charity Developing Patient Partnerships asked GPs about missed appointments. The total was 12.6 million per year. There were 4.3 million missed practice nurse appointments, half a million in London. A BMA spokesman commented that fining patients "Goes against the ethos of the NHS" despite the fact that 70% of GPs back a fine for patients who fail to turn up. Why is it that the BMA just like the RCGP are the GPs' national representative bodies but fail to actually represent their views and opinions on most matters of organisational politics? Interestingly one doctor in the correspondence related to the DNA article said he had cured the non attender problem in his practice by seeing all the 91% of patients who wanted to be seen on the day, on the day. Interesting.

Again, this is what it was like when the NHS began. You went to the surgery and you waited to be seen.

Why has every news item on the NHS for the last decade or so been so relentlessly negative? All that patients in General Practice want is a doctor they can get to know and trust and who knows them. A named GP they have relationship with and who stops the buck. Ideally they would like the out of hours service to be staffed by local GPs and not by overstretched, often unrecognisable locums. They want the soft politics out of medical care and some sense of vocation and commitment and of caring for the patient, yes – perhaps of self sacrifice, back into it. Just like it was from 1945 until got messed up ten years or twenty years or so ago.

And all that patients needing hospital care want is enough spare (empty) beds to accommodate the wholly predictable fluctuations in emergency admissions, sufficient staff to avoid last minute cancellations of routine lists and procedures, nurses who have the freedom and time, the flexibility to react to the patient's needs, doctors trained to the equivalent of British standards and able to speak with and relate to the average British patient, and again they want doctors and nurses who they can respect and who respect them and who make a good fist of **caring**.

We got it right for decades. We had a vocation, we worked all the hours God sent, we respected the patient and each other, and we cared about the system. It was the politicians not the doctors and nurses who changed it and put the dogma and the organisation first and the patients' needs at the bottom of the pile. If you were to allow me, or anyone to put the patients' needs above every other consideration, bogus financial and clinical targets, Equality and Diversity law, Human Rights and discrimination law, the vested interests of unions, E.U. employment and Language rules, the over education of nurses and the under education of doctors, the entrenched feminism of medical schools – all of which actively harm patients and allow me to ensure the only consideration is how the patient will be affected then we **could** turn the NHS around.

Wish me good luck with that, but until that day comes, there is still no out of hours quality care: the new generation of GPs who are mainly female, want a work life balance, don't feel they owe the state anything back for their exclusive education, and certainly wouldn't want to be involved in the best on call system that we had: The GP Cooperatives organised and manned by local GPs on a rota in every area of the country with everyone taking a share in nights and weekends. But then I suppose manned was, for the most part, the appropriate term.

We almost need to start from scratch because even the latest "back to basics" suggested by the Health Secretary in 2013 was half hearted (only the over 75s will have a named doctor, the GP will be nowhere to be seen at midnight or Sunday afternoon, most GPs being women will not want to be full time or partners in practice and so they will not be able to provide what the patient craves and the Government belatedly values: continuity of care.)

Our much vaunted and once respected system was, of course "much admired throughout the world but never copied" and the best aspects of it, which depended on the good will and dedication, long hours and sacrifice of its medical staff are now lost in tiers of reorganisation.

It is time to rethink the National Health service. We have let it get out of hand. Like a traveller who goes equipped for every terrain, climate and every eventuality the NHS is too cumbersome to be responsive or flexible at all.

Surely all political parties should now get together with representatives of the medical, nursing and other allied professions and decide on a twenty year plan. We need tough rules and we need to back up the staff who apply them. All politics should be expunged. Strikes made illegal, compensation claims restricted and limited in value – the patients' wider needs being the sole consideration. "Needs" being the important but difficult concept. We should decide on what services will be funded and the level of staffing that is necessary to provide a safe service.

It was only in the Summer of 2014 that hospitals in England were given guidelines on safe nursing levels – 8 patients per nurse on standard wards during the daytime. Even these "stopped short of absolute minimums". This should be available everywhere. Surely the whole care structure depends on this basic accepted provision. NICE said that this ratio, if exceeded should act as a trigger for a check to see if general care was being compromised. Other "red flags" were delays in pain relief, giving of medication or such things as not being helped to the bathroom.

We have to bang politicians' heads together to conclude what can the NHS provide? What will it stop providing?, Who will be allowed to provide it, what will their contracts say, how will they be regulated, disciplined and nothing, excepting a national economic meltdown, a national medical emergency or a completely revolutionary advance in treatment will be allowed to mess around with how the service is provided.

Well that is a dream. But how is it provided now?

The Structure, History and Partnerships of the NHS

Is it beyond the wit of politicians to agree the level of services we must provide for all and the clinical areas of those services? Do we need to pay for infertility treatment and inves-tigations, smoking cessation, bariatric surgery, erectile dysfunction, gender reassignment, any treatment of foreign nationals who turn up on the doorstep, the perinatal care of extremely premature babies, – well perhaps we do? Should we charge for non serious consultations in A and E and for all out of hours consultations? Should GPs charge for house calls to the non house bound?

Should anyone who consults more often than the mean pay a contribution each time, which is assessed and refunded if they suffer a genuinely unstable or serious chronic condition? Can we make the system FAIRER?

Whatever we decide, we need a consensus across politics and we need to stick rigidly to it. Then we might start removing the politics and letting some of the original goals of the NHS back to centre stage. Part of this involves changing the attitudes and standards of nursing and medicine. Giving back clear responsibilities, clear demarcation of roles and in my opinion going back to doctors making clinical decisions and nurses doing nursing. In short, giving CONTROL back to doctors and to nurses at ward level.

I emphasise however that doctors should have control over medical decisions (admissions to hospital, clinical decisions, prescribing and management, service provision) and nurses should have control over nursing issues (staffing levels, routine management of stable patients, patient supervision, record keeping and bureaucracy, visiting times, even management roles). Problems and conflict arise where these responsibilities and roles become confused or overlap.

Well that is a dream. But how is it provided now?

Basic Workforce figures 2014-5 from the RCP Census:

	Consultants	Registrars
Geriatric Medicine:	1,300	570
Gastroenterology:	1,152	567
Cardiology:	1,130	729
Respiratory Medicine:	1,100	624
Haematology:	903	484
Endocrinology:	800	428
Neurology:	756	293
Dermatology:	740	206
Rheumatology:	732	262
Renal Medicine:	567	379
Palliative Medicine:	500	222
Acute Medicine:	500	325
Medical Oncology:	422	222

Intensive Care Beds/100,000 population

Germany:	25
Belgium:	22
Croatia:	20
USA:	20
Canada:	13
France:	10
Netherlands:	9
Spain:	9
RSA (private)	5
China:	3
RSA: (Public)	3
UK:	3

No wonder it is so difficult to find an intensive care bed in the UK when we provide an eighth of those in Germany and a third of those in France and only the same

proportionately as public beds in South Africa and China.
(Adapted from Future Hospital Journal Feb 2016)

GP Consultations:

1n 1995 there were 4 consultations per head of population per year for each GP. By 2005 this had become 5 each. See below: it is now 6-7.

Roughly speaking there are 336m GP consultations a year in the UK. In 2014 the RCGP did a survey and publicised the fact that 28% of patients were unable to get an appointment in the same week, 40% saying this would adversely affect their health (-why wasn't that figure more? – were too many people asking for trivial appointments in the first place then?) It was estimated that approximately 50m patients would be declined appointments in 2014. 62% of GPs said the large number of consultations were risking the standard of care they were giving. We are now in a situation where immediate access, on the day appointments, both given the political status of human rights a few years ago, clog up surgeries and together with NICE guidelines, disease management and QuoF follow ups have all but strangled primary care. GPs cannot cope with the demand for appointments, one twentieth of which are defaulted on the day. Those patients who feel they cannot wait just go to overwhelmed A and E units, where a large proportion are sent home without treatment. To be honest, if there were a simple filter, say a fee of £25 per appointment, how many of those patients would still feel such a burning desire to see their doctor so quickly? I can't count the number of indignant patients who told me in a wasted appointment that had I not been so busy, they might have been able to see me a few days earlier when they were ill, before they had frustratingly got better.

I audited a year's worth of my out of hours calls about twenty years ago and found, in the absence of a chronic or debilitating illness, the average patient really needs to see their doctor within 24 hours about twice in a lifetime and within a few days about once every four to five years. About 75-80% of out of hours requests for visits were unnecessary medically. Clearly we are now a very dependent population who cannot take the slightest sensible decision about our own health or that of family members. We are all totally "Risk Averse". GPs do 90% of the NHS' patient contact with 8% of the budget and we are as a population, used to an incredibly indulgent and over accessible primary care service. General Practice is now failing the genuinely ill patient of course, who gets elbowed out by the "you can't be too careful"patients.

I have heard a figure quoted of significant medical errors taking place in 1:120 consultations. Given the fact that general practice is the management of uncertainty and endless trivia with atypical and inconsistent presentations, unreliable histories and witnesses, I am amazed that this comes to only 2.8 million mistakes each year. Especially with the current out of hours system of back up cover.

There are 580,000 deaths each year in the UK.

In 2014 we had reached, as I have said, some sort of crisis in offering sufficient appointments for consultations. GPs will say this is because patients consult far too readily (-the "you can't be too careful culture") encouraged by a Nanny State and risk averse journalism. Or otherwise because of the routine screening, guidelines and follow up responsibilities that we GPs of 20 years ago simply did not have. Certainly our role has expanded well beyond just seeing, diagnosing and treating ill people. There were calls in the medical literature to end QuoF in August 2015 as these administrative checks on healthy patients imposed by our contract, hugely distracting and time consuming have now become a predominant and irrelevant part of a GP's consultation work load.

We offer Midlife MOTs which are Public Health England's flagship screening programme. These too take up lots of time and seem pointless to most of us and the patients. A study in September 2015 suggested that since its introduction in 2009 it was also a waste of £450m/year, failing to achieve its goals of preventing heart disease etc. Various other studies had shown the project to be no better than opportunistic GP case finding. This is certainly my opinion. New research in 2016 (BMJ open, Jan 2016, Queen Mary Uni. London) was less negative and however suggested 2,500 cardiovascular events had been prevented over 5 years. This because high risk patients had been found and given statins. Only a half of the 15m eligible patients in England took up invitations to be screened in 2015 however. This latest (encouraging) study suggested that one case of hypertension was picked up per 27 screening appointments, one diabetic every 110 and one with CKD every 265 appointments. I suggest that if GPs were not bogged down with the other 26,109 and 264 wasted screening appointments, QuoF, computer generated red flags and so on but free to see patients with their own agenda and with a consultation centred on what they want to ask then we would almost certainly opportunistically pick up the very few abnormal at risk patients ourselves.

For patients, it can be incredibly frustrating trying to get to see a GP if you are genuinely ill and you know – even if they are "nominally full time" (which is never 10 sessions a week for GPs like in the real outside world and many GPs for some reason tell me it is 8 sessions, or four days*) they are probably not actually seeing other patients. Instead they are wasting their time with diabetic or hypertensive patient screening, being appraised, teaching, attending prescribing committees or CCGs, Equality and Diversity training, practice Away-days, Health and Safety Training, QuoF or CQC inspections, yet another Trainers' Residential meeting, going on a course to do a post graduate degree in Medical Education, doing part of their compulsory 50 post graduate learning credits, or any of the dozens of irrelevant diversions that GPs escape real work with these days. My GP in the 1950's just saw sick patients. He was always available. He had continuity.

When I qualified, of all these things, only doing the training of the "trainees" existed to distract me from patient care and usually this was done as you were seeing the patient, not in separate sessions.

Almost no practice I know has a really fair or accessible system for sorting and seeing the genuinely needy patient right up to the last minute of cover. Telephone and nurse triage, skype and E mailing are all dangerous and exclude a significant number of really sick patients. The first come, first served, grab the few reserved on the day appointments early, Screwfix "once it's gone it's gone" is the least fair of all – and it is the commonest current system. Unless you run an open house and see everyone who turns up on the day which is probably the safest and fairest system. Certainly it is the one with the fewest "no shows". Most practices are, quite frankly, inaccessible and dangerous to the acutely ill and the least pushy.

*When GPs actually did night cover in between working days they were allowed to have a half day a week off. This was theoretically in order for them to catch up with the sleepless night they would have had the night before. Many GPs, over the years found that they could, with the aid of an appointments system and mutual cover, take a whole day off a week and yet still regard themselves as full time. This continues today even though almost no GPs do their own out of hours cover or work late evenings regularly. Therefore we should all be doing 10 sessions if we call ourselves full time today. At one appraisal I had a female partner call 6 sessions "Full Time".

A RCGP questionnaire in April 2014 found 28% of patients could not get an appointment in the same week, 40% said the wait adversely affected their health. There was a marked post code variation. As for GPs, 62% said the number of consultations they were doing risked the standard of care. You will remember that GPs do 90% of the patient contact of the NHS. Anyone in their right mind would conclude that with the third and fourth generations born with a free NHS that "Free at the point of demand" was a nice but naive political idea which has had its day and no longer works.

The average patient saw their doctor 4 times a year when I entered GP a third of a century ago. The RCGP says it is now 7 times a year, a million patients seen by GPs each day. I can't remember the last time I had any empty slots. These numbers can vary between 14 and 20 appointments per session; if I am on call or during times of high demand, I will see many more.

There was a call in 2017 for appointment times to be increased to 15 minutes. This was because so much relatively complicated traditional secondary care work had been off loaded into Primary Care. Add to this the multi-morbidity of so many elderly, the time it takes old people to undress and the increasing complexity of today's treatment guidelines and consultations simply take longer. My consultations have been seven and a half minutes for decades. This is because at ten minutes there could be occasions when I might be waiting for patients to turn up and three to four hour surgeries leave precious little time for admin, phone calls, visits and refuelling. Life as a GP is always rushed so there is nothing more frustrating than working flat out then waiting for traffic delayed, feckless or forgetful patients to turn up.

The number of consultations in the UK has increased by nearly a quarter in the 5 years to 2017. Perhaps Brexit will ease this. Research from the Health Foundation based on information from 11 countries in Europe, Australia and the US suggests time spent consulting by UK GPs is the lowest in the developed world. 92% of consultations in the UK are done in less than 15 minutes compared with 27% in other countries.

From teenage to the age of 70 there is an enormous female bias in consulting rates with the biggest bias between the ages of 20 and 40 when men on average consult proportionally twice a year and women five times. Consulting rates between the sexes only actually equalise at about 80 to 85years of age so it is hard to attribute all the consulting propensity of women to pregnancy and contraception.

Broadly speaking, surgery appointments are 85%, telephone consultations make up 10% and visits 5% of the total consultations. (In other words home visits are roughly 35-50/1000 population/year) I audited the number of evening and night visits once when I covered a lot of other local doctors out of hours and it was clear that I was visiting patients from some doctors' lists far more often than others. Obviously the age and decrepitude of the list and number of nursing homes covered will influence the number of visits. But the threshold for expecting a home visit OOH also varied a great deal – with the patient's perception of the severity of the illness, the patients past experience of illness and their doctors' behaviours OOH, the patient's social attitudes, their personal self confidence, the quality of the other doctor's daytime practice and the accessibility of short notice appointments during the daytime, the opening hours of the other practices, the clinical skills of the other doctors on the rota, whether they personally did sessions in the rota (in which case they were less likely to advise the patient to call later if not better) and so on. Few things caused greater resentment in a shared rota than knowing it was impossible for patients to get to see their own doctors as "an emergency" in the afternoon and finding that their patients needed to be seen far more often in the evenings and at night with emergency problems that could have been pre-empted had their own doctor been a bit more accessible in normal hours. I also worked out that by my definition of an emergency, (the possibility of a significant real deterioration in health or risk to life if a consultation is delayed) in someone not suffering from a recurrent paroxysmal deterioration in a chronic illness, happens no more than 2-3 times in a lifetime. Some patients in our out of hours cooperative, without a life threatening illness or serious disability were being visited 30-40 times a year. So much for Care in the community, The Patient's Charter, free at the point of demand and so on and so on. You can often blame the doctors at the front end who have been trained to avoid confrontation at all costs for some of this but the politicians and the lawyers often make the rules and create the atmosphere in which common sense and priorities in front line General Practice no longer apply. Many doctors just visit in preference to a telephone confrontation about the inappropriate use of an emergency service therefore encouraging its future misuse.

Nurse Practitioners, phone consultations and other ways of consulting.

Can non doctors do consultations on behalf of GPs? Prompted by the endless complaint that we are over worked and that patients just can't be fitted in, on demand within a reasonable time scale, various solutions have been discussed in recent years. There was a great deal of media chatter (2015) regarding non doctors in various guises substituting for GPs as a first port of call to take some of the demand away from GPs in order to reduce waiting times in Primary Care. This is cheaper than building medical schools and less sensible than addressing the real problem that half our time is spent on administration. Practice Nurses, Nurse Practitioners, Primary Health Care Assistants, Occupational Therapists, Practice Pharmacists, all have been suggested as being suitable triage assistants or substitutes. Patients however generally want to see someone they know, with whom they have personal and therapeutic trust and continuity and someone with authority, with whom the buck stops. Otherwise they rightly feel short changed. Ask **them**: they would rather see a doctor for five minutes than a nurse for fifteen. They often have to come back and see the doctor after doing the former anyway according to the research evidence. A study in the BJGP, (Bostock Feb 2016) found the following, none of which should come as any surprise given doctors' and nurses' respective day jobs and responsibilities, our patients' needs and expectations and how doctors and nurses are trained to think:-

Telephone triage systems in GP practices do not reduce workload or the overall time clinicians spend with patients. GP telephone triage contact with patients last 4 minutes while nurse triage calls last 6.6 minutes on average. Telephone triaged patients are more likely than those who come to the practice to need seeing again in the next 28 days. Overall, **total clinician time is higher** in practices using telephone triage systems.

Patients seen without previous phone triage take on average 9.6 minutes of clinician's time,

Patients seen who had been previously triaged by a GP take 10.3 minutes

Patients seen who had previously been triaged by a nurse take 14.8 minutes.

So found the BJGP study.

The authors concluded there was no health economic saving and the workload was just redistributed..

It seems to me that bringing in any number of relatively unskilled assistants is dangerous and missing the point. What General Practice needs is an end to the interminable patient administration, audit and screening related distractions which have appeared as part of The GP's job in the last 40 years. We need to refocus on the agenda that the patient brings in not the one the computer posts up for us.

I attended a meeting some years ago about clinical nurse specialists/practitioners and I went fully supportive of an expanded professional and prescribing role for practice nurses. I thought that many nurses I had worked with could easily work within protocols, make some diagnostic and prescribing decisions independently and thus improve accessibility for the patient and reduce my work load. As long as they were in cooperation and not in competition or conflict with the doctor and as long as I employed them. Especially for mundane and relatively trivial cases. I would be next door in the ?rare event that she would want a second opinion. Half the audience already had a nurse practitioner and half didn't. We took a show of hands – "who is in favour and who against?" before and after the talk. Then a speaker in favour and a speaker against gave their talks.

The gist of the arguments for me came down to the average length of each nurse's consultation (which it then turned out was 20 minutes +) The cost (the nurse was more expensive per patient than a locum GP) and the number of patients who were referred to the doctor after seeing the nurse (actually over half). The work load was therefore not reduced, most patients were not satisfied and still only reassured by subsequently seeing the doctor. Most nurses were seen as risk and decision "averse" and trained to follow clear instructions and protocols – not to make their own diagnoses or follow independent appropriate lines of enquiry. They avoided reasonable decisions based on limited evidence and were unprepared to take clinical risks when there was no obvious management tool or protocol to guide them. The management of risk and the acceptance of responsibility. That I suppose IS the difference between a doctor and a nurse in a nutshell.

At the end of the meeting the initial 50/50 vote had gone 90% against 10% in favour. I mention all this because a 2014 study showed that phone consultations rather than face to face consultations do not reduce GP work load (Lancet, July 2014, 42 practices) and the 2016 BJGP study just confirms it. In this attempt to take some strain off the GP a lot of patients were eventually seen in any case said Prof John Campbell, University of Exeter. The average practice has 20 patients who need to be seen on the day and researchers at Exeter found that if a doctor phoned the patient, the number of patients dealt with by practices increased by 33% and if a nurse phoned it was increased by 48%.

If the first meeting was in person, 50% of patients needed a second visit but 75% of GP phone calls and 88% of nurse calls required a later visit to the doctor, "**This is not the silver bullet** to dealing with work load" – Not at all. As far as silver bullets are concerned, GPs are still Lone Rangers when it comes to the front line of General Practice and Tonto isn't a nurse practitioner.

Some History:
We may be going through a decade of disbelief and disappointment with the NHS, – the Bristol Heart scandal

The Mid Staffs, Morecambe Bay, Cardiff and other nursing scandals,
The GP out of hours failed alternatives,
The inflexible application of The Liverpool Care Pathway
NHS Direct problems and then NHS Direct pulling out of 111. Poor 111 staffing and response time,
The A and E chaos,
Frequent reorganisations (eg Commissioning outcome framework COF, replacing QOF)
Increased complaints regarding doctors before the GMC,
The corrupt practices at The CQC, gagging whistle blowers, inspectors not fit for purpose,
The appalling treatment of whistle blowers in the NHS,
the junior doctors' strike,
but it was not always so:

The Evolution of the N.H.S:

To quote the excellent Civitas critique of what is wrong with the NHS by multiple authors – "The Health of the Nation" 2016: The returning troops from the second world war had experienced the depression of the twenties and thirties and had seen off fascism. "They were fired up by the need to create the conditions which would prevent a recurrence" The enemies were now want, ignorance, idleness, squalor and disease. The weapons were social security, universal education, employment exchanges, town planning, a massive house building programme and the NHS.

1948 The NHS launched by Health Secretary, Aneurin Bevan
1952 Prescription charges introduced
1953 DNA structure discovered (Deoxyribo etc etc Not Did Not Arrive)
1954 Smoking linked to cancer, Children in hospital allowed daily visits (not just weekends)
1958 First mass vaccination. Polio, Diphtheria.
1960 First kidney transplant
1961 The contraceptive pill – free on the NHS
1962 Porritt Report results in Enoch Powell's Hospital Plan – District General Hospitals, Post Graduate Centres, The NHS in 3 parts. Hospitals, GPs and Local Health Authorities.
1967 The Abortion Act (Legal up to 28 weeks, lowered to 24 weeks in 1990) Abortion on demand.
1967 The Salmon Report – The development of Nursing Staff Structure
The Cogwheel Report regarding the development of medical specialities and how hospital doctors to be organised
1968 First UK Heart Transplant
1972 CT scans introduced
1978 In Vitro Fertilisation
1979 Bone marrow transplant on a child, GOS (Bone marrow transplantation was started in the 50's in the US)
1980s MRI scans introduced, Laparoscopic surgery, AIDS (Health campaign started 1986)
1988 Breast screening. The Black report looked at inequalities in Health Care (as did

The Whitehead Report 1987 and the Acheson Report 1998)

1990 NHS and Community Care Act – The Internal Market, Health Authorities with own budgets.

1991 NHS "Trusts" start (independent providers of health care services with their own budgets and managements supposedly challenging the monolithic dominance of hospital based services)

1998 NHS Direct. Nurse led. ("You don't know what you got til its gone" – Joni Mitchell)

2000 NHS walk in centres managed by Primary Care Trusts, mainly nurse run, no appointment necessary

2002 Primary Care Trusts. A choice of providers if you are referred to secondary care. (this continues today with a local choice of hospitals as well as NHS Foundation Trusts elsewhere and some private providers)

2008 "Free choice" introduced – referral to any hospital that meets NHS standards

2009 New NHS constitution

2010 Equity and excellence – liberating the NHS (White paper)

2011 Health and Social Care Bill

2012 Health and Social Care Act – Abolishes NHS PCTs and SHAs. Sets up Clinical Commissioning Groups. A new Dept Health executive Agency, Public Health England.

2013 New NHS Structure

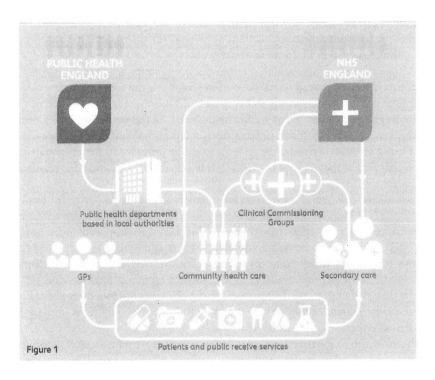

Figure 1

There have been fifteen major reorganisations of the NHS in thirty years (Goldacre "I think you'll find it's a bit more complicated than that") – Including GP Fund holders, (which, despite the accompanying fanfare and the profits made by the participating practices has never been shown in any research to have improved patient care, (Kay 2002, Greener and Mannion 2006, Coulter 1995, Petchley etc) GP Multifunds, Primary Care Groups, Primary Care Trusts, Family Practitioner Committees, Purchasing Consortiums, etc.

The British Health Service was founded on the 5th July 1948. Following the destruction of swathes of Europe and the political and social turmoil that followed the social reformer William Beveridge wanted to slay his "five giants":
Want
Disease
Squalor
Ignorance
Idleness.

Some would argue that today, excess demand, directly because it is so freely accessible, has ruined many of its fine objectives. Indeed, the problem may be that there is too much "want" for its services and too much of the service coping with the effects of idleness rather than disease. Perhaps also not enough defining what "disease" actually is.

It seems obvious in retrospect that this admirable plan of free health care for all could only work if as well as having the original role of the GP as patient's advocate, it also included a role as the patient's quarter master.

Did William Beveridge envisage that treatment for Erectile Dysfunction, Gender Reassignment, Infertility, the complications of idleness (Diabetes, Obesity, Cardiovascular Disease), the preservation of 23 week gestation babies, or 100 year old men and women with multiple disease complications, the provision of interpreters and treatment to the world, the provision of psycho sexual counselling for all, or the addition of a myriad other accessories to core "Health" services as being part of his brave new, disease free world?

Some might argue that "want" rather than "need" is the very reason why free state health care can never be affordable or fairly distributed, without rationing. – That too many states of being or lifestyle choices are now managed by doctors and therefore redefined as illness. – That free at the point of demand is only possible if the demand is reasonable in the first place.

If no one says "no" then it is everyone for themselves and the devil take the hind most.

When the NHS was set up, Family Doctors, Opticians and Dentists were self employed and sub contracted to an Executive Council. The GP was **supposed** to be the "Gate Keeper" to the secondary care services, referring where appropriate to hospital specialists and prescribing drugs which were dispensed at local pharmacies or by the dispensing GP himself. Finance became available in 1955 to set up group practices and this basic model has persisted until today. Things may now be changing but two things have kept the system the most patient accessible and the most (up until now) efficient primary health care system anywhere.

1) Practices run as **Partnerships** with doctors and their paid managers committed to the running, organisation, staffing and financial efficiency of their small business and

2) The **Personal List System** where patients develop a personal long term relationship with one doctor who they learn to trust and become familiar with and with whom they experience a degree of familiarity, empathy and understanding.

Various studies have shown the value and popularity of a personal list system over an anonymous walk in and be seen system in all population groups other than the younger mobile patient with an acute transient illness.

Despite the fact that both these mainstays of Family Practice make it patient friendly and more efficient, they are under attack from politicians and health economists who find it convenient to regard health care as impersonal, easy to standardise and therefore ripe for impersonal cheap providers. This devaluation of medicine is similar perhaps to the changing ethos that has seen more young doctors preferring salaried, sessional jobs rather than partnerships, part time rather than full time commitments and the increased willingness to take time off when not really sick – The cheapening, packaging and standardisation of healthcare.

The Feminisation of Medicine:

One of the elephants in the parlour is the tidal wave of female GPs who are washing over the profession and who have or soon will have young children and who place family above professional commitments. This is due to the A level grade bias of girls and the blind selection procedures of medical schools which act as if they have no social, professional or economic responsibility at all. It is having a profound effect on the character of Family Practice. I was recently at a post graduate meeting on hip replacements. Half of the audience were female GPs and, as they often do, they all (about seven or eight of them) stayed to chat after the talk finished. Two thirds of them were currently on maternity leave from GP jobs or registrar years and the conversation was entirely about their children and how they were "dreading" "returning to work". Just think of the chaos and disruption that their lifestyle choices, their statutory rights and their gender had imposed not just upon their careers and their professional partners but most of all on their patients.

Why did this not happen when I first became a doctor and why is it such a huge issue in Britain now?

In 1970, about 15 of my year of 90 were women and they subsequently took no more than an average of a few months off for maternity leave. They then came back to full time work. The same was true of every female hospital doctor I worked with throughout the 70's and 80's. But now it seems that every female registrar and SHO equivalent has the maximum she can possibly take away from her patients. This often amounts to half of her first five or more years off having her family with all the disruption that this causes, returning part time if possible.

Now as then there is a grade bias towards girls at A level but now up to 70% medical students are female. Very few medical schools admit an equal sex ratio. This is not only unfair toward the late developing male aspiring doctor but financial idiocy when medical careers are viewed overall. Who can blame young women GPs for not wanting to do 9 sessions a week, or late surgeries, or go to practice evening meetings, practice away days, informal late networking or for finding cover hard to provide during seasonal family illness?

There is a constant complaint at appraisals by part time female GPs that they feel less consulted, less listened to, that they find practice meetings a challenge to attend, to prepare for, that their other commitments take precedence and there is a common ethos of grievance about this. They are "less involved" although I am never quite sure whether to be involved is a passive or active verb.

Overall on average, in a career, however, female GPs give back 15 years of full time work and 7.5 years of part time work i.e. less than a total of 22.5 years work instead of the 30 years of mainly full time work that the average male gives. (or 37 1/2 in my case).

Compared with a GP of my generation, female GPs today are almost half time throughout their career and give only 2/3 the hours of their male colleagues.

If we really want a cost effective health service then we would have to conclude that men give better value for money over the course of their careers as they cost the same to train. £500,000 for a GP and £850,000 (roughly) for a consultant.

Research by the RCP suggests that by 2013 female GPs outnumbered male. **Apart from the cost, does this matter?**

- My own research shows that men with urological/perineal/erectile/psychological and other personal problems are 4-5X as likely to want to see a male GP as a female GP. On the other hand, exactly 50% women with Gynaecological/ Urological conditions will want to see a woman GP. It is quite wrong that most women want to see a woman doctor but on the other hand, most men with "personal problems" **do** prefer to see a man. We have already mentioned the "manpower" considerations of a group of workers whose career, seasonal and daily hours commitment are likely to be less than their male counterparts. If there may be a slight overall patient preference for a male doctor as well, the resource and manning implications of a female takeover of General Practice are significant.

How many of us are there and are we male or female?

IN 2011 there were 230,000 licensed doctors in the UK, 240,000 registered and 30,000 working overseas. This number is rapidly growing. This is 2.8/1,000** – up from 2.3 at the turn of the century. The average in OECD countries is 3.3/1,000. (Greece, Austria and Russia are at the top and South Africa, India and Indonesia at the "lower end." Clinical Medicine 2016 Vol 16. N0 1. 3-4)

In March 2012: The figures for General Practice were: 35,500 FTEs (increased by 25% in 10 years). Excluding registrars and retainers, there were 27,000 "Headcount GP Providers" and 8,500 salaried practitioners. Women constituted 16,300 of the total (increased 66% in 10 years) – and as you might expect, women were 40% of the "providers" but 68% of the salaried GPs.

Since 2001 female practitioners have seen an increase of 6,473 (66.0%) from 9,812 in 2001 to 16,285 in 2011.

By 2015, women were just over half of GPs (Pulse Aug 2015) 20,435 women vs 19,801 males. Women GPs had gone up by 3% and males down by 3% in the previous year. In the last decade, female GPs had increased by 50%. The overall headcount of GPs was by 2015, 40,236 (40,697 – different source) with 36,294 FTEs. (34,055 FTEs). There were 7,962 practices in England with an average list of 7,034. These figures were in August 2015 and differ slightly from figures published a little earlier in the year*

Registrars?

In 2012 there was a 3:2 gender split in favour of women. 62% are female and 38% male. **The very latest figures available: (April 2015) are*:**
GP numbers:
36,920. One in five is over age 55, 52.2% female. A 260.5% rise in salaried GPs from 2,742 in 2004 to 9,885 in 2014 – presumably because of the well recognised reluctance of female GP applicants to be full timers and partners.

There are 7,875 GP practices in England, 7,171 patients per practice, (compared with 6,149 in 2004) and 66.5 GPs per 100,000 in 2014 compared with 62.9 per 100,000 in 2004.

In the same issue of GP magazine that these increased numbers of GPs were announced, the GPC warned that "GP numbers were not keeping pace with demand"

Where did we come from?

If you want to know where your colleagues in General Practice and hospitals were trained, much is changing within the medical demography of the UK. Not all of it is reassuring. In terms of the **overall** medical work force, the white male doctor, the back bone of the NHS work force since 1948 now constitutes just 20% of the new work force. There is a clever and somewhat **disturbing workforce calculator website "The state of medical education 2012" from the GMC which** will give you almost any permutation of doctors' backgrounds you ask it. I remember an impassioned editorial from the Royal College of Physicians a few years ago in which the plea was made for the profession to reflect the society of this country. In 2015 Theresa May, the then Home Secretary made a demand of the Police Service that it reflect the ethnic mix of the population it polices. I have never heard a Health Secretary make an impassioned speech demanding, like many senior doctors and so many of my patients that the Health Service do the same. Currently (2015) 41% of doctors come from ethnic minorities compared with 14% of the population. Up to 70% of medical school output is female compared with 50% of the population. When do we hear our politically correct politicians sounding off for white males? The fact that three quarters of doctors struck off had been trained abroad became first item news on radio 4 in December 2012. There was little surprise at this amongst many British trained doctors from all ethnicities. The differences in skills, attitudes and what I call cultural availability of some foreign doctors has been backed up by what are now endless private anecdotes and personal conversations regarding cultural alienation and diffidence between British patients and some foreign trained doctors. Trained abroad is not the same as "Ethnic Minority" of course. Not at all – and huge numbers of doctors from ethnic minorities are amongst the best in our country. Some have been my registrars, colleagues and partners. However, the GMC website makes disturbing reading for any patient who wants the profession to reflect the society that it serves notwithstanding the views of our politicians.

As I mentioned before a former Royal College of Physicians President gave a speech a few years ago in which she emphasised the importance of the medical profession reflecting the population it serves. It would certainly seem ethical and reasonable for doctors, the most expensively trained public servants with amongst the highest expected income to reflect the public that paid the bills in general terms of identity, race, culture, class, attitudes, background, religion (or none) and history. To understand and relate to their patients. Is that unreasonable?

Pictured over is the first batch of Senior Representatives the "Chief Registrars" of Junior Hospital Doctors chosen by the Royal College of Physicians in 2016 to feedback to the College on daily working conditions. Most of the public in these days of financial constraints would also prefer doctors to commit to *full time* work once qualified in order to repay the £500,000-£850,000 cost of training. Bear in mind that female doctors today will put in two thirds the career hours of their male colleagues.

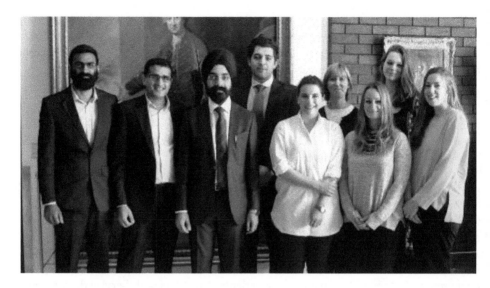

Doctors by World Region of Primary Medical Qualification (PMQ) (GPs only)

The World Region of PMQ (Primary medical qualification) refers to the region in which a doctor gained their initial qualification and therefore does not necessarily reflect the nationality of the doctor.

	No. of GPs	%
EEA (excluding UK)	3,904	6.2%
International	10,232	16.4%
UK	48,390	77.4%
Total	**62,526**	**100.00%**

Over 30% of London GPs qualified abroad, fewer than 10% South Western GPs did. Overall (in 2013, **RCP Journal, 2016**) 28% of all UK doctors were trained elsewhere, 48,000 individuals in all. A third from India, a tenth from Pakistan, 20% from other EU countries. Other developed countries share this dependence on foreign doctors: Our 28% is exceeded by New Zealand's 43% and Australia's 30%. Presumably a large proportion of these will be British. The US is 25% and Canada 23%. We are in fact training more medical students than we did, despite bulldozing historic medical schools. Between 2000 and 2013 the number of new medical graduates doubled and we have one of the youngest medical professions in the world. Only 15% are over 55.(33% is the OECD average) You could argue that this is one of the reasons they have been so willing to strike over conditions of work and to not regard medicine as a tough apprenticeship that demands a great deal of personal sacrifice.

Nearly 20% of the UK's doctors are however not on a register OR in training. Not engaged in treating patients at all. This has by far the highest proportion of international graduates (Non UK, Non EU).

In terms of the specialist register in 2013, 5,000 doctors joined of whom 2,500 were from UK specialist registrar training posts but in the same year 3,500 doctors left. Under the age of 50, 1,500 left, 85% going to overseas posts. 312 were UK graduates. In other words UK graduates leave at 10% of the rate that UK graduates enter the specialist register. The GMC report on medicine in 2016 states that the UK is supplying Australia with 22% of its specialists and 13% of its GPs and our work force is dependent on foreign trained doctors, including EU graduates as well as a growing group of over 50 year olds.

So we have a young, readily emigrating work force, our patients make do with a disproportionate number of foreign trained doctors while many of ours take their expensive and quality training and donate it to the Australian public. Hardly grateful, fair or loyal is it?

Are foreign trained doctors equivalent to the UK doctors who are heading for an easier life, more money and a better climate in the Antipodes? Over half of my registrars and partners have been trained abroad and almost without exception, I would trust them with my life. But many doctors I have appraised have not been up to their standard.

After complaints, more than twice as many overseas doctors are referred to GMC hearings and are struck off.

The USA seems to have a similar problem:

Marcella Nunez-Smith, Assistant Professor at Yale University School of Medicine, says that given the rise in the dependence on foreign-trained doctors in countries like the UK and US, it is essential to determine "whether international medical graduates offer the same quality of care as doctors who train and practise in destination countries."

The quality of training abroad and the types of patient seen during their training is one area that may be of concern but there are constant complaints from unbiased and tolerant British patients about the cultural and language readiness of many foreign trained doctors from within and outside the EU. "He was very nice but I couldn't understand a word he was saying" is a common report to GPs after outpatient appointments. I frequently phone our local DGH to enquire about my patients who have been admitted. I am often handed over to a British nurse by a foreign colleague who I could not understand and who could not follow even my slow, patient, standard received English. This is almost as hard when I try to admit a patient via some on call junior doctors.

So this is another elephant in the front room and one which no one in the new NHS seems brave enough to consider openly, let alone discuss. Doctors trained abroad, despite General Practice's clear reliance on instant understanding and communication during brief consultations are likely to suffer disadvantages in:

1) Communication skills, formal and informal, verbal and non verbal.

2) Particularly spoken English skills, including colloquial expressions, recognition of regional accents and expressions. The ability to speak to and be clearly understood by the great majority of British patients without the disadvantage of a heavy foreign accent.

3) Cultural communication norms, irony, cynicism, humour, affectionate rudeness etc

4) Familiarity with the patient's history, cultural expectations, traditions, when to touch, how much eye contact, the tone and intonation of instruction or advice.

5) Family, Social and Class attitudes which are complex enough to occasionally tax people who are born here let alone those brought up in cultures where professionals are handled with diffidence and respect.

6) The personal experience that the patient has had of other people from ethnic minorities and their willingness to engage fully in cultural integration may have led to a pre

existing apprehension or expectation in the patient of being misinterpreted or misunderstood or not being sympathised with. For instance: Attitudes to women, sexual identity and development, attitudes to children, miscarriage, homosexuality, substance abuse etc.

7) Appearance and clothing. Many British patients find the Hijab, the Yarmulke, to a lesser extent the turban and other cultures' traditional clothing may be an overt sign of separateness or a marker of attitude or personal inaccessibility. This may not turn out to be the case but since most British people know Sikhs, Jews and Muslims who do not choose to wear these outward markers of separateness, they **can** be seen as a desire to remain "apart" from the patient's majority. One patient likened a headscarf to an eyebrow ring or a facial tattoo. These were markers worn by people as an overt sign that the wearer was establishing a desire to separate themselves from a "willing understanding of" or "belonging to" of the patient's majority culture.

There was a debate on Radio 4 in 2014 where a representative from The RGN defended its decision to permit the training and qualification of nurses wearing full face veils.

The Niqab and other full face coverings prevent the communication of facial expression. Two thirds of communication is non verbal and most non verbal communication is by expression. Covering the face and mouth can inhibit clear speech and always puzzles, offends and frightens western patients in equal measure. It is a rare sight in hospitals and practice as yet but may well become more common and, like other cultural issues currently foreign to most of us be the source of potential difficulty and conflict in future. Imagine being a hospice patient slipping away and your nurse is wearing a full face covering. The only (Radiographer) I heard of wearing one refused to touch the skin of any male patients so it is hard to see any role in which such a nurse would be of practical use in an NHS hospital. Fortunately the GMC has now quoted case law stating that any face apparel interfering with important communication (which by definition it must) should be removed on request without the defence of human rights.

Are all doctors equally good?

Increasingly the press, the profession and public think not. This is taken from The Daily Telegraph January 2013:

"Doctors trained overseas are five times more likely to be struck off than those trained in the UK"

The country with the biggest single number of doctors who have been removed or suspended from the medical register is India, followed by Nigeria and Egypt.

In total, 669 doctors have been either struck off or suspended by the GMC over the last five years.

Of those, only 249 were British (37 per cent) while 420 (63 per cent) were trained abroad – whereas one-third of doctors on the register were trained abroad, and two-thirds in Britain.

and from GP magazine May 2015:

"Black and minority ethnic doctors are less likely to be offered GP training places than white doctors" – although UK trained BME doctors are more likely to be offered a place than white doctors trained abroad.

Black GPs are twice as likely to have their revalidation deferred as white colleagues. This is from GMC figures which show white GPs "less likely to push back their revalidation date than black, Asian or mixed ethnicity GPs". 10% of white GPs had deferred the process by mid 2015 compared with 18% of black GPs (this figure includes British and overseas doctors working in the NHS). Over the same period, 14% of Asian GPs, 14% of mixed ethnicity and 16% from other ethnic groups had to defer. In terms of where the doctors qualified, GPs trained in the UK were the least likely to defer, (10%). Of those trained in the EU the figure was 15% and it was 16% for international graduates. One in five GPs working in London defer the process but only 6% working in Scotland. Those over the age of 65 are the most likely age group (20%), female GPs in their 30s are twice as likely as male GPs at the same age to defer.

The conclusions you draw will depend upon your experience of the competence of a range of doctors within the NHS and your assessment of the value of Appraisal and Revalidation. But list size, (small in Scotland), quality of previous training, work/life priorities (female), language skills, time commitment to work, cultural and other factors are bound to influence an individual's ability or willingness to become engaged in a formal and standardised process such as revalidation.

What are we like?

The truth is that many patients would be happy to consult a computer terminal and intelligent software for a sprained ankle or a sore throat. For real Family Medicine however, a consultation which involves a connection, knowledge, history, familiarity, continuity, people generally want to see someone they can communicate easily with, who will listen and understand and preferably someone who knows them.

Time and time again I have heard people of my age (late middle age) and cultural background (white British) say that they want a doctor who they can talk to but respect. A mixture of accessible for their own problems but with authority and distance in terms of their superior knowledge and experience. They still want the doctor to maintain that aura of mystique and separateness that knowledge, experience and wisdom gives all professionals. NOT chummy, familiar and not their new best friend.

This may seem obvious but there has been a slow and unwelcome cultural shift that became clear to me when I spent some time visiting my wife who was an inpatient recently. Due to the working time directive and the resulting inevitable weekend lack of continuity, she was visited by 3 different surgical teams over one weekend and given a discharge time which was contradicted then reinstated several times in the space of 36 hours. There has been a recent (2013) disclosure that you are 44% more likely to die these days after a Friday operation than a Monday one. Could this be at least partly due to the lack of continuity, consistency, communication, and competence – because as well as fewer doctors out of hours they have fewer hours and less experience under their belts than their recent forebears? I was reminded of my 80 hour weekends on call. No continuity issue then.

I asked my wife who the various doctors visiting her were. She did not know and they had not introduced themselves. Being an intelligent able and articulate woman did not help when she was out of her environment, in her night attire, on a ward of sick strangers and visited at unpredictable times by unlimited nameless, over confident and entitled strangers. The next day she asked the name of the visiting doctor and the reply was "Shammy". I subsequently discovered that this was the Christian name of one of the surgical registrars. As well as a couple of other doctors in the hospital.

Later in out-patients I asked one of the house officers how he introduced himself to patients and he replied "Ben".

Everyone I have asked over the age of twenty five deplored the use of first names by doctors and replied to a man (and woman) something like: I would like them to say "I am

Dr Smith, I am Mr Brown's registrar....etc You may have heard of Dr Kate Granger who died in 2016 after starting The ""Hello My Name is" campaign to encourage doctors to introduce themselves to patients. She sounded like a really nice person and I fully support her campaign to get all doctors to say who they are to each patient they meet. I think Hello My name is Doctor Heath and I am the Geriatric Registrar, Paediatric Houseman, a local GP, etc would be far more welcomed and respected by most patients than Hi I'm Chris, your doctor tonight".

Doctors do not wear obvious name badges and have dispensed with white coats and ties in Britain on the specious and unproven grounds of infection control. There is actually precious little proof that these changes would have or did make any difference to cross infection. Doctors still carry unsterilised stethoscopes draped ostentatiously around their necks au George Clooney and these are as much of an infection risk as cuffs. Far worse than tucked in ties. It is noticeable that most advertising medical websites in the US show male doctors with ties, many with white coats and when famous sportsmen or politicians are injured in Europe the surgeon appears to comment to the press in a white coat and tie.

You can make up your own mind why British doctors are happy to look like a bunch of party goers and far less professional than most phone and carpet shop assistants.

How do we appear?

I readily admit I looked about seventeen when I qualified. I went straight to medical school from school, I had no gap year or time off so I was a doctor at 22. It was a decade before I felt I looked to a stranger like I knew what I was talking about. By then I had delivered dozens of babies, operated on hundreds of people, anaesthetised several hundred (at least I could hide behind a mask), some at death's door, resuscitated many who most doctors would not have been able to- (because I became quite good at intubation and CVP lines), I had supervised dozens of comfortable and dignified deaths, resuscitated dozens of tiny babies, run an adult and neonatal ITU and become the sympathetic friend of many bereaved strangers. Initially in the 70's we wore white coats – through ease of identification, practicality and because I always carried my own notebooks, instruments, bleep and personal possessions with me. There were a lot of things to have to hand. Junior doctors nowadays do spend a lot of time looking for the ward ophthalmoscope or the MIMS and despite the stethoscope, draped George Clooney style over their neck which acts as a badge of status now the others have been socialised away, they carry no other useful medical instruments or small reference books as I did. They look unencumbered but they are a bit like a plumber who turns up to your house and asks if you have any water pump pliers and a Stillson wrench.

I always wore a shirt and tie, the latter tucked into my shirt if I were over a patient, I always tried to look what I regarded as respectable-worthy of respect. Someone a stranger could trust, at least be willing to give a chance. I was a Paediatrician for several years and wore ties with dinosaurs and teddy bears, changing these if I knew I was giving someone bad news or turning off a ventilator. Like it or not we judge others by their appearance. Especially by first appearance, especially if we are stressed, worried and vulnerable. Clothes, costume, hair, earrings, piercings, shoes, hands, finger nails, jewellery, all these things are important pointers about you, who you are, what you attitudes and background are. You can make life harder or easier for yourself by sending out different signals. The wrong initial impression can be impossible to counteract.

I have worked with female GP colleagues with nose rings, male GP colleagues with ear piercings, and whatever they may think about their own right to be individual and idiosyncratic, I bet none of them have ever asked in their PSQ "What do you think about your doctor's appearance? Does this matter?

I appraised a very competent female doctor in her early forties a couple of years ago. She had a bright green dress which ended three or four inches below her perineum. In a different context she would have been quite sexy. She had light tights and as she sat, seriously discussing her patient feedback and audit results, kept pulling her skirt down ineffectually, only drawing attention to its brevity.

It was impossible to take her seriously as a doctor and as a professional even though I knew how serious and respected she was. I can only imagine how distracted the majority of male patients would have been and how any serious conversation with her would have been undermined by her clothes. I was surprised none of her partners had mentioned this sort of thing as an issue in her MSF – but then would I? How would that sort of feedback from a male partner have been interpreted and what can of political worms would have been opened by it?

I mention elsewhere how my family has been on the receiving end of NHS care over the last year and how many thoughtful friends, colleagues and relatives have asked me why "standards have fallen" so much in the last decade or two. Doctors who give their first names when asked to identify themselves may not bother the under twenties, male doctors who do not (in the NHS anyway) wear ties because of the supposed infection risk (-so why not tuck them in, and why is there less cross infection in the private sector where ties are worn, are they bacteriocidal ties?) But I do feel the loose floral party dress and pink pumps as worn by the SHO called to an elderly collapsed lady on a chemotherapy unit I was observing, the microskirt I described and the open necked party shirts I have seen on registrars attending to bereaved relatives are disrespectful, inappropriate and just **wrong.**

Clothes are important. When you are out there being a doctor, you are undertaking a role, playing a part, you are acting, giving something back – you are paid to fulfil the expectations of the people who paid for your expensive education and so I believe you owe them some respect. It is called being professional.

Partnership

The original model of much of General Practice may be coming back into fashion: GPs needing to be involved in out of hours cover, patients with a "named GP" again (in other words, the list system), research that shows telephone consultations and nurse practitioners don't save time or money, even the newest proposal that appointments should be scrapped and patients encouraged to turn up and all patients be seen on the day they phone and just wait. All these things were familiar to my parents when they first encountered the NHS and most were how it was when I first started work in it in the early 70's. The full time GP in partnership.

Jeremy Hunt the Health Secretary at the end of 2014 made a series of speeches praising the GP based model of care, the Gate Keeper role, the "First instinct of the patient to go to the GP" and "Other countries are grappling with how to set up this model of care" He also decried the relative increase in the proportion of NHS funds spent on secondary care where a small fraction of the total NHS work is done. He called for a culture shift so that GPs felt that the patient was at the centre of health care, not the organisation. In other words what he and the patients seem to want is to turn the organisational clocks back 30 years. I have to say I agree wholeheartedly. A friend of mine, a dentist, tells me he asks all his patients who their doctor is and "90% don't know anymore". This is a disaster, a form of organised neglect. But it has been politicians, vested interests and political considerations that have sabotaged the once patient responsive and patient centred system in the first place.

But to begin with we will have to bolster full time GP partnership.

The partnership model has been the heart of General Practice since 1948 but since the new contract in 2004 practices have taken on more salaried GPs rather than partners. You don't have to share profits with a salaried partner but there are many extra, hidden costs and the GPC of the BMA is right to believe that the gold standard of General Practice and the one that gives best care to the patient is the partnership independent contractor structure. The BMA "Fears that the future of General Practice will be undermined" by the erosion of this system. They are right.

The salaried GP has contractual maternity leave, sickness and redundancy pay as well as one paid session of CPD per week built into their contract. The true cost of a salaried partner is 40% more than their salary (BMA Focus on taking on new partners) of around £90,000 FTE (Including 12.8% NI and 14% Superannuation)

The advantages of a GP partner are continuity, ownership, new skills and ideas, investment and risk management, greater influence and control, professional autonomy, ability to influence patient services, recruitment (over half of salaried GPs become profit sharing partners at some point), working hours (no working time directive) and the sense of ownership within the practice and, of course, belonging.

Many GPs favour the personal aspects of involvement, commitment, control, higher income and tax advantages of partnership too. It is said that the new generation of GPs prefers a 9 to 5, no financial responsibility for premises or staff, uncommitted freedom. It is interesting that, having appraised GPs for 10 years, in many cases (just like in the teaching profession) the main emotional stresses are linked not to unreasonable behaviour by patients but to perceived unreasonable behaviour by partners.

The main complaint is a frequent belief that work load is unevenly distributed and that the partner spoken to is being taken advantage of. True or not, this is often difficult to quantify as we rarely put a financial value on the non clinical activities that each of us undertakes and we don't have a generally accepted way of bartering one activity within the practice for another. Often one partner will feel that another's training activities or other outside responsibilities are not generating sufficient income to justify the time away from the appointments conveyor belt. Sometimes resentment develops over the fact that the less popular doctors have smaller lists, shorter surgeries, fewer extras, house and phone calls but still earn the same as the popular, conscientious, harder working partner(s).

It has always puzzled me that G.P. partners generally have

1) Profit Sharing practice agreements – whereby however many patients seen, however many days a partner is away to train or to do non clinical activities (this depends on practice agreements), however little the pooled income makes up for the absence, whatever the individual's earning aspirations at their stage in their career, each partner takes home an equal sum. Compensation for extra sessions or responsibility (eg staff training, Saturday surgeries etc) can be negotiated but the basic assumption is that every partner gets the same take home pay come what may.

This is not the case in our fellow professionals the Dental profession who have the fairer system of pooled expenses and individualised income.

2) Cost Sharing practice agreements: If one partner stays late to see more patients, he will earn more money. If he covers a partner who goes off to play golf, he earns more. They pool all the reception and running costs with some adjustments – but surely this, with its in built incentives and rewards for hard work is a much fairer system than ours?

The Partnership agreement:

Should be negotiated, agreed and signed as soon as any new doctor joins a practice or any significant reorganisation happens. It is superfluous while each partner feels the others are sharing the work load equally, their outside commitments are benefiting the partnership enough to justify their absence and their teaching and GPSI commitments aren't just a way of avoiding the grinding demand of the coal face. But in my experience true generosity and compromise are rare in partnerships when hours and income are involved. Throw into this mix the inevitable variation in popularity (and therefore extra patients slotted in, phone calls etc), variable clinical thoroughness and poor history recording, the frequent minor illness absences or childcare issues or leaving early to pick up the kids of some partners and you realise a clear list of duties and responsibilities written in black and white is an important prerequisite for a contented practice. The mentoring discussion at appraisal is often an emotional or frustrated diatribe from a doctor who feels they are doing more than their fair share of the clinical duties. Appraisal can often be all about getting on with difficult partners rather than difficult patients. Certainly, it is rare in our income sharing partnerships for each partner to feel all the others are pulling their weight.

A typical practice agreement:

Is a fairly standard document and can be added to at any time. Thus:

PARTNERSHIP AGREEMENT
Relating to **Riverbrook Surgery,**
Bartholomew Square,
Hersham,
W.Sussex.
RH 15 7ZE

Dr Jonathan Coldley
Dr Paul Forest
Dr Ajaz Rattle
Dr Ann Ferrari
Dr Hwa Lon Loan
Dr Christopher Park

Covenants

The parties (each a 'partner') covenant with each other from the date following that they shall be partners in the said general medical practice on the terms contained in the following clauses. References to the masculine gender shall wherever required include references to the female gender. The partnership shall be known as 'Example Surgery'.

Duration and Name of the Partnership

It is hereby agreed as follows the partners will carry on in partnership ('The Partnership') with effect from.................. as general practitioners practising in their own premises, Example Surgery, Example Road, Example ('The Premises').

The Partnership shall continue during the joint lives of the partners or any two or more of them

The bankruptcy, death or retirement of one partner shall not determine the Partnership between the others

The name and addresses of the partners shall be in Appendix 1

The Accountants of the partnership shall be.....

Nature of the Business

To carry out the profession of General Medical Practitioners

The partners shall use 'the Premises' primarily for the provision of General Medical Services or reflect any change in the nature of the general practice contract with the NHS. Any other medical use of the premises shall be allowed with the agreement of the partners.

The partners shall at all times comply the provision of the Business Names Act 1985 and of any regulation, instrument rule or order from time to time made there under.

All partners shall be duly registered under the Medical Act 1983 and their names appear on the medical list maintained by the relevant NHS body.

Assets of the Partnership inc Profits and Losses

Assets of the partnership will comprise of the surgery premises, drugs, money in the various accounts, medical and office equipment, fittings and furniture and any other sundry items. These assets will be owned by the partners in the agreed profit shares. This will form the capital of the partnership.

Any further assets that are required for the efficient working of the practice will be purchased out of the funds of the Partnership with the consent of the Partners and become the property of the partnership.

Any finance required by the practice shall be agreed, contributed to and guaranteed by the partners in the proportions in which they share the profits.

The capital of the partnership at the date hereof shall be defined by the appointed accountants and will belong to the partners in the agreed profit shares.

The premises are owned by the 'property owning' partners in the proportions recorded in the Premises Agreement/Deed of Trust relating to Example Surgery dated..... The partners personal property contained in their consulting rooms remains their property.

Proper books of accounts should be kept and promptly posted and should be available at all times for inspection by each of the parties and by the Partnership accountants. An annual account shall take place on the 31st March by the Partnership accountants and shall, once approved, be signed by the Partners and shall thereupon become binding except upon discovery of any manifest error which becomes apparent within six months of signature.

Partners Individual Expenses
Each partner shall be personally responsible for:
Superannuation, added years AVCs and any other personal pension contributions
The provision and maintenance of his own medical instruments
The provision maintenance and running expenses of one or more motorcars used in the practice
The telephone at his residence and mobile telephones
The cost of membership of certain professional bodies, as agreed by the majority of partners
Course fees unless otherwise agreed with the partners
The full cost of locum replacement during periods of sickness exceeding 6 weeks of absence
Each partner shall be responsible for his own permanent health insurance arrangements

Partnership Expenses
The expenses chargeable to the Partnership shall be:
All expenses of the surgery at 'Example Surgery' aforesaid
The cost of all medicines drugs, dressings, instruments, apparatus, files and other things necessary for the carrying on of NHS General Practice
The salaries and expenses of Partnership employees
The Partnership accountancy fees. Partners' personal accountancy fee will be covered in part by the partnership, or pro-rata for part-time partners, this will be based on the lowest amount each financial year. Partners will be responsible for accountancy fees exceeding this amount.
Such other expenses and outgoings of whatsoever kind incurred incidental to the carrying on of the Partnership practice as the partners may agree
Defence organisation fees for NHS work

Partnership Bank
The Partnership Banks are: ....

Bank or banks may change as the Partners shall from time to time determine.
All partnership monies not required for current expenses and all cheques shall be paid promptly into the Partnership bank account and all securities for money shall be promptly deposited in the name of all parties.
Cheques drawn on these accounts shall require two signatures, one of which may be the practice manager
All partners are to have access to view the accounts
No individual partner shall without reference to the practice as a whole incur debt or write a cheque for a sum in excess of £5,000.

Earnings
Individual payments intended as gifts and not expressed or implied to be in payment for professional services, sponsorship or compensation to individual partners for work carried out in spare time or holidays, personal insurance policy payments and personal income received when not acting as representatives of the Partnership may be kept by the individual partner. Earnings from such work in a partner's personal time will be allowed provided that the Practice as a whole has not deemed this to be a disadvantage.

The Partnership earnings shall include ALL payments to a partner under the NHS by way of reimbursement for providing professional or ancillary services. This will include such items as training allowance and other fees paid by the NHS. Also earnings from private medical work undertaken on behalf of the practice, eg. nursing homes, occupational health work, private medical reports and Part 2 cremation fees.

The individual earnings to be kept by an individual partner shall include:

Any gift from a patient specifically intended for one partner

Postgraduate Education Allowance

Seniority Allowance

These lists are not exhaustive and for some earnings clarification should be sought by partnership discussion and agreement. Any gift which has a value in excess of £100 shall be recorded.

Shares of Profits and Losses

The profits of the Partnership including profits of a capital nature other than capital profits relating to the premises shall belong to the partners in the agreed profit shares of the partnership, unless otherwise unanimously agreed in writing and in return for demonstrably different duties or responsibilities. Capital profits relating to the premises shall belong to the property owning partners in proportion to the shares owned.

The losses of the partnership including losses of a capital nature other than capital losses relating to the premises shall be apportioned in the same shares as the partners from time to time share profits. Losses relating to the premises shall be apportioned to the property-owning partners in proportion to the shares owned.

New Partners and Parity

New partners joining the partnership shall have a period of no longer than 3 years to reach parity.

Incoming partners will be subject to a period of six months mutual assessment after which they will be expected to purchase a share of the premises and/or assets in accordance with their profit sharing ratio as calculated by the practice accountant, by unanimous agreement of the existing partners. The purchase of such assets to be completed within one year of the succession date agreed by the partners.

Partners' Obligations to Each Other

Each partner shall:

Provide general medical services to his own patient list and to his partners patients at their request or when they are not available. The general medical services provided shall be those traditionally offered by General Practitioners with extra services as agreed by the practice as a whole. All partners shall provide comparable or equivalent professional services to be agreed by all partners unanimously and regularly reviewed. Each partner shall provide/arrange out of hours emergency cover by whatever means is unanimously agreed currently by the Partnership. These out of hours services shall be in proportion/equal to their day time commitments and profit share.

Endeavour to do his utmost to further the interests of the Partnership

Be just and faithful to the others and to each of them

Conduct himself both personally and professionally in a manner becoming a medical practitioner

Make good to the Partnership any loss occasioned by his negligence or misconduct

Be a member of an appropriate and approved Medical Defence Body

Furnish to the others and to each of them when required full information in writing of any matter undertaken by him on behalf of the Partnership

Promptly and regularly make entries of all matters which should be recorded by any Act or Regulation made by a competent authority respecting the general and pharmaceutical service of the National Health Service

Allow the other partners and each of them free access to the Partnership accounts and to the records of patients

Maintain his patients' notes in good order to the standard required of a training practice and ensure that all computer entries comply with the 'Good Practice Guidelines for General Practice electronic patient records'

Discharge his own debts and liabilities and indemnify the partnership against them

No partner shall without the prior consent of a majority of partners:

Restrict the services given by him as a general practitioner under the National Health Service or assign or change his interest in the Partnership or any part of it.

Retirement

Partners must retire at 65 unless specifically invited by unanimous vote to continue. Retirement may be at 60 or earlier with the consent of the remaining partners

Six months' notice must be given by the Partnership or individual partner of retirement

Retirement must occur at the end of a Health Authority accounting period and the Accounts requested from the practice accountant at that time.

Decision Making

Each partner will be entitled to one vote irrespective of whether full or part-time.

The following decisions will require a unanimous vote:

The admission of a new partner

The alteration of any of the terms of this deed

The dismissal of a member of staff (unless the individual is considered guilty of bringing the practice into disrepute or serious professional misconduct)

The development or purchase of premises

The opening of a new branch surgery

The increase in partnership capital or the borrowing of any sum in excess of £5,000

The giving of any guarantees for the benefit of the Partnership, or any of the partners, or any third party

The pledging of the credit of the Partnership, or incurring any liability, or the loaning of any money, or the giving of any guarantee on behalf of the partnership

The placing of any order, the incurring of any obligations in excess of £10,000 and/or continuing for more than three months from Partnership funds

The entering into a contract or hire purchase agreement involving the partnership or other partners individually or severally and so that commitments or expense entered into without prior unanimous agreement shall be paid back to the Partnership bank account by the relevant partner immediately, or by agreement within a period not exceeding six months.

Except:

Decisions may be made by a majority vote such as the expulsion of a partner and the dissolution of the Partnership

The partnership may expel a partner under the following conditions:

If any partner shall become bankrupt or insolvent

Shall grossly neglect the practice of the Partnership

Shall commit any grave or persistent breach of the provisions herein contained

Shall be guilty of addiction to drugs or alcohol or of flagrantly immoral behaviour or of any other behaviour or conduct likely to have a serious adverse effect on the Partnership practice

Shall be guilty of any grave or persistent breach of the ethics of the medical profession

Shall have his name removed from the local medical performers list

Shall have his name erased or suspended from the Medical Register

Shall be compulsorily detained in hospital or received into guardianship under the Mental Health Act 1983

In the event of a partner absenting himself through illness or accident, and as a result that partner is unable to perform their fair share of the work in the practice, for a period of absence which continues for more that 12 consecutive calendar months or for a total of more than 300 days during any 24 calendar months

Then and in every such case the other partners may terminate the partnership as regards such partner by service of a notice in writing and immediately upon the service of such notice such partner shall cease to be a partner of the Partnership PROVIDED that if any question shall arise concerning the existence or exercise of the power conferred by this Clause, such question shall be referred to arbitration under the provisions in that behalf hereinafter contained.

HOLIDAYS

Six weeks (the equivalent of 54 sessions) for full-time partners and pro rata for part-time partners is allowed for leave per calendar year. In addition there will be one week (9 sessions) per full-time partner and pro rata for part-time partners for study leave per year. Each of the partners shall take turns to have first choice in fixing the time of their holidays, provided that at normal school holiday times, preference wherever possible shall be given to partners with children at school to allow them to take a holiday at that time. The partners shall choose in rotation according to the order of names in this agreement. Holidays shall take priority over study leave and no more than two full-time partners shall be absent at one time except during the months of November to February where no more than one and a half partners shall be absent. No more than two consecutive weeks may be taken unless agreed by the partners and part-time partner's allowance will be on a pro rata basis in accord with the number of sessions that they would normally work.

MATERNITY LEAVE AND SICKNESS

The absent partner shall be paid the full partnership share but will find a competent locum after six weeks. The absent partner shall receive any locum payments paid by the Health Authority. The total period of absence will not exceed 12 months.

In the case of maternity leave, the partner should not lose her entitlement to pro rata holiday and sickness leave in respect of this period

It shall be the practice's responsibility to engage a locum at their discretion. The locum should cover normal duties.

OTHER LEAVE
Paternity and Adoption

Under the Statement and Fees Allowances, payments are available for 2 weeks paternity leave within a maximum of 18 weeks of the birth or the partnership will allow 3 days leave. If the partner chooses to take the 2 weeks, the payment received will be paid to the absent partner who will be responsible for the engagement of a competent locum to cover the absence.

Compassionate leave for crises involving immediate family. 3 days shall be allowable. This may be extendable in certain circumstances

Other Leave may be granted with the consent of the remaining partners

EFFECT OF RETIREMENT, BANKRUPTCY OR DEATH

Upon the outgoing permanent retirement from the Partnership or death of any partner, The Accountant to the Partnership appointed pursuant to this Agreement (the 'Accountant') shall draw up Accounts of the Partnership on the usual basis for the Partnership valuing assets at net book value (the 'Termination Accounts') as at the accounting Partnership date next following the date of such outgoing or death. The profit shall be time apportioned by the Accountant in respect of the former partner subject to and in accordance with the provisions of this Deed.

The continuing partners shall pay to the former partner, a sum in cash equal to the capital account of the former partner in the proportion in which they share profits. The sum will be as shown in the Termination Accounts. The continuing partners shall be allowed a period of up to one year from the date of the Termination Accounts in which to effect payment thereof. The former partner shall be entitled from the date of outgoing to interest at the rate of the Base Rate of National Westminster Bank plc plus 1.5% per annum on the balance thereof outstanding from time to time.

COST RENT AND BUILDINGS

The partners shall be able to own a share of the building in proportion with their profit share, this will include a share of any mortgage and any profits made in respect of the premises. Property owning partners will be party to a Premises Agreement/Deed of Trust dated............. Cost rent payments will be apportioned to the property owning partners in proportion to their shares.

Incoming partners will, at the discretion of the remaining property owning partners, be required to purchase a share of the current market value of the building and land in proportion with their profit share. The valuation of the premises shall be carried out at the current market value, such value to be agreed or in default of agreement fixed by an independent valuer.

Purchase of a property share if agreed by the outgoing and remaining partners shall be after an independent current market valuation for use as surgery premises by a mutually agreed valuer. Purchase to be completed within one year of the succession date agreed by the partners. Goodwill is excluded from any valuation.

The outgoing partner will be entitled to the appropriate share of assets (and, if a Trustee), to their share of the current market value of the building and land.

All partners will be liable for repairs and renewals to the buildings and contents that are necessary to continue the business of general practice, the property owning partners will be liable for all other costs relating to the fabric of the building and grounds.

SABBATICALS

These will be permissible for a period of three months at a minimum interval of five years, as long as a locum who is acceptable to the other partners is provided at the expense of the partner concerned.

PATIENT LISTS AND DUTY COVER ARRANGEMENTS

Patients at Example Surgery will be registered with a 'preferred' GP. The number of patients registered at the practice will be shared on the basis equal to the profit sharing arrangements at the time. The partners will be expected to provide the necessary medical care including appointments and visits for his or her 'preferred' patient list.

The partners are responsible for visits to their own patients between 8.30am and 5.00pm except on half days or by mutual arrangement. All partners shall comply with the current regulations on minimum availability that shall apply at any given time.

On weekdays, emergency cover for all the practice's patients will be allocated on a rota basis proportional to each doctor's partnership share. Each partner shall be responsible for informing the administrative staff of any rota change made so there is no doubt who is providing emergency cover.

Day time emergency duties will run from 7.00am-8.30am, 1.00pm-2.00pm and 5.00pm-7.00pm on each weekday. The duty partner must be available during these times or have made suitable clear alternative arrangements with another partner.

Saturday morning duties from 7.00am-12.00pm with a surgery for emergencies will be provided on the same equitable rota basis.

Each fulltime share doctor will be entitled to a half day away from the practice each week. Half days will run up to or from 12.00pm provided emergency cover for the absent partner's patients is available. Administrative staff must be aware of alternative cover arrangements. Partners must be available for all their duty periods and able to visit or respond to medical requests at short notice.

Surgeries, visits, night, weekend and all other duties shall be shared by the partners in the same shares as they from time to time share the profits in the Partnership. In the case of any dispute, the majority decision will be final.

20. ARBITRATION

In the event of a dispute relating to this agreement and where appropriate, the Partnership shall refer to the Secretary of the British Medical Association who will be responsible for appointing a suitable arbitrator.

ACCOUNTS

.... or any other firm of Chartered Accountants, which the practice may vote to appoint, will prepare the accounts. The partners will cause to be prepared accounts made up to 31 March each year and these will be signed as approved by all partners. In the absence of any manifest error discovered in the next six months after signature, those accounts become binding on all parties. All partners are entitled to access the practice books and records of account and outgoing partners will have such a right within six months after leaving.

DRAWINGS

The partners' drawings will be withdrawn on the 26th day of each month in amounts that will be determined unanimously from time to time by the partners, having taken advice from the Partnership accountants. It will also be permissible for each partner to withdraw from the Partnership account any excess outstanding to his credit over and above the amount required as retained working capital. Conversely any partner whose account balance is less than his required share of working capital shall be required to pay in the difference therewith. The partners shall be entitled to withdraw the leave advances paid in their names.

The partners shall be entitled to draw upon the partnership bank accounts such sums as they shall unanimously agree on account thereof or in default of agreements such sums as the partnership accountants shall recommend provided that:

Additional drawings shall only be permitted after quarterly payments have been received from the XXXXXXX Health Authority and leaving a sum for working capital advised by the accountant.

If at the taking of an annual account the aggregate amount drawn out by any partner exceeds his entitlement to a share of the profits from the Partnership, he shall forthwith repay any such excess.

TAX

An income tax reserve account is to be maintained and amounts are to be withheld from partners' drawings and paid into it each month. Such amounts are to be determined from time to time by the partners after taking advice from the Partnership accountants.

Dr....... is the nominated partner for the Partnership tax return and he shall have the final say over items contained within that return, including practice expenses paid personally by the partners. Any additional tax, interest or penalties arising from individual partners' acts or omissions will be borne by the partner in question.

We the parties of 'Example Partnership' agree to the terms and conditions set out in this partnership agreement:

Names of each individual partner plus a witness to each signature

While we are on the subject of doctors taking expensive time away from the coal face, it seems ironic that the

The Working Time Directive

An EU directive stating the right to a minimum number of paid breaks and paid holidays per year, a rest period of at least 11 hours in any 24 hrs, restricting excessive night work, and limiting a week's work to 48 hours has had at least two highly damaging effects on health care provision. This is compared with the almost unlimited (and admittedly sometimes dangerous) 90 to 130 hour working weeks of doctors in all parts of the health service a few decades ago.

The two most obvious **effects of the WTD** have been

1) A tripling of sickness absence amongst junior doctors ?due to an increased sense of "job" rather than "vocation" or possibly a 21st century "salaried" mind set, the feminisation of medicine, (female doctors take more time off with both physical and mental ill health according to official figures), a lack of personal commitment or a loss of the apprenticeship ethos?-No longer a sense that doing is learning and learning is the whole point of the apprenticeship. Or possibly a societal trend towards rights rather than commitment, a European 20th/21st Century cultural association of doing hard work with being abused amongst the baby boomers' babies?

When I qualified nearly 40 years ago the sickness absence figures showed that doctors took between 1/3 and 1/2 the sickness absence of nurses and nurses about 2/3 the sickness of ancillary workers. For someone of my generation who regularly worked one in two rotas for years on end: Which meant an average on call duty week was:

Monday 24 hours
Tuesday 10 hours
Wednesday 24 hours
Thursday 6 hours
Friday 24 hours
Saturday 24 hours
Sunday 24 hours

----

136 Hours a week. –

it is bizarre to read the GMC feedback website with comments from junior doctors today saying how hard their 48 hour week is.

2) Also the quite obvious (to the approx 5000 GP trainers anyway) relative lack of experience and maturity of GP trainees and junior doctors at all grades compared with their peer group of, say 2 decades ago in dealing with a wide variety of patients or illnesses. How could it be otherwise when their clinical training has encompassed less than half the hours of a traditional 1 in 2 or 1 in 3 HO or SHO job?

Consultations: The Size of the problem:

There are roughly 310m GP consultations a year with an average consultation taking between 10 and 15 minutes. List sizes vary considerably and have gradually increased over the last few years. Most estimates suggest that systematic education of the public perhaps together with the local pharmacist could prevent 20% of consultations. (eg Civitas The health of the Nation: A Public Health Perspective 2016 p31)

The figures:

1) 90% NHS Consultations are in General Practice

2) There are approximately 310m GP consultations a year. Roughly 10% result in a referral to secondary care.

3) The average patient sees his GP 5X per year. Perhaps this should be sees HER GP as women are far more likely to consult with any condition at any age other than up to 4yrs and over 75 years. In the first group, babies and toddlers are booked in and brought by women and in the second group, older men tend to be less healthy!

Men's usage of the health service

Consultations per year

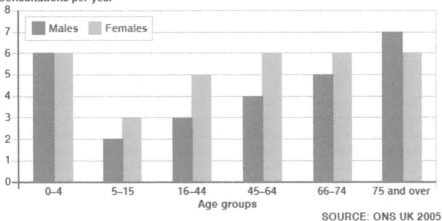

SOURCE: ONS UK 2005

4) The prescription bill in GP in 2007 was £8.7Bn – that is 1/4 of the total cost of primary care. In August 2015 the radio news proclaimed that one tenth of the NHS primary care drugs bill or £900m was being spent on antidiabetic drugs – a lot of money to pay as the wages of gluttony and sloth. The official total NHS bill for drug expenditure seems to be £14.4Bn. (£5.8Bn in secondary care) (2015)

Since 2011 the public have been able to access (on line) the following prescribing data related to their own GP practice:

All prescribed and dispensed medicines (by chemical name), dressings and appliances (at section level) are listed for each GP practice.

For each GP practice, the total number of items that were prescribed and then dispensed is shown.

The total Net Ingredient Cost and the total Actual Cost of these items is shown.

Last year the total healthcare budget was £112 billion. To put this in perspective, that is more than the whole of agriculture generates each year in the UK and more than the cash circulating in the economy.

Around 11% is drugs budget (8% primary care, 3% secondary care).

Interestingly 68% is staffing (salaries/wages/etc).

This leaves only 21% of that £112billion to spend on patients.

In terms of named drugs and generics, GPs sit around 65%-75% generic prescribing/dispensing.

13.5% practices were dispensing practices in 2012.

So it can easily be seen that GPs do the overwhelming majority of the Health Service's General Medicine, Gastroenterology, Paediatrics, Dermatology, Rheumatology, ENT, Gynaecology and virtually all of its Psychiatry. The ONLY areas GPs don't dominate the work of the Health Service are in purely operative Surgical specialities, Intensive Care, invasive investigations and Obstetrics.

General Practice's funding is (2016) 8.1% of total NHS funding, down from 10% in 2004/5. Total funding, for GP including drugs reimbursement comes to £9.45Bn. Pretty good value.

Jam tomorrow? It is promised that Primary Care will have its share increased to 11% of NHS funding by 2020. GPs do 90% of the patient interactions of the Health Service and we are going to get a raise from 8% to 11% for that by 2020! Scottish GP will receive 11% of their NHS budget by 2021 despite having some of the smallest lists in the country. Perhaps this is negatively compensated for by the nation being the current sick man of Europe due to diet, smoking, alcohol and lifestyle.

Patient Lists and List sizes:

1) The average practice has increased in the last 10 years from 5,753 to 6,650 patients. Practices are getting bigger.

2) And there are fewer of them. There were 8,230 practices in England in 2007, by 2011 there were 8,300, by 2,014 there were 7,962. The number of single-handed practices (1,740) were then and are now diminishing – partly because of historical PCT distaste for them partly because old style, all day, full on G.P. is becoming less interesting to newly qualified GPs.

In the UK as a whole, in 2010, there were 41,349 GPs (34,101 in England) 34,000 partners and 7,260 sessional GPs. In the UK as a whole there were 10,112 practices. (BMA Briefing paper)

3) The number of GPs varies per head of population by up to 100% (43 to 88 GPs per 100,000 population over the decade) around the country. The average is currently 68 GPs/100,000 population. London has 69.5/100,000. The East of England is poorly served (62.8/100,000) but if you want a small list, "Go West young man" (actually,"Woman", see above), with 77.2/100,000.

4) But the average list per practitioner has gone down from 1,780 to 1,562 over the last 10 years.

Large Scale GP Providers:

In more recent years there has been a trend towards (2014 onwards) the large scale GP provider organisations. These were supposed to provide more extensive services, better access and a new range of primary care services to the huge numbers of patients on the anonymous lists of these GP factories.

They were popular with some newly qualified part time and sessional doctors, entrepreneurs and the sort of doctors that do not want to offer cradle to grave or named doctor registration personal services. But the justification for them was always efficiency, income and access. The patient would never really have been expected to enjoy being registered in these "never see the same doctor twice" conveyor belts of primary care. Many CCGs and many younger GPs saw them as the way forward. To me they sounded the worst possible impersonal third world, cheap and nasty, impersonal, 1984, bare minimum, primary care. Unsurprisingly the first large scale study, over 15 months, published in July 2016 said the obvious, – that patients preferred to be treated as individuals. 15 care quality indicators in large scale organisations across England found NO EVIDENCE of consistent improvement over time or reductions in organisational variation between practices in large GP providers. Patients however decried the loss of personal relationships with their GP and patient satisfaction deteriorated progressively. The researchers FOUND THIS SURPRISING – !!!! The research did find the large scale organisations maximised GP income and deployed "technology". (-From a patient's perspective neither are positive factors!) The lead researcher for the Nuffield Trust publishing the paper said "It is important that political and NHS leaders don't let expectations of these new organisations run away from reality". **Indeed.** The reality appears to be DIRE.

The reality is that they were designed to make like easier for sessional GPs, to maximise income, to depersonalise General Practice and patients know when they are being ripped off. Yet another example of someone trying to dismantle the ideal structure of General Practice which I have described so many times and has been shown to be popular and successful and consists of small practices of less than 8 partners, all or nearly all full time, named patient lists, few out of practice commitments, plenty of on the day appointments and partners committed to the life of General Practice. Willing to cover dying patients at night, to carry strong painkillers even. They do still exist. It can be done.

Sustainability and Transformation Plans. STPs

These were to be developed across the NHS from 2016/7 with the goal of building services "around local areas not institutions". NHS England has created 44 STP areas (or footprints) each of which combines an average of 5 CCGs covering populations of between 1m and 2m people. The groups will incorporate all health and care systems in each area. It is hard to see why another administrative reorganisation will improve the actual receipt of caring that sick people experience. Particularly when CCGs are yet to prove themselves in any arena other than generating income for relatives of board members. To anyone who has worked for several decades in the NHS there are many long forgotten such realignments of the toys. It is hard to think of one administrative change that made much of a difference. To patients.

Staff:

Practice Nurses;

There are 21,600 practice nurses, (15,600 FTEs) – this number has gone up a fifth in 10 years – no doubt due to disease management, QuoF management and Nurse Practitioners etc.

Other Staff:

There are now 101,200 practice staff (64,000 FTEs)

Since 2008 and the new contract arrangements, most GPs have taken up the opportunity to off load out of hours (night and weekend cover) to deputising services. Originally these were non profit making Cooperatives staffed by local GPs, now they are more likely to be larger regional or national commercial organisations. The employed doctors are far more likely to

1) Have little actual experience of British General Practice

2) Have limited knowledge of local practices, secondary care units and consultant skills and services

3) Be more likely to be exclusively or largely OOH doctors with little daytime experience. (GP OOH may eventually become a subspecialty with training and qualifications of its own) They may be retired, portfolio doctors or trained abroad. Language skills, local knowledge, quality of training and experience are, logic would suggest, even more important in the sometimes isolated, stressful and confused medical environment of OOH. As we all know, the public and even the government are beginning to realise that the current out of hours system is not working. Daniel Ubani, a German doctor, killed a patient in his care with a morphine overdose while working for an out of hours service and there are many other examples of poor out of hours care that come to light regularly.

- Overwhelmed A and E departments, ambulances queuing outside, one over-stretched doctor covering an impossibly large area for a commercial company. – That is the reality of 21st Century OOH cover in the UK. The service is supervised now by profit making out of hours services in most areas. Their role is often to advise patients who I would have gone out to see at home a few years ago to call an ambulance instead. Why was the profession able to predict all this but not the politicians? The Prime Minister is talking about compelling GPs back to doing OOH. Well, we'll see. The huge number of female part timers in GP mitigate against extended hours (as explained above, they all seem to want 9 to 5, family friendly hours when I appraise them), – and of course they will put back no more than 60% of the hours over their careers that male medical graduates will – There won't be the "manhours" soon to cover days let alone nights. The day time demands on GPs have ratcheted up with the endless routine healthy screening, QuoF and rapid access of the last 10 to 15 years (the best political intentions ALWAYS have negative unforeseen outcomes in medicine) so the days are BUSY. After my 13-14 hour full on days, I don't feel like doing evening or nights anymore. The ridiculous Working Time Directive set the slaves free and the new generation of doctors, as well as being less experienced, really don't want to work the long hours that my generation and the country took for granted.

- So it was a series of well meant but naive political decisions that decimated the OOH service and the cure would involve some politically very unpalatable restoration of common sense.

- We could start as I have said before, with cutting the number of female medical students, ending the Working Time Directive, signing all medical students up in their first year to a contract committing them to working in the UK for at least 5 years and at least 3/4 full time. Does all that sound a bit harsh? Well, unless we import tens of thousands of relatively undertrained (if passing British exams is a guide) or badly performing (if referrals to the GMC and removals from the register is a guide) foreign doctors or otherwise reduce vastly what services the NHS is currently offering, or rapidly build twenty fast track medical schools, what choice is there?

QuoF:

(Roland (who advised the government on QuoF at the outset) and Campbell in NEJM May 2014)

The Quality and Outcomes Frame work was imposed on General Practice in 2004. It was one of the world's largest pay for performance programmes with a quarter of GP's pay linked to various performance targets. There have been 20 systematic reviews of the effects of QuoF since then and a great deal of information published about how the system has affected General Practice at the front end. This is a summary of them.

The results on doctors and patients have been mixed. There were some short term clinical benefits of limited scale and some significant unexpected negative effects.

Apparently it was initially introduced in order to boost GP pay and recruitment. It certainly worked at boosting pay. Almost overnight mine went up nearly 50% but very soon and ever since then it has dropped progressively year on year as governments realised the error and got their financial revenge.

From the patients' point of view, and increasingly from that of objective GPs, the fact that the doctor was concentrating on a points scoring agenda, rather than the needs of the patient was seen as being a major distraction in consultation and to practice organisation. A diversion of focus onto limited parts of clinical practice – thus short changing the patient whose doctor was now more interested on a computer screen and asking irrelevant questions than what the patient had made the appointment for.

The pay for performance part of GP's pay has recently been reduced by a third and redistributed – for instance back into capitation payments. So instead of training and attracting more GPs, as was the original idea of QuoF the message is now big lists will be rewarded (2014)

Systematic reviews of the effects of QuoF show that when performance related pay exceeds 10% the risks of "unexpected or perverse consequences increases" but also that clinical improvements which do result may be short lived and only as long as the incentive continues to be paid.

Rapid practice change followed the start of QuoF. Electronic records became universal, more nurses were employed to do the chronic disease management via protocol driven clinics and administrative staff numbers increased. As time went by, more checks on more conditions were added and doctors found consulting became punctuated by a check list of items to be got through before finding out why the patient had come or beginning to relate to them as a real person.

A systematic review of the system showed:

Clinical Care "probably improved although the effects were not compelling and were difficult to entangle from other initiatives..." For chronic conditions, the incentive "maintained or increased pre existing trends but the effect plateaued as soon as GPs gained the maximum rewards available." Hardly a ringing endorsement of short or long term benefits of this sort of pay for performance system.

The use of the PHQ9 as part of depression screening was seen as intrusive and sometimes counterproductive by most GPs. If there is any group of doctors anywhere who can quickly judge the severity of depression with reasonable reliability in MOST patients, it must be the "Good, experienced GP". I decided not to play the QuoF game in these sensitive consultations but to guess PHQ9 scores based on my subjective assessment of the degree of depression after interviewing the patient. So most patients scores were either 8, 15 or 20. (on a scale of 0-27). I felt it was wrong to let an intrusive, detrimental, academically driven and unnecessary questionnaire upset my patient or, of course me suffer for it financially. Subsequent published reviews have shown that the questionnaire works as a screening but not a diagnostic tool, that it works fairly well and that it over diagnoses depression in the hands of Gps! So much for its consistency and reliability. – Anyway, I felt a few minutes of relevant, sensitive, personal conversation worked better and I could then spend the extra time counselling, empathising, relating to and treating the patient. The published reviews say the obvious: **That not everything of value can be measured.** I think this should be written in large red letters on the walls of every CQC inspector, GMC, Royal College, Prescribing Committee, Appraiser, Local Commissioning Group and Deanery office.

As far as patient experience indicators go, at about the same time, largely because of the previous quality indicator of 48 hour appointments and "Advanced Access" schemes, patients were finding it (as now) hard to get booked future appointments (or for that matter on the day appointments as well – unless you were lucky with the phone queuing system). So the quality target was met and paradoxically patients found it harder to get appointments! Even worse, a subsequent attempt to link pay to the ease of getting appointments assessed by a large national patient survey, incorporated a misjudgement in the formula which linked payments to survey scores and led to large and unpredictable fluctuations in reimbursement.

There is some faith expressed through incentive schemes in the patient participation group and incentives for setting up these. Most GPs though, will say that the same tiny proportion of the same individuals always come or respond to PPG meetings and that as a tool for education and information spreading they are of limited value.

A recent assessment of the whole system ((Univ. Manchester, April 2015) looked at 8000 practices' all cause mortality data and data on premature deaths to compare framework performance with local community health. They found "overall quality of care provided by practices – as measured by achievement across all clinical QOF indicators – was not associated with mortality rates in their localities for conditions covered by the QOF. Improvements incentivised by the QOF were not associated with an improvement in premature mortality suggesting that the impact of the incentive scheme has fallen far short of previous estimates". In other words QUoF doesn't work.

So: criticisms of pay for performance are that there is a limited number of useful things in GP that can actually be quantified and scored, that holistic care soon suffers when doctors are incentivised to spend their very limited consulting time asking questions and checking factors on a QuoF tick list, that quality of care for unincluded conditions gets worse, GPs are aware of public access to data and also want to maximise their earnings, so a lot of energy is spent maximising scores to the detriment of all other areas of GP care.

Doctors were always at best ambivalent about QuoF. The big unexpected hike in income was a bonus that neither the profession or DoH expected – although salaried doctors and practice nurses sometimes saw themselves as "cash cows" for the partners and resented that. The loss of autonomy and professionalism, the deskilling in clinical areas handed over to nurses (especially true of diabetes which has seen huge therapeutic changes in recent years), the below inflation pay rises for most of the subsequent ten years or so as part of the "claw back" are all negative features. The annual addition of more and more checks to be done from the same budget became a yearly cross to bear, but for me and most doctors the worst features were the incredibly intrusive prompts and requests to record data which disrupted the natural flow of every consultation and led, continue to lead, to a subconscious clash. This clash is: to generate income or to respond to the patient's agenda. To concentrate on the patient or the computer. In other words: Under QuoF, spending time responding to a patient led consultation costs you money.

A third of the QuoF budget was withdrawn in 2014-15 and there was a return to weighted list size payments. London GPs shared QuoF incentives (for instance to open routine surgeries on Saturdays) across large groups via an APMS deal planned in 2015. Scottish GPs will no longer use a pay for performance National QuoF after 2017. – What goes around...

Screening:

I could never see the point of screening large numbers of the healthy population for diabetes, blood pressure or raised cholesterol. These time consuming activities became part of our contracts under QuoF and were looked upon as some sort of quality marker for the practice. To those parameters my experience and knowledge would have me add PSA in asymptomatic men (probably). I can hardly think of a diabetic or genuine hypertensive in the last 10 years who I wouldn't have picked up in another way without the formal Government population screening. But I can think of many patients with borderline lipids and blood pressures who suffered a great deal of worry, extra testing, taking of medication and probably no real benefit. Screening the healthy is not a medically motivated initiative but always political one and screening the well is one a way a government shows the population that it cares about them.

The truth is that it isn't a very good way. Several (18) studies, now linked and published together in Denmark have shown that screening the healthy population has nothing but downsides and absolutely no health benefit to the population in the short or long term. On the basis of this scientific analysis of screening the healthy, Denmark has ended healthy population screening.

Over here **Public Health England** still defends screening (August 2013) saying "Screening isn't primarily aimed at detecting disease but at making changes in lifestyle to improve health" and The RCGP disagree saying GPs have better things to do with their time than tell fat people to lose weight otherwise they are at risk of heart disease, diabetes, strokes etc. The latest data (2016) suggests the pick up rate is, as I suspected, so low as to be a waste of our time. (See the appropriate sections)

What do Health Visitors do?

For many years I would have been completely unable to answer that and indeed for five recent years I did not even know who our practice Health Visitor was or if we had one.

The official list of roles, some of which do sound like classic bland newspeak are as follows: For instance: "Building capacity by supporting the development of services that communities and families can provide for themselves. Universal partnership plus: For particularly vulnerable families who require a multi agency approach to meet more complex needs". I can imagine that they help the particularly weak, dependent and vulnerable but does it have to sound so mystical, unworldly, vague and new agey?

Officially the list goes: The Health Visiting Team provides Information on all aspects of Healthy Living, for preschool children and their carers.

They offer 4 levels of service from
1) "Community" – promoting Sure Start Centres and Family Centres
2) "Universal" Contact with families: Pre birth, within 10-14 days, 10-12 weeks, by

1 year, by 2 1/2 years. At these meetings child development and health promotion are discussed.

3) "Universal plus" Extra support can be given to some families regarding breast feeding, parenting, emotional support, relationships, lifestyle issues, immunisation, growth and development, healthy eating, behaviour, sleep, toilet training etc.

4) Universal partnership plus: Working with other professionals when there are drug alcohol or mental health issues.

5) Safeguarding: Health visitors assist when children in the family are at risk of harm. So have you got that now?

PMS or GMS? – or APMS?

In 2005, following the introduction of the new GMS/PMS regulations nearly 60% of practices held the 'traditional' General Medical Service contracts but 40% had gone to the selective PMS status. In 2006 37% were PMS. By 2011 there were 3,381 (40.7%) PMS contracts. Having remained at about this level, this system was due to be phased out by 2015. PMS allowed GPs to be salaried and to offer limited services tailored to local needs but they were considered poor value for their cost. They were symptomatic of the demise of the full time, jack of all trades GP that patients had grown up with from the start of the NHS.

GMS had been introduced in 2004, ending payment by the Red Book.

Now the payment system works like this: There is a "Global Sum", based on list size, weighted for the more demanding patients – the female, elderly and children. There are adjustments for rurality, staff costs, morbidity and all this is buffered by a Minimum Practice Income Guarantee (MPIG).

There are a total of four contracting routes (by 2014) to enable PCOs to commission or provide primary care in their area. They are in all: General Medical Services, PMS – Personal Medical Services (aimed at "specific needs of the local population" including Specialist PMS), Primary Care Trust Medical Services (where PCTs provide services) and Alternative Provider Medical Services.

APMS allows local contracts between PCOs and non NHS bodies (voluntary or commercial sector organisations) to supply enhanced or additional primary medical services. PCOs can enter into APMS contracts with any individual or organisation "as long as core NHS values are "fully protected and secured. Some see this as the start of dismantling the way traditional NHS General Practice has always been delivered as it allows non NHS and private providers to bid to run practices.

There was growing concern from the BMA (Sept 2014) that NHS England was opening up all GP contracts to competition in the form of offering them as APMS contracts.

In 2016 a new multi speciality community provider (MCP) "new care model contract" was announced. Practices opting for this will be able to continue as GMS practices but drop QuoF. They will be very large practices despite the distaste that patients have for the anonymity and impersonality of these. As discussed elsewhere, they do facilitate the introduction of technology, also generally unwelcomed by patients and increase GP's income. Something to which patients are at best neutral. Interestingly one of the other supposed advantages of large practices, economies of scale, was dismissed by NHS Digital in August 2016.Practice expenses per registered patient, it was found actually got more the bigger the practice. Average practice expenses per patient in 2013/4 were £88.50 for single handed practices, £91.11 for practices with 2-3 partners, £95.82 for 4-5 partners, £98.45 for 6 or more partners.

Revalidation:

GPs as individual professionals are also subject to a revalidation process, which has two elements. First, from autumn of 2009 all doctors have been required by law to hold a licence (subject to renewal every five years) from the General Medical Council (GMC 2009) and there has been a mechanism for re-certification for doctors on the specialist or general practice registers – this will be carried out by the relevant Royal College or specialist society at least every five years.

Compared with physicians, surgeons or other medical specialists, most GPs are relatively reluctant members of their Royal College. Although membership has gone up exponentially of late, participation and a sense of "belonging" is unusual amongst my colleagues and this is because many college attitudes, decisions and rules seem distant, politically left wing and naive to those who are full time Family Practitioners. College spokesmen and women are almost never intellectually representative of general GP opinion on public health issues or even organisational work issues. They do not seem to try to find out GP opinion either. In 40 years as a doctor the RCP has sent me referenda and questionnaires on many issues, the RCGP hardly, if ever. Many doctors take the exam, these days – it is compulsory and there is talk of allowing up to five attempts so that everyone can now scrape through.-This in response to criticism regarding the poor pass rate of the AKT section by foreign graduates. It is still described as a marker of excellence despite this contradictory "keep trying until you get it" ethos.

Many GPs were disappointed that our Royal College was allowed to take control of our profession's revalidation process. A major expansion of kudos and power and not one it had demonstrated either its suitability or ability to provide. What resulted was what you might predict when a distant academic organisation takes on something a little more than it can cope with. A standardised, rigid, clip board de-individualisation process with easy to count scores which, in the end allows an un-nuanced pass or fail assessment. It is a bit like asking the Arts Council to run the army selection process.

Revalidation was planned to have four layers:

The professionalism of the individual. – Try to think hard about what "professionalism" means – A body of competence and skills, yes but also isn't it also a "professional attitude" a thoughtful, serious, dedicated, considered one, worthy of respect – and this all implies an uncommon skill and a certain distance from the patient? Something many patients feel we may have lost over the last twenty or so years.

Constructive self assessment within the clinical team – something which I always thought, along with constant self education was part and parcel of a professional attitude toward medicine. – Who amongst us would see a patient with blue urine and not want to find out the potential causes and treatments? Or would allow an area of therapeutics which has altered rapidly, like the management of diabetes to become a mystery to them?

Effective clinical governance and

Quality improvement within the organisation.

There are 218,000 doctors overall who will need a licence to practice. The GMC says the process is to "affirm good practice" not to detect bad apples".

I go into whether this is what he public wanted, expected or deserved after Shipman elsewhere. Appraisers now have to do equality and diversity training twice a year (twice as frequently as trainers), appraisees have to do MSFs, PSQs, with all their inherent bias and confusion, and of course, until recently a dreaded audit. Ask yourself what purpose all this serves and note the phrase is: *equality and diversity* not **quality and uniformity**. Which would it be if we were genuinely putting the patient's interests first?

Practice-based commissioning (PBC) was supposed to give GP practices the opportunity to use funds to 'purchase' or 'redesign' services (including hospital care) for the benefit of their patients (Department of Health 2004b). This was supposed to be undertaken by practices coming together to form local consortiums. PBC was intended to make care 'more responsive to patient needs' and to encourage investment in community-based alternatives to hospital care as well.

This has now been taken over by the developing **Locality Commissioning** system. Well, we will see if out of hours care, local mental health beds, Child and Adolescent Mental Health Services, Substance Abuse, Health Visiting and the other often half hearted or absentee services start to improve.

Clinical Commissioning:

In 2012 the Health and Social Care Act became law. It had been in development for the previous 20 years, and was considered to be the most significant reorganisation of the NHS since its inception in 1948.

Clinical Commissioning Groups, CCGs (or corrupt commissioning groups as they will soon be known) to some extent replaced the PCTs, though some staff and responsibilities moved to Council Public Health Teams when PCTs ceased to exist in April 2013.

The point was to give General Practitioners the responsibility for the commissioning of NHS services in their localities and the accountability for a large part of the £110 billion (The BBC in one year, 2014, quoted both this and £130 billion) cost of the NHS. From April 2013 all GPs would have to be part of a Clinical Commissioning Group (CCG) and the previous arrangements for commissioning by Primary Care Trusts – generally covering larger areas such as an entire County – would cease with the PCTs being abolished. The new way of commissioning would henceforth be considered "Clinically led, managerially enabled". This had been tried before but without actually making the GPs accountable and responsible for the NHS services in their area. CCGs include all of the GP groups in their areas with the aim of giving GPs the clinical commissioning authority in their own areas. CCGs would be overseen by NHS England (Regional Offices and Area teams). These structures would henceforth manage primary care commissioning including holding the NHS contracts for GP practices.

The Act also stipulated that the CCG would engage and work with Patient Groups and the wider public, Local Authorities (locally and at County Council level) and with Public Health. This would try to make the NHS much more accountable to the public it served, work closer with Local Authorities and improve working between Health and Social Care – an area where the previously separate budgets usually resulted in disjointed provision particularly concerning frail elderly patients – especially when ready for hospital discharge. Pooled elements of the Health and the Social Care budgets could for example reduce delayed discharges from hospitals and create a more "joined up" service in the community in order to avoid some admissions to hospital.

At the same time, from 2010 there was a program called **QIPP** (Quality, Innovation, Productivity and Performance) which planned to produce efficiency savings of £20 billion over 4 years; All sectors of the NHS were in effect to achieve a 5% efficiency saving every year. This was needed for 2 reasons; the true rate of inflation in Health Care runs at about 7% (due to increasing needs of an aging population and greater demands on the system generally) and because of a weak economy, central funding from taxation was unable to afford more than a 2% annual increase in funding for the NHS. Producing these QIPP efficiencies as well as undergoing major reform was a considerable effort for the NHS but it "opened up opportunities" for different and more efficient working. For most GPs QIPP meant Simvastatin and Pravastatin were substituted for the still patented Atorvastatin, Naproxen for Diclofenac and ACEIs for ARBs – you get the idea. Cheaper, not necessarily better. Questionable improvements, parsimonious pharmacology.

By 2015 many examples of conflicts of interest and extravagant spending on superfluous advisors had been exposed within CCGs where GPs had commissioned services from organisations or businesses in which they or close family members had a personal vested interest. This seems inevitable given the "entrepreneurial" type of doctor that often gets involved in managing budgets in any reorganised area of medicine. I have seen money made indirectly by individual doctors with almost every reorganisation and incentive that the NHS has undergone for decades. I have to admit it goes against the grain to see personal profiteering from the NHS like this. But in late 2004 the risks of this were diminished somewhat when tougher measures to guard against conflicts of interests were proposed. These included enhanced training for lay board members, public registers of interests and decisions and observer rights. There would also be a "Lay chair" and a "Lay and executive majority". We all hoped that these controls would curb some of my more innovative and ambitious colleagues.

The front page of the Times Nov 11th 2015 gave us the depressing answer "GPs award £2.4Bn deals to their own companies". A total of 400 contracts and the funding for these had gone to family businesses of the board members of CCGs. Patient leaders "Condemned the process as a free for all" and how could we see the doctors involved as anything but corrupt?

How is the current NHS organised?

NHS England

CQC Inspects practices and all other providers		
"Monitor"		Hospital Trusts
(Independent financial	Clinical Commissioning Groups	
supervisor and regulator		
for NHS providers) makes		Community Trusts
"probity visits" to practices	GP Practices	(H/Vs, D/Ns etc)
		Mental Health Trusts
		Local Councils commission some services – smoking cessation, contraception, weight, alcohol, drug misuse, via GPs.

Care Quality Commission:

As with many health related organisations you will begin to appreciate the total irony in the name of the organisation as you read a little about how it has been run and organised up until now.

The recent history of the organisation shows a complete lack of patient care and a failure to pursue any kind of genuine quality.

Its various executives have excused this by complaining it was underfunded and asked to do too much from the start. (Jill Finney, Today Programme)

This official body was established in 2009, replacing the Healthcare Commission and Commission for Social Care Inspection and based on the Health and Social Care Act of 2008, to inspect providers of health and social services. There are 40,000 providers of care that need inspection by the CQC. So you could argue they have a difficult task.

Intended to improve health and social care integration, all health and social care providers have to register with the CQC. The Commission inspects care providers and has and uses various enforcement powers if it regards "standards" are inadequate. (e.g. care of mental health patients, infection control in hospitals, GP and dental surgery services etc). Although it has uncovered many abuses in care homes, it has also failed to uncover serious systematic failures in other areas. In fact it missed 9 out of the 11 failing organisations now in "Special Measures" since the advent of "Chief Inspector of Hospitals", (Professor, Sir Mike Richards, the ex cancer "Tsar", a **doctor**, with a team of doctors, nurses and patients. -Hurrah).

Ironically Cynthia Bower the Trust's one time chief executive, failed to notice Mid Staffordshire's mortality rates when she was the responsible strategic health authority's chief executive there before being appointed to the Commission and more recently, has been accused with her deputy Jill Finney of gagging the seemingly only honest member of the board at the time. This was Kay Sheldon – who wanted and tried to publicise failings in the inspection of the Maternity Unit at Furness.

Until recently, amongst GP and Dental staff the CQC had a reputation not for incompetence but for pettiness and nit picking – for instance water tanks in the attics of dentists have to be labelled hot or cold, etc.

GP practices have to register, comply with core standards, ensure ongoing compliance and pay an annual registration fee. In November 2014 they missed the Nottinghamshire dentist Mr Desmond D'Mello who didn't wash his hands, change his gloves or sterilise his instruments between patients and prompted the biggest recall of 22,000 patients in NHS history for check serology. This was after a whistle blower filmed him seeing patients and the CQC had previously visited his practice unexpectedly the July before and found the surgery "Did not meet cleanliness and infection control standards"

The CQC inspects GPs, dentists, hospices, hospitals, nursing homes, urgent care services, prisons, ambulances stations and care homes etc.

More recently the new Chief Executive, David Prior, on the Today Programme (19/6/13) apologising for the cover up of a critical internal report on its failings regarding **Morecambe Bay/Furness maternity services** explained that the inspections of hospital units and subsequent reports had been done by police officers and firemen. He went on to say that the CQC leadership at the time had been dysfunctional and you've guessed it, "not fit for purpose" and had all gone now. So: Mothers harmed and one dead and at least 11 babies lives lost, through nursing incompetence at a bad maternity unit, official inspectors not knowing what to look for or to ask about, having no experience of what they were asked to do, then hoodwinked into writing a positive report which was subsequently rubbished by another, honest employee of the Commission who recognised the unit as dangerous and said so. Amazingly that report was then actively suppressed by the CQC to save embarrassment of the organisation whose purpose it was to protect patients. This all finally came out in 2015.

The Morecambe Bay Enquiry (2015) was an object lesson in how NHS self interested, culturally different, professional groups can put themselves, or at least their narrow professional goals hubristically before the needs of patients. The midwives seem to have been the main culprits at Morecambe Bay, regarding themselves as "The Musketeers" and forcing mothers to have a "normal birth" even if it killed their babies and in one instance the mum as well. They had no functioning relationship with the obstetricians, no professional standards, the CQC inspections were botched and the managers were, it seemed, so determined to become a "Foundation Trust" that they wilfully ignored the intolerable and dangerous behaviour of the midwives. This is a conflict that could and might well happen daily in midwife run maternity units everywhere – when the skill and the risk is knowing when to ask an obstetrician to intervene. – And, by the way, having rapid access to an obstetrician who is available at the drop of a hat. Obviously this is a structure that has an inherent design flaw. This is not something that was generally broadcast. Unfortunately, because delivery is a joint area of responsibility, the historic and traditional obstetric arena has always been a potential conflict zone between doctor and nurse where the patient can be made to suffer for the professional hubris of the midwife. I am afraid this is the classic doctor vs nurse-in-control-of-patient-management-decisions conflict zone.-where the patient always finishes as a potential victim.

I heard about this CQC chaos shortly before reading the NHS Sussex leaflet "What to do if you have concerns about the performance of a colleague" which advises "Failure to act may be considered serious professional misconduct which could put your own registration at risk" – obviously the reverse applies to senior administrators and potentially to nurse led delivery units. (?)

Why has this sort of story been repeated time and time again within the NHS over the last ten years? A system which is supposed to be a caring system devoted to patients' wellbeing, systemically, from nurses on wards to nursing managers supervising them and senior managers in hospital to inspectors, Chief Executives and regulators – all seem to conspire to ignore patients' needs, pain and suffering and to act as if their own priorities are more important.

Robert Francis QC, who ran the Mid Staffs enquiry said on The Today Programme (24/6/13): "There was a crying need for candour, openness and transparency and that the management of the Health Service needed to include patients, doctors and nurses more". What a surprise! One of his other absolutely right to the heart-of-the-problem conclusions was that **the more you supervise and organise the role of nurses and doctors the less personally caring they become**.

I have highlighted this because it is the heart of what caused the breakdown of compassion in every unit where patients were ignored, subordinated to gold standard protocols or lost behind work sheets and tick boxes. Tragically, it looks like the same miserable process may be starting up again with The Royal Shrewsbury Maternity Unit and baby deaths between 2014 and 2016. What does it take to change the mind set of some of our colleagues?

When politicians constantly make changes to what is now an impractical (free to all, all our health care needs, everywhere) structure and professional managers with no experience of medicine administer hospitals, all they recognise are costs, deadlines and targets. To them the patients are, to be honest, an embarrassment. A problem and not the purpose of the exercise.

The CQC gives the following areas which they call "Essential standards":
Respecting and involving people who use services
Consent to care and treatment
Care and welfare of people who use services
Meeting nutritional needs
Cooperating with other providers
Safeguarding vulnerable people who use services
Cleanliness and infection control
Management of medicines
Safety and suitability of premises
Safety, availability and suitability of equipment
Requirements relating to workers
Staffing
Supporting workers

These are all organisation and management issues and none relate to how competent, safe or effective the medicine, dentistry or nursing is.

The CQC does not get involved in the professional competence of doctors, nurses and midwives, but leaves this crucial aspect to the regulating bodies. Like so many politically and judicially crafted official bodies appointed to supervise and control our work and which did not seem necessary at the start of the NHS, the CQC has political objectives rather than the real health, comfort or happiness of patients.

Listen to its "executives" discussing their role and they have the usual (and sometimes freely admitted) "Tick Box" mind set. They avoid concepts of control, sacking and disciplining bad staff, and they are wedded to management concepts and attitudes and catch phrases like "Delivering" care, even of introducing "caring" into the nursing curriculum (the Today Programme 27/3/13)

Look at their "Guidance about Compliance" book, a copy of which every GP and dental practice has to study and "comply with". – It has 28 "Outcomes" from Involvement and Information, Personalised Care, Treatment and Support to Suitability of Management.

Nowhere does it say:
There will always be a fresh jug of water on the bed side table

And if the patient can't feed or drink themselves they will be offered help every hour and every mealtime.

All patients who request the loo or cleaning up will be helped within 10 minutes.

All staff will be polite and have achieved clear, articulate, comprehensible English language skills, whether they come from Surrey, Glasgow or Somalia-and be regularly reviewed.

All patients will have regularly, a confidential questionnaire on the personal attitudes and skills of the medical and nursing staff and these will be acted upon if consistently negative.

All patients' relatives will be able to book an appointment with the Medical Registrar responsible for the patient at least once a week and the senior ward nurse at least twice a week if requested.

No hand over period for nurses will take more than 20 minutes and during that time at least half the ward staff will be on the ward, (two hand over shifts, obviously)

Other than at hand over times all nursing staff will be on the ward except one individual, delegated to answer the ward phone and coordinate administration tasks.

Every nurse with have responsibility for every patient on the ward at all times they are on duty.

No nurse will ever refuse any reasonable request for nursing assistance.

At night, most lights will be switched off unless clinically necessary and all conversations between staff and with patients shall be only as loud as needed for clear comprehension.

Noise will be kept to a minimum and noisy visitors and disruptive children will be asked to leave.

I think in return for this patients, staff and relatives must understand that the health and care needs of the patient-majority on a ward often trump the vague ideals of political human rights, working time directives, the rights of all relatives to see their loved ones at any time, the rights of visiting children to make noise, the endless crying, screaming or disturbing confusion of one disruptive patient who MAY for the benefit of everyone else, on occasion, despite NICE and GMC guidelines need to be calmed, sedated and settled with drugs.

One other small point which you can take any way you want: The CQC hand book "Essential standards of quality and safety" is 274 pages long. It is peppered, like most modern day government publications with pictures of "Health Care Providers" and "Health Care Users" having a mutually respectful but jolly time together..

For some reason, of the 17 faces visible in the photographs, 9 are of people from ethnic minorities.

Does this mean the authors think that Ethnic Minorities disproportionately use Health Services or that most Health Care is provided by people from ethnic minorities or perhaps, only what happens in London matters, or, our politicians assume that London IS Britain, or as is always the case in any health literature from a public body these days, the desire to be politically correct supersedes common sense, accuracy, reality and by doing so can subtly distort the message it tries to convey?

The CQC and General Practices:

Special measures as applied to failing hospitals were as of 2014 extended to GP practices. This was the first time a "national failure regime" has been instituted for the profession. The lowest, "Inadequate" rated practices it was suggested would be given six months to a year to "resolve problems" or be shut down. The rating system will be: outstanding, good, requires improvement or inadequate.

The proposal is that after a defined period of trying to sort out their own problems they will be placed in "Special Measures".

Failure to improve by the end of this time will result in the CQC withdrawing its registration or NHS England terminating the practice's contract. In this event it is suggested that new GPs will be found (from where? – there is a national shortage and none are going to WANT to work in the sort of failing practices that we are probably talking about) or alternative local surgeries found (Oh yes? all our local surgeries have big lists already and find it hard to cover the patients they already have let alone another practice's). The first assessments (Jan 2015) put three "inadequate practices" in special measures. The accompanying announcement said that these practices had a twelve month deadline to improve care or have their registration cancelled and be forced to close. If in "special measures" the practices can pay half the costs of an intensive peer support program from the RCGP and NHS England.

Initial assessments by the CQC of 69 GP practices came up with: 3 outstanding, 56 good and 10 required improvement. An interim report in September 2015 after 2000 practices had been inspected, announced 4% of practices were outstanding and 4% inadequate. The 4% of failing practices covered 330,000 patients, "chaotic and disorganised" "with a poor culture of safety and learning, deaf to complaints and with no outcome measures".

Steve Field, the Chief Inspector of General Practice at the CQC said that these practices had been known about for years, why had no one intervened? Why indeed?

Other matters:

The Visiting Bag:

When I qualified nearly 40 years ago, the average G.P. was the boy scout of medicine. Prepared to deal with every medical situation that work and life could present. Even in commuter belt England in the second decade of the 21st century, all my experience tells me that neighbours still fall off step ladders, neighbour's children fracture collar bones, you come across men with broken necks in wrecked cars on the way home from work, people in pubs have fits, friends and their guests have asthma attacks and that the out of hours service does not provide adequate immediate home care. Certainly the ambulance service, burdened as it is with ferrying patients to casualty out of hours that we GPs used to see and reassure does not arrive promptly at any time of day or night anymore.

So you have a choice as a G.P. – You can turn away and pretend, as many do, that General Practice is all elective and desk bound or you can do what the public expects of you and treat pain and illness and give sensible referral advice based on the response. You can put only a prescription pad and a stethoscope in your handbag but to do the job properly you do need a proper set of tools. I carry a routine visits bag (9.7kg) everywhere and a second bag (6.6kg) with starter packs, ear syringe, foetal heart monitor and various spare equipment to selected homes. The resus. case, nebuliser, drips etc usually stay in the boot (trunk) of the car.

My visiting bag contains:

Tongue depressors, a bright pocket torch, nasal speculum, Band Aids and Medi Swabs, an adult Guedel's Airway, a Resusciade, a selection of syringes (5mls the most useful) and needles (21g, Green Needles are the most useful), latex examination gloves, KY jelly or similar, glycerin suppositories and Micralax Micoenemas, (Micolette), Voltarol 100mg, Motilium 30mg and Paediatric Paracetamol suppositories (Alvedon 125mg), 75mg Soluble Aspirin, GTN Spray, (Coronitro is small, but keep an eye on the expiry date), Glucogel.

A MIMS – Although this is now available as an App in my iPhone, which is much lighter to carry, A variety of changing Aid Memoires in the form of an old PDA (Psion), my prescription pad folder with FP10s, a pad of Med Certs, A few private prescriptions (never used) and compliments slips (I always put through the letter box if I call in on a "house bound" patient who happens to be out).

Paper instructions on:

Parenteral doses of emergency drugs,

Adult advanced life support algorithm

Mini Mental State Examination.

Treatment of Anaphylactic Shock algorithm

A list of symptoms and signs of specific diseases in children as well as the Traffic Light System for identifying the likelihood of Serious Illness in Children.

Guidelines for the management of Infection in Primary Care from our Local H A.

My own protocol for missed pills and Contraceptive Advice as this seems to change frequently.

Guidance on the use of anti flu treatment

A Risk Assessment Tool for the evaluation of Occupational Exposure to HIV

The ABCD2 scoring system and the CHADS scoring system of strokes and AF

Algorithm of treatment of patients with Acute Stroke and TIA

Algorithm of Adult Choking Treatment

Summaries of the law on clarification and confirmation of Unexplained Deaths, the Eligibility of Overseas Visitors to receive free primary care.

Phone numbers of OOH and Unregistered Dental Services

Phone numbers of all my partners, local surgeries, D/Ns, CMHT, local hospitals, ambulance services etc etc

My cover rota.

Surgery headed note paper, envelopes, EDD calculator, Drug Interaction Alert, a "Guide to Drugs in Breast Milk" (the iPhone can usually access "Safefetus.com" which does much the same thing) A list of Tubigrip sizes, spare pens, a "crocodile" which is a device for safely cutting off the tops of ampoules) and (because I once fished out a beer can ring pull from a croupy child's hypo pharynx), a pair of ENT elongated forceps, as well as sharp scissors, a pair of splinter forceps, a scalpel and blades (disposable scalpels are poor substitutes for the real thing), a Jobson Horne probe (lots of aural foreign bodies over the years) and suture material. You look really feeble if you can't stitch a neighbour's cut at the weekend and they have to spend 6 hours in casualty with the drunks.

Stethoscopes, adult and neonatal, a sphygmomanometer, a patellar hammer, a mini auriscope/ophthalmoscope set (even though the later has NEVER significantly contributed to the decision as to whether to admit a patient from home or not), a urine multitest Dipstix kit, (10 tests). A digital thermometer, transcutaneous oxygen monitor (very overrated as this depends as much on peripheral circulation and temperature/hydration as it does on oxygenation) tourniquet, a selection of butterflies and Venflons, cotton wool balls, micropore tape.

Drugs:

I carry:

For the nebuliser: Salbutamol, 5mg in 2.5ml, Atrovent 500mcg in 2mls, Pulmicort 0.25mg/ml 2ml nebules (for croup etc).

Oral: Penicillin V, Erythromycin, Cefadroxil and Co Amoxiclav (my antibiotics of choice for OOH UTIs or LRTIs), Norfloxacin (Prostatitis), Timethoprim, Solpadol Tabs, Half Inderal LA, EC Prednisolone 5mg. Soluble 5mg Prednisolone. Propranolol Tabs

40mg, Furosemide tabs 40mg, Cyclizine tabs 50mg, Diazepam 5mg Tabs.

Co Dydramol, Co Codamol (500/30), Codeine Phosphate 30mg, Dihydrocodeine 30mg, Tramadol 50mg, all have different uses. Unfortunately the far more useful and side effect free Co-Proxamol is effectively banned by the NHS these days. Lormetazepam 1mg, Maxalt Melt (Rizatriptan), Ranitidine 150mg and Omeprazole 20mg, Chlorpromazine Tabs 50mg, Haloperidol Tabs 1.5mg, Diazepam 5mg.

Minims Tropicamide, Fluorescein, Amethocaine.

Controlled Drugs: MST 10mg Tabs, Diconal Tabs, Pethidine 50mg Tabs.

A one drop blood glucose testing kit, lancets and test strips. (e.g. One touch Ultra).

Rectal Diazepam 10mg (Stesolid).

Injectables:

Naloxone (short shelf Life, but still works long after the expiry date), Water for injections (2x10mls), Benzyl Penicillin 600mg dry Powder, Cefuroxime, (Zinacef) Injection for the supposedly penicillin allergic, Adrenaline 1:1000 at least 2 in date ampoules, Glucagon 1mg (oral glucose gel just isn't enough sometimes), Chlorpheniramine 10mg in 1ml, Hydrocortisone 100mg in 1ml (at least 2 ampoules), Buscopan 20mg/ml 1ml amps, Atropine 600mcg in 1ml, Hypnovel/Midazolam (terminal Care, aggression, panic and anxiety states), 10mg in 2mls, Nozinan 25mg in 1ml, Haloperidol injection 5mg in 1ml, Chlorpromazine inj 50mg in 2mls, Depixol inj 20mg, (you might not expect these to be present in an emergency bag but the domiciliary psychiatry services I have had contact with over the last 30 years have been so inaccessible, so inconsistent and often so unhelpful that after they have finally come, deliberated and gone, a systemic injection of one of these drugs has been of huge benefit to the patient and relatives and avoided both short and long term harm to all involved), Diazepam inj 10mg in 2mls, Stemetil 12.5mg in 1ml, Metoclopramide Injection 10mg in 2mls (avoid under 14-15 years old because of dystonia), Cyclizine 50mg inj. in 1ml, Furosemide 50mg in 5mls, Sodium Chloride inj 0.9% 2ml amps, Glycopyrrolate 200ug in 1ml (terminal care), Kemadrine 5mg/ml, and Aminophylline 250mg in 10mls (which I haven't used in over 10 years because the nebuliser is usually so effective). IV Glucose 10g in 20mls (50%),

Systemic pain killers: Diclofenac, Voltarol Inj 75mg in 3mls.

Controlled Drugs: Pethidine Injection: 50mg in 1ml, Diamorphine 10mg Dry Powder amps.

You may think that all this is GP overkill but the VERY LEAST a real GP carries with them at all times in terms of systemic drugs are: Benzyl Penicillin and Water for injections, Adrenaline, Hydrocortisone, Diamorphine, Diazepam, and Furosemide. I just don't see how you can pretend to be a doctor without having these basic systemic tools at your command.

GPs and Systemic analgesic Drugs:

(Non controlled alternatives: **Tramadol** injection 100mg in 2mls. Tramadol is an opioid agonist, not fully antagonised by Naloxone, more effective in surgical than dental pain, in terms of strength 50mg orally = Co codamol 30/500. Parenteraly *it is said to be* equivalent to Pethidine, approx 1/10 that of Morphine. Can increase seizures and per operative recall but causes less constipation than codeine. I don't find it a very effective pain killer despite its addictive potential.

Meptazinol injection is likewise not controlled but not very strong.

Other systemic analgesics (controlled): Morphine, Diamorphine, Methadone, Pethidine, Dihydrocodeine, Buprenorphine, Oxycodone, Pentazocine, Fentanyl.

Harold Shipman:

Was a British trained GP, who as a junior doctor killed approximately 15 patients including a 4 yr old and was known to have been "cavalier" with the doses of systemic drugs (including Diazepam) that he administered. As a GP is thought to have killed 250 of his patients. His "unlawful killings" took place between 1970 and 1998 when he was finally arrested. Altogether 800 of his patients died during his medical career and were investigated, I presume this number is related at least partially to the practice age demography and the type of hospital jobs as to his murderous behaviour. His victims were mainly previously well elderly women who he killed by administering intravenous Diamorphine. He was known to have been a Pethidine addict in his early career when he had forged scrips which led to his being expelled from one GP partnership. He was treated for his addiction before the GMC permitted him to start practising again. He became a partner in Hythe, Manchester, killing 70 patients, then a single handed GP – by all accounts very popular, **many patients spoke in his defence** at his trial, so he would have had excellent patient feedback, he had a good practice prescribing profile and a huge list of 3,500. He was at one time secretary of the local LMC and there was a 1 year wait to get on his list. I don't doubt that he was good at audits and SEAs as well. This just demonstrates that the worst British doctor in history would have scored highly on our standard ways of assessing the quality of GPs today. **He would have done a brilliant Appraisal.** So surely there is something wrong with our ways of assessing each other isn't there? Like MCQ examinations, the ease of administration builds in an inherent fallibility.

The high death rate amongst his patients and the suspicious circumstances (previously well patients, he had visited earlier in the day and had left the door on the latch so that he could return to "discover them" etc), led to suspicions being raised by another GP who was asked to sign Part2 cremation forms and by a local undertaker. The police undertook a superficial investigation and found insufficient evidence to proceed. He then forged a will and this was instrumental in his final detection.

Harold Shipman denied the murders until the end. He hung himself in prison.

The subsequent enquiry under Dame Janet Smith addressed the question why no one in authority had noticed what Shipman had been doing despite the existence of numerous concerns being expressed by various colleagues both medical and non medical during his career.

The net result of the enquiry was a series of recommendations. The bottom line for the practising GP is that Shipman has resulted in

1) Appraisal:

This is an annual "Cornerstone of Revalidation". This was a political response to address the public revulsion at what had happened and to regulate a previously self regulated profession. It didn't really construct a system for detecting dangerous doctors early or improve the quality of consulting skills but resulted in a way of managing post graduate training and formalising professional reaccreditation of GPs. Not really the point in Shipman's case. It consists of the recording and "reflecting" on the appraisee's year of learning activity by discussing the varied forms of personal development undertaken. It is frequently a mentoring and support session and highly unlikely to uncover occult rogue doctors.-The most positive thing that can be said for appraisal is that another doctor meets the appraisee formally and suggests alternative ways and means of keeping up to date, coping with difficult patients and partnership challenges. It has also led, not surprisingly, since it is time consuming, largely standardised, ritualistic and mostly without a positive benefit (in the opinion of most older doctors) to the early retirement of a disproportionate number of older GPs (Biomed Central Study July 2016). Three quarters of GPs who complained about Appraisal were over 50 and were twice as likely to have had over 20 years experience. The more you know about General Practice the more you realise the pointlessness of Appraisal. In the only published study on attitudes to appraisal (August 2017, GP Magazine,) 16% of GPs found it useful and 67% a waste of time. The Royal College of General Practitioners and its academics now own Appraisal and you know what they say about teachers.

It is, predictably, exactly what many of us hoped it would not become. Royal Colleges and Deaneries setting the agendas and standards for what makes a good doctor. It is in practice based on one of three electronic standardised Toolkits which stop you in the event of you try to demonstrate your individualism in any way. It includes the recording of fifty hours of personally chosen study, the highly dubious and often totally pointless multi-source feedback questionnaires, some form of uninterpretable patient feedback, SEAs and, until recently, standardised audits amongst a series of other data recording tasks and plans for next year's learning. Nothing that really assesses the consultation skills or the doctor's abilities. What could have been a more useful assessment process would have been a flexible, less frequent, more intense analysis of the doctor's consultations, referrals and complaints. Patient centred, over a couple of days, every few years. What we got instead was a computer centred, form based, standardised national format of measurable tasks forced into pretending to do something it can't. And something that most experienced GPs felt was a burden and resented.

Why is there an establishment compulsion to standardise and to make compulsory only those things that are easy to record – not the things that actually reflect and indicate good practice?

Go to a course on appraisal or revalidation and the party faithful will use terms (and I quote) like:

"Appraisal is part of a drive for quality in our healthcare systems,

-it is about improving the governance of medical practice

it is intended to bring doctors into a structured process and encourage self reflective practice

or it must be a positive affirmation of a doctor's professionalism" – BUT

"It is NOT a new way to raise concerns about a doctor" – Well, given the fact that the Francis enquiry about the Mid Staffordshire cruelty concluded that: "the more box ticking there was and management supervision of previously independent medical professionals the less committedly and caringly they did their job", you have to wonder why appraisal and revalidation are supposed to improve standards in this form. But more importantly why all the academics who now control the process fall over themselves to emphasise how it isn't a way of weeding out bad doctors. Don't the patients have the right to expect exactly that for their £550 a doctor a year?

Over a five year appraisal cycle, five separate annual files (each recording 50 or more one hour periods of documented "learning") will be considered sufficient for a 5 year Revalidation and Relicensing – Reaccreditation, before the granting of a Licence to Practise for another 5 years.

If it were designed to detect a psychopath who was murdering his patients, it would have missed Shipman by a mile.

2) A longer and more intrusive Part 2 Cremation Form and its associated bureaucracy.

The most intrusive and harmful part of this is the necessity to telephone the grieving relatives and to try subtly to find out if they had any suspicions about the death itself without upsetting them further. If the death took place in a nursing home there is likewise a duty to talk to the nursing team involved (although this is often impractical given shift rotas, team responsibilities, holidays and so on so the information is second or third hand). Either way it is a profoundly awkward process without raising unfounded suspicions and pointless distress in the relatives and no little resentment in the other doctor. ?Why on earth did you ask the family that?

It appears (July 2016) that all death certificates are now to be scrutinised by a medical examiner and discussed with the family members of the deceased to ensure the information is correct and to flag any "Indications of malpractice or clinical governance issues". Medical examiners will assess the medical certificate and the medical records to "Pinpoint inaccuracies". If they "Deem something is incorrect" they will discuss it with the doctor who signed the death certificate. This is all because the DH has concluded the "Existing arrangements are confusing etc etc" Just imagine the impossibility of doing this job conscientiously: – Indications of malpractice? by whose standards? Inaccuracies? How often in a rapidly changing and deteriorating clinical situation have I forgotten to keep contemporaneous and perfectly accurate notes (especially about what doses and when drugs were administered to distressed, deteriorating and suffering patients). Deem something is incorrect? Again, by whose standards? Who are these inspectors going to be and how much experience of caring for dying patients in the community will they have had?

Surely the solution, since Shipman would have side stepped all these barriers is to examine in detail every death where the GP was the last person to see the patient alive alone.

3) More intrusive controlled drug management.

The more rigid stock control of CDs has been potentially the most patient-harmful result of the Shipman aftermath – and, by the way, unlikely to prevent CD hoarding if the doctor is determined to do it. When I entered General Practice 30+ years ago, every GP carried controlled drugs as a normal tool in their bag. I have asked colleagues from my own and other local practices and at two recent post graduate meetings who had injectable controlled drugs in their bags. I was shocked that only 10% of my colleagues now carry Pethidine or Diamorphine with them. This is in my opinion a professional act of mass cowardice and patient betrayal which is beyond precedent. It must be as a result of "burdensome" new CD regulations and the fear of being misinterpreted as a murderer not a carer by relatives and administrators. The suffering, pain, fear and distress that this has already caused is immense. We seem to have forgotten that we are supposed to put the patients' needs uppermost, not our own sensitivities or misplaced concerns about the potential suspicion of relatives or officious administrators.

The new Strengthened CD audit Trail includes:

An **Accountable Officer** who now asks every the GP to fill in a form (a "Declaration and Self Assessment Form) regarding his or her use of CDs.

Typical questions: Do you prescribe, hold stock, dispose of CDs, do you have SOPs for CDs, do you have SOPs for significant events involving CDs, have there been any complaints about your prescribing of CDs, have there been any significant events involving CDs, are returned medicines ever reused, do you supply addicts, do you maintain records of administration, are all CDs kept under lock and key, do you keep CDs in your bag, how often do you date check your CDs, do you keep an up to date CD register, do you keep unused patients' stock etc.??

Every practice has to write up a **SOP for the use of controlled drugs at the surgery. The Safer Management of Controlled Drugs (Record Keeping) Oct 2006 includes:** Strengthened record keeping ("The audit trail") throughout the NHS and private sector. There are now computerised systems for monitoring excess prescribing (eg the ePACT system) and whether maximum licensed doses are being exceeded, more than 30 day prescriptions are being issued and whether the CD is routinely prescribed in GP.

Records for schedule 2 drugs (Opiates, Amphetamines, Barbiturates) to be kept in a Controlled Drug Register, a CDR – All "Healthcare Professionals" who hold a personal stock of CDs must keep their own CDR and maintain it. All GPs should always have done this anyway. These records must include the date the supply was obtained, name and address of the supplier, the amount obtained, name, form and strength of the CD.

For CDs supplied to patients or practitioners, the register must include the date, the name and address of the recipient, the quantity, the name, form and strength of the CD supplied.

The following information is likely to be necessary later: Running balances, (this was recommended by the Shipman enquiry and is considered good practice), prescriber identification number, or the name and professional registration number of the dispenser.

Regular running balance checks should be made – I tend to do this every time I give an injection of a CD, the responsibility being that of the GP not a non clinical member of staff.

The paper records must be kept for 2 years, 11 years if on computer.

Other requirements upon dispensers are to obtain proof of identity of the person collecting the drug, to record this in their drugs register etc.

There are denaturing kits available for the destruction of old CDs.(Usually from the Medicines Safety and Controlled Drugs Manager at the PCT. – Now I assume the Commissioning Group) but the list includes

A Chief Dental Officer

Supervisors of Midwives

Senior Officers in NHS Trusts

Chief Executives of NHS Trusts (!)

A Primary Care Trust Chief Pharmacist

A Registered Medical Practitioner

Medical Director of a Primary Care Trust/CG

etc

This role used to be performed by a Police Controlled Drugs Liaison Officer.

The proposed Patient Drug Record Card is not yet a legal requirement.

All this is particularly applicable to Diamorphine, the most useful Terminal care drug and Harold Shipman's murder weapon of choice.

Up until now the fate of every ampoule of Pethidine and Diamorphine in the possession of a GP should have been recorded in a Controlled Drug Register. Mine goes back to 1984 when my trainer gave me two ampoules of Diamorphine which were duly recorded at the start of the book. So far I haven't been inspected by the Drugs Squad officer during my career but perhaps Shipman will change the frequency and intensity of that like he has changed nearly every other aspect of the CD GP/trust/self regulation environment that existed before.

The practical Rules for Controlled Drug use in practice are (MPS)

1) Keep CDs in a lockable cupboard/safe

2) Maintain a CD register (written (2 years) or electronic (11 years)) which includes

3) A running balance of stock and

4) Entries on the correct page (separate sections for each CD, Pethidine, Diamorphine etc).

The CD register must be bound, contain class sections for each CD, have the name of the drug specified at the top of the page, entries in chronological order, no blank lines, in ink without cancellations/alterations, be kept for a minimum of 2 years after the last dated drug was given. This can be computerised.

New CDs entries must record the supplier, the date, the amount, name, form and strength.

For CDs supplied to patients, the record must include the date, the name and address of the recipient, the amount, the person collecting the drug if not the patient, plus or minus proof of identity of the person collecting the drug if not the patient.

5) Try to have 2 members of staff (at least one clinical member) to check the stock that comes and goes. This can be done monthly.

6) Keep individual registers for your bag CDs. Given that so few of us carry CDs now most practices leave the CD book to the individual doctor and let him obtain, store and dispose of stock.

7) Check expiry dates regularly as with all other injectable drugs.

8) Have expired stock disposed of by an authorised witness.

Why do most GPs think General Practice has deteriorated over the decades?

Every GP I have met who, like me, has spent a few decades devoting their lives to family practice gives it up without much regret. A third of GPs are said to be about to retire within the five years following 2015. With up to 70% of medical school output being female and therefore likely to be part time, there will be an inevitable crisis of commitment and "manpower". The willingness to leave is not because the discipline or medicine has become harder but because

1) The freedom to choose what to prescribe, probably the greatest token of independence of GP is now so limited by national and local guidelines and by cost constraints that a GP's therapeutic choices are becoming as regimented and limited as those of hospital doctors.

2) We are now unable to monitor and regulate our own performance and be trusted – and all, it seems, because of one psychopath amongst us. The great irony, of course is that Appraisal and Revalidation are specifically designed not to detect dangerous or underperforming doctors, just to formalise a structure of learning behaviour.

3) The ability to discipline unpleasant rude or aggressive patients with whom we can never have a good, constructive relationship has been removed from us by the GMC. We cannot remove patients from our lists with whom we cannot get on due to their difficult,

unreasonable or unpleasant behaviour. Despite the fact that all good GPs offer a personal as well as a professional relationship to their patients and this is not possible with antagonistic, aggressive, mischievous and unreasonable patients, we are prevented from ending the relationship now. A meaningful and productive medical relationship is always at least partly, personal – and personal relationships have to be two way.

4) The constant and relentless payment by statistics and scores, local and national guidelines, some self defeating, – of QuoF, " good prescribing" protocols, QIPP (quality innovation productivity and prevention) and so on. It is doubtful that this adds up to good, patient-first practice. The intrusive, distracting and often harmful QuoF incentives (see PHQ9, depression section) are now seen as excess baggage by the profession with national conferences north and south of the border calling for their end (Aug 2015).

5) Frequent political reorganisation of the structure and funding of General Practice as well as the demography and commitment of GPs themselves. I can see no evidence whatsoever that the face to face service has got anything but worse for patients over the thirty years I have been part of it firsthand. Certainly, the threatened loss of the personal list system and partnerships based on full time doctors working every or most days, the problems with getting appointments with your own doctor, any doctor, soon, the end of doctors doing or contributing to their own out of hours service, the huge number of outside commitments that GPs now spend time at and the part timism and sessionism of so many doctors, GPs no longer doing their own domiciliary terminal care, GPs not living IN the practice area, – all these things diminish the quality of the service from the patient's point of view. Just go and ask an older patient.

6) The dissociation of those in the training establishment of General Practice, the Royal College, The Deaneries and so on from the day to day reality of the great mass of G.Ps who regard training, education, assessment methods and attitudes with bemusement and sometimes disbelief.

7) The often pointless and self defeating assessment and reassessment of practices by inexperienced, unrespected, self important officials who by virtue of their titles (infection control officer, CQC, QUoF panels etc) hold the power of control, authority and payment over long – standing, experienced, safe and effective doctors and nurses.

8) The seemingly endless NHS complaints procedure which is balanced heavily in favour of the mischievous and manipulative complainant and which causes such distress and real harm to the doctor. He or she meanwhile has very little help or support and has to carry on working and smiling and (usually) treating the complainant before during and after the person should be and used to be (*but probably no longer is*) thrown off the list.

9) The poor state of Out Of Hours cover with understaffed, unqualified 111 call handlers, overstretched doctors and the overuse of "Call 999".

The GP is of course, paid by results. Not the result of having a satisfied, long lived, healthy list who trust him and are willing to wait a few days to be able to see him but by the percentage of cheap drugs, the number of patients for whom smoking habits, weight, cholesterol, or other blood tests have been recorded and submitted, the sterility of his or her consulting room (sterile in terms of personality and character because family photos and children's toys have now been banned) and the number of national guideline hoops that he has jumped through. All these boxes could be ticked of course – and yet the GP could still be the most miserable, unapproachable, unfriendly, negative, self important, self righteous, dangerous, and incompetent pain in the neck.

Familiarity:

All patients who have more than a sore throat or a Temporary Resident morning-after consultation will value the possibility of getting to know, to trust and to like you. Indeed, it is more than likely that the good GP will want to get to know the morning after patient and offer a bit more than the post coital contraceptive as part of the consultation.

I call the patient in to my consulting room over a loud speaker although many doctors go out into the waiting room to collect them. I try to sound welcoming on the PA, I offer my hand to all patients, especially children and I try to perform a brief examination, whenever clinically indicated, if possible. I profoundly believe in the importance of touch during most consultations. I cannot see how it is possible to prescribe an antibiotic for a cough without examining the chest or in low back pain to give analgesics or arrange an XR or physiotherapy without a brief formal examination of the spine.

However, even trusted and respected colleagues do take these short cuts. I can only assume out of laziness or boredom. The pick – up rate of something altering a management decision is, I admit, low, but patients genuinely appreciate the thoroughness of even a brief retinal examination, straight leg raise, chest percussion, palpation of the abdomen, etc. where appropriate. Perhaps the examination is not JUST to find new medical information, but also to do something else: to cement a bond of trust between you and the patient for the next consultation, to help confirm a therapeutic relationship, your competence, thoroughness and reputation. To contribute to the doctor's mystique?

To all this I would add that all patients over 16 years of age will want to call you "Doctor Smith" not John or Suzy or Shammy. There should be recognition of your superior wisdom, experience and knowledge. You should be accessible and articulate and explain things in ways that the patient can understand but false familiarity diminishes your authority and makes the job much harder for both the patient and doctor. Being a Family Doctor doesn't always involve constant friendliness and pleasantness to patients or having all patients be nice to you. Some of your responsibilities will involve confronting difficult patients and facing awkward or threatening situations.

So If there is NO clear respect demonstrated for your greater experience and knowledge, no tacit recognition of the years of study, the continual self analysis and improvement, the continual striving to improve, the self questioning, the suffering and the sacrifice that you SHOULD have gone through to do medicine and to stay in it, or for the recognition that you have seen more of birth, living, suffering and dying than the patient can imagine, then either you are not worth consulting or the patient deserves who he gets.

Who has decided it should be like this? Where is the representation, the democracy? For instance: Prescribing for the family or yourself:

I recently did an appraisal on someone who I regarded as a good GP but who had been suspended for a year pending the GMC's review of her case. To summarise her situation:

Her sister had come to visit a year before from France, dying of breast cancer and had run out of Fentanyl patches, – My appraisee prescribed her two. At this time the practice had a part time partner who tended to be away on maternity or other forms of leave more often than she was at the surgery and a new full time partner who's past history had been taken on trust. Probably he had mild Asperger's syndrome. Once appointed he turned out to be unpopular with the staff, unliked by the patients and unconstructive at practice meetings. They kept him on because full time partners were hard to come by. Suddenly after running a popular and successful practice for years, my appraisee found herself suspended by the GMC for having prescribed her dying sister pain relief. It appears that the new partner may have reported her. She was unsupported and rejected by a practice she had set up herself but from which the new partner had now alienated her with mischievous enthusiasm. She started drinking and became seriously depressed.

My question is this: What did she do to deserve this chain of events? Why was prescribing pain relief to a terminally ill patient who happened to be her sister wrong? How would it have helped her, her sister, or anyone else to force her own kith and kin with a straight forward and genuine medical need to travel 30 miles to the nearest out of hours centre to negotiate with a complete (and usually inexperienced) stranger a top up of her pain relief? The doctor had no accessible partner at the time, to call upon. Unlike her, the other partners lived outside the practice. Not everyone works in the centre of a big city with colleagues on hand.

Why is it always wrong to prescribe for oneself or one's family? Is it ethically any more honest to ask a partner to write a no questions asked scrip for whatever you want and why should the vast majority of sensible, ethical doctors and their families be punished because of the actions of the miniscule number of addicts and abusers amongst us? Will these rules prevent them abusing drugs anyway? Of course not.

In 2009 a Canadian survey showed 75% Canadian physicians were happy to self prescribe. In 2005 a similar survey showed half of Norwegian physicians did, as did a similar number of American doctors in 1998. In a British Survey (Pulse 2007) 43% of British GPs self prescribed but the GMC "tightened" its advice from "should not prescribe" for relatives, friends and yourself to "must not prescribe" in 2013. The GMC had trebled its fitness to practice prosecutions in the preceding two years related to self prescribing but if you read its literature on the subject and you will be hard put to find the justification for this sudden self righteous crusade. Could it be another knee jerk reaction to Shipman who was a Pethidine addict and the resultant desire to demonstrate to all the other London based legal and political authorities that the medical profession was cleaning up its act?

And anyway, who elected the GMC members, what particular credentials do they have to represent us and who voted for or agreed an ethical system that says it is always wrong for a doctor to treat his or her own family? Why is our profession ruled and dominated but never consulted by this undemocratic and unrepresentative sort of dictatorship? And it charges us a compulsory, ever increasing non negotiable subscription annually which is anything BUT value for money. Who sets the ethical standards and rules that dominate the profession and why don't they ever ask the real people that do the real job if these ethics are reasonable? I have never met a doctor who was consulted by the GMC Ethics Committee, or come to that The Royal College of GPs on what is "Good Medical Practice" or ethical medical behaviour. Since both these organisations are so obviously unrepresentative of the doctors who do most medicine in Britain (there is now one GP on the GMC Committee) and most GPs feel the College is an academic and isolated "law unto itself") what right do they have to make the rules that control us? All GPs feel the GMC's disciplinary processes are at best out of touch with reality, unresponsive, unfair, its decisions often inexplicable and always glacially slow. An increasing number are so despairing at the unsympathetic "guilty until proven innocent" nature of the process that they take their own lives during the investigation.

The GMC's response? In May 2017 The GMC proudly announced that "We need a bit more emotional resilience".

To be or not to be: Depressing doctors

British suicide figures for doctors are hard to find but self poisoning is the commonest method, anaesthetists using anaesthetic agents other doctors using what drugs come to hand or cutting methods. Depression, drug and alcohol abuse, work, relationship and financial problems are common co factors. (Quart J Med 2000 93. 351-357). The suicide rate in female doctors is higher than the general population, in male doctors it is lower than the general population. This difference is statistically significant. A diagnosed psychiatric illness is present, not surprisingly, in the majority. The specialities at most risk in the UK are anaesthetists, community health doctors, GPs and psychiatrists. All these having increased rates compared with "general hospital doctors". The seniority is not significant but female gender **is**, the paper saying "This requires monitoring in view of the very large increase in the numbers of women entering medicine". Surely this is another reason for a reduction in the overwhelming numbers of women who are now dominating medicine?

In the US, a doctor commits suicide each day on average (300-400 per year) This is thought to be due to the combination of sleep deprivation, relocation, feelings of isolation as well as the emotion demands of dealing with sick, worried, suffering, dying, depressed sometimes aggressive unreasonable and unpleasant people. And then there are the patients...

The incidence of depression amongst 740 interns rose from 3.9% to 27.1% in the first 3 months of their intern year and then interns' thoughts of death increased 370% (Arch Gen Psych 2010 67, 557-566). Male physicians are 1.41X more likely and female 2.27 times more likely to die by suicide than the general population. This confirms the female dominant suicides in the British literature.

As I mentioned, the GMC has (December 2014) publically suggested that medical students should be taught **"emotional resilience"** – whatever that may be, at medical school. This after it became public that 28 doctors under investigation by the GMC had probably committed suicide between 2005 and 2013. They do not say what proportion were women doctors. I assume proportionately a majority given the published data on doctors' suicide. I would suggest emotional resilience used to develop on its own with the tougher medical training, the sort of candidate selected by medical schools and with the long hours of the apprenticeship.

At a 2016 GMC conference on Medical Professionalism, the subject of resilience was discussed at length. The GMC report said: "Some of the doctors we spoke to believed resilience came with the territory. In our survey 38% felt that doctors were already resilient (-Could these be all the males?) – so did not require further training. 6% felt it came from experience. Most believed it could be learned". It went on: "Doctors regret the loss of fixed teams with colleagues who they know resulting in less camaraderie than in the past". This is an obvious result of the current short rotas and short Working Time Directive decimated working week. If the juniors want stability on the wards and camaraderie, they can work longer hours. Simple. Then they would get to know their colleagues and their consultants would get to know them (See "Do no harm").

RDA (NO, not Recommended Daily Allowance)

There was a whole article on "aggressive communication between doctors" in the RCP journal entitled "Sticks and stones" in December 2015. This is apparently called "rude, dismissive and aggressive communication" and goes by the acronym RDA. A slight feeling of despair came over me akin to that when I listened to the Royal College Of GP spokesperson say it was "Society's fault that fat people ate too much and smokers smoked".

I doubt when I was training and 85-90% of the work force were male, RDA would have been considered so serious an issue that it warranted an acronym or a journal article. Possibly we would not have interpreted much of the less sympathetic communication between us so personally then. I never remember any male or female colleague complaining about their thoughtless or rude colleagues 40 years ago. Perhaps the emotional resilience and the RDA were all accepted as part of what was a much more thick skinned profession. But now, with the work force becoming largely feminine, chosen for academic prowess and personal statements not life skills or experience, unhardened by tough training and long hours it is all different. Demanding a life/work balance, a protracted, unfair, alien and out of touch with reality GMC investigation must seem quite an incomprehensible shock. No wonder many doctors hit the emotional buffers when under investigation by a distant organisation like the GMC. Indeed this new sensitivity has now become manifest even earlier, at medical school. 1600 medical students have dropped out early in their training the last 5 years costing the taxpayer millions and this tidal wave of medical drop outs was said in a Sunday Times article (Aug 27 2017) to be due to "mental health problems".

There are several important issues here: Medicine is not a job for those without thick skins, self confidence and determination. Anyone who is too sensitive, who expects or is used to a support network of colleagues or who wants to have time care for their own family as well as their patients will flounder. Anyone who is too naive to accept how challenging, demanding, sometimes threatening, abusive and unappreciative many patients can be will do badly. Likewise anyone who expects fair appreciation and praise. The resilience needed probably can't be taught.

My medical school year and every cohort I worked with for well over forty years after were not offered any emotional support that I remember, by any agency, ever and we didn't seem to need it, despite the 2-3X longer hours than student doctors today. I remember one student in the year above me "having a breakdown" but no others, no housemen, registrars, no hospital doctors at all. And precious few GPs of my generation. All the more surprising that our contemporary students and doctors seem to be so sensitive. In the Sunday Times article "300 student doctors quit a year" - "an epidemic of mental health problems is being blamed as a large number of would be medics fail to complete their degrees" -there is a picture of a pretty female student who "Dropped out of UCL, saying she did not receive enough support". Surely the mental health problems are the result- not the cause of whatever the basic problem is? And this seems to be: The wrong people going into/ being selected for medicine, or misunderstanding how tough a medical life and degree is. Shouldn't medical school selection processes try to assess candidates' emotional toughness, determination, not just intelligence, empathy, dedication, caring and enthusiasm as all these virtues will offer little protection in the hard real world of sickness, pain, too many patients and too little help from colleagues.

The new GMC recommendations are that doctors under investigation should be considered innocent until proven guilty. An amazing idea. They are also suggesting a change to the way they investigate complaints (April 2015). Perhaps even the GMC is beginning to appreciate that for the 90% of consulting work done in the NHS (by GPs) and the number of doctors with real experience on the GMC governing body, there is a catastrophic, not fit for purpose and unethical mismatch.

The recommendations include:

A reduction in the number of health examiners' reports required for health assessments.
The appointment of an SMO in the GMC for overseeing "health cases".
Case conferences for all health and performance cases.
They should set out pre qualification criteria for referrals from NHS providers and independent employers.
Medical schools should make "emotional resilience" part of the medical curriculum.
GMC investigation staff should be exposed to front line clinical practice.
They should develop a GMC employee training package to increase staff awareness of "mental health issues".

Read between the lines and it is quite clear that the investigation staff have, up until now assumed the guilt of the doctor they are investigating, been ignorant of the huge emotional toll the investigative process takes on the doctor's health, that the GMC staff have not been equipped to understand, recognise, treat or support doctors in this vulnerable state and that they have been handled with far less care than a patient or even a criminal in the criminal justice system. It is amazing that the relatives of the 28 doctors who killed themselves haven't so far sued the GMC for contributory negligence.

Nevertheless there does seem to have been an increase in the emotional vulnerability of the medical professions in the U.S. and U.K. over the last 20-30 years compared with the thicker skinned graduates of the 70's and 80's. RAF Bomber Command about whom I have been reading recently would have had another acronym for its pilots and crew who found the stress of flying over Germany intolerable and couldn't carry on. LMF, lack of moral fibre. The NHS may have been set up in the same decade as Bomber Command flew nightly raids over Germany but our attitudes to coping with stress have changed completely since the 40's.

Boundaries:

One of the exercises that the PCT set for my suspended appraisee and is often raised at College and Deanery assessments was to send her on a course about Professional Boundaries. This means knowing when you are becoming too personally involved with a patient and needing to back off. The doctor practiced in a rural village where she was known by everyone, as were her children and husband who was also a doctor. Her children went to the local school, she was part of "the school run", presumably the kids were in the Brownies, the Scouts, she was in the PTA, probably in the church choir and church flower arranging rota (it was that kind of village). She was expected to be involved in community activities and organisations and where the boundaries between her personal and professional life were somewhat different from urban 9 to 5 job-share, switch off when you get home doctors. The rules about this kind of community General Practice are now made and supervised by urban, often politically fairly judgemental and rigid doctors with no idea of real Family Medicine in smaller communities. This applies to The GMC, The RCGP and the BMA. These of course, are all London or city based, undemocratic, alien, authoritarian bodies, none representing or referring to the work force for direction or opinion but each with total power and control over it. Think of the attitudes and demographics of professional, public and political London and they are reflected by the attitudes and decisions of the organisations and professional bodies that are based there. But not by most of their members. Clapham West Sussex and Clapham South London demand different attitudes and approaches to medicine.

I suspect the thought that a GP might accept an invitation to dinner with a patient, or play squash, or pop in for a coffee and a chat after that patient's spouse had died as they had struck up a personal friendship, or that the GP might in the course of a consultation admit to having got over cancer or alcoholism themselves and to "know what the patient must be going through" would be anathema to the thought prefects of the urban medical supervisors. Even worse, that the GP might be supported or nurtured in their hour of distress by their patients. But amongst my **most** grateful patients have been the ones who told me long after I had forgotten the consultation, that the thing that helped them most was knowing that "you had gone through the same thing as me and you had survived."

This is what real family medicine CAN be like, to the mutual advantage of doctor and patient. It is based on familiarity and trust.

But there are many new factors in medical culture that mitigate against that immersion of the GP in the community:

Increasing job sharing and part time GPs, due to the success girls have at A Levels compared with boys.

Doctors living outside the practice area and not being as personally recognised, committed and familiar with it.

Lack of 24 hour cover.

GPs of varying cultural backgrounds, perhaps not integrating into community life in quite the same way as the GP they may have succeeded,

A genuine change in doctors' attitude to work encouraged by the politics of salaried 9 to 5 doctoring.

The de-vocation of medicine borne of the end of long hours of on call, the hard apprenticeship.

The Working Time Directive outlook rather than that of a vocation and a way of life.

The pervading fear of overstepping a "Professional Boundary". I see this with registrars who would rather not examine a sick patient than perform an examination without a chaperone. We are rapidly losing something priceless we didn't know we had. Junior doctors take far more time off sick now than two or three decades ago. Have we forgotten that job satisfaction is proportional to job commitment, generally speaking, you get back as much as you give.

Are all patients equally as good?

"Attention to health is the greatest hindrance to life"

Plato

James Groves wrote about Hateful Patients: (NEJM 1978 Apr 20)

He identified four types of challenging patients although I am sure you and I can think of many others than:

Dependent clingers

Entitled demanders

Manipulative help rejecters

Self destructive deniers.

There is an injustice at the heart of the National Health Service. It is that those patients who suffer in silence and self medicate at home or who are hardy, self reliant or stoical and therefore rarely go to see their doctor, still pay just as much in tax as the frequent attender, the hypochondriac or overly anxious patient. The demanding patient is not usually the sickest. In other words, those who are ill and suffer in silence subsidise those who demand attention but who often have no serious ailment. There is no sanction against the time waster, the neurotic, the "entitled demander."

It is the inevitable fault of our free at the point of demand system that it encourages and allows over consulting, dependency, easy medicalisation and over treating. The interposition of a simple fee would change these dynamics completely. This is where politics and psychology, funding and public health all get conflated by the system. The design of our structure of administering health care assumes an essential reasonableness in all people, that we are all part of a fair and civil society. However some of the most frequent attenders regularly consult and consume up to 5 times as much as the average patient and yet usually have no serious illnesses to show for it. Up to one in seven patients is classified as a frequent attender. There are some patients with no serious illness who contact out of hours services most nights and who try to manipulate a visit several times a week.

(Smits FT Brouwer etc Epidemiology of Frequent Attenders BMC Public Health 2009 Jan 24 9:36).

Some patients, as we know, even attend casualty 200 times a year now.

In a poll by Pulse Magazine in 2014, a small majority of GPs now think that all patients should be charged for each consultation – as patients with self limiting and trivial demands are overwhelming the system. This is the "Well it said it was a walk in centre, so I walked in" and the "You can't be too careful can you?" era of the NHS. Doctors are basically nice people who rarely challenge unreasonable or demanding patients and probably should, more often. This is for the sake of their own peace of mind but these days all doctors seem to be constrained by an overwhelming fear of missing a serious condition and subsequent litigation. The law seems designed to create and encourage health related neuroses, reflex investigations, unaffordable expense for the healthy majority because of the tiny risk for the exceptional, rare, unlucky patient that the average doctor poses by taking rational and sensible diagnostic guesses. The law should recognise this and being able to sue the competent doctor should be almost impossible.

But now the system is at some kind of turning point where all doctors are aware of a huge weight of unreasonable and pointless consulting in General Practice and Casualty Departments which is for the first time overwhelming the system for everyone.

There have been many analyses of the "Frequent Attender" or "Heart Sink" patient. This is someone who I think of as attending frequently, having no clear or single defined diagnosis, being depressed or chronically anxious and having little or no objectivity about their own behaviour or symptoms. They may have a clear sense of entitlement and are therefore demanding and self focussed. They usually have no sense of humour or a self victimising sort of humour or no amiable redeeming personality features. This is obviously someone who often elicits little anticipation in the doctor except a sense of resignation and impotence. Putting aside patients with serious or chronic illnesses – and some heartsink patients undoubtedly do have serious conditions, those with social, emotional or psychiatric problems tend to consult more frequently and with a variety of complaints. If you think about it though, a good half of an average list will be patients with either psychiatric or social problems or both and yet frequent (unnecessary) attenders are probably no more than 10 – 15% of the total patients on a list. Indeed, the most demanding 10% of any list take 30-50% of the appointments.

The common patient characteristics of frequent attenders are therefore:

In the case of frequently attending children, anxious or depressed parents, in the case of adults,

Female,

Lack of trust in the doctor (an endless need for second opinions),

Susceptibility to mass media influence,

A "conflictual relationship" with their disease, (not "fully convinced their disease is lifelong") – as in hypertension, diabetes, bipolar disorder or arthrosis.

Coexisting psychological and social problems with or without a "genuine" physical complaint.

"Medically unexplained symptoms" but beware one study showed 12 out of 28 "heartsink" patients developed serious medical problems eventually. That's 43%. HOWEVER I am not sure how many asymptomatic individuals (NORMAL PEOPLE) will develop a serious condition "eventually" – about the same number?

The frequent attender is more likely to be divorced or widowed, female, unemployed, of a lower social class and the frequency of consulting increases with ageing. I also find they have few educational achievements. Interestingly these, apart from the age, are the features which are associated with having a child in trouble with the police **and** having an abortion.

There are doctor related factors too: a personality that wishes to avoid confrontation, a non taking-control style of consultation and in General Practice of course you are "stuck" with your patient in a way that a junior hospital doctor isn't. Hospital consultants can transfer the care of frustrating or unrewarding patients to their own transient (fresh and freshly lit, not yet burnt out) junior staff – an option GPs do not have. Add a tendency to allow or encourage emotional dependency, a desire to be needed or wield power and all these factors encourage a functional attachment. The issuing of a prescription or a set of investigations may perpetuate and medicalise a self limiting condition and although I have previously mentioned how modern doctors often seem reluctant to offer reasonable "follow up", the constant offer of an inappropriate further appointment may cement a minor ailment as an established medical condition. This is the passport they need to keep coming back.

The patient on the other hand may have related to all sorts of people in a dependent way, a behaviour that has been learnt in childhood and often reflected by the rest of the family. Loneliness and depression also increase the frequency of consultation.

Patients generally like a smaller practice and one running a personal list system if they value a continuity of relationship with their doctor. I assume any attempt at reducing or even addressing the frequency and reasons for over consulting must be immeasurably more complicated for the practice and patient in non list practices, especially large ones. This is because the key to addressing the issue is that the doctor and patient each has to take responsibility for their own role and for the fact that there is a problem in the first place! Certain cultures may find some conditions, (rape, epilepsy etc) embarrassing or shameful and this can lead to an attitude of dependency.

The characteristics of the frequent/heartsink/medically unexplained (although these are not necessarily all the same) patient tend to be lonely depressed women but some frequent female attenders in my experience who I have seen were charming, light hearted, required brief reassurance and occasionally brightened my day! Although they might come back with a new symptom every few weeks over a decade or so we developed a friendly but professional relationship and each time I did the minimum necessary to reassure them and satisfy an objective observer that I was missing nothing serious. Often this would be the only enjoyable consultation in a surgery. (Discuss.............)

The cost and extent of investigations for frequent attenders should be limited but bearing in mind that figure of up to 12/28 "heartsink" patients developing serious conditions at some point, do not exclude all secondary investigations in principle on patients previously investigated but who have new symptoms. I must say my experience of serious illness in frequent attenders is much less than this. I have had a patient with 4 decades of IBS present one morning just like every other but this time with colonic cancer and a liver full of secondaries, also a woman of 70 with monthly abdominal pain for 20 years who developed rectal cancer, missed by me and the gastroenterologist at first and which had already spread to the pelvic nerves, – but it is hard to think of many others. ALWAYS be ready at every consultation to examine every patient however. I felt my patient's rock hard liver edge and my heart sank with surprise and disbelief as soon as he said his longstanding pain felt a bit different.

Various techniques have been proposed for dealing with frequent attenders but the worst thing you can do is pretend they don't exist and ignore them.

One possibility is a detailed summary listing their chronological attendances, investigations and results (I print these out as I find them easier to refer to with the patient) then arrange a half hour appointment to go over the history, underlying health beliefs, fears, your interpretation, what to do next time, perhaps discuss post dated prescriptions at the next consultation, information leaflets, (although these have NOT been shown to reduce attendance rates), even CBT, discuss depression, anxiety, family influences, encourage methods of self care (although I do not find this works very well either), offer to "Let another partner see them as I don't seem to be helping you much" – this often produces and interesting result for both the patient and me. One aggressive and manipulative self destructive diabetic who I was being asked to visit almost weekly in the end told me not to be "Such a xxxxing xxxxhead, who do else do you think would put up with the likes of me?" !!, Even discuss regular ten minute appointments but no others "Unless you genuinely think you are dying."

The truth is they will keep coming back and you do have to learn to live with them and keep smiling.

Uncertainty:

It has been said that General Practice involves the constant management of boredom, repetition and uncertainty.

Uncertainty in this context relates to an environment in which the doctor is willing to make diagnosis and management decisions based solely on assumptions, subjective conclusions and his own experience. Without a strong evidence base or the results of investigations or objective observations over a time period. He often has no reasonable objective proof – and uses subjective rather than objective factors to come to his conclusion – some might say "guess". Uncertainty is something medical science has previously sought to exclude from the medical model, certainly not to accept or embrace.

To some degree the combination of these frustratingly unquantifiable factors – (inaccurate histories, timescales, descriptions, uncertainty about previous treatment, current medication, etc) can lead to burn out and fear of litigation as well as professional and personal insecurity. Uncertainty is one of the constant features of life in General Practice and the natural GP is someone who is at home with it.

Contemporary medical training does not prepare new doctors for risk taking, vagueness of diagnosis, accepting the managed progress of a disease or the encouragement of educated guesswork in medical life.

The uncertainties that are part of consultations in General Practice are many fold: Let us start with factors that involve the doctor:

GPs are the only true generalists in medical practice these days. Physicians now all sub specialise and in any case, even they don't see the variety of medical, surgical, Paediatric, Psychiatric, psychosocial and all the varied socio-medical presentations of modern general practice. It is impossible to be completely familiar with or be prepared for everything that might present on every average day to a family doctor. GPs have no firewall or filter to triage the different types of patients, complaints and presenting formats (-while I am here, would you look at the baby, he's 14 months shouldn't he be talking by now?, my husband won't come to see you but I am very worried, ever since he had that temperature he has been behaving very strangely, I know you are not on duty but would you pop in if you aren't too busy? etc) that present without warning to the family doctor in or out of the surgery.

GPs **are** the triage, the gatekeepers, the initial assessors. There is never a clear history and all the relevant information is rarely offered at presentation. Leading questions have to be used appropriately, clues and cues are sifted, followed and discarded. GPs therefore, very early in every consultation have to decide on the potential or actual medical significance of every presenting problem. – Not just accept each raw symptom at face value. They discard and ignore much that is presented for consideration in each consultation through a process of learnt value judgment. But also of "gut feeling". This is the art of General Practice. (In a world where relatives, lawyers and colleagues assume it is a science). This involves not only a personal knowledge base but a risk assessment derived from an awareness of the patient's previous help seeking behaviour, a knowledge of that patient's help seeking threshold, their stoicism, their reliability, their experience of ill health and so on – for instance: first time mothers, a friend who has just had a coronary, the patient's personality and anxiety and so on. The so-called personal "Health Beliefs" may be part of this assessment.

Several studies have shown the reliability of the "gut feelings" of experienced primary care physicians in the absence of objective demonstrable evidence, in assessing complex symptoms and getting an accurate diagnosis.

The GP must also factor into this risk assessment a knowledge of prevailing illness patterns (-Is there meningitis, "flu", etc in the locality?) and a host of other factors including their own mutual relationship.

In previous years, the GP would be familiar with the families, history and background of the patients on his "list". There would have been the cushion of extended families, the reassurance of a stable culture and tradition within his community. The consistent and self confident patient. Add to this the bonding factor and familiarity of the list system (or panel) and familiarity, reliability and mutual trust tended to be the norm.

Today's populations are transient, mobile and of mixed culture. The demography of the standard nuclear family has changed and the overwhelming politics of today is to loosen the bond between individual patients and a specific individual doctor. Patients often now register with a practice not an individual with whom they might develop familiarity and trust.

This mutual unfamiliarity can lead to less confidence in the diagnosis and management of an event and even a safety culture of over treatment and more frequent admissions.

Factors involving the uncertain diagnosis:

Medical training begins within a hospital and is thus taught in a highly scientific way. Rational and evidence based, – the diagnosis of illness and disease via the step wise exclusion of alternatives. This involves a logical system of questioning, then examination and if possible applying investigations to the patient. This standard and successful evidenced based system is partially and half-heartedly adapted these days to include social, cultural and psychological modifiers, health beliefs, expectations and other social issues. It has been at the developing heart of western medicine since the discovery of the circulation, microbes, effective drugs and treatments –in other words–for centuries.

It is based on observation; asking questions, evidence gathering and getting information – upon which a reasonable diagnosis and a course of treatment can be based. –Ask, observe, examine, conclude, agree and treat/prescribe. Above all, be objective. The basis of all medical consultations. It has been so successful that it has been universally adopted by all cultures and traditions.

One uncertainty of general practice however is that much of the proffered information is inaccurate, biased, subjective or wrong. Personal feelings, experience and interpretation of the "presenting complaint" in both the patient and the doctor dictate the emphasis which will be placed on which parts of the "raw data". In the real world of general practice, subjective not objective factors are of crucial importance. There are no golden rules.

Personality and confidence, age, experience of risk taking and litigation, psychological and personal factors are far more important to the general practice assessment than that of a hospital or outpatients consultation.

The absence of attached staff, the unavailability of regular objective monitoring, or of accessible biometric data, or even of a reliable four hourly pulse and temperature dictates that diagnosis and prognosis will always be a "best guess" in the world of General Practice.

The uncertain patient:

The patient presenting to a GP doesn't come with a referral letter. He or she has not been seen, assessed, triaged and referred appropriately by another professional. The initial assessment in general practice includes factors unknown to hospital colleagues: How ill (or otherwise) is the patient, why have they presented in this way, here and now, even factors such as do they actually need to be seen, why are they actually asking for help?

This is compounded by "Tesco" attitudes of consumerism in the supply and availability of medicine and of modern political attitudes. Patients' charters, the entitled demander and so on.

The net result is that there is no longer a mutual assumption of reasonable consulting behaviour between doctor and patient. The tacit understandings of the early NHS have gone.

The patient has been trained to consult early "just in case", to regard the doctor as like any other supplier of goods and services. "I want an MRI just to be sure." The media sometimes exaggerate the risks of self-diagnosis and treatment but far more so the risks of missing early symptoms of illness. The ever-present fear of a rare serious illness combined with the ease of modern consulting has led to much "inappropriate" and early contact. We have all seen the 3 hour backache and sore throat.

Mutual consideration of the roles and responsibilities of doctor and patient have become a thing of the past.

Transience: Even in relatively stable social environments, families are now temporary and often uncommitted to a place, a practice, a doctor. In many environments even where stable family groups are the norm, modern work practices and temporary relationships mitigate against social stability. The average GP loses and gains 10% or more of his list per year. In cities it can be many times this. Patients often don't know how best to use local medical services, are unfamiliar with an experienced doctor and some individuals simply do not even have the tradition of trust, consistency and familiarity with the family practice structure.

Accessibility: GPs are encouraged to offer ready appointments to all patients – registered or not, who feel they need to be seen. As soon as possible. In practice this can't and doesn't happen, the demand is too great. But the ever-present worry of litigation can lead to GPs over treating and over investigating to reduce uncertainty. The long-term result of this is a second rate service for the patient, an expensive one for the tax payer and further anxiety for the doctor.

Uncertainty and the management of risk occur at every out of hours consultation now that emergency general practice is done by a different population of doctors with no knowledge of the patients they might see. Sometimes with little or no contact with the patients' GPs either.

The statutory lowering of the availability threshold, consumer attitudes and patients' rights are leading paradoxically to an overmedicalisation of society as confidence, reasonable self reliance and the risk benefits of treatment (ie antibiotics) are no longer part of the routine consulting agenda.

There is, of course, a cost issue in the increasing reluctance of patients and doctors to manage uncertainty.

General practice remains an area where the management of uncertainty is partly mitigated by personal knowledge, experience and familiarity between doctor and patient but the consultation is by nature brief, focused, selective and risky.

Politics in General Practice: and why we have no democracy

In 1979 a questionnaire was sent to 60,000 American college and university professors, research and teaching staff asking a gamut of questions about their attitudes, affiliations, politics and beliefs. The results, published three years later shed what I think is an entirely predictable light on the political beliefs held by men and women who are intrinsically suited to various academic disciplines **or** who become changed by working in those disciplines:

The study showed that there was a clear correlation between your political orientation, your specialism and your career role in it. We can argue chicken or egg but the results showed:-

The Social Scientists and Humanities specialists were mainly liberal and politically left wing while the other scientists, particularly the Physical Scientists were more conservative, – politically right of centre. The engineers being the most practical and down to earth of the specialities were the most conservative of all.

The interesting thing to me is that the medics were naturally more conservative than geologists and chemists and only slightly less so than the engineers themselves. It's like we are the most down to earth of all the biological scientists.

The range was:

Liberal (Left wing)   Mathematicians
Physicists
Biologists
Chemists
Geologists
Medics
Conservative (Right wing) Engineers.

The analysis of the data found that the academics, lecturers and teachers in any discipline were more likely to be politically liberal and left leaning. The educators, opinion and rule makers therefore tend not to represent the majority of front line practical scientists and medics. The ideologues of a profession or discipline, the group that draws up, imposes and teaches the ethics, rules and guidelines, -its teachers, are drawn from a small and highly unrepresentative group. All this bears out the experience of the average doctor when faced with the guidelines and professional rules issued by the GMC, RCGP, Deaneries, those formulated by goodness knows who for appraisal, those who wrote "Good Medical Practice", the political requirements of appraisal and training (such as compulsory Equality and Diversity training), even the unwritten guidelines for the selection committees of medical schools with their racist and sexist bias against white male candidates. You can see that the politics of minorities has been written into the rule books of medical training and professional discipline and why the profession as a whole is never consulted in anything like a democratic ballot on matters that profoundly affect us all. Presumably because most of us would never agree.

The pale male doctor built up and made the NHS with 100 hour weeks, self sacrifice, a code of **the patient comes first** and some help from commonwealth doctors, again, mostly male. Today with part time working, the 48 hour full time week, striking without even emergency cover, family friendly rotas, and "my own children come first", (See "Do no harm") almost no junior white males visible these days on wards in medical schools and certainly on picket lines, you *could say* the FEM BEMs are slowly dismantling what the Pale Males assembled. The latest census said 82% of the population was white. 41% must be white males but only 15% or so of many or most medical schools are white male. The Presidents of The RCP, RCGP, the Chief Negotiator during the strike of the BMA, the next president of the RCGP, at least 9/10 of the RCP's first chosen representative Junior Doctors, the Chief Registrars, 85% of virtually all medical school students are not white males. Is this an underlying cause of the NHS malaise or a result? The politics and the ethos of the NHS and its doctors have changed and not to the patients' advantage.

Why?

In America many commentators have been aware of the feminisation and left wing shift of their medical profession for a decade or more too. The latest study looking at medical specialities and political affiliation was reported in the New York Times in Oct 2016. (Hersh, Goldenberg, Dept Psych/Political Science Yale Uni. NYT). This was a study of all US physicians (!) (Medscape Oct 2016)

They found that most
Infectious Diseases specialists,
Psychiatrists,
Paediatricians and
Geriatricians were Democrats (Liberal/Socialist/Left Wing/higher tax/pro welfare

state) and most

Surgeons,

Anaesthetists,

Urologists and

ENT specialists were

Republicans Conservatives (Right wing/Small Government/low tax).

Overall physicians were fairly split between the two parties. "Dr Hersh said patients already think a physician's gender and medical school, facts readily available online, are important in their personal provider choices and party affiliation is another piece to consider". Clearly, American patients, in the home of consumer choice, can exercise a great deal more personal preference in choosing doctors of preferred gender and training than UK patients.

The authors found that Republican physicians were more likely to discuss the risks of marijuana while democrats were more likely to discuss the risks of guns at home. So the doctor's politics affected attitudes and care. Since neither guns nor marijuana are legal here I suppose the equivalent would be the doctor's attitude to claiming benefit or "going sick" for minor illness, or whether to work through such conditions as CFS or post viral malaise (??) The researchers said that 25 years ago most physicians were Republicans but a study published in 2012 (Bonica, Dept Political Science Stanf Univ) showed donations to the Republican party dropping from 70% to 50% amongst US physicians. They attributed this to the feminisation of medicine and the decrease in small and solo practices. Party affiliation was linked to income and gender! "Women surgeons were not as democratic as women paediatricians but they were more democratic than male surgeons". Also the researchers found that hospital employed physicians were more likely to be Democrats and those in independent practices were more likely to be Republican.

So: translating this to the UK,: Male, full timers, surgeons and the self employed in Primary and Secondary Care, especially those with their own practices, Owner Occupiers, Small Practices, tend to be right wing, The part time, salaried, female and those in certain medical specialities, particularly educationalists, and sessional doctors in big practices, tend to be left wing.

One of the ironies about General Practice is that it has been the most accessible and popular part of the NHS since the NHS began from the public's point of view. It was a personal, personalised and personality based service where long term familiarities and relationships developed and were the basis of the care. It has been the part of the NHS that has always been the most cost effective and valued by the tax paying customer. Most developments in General Practice over the last ten to fifteen years have however, deliberately or inadvertently dismantled the personal nature of primary care. If you find a patient who has been around long enough to experience how family medicine has changed and give them a chance to discuss the last ten to twenty years they will mourn the loss of something valuable and exceptional within the Welfare State. Whether it is the reduction in full time committed family doctors who live and work in their practice, the end of personal registration and the list system, the end of out of hours continuity of care, the vast increase in foreign trained doctors unfamiliar with nuanced British cultural attitudes and often the English language, the end of the boy scout GP who treats everything, including terminal illness, or even the demise of the GP who simply carries strong pain relief. 90% of patient interactions within the NHS are done in General Practice – where doctor patient relationships are closer, less formal, continue outside the consulting room and are often long term compared with hospital consultations. And yet there are usually no GPs on the whole GMC council. This is the group that considers complaints against doctors and is therefore particularly ill qualified to judge the context and working environment of most of them!

GPs are misunderstood therefore by the disciplinary authorities who know little or nothing of this, – the vast majority of the NHS workload.

G.Ps have never been liked by the right wing of politics as they are expensive and independent employees of the state or by the left wing as they are the front of house of the Welfare State, middle class professional high earners, self employed and yet paid for by the Treasury.

The system worked pretty well for a few decades because it relied on dedicated doctors and was designed around the patient but as you will see from my various descriptions here and elsewhere, we now have a system that suits fewer, is less caring and certainly less popular thanks to political interference.

It has been an endless source of fascination to me how out of touch many medical "leaders", managers, teachers and policy makers are with working doctors and sometimes with reality. I listened with disbelief to a BMA spokeswoman saying on a radio debate recently how individual patients should not be held responsible for their own obesity, drinking, smoking or other harmful behaviours as these were learnt from family or environmental influences and it was, in the end, society that was to blame for all an individual's ills not the patient. This is the sort of drivel some of our medical leaders actually believe. That patents aren't responsible for smoking themselves or eating themselves into ill health and that if we sort out a utopia then they wouldn't need to overeat or smoke. That type two diabetes isn't usually due gluttony and sloth.

I was a trainer of GP registrars for 6 or 7 years before giving it up and then became an appraiser of other GPs. As a trainer, I found that most of my registrars who had trained abroad were excellent doctors and very likeably individuals. But I became aware as an appraiser that there was a major problem with some GPs due to their cultural upbringing and attitudes which prevented them from fitting into the modern liberal consultation ideal of British GP Training. Some foreign doctors found it impossible to accept challenge or cross questioning from patients, especially some male doctors from female patients. There seemed to be endless time devoted at trainers' meetings to discussing the difficulties some male Asian and Arab registrars were having taking advice and instruction from female practice administrative staff or challenges to their opinions from female or teenage patients. In many cultures a challenging question from a patient is still perceived as disrespectful or a personal threat or a criticism of their status or authority. Many foreign trained doctors from the EU and elsewhere in the developing world, which we drain of scarce medical staff are not masters of the English language let alone familiar with British culture, irony, regional dialects, self criticism, humour, sarcasm, all the things that make up our identity and are so important in effective consulting and bonding relationships in British General Practice.

Why is it then that every trainer is compelled by some un discussed dictat to go on Equality and Diversity training? It must be obvious that diversity, if it means inconsistency and variability in quality (which it often does), is harmful to patient care and causes resentment amongst patients and colleagues alike as well as a lowering of standards. It results in a reluctance to challenge poor standards in some doctors who have been trained abroad for fear of our motives being misunderstood. I saw this frequently in the context of Training and Appraisal assessments. It is also obvious that there is no such thing as equal opportunity in medicine. Western science is based on a philosophical approach called Empiricism. This is Truth from Experience. This is the opposite of what "Equality and Diversity" stands for (– that we must make the initial assumption that we are all equally able despite having very diverse medical backgrounds). Instead we should be undertaking "Quality and Uniformity of skills" training.

If I were having a C.A.B.G. I would want it done by the person who was the very best at grafting coronary arteries and had beaten all his contemporaries to get there. I wouldn't want anyone who was reasonable at cardiac surgery offered the job by virtue of positive discrimination. The job should be gained on personal ability – which is obviously a meritocracy. What we should have is meritocracy and uniformity of excellence training irrespective of background. Most trainers go to equality and diversity training sessions bored and resigned. This indoctrination, generally considered political and pointless by its recipients was introduced (summer 2013) biannually to all appraisers as well as trainers. It goes without saying that there was no consultation on its relevance to clinical governance or professional development and as with all political interference in medicine of the last few years is misplaced, undemocratic, irrelevant dogma which will have unforeseen negative consequences for patients. If you are liberal and politically left wing (like the high flying educationalists who make the rules) you won't need the reinforcement. If you are conservative, practical and in the engine room of general practice you won't believe it. Or you will be intelligent and objective enough to make up your own mind about the abilities of each of your colleagues.

Isn't it an irony that everywhere else in medicine not dominated by political ideals we are improving standards by removing diversity? We make everyone wash their hands between examinations, we have strict rules on access to patient data, treatment guidelines and protocols, national codes and laws governing rules of behaviour and ethics, we expect everyone to pass the same exams to prove they are at a certain level of competence. But ironically we force trainers and appraisers to undergo dogma training in language, cultural, experience, training and attitude DIVERSITY. We have standard protocols and pathways governing birth and death. We have NICE guidance in every conceivable clinical situation, there are ethical guidelines on everything from writing prescriptions for your family to taking gifts and the limits of affection for a patient. We impose uniformity for the sake of the patient. No diversity anywhere except in the most potentially important and harmful area, that of the consistency of the doctor and that doctor's own personality, attitude, training and therefore, ability. This is, of course, the most important factor in any medical equation.

The complaints procedure:

A complaint: "An expression of dissatisfaction that requires a response". The GMC's annual State of Medical Education and Practice in 2016 showed that 5% of all GPs were complained about in 2015, slightly more than the average for all doctors at 3%. However, GPs have the lowest proportion of complaints investigated (27%) resulting in GMC action. For doctors overall, 32% of complaints were investigated.

76% of complaints against GPs came from the public compared with 66% of complaints against specialists who were twice as likely as GPs to be "flagged up" by other doctors.

Outcomes: 69% were closed with no further action, 14% were closed with advice given to the doctor, 5% leading to official warnings, 6% resulting in undertakings or conditions, 7% leading to suspension or erasure.

Surprisingly, there were 8,269 complaints received by the GMC in 2015, 7% LESS than in 2014. In fact during the preparation of this book a sea change took place at the GMC. Between 2012 and 2017 the number of suspensions and erasures after hearings increased (82% in 2016, 69% in 2015, 54% in 2012) and the number of investigations went down from 3,000 in 2013 to 1,400 in 2016. They say this indicates they are only now investigating serious complaints. In 2017 the GMC, perhaps recognising the new emotional sensitivity of the profession and its own procedural insensitivity, announced it was only pursuing action against doctors guilty of more serious offences. Thus 82% of doctors who faced a hearing in 2016 were now suspended or erased. This was the highest proportion in ten years. In 2015 69% of hearings had resulted in action against the doctor, 54% in 2012. The number of investigations had halved from 3,000 in 2013 to 1,400 in 2016 so perhaps it had listened to some of the decade of criticism.

Generally there are three stages of what can, from the doctor's point of view sometimes seem an endless, interminable and indulgent complaints procedure. I have no doubt that if you are a patient however and you have one of the distant, self opinionated and self righteous doctors that fill the NHS or, worse, one of the incompetent, incomprehensible ones; it can seem an unbalanced, arcane and complicated process.

If verbal complaints can be resolved informally then it may be that a meeting between the GP, the patient and PM may suffice. If not:

There are three further stages:

The practice based Stage 1, "Local Resolution". This must comply with national criteria – one person is nominated to handle the complaint, the practice must acknowledge the complaint in 3 working days and write a reply in 10 working days.

After the complaint has been made to a member of staff, a copy of the practice complaints leaflet must be given to the complainant and they must be referred to the "Practice Complaints Administrator". A meeting must then be organised in private, notes taken etc.

The practice Complaints Administrator gives information at this meeting such as:

How the complaint will be dealt with, the purpose of the procedure, the timetable anticipated, the confidentiality rules, help from the Local Authority, how to pursue a complaint with the H.A.(etc) the time limit (6 months after the incident) etc.

The Complaints Administrator will wish to discuss or investigate the complaint by meeting with the team members involved, HA (etc) complaints Manager, LMC etc where appropriate. The LMC and your medical insurer can be great sources of support and advice. The Administrator will usually then discuss a plan of action with a responsible partner/ Practice Manager before making a formal response. Sometimes resolution may require a meeting between the complainant and the member of staff. My experience of the value of these depends entirely upon the attitude and reasonableness of the person complaining. I say this in all humility. Some patients genuinely do complain about every doctor, practice nurse, midwife, receptionist and member of hospital staff they come up against. About 1% of the population are deeply unpleasant sociopaths who are serial and career complainers. Some complaints are regarding attitude and I am sure these are probably unprovable and irresolvable and the complaint is by way of vindictive punishment. Sometimes the facts of what happened are disputed and it is usual for the complainant's spouse or attendant to provide unqualified support, – of whatever is alleged. I know that I have been accused and quoted by a husband and wife of having used a phrase I have never used in my life but hey, you only have my word for that. Their particular complaint was regarding my denying him a long term sickness certificate. I knew he had a lucrative part time window cleaning job, cash in hand and he didn't actually have the time to work. Their letters about me were vehement, personal and nasty. The complaint went through each available stage of the process and up to the Health Service Ombudsman, it took a dozen letters from me over 10 months, about 30 sides in total saying the same thing in different ways regarding 10 minutes of an unmemorable consultation and soured my attitude towards General Practice, all patients and life in general. 18 months after the first letter, the case was finally dismissed. I then took fate in my hands and threw the manipulative and lying couple off my list. This is something the GMC tells us we can only do if the relationship has "irretrievably broken down." Well I suppose you could say that if the patient feels justified in making a significant complaint then he has every reason to lose faith in you and if he has made a mischievous, manipulative and dishonest complaint then you will have lost your faith in him. You need both, Dear GMC, for the relationship to work.

If any significant number of the GMC had ever done any General Practice, they would already know that.

The official **NHS England** guidance goes:

A patient can complain either to the service direct (in this case the GP practice) or to the Commissioner – not both.

Complaints should be investigated and a response provided with the findings of that investigation along with an appropriate apology and information regarding any learning or changes made as a result of the complaint. As part of the local resolution process, it may be appropriate to invite the complainant to a meeting, however the outcome of that meeting should be recorded in writing and may form part of the response. (If the complaint is made to NHS England we acknowledge and forward it to the practice for investigation and response to NHS England. Following our own investigation a response is sent to the complainant usually enclosing the practice response).

When local resolution is complete, if the complainant remains dissatisfied they should be referred to the Parliamentary and Health Service Ombudsman. This means if the complaint is made to the practice, the complainant should be referred to the Ombudsman and not to NHS England. (My thanks to: Dr Alison Taylor, Assistant Director (Revalidation) Deputy Medical Director, Surrey and Sussex Area Team, NHS England for the above summary).

The assumption, from the "appropriate apology" reference is that the GP is guilty until proven innocent and when there are usually only two witnesses I would have thought the doctor's human rights were being ignored here. Don't we have a right (especially if we have an average or better track record of complaints) to the benefit of the doubt particularly given the highly selected group of the public that we are dealing with? – in other words: Patients who quite often demonstrate emotional oversensitivity and lability, personal vulnerability, dislike of authority, complex psychological histories and a willingness to attribute blame to others, all contributing to their complex emotional state.

Anyway, after the in-house response and the in-practice supervised meeting used to come stage 2:

Stage 2: The Independent Review: This was done at the Health Authority by a senior member of staff who worked with a "Convenor", a non executive director of the HA. They decided if the complaint warranted an independent review.

They could refer the complaint back to the practice for further action under local resolution, arrange conciliation, set up an independent review panel (2 lay members and the Convenor), take no further action, advise the complainant of his right to approach the Ombudsman. If the complaint was clinical then 2 independent clinical assessors could be appointed to advise the panel.

Now the system is slightly different at this stage:

Now Stage 2 is direct to the Parliamentary and Health Service Ombudsman.

The local Patient Advice and Liaison Service, PALS is usually impartial, practical and constructively helpful (to both sides in my experience) and they are often involved at this stage.

Local Authorities have to provide a support service to the patient now, – an independent advocacy service, the **NHS Complaints Independent Advocacy Service** to give them independent advice and help with the complaints process.

Stage 3, The Ombudsman: (Health Service Commissioner) PHSO, (Parliamentary and Health Service Ombudsman). The patient, if the complaint remains unresolved at stage 2, can decide if he investigates the complaint. The Ombudsman is independent of the NHS. My experience is that the Ombudsman sends a representative to listen to your side of the complaint and likewise that of the complainant and in my case anyway, was fair and reasonable.

You will have to trust me on this.

The Ombudsman (who is currently an Ombudswoman) has come in for a great deal of criticism for not investigation the vast majority of serious and reasonable complaints, for being too close to the CQC and for not recording and justifying decisions. I heard an interview with her recently and the explanation was, of course, a lack of resources.

My only personal contact with them was that they spent an inordinate amount of time and money on what was clearly a trivial complaint. One which I knew but they did not, was malicious and manipulative and in which no one was hurt but political correctness was at stake. Both the complainant and wife had learning difficulties.

There are various bodies that can facilitate or act as intermediaries in the complaints process and these include ICAS, The Independent Complaints Advocacy Service etc.

Anyway, putting aside the fact that new doctors and foreign doctors from a handful of countries and doctors with a poor grasp of English and doctors with a God complex all get more than the average number of complaints, patients want competence, accessibility and friendliness more than anything from their doctors. Various studies show as few as 3% of doctors cause up to 50% of complaints.

The main reasons for complaints are:

The wrong diagnosis, delay or failure of diagnosis (25%). – It is salutatory to note that diagnostic accuracy as measured by post mortem hasn't improved in 80 years.

Inadequate management/treatment 14%. Difficult this, -as I constantly hear the opposite as well, –

"Why don't they just leave the old lady alone, keep her comfortable and stop prolonging her pain, ? You wouldn't let a dog suffer like this".

Delay or failure to refer 13%

Delay/Failure to visit 12% – The bête noire of all GPs especially those that did or do OOH cover. You KNOW the patients who are genuinely bed bound and you also know the patients who expect and demand a house call but are capable of visits to their precious hair dresser and are often out if you call in unexpectedly. You also know that for many, – doctors and patients alike, life and decision making would be far safer if, as in America, house calls were banned (save perhaps for an agreed few, – say the terminally ill or the single unsupported genuinely disabled who could not get into any form of transport).

Attitude 10%. This must be growing for a number of patient and doctor based reasons but unless one doctor is disproportionately complained against, how and what do you do about his or her attitude?

Outcomes:

Until recently more than 90% of complaints were dismissed or resolved but they could take months and months and be very draining to the caring GP. The sociopathic GP (and I have worked with a couple) isn't affected by the complaint's rights or wrongs or the process of resolution and will no doubt continue to behave in the same way.

Only 6.5% progress to an adverse outcome for the GP.

If over nine tenths of complaints are in effect without censure to the doctor then they must serve another purpose: to make the system **appear** responsive to patients feelings, to allow patients to express or expunge feelings of resentment, guilt, disempowerment, anger and frustration by hitting out at the messenger of the bad news, to make the politicians sound good at interview, or to perpetuate the myth that the juggernaut of the NHS listens to each of its customers – which of course is impossible. Often the complaint is because we are doing our job properly. Just after my patient complained about "my attitude" (in not giving him a repeat sick certificate") and the complaints process continued for 18 months, the Secretary of State was on the radio criticising what a soft touch GPs were in handing out sick certificates to all and sundry. Either way doctors are made to suffer a protracted, often highly traumatic, unsympathetic and in the end unapologetic admin- istrative process designed by politicians and run by administrators from the blunt end of clinical practice. Complaints can knock the stuffing out of you, even if you have emotional resilience. The 2015 tirade of criticism of GPs for "dishing out antibiotics on demand" is likewise pointless when governments for decades have blessed a well worn legal process whereby doctors who miss a fatal infection after a proper examination are sued for huge sums of "compensation" with the enthusiastic help of lawyers who advertise their services: "No upfront costs and nothing to pay if you lose."

As a trainer, one of the first tutorials I gave to each new registrar was on how receiving a complaint made you feel, how you coped with it and the personal and professional aftermath. We all want to be liked and respected by our patients. More in General Practice than in Hospital Practice because we are more deeply embedded in our lists and the community, we see the patient more frequently, often outside of a medical context and for an open ended commitment. We are more personally involved or should be, as part of the community ourselves and we take complaints as a criticism not of our work but of ourselves. This is in a way that the outpatients doctor would not readily understand. According to an Imperial College/University of Leuven study (BMJ open 2016) expanding on research done by Bourne (2015), patient complaints left doctors with considerable morbidity.

Surveying 8,000 doctors about the impact of complaints, doctors who had suffered a recent complaint had significant risks of moderate to severe depression, anxiety and suicidal thoughts. Complaints led to defensive practice which included avoiding taking on high risk (previous complainers, over anxious, multiple morbidities) patients. Well, why would you go and ask for trouble?

What we need above all is to streamline and speed up the complaints process so that it has fewer, clearer stages and is over quicker and I have to say, with the possibility of some sort of patient penalty for what is clearly currently a patient indulgent process with no downside to them. After all, 90% of complaints used to end in no significant professional criticism, so were probably unfounded, mischievous, subjective, trivial or malicious – but even so, result in a huge amount of emotional harm to the doctor. At each stage the patient is encouraged to proceed to the next, even if their complaint is not confirmed and huge amounts of time, money and worry are expended on pointless, frivolous and manipulative complaints that either can never be resolved or proven or are clearly motivated by ill will. There are of course bad doctors and over the last few years I have become more and more aware of some of them. Here I suspect the Appraisal process and Responsible Officer should become more involved in the process as the supervisor and head master who knows the GP's track record and the previous complaints history. Human Rights, Diversity and Equality Laws, Data Protection and all the other 21st century politics that confuse so many medical issues for patient and doctor have no place here in obfuscating what is best for the patient or for the NHS.

In a press release in October 2014 The GMC confirmed the increased likelihood of black and ethnic minority doctors being the subject of complaints compared with their white counterparts. They said that they were 50% more likely to be complained against irrespective of their gender. But overall, male doctors were twice as likely to be complained about and older women over 50 twice as likely compared with younger women. This is as I have said, probably to do with the different specialities and the longer hours worked by male doctors. Older female doctors who qualified before the working time directive are not quite so protective of their work life balance and probably work more hours and see more patients, who then complain more.

In 2013 the GMC received complaints about 7.7% of all female doctors and 15% of male doctors. Regarding the female complaints, 3.6% resulted in a warning or sanction, 6.4% of the male complaints did. Over the age of 50, 14% of female doctors were complained about in 2013, for men over 50, 23% had a complaint. This again might reflect the number of patients seen.

In 2015 an American study confirmed the higher rate of complaints against male doctors over there. However the authors went a long way to explaining the discrepancy by suggesting that it also was due to the greater hours worked and the higher risk occupations (ER departments, General Surgery, Orthopaedics. out of hours cover etc). undertaken by male doctors. So we are not comparing like with like.

It is true to some extent that we now have a part time (largely female) and a full time (largely male) work force of doctors developing in the UK. Those that accept long out of hours on call rotas and those that do physically and developmentally arduous careers (often predominantly male) and those that job share and are part time GPs and consultants (mainly female). This was demonstrated in the latest RCP Census. As of 2015 the greatest percentage of UK female surgeons were Paediatric surgeons at 25%. Altogether women make up 11%, 800 of the total number of surgeons. A 2013 survey of newly qualified doctors suggested 68% of the women thought surgery was not a career that welcomed them. Or could it be, what with tough rotas, physically and emotionally draining jobs and family unfriendly careers that demand full time dedication it wasn't a case of the career not welcoming women but possibly the other way round? So we do seem to be developing two health services – a male run one and female run one.

BME doctors who are 39% of the workforce in the 2014 report were "more likely to face complaints and 50% more likely to receive a warning or a sanction after"

Apart from the uneven distribution of complaints which are due to a multiplicity of factors, some politically undiscussable and covered elsewhere, isn't it clear that if one in four male doctors over 50 have a complaint against them annually, either we have become a pathetically complaining culture, huge numbers of older male doctors ARE hopeless, or the complaints procedure is just too easy and unfair to doctors?

Underperforming doctors:

There will be a **Lead Officer** of some kind coordinating any "concerns" expressed to the LMC, local "Responsible Officer", the Lead Officer themselves, appraisal administrators or, presumably, the Commissioning Group Clinical Governance Representative who will take over (?) the previous PCT Board "Referral Committee's" coordinating role.

"The process" is:

The Referral Committee sets up a **Performance Support Group** and makes the decisions about the case. They have the power to suspend and to recommend remedial or other "corrective" action by the GP. They can, if the situation is considered serious, refer on to the GMC, seek help from the NCAA (**National Clinical Assessment Authority**) and get the local **Professional Advisory Group** (PAG) representative to see the GP and or his/her practice.

These various roles may be taken on by a **Clinical Adviser for the practice, The Performance Steering Group, The Performers List Decision Panel** and **The Area Team** these days. It took five years to write most of this book and during this time the process, titles and organisation of investigating "underperforming doctors" changed twice. I have tried to include most of the titles. I hope this assists in clarifying the process rather than the reverse.

As a PAG "expert", I was once parachuted into a practice as part of what was in effect a show punishment of a very good GP. I was there to assess his record keeping and general organisation (which was at least as good as most GPs) after an episode on Friday afternoon, when he had been tired and inconsiderate – and very offhand to a bereaved relative over the phone. He was under intolerable pressure at the time and trying to cope with too much when a distressed relative was put through by a receptionist without any warning. The GP was unaware a patient had just died. It seemed to me that the process felt it ought to exert its authority over the doctor and an example should be made of the GP. Muscles being flexed etc.

The system was unwieldy and heavy handed and caused him far more distress than I thought the relative had originally experienced. There was no lightness of touch once administrators and "my pound of flesh" and "justice being seen to be done" got involved. I did my best to soften the blow with my sympathetic attitude and personal anecdotes and "there but for the grace of God conversations" but I do think the whole complaints system for minor misdemeanours is designed to satisfy a consumer culture and sometimes it can be distant from real life for the full time overworked GP. Take for instance the ludicrous

GMC assertion that making an apology is a fair, reasonable, cost free, emotionally tolerable, psychologically acceptable first response to some perceived patient "harm". Say a hard working motivated and caring doctor who has done their best finds a mistake or accident has befallen their patient. Something that they are as upset about as the patient and did everything reasonable to avoid. The imposition of an inappropriate apology can destroy that doctor's sense of fairness, justice, morale, confidence, love of his job and his patients, leading to self doubt, resentment, depression.

Anyway, the PAG can be used if some sort of practice/partnership level investigation or reorganisation (with the appropriate help from the team member at the Trust/Commissioning Group) is inappropriate and The Lead Officer may then take the issue via the Referral Committee or PSG or even via a newly convened "**Diagnostic team**" to gather and collate information regarding the doctor and the practice.

The PAG may then look at the "Diagnostic Team's" assessment, possibly using advice from the NCAA and set up a support package.

This may include Occupational Health, Deanery (educational), managerial, time off, mentoring, etc. support.

The PSG decides when the GP can restart normal activities and when monitoring is no longer required.

If the complaint is very serious the Referral Committee can remove the practitioner from the Performers' List and/or refer them to the **GMC/Fraud Authorities/Healthcare Commission/Police.**

Considering how we work in lonely professional and personal isolation in General Practice and how little support colleagues and partners traditionally offer one another, it is dizzying, the variety of different teams, organisations, authorities and groups which are now available to judge, discipline, educate and censure the errant GP from their various exalted positions of expertise.

2: Administration, Training, the Consultation and Teaching

Medical School:

Most medical graduates today, due to a combination of asymmetrically early emotional and academic maturation are girls. There are 34 medical schools listed in the UK today. At least 2/3 of medical school graduates are now female and a moment's thought will show this to be short sighted, sexist, un-demographic, undemocratic, organisationally unrealistic and suicidally expensive. When I qualified, 18 of the 84 in my year (21%) were female and only one of each sex dropped out by the end of the first year. Everyone else completed the course and most of the women who qualified became full time doctors in their specialities. Five years later I think they were all or nearly all still full time. Now things have changed. Two thirds of the medical workforce is being specifically selected to work only 60-65% of the hours of the other one third, to take more time off for psychological and physical illness – often at short notice, to want to job share more often or work part time, to retire early and to be willing to work in a relatively restricted number of specialities. In other words, women. A question asked about the restricted career choices and the **life/work balance** of women doctors drew "poisonous looks" on the January 2015 Women's Hour programme. This was discussing women in British medicine. Poisonous looks but no answers from the all female medical panel. It is obvious to anyone without a purely political and feminist agenda that from the patient and tax payer's perspectives, quality, choice, continuity and value for money have been sacrificed in giving young women this huge new numbers advantage over men in the career of medicine. They don't make better doctors. The evidence shows that female doctors are less intuitive, take fewer of the "inspired guesses" and risks necessary for independent working, primary care, emergency and front line medicine and refer a greater percentage of patients for second opinions. But there are now more of them in the UK work force and in many other advanced countries. This is rampant sexism. I cannot see any advantage for patients, the profession or the paying sponsors (you and me, the unconsulted tax payer) in making medicine a predominantly female profession. So why is it happening? Concern is likewise being expressed in the USA about the limited career choices that women make. The concern there, as here, is what happens when all the male general surgeons, specialist surgeons, orthopaedic surgeons and casualty staff retire? Who will replace them? Headlines in the national press throughout one year (2015) outlined the problems of this feminine bias: How the overwhelming numbers of women in the contemporary NHS have shut down Casualty units by their reluctance to do that particular speciality but how they have also shut down Paediatric units by their domination of child medicine (70% of junior staff) and their extensive and unprecedented time off for maternity leave and propensity for part time work as soon as they are appointed.

Selection for the career of medicine has for years been hopelessly scholarly and based on A-level grades. This ensures further generations of academic, intellectual doctors who may not be good at communicating, sympathising or relating to the complexities of real people in distress in real life. Abstract intellect and the ability to pass exams may be useful in some research, academic and educational arenas. It might be good to have in the spheres of basic genetics, pharmacology, molecular medicine, biochemistry, pure sciences and so on but it is emotional intelligence, sympathy, listening skills and the ability to articulate and explain that are more useful in most face to face medicine. Here the very brightest don't always outshine the rest. Obviously most doctors need a bit of lustre in both areas. Some may say that the female personality is the more programmed for caring but my forty years in medicine have not borne that particular assumption out. The complete opposite in fact. I heard with disbelief that "most" patients preferred consulting women doctors at a meeting recently – as if this were a "given". Which patients? Not adolescent boys or young men who need to be intimately examined, not males with erectile or urological abnormalities and frequently not men with depression, anxiety, men from a variety of cultural backgrounds or many men suffering a crisis of confidence loss of self esteem. I was visiting a relative in a midlands hospital recently and telling him about the female bias of medical schools and how it could disenfranchise some male patients. The curtains of the next door bed were then suddenly pulled back by an elderly Muslim man who, with his sons gathered around visiting him, enthusiastically agreed. None of them would consult a female doctor he said, with a personal, emotional, stress or "sensitive problem" (he said, pointing between his legs).

So medical schools currently seem to be selecting huge numbers of female academically gifted A – Level students for medicine today. Life experience, emotional resilience, genuine caring skills and empathy are difficult to display, to judge and to grade. Increasingly there seems to be a realisation, not least from the GMC, that a degree of personal toughness is necessary to withstand the emotional and personal traumas of a life in medicine. "Emotional resilience" is what the GMC calls it. These characteristics are not selected for or encouraged and probably not much in evidence in the average modern medical student or doctor or the modern medical curriculum. So where do we stand and what can we do to make doctors more relevant to a tough life in medicine and to caring for patients?

In an article: "UK medical selection: Lottery or meritocracy?" in the Royal College of Physicians Journal, Clinical Medicine, Feb 2015, there was a review of "non knowledge based tests" which are used, supposedly to improve medical student selection above that of just A Level grades and ghost written or coached personal statements. They mention the new UK clinical aptitude test UKCAT as well as Situational Judgement Tests, (SJTs), The Biomedical Medical Admissions Test (BMAT) and the Graduate Australian Medical School Admissions Test (GAMSAT).

The authors mention that the attributes of scientist and scholar (A level grades followed by an interview) on their own are not enough to be a good doctor. You also need the "social attributes" of empathy and communication skills. The problem is how to assess these fairly and what combination of all these things is needed to make the best doctor.

The three parameters currently used by UK medical schools to assess candidates are: The UCAS Form (academic achievement and commitment to medicine) followed by selection using one of the above non knowledge based tests:

The UK Clinical Aptitude Test (UKCAT), The Biomedical Medical Admissions Test (BMAT) and the Graduate Australian Medical School Admissions Test (GAMSAT) – the scientific knowledge components in these being: 0%, 33% and 50% respectively. Finally medical students are assessed with their personal statements via traditional or multiple mini interviews (MMIs).

Unfortunately it turns out that these non knowledge based tests do not correlate well with the subsequent medical school performance of the student. Indeed, UKCAT actually correlates worse than A Level results. In fact A-level performance itself is a pretty good predictor of medical school success and beyond (BMC Med 201311: 243). UKCAT does increase the numbers from lower socio economic groups but it isn't clear whether these candidates are those who actually go on to make good doctors. It sounds like you might as well draw names out of a hat if all you want is diverse backgrounds for your doctors. Surely, how good they are at looking after patients should be the only gold standard?

BMAT and GAMSAT have similarly poor predictive abilities and correlate good medical school performance with their scientific components only.

So A levels and interviews are the best determinants of success at medical schools-and the quality of doctors. This is exactly what medical schools used in their selection process forty to fifty years ago. As in so much of this book it turns out that change for change's sake has reduced standards and in the end has harmed patients.

American medical schools use the undergraduate's grade point average and the National Medical College Admissions Test (MCAT) (which has three sections: biological sciences, physical sciences and verbal reasoning). Like here, the best predictors of Medical school performance in America are the scores in the scientific knowledge sections. **Basically, exams testing abstract qualities have not been shown to have any predictive ability of medical school performance at all. Anywhere.**

Although I am not clear that performance at medical school – presumable assessed by further imperfect exams is the right way to assess the quality of a future doctor. I was virtually last out of 90 students in the Paediatrics MCQ at my medical school. I loved looking after children, I hung around on the Paediatric ward in my spare time, helped out the nurses, I loved Paediatrics but hated and never got the hang of MCQs. Later I got Membership in Paediatrics and eventually lectured it at a famous university medical school, I taught it and saw it as my life's focus until I changed horses. The point I am trying to make is that exams aren't infallible. I was always hopeless at MCQs. Clearly the introduction of non knowledge based tests is doing nothing but vary the background of medical students without necessarily improving the quality of the doctors they become. You wonder whether this diversification, like the mass feminisation of the workforce, is just another attack on the traditional organisation of British medicine for the sake of it. The article in "Clinical Medicine", which has 46 references, ends with this statement: **"Therefore let us halt this fashion based approach to medical selection and focus our attention on the evidence and what really matters, diagnosis, management and patient CARE.**

Amen to that.

Until that Nirvana occurs, patients will just have to wait.

This is the social engineering that British medical schools are currently engaged in:
I wrote to all the country's medical schools under a "Freedom of information request" and asked them for the demographics of their students. The figures surprised me bearing in mind that the medical profession has an obligation to reflect the population it serves. The population it serves is 86% white and 50% male:

Queen Mary, London (they explained their figures by saying they have an ethnically diverse catchment area but surely, given the concentration of medical schools in cities, especially London, they have no right to represent only their LOCAL population?) had the fewest white students. As you can see, many medical schools had had no problem selecting only a third of their students from male applicants.

As anyone who has tried using it will know, the idea behind the FOI act and the actual accessibility and interpretability of data you obtain are two completely different things. Some medical schools were far more willing to part with information on demography of students than others and in the end some didn't share their data at all. I wrote to every single medical school in the United Kingdom twice. Here are the results:

	2011/12		2012/13	2013/14
Birmingham:				
White:	66%		64%	55%
Male:	38%		38%	36%
Queen Mary London:				
White	43%		35%	33%
Male	53%		56%	48%
Newcastle:				
White	79%		75%	82%
Male	50%		50%	48%
Cardiff:				
White:	77%		77%	72%
Male	37%		33%	37%
Swansea:				
White:	84%		85%	82%
Male:	47%		58%	55%
Bristol:(Roughly one tenth are overseas applicants)				
White	80%		74%	67%
Male	41%	36%	36%	
Manchester:				
White	61%		60%	60%
Male	46%		49%	49%
UCL				
White	59%		48%	46%
Male	51%		49%	54%
Brighton:				
White:	66%		70%	70%
Male:	45%		45%	45%
Oxford:				
White:	76%		83%	74%
Male:	47%		48%	48%
Cambridge Preclinical Years				
White	62%		59%	57%
Cambridge All Years				
Male	51%		52%	53%

Hull/York

White	72%	71%	64%
Male	44%	39%	52%

Leeds

White	67%	62%	67%
Male	40%	34%	33%

Nottingham	2010/11	2011/12	2012/13
White	76%	78%	77%
Male	49%	50%	49%

Leicester: "Elite without being elitist"*

White:	53%	57%	62%
Male:	46%	42%	42%

Liverpool:

White:	58%	59%	61%
Male:	39%	29%	25%

Edinburgh:

White:	81%	76%	69%
Male:	44%	43%	52%

St. Andrews:

White:	84%	82%	80%
Male:	41%	42%	42%

Peninsula School of Medicine:

White:	67%	66%	62%
Male:	45%	54%	48%

University of East Anglia:

White:	67%	63%	53%
Male:	42%	45%	35%

Keele University:

White:	66%	65%	64%
Male:	46%	45%	46%

Exeter:

White:	N/K	71%	72%
Male:	39%	46%	46%

*Leicester's response to "Who is the selection Committee?":

We have a selection committee which decides on the admissions policy and the way that students will be selected. This committee consists of 3 Admissions Tutors, 3 Admissions Administrators, the University Director of Admissions, the Director of Undergraduate Medical Education, a Deputy Director of Undergraduate Medical Education, a student member, 2 patient representatives and the Head of School & College Services. As to answering the question "Why is the makeup of your medical school intake so different from that of the British public, given the profession's often publically stated responsibility to reflect the population it serves" They replied "Matters of policy are not covered by the Freedom of Information Act."

So there.

The Peninsula Medical School answered:

There is a separate and distinct Admissions Advisory Panel (AAP) for the Bachelor of Medicine, Bachelor of Surgery (BMBS) programme. The membership of the AAP includes the Associate Dean for Teaching and Learning, the Head of Administration, the Admissions & Student Support Co-ordinator and the University's Admissions Manager (undergraduate programmes) along with clinical representatives and the Selection and Admissions Psychometrician.

The AAP is responsible for making recommendations to the Dean or his/her nominee on:

- The number and identity of applicants to be selected for interview in each application cycle.
- The threshold interview score to determine which candidates should receive offers in each application cycle.
- The number of offers to be made to candidates.
- The confirmation of students following the publication of examination results.
- All information from self-declaration forms and disclosure and barring service enhanced disclosures which may be deemed significant in the context of the College's fitness to practise procedures.
- All information received from the Occupational Health & Wellbeing Service which may be deemed significant in the context of the College's fitness to practise procedures.

Our students are selected using academic criteria, the UK Clinical Aptitude Test and interview performance. Ethnicity data is not made available to Medical Schools/Universities at the application stage (indeed this is only passed to Universities after enrolment) and so this plays no part in the selection process. Interview panels receive no prior information about selected candidates prior to the interview. As such, our student demography will be reflective of the range of applications received during any particular cycle. (*I wonder whether the Metropolitan Police Force or The BBC could have used the same argument when they were instructed to positively discriminate in favour of ethnic minority candidates?*)

No medical school comes anywhere near reflection the true ethnic mix of Britain and most white parents would find these figures puzzling or unfair at the very least. Most medical schools under represent males too. UCL and Queen Mary have half the number of white medical students you would expect from population data and as ethnicity is not known at the application stage it is difficult to see how the nation's frequently patient-expressed and the Royal College of Physician's occasionally publically expressed concern that the profession should reflect the public it serves can ever be met.

The result is sexism and racism against white male applicants in the selection of medical students and the future medical profession will certainly neither resemble the UK population or offer it value for money. It will also be increasingly difficult to fully staff many specialities and reflect our population properly despite an increase in doctor numbers unless there is some definitive white/male positive discrimination for many years.

Elsewhere I explain research that shows teachers and academics in many careers have a left wing/liberal political bias. Assuming medical selection committees are drawn from medical school staff, rather than front line GPs or hospital doctors as a whole, could this be why a feminist and ethnically biased agenda is secretly changing the face (literally) of the profession? My dentist friends tell me that same is true for dentistry.

You could argue that some medical schools take applicants from all over the world and that a little foreign weighting is inevitable in these figures but given the UK's huge and growing dependency on foreign trained doctors to provide the work force, increasing concern that foreign qualified doctors are more likely to be complained about and struck off (see later) and recently published data on competencies of foreign trained doctors and examination failure rates, one has to wonder why these places at our tax subsidised medical schools aren't being reserved for more badly needed UK doctors. Indeed, in a 2016 Civitas report, it was made public that our medical schools, by training so many foreign students, not only deprived our young men and women of the chance to become medics but cost our tax payers huge sums of money, never to be repaid. They suggest a differential charge on students, thus:

"Tubbs points out that another problematic element of current recruitment practices is that foreign students are given their placement fees (at £34,000 per placement year); the same as any UK national student. These fees come out of the NHS's training budget, meaning the NHS is paying up to £12 million per year for overseas students to study here with no guarantee that they will stay beyond the end of their studies. The proposed placement fee loan would ensure that such students either remain and work for the NHS after graduation or fully pay back their placement fees if they wish to return home."

According to the 2011 census the white population of Britain was **86%** (black, minority ethnic population therefore 14%) and male **50%**.

I have now followed up my initial enquiry more extensively and all medical schools seem to be acting as if this racist and sexist bias against the white male is a secret national agenda.

No single medical school is taking its responsibility to reflect the British population seriously. All are, it seems busy sexually and ethnically engineering an unrepresentative medical workforce and one that has a variety of implications for the British population which I am fairly sure it would wish to be consulted about. The cost, the unfair and unadmitted sexual and positive racial discrimination being but three.

The President of The Royal College of Physicians gave a speech a few years ago saying that the medical workforce should represent and reflect the society it serves. If 60%+ doctors are to be female and in many parts of London and many regional hospitals 70% or more medical staff are from ethnic minorities then we need to do some serious positive discrimination for white male doctors for many years to come to redress the balance. I have a friend who's brother in the Midlands goes to a district general hospital where every single doctor was trained abroad and has English as a second language. There are GP practices a few miles from mine where a male patient with testicular swelling, prostatic symptoms or erectile dysfunction would be forced to see a female GP. This is because they only have female partners there and this is an increasingly common situation. 90% of men with these type of problems prefer to see male doctors in all the audits I have seen. Why are we disenfranchising the very people who will have paid, over their working lives, proportionately the most towards the NHS? – the full time working male tax payer.

In passing, the same audits that showed most men prefer male doctors for personal medical problems also showed women consulting with gynaecological and urological problems were generally not as bothered by the gender as they are by the personality of and their relationship with their doctor.

In Pediatric Emergency Care 2005 "Doctor or Doctora" 60% parents preferred their child to see a male doctor, 19% a woman and the rest a doctor with "the most experience."

In: Male/Female Obstetrician – Gynaecologists ? A study of gender preference: JAOA ISSN 0098-6151

80.8% patients felt the gender of the physician did not influence the quality of care. Two thirds of (female, obviously) patients had no gender bias as to what sex their Obstetrician or Gynaecologist was.

A University of Montreal study found female doctors spent longer with patients, referred more on for further care and prescribed more medication, but male doctors performed 1000 more procedures a year than women and the differences were greater among older doctors (Oct 2013 Mail online). Men are more efficient and the more experienced they are the better they get.

A New Zealand study on the care of elderly diabetics found male doctors got through more patients with the same clinical outcomes but without the same diligence at recording data for audit.(?)

So there **Are** differences between male and female doctors-as if you didn't know. Men are more efficient and intuitive. Women take more notes.

I think these are the sort of questions we should be asking at audits: "Would you prefer a different sex doctor for some consultations?" "Has ethnicity or cultural background, sex, race or nationality ever adversely affected the doctor's ability to communicate with you or your family?" Imagine if medicine were so free of politics that it could actually ask questions like this and even more unimaginable, do something about the results?

So there are differences in how male and female doctors work, what we do and what sex doctor that individual patients may want to see – whatever the soft politics and the sleep walking choices that medical school selection committees may be leading us towards. Patients should have a say in this too.

Finally, and to quote Kevin MD:(From the website on "Gender preferences":)

"The issue has been mostly resolved for women with the entry of large numbers of women into medicine. But large numbers of men still avoid medical care because of embarrassment. Statistics on this are difficult to obtain as men are loathe to admit that the presence of women may embarrass them. Study questionnaires on this topic will have to be filled out in private; frank answers will not be obtained if questions are asked by women."

Putting aside the communication and cultural difficulties that many patients (and my friend's brother who never sees a British doctor) have at outpatients appointments, we are the sixth largest economy in the world. Can we not educate a home grown medical profession that reflects our population – in terms of cultural background and sex? Heaven knows there are enough 18 year old boys who happen to be from the majority community who would jump at the chance of a place in medical school if the selection were fairer.

The Dumbing-down and Devocation of medicine:

So that is where we are and where we are going. You will see time and time again as I continue this description of modern General (and Hospital) Practice that the quality of doctors and doctoring, nursing, education, administration, medical care and much of what the NHS does for us have been negatively affected by a variety of factors over the last two or three decades. This is primarily because of politicians, ingrained political attitudes and soft politics interfering with health care. Whenever a change in organisation or process has been introduced no one seems to have thought "How could this affect the patient?"

The secret but progressive remodelling of the profession through selection committees of medical schools and the political bias of professional colleges and examinations,

the dumbing down of the culture of the medical profession through a concentration on social attitudes rather than diagnostic rigour in clinical exams, (even the MRCGP was being challenged in 2014 in court by Indian doctors who have a higher failure rate, not because it is too rigorous but because they wanted it less **culturally British**),

spurious dress codes, the wear what you like chaos, the specious rolled up sleeves and dispensing with ties in the NHS but not the private health care system. Something that has never been shown to reduce infection and if you compare the two systems using evidence based medicine, actually increases it.

The first name informality amongst young doctors, which far from making them seem accessible, just makes them appear unprofessional.

The elevation in status of specialised nurses, often in day to day conflict with more experienced doctors,

the removal of the professional independence of doctors via contract negotiations and cost obsessed committees, QuoF, the targets focus of the last two decades – it goes on and on.

All serve to weaken, cheapen and de-professionalise doctors.

You can't help wondering whether that indeed WAS the whole idea.-to knock doctors off their professionally independent and therefore powerfully elevated pedestals.

Much of this has been indirectly, through soft politics and has had negative, predictable but **apparently** unforeseen consequences – at least from the point of view of the patient. – The quality of care for them has just got worse.

Put simply, when the NHS was founded, doctors and nurses had their own code of ethics and were trusted to put the patient's interests above all else. This they generally did. To the detriment in fact of their OWN health, longevity and indeed of their own families. Now ask yourself if direct political influence and considerations – from the 48 hour Working Time Directive, Equality and Diversity legislation, some lowered academic bars to jump, data protection issues, prescribing controls on controlled drugs for seriously ill patients, (as an exaggerated and inappropriate response to Shipman), petty alteration of dress codes in the name of infection control, the wholesale feminisation of medical staffing, increased part-timism etc have really improved standards of care or worsened them? As I show later most items of news regarding the NHS over at least the last 5 years, except perhaps the progress in genomics and the slight reduction in cancer mortality in the UK have been depressing, to the patients' detriment and whole-heartedly negative.

The quality of doctoring is, of course, affected by the quality of medical education but also the hours put in and the dedication that each trainee doctor brings to it (-their "vocation" as well as their total patient contact time). I went to medical school in the 70's and trained in what was often a more than 100 hour week. These were standard "one in two" or "one in three" working rotas – an environment dedicated to learning and getting through the workload – not to the comfort or human rights of the doctor. It was a hard apprenticeship. A very steep learning curve.

The junior doctor today will work fewer than half the hours per week, per medical or surgical job and per grade that I did. **She** will see fewer than half the cases and have half the experience at the same point in training. At the same stage of training she will be less competent, less skilful, less safe. She will also take two to three times longer off sick for some reason. Increased sickness absence is a characteristic of both a feminised work force and the post Working Time Directive work force. (Feb 2014, Nat Off. Statistics, women are 50% more likely to take time off sick: BMJ Careers 7 Apr 2010. Junior doctors' sick leave more than doubled after the introduction of the WTD). Over the 40 years since I started my apprenticeship with house and SHO jobs, I have seen the loss of that ethos of commitment – the tacit acceptance of long hours to earn and gain experience quickly, the working when you were unwell because you didn't want to "dump on" your overworked colleagues (now called "presenteeism"), missing out on family life because you prioritised the safety of your patients and wanted to gain as much experience as quickly as you could.

So that this is what we often seem to have now: A medical student body and junior medical workforce with significantly less experience and competence and sometimes without genuine confidence. Graduate doctors were reported to be "Too nervous to do basic procedures, blood taking, ECGs and even prescribing" in a Times article, Feb 1st 2017. A third of the 7,500 newly qualified medics were said to be unready to see patients. Presumably due to restricted contact time with patients and emotional immaturity not common in their forebears. This has now resulted at long last in a standardisation of finals exams across all British medical schools in five years and which will be compulsory for foreign graduates at last. "The Medical Licensing Assessment". Half of GP trainees now report being faced with problems that go beyond their competency level during training according to a GMC survey in Jun 2014. Less Esprit de Corps, less vocation, less skill, less confidence. This according to the RCP apparently extends as far up as some young consultants when compared with their predecessors.

If doctors are less able than they were, the intellectualisation of nursing often hasn't delivered a better quality of care for the patient to compensate. Nurses, some of whom are graduates often seem "too clever to feed, clean up or attend to the bodily needs of sick patients". Rightly or wrongly this has been blamed for some patient neglect scandals and increasingly, conflict with doctors in decision making. Less skilled doctors and over skilled nurses, both the result of politics interfering with training that WORKED. My medical students and GP registrars sometimes shock me not only with what they have never seen before but with their unwillingness to stay late and see a few emergency extra patients because of family or social commitments. They take time off for relatively minor ailments, which are, of course constant and recurrent occupational hazards and for which I would have swallowed a couple of paracetamol and kept going. Bred with the working time directive, with family friendly working conditions, with a far gentler educational and working environment, – in other words the emasculation of medicine, their commitment and enthusiasm often seems less than it would have been a few decades ago. Patients suffer as a consequence. I am amazed at the lack of experience of many doctors at qualification and on completing their GP training – many never having managed a patient with acute heart failure, acute severe asthma, a choking child, status epilepticus etc. All these were the bread and butter of my generation. This is because we would have been on the wards for perhaps 50% more hours than a modern medic, hanging around after hours as students and doing 80-100 hours cover a week as housemen. By the time we qualified or registered we would have done dozens of red-eyes and long weekends. We had simply seen, done and taken on and taken in more than young doctors are allowed to or *want to* today.

One other frightening fact from the point of view of the poor old tax payer is that not only do nine tenths of medical students say (2017, January) that they plan to go part time permanently but at least one in seven or eight of these relatively under stretched, expensively trained medical students intends to leave the country for Australia or New Zealand once they have completed their training for General Practice (August 2014). The cost of training a GP is now (2015) approximately £500,000 and a consultant £560.000-£650,000 (Later estimates during the doctors' strike of 2016 put a consultant's training at up to £850,000). Some political parties are so alarmed at the prospect of large numbers of British doctors taking their British training to warmer climes that they have proposed a written contract to stay for a compulsory period after qualifying rather than the moral one most of my generation seemed to have. (UKIP Manifesto waives tuition fees for doctors staying in the UK for 5 years after qualifying, 2015).

Could this lack of rigour, this weaker commitment and this new half heartedness be an inevitable consequence of the feminisation of British medicine, restrictions on working time, excessive tolerance of minor illness and an over acceptance of stress in the work force? – all virtually unknown forty years ago. What about the universal acceptance of inevitable long breaks for maternity leave at the start of careers, almost always disrupting the establishing of patient relationships, continuity and forward planning with their colleagues? As I mentioned, one of my own audits, of 200 random patients, 15 – 80 years old, showed 90% of male patients want to see a male doctor if they have a urological, psychosexual or an ano-rectal problem and are becoming disenfranchised by the increasing lack of choice – offered by all female or nearly all female GP practices. Fewer than 50% women preferred a woman doctor for these same conditions and for gynaecological complaints.

As I said, I know already of GP practices where there are no male doctors and this situation is just going to get worse unless we start restricting the number of female entrants to medical school.

The Consultant Census

In April 2014 The Royal College of Physicians published the latest annual Consultant Census. This is a summary of the numbers, demography, specialities, attitudes and other work force details of all the Consultant Physicians in the UK.

You can read a great deal between the lines in this publication and not all of it is what patients, the tax payer or the concerned citizen might hope of its senior medical staff.

As I have previously mentioned, we know that female doctors as a whole do not like the life or training involved in an A and E and most surgical specialty careers. Their failure to apply for work in casualty departments was the reason many went unstaffed in 2014/5. They do like certain other specialities – particularly Obs and Gynae, General Practice, community work and Paediatrics. Their concentration in Paediatric units (75% of doctors in Paediatric training posts in 2015 were female), combined with the maternity and part-timism of female medics, led to a crisis in staffing in this speciality in 2015. Medical schools have what seems to be a gross female intake bias at the moment. We also know that female doctors tend to give back fewer hours – often half as many career hours as men. Just in passing and in case it has been forgotten, the population of the UK, which the medical profession is morally and duty bound to reflect, is currently 50% female and just less than 15% from an ethnic minority.

If we start with the front page of the report we find what seems to be a consultant physician and his team on a ward round. If you are a tax payer who wants value for money in medicine, if you are from the majority, host population of Britain or if you have traditional values, the disappointment starts here (see first chapter page 33 for the picture). The consultant's team appears to consist of 60% female doctors and 40% appear to be (I could be wrong) from an ethnic minority. Agreed, they may all have qualified in the UK and have high quality training and perfect language skills but given the higher complaints and striking off rates for foreign trained doctors, there could be a sense of disappointment and resignation from the NHS experienced patient on seeing this. Certainly, the feedback from my patients over the last few decades would suggest so. Just like I have mentioned regarding GMC publications, the Royal Colleges and Department of Health fall over themselves to show in their publications their own enthusiasm for multicultural medical staffing, not always shared by the patients – at least as demonstrated by frequent informal feedback related to language skills and sometimes attitudes that I hear from my patients. Objectively this conflict is demonstrated by disciplinary hearings, the numbers of complaints and so on. The dominant numbers shown of cost ineffective women doctors and the casual dress and untidy hair (particularly of what I take to be the consultant) are an added frustration to the thinking observer who might remember and long for a cost effective, representative health service with doctors who look and behave professionally. The fact is that this picture represents modern medicine but not modern British society generally (outside London or Birmingham) or even what most patients really want from the medical profession if **given a choice**. Whether the profession gives value for money is not discussed in the report. It talks about what happens now, not what should happen or what the patient and tax payer would like to happen in hospitals if they were ever consulted.

These are the figures:

The ratio of Part Time female physicians to male is 7.4: 1 (39%: 5.3%) so as elsewhere in medicine, they are not good value for the tax payer who, of course, put up hundreds of thousands of pounds to train them – up to £850,000 at **some** of the latest estimates (2016). Part time means a poor return on the cost of training. Women cost the same as men to train and then seven times as many work part time.

In **2013** the figures for the cost of training from the BMA were:

	Pre registration			Postgraduate	Totals
Tuition	Living Exp	Clinical Plac't	Tuition etc	Total investment	
Foundation Officer 1	£57,433	£60,301	£151,702	N/A	£269,527
Foundation Officer 2	£57,433	£60,301	£151,792	£24,637	£294,164
Registrar Group	£57,433	£60,301	£151,792	£73,924	£343,451
Associate Specialist	£57,433	£60,301	£ 151,792	£113,951	£383,477
GP	£57,433	£60,301	£151,792	£228,962	£498,489
Consultant	£57,433	£60,301	£151,792	£275,182	£564,112

Some reports now put that top figure at between £600 and £650K (2015), £850K

(2016) but there are suggestions that the government (2015), following a training review, wants to increase doctor numbers simply by cutting consultant training time by two years. The Royal Colleges in view of The working Time Directive, Maternity leave absences and the deteriorating practical skills of senior registrars in training compared with previous generations, seem to want to **extend** training by 2 years. In my opinion cutting consultant training by two years will bring them down to what was an SHO level in the 70's and 80's. A Department of Health spokesman was quoted as saying (Jan 2015) that Professor David Greenaway's recommendations on changes to consultant training would only be made if they were in the patient's interests. "The shape of training review" made its 19 recommendations in 2013. One idea was to shorten consultant training from its current 8-10 years to 6-8 years while another was to allow doctors to be registered to practice when they left medical school – not a year later as now. In 2016 the papers were quoting an all out cost during the strikes of £500,000 for GPs and £850,000 for Consultants. This was in the context of the one sixth of doctors who told interviewers that they were going to emigrate to Australia or New Zealand "For an easier life"!!

Given the inexperience and lack of confidence of newly FULLY qualified doctors now and the relative lack of skills of new GPs and consultants compared with their prede-cessors (see elsewhere in this section) this is just asking for trouble. Unless you improve (extend) the patient contact time, training and experience of those years.

As recently as June 2016 the Royal College of Physician's own Journal published a paper from Imperial College regarding the service contribution of specialist registrar grade junior doctors. This is one of our best teaching hospitals and specialist registrars are moti-vated, specialised and ambitious to succeed in their chosen speciality. This quoted: "With the adoption of the EWTD in 2003 and the increasing complexity and subspecialisation of medicine and increased consultant delivered care,

THERE IS A PERCEPTION THAT SPECIALIST REGISTRARS ARE NOT AS SKILLED, AUTONOMOUS OR CAPABLE AS THEY WERE IN PAST GENERATIONS" and "THERE HAVE BEEN CONCERNS IN THE UK THAT SINCE THE INTRODUCTION OF THE EWTD, TRAINEE'S EXPERIENCE OF THE PRACTICE OF MEDICINE HAS BEEN REDUCED SIGNIFICANTLY." "It has been estimated that presently trainees can expect to receive a total of 6,000 hours of training on average compared with the 30,000 hours they would have received in 1993"." A comparison of log books found that the proportion of theatre cases operated on inde-pendently by specialist registrars more than halved after the introduction of the EWTD".

How can higher grade junior doctors possibly be as competent, experienced or as safe as their forebears if they are seeing a fraction of the patients, doing less than half the hours and meanwhile complaining during their strike (which was about weekend and night working) that huge numbers of them were planning to emigrate for an easier life? I am sorry, but the hours that juniors currently do just clearly are not enough to learn their trade. 48 hours is in fact the AVERAGE working week of Londoners.

My prescription wouldn't be as cheap but it would be safer for the patient:

End the Working Time Directive which has been responsible for halving doctors' patient contact and experience throughout their training grades.

Build at least 5 new medical schools in the UK, as time and time again, even with their faults, British trained doctors out-perform most foreign trained doctors at all objective assessments of competence. Especially Membership examinations. Every government since the start of the NHS has filled its gaps with cheap foreign doctors. Why are we not prepared to train enough to supply our own NHS?

Restrict the number of female medical students to no more than 25% of the intake, as they do no more than 2/3 of the career hours, tend to be part time, want a restricted number of career options compared with male doctors and are not good value for money (see below, etc). We as a country have more and younger doctors today than at any time in history. They work fewer hours, are less experienced and take more time off for physical, emotional and stress related illness than when we worked up to three times the hours. They take infinitely more time on pregnancy and maternity related leave. As a consequence of this soft skinned and home focussed generation and despite their numbers, services are constantly restricted at short notice (paediatric units with 70% female junior staff, most on maternity leave, casualty units unable to afford agency locums as there are no male doctors in the standard employment pool and women don't do casualty) – see elsewhere.

Insist on a medical school entry contract committing that the doctor works in the UK for at least 5 years after qualifying. Full time.

I would also, before entry to medical school tell prospective students that medicine is a vocation, a life, something you have to dedicate yourself to heart and soul, not squeeze it in between social or childcare commitments. It is an apprenticeship and the more time you spend hands on patients the safer and better you become as a doctor. The patient comes first, if your on call session ends at five you should never, never, expect to be home before seven. Your family IS going to suffer and you won't necessarily be home to read the bedtime story or help your spouse when they are stressed. It can be a very rewarding, fulfilling job, which brings you closer to your fellow man, even perhaps to why we are here but it is often a deeply unpleasant, frightening and upsetting job. Now do you really want to do it?

Then slowly, probably over 5-10 years, we will start to have enough competent committed doctors to staff the NHS again. Even perhaps, to staff it with adequate weekend cover.

The Consultant Census showed that there are 1,221 consultant General physicians in the UK.

The largest speciality is Geriatric Medicine (1,252).

Acute Medicine had expanded the most in percentage terms at 33% but there were still only 393 Acute Medical consultants.

The largest expansion in actual consultant numbers was in Cardiology (to 1,066 consultants).

Various specialities got smaller and these included Audiovestibular Medicine, Endocrinology, Diabetes, General Medicine, Metabolic Medicine and Paediatric Cardiology. Given the diabetes time bomb currently exploding around us this is a little difficult to understand.

Various areas are short of consultants but not London. There are no specialities with low numbers in London. Outside London and especially in rural areas, some specialities are hard to fill but women now make up over half of the youngest age group of consultants (51.3% of the 34 years and younger). The report comments that "This changing demographic has transformed the working practices of consultant physicians with 17% of physicians overall less than full time, **39% of women part time – but only 5.3% of men part time.**

They don't comment on the negative effects this has on departmental organisation and planning. Part time availability of a consultant will clearly affect both junior staff and patients, have out of hours implications, increase overall cost (with two part timers doing the work of one), damage patient continuity and consistency of care and affect accessibility to her colleagues as well as ongoing relationships with patients. If she is unavailable half the time how can it be otherwise?

Do two job share doctors always share the same approach to managing the same conditions or even the same patients? The answer in my experience is a frustrating NO.

Most consultants are contracted to work a 42 hour week but actually worked slightly more.

Interestingly there is a slow move towards "Generalism" from Specialism (These should read "Generalisation" and "Specialisation") in the provision of medical care.

2% "never" enjoy their jobs, **more female consultants plan to retire early** (67.2% compared with 56.5% of men) and the reason commonly stated was "pressure of work."

So, overall we have women flooding into the consultant grades just as we do in General Practice. They are becoming the majority of younger consultants because of their dominant numbers but are being selective and restrictive about the specialities they are prepared to work in, the hours they work, the out of hours they do, having far more time off for a variety of reasons, including stress, other illness and family commitments, having a shorter career duration and retiring earlier. Just as in G.P. you have to ask who on earth is responsible for this, have they thought it through, what are the implications for service provision, what do the patients think about the new part time doctors (I know the answer) and can we actually afford it?

But mainly, how does this affect the care given to patients?

Medical Training:

Typical Modern Medical School Curriculum: MBBS

	Aug	Oct				June	July
		Clinical	Practice	1	(30 credits)	(Level 4)	
Year 1		Foundations of Health and Disease 30 credits Level 4		Heart Lungs Blood 30 Credits Level 5		Nutrition Metabolism and Excretion 30 Credits Level 5	

Phase 1

		Clinical	Practice	2	(30 credits)	(Level 5)	
Year 2		Neuroscience and Behaviour 30 credits Level 5		Reproduction and Endocrinology 30 credits Level 5		Musculoskeletal and Immune Systems 30 credits Level 5	

Year 3	Clinical Foundation Course 20 credits level 5	**Scientific Basis of Medicine** Medicine Surgery Reproductive and Child Health	**30 credits** Elderly Medicine and Mental Health	**Level 6** Revision and exam
	Clinical Foundation Course continued	Student selected components 10 credits Level 5		

Phase 2

		Specialist Rotations 60 credits Level 6	
Year 4	Clinical Elective 30 credits Level 6	General Practice and Population Medicine 30 credits Level 6 Individual Research Project 60 Credits Level 6	

	Regional attachment 1 40 credits Level 7	Regional attachments 2 and 3 80 credits Level 7	Revision Integrated Medicine Finals 60 credits level 7	Emergency Preparation for practice and student organised clinical experience
Year 5				

Phase 3

	Professional	Studies	online
	....................................Seminar programme..		

My only comment as an appraiser and trainer and a GP of 30 years is this: Most medicine in Britain is done by GPs. Often it is not done well because the complexity and breadth of General Practice is underestimated by all but those who are its full time practitioners. It is probably the hardest speciality to do well. Research on the other hand is done by no more than a few percent of doctors and very rarely in General Practice. Why on earth the research project module which will be of little long term real use to the student and will probably be spent aimlessly, is given double the credit value of the General Practice section just indicates how out of touch medical educators are with the reality of patients' and doctors' needs. It also indicates how little they value General Practice.

Typical modern Medical School Curriculum MBBS

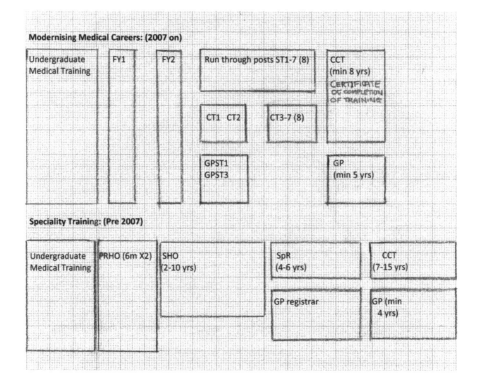

Modernising medical careers

At medical School and after the typical curriculum is:

MMC training (2007 onwards) (Modernising medical careers but could also stand for mostly maternity care, most men cancelled, medicine minus commitment),

Undergraduate medical training>FY1>FY2>Run through posts ST1-7(8)) >CCT (Min 8 yrs)

>CT1, CT2> CT3>7 (8))

>GPST1)

>GPST3-The "Stage of commitment to higher specialist training")...........GP (Min 5 yrs)

(Which stand for: Foundation year, Specialist training, Core Training, Higher Specialist Training, Certificate of Completion of Training)

So:

Preclinical 18 months,

Clinical

F1: 1 year with 4m rotations (House Officer equivalent)

F2: 1 year with 4m rotations (SHO equivalent)

ST1 (SHO) 1 year

ST2 (SHO) 1 year

ST3 1st year registrar

All the way to ST7

Consultant.

This may all change if the new structure of "The Shape of Training" comes into being.

Speciality Training (Pre 2007)

-This was when a working week often meant 72 hour work periods without a break, – in a total working week of 100 hours or more but the total patient experience gained by the doctor was hugely greater than now and doctors inevitably learned more and became more competent (better, safer) quicker.

I remember when the teaching profession was thinking of striking to cut its working week to less than 40 hours. My hospital colleagues and I used to laugh at their cheek. If we did a one in two, our working week was 136 hours, we could have done their 48 hours during part of the weekend between two standard working weeks.

Obviously it was harder, more stressful and tiring for the doctor and their social and family life was often absent. Perhaps people were just made of sterner stuff then. Most of us considered ourselves fortunate though to be in a flexible well paid profession, to be respected, to know that this phase would be short lived and that we owed the sponsors of our expensive education, the tax payer, some return on their investment. At some point we knew we would start to make a decent living and our own junior staff would take over some of the burden. There was some pride in coping with the arduous nature of the apprenticeship.

The Working Time Directive

The reduction of the working week from the already historically low 56 hours to 48 hours in 2009 resulted in 1400 hours lost from the average consultants' 5 year training. Sickness rates were now historically high, running at between 1.5 and 3.5%, with much higher rates in the FY2 year. They went up 300% with the introduction of the WTD and a good night's sleep. I regularly hear consultants who qualified 10-20 years ago complain about the quality and experience of other new consultants. This is said to be particularly evident in "practical procedures" such as endoscopies. GP trainers feel the same. I was amazed some of my registrars had never seen (or heard of) Status Epilepticus, or managed acute LVF. The RCP magazine now regularly runs articles on the fitness of newly qualified consultants and the suitability of their training. Hospital trainees were available "to train" only 66-80% of the time in one published survey. There were puzzling greater sickness absences with the reduction in the working week each time a further working time restriction was introduced. You can only explain this sea change in my opinion by an alteration in the personal psychology of medicine from a way of life to an occupation, a job. By a reduction in commitment, in dedication. From someone **you are** to something **you do**.

Newly qualified doctors seem to constantly complain about their long shifts and long working weeks these days. This was a constant self justifying refrain in the strike related medical correspondence in 2015/6 when increased weekend working (the 24/7 NHS) was being proposed by the government and vehemently rejected by junior doctors, on line, in the press and in every medical journal. The letters from junior doctors defending their weekend time at home with their families sounded like spoilt children who were going to be forced to help their parents with the housework. Their catch phrase was "Not safe/Not Fair." The first thing we teach our children about growing up is that real life as a responsible adult isn't fair. Two married doctors complained bitterly on Radio 4 about how hard it would be to find child care and to study if they had to work at weekends.

They lost almost the last ounce of my sympathy when I heard this. The final shred of sympathy was lost when the strikers refused care even for emergencies, for neonates, for women in labour and for ITU patients. This was something we would never have dreamt of when my generation struck in 1975, the year I qualified. In that year, on a one in two rota, my standard working week would have been 136 hours during my long week on call. The WTD restricts today's doctors to a third of those hours with the resulting reduced competence at all grades, reduced safety at practical procedures, reduced continuity on the wards (and clinical consistency for patients), poorer training for specialists and GPs in training grades, (which is so obvious that it has been suggested that medical training in various specialities should be extended), a junior work force that takes 3X the sickness leave and in the opinion of me and many colleagues, a far less dedicated and committed medical work force: Presumably despite their increased sickness absence and both physical and psychiatric ill health they would claim a better quality of life. Otherwise the shorter working week seems to have gained them nothing.

The brilliant neurosurgeon and author of "**Do no harm**" Henry Marsh put it like this: "It was at the time when the government was starting to reduce the long working hours of junior hospital doctors. The doctors were tired and overworked and it was said that patients lives were being put at risk. The junior doctors, however, rather than becoming ever more safe and efficient now that they slept longer at night had instead become increasingly disgruntled and unreliable. It seemed to me that this had happened because they were now working in shifts and had lost the sense of importance and belonging that came with working the long hours of the past." (*and lost their sense of commitment*) my itallics.

-He goes on to criticise the rapid turn-over of doctors holding the bleep in one 24 hour period on his neurosurgical team. He used to know his junior staff by name but no longer, they worked short shifts and weren't there long enough to build up a relationship with. "5 on call SHOs – Handing over to each other every four point two hours!" It's utter chaos. "

Utter chaos indeed. My wife was an in-patient over a weekend two years ago and asked four sequential registrars over the four days, Friday to Monday when she would be discharged. She received four contradictory answers from the four doctors, all of whom gave only their first names as identification and all it turned out each was wrong about the discharge. I assume they got their names right although I tried to contact one via the switch board and the telephonist couldn't identify the doctor. This was because at least three doctors in the hospital had the same first name. So much for reading the notes, continuity, communication and hand over. On my weekends on call I would have been the registrar on call each day Friday morning through 'til Monday night so NO problem with handover or continuity. And I would have given my full name.

Henry Marsh again:

"Junior doctors work such short hours that they are desperate for even the most basic surgical experience and I feel obliged to leave all of the opening and closing (of the skull) to them...... The intense anxiety I experience when supervising my juniors however, so much greater than when I operate myself means that I find it quite impossible to leave the theatres when they are operating on anything but the simplest of cases." He goes on to describe a junior whose inexperience leads him to mistake basic spinal anatomy and sever a lumbar nerve root during a simple spinal decompression procedure, which Mr Marsh thought was an easy, basic, foolproof operation but left an athlete permanently disabled. "The juniors are so inexperienced now, on the few occasions they are actually in the hospital that is......"

Average hours worked in various specialities also vary a great deal. For instance in one review, Palliative care saw an average of 38 hours a week while Cardiology was 54 hours. (EWTD etc Clinical Medicine 2011)

In General Practice in early 2017 the papers were full of apparent surprise at the number of GPs shutting up shop during normal working hours. GPs used to have a half day off in the week in recognition of their nights on call. Almost no GPs do nights on call covering their lists today but even full timers take a day off as their right. And call themselves full time! The National Audit Office found however that in the week that 40% of hospitals called a major alert, the first week in January, 46% of GP surgeries closed at some point during their core hours with 18% closing before 15.00 at least one weekday. Three quarters of those received extra funding in 2015-2016 to provide access outside of core hours. According to the Director of Acute Care for NHS England 30% of Casualty attendees would be better cared for elsewhere-presumably in their GP surgery if it were open.

Anyway, most senior doctors, in confidence if not on microphone accept that medical training and on call for junior doctors are far less rigorous and intense these days, that they certainly are not the test of emotional resilience as well as clinical competence that they used to be, that junior staff are probably less committed, heart and soul to the life of medicine compared with previous generations and that the NHS and patient safety are the worse off because of it:

The current GP training system:

The Trainee Year:

The Registrar now maintains an e Portfolio on the computer up to date throughout the year with a theoretical 2-3 entries per week. These should show their development/ progress and the Trainer gives constructive feedback on these entries.

There is a common set of guidelines and regulations covering all medical training including GP. This is commonly called the Gold Guide 2010 though formally titled "A Reference Guide for Postgraduate Speciality Training in the UK".

All GP trainees have to do 3 years of an approved training programme of which 18 months has to be in GP. The years are often referred to as ST1, ST2 and ST3 (ST = specialty training year). When a trainee joins a programme, they are given a National Training Number (NTN) which stays with them until they complete their training.

During the three years the trainee is clinically and educationally supervised. Clinical Supervision is about helping them to acquire clinical knowledge, skills and attitudes (and gain competence) whilst educational supervision focuses on their educational development and making sure that learning gaps are identified and worked on. That is the theory anyway.

Throughout the training programme, the trainee is assessed using Work Place Based Assessments (WPBA) – things like Case Based Discussion (CBD), Multi-Source Feedback (MSF) from colleagues and Direct Observation of Procedural (clinical) Skills (DOPS), Patient Satisfaction Questionnaires, (PSQs) and COTS (Case Observational Tools) and so on. The trainee needs to demonstrate "competency progression" throughout their training period through these WPBA assessments and a log of their learning/clinical experiences. All of this is kept in an electronic folder called the e-portfolio. They obviously need to satisfy their educational supervisors.

Every ST year, the trainee's e-portfolio is assessed by an independent panel called the ARCP (Annual Review of Competency Progression Panel). If progress is good they will give an "Outcome 1" though there may be comments on this that need to be followed. If the panel has some concern but progress is good enough for the next job to be taken up then an "Outcome 2" is likely to be given. On the other hand if there are concerns that not enough progress has been made, the trainee will have to repeat a period of training and "Outcome 3" is given. By the end of training the trainee needs to have taken two examinations. One is a multiple choice paper testing knowledge (called the Applied Knowledge Test or AKT) and the other is a special OSCE type exam where they are tested on a variety of clinical and communication skills. This is called the Clinical Skills Assessment or CSA, using simulated patients.

Communication and culture:

The British Association of Physicians of Indian Origin, BAPIO, called for the CSA to be made "Culturally Neutral" in June 2014 following public concern at foreign doctors' high failure rates in the MRCGP exam. This begs various questions: Should the goal posts be moved to suit one particular sub group of examinees? Can any country, any patient, any set of partners or any consultation ever really be "Culturally Neutral"? Is General Practice culturally neutral? Is any patient culturally neutral? Is it a doctor's job to be as adapted as possible to the patients he works with or the country he works in so that communication is optimised and misunderstanding minimised? You might expect travellers to a new country working in medicine to be obliged to make stringent efforts to improve communication and compromises to that country's traditions and norms (when in Rome) but the Association's president also went on to say: **"The question is of their language skills, communication skills and the cultural differences. We think that is the problem, we don't believe there is any problem regarding their competency to practise as GPs."** **(GP Online 27th May 2014)**

Did I hear that right? So GPs don't need to communicate, to understand English fluently? They don't need to relate at a personal identity, cultural background level with their patients? What??-How can you be so out of touch with the real feelings, the background, the whole purpose of the consultation? Don't family doctors have to try to relate to their patients, to understand them, where each patient is "coming from", what "makes them tick", what has prompted the consultation, the why this, why now?, to pick up subtle clues and cues?

Well of course they do. GPs almost more than any other kind of doctor. A consultation is a complicated interaction. When I have had patients talk about unsatisfactory consultations with foreign doctors it is exactly their misunderstanding of spoken and colloquial English, affectionate cheekiness, their failure to understand or accept humour, sarcasm, irony, informal social and professional challenge, often misinterpreted as a personal criticism, the tendency of some foreign doctors to default to "literalism" and their cultural and linguistic distance that alienates them from the patient, not their medical knowledge. In a Maslow's hierarchy of General Practice, language and culture are even more basic than personality and attitude. Ironically, I know and have worked with numerous Indian and Pakistani doctors who get this completely right and fit in personally, socially and culturally, perfectly. One of my best registrars and I had a long running joke about his love of gardening which he regularly "deweeded" – so much more rational than "weeded" when you think that "seeded" means putting down seeds not pulling them up. I would have trusted him and many other foreign trained doctors I have worked with, with my life. But I estimate about a quarter I have known or appraised just don't get the huge importance of British culture and the nuances of the English language in doing medicine. Nor I may say do The GMC, The RCGP, The DoH, the Appraisal authorities or apparently, BAPIO.

The British Association Of Physicians of Indian Origin took the RCGP to court over the alleged racism of the MRCGP examination CSA test based on the number of Indian candidates failing the exam. They lost the case but got a sympathetic summing up from the predictably liberal judge and the, to me, inexplicable advice to try again. In July 2015 it was announced that candidates would be given not four but five attempts at the CSA and AKT sections. This was after the RCGP lengthened the exam so that those not proficient in English were not disadvantaged (Oct 2014). July 2015 was the same month that a major medical school entry exam scandal broke in India where blank MCQ forms were being handed in to be filled in by paid insiders, substitute imposters were taking entrance exams, questions were being handed out in advance and several whistle blowers had been murdered. Over here we are easing up the requirements of the already basically fairly straight forward CSA and AKT exams. What are patients going to think now when their new GP has scraped through the membership exam on the 5th attempt and just doesn't seem to understand what is being asked in a consultation?

How about taking the politics out of this quality selection process? From a patient's perspective and a safety point of view, the racial and ethnic sensitivities of the doctor regarding the professional assessment of his ability should be irrelevant. The only thing that matters is competence. Why shouldn't we let some impartial patients' representatives rather than lawyers, vested interest groups, politically motivated doctors and academics take a look at the skills and background of some of our doctors and how they are assessed-how about that for a change? Forget Equality and Diversity if it means dumbing down. For the patients' sake give us Quality and Uniformity.

When the ST3 trainee has successfully done everything and is deemed competent, they are given a certificate to "signpost" that they have reached the competency level required for independent safe general practice (called the CCT – Certificate of Completion of Training also known as ARCP "Outcome 4").

The Gold Guide[4]

This is a reference guide for postgraduate training in the UK for all medical specialties including general practice. Written by the UK Scrutiny Group (led by the four UK Chief Medical Officers – England, Scotland, Northern Ireland and Wales). The first edition came out in August 2007 and has been updated periodically ever since through an iterative process of feedback from various stakeholders. The standards and requirements set by the General Medical Council (GMC) are extensively quoted in the Gold Guide to ensure that its recommendations are underpinned by them and the GMC's other publication Good Medical Practice.

It sets out the arrangements for competency based specialty training and primarily deals with the operational side of things – providing recommendations for things like approving training programmes, flexible training, Educational Supervision, ARCP panels, remedial training and so on. In short, if you're uncertain about anything in relation to training, look it up in the Gold Guide first (although it is primarily aimed at Royal Colleges, Deaneries, Local Education Providers and TPDs).

The Gold guide is available online on the MMC website: http://www.mmc.nhs.uk

What happens after training?

The First Five Initiative

This provides educational and peer support for newly qualified GPs up to five years. They usually run conferences, meetings and social events to help new GPs "network" and find their bearings. Contact your local RCGP office to find the nearest one to you.

After that?

The education available to all well established and new GPs is variable and depends on what your locality trust provides. For example, nearly all trusts provide an educational afternoon periodically where medical cover is provided for your practice. You are also expected to engage in practice based learning on a regular basis – where your practice comes together to learn from and solve local problems and issues in a collaborative way. Then there are evening courses – some sponsored, others not. And let's not forget the RCGP – local RCGP offices are now becoming more and more proactive. Most local faculties now have an educational programme of events – check out what yours provides now. Go to www.rcgp.org.uk and scroll to the bottom right where it says 'Find your local RCGP'.

The configuration in different Deaneries can be at variance with this map. For example, Scotland does not have APDs and TPDs – instead, they have Associate Advisors who seem to do both of these jobs. The presence of Deputy Directors depends on the size of the deanery. Some deaneries will e.g. have a team of Associate Postgraduate Deans whose overall specialities including GP. It would be impractical to present an array of different map configurations and our aim here is to give you some sort of idea about how things might look – which is better than nothing.

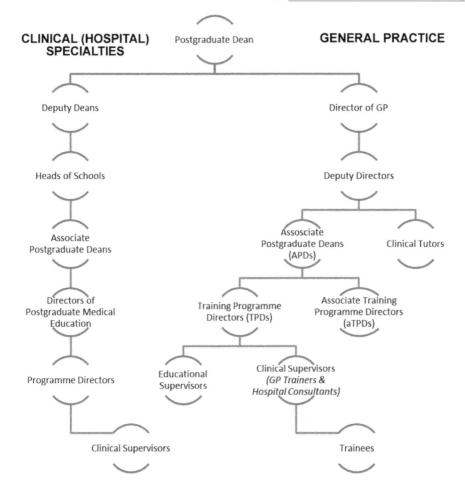

Caution 2: Some of the terms may be different in different Deaneries. For example, some areas use the term Course Organisers for TPDs – both having the same role and responsibilities.

MY THANKS TO THE BRILLIANT BRADFORD TRAINING WEBSITE AND TO THE INCREDIBLY HELPFUL RAMESH MEHAY FOR HIS PERMISSION IN REPRODUCING THIS.

What is General Practice?:

GPs see more than 300 million patients a year. The number of consultations per patient per year and the reasons for coming have grown inexorably since the NHS was formed in 1948. The role of the GP is now not just Gate Keeper to the panoply of NHS services but also counsellor, general medical expert, the main NHS provider of psychiatry, paediatrics, dermatology, ENT, gynaecological, family planning, rheumatology, sports medicine, preventative services, dietary advice, child guidance, lifestyle advice, indeed every medical speciality there is – apart from surgery and a few rarities like Nuclear Medicine and Imaging. Indeed in my region over the last ten years we have had virtually no effective secondary care psychiatry or adolescent mental health services, no Family Therapy, no

Psychology, Educational Psychology services and next to no Health Visiting – so GPs were primary and secondary care in these areas too.

The work load is changing and increasing but I don't remember a time in the last thirty years when we as a profession weren't "at breaking point". GPs already do the vast majority of NHS patient interactions. There was a 95% growth in the consultation rate for people aged 85-89 in the 10 years up to 2008. These, of course are the group with the most complex and multiple medical "needs", (hateful word) treatments, complications, side effects, drug interactions and symptoms. General consultation rates are rising: From 3.9/patient/year in 1995-96 to 5.5 consultations/patient/year in 2008/9. In 1995/6 10% of GP consultations were in the patient's home, but by 2008/9 actual house calls had dropped to 3%.

In the last couple of decades though we have begun treating more and more complicated demanding patients in the community. End stage heart failure, salvaged stroke victims, elderly diabetics and cancer patients, severe COPD, those with multiple conditions now survive at home partly because there are new treatments for their conditions, because of the off loading from secondary care of patients that were traditionally their domain and partly because of the catastrophic reduction in hospital beds over the last two decades.

GPs act as legal advisors, providers of signatures, legal and statutory permission granters and guarantors of everything from certificates for the performing of children on stage at Christmas, for teenagers embarking on outward bound courses, insurance claims and so on. Official countersignatures now seem essential for the simplest process, to attend nursery school – free of infection, for licences to do dangerous sports, to dive, fly, even to go on some school trips or "week at work" experience attachments (can you believe it?) The Primary Care Physician has to be expert in social care services and nursing homes, interpreter of the medical terminology (and sometimes the actual language) spoken by hospital doctors, an expert on personalities, skills and services of secondary care doctors and providers. They are the giver of the best terminal care for patients-that of dying with dignity at home supervised by an expert family friend who is available 24 hours a day. This is now more important than ever. It is, as with so much, influenced by the commitment of the GP you are lucky or unlucky enough to have. The GP gives personal, medical, social, family and psychological advice in a "what would you do if you were me?" format and is the bearer of blame for a huge number of factors over which he (and increasingly she) has no control.

General Practice is a culture shock for junior hospital doctors who are protected and supported by their extended professional teams, Consultant down to Houseman, their 24 hour nursing support, reassurance and feedback, investigations on hand, the relatively stable environment, bright lights, reliable observers and the reasonable hope that their instructions on treatment and care will be carried out. No so in the community.

It is all a bit more nebulous and frustrating in General Practice. It took me years to control my frustration and disbelief at patients who returned a month after a consultation or who phoned a week later complaining they were no better but saying that they hadn't taken the prescribed medicine and therefore ignored everything that I had said to them because they had read the potential side effects on the drug data sheet. The inference was that I was trying to harm them.

Once I made the mistake of mentioning my view that these inserts did more harm than good to one patient. I had always thought that I got on well with him before this. I received through the PCT a formal complaint from him about my dangerous lack of professionalism a week later. It turned out his job was to write patient data inserts for one of the local pharmaceutical manufacturers.

The relationship, the trust in and the interdependence between doctor and patient is much closer in General Practice than hospital medicine, far more personal. Indeed I firmly believe that the GP has to be able to trust the patient as much as the other way round and if the patient is free to leave the practice when trust "breaks down" then the doctor should just as readily end the registration when the patient makes an unreasonable complaint or shows no empathy with the doctor. At present the GMC says this is not ethical. But then there are virtually no GPs on the GMC despite 90% of doctor patient interactions taking place in General Practice. This is a bit like the Professional footballers' Association being staffed, managed and run only by the turnstile operators isn't it? The turnstile operators say you cannot remove a patient from your list if you find it impossible to have a trusting confiding relationship, don't get on, can't get through to one another or just plain dislike each other.

GP wasn't my first choice in career. I spent 5-6 years following a Paediatric hospital career, finally lecturing it at a teaching hospital and doing locum consultant jobs in peripheral hospitals. It was at this point in my career that I took a sabbatical to do a trainee year in GP.

Although I loved Paediatrics, I realised that I didn't want the quality of my care to be based on the number of beds, the training of and number of the nurses, the quality of the junior doctors, whether you had a registrar on with you – not all district general hospitals did in those days outside teaching hospital rotations. Would the SHOs be career Paediatricians or GP trainees? Would they need to be baby sat 24 hours day every few months when a fresh batch with no Paediatric experience arrived? There would be a multiplicity of factors outside my control influencing the quality of my care. The lack of independence came home to me when I wanted to prescribe a new antibiotic for a sick child, this was Co Amoxiclav – a new drug at the time and I was told I couldn't as it wasn't on the hospital pharmacopoeia. Local GPs had been using it for months and the alternatives available were far less effective in my opinion. This was decades before the current preoccupation with super infections, back when the greater concern was death from sepsis and Scarlet Fever was a rare condition.

As I did my GP trainee year, I began to realise that I valued the personal and individual ethos of GP and particularly the independence to refer and treat in my own way when I only had the patient and my conscience to answer to – and this was actually the essence of real personalised medicine.

But the independence of General Practice is also the isolation of General Practice. We are not team players and if we don't want to, we don't have to refer to or confer with partners and colleagues – and that can be a very lonely place to work.

I had taught paediatrics to students and junior staff at a busy hospital/medical school before going into General Practice. This was a University Academic Department of Paediatrics. The teaching and ethos there was focussed on the practical problems of recognising, diagnosing and treating ill health in babies and children. It was a practical discipline and directed at diagnosis and cure. It was completely unlike the largely theoretical, hands off, academic and class room based training that GP trainers are given and instructed to give their registrars. This I soon found was the downside of General Practice – the apparent irrelevance, disorganisation and unworldliness of much *academic* General Practice and GP academic staff compared that of other, older medical specialities.

When I became a trainer of GPs and started the trainers' course (one year of education theory and various assessments of practical and theoretical knowledge) I thought that GP was par excellence the medical speciality which should be learnt by practical apprenticeship and not hypothetically. All my experience of medical education has confirmed that impression since. I remember my own trainee year attached to a brilliant, unpretentious GP who was kind and humane and taught me common sense, managing risk, living with uncertainty and developing patience. He would have laughed at the thought that you needed a Membership examination to call yourself a GP. My abiding memory – and this was pre Shipman, was one that had a huge positive impression on me and was of us visiting a new resident in a nursing home. She had been sent out of hospital to die alone – probably because they needed the in-patient bed. Semi conscious and riddled with metastatic cancer she was 7stone, dehydrated, confused, in awful visceral pain and incurable. I have no idea why the hospital had shipped her out in this state. My trainer read the notes, spoke soothingly to her and the nurse, examined her gently and took from his bag some injectable Diamorphine. It was only 5mg, – a small dose. He told her what he was doing throughout and he wrote her up for some oral pain relief to take over once the injection had worn off. He and I returned 2 hours later but she had already died peacefully. I was shocked and simultaneously impressed with the rightness, kindness, care and empathy of what he had done. He had relieved pain and ended her life when nothing else was possible. In hospital and these days particularly, the process would have been inhumane, bureaucratic, taken days, followed some sort of rigid protocol and led to profound misery of the relatives and the patient. This institutionalised regimented inhumanity inevitably leads to the depersonalisation of the staff and the despair of relatives who often comment on the relative and ironic **humanity** of the vetinary care they have witnessed compared with human terminal care. How often we hear: "You wouldn't let a dog suffer like this" and no, we wouldn't.

How having to cope with so much suffering and death in their professional life can often blunt the emotions of doctors and the way they deal with suffering in their own families is a subject completely ignored at medical school and afterwards. But it does have a profound effect on each of us. The GMC now wants "Emotional Resilience" taught at medical school after a series of doctors committed suicide while under investigation by the GMC itself. The GMC is taking measures to address this (2016) at long last. Are doctors today less resilient now than we were a few decades ago? Has the easier training, the freedom from "training by humiliation", the far less testing maximum 48 hours a week, the constant supervision and feedback, the 70% feminisation, the human rights preoccupation, the Occupational Health support (nonexistent when I was a hospital doctor) changed the mind set of doctors from "It's a tough career and I am no use to anyone if I crumble" to "If I am uncomfortable with this, it isn't fair, I will get more support".

As a post script, and by now after the Shipman scandal, I mentioned how the ending of a hopelessly ill patient's life can sometimes be a correct, loving, ethical and humane act at one of the trainers' meetings saying that it exemplified the independence, professional freedom, common sense, humanity and closeness to the patient's best interests of GPs at their best. At the end of the session I was taken aside with great seriousness and cross examined by a course organiser. He had missed the point completely and a week later I was summoned to an interview with the Dean of our Deanery asking me to explain myself. Neither of them had understood the essence of what I had said, neither of them had stepped outside their institutional instruction book of what Family medicine is and how it should be taught. I certainly hope they were better doctors than they were teachers or lateral thinkers. That inflexibility of thought is one difference between the teachers and the doers in medicine – the academics and the practitioners. It was the first of many instances for me of how out of touch many doctors "in authority" have become in medicine-especially in General Practice. Especially in General Practice education.

How is GP different from every other realm of medicine?

Think of the following Family Medicine issues:

Ending life at home, compared with hospitals or hospices. It is far more involved and personal. If you are a good GP you may give the patient's family your home phone number. I don't believe you can really do Family Medicine properly, committedly, and live outside your practice area. Home IS where we all would prefer to die and it is facilitated and at best managed 24 hours a day at home by a good GP. Consider how the part-timism, job sharing, port folio careers and the feminisation, sorry to harp on at this, – all overtaking GP now with a direct negative effect on continuity of care have affected this particular bench mark of good practice. I was at a medical evening meeting recently where I asked all the other doctors (about twenty in all, two thirds of them female, – how many carried controlled drugs in their bags? (the answer: only one doctor, me), who would offer to be available to a terminal patient 24 hours a day? (three doctors, all male) how many worked part time? (about half, all female). Who, I thought, would be of any use to a terminally ill patient who wanted to die at home?

While we are on the subject of the overwhelming but surreptitious negative change that the **Feminisation of General Practice and medicine in Britain** is having on the provision of health care, there was a debate in the broadcast media about the "Crisis in General Practice" in June 2014. It was said that the "perfect storm" of a reduced funding share of GP and increased patient and contract demands would result in longer waiting times to see the doctor:

A doctor commenting on The Today Program was a West Country female GP. She said that she and her colleagues were planning to retire as soon as they could and there were very few applicants for the jobs advertised. But the most interesting questions were not asked: How many career years had **she** done and were they full time, how many years had she had off, how much sickness and maternity leave, had she been a full time partner? – How many of her local vocational training scheme's output were full time male doctors, what percentage of her local medical school's output were female and therefore destined to be part time and not interested in partnership anyway? These are all issues related to the sex of the doctor and the quality of the care they give the patient. But most of all to the **availability of care.**

It turns out that in recent years salaried GP numbers have increased by 400% mainly because fewer doctors want to become full time and take on the extra duties and responsibilities of partnership if they are the main family carers. In the same radio debate, although the government announced they had increased GP numbers by 1000, GPs as a percentage of all NHS doctors had fallen from 34% to 25% over 5 years. Don't forget that GPs do

90% of the work of the Health Service. What no one in the debate, or in the coverage or discussion of it ever seems to highlight is that medical schools with their feminised intake and output and the tidal wave of female doctors with their inherent and voluntary career restrictions may contribute to the total numbers but they don't contribute proportionately to the hours worked, the career choices or the continuity of care as compared with the shrinking male medical population.

Even the politically correct GMC announced in its **"State of Medical Education and Practice in the UK"** Report in Oct 2014 that 44% of registered doctors, 54% doctors in training and 57% medical students are female. They say that female doctors are breaking into more traditional male areas like surgery and emergency medicine (-well not really, looking at the figures) and more European doctors are coming to work here (-not necessarily an unalloyed benefit to our patients, – see above and more of this later). This was, of course, pre-Brexit.

The particular problems of Family Medicine:

Acute Care In the Community:

One major and harmful result of this demographic change to part-timism has been a slow and progressive withdrawal from **providing any acute care** in General Practice. The hammer blow was the Blair/Brown opt out of OOH and the subsequent end of the mostly excellent Cooperatives but most GPs have now undergone a change in mindset over their predecessors too. This is best exemplified by the fact that 90% of GPs are now unwilling to carry strong pain killers like Diamorphine, essential in the management of acute coronary syndromes, heart failure, terminal breathlessness, a multiplicity of acute accidents, injuries and severe pain. Perhaps it is unreasonable to link femininity to an aversion for acute or emergency medicine but I have worked with doctors who did house calls with no more than a prescription pad, auriscope and a stethoscope and I have heard colleagues say that GP is not an acute service and their management of chest pain is to dial 999. They have all been women. There are now many reports from cancer charities on the poor pain control in community settings at the end of life. Again, if your GP doesn't "do Diamorphine", doesn't live in the practice area, isn't used to night calls, even for the rare terminally ill patient at home and makes no exceptions due to (her) family commitments or her part time contract then you will know what the loss of the full time, committed GP really means to patients. Unfortunately for the doctor, she is missing the most rewarding part of Family Medicine too.

Becoming involved personally in families: Something the GMC specifically warns against but personal friendships and the building up of relationships within communities is inevitable and I believe beneficial when the GP lives and works surrounded by his or her patients. Unless he or she is a robot.

Likewise, becoming involved in community life – schools, churches, politics, Brownies, Beavers, choirs golf clubs and so on. Good or bad, pros and cons? How do those relationships, irrelevant to most hospital doctors, certainly junior hospital doctors, affect your objectivity to the patient?

How to behave in public when everyone knows who you are. Do you use the local pub, do you express political views, run for the council?

How often do you get the patient to come back?: – To see you? Some GPs will go out of their way not to invite the patient back after *any* acute illness. They may fear causing dependence, adding to their workload or setting a precedent. GPs already have busy surgeries without making them worse. But for the patient this is a crucial test of the quality of the doctor and often a stamp of reassurance. "Come back if you aren't better, if the swelling hasn't settled, If you are still in pain but give it one week, two weeks, etc." Do you suggest that the patient makes a phone call and when do you suggest that they can make it ? – All these are considerations which will be new to most hospital doctors who have a more formal appointment and follow up system than the threadbare safety net of the GP.

How do you avoid taking sides?: In divorce situations, when the parents drag in a recalcitrant teenager with "behaviour problems", when one individual wants cosmetic surgery, sterilisation, or in other family conflicts and when you are used as the family's objective expert? How do you avoid, or should you avoid personal anecdotes, personal involvement or relating your own similar experiences in reassuring patients who are worried or even having an **emotional involvement** in a patient's predicament? There was a recent radio debate about psychiatrists who cried during difficult consultations (they were American) and generally this was shown to be unhelpful, not to say harmful to the relationship and outcome. Enough empathy is good – but not too much.

Death at home:

One of the most emotionally rewarding moments in your professional life is the cup of tea at 3 in the morning and the hug in the kitchen after you have certified the parent or relative who has just died upstairs. If this happens to you, hopefully you have been available and supportive, you will have helped to keep a known and familiar patient out of the Hospital or Hospice and in the heart of their family. With any luck you have been an extended part of the family and enabled a dignified home death. A hug and even perhaps a few tears if you feel like it, might be acceptable then. Never mind the GMC forbidding personal involvement, virtually none of THEM have done family medicine or ever been in this situation. (There is only one person with GP experience on the GMC council.)

Some Sacrilege:

It might be worth mentioning that the Hospice team, universally admired and generally very caring and supportive to patients and relatives at home at the end of life can **sometimes** be bossy, over controlling and rigid especially regarding drug doses and administration. They can forget that the good GP is the first port of call and a familiar face to the patient and you, the family doctor, must try to retain overall control clinically. This must be without disturbing the apparent unity of purpose as far as the patient is concerned. Never air differences of management or treatment in front of the patient or the relatives. Obviously.

I have certainly been involved in terminal care situations where hospice doctors and nurses have paradoxically been protocol driven, inflexible and insensitive and in my opinion emotionally drained and lacking empathy.

Do you ever moralise?: I find it difficult to be as openly empathetic with people whose immoral, violent, selfish, self destructive or abusive behaviour I disapprove of – despite ethical guidelines against being judgmental. Recurrent child abusers, the regularly violent or drug dealers being examples. I am not a machine, I would be useless in some GP roles if I were, but I try hard not to let my internal disapproval influence my medical decision making. Even if it sometimes stops me showing my normal universal sympathy and friendliness. Even GPs are allowed human feelings and sometimes you have to voice these in some way for your own mental health. I believe somewhere in the Human Rights Act is a clause saying we are allowed to resent and disapprove of people whose actions harm others. All caring people are allowed to have feelings.

"Denying reasonable feelings leads to their repression, repression leads to conflict, conflict leads to anger, anger leads to hate, hate leads to the dark side"

Yoda

How hard is **being "professional" with unpleasant people:** in awkward, threatening or difficult situations and what does professional mean? I am still trying to answer this after 40 years.

The **Art rather than the Science of General Practice**: The "instinct" rather than the clever signs and the theory. Much of what I do "Just works". It has no evidence base and is hard to teach and justify. This is why GP is an apprenticeship, cannot be learnt in class rooms and has as much to do with personality as intelligence.

You could argue that the obsessional 3 or 4 A-star student who passes all the exams and who tends to have little emotional intelligence or warmth by virtue of their personality would make the worst possible GP. You need Dr Watson not Sherlock Holmes. Indeed Arthur Conan Doyle was a GP in Portsmouth before he became a successful crime writer. Apparently he wasn't a very good GP – at least not a financially successful one.

Managing boredom, sameness, trivia and repetition: while maintaining a reasonable index of suspicion for the rare hot child with meningitis or the odd abdominal pain that is early appendicitis or ovarian cancer-This is probably the hardest part of being a good GP.

Communicating with the increasingly naive, unreasonable, **inexperienced and distant hospital junior doctors** who have a limited set of reasons for agreeing to see the patient that you are worried about and know nothing about GP. Even worse these days is **the gate keeping educated nurse**. I know of many examples where a GP's concern for a patient, based on actually having SEEN the patient and on the experience of decades has been dismissed by a specialised nurse working to a set of admission guidelines. This is a system sanctioning and encouraging risk. The GP then has to put the facts in a synthetic language that the admitting "health professional" can digest, understand and accept. Even if all of what he says is not completely true. The nurse or SHO won't these days accept the fact that you have done the job for 30-40 years and, for instance, the baby is a bit floppy, unresponsive and sickly and you are worried about it. You have seen this before, it can end badly for the patient if you don't act on your gut instinct quickly and by the way, you don't send in every sick child you see like some doctors. The receiving doctor is never in post long enough to get to know the local GPs that they **can** trust. I do admit that there are experienced, confident and competent GPs on the one hand and there are also insecure, frightened and over referring GPs on the other. It would be nice if we could say that the more experienced of us were Consultant or Senior Registrar GPs and just expect to have our opinions trusted but MRCGP and FRCGP don't these days represent clinical excellence especially if you can take parts of the exam 5 times so how do you differentiate the clinical skills of one GP from another if you are a temporary hospital doctor?

Sometimes as the admitting GP you will have to say the child has a capillary return of 4 seconds, 5-10% dehydration, respiratory indrawing and so on. Even if these things are not strictly true. They will usually understand why you sent the child in when he or she arrives at the hospital. I am afraid this is the new NHS and it is one designed by educators and academics with very narrow clinical perspectives and very few beds. It is one that does not take account of experience, knowledge or mutual trust or one that puts the interests of the patient in front of the system. **Gut instinct**, by the way, has been shown on a number of occasions to be an objectively reliable indicator of occult serious illness or impending ill health in a patient with ill defined symptoms – when the gut belongs to an experienced GP.

Dealing with **unreasonable patients, unreasonable expectations**, demand, rudeness, being nice to people you would never want to have round to dinner. That is probably one of the hardest parts of living and working in the community.

Knowing your own limitations, dealing with professional and personal **isolation and loneliness**, communication and **partnership problems** – often the main issues raised at Appraisal, cultivating an apparent bonhomie with patients, maintaining a genuine empathy and keeping a protective professional detachment with the patient all at the same time. You are a problem solving actor, counsellor, advisor, friend, eternally optimistic and ever knowledgeable, friendly and caring but not too affectionate. Supportive and understanding you are always aware of "professional boundaries". Well that is the theory.

These are some of the issues of day to day General Practice which hospital doctors are unprepared for.

Training: The Consultation:

"**Where many ethicists go wrong in promoting patient autonomy is as a kind of ultimate value in medicine rather than recognizing it as one value among others. Schneider found that what patients want most from doctors isn't autonomy per se: it's competence and kindness.**"
Atul Gawande "Complications"

The trouble with doctors today compared with when the NHS started is that most doctors, especially GPs, think they can do the job without getting off their backsides. They consult with their ears, voices and their prescription pads. It has become a sedentary occupation. Their eyes are mostly on a screen and they rarely touch the patient because that means a hypothetical risk of being blamed for assault or spreading or getting an infection – and getting out of their seat. They ask, listen and talk. They rarely examine and even more rarely examine adequately. Good doctors don't just consult with their ears, they use their eyes, hands, stethoscopes, ophthalmoscopes, tongue depressors – any relevant instrument and sense that they have available. They also know that the patient often has to get undressed.

The Consultation:

There are as many styles of consulting, as many relationships between doctors and patients as there are doctors. Personality, experience, gender, culture and mood are more important factors than consulting styles or techniques. There are however three basic approaches to how you can impart caring, advice and information in any consultation more complicated than a brief interaction and these are:

The Paternalistic Relationship: This is the traditional old style experienced doctor and the dependent patient. The doctor knows best and the patient seeks enlightenment in the form of information as to what is wrong and how to get better. The doctor tells the patient what medicine or treatment to take and if and when to come back. This is how all medicine has worked for everyone except royalty since the concept began-except for the last 5-10 years.

The Informative Relationship. The patient gives a list of symptoms, the doctors says what is the matter or what must be done to elucidate the cause and asks what the patient wants to be done.

Most modern doctors like this approach as they believe it does not patronise the patient. Many patients reply by saying what would you do if you were me doctor?

The Interpretive Relationship: The patient gives the doctor his symptoms, the doctor helps the patient interpret what they mean and then work out his needs and wants in the light of that.-What is most important to you? Many patients will reply "Getting better."

The truth is, like every analysis of consulting, the rules are there to be ignored or bent. You will start off with Informing, then Interpreting and if you start overrunning your 7 1/2 minutes you may well resort to being paternalistic – I would.

When I retired from full-time practice, my patients remonstrated with me about "doctors today" (meaning new GPs, registrars and locums) and how they don't listen but seem to be distant, preoccupied, self absorbed.

Much of their dissatisfaction was that it takes years, even decades for patients on a list to get used to the personality of their doctor. Once this bedding in has taken place however, the structure of care is one valued highly for its continuity, familiarity, unspoken understanding, empathy, inherent short cuts and shared experience. Conversely, the doctor accommodates and adapts to the personality of the list. But many patients are increasingly frustrated with their inability to "get to know" part time, sessional and locum doctors. To get to like them. "Alright for a sore throat but what if you actually want to talk to them?" said one mature for his age teenager. This is much worse in the increasing numbers of very large practices, a trend that many part time doctors and medical organisations espouse but patients *well*, **hate.**

In an half page Sunday Times critique subtitled "Sickened by the bedside manner of many doctors, a new vice chancellor will shake up medicine by teaching students mind-fulness", Sian Griffiths wrote about Sir Anthony Seldon in May 2015. He was the Head of Wellington College who was about to take over as Vice Chancellor of Britain's first private University. (£35,000/year fees for the medical degree). He had seen a lot of doctors, having had parents and a wife who had suffered cancer and many sick or injured students over the years. He had been struck by doctors' "Worrying inattention, – there are lots of doctors who are simply not present when they are in front of their patients, they are all over the place, thinking ahead to the next thing.""-They do not connect with their patients, because their minds are very often elsewhere." To me this is the too important, too busy syndrome, made even worse now by the ironic patronising universal use of first names and slovenly dress. **Doctors today: too important, too busy, too informal, too scruffy, too alien.**

Seldon wanted to change this by introducing reflective meditation (mindfulness) for medical students. He said "You cannot be good doctor until you learn to be mindful, calm, present, attentive, listening to the patient, so they do not come back with the wrong treatments." He blames the curriculum of medical schools for the disconnection from the patient. "Because it is not in the culture of the teaching hospitals-the curriculum is very cerebral. If you do not have doctors and nurses who are showing **a sense of loving and dedication to the patient,** you may as well be wired to a computer." Hear Hear.

I think the very selection criteria for medical school, the three A stars and the academic bias prevents those with more empathetic and emotional qualities coming to the fore. It may be oversimplifying but we talk of intellectual and emotional intelligence, head and heart. We have been selecting doctors without heart for at least two decades now. Perhaps we need a better way of selecting candidates for medical schools than we do now. Don't we realise yet that at least 90% of doctors do not need to be particularly intelligent to do an excellent job?

You could also argue and I do, that many new doctors are self important and distant or appear so because of many reasons:

Let's look at some:

Modern medical practice (apart from rolled up sleeves and the absence of ties) is based on hard evidence, – or it is supposed to be. However, some things just work: A prescription for high dose multivitamins may make a Glandular Fever or flu ridden teenager get some energy quicker if prescribed with care, suggestion, support and encouragement. Steroid nose drops in infants stop the cough of post nasal drip and the deafness of glue ear. Plain oral Penicillin will improve many sore throats quicker than just waiting – so if a patient has suffered severe tonsillitis in the past and is desperate to avoid the same misery again, it is one of the safest and most appreciated responses we as doctors can make. It also prevents, or would have prevented the current tidal wave of Scarlet Fever and Tonsillitis. But the evidence based scientist just out of GP training hasn't got the sense to realise that there is far more to the consultation and the therapeutic relationship than a pure, rigid evidence base. Sometimes vitamins or Penicillin do more in vivo than in vitro.

I have had three miserable hospital admissions in thirty years with maxillary sinusitis. A week of uncontrollable vomiting, lancinating pain in one eye, dehydration and sheer misery each time. Gallons of IV fluids before my kidneys started functioning. Each of these infections followed a simple cold and went through a predictable course of increasing congestion, facial discomfort, worsening pain and then a stiff neck, headache, paroxysmal vomiting, wanting to die etc. There are only two standard antibiotics that stop this happening once I get to the facial pain stage – so there are, for me always two sides to even simple stories, like treating "colds" with antibiotics. The current witch hunt against all doctors "who prescribe powerful antibiotics for self limiting infections" is not as straight forward as it seems. The Scarlet Fever epidemic shows that we don't often know a self limiting from a self perpetuating infection. Doctors should NEVER be rigid with individual patients about any condition, however commonplace. Almost no patient with an agonising painful throat I have spoken to in the last couple of years has had it examined properly and their glands properly palpated – so convinced are today's GPs that they are not going to treat "sore throats". I am glad to say the new American guidelines for managing sinus pain at least recognise that the patient's view and experience should be accommodated in the decision making on when to treat and when to use "second line antibiotics".

The computer is a tool for documenting, auditing, reporting, claiming money, – all those relatively unimportant but time consuming things the modern age has interpolated between the doctor and patient. So these days we sometimes pay more attention to the screen (or in my case the keyboard) than the patient. And we miss so much as a consequence. Empathy, availability, accessibility, friendliness, openness, understanding, eye contact, communication, awareness, even sometimes making the diagnosis. American doctors feel much the same way about the negative effect of the computer and computerised medical notes. Indeed over half of the American profession came within a hairsbreadth of being fined at the start of 2015 for failing to make their first Medicair and Medicaid data recording targets. Such was the furore that the targets were changed! God bless American Primary Care Physicians. Compare that with the Blair/Brown shock at the overclaiming of the first year's QuoF points by the British profession, all shamefully chasing every computer based box they could tick when points meant prizes and prizes meant money.

As part of modern GP, doctors are supposed to score annual target and Quof Points. To ask and to record selected data information. This is like asking Van Gough to forget what he is trying to paint and instead to count the number of petals and make sure the sunflowers are exactly in the same position on the canvas as in the vase. All this distracts and diverts the doctor from the whole point of the exercise, the caring and curing, from the quality of the interaction and towards the administration. It takes the patient away from the centre of the whole process and puts the process at the centre of the process.

The new doctor (as I once did) doesn't realise that patients often WON'T DO AS THEY ARE TOLD. They will not take the medicine, they will ask if the doctor is sure of the diagnosis or the treatment, because their friend, their hairdresser or their mother in law has a different opinion. They will come back and say the pills gave them side effects so they stopped them. The doctor has to pretend to have the self confidence not to be offended and not to react negatively to this.

The doctor has to smile and appear welcoming, to offer a hand and to touch the patient at some point within a therapeutic context in the consultation. All mature and experienced GPs agree on this. Many new doctors stay rooted to their seats and act as if consulting is just paperwork (now screen work) and just talk. At some point in the development of a good GP he or she realises that professional maturity involves a great deal of smiling tolerance and that respect, compliance and admiration are not universal. You must have the confidence for your advice to be ignored without being upset. Or without *appearing upset*. This perhaps is the hardest bit of the process. The *acting*.

So whether we are mindful or empathetic, patient focussed or just acting well, what the patient wants most is a doctor who seems to listen, has some time and thought to devote to them, wants to help, knows what they are doing and above all likes them (or at least is pretending to). Competence and kindness.

The consultation is **the unit** of General Practice just like a fare is a unit of taxi driving or a sale is a unit of retail management or a boiler repair is a unit of plumbing.

There are acres of text on how to consult with patients but the truth is that we all work out a way that suits our own personalities, depending on where we are in our career, our knowledge and attitude and these change with each patient, their type of problem and over time. There is NO one type that fits all. Dozens of reputations have been made promoting a new spin or format and there have been endless ways of emphasising current political or social attitudes and cramming them into the complex interaction that is the consultation. So often, an approach that is influenced by fashionable politics or social engineering can subordinate the whole point of the consultation, which is to find out what ails the patient and to make it better. Not primarily to assess their health beliefs, or to show respect for their cultural or religious diversity. These are side issues on a par with which political party they voted for. What price prayer or cultural healing traditions when they need an abdominal USS, HIV test, anti-malarials or penicillin?

The consultation is the unit of GP work by which we are judged. We don't make pots or paintings, we don't compete in races or sell shirts, we consult – and that is how we should be and are judged. You just have to think how the last twenty years have seen social and political anti-elitism, an anti-establishmentism, the growing mistrust of authority and the increase in unearned general entitlement. Then add that to the ever increasing availability of often wrong information on the Internet and you can see how the consultation can be at best unsatisfactory and often confusing if not managed sympathetically, clearly and decisively. At worst it can be a flash point of conflicting attitudes. Indeed, this came up in a (2014) radio discussion regarding a child with a medulloblastoma taken from Southampton General Hospital by its Jehovah's Witness parents, believing that proton beam therapy abroad might be helpful. The discussion revolved around all parents wanting the best for their child, the Internet being an unreliable source of medical information and full of false hope and claims of cures. Add this all up and a good doctor these days should be someone who is willing to consider and review all alternative options and therapies presented by patient and relatives without dismissing them because of a narrow minded conventional bias. After all, some alternative therapies **do** work.

A study presented on the Today Programme (2/9/14) suggested that given the huge amount of unreliable information available to patients these days about treatment options,

a third of patients or parents want the doctor to tell them what to do,

a third want to make the decision "with the doctor,"

and a third want the doctor to lay out the options and leave it to them to decide.

In the situation above: I can't help thinking an informal, accessible, non authoritarian, friendly, non Asperger doctor and a couple of fair minded, reasonable, open minded parents or relatives will come to a sensible conclusion most of the time. The problem is that this combination often doesn't exist.

But don't be fooled into thinking the models of consultation given below mean that consultations must follow a pattern. Everyone is different. I am frequently fascinated by how an appraisal I am doing turns into a consultation, (by way of a mentoring session), or by how a conversation in a gym, a drink with a friend or a relative or a loved one can turn into a serious consultation in a flash. – And isn't it interesting how poorly the vast majority of actual consultations in the surgery or outpatients are handled despite all the effort and theory that go into this part of GP training?

I have been given mutually contradictory advice in two consecutive sentences in outpatients about the prognosis of a loved one by a consultant. Someone very close to me in my family awoke from an anaesthetic after an exploratory laparoscopy recently to be greeted by a registrar with the unbelievable "– You are Mrs xxxx, the lady with the ovarian cancer?" This was her first confirmation of a much feared but until then unknown diagnosis. You would hardly believe the effort that goes into teaching empathy, communication skills, breaking bad news and trying to relate to a patient's feelings." Clearly, with some junior doctors it isn't getting through. But it isn't just junior doctors.

Having had the diagnosis broken in that way, the subsequent first oncology outpatient appointment was supposed to be with the consultant to discuss treatment options. When ushered in to the consulting room my relative and her husband found themselves in a large room, surrounded by two dozen students, doctors and unidentified other people only to be introduced by someone who it turned out was the consultant. He described her advanced disease to his audience, all of which my relatives understood, but had not known, being very intelligent people who had researched the condition in the mean time, without any introduction, preamble or permission. At this point my relatives told him what they thought of his lack of professional and personal skills – which I hope humiliated him in front of his team, got up, left and were re-referred to a different hospital.

Forget the ubiquitous political values of equality and rights that are prioritised in medical education, training and appraisal supervision these days and concentrate on the far more valuable and patient friendly human values of thoughtfulness, friendliness and empathy. or as Schneider says, **Competence and Kindness.**

Everywhere in this book I talk about the doctor maintaining a knowledgeable professionalism, being confident, entirely ready to be challenged and questioned and to explain in simple language, of being accessible to every patient but on the other hand, not trying to be the patient's best new mate. Not his or her first-name-terms-buddy. Generally I believe that is **not** what patients want. But instead, be aware of the responsibility that knowledge and the power and exercise of that knowledge may sometimes have over people's lives. Serious but friendly, thoughtful, confident, decisive and sounding definite in our very grey area speciality of Family Medicine. That is what patients want and need.

The single most important factor in determining whether a consultation is successful is not the experience of the doctor, the duration of the consultation, the age or sex of the protagonists, the presenting complaint, the possession of MRCGP or any higher GP qualification, it isn't the structure of the consultation that the doctor uses, it isn't even how long the doctor and patient have known each other. **It is the patient's perception that the doctor likes him (or her).** If you think about that for a while and if you have ever consulted a doctor who was unaware that you yourself were a doctor, you can see why a personal relationship, a rapport, an empathy, basic friendliness is the key to proper consulting. That is a feeling for the patient and an attempt to like and be accessible to the patient – but it is not the same as giving the patient's beliefs and attitudes equal value to your own. Never forget you are the expert. Accessible, open to any question or challenge. Be patient and understanding but in the end you do know best.

You will see what my opinion of some consultation guidelines are by my brief and somewhat out of date article on "The MRCGP Video". Also how some of my practice's most uncommunicative and less competent registrars gained a RCGP *merit* by ending each video consultation with "What will you tell your wife we have discussed today?" My patients were too polite to say "anything but the real reason I came" but that IS what they told me when the camera was off. They saw the doctor and then went to reception and booked an appointment straight away with one of the other "real partners who wouldn't ask them bloody silly questions".

In "What do you expect from a doctor?" (Six habits for healthier patient encounters), Annals of Family Medicine, 2013, Dr David Loxterkamp made some basic and honest suggestions. I read this recently and found that it echoes much of what I have already written about eye contact, the importance of touch in an appropriate way and identifying clearly who you are at each consultation. Anyway here is a contemporary American Family Physician talking about a good doctor patient interaction:

Patients don't expect perfection or cures but do hope for a connection with someone who cares about the clinical outcome. The sense of connection, the bed side manner, face to face time (-this implies looking at each other) all matter – at least as much as the services delivered. So much for the computer based consultation or the suggestion that a nurse can do her job behind a niqab.

The factors he suggested that the patient values highly are:

1) Identify yourself. "I am Dr so and so and I do this or that job". This is crucial if the patient is not your usual patient. Tell the patient what they can and can't expect from you including your level of responsibility and decision making. Not, as my wife discovered during a recent long week in hospital, a series of first names from junior doctors, without explaining who they worked for or why they were calling in to see her. Even more importantly, if the patient asks you a question and you say you will try to find the answer COME BACK TO THEM WITH THAT ANSWER when you promised.

He makes the point that in the USA, with the presence of Nurse Practitioners, Physician Assistants, Medical Students, Residents in Training, etc, etc, the patient no longer recognises the doctor by sight or voice. It is the same in the UK, which has a growing number of "Physician Associates" - getting histories, doing examinations, interpreting results, performing diagnostic and therapeutic procedures and making diagnoses (Clin Med 2016 16/6. 511). Given the destratification of medicine exemplified by the specious loss of status white coats and ties for men and loss of formal clothing for female doctors (-my wife thought the female SHOs and registrars dressed like they were just coming home from a late night party) patients need absolute clarity from the moment you see them about who you are. This is a constant and unwelcome danger when other staff step in and act as pseudo doctors. It may solve staffing and funding crises in primary and secondary care but it confuses the hell out of patients. Perhaps also a little more effort with clothing and hair also a bit of backbone when it comes to some of the nonsense from the infection control staff about wearing ties and rolled up sleeves. The lowest infection rates are in the private system and GP where, generally, we still wear ties and long sleeves.

2) Listen. Patients know that just talking to a sympathetic listener is therapeutic. Instead doctors interrupt within 12 seconds. Listening also involves eye contact (at the same level) and non threatening face contact. If the doctor is concentrating on a computer screen for more than a fraction of the consultation then he has lost the confidence of the patient and failed. All my friends tell me that the new doctors they have visited resent questions, fail to look at them, don't smile, don't welcome them, don't appear to pay attention or credit them with common sense. Why are doctors so distant and unfriendly now, is it lack of self confidence, or could the A in "A star at A Level" stand for Asperger?

I have believed that medical school selection committees have for a decade or so been doing the public a double injustice by placing the huge emphasis they do on academic grades. Sure, it makes selection easy for them: Almost no interviews. The three A star pupils elbow out those with caring personalities, common sense and with practical skills. So we now have a profession packed with public school products and brain boxes, unbalanced in favour of ethnic minorities and those from private schools, life experience-light teenagers, mainly early achieving girls. When they face the tough world of long(ish) hours, challenging life events and unreasonable patients, with the need for emotional resilience and good empathy they don't communicate well with the patients or with other staff and they crash. They are not prepared for the real hardship and the demands of a medical life. They only want to do restricted hours in a restricted list of specialities. The double injustice is that the profession is fast becoming "manned" by part time women with prioritised family commitments and unrepresentative, often unenthusiastic and unhappy high achievers many of whom are in the wrong profession. Net result: A worse service for the patient and a more expensive one for the tax payer. Also mental health disorders amongst doctors, particularly stress and depression are up many times the rate of two decades ago.

I was interested that, at long last, GP leaders were coming to this conclusion too when in June 2015, Charles Alessi, Chairman of the National Association of Primary Care commented that the brightest pupils were not for General Practice. He said that "The way medicine was developing meant that communication skills were vital to new doctors". He said that academic entry criteria needed to be relaxed. Two points: All doctors have always needed to communicate, it has nothing to do with "The way medicine is developing" and every doctor in every speciality, except perhaps morbid anatomy, pure academic research or histology has to talk to other doctors and to patients.

3) Touch: A careful physical examination often provides clues as to what is wrong, even if the history does not strictly indicate the need for one. It is called "performing" an examination for good reason. The consultation is an entertainment in some ways with anticipatory anxiety, a varying audience of patient, relatives and others, an uncertain reception and the need to vary the act to suit the house.

I remember being called to a meeting of The British Legion one evening in my Trainee year where an 80 year old lady was feeling faint but refusing to leave the company of her friends. I offered a side room for "confidentiality" but she refused and so I went through a formal examination (modified) with an audience of a hundred well meaning and smiling onlookers. That really was a performance, one of the most stressful I have ever done and worthy of best supporting actor.

The performance of an examination shows a "commitment to thoroughness" even when it isn't strictly necessary and this often helps to improve and establish the relationship between doctor and patient. Touching establishes a physical connection, a sense of intimacy and encourages communication – provided it is done sensitively and appropriately. It is a private bond that doctors have with their patients that no other profession has. Apart from possibly the oldest one. What is also crucial is confidence. If the doctor approaches the examination diffidently with "I could examine you but would you rather I didn't?" or "I think I might need to examine you, would you like a chaperone?" The patient will lose any benefit and advantage from the examination and any sense of confidence in the doctor. The examination must be done with calmness, gentleness, sensitivity, confidence, steady hands and no chaperone 99% of the time (-unless the doctor himself/or herself feels threatened). To quote the Science Fiction writer Robert Heinlein (Stranger in a Strange Land) "Audacity, always audacity-the soundest principle of strategy. In practicing medicine I learnt that when you are most at a loss is the time you must appear confident". You should listen to the chest of everyone with a cough, you should feel the temporal arteries of everyone with a headache, you should lie the patient down and straight leg raise everyone with back ache every time you see them. Need I go on? General Practice, like gold prospecting, is boring and repetitive but you never know when you are going to find that nugget.

4) Look: Look at the patient and not "the computer, the smart phone or the clock". My experience is that fewer than 10% of GPs have sufficient keyboard skills to touch type. But the screen demands your attention: Red flags and messages as well as the highly

condensed two finger summary of what you are writing (-no wonder the defence organisations despair). These are all a continual distraction. In my opinion the best way to improve the quality of consultations would be to install software that would switch off the computer as soon as the patient sat down. This is effectively what we did a couple of decades ago. We concentrated on the patient and scribbled some notes when we could. This was for the most part briefly at the start, as they undressed, got dressed or left. When they were talking we tended to pay attention to them.

5) Plan: After the History, examination and assessment the doctor "Outlines specific steps to recovery." Although the patient may want to be involved in helping to create or decide on a plan they are happy to leave the actual plan, the details and final choice to the doctor.

Don't you love the honesty of this American approach? No soft politics, just a straight forward concern to put the patient's interests at the heart of the consultation. This is absolutely true and has nothing to do with outside influence, control or paternalism but knowledge, experience and trust. Compare this with "The Appropriate Management Plan and Sharing Management Options, Patients Health Beliefs, Exploring Health Understanding, Social and Psychological Context" and all the new – agism student politics of The RCGP MRCGP video of a few years ago and that still persist today.

6) Follow up. The diagnosis is not the end. The patient often also needs a prognosis or a likely timescale. In GP this can be "You won't get better straight away, but if you don't feel significantly better in.... weeks see me again". It is important to give a plan. – To ensure that they are not back tomorrow as much as that they will come back if not better in the right time scale. But it **is** important to offer a follow up.

The article states that the American primary care physician has administrative contact with 5X as many patients in a day as he or she actually sees personally (-with pathology results and phone calls etc). I would say it is roughly the same, perhaps slightly fewer, in the UK with letters, in and out, path results, calls to and from hospital doctors and relatives.

The article ends by saying something interesting in relation to the consultation: That "The doctor wants to be understood and respected as badly as the patient does". I am not sure that this is true of all of the GPs I have appraised and worked with. Perhaps they select them differently in America.

Needless to say the consultation is a very personal, some might say a secretive activity. I have often wondered why some of the best doctors don't want to become trainers and at least one told me that his style was too personal to share, that being studied cramped his natural relationship with the patient – It was ruined by a third party, an observer. I call this a Heisenberg consultation. Sometimes the very fact that a video camera or a third party is present, be it another doctor or another of the patient's friends or relatives can dramatically change the behaviour and the comfort and accessibility of each protagonist and the whole thing becomes strained and artificial. A bit like Heisenberg and uncertainty, you change things simple by observing them.

You can regard consulting as being transected by various axes (for instance task and behaviour) as having various centres (doctor and patient) or as various models (Health Belief, Disease-Illness, etc, etc.) There are many standard ways of analysing Consultation Models.

Consultation Models:

Anyway, the standard models (The Newtonian consultation theories, if you like) are:

Medical School model:

History of presenting complaint, past history, medication history, family history, social history, direct questions, clinical examination, investigations, presumed diagnosis, suggested treatment, follow up. This is longwinded, familiar and a bit formal but misses little of importance.

Byrne and Long:

In this model, which is descriptive, vague and very general in its structure, you establish a relationship and the reason for the consultation, then perform the examination – verbal or physical or both, then doctor and/or patient consider the condition before the treatment and investigations, and finally the doctor ends the consultation. The focus here is on the patient's perception of the condition and is often actually therefore irrelevant to making them better. The patient may be there to consider: some *better indigestion treatment than he can buy over the counter.* Your job could be to show him that he actually needs an *exercise ECG, a statin and aspirin.* There can be a great danger in all patient centred approaches (ie considering the wishes and worries of the patient) – which you should, that the concept is confused with patient dominated approaches (ie considering that the patient knows what is best for them and letting them have control) – which you shouldn't.

Stott and Davis:

(from their paper "The Exceptional Potential of Each Primary Care Consultation.")
The Management of Presenting Problems,
Modification of Help Seeking Behaviour,
Management of Continuing Problems,
Opportunistic Health Promotion.

If Byrne and Long let the patient take the lead and the doctor had to consider the patient's thoughts and feelings (however unconstructive they were) this model is basically how the doctor structures and organises the consultation towards different ends. – Thus: "Next time this happens, do this, and by the way should we talk about..... while you are here, and when WAS your last smear?" etc – Doctor directed.

Pendleton:

Ironically this was first promulgated in 1984, a consulting brave new world being devised by a psychologist and putting the patient's perceptions and feelings about illness centre stage with all the potential for confusion and reinforcement that this entails. My problem about this is that it is fine to ask what the patient thinks and feels but they are often then frustrated at this back to front consultation and their feelings are often secondary to the cause of their problem not the problem itself. After all, they have come to seek advice FROM the professional and are insecure if given credit for too much understanding – and far from appreciating it, become confused. Audi never ask me to tell them why I think my car isn't running properly and if I did they would ignore it. I want a safe and competent surgeon and anaesthetist when the time comes not someone who asks me what I think they should do. I want a GP who tells me what is wrong and makes it better from his experience and wisdom. Someone who gets the diagnosis right. Putting it across sympathetically in words I can understand comes next but considering my feelings and misperceptions and taking them into account is a long way down the list.

So:

Reason for attending (nature and history of the problem, aetiology, patient's ideas, anxieties, expectations, effects of the problem).

To consider other problems (continuing problems, at risk factors).

Doctor and patient choose an action for each problem.

Sharing understanding.

Involving the patient in management, sharing appropriate responsibility.

Use time and resources appropriately.

Establish and maintain a positive relationship.

Also of course, does Pendleton realise we have (in my case) 7 1/2 minutes per consultation and we have to balance what is an almost infinite demand with an exhaustible supply?

There is another "Pendleton" which crops up in teaching circles and these are

"Pendleton's Rules of Feedback":

This is how a tutor and trainer group feed back to a registrar about a video consultation (etc) that they have just watched.

It is a classic example of how teachers justify their existence by making simple things over complicated and how authors writing on educational subjects make reputations by dismantling something so that the whole point of it is eventually missed. It is the emperor's clothes in GP education.

Rule 1 Briefly clarify any matters of fact.

Rule 2 The Doctor on the video discusses what he did well.

Rule 3 The observers then discuss what he did well.

Rule 4 The Doctor on the video then discusses what he didn't do well and would change.

Rule 5 The observers discuss what he didn't do well and should change.

Pendleton's Mona Lisa:

Now Mr Da Vinci, you have painted an oil painting in oils, on canvas, yes and this is it? You say you have covered the whole canvass and technically you have the paint fairly evenly spread. You say it is a good likeness of the woman of about thirty, the one you were painting. She is not particularly pretty and totally unknown, yes? You say she Is in the middle of the picture, light and shade isn't too bad and she is looking interestingly enigmatic I suppose. She isn't really looking at the observer is she though? and yes she isn't smiling or looking particularly happy either. Also the picture doesn't tell a story an isn't a standard allegory is it? There are some pointless rocks in the background too. So some of it is quite good as far as it goes, – Now how would you do it better next time? What about a nice vase of flowers?

Neighbour:

"-With a little understanding you can find the perfect blend"
(From" Neighbours" by Tony Hatch/Jackie Trent)

Roger Neighbour described a system of thinking about consultation in the late 80's in **"The Inner Consultation".** He was a London GP who said the doctor was both an Organiser and Responder – as if we acted in two different roles rather than the dozens of changing roles we actually do simultaneously during a consultation. He also described performing 5 main activities in the consultation:

Connecting – establishing an understanding of who the patient is and why they have come.

Summarising, – focussing the discussion – going over information coming to a conclusion and a diagnosis.

Handing over. Giving responsibility back to the patient with the information, diagnosis and advice after the main consulting is completed.

Safety netting. This is what to do if you don't get better....

and Housekeeping. This is actually self care for the doctor and is sometimes the least practical aspect of the list, depending as it does on so many unpredictables. But at least it does consider the doctor as a vulnerable and important part of the interaction. High time too since the value and quality of each consultation depends entirely upon the quality, skills, personality, patience, dedication, experience, enthusiasm and effort of the doctor and in my opinion has very little to do with the consultation model they subscribe to.

(The Inner consultation has 5 categories but 169 suggested tasks).

Calgary Cambridge:

This is probably the most practical text book description of what happens between doctor and patient, albeit somewhat longwinded (70 tasks). Thus here is an edited summary:

Initiating the session: establishing a rapport, identifying the reasons for the consultation.

Gathering Information: Exploration of the problems, understanding the patient's perspective, providing structure to the consultation.

Building the relationship – developing rapport, involving the patient.

Explanation and planning-providing the correct amount and type of information, aiding recall and understanding, achieving a shared understanding, incorporating the patient's perspective, planned and shared decision making.

Closing the session.

There are the **Cambridge Calgary 55 consultation (communication process) skills** (!): Some of the most important I have included here:

It is called the: CALGARY – CAMBRIDGE OBSERVATION GUIDE:

INITIATING THE SESSION:

Establishing Initial rapport, identifying reason(s) for the consultation, greeting the patient and obtaining the patient's name, the opening question, introducing self and clarifying role, listening to the opening statement, demonstrating interest and respect, screening, agenda setting.

GATHERING INFORMATION:

Exploration of problems, understanding the patient's perspective, the patient's narrative, ideas and concerns, question style, listening attentively, facilitative response, clarification, cues, internal summary, providing structure to the consultation, sign-posting, timing.

BUILDING RELATIONSHIP:

Developing rapport, involving the patient, non-verbal behaviour, sharing of thought, use of notes, acceptance, examination, empathy and support. Sensitivity.

EXPLANATION AND PLANNING:

Providing the correct amount and type of information, organising explanation. Using explicit categorisation or signposting. Using repetition and summarising. Giving explanation at appropriate times. Using visual methods of conveying information. Checking patient's understanding of information given (or plans made). Achieving shared understanding.

Planning: Shared decision making. Sharing own thoughts. Encouraging patient to contribute. Picking up verbal & non-verbal cues. Eliciting patient's beliefs. Negotiating. Offering choices. Checking with patient.

CLOSING THE SESSION:

End summary, contracting, safety netting. Final checking.

"BARD:"

Role based:

Behaviour, how the GP acts with the patient.

Aims: What needs to be achieved this consultation?

Room. A bit odd this: The space and furnishings we surround ourselves with. Recently in my case under assault by the non evidence based infection control police. With the removal of personal artefacts, just in case they encourage cross infection (!) All our spaces are becoming soulless and sterile in more ways than one (-prompting my writing an article: An end to the surgery toy box?)

Dialogue: How do you communicate – your personality, communication, English skills etc.

Flanagan's CSA Model:(ten minute target:)

Welcome, open question.

Golden Minute (Be quiet and let the patient speak uninterrupted).

Exploration of ICE (Ideas concerns expectations) – not in car entertainment.

Medical data gathering including red flags.

Summarising.

Examination.

Summarising.

Explanation.

Option sharing.

Shared management plan and safety netting.

The Golden Minute has various medical contexts. It can be the period after the patient sits down when he or she is assessing you, the doctor, your mood, willingness and ability to listen and understand and not impose your own agenda. So from the perspective of trendy consultation theory it is the time to be passive and let the patient lead the conversation after your "what can I do for you?" introduction. It is also the phrase attached to the 60 seconds after an apnoeic baby is born when priority is given at all costs to oxygenating the baby's brain – as it is this time, once lost, that cannot be made up by any intensive care.

Disease/Illness Model:

This is of course, two ways of looking at the same problem, one from the inside, one from the outside:

Thus:

The patient tells you he/she is not well: Looked at from the

Patient's point of view, the Illness Framework, or from the **Doctor's point of view**, the disease framework:

Ideas, concerns, expectations.   History, symptoms, examinations, signs.

Feelings, thoughts, effects.

Understanding the patient's unique
experience of the illness.

Investigations.

Underlying pathology, differential diagnosis.
Integration of the two frameworks.
Explanation and planning, shared understanding and decisions.

You could throw in a Health Belief, Balint or Transaction Analysis approach which may modify how you approach the patient once the consultation begins.

You can consider the

THE SIX INTERVENTION CATEGORIES,

Doctor centred – prescriptive, informative and confrontational and

Patient centred-cathartic, catalytic and supportive.

This is how some people look at consulting:

TASK ORIENTATED

Stott and Davies

(Exploration of presenting and
continuing problems

Modification of health seeking behaviours, opportunistic
health promotion)

Byrne and Long

6 Phases, relationship, discovery, examination, consideration,
treatment, investigation, termination.

Pendleton

7 tasks, the reason, other problems, action, shared
understanding, management, use time appropriately
Establish relationship.

Helman

Folk Model, What has
happened, why me, why
now? etc

Health Belief Model
Ideas, concerns,
expectations.

DOCTOR CENTRED

Byrne and Long

Patient explores at own
pace

6 Category Analysis, Heron.

Prescriptive, informative, confronting, cathartic
catalytic, supportive.

Transactional analysis:

Parent, adult, child

BARD

PATIENT CENTRED

Counselling

Bendix

The anxious patient, 7 rules
of thumb.

Balint

Dr/Pt relationship, Dr as
Drug, transference, counter
transference.

BEHAVIOUR ORIENTATED

And: **Neighbour** is:

Connecting, summarising, handing over, safety netting, housekeeping, 2 heads, the organiser and responder with an internal dialogue.

Well that's enough of that. As you can see, whole careers have been made, tens of thousands of tedious tutorials and endless teaching careers have been forged on the interaction between doctor and patient. Something that in the real world is time limited and depends more on personal warmth and the ability to communicate than analysis of what is going on, role playing, politics or such ludicrous things as the examination of health beliefs. It all makes your head spin.

How should you conduct a successful consultation?

Nor bring, to see me cease to live, some doctor full of phrase and fame, to shake his sapient head and give the ill he cannot cure a name.

Matthew Arnold

This is how the average patient approaches a consultation:

Most patients who have seen several different GPs over their life assume doctors come in a few standard categories: Thus, either:

1) Young, jumped up, full of themselves, expensively educated and without real maturity. They make up for inexperience with bluster and self importance, constantly asking pointless standardised questions from their General Practice for Dummies textbook. New doctors are obsessed with narrow evidence based dogma which makes up for their lack of life experience, lack of real confidence and maturity, inadequate common sense and friend-liness and instead work to protocols and rigid rules. They are good at refusing. No you cannot have another smear, it is too soon, no you haven't earnt a second opinion, no you can't have an ultrasound, you don't need antibiotics, antidepressants, hypnotics, PPIs, they are expensive, not indicated, against guidelines and so on. That is their security-they feel safe. Their focus may be Nice Guidelines, local, national or practice prescribing protocols or costs, national recommendations as applied to populations, all sorts of cost constraints and public health recommendations but it isn't flexibility, *empathy* or responsiveness or the patient's real needs. or

2) Doctors who have been around a while, who are self important, old, tired, bored and disinterested, totally unchangeable in their approach to everything, spent and unengaged, they know everything on any subject and you can't tell them a thing. or

3) Doctors who are disengaged through culture, language or personality, and just passing the time, prone to easy resentment and misunderstanding and they don't want to become personally involved if at all possible. For them this is just a job. or

4) They are intellectually superior, a 4 A star A-level student who didn't really think medicine had to do with empathy but thought each case would be a diagnostic conundrum so that talking to worried people is now just a frustrating distraction. Instead they ignore the obvious and make complex and structured diagnoses or give all patients scientific analyses and seemingly rational drugs and explanations to their problems ignoring the real reasons for the consultation. Or

5) Many doctors are locum, part time or job sharing and therefore so uncommitted to the life, continuity or the role of GPs that are unlikely to see you again and face the consequences of anything they suggest or decide. So they reason that Family Medicine is simply the management of a brief episode of one presenting complaint after another and requires no actual personal engagement or, possibly the worst of all,

6) Doctors who want to be your best friend as soon as they see you and so ask you what you think is wrong and give you a prescription out of misplaced friendliness or laziness or the avoidance of conflict. Some doctors just want to be liked and popular and assume the best way to be a good doctor is to be all things to all men.

Anyway if you get to see a doctor who is old enough to have done, say ten years or more in general practice and has had the "this is a doddle" attitude disappear – so he or she realises they don't necessarily have all the answers and may have gained a reasonably broad experience so that they can make a decent stab at the unknown, then you are fortunate. If he or she hasn't yet burnt out, is not intrinsically over confident or under confident (both disastrous), is approachable, open to direct questions without feeling threatened, hopefully able to understand colloquial English, possessed of a friendly and open personality, count your blessings. If you are very lucky and of the same age, sex and background as the doctor (or they can relate to all those factors) you are extremely lucky. Then you are likely to want to see that doctor again. In fact you will want to be on his or her list.-And you will want them to be the sort of doctor who believes in personal lists.

By the way, the really thoughtful patient who analyses how the modern NHS has changed might tell you as my patients did:

"Very few GP s these days ever seem cheerful, interested or genuinely engaged with the patient. They are somehow "disconnected". Fewer and fewer are full time and therefore few will bother to follow you up to see how you are or if you are better. Many who are just filling in have a temporary mentality and don't live locally and they won't be around to establish any sort of relationship with you. Some who trained abroad are not very close to how "we think and feel". There are large numbers who even have language or cultural barriers and misinterpret friendly questions as challenges and so the best you can expect is a person you probably won't be able to see again who is not really worried about a long term relationship with you and doesn't have a genuine interest in your outcome."-"And anyway all GPs would rather not be dealing with the endless trivia that they do (because they are too bright) and are not likely to give the rare serious illness hidden in the rough due care and consideration. Few GPs examine the patient sufficiently and none think outside a very limited collection of standard diagnoses for a potential alternative." That, I am afraid is what intelligent patients have told me is how they find many GPs to be like today.

On the other hand:

Thus there can be a fairly low expectation from the travelled, experienced patient, particularly of the busy urban GP in a big practice. It is different, I believe, for the patient who is registered with a personal GP, actually feels they are on one doctor's list and this doctor is full time or nearly full time, especially in a smaller practice, as a named doctor they normally see and especially in a smaller community. General Practice is done differently in urban and rural practices, in partnerships with fewer than 6 partners, with fewer than 1/3 of the doctors being assistants or sessional – so that more doctors are available for longer hours and dare I say it, with smaller proportions of female (part time) doctors there may well be more continuity, choice and availability. More full time partners.

So expectations can be fairly low amongst many patients. This is why I sometimes differentiate between "Family Medicine" with practices running personal lists where each patient has a named doctor on the one hand whom they **usually see** and those where you see any partner (or assistant) and where you have no real sense of belonging, continuity or commitment in the more impersonal "General Practices". The new mega (very large industrial) practices fall into the latter group.

So what about the consulting?

The consultation begins before you see the patient with you summoning the patient over the loud speaker or going to greet them in the waiting room.

I once attended a lecture about Data Protection where I was told that we should say

"Next patient for Doctor Smith please" when we summon our patients rather than "Daisy Brown for Dr Smith please" – This was to protect their identity and maintain *confidentiality* for some reason. What utter idiocy. Should we insist all patients wear paper bags on their heads in the surgery too, just in case someone recognises them or have our receptionists whisper across the front counter to all patients checking in? Complete confidentiality in the real world of medicine does not and cannot exist.

Sit in a waiting room with a relative and you will soon realise what absolutely dire places they are. Screaming, badly behaved children, loud, obese and smelly mankind, all talking loud banal rubbish, a disproportionately high percentage of emotionally and mentally unwell or unpredictable, impertinent and frightening sociopaths or even psychopaths, vomiting babies, men and women coughing without any concept of how droplet spread takes place and you will realise why no one likes to be there – let alone be kept waiting there.

No wonder everyone has hypertension when they have it checked in General Practice. It is amazing there are so few strokes and infarcts in the waiting room.

Remember you are **managing** the consultation, organising and steering it – not waiting for some indefinable spontaneous magic to take place. **You** are making the magic happen if any happens at all. To quote the late great Terry Pratchett speaking as Granny Weatherwax the local village witch/shaman/medicine woman: "I saved a man's life once: Special medicine, twice a day. Boiled water with a bit of berry juice in it. Told him I bought it from the dwarves. That's the biggest part of doct'rin really – most people get over most things if they put their minds to it, you just have to give them an interest." So remember you are part of the cure, part of the placebo is you.

Thus my first rule of the consultation is:

Welcome the patient. Do this with an attitude of friendly confidence. You are open and accessible but **you** are being consulted and it is you who is being asked for your experience and opinion. Act like you have the first and the second **will be** of real value. The welcome is important. – By which I mean call them by name. I use a Tannoy but you can go and get them if you prefer – getting up out of your chair is important at least once during the consultation for your own health and for the patient's respect. More and more studies are demonstrating the health dangers of a sedentary lifestyle so get as much personal movement into each consultation as you can. You must greet them positively and smile. When sitting in waiting rooms I have heard endless depressed sounding doctors calling patients into their rooms as if the world were resting on their shoulders. Indeed I used to sound exactly the same as this until I realised how self destructive it was – The "I am depressed and overworked, and not going to like seeing you – nor you me, so give me a break and don't expect too much" voice, – reasoning I would gain sympathy and the patient might shorten the consultation or withhold a few symptoms and let me off lightly. Perhaps they would realise I was tired and had had a hard day. Of course, exactly the reverse happens. The patient is angry that the doctor can't be bothered to make an effort. The doctor is treating them as a faceless number NOT an individual, just the next on the list. All those pre-conceived entitlements and resentments surface, the unpleasantness of the symptoms, the smelly waiting room and the long wait for the appointment, the obstructive receptionists and the depressed sounding doctor just makes his own job worse in the end. The patient is more than ever determined not to be fobbed off by a privileged functionary who is just going through the motions. So sound welcoming and smile even though you both know from previous encounters that you are playing a game, putting on a performance. Look welcoming and cheerful. You **are** acting after all. That is what we do for a living day in and day out. We go out on stage and act. The second rule is:

Shake hands and greet the patient. This is whether they are adults or children. In fact children get used to shaking hands and it becomes a game which is part of the ritual of seeing the doctor. An expert in a lecture I attended recently said what a bad idea shaking hands was because of "Infection control". The same expert who wanted the toy box, flowers and family photos removed from the surgery. More short sighted idiocy. Not only are most of the living organisms on the planet potentially infectious micro organisms and cover everything we come in contact with, unless it has been sterilised, but most of the individual cells (in terms of numbers) in a human body are already bacteria, not human and not genetically our own. We are all contaminated all the time. Indeed our health depends upon us being recolonised and our microbiome (biota) constantly being replenished. We can't avoid bacteria by not shaking hands. Avoiding further contamination is impossible. – Don't patients leave the surgery and pay for their prescription with money touched by hundreds of other potentially "infected" people, don't they get on buses and touch hand rails, push lift buttons, hold escalator hand rails, take Sainsbury's Car Park Cards from the dispenser which have been in the hands (and between the teeth) of hundreds? And actually isn't that in the long run what our immune systems learn to co exist with and learn from? Indeed, RELY ON?

Shaking hands is an essential skin on skin primeval signal of trust, friendship, contact, integrity, a bond between individuals and in my opinion no consultation, however trivial should ever take place without the doctor touching the patient in one way or another.

The greeting must always appear cheerful. I have done it over a third of a million times in my medical career. Roughly 100,000 in the middle of that time as a doctor might have been blank, negative, distant, neither welcoming nor off putting but a reflection of my sense of "resignation". I was unhappy with my practice, disenchanted with life as a doctor. No longer excited by my status, the human contact, the secrets of people's lives or the variety of behaviour I saw. I felt resentful and overloaded, bored and burnt out. I had come to realise the hardest things about being a GP were being personally pleasant to endless self destructive and self pitying people and trying to maintain a high level of concentration for the rare serious symptom lost in the haystack of trivia. I did not have novelty and curiosity to stimulate me as I did for the first 100,000 consultations and somewhere in my psyche I thought the general goodwill of people would recognise my lack of sparkle meant I was emotionally drained and I would garner some sympathy. Of course it didn't. My unsmiling face and unsympathetic questioning prompted immediate resentment and distrust and simply produced a more prolonged and antagonised consultation.

So: for the last third of my career (13 years, 100,000 patients) I have pretended to be cheerful, always smiled and looked happy to see even the most miserable, self absorbed and unlikeable patients – unless I knew that the patient was in severe pain or bereaved and have always, where not totally inappropriate, tried to introduce humour if possible. This, oddly, is often very helpful in coping with serious illness, misery, even death.

And when you introduce yourself to a new or unfamiliar patient you will lose respect and half of your potential credited IQ if you introduce yourself without the title "Doctor" (or "Mister" if you are a surgeon in the UK) or call yourself by your first name.

Constantly observe:

Neighbour and others talk about the doctor performing different roles during the consultation – organising and responding or doing different parts of the same process like explaining and agreeing, confirming understanding. These things aren't of course separate and distinct unless you are a registrar making your consultation video. You do all this constantly without clunkily going through a check list. Consulting is the ultimate multi-tasking. – Which is why it is odd that men are so good at it. Also you do not do things in order. I have started with welcoming the patient and I will end with terminating the consultation but observation and the willingness to interrupt with "Are you OK?" or "Is that really why you are here" or putting your hand (appropriately) on the patient's forearm and saying "Poor you" etc. etc. can be introduced at anytime from the moment they (or you) enter the room. So observing for obvious things like gait, jaundice, cyanosis, clubbing, dyspnoea, – these are all straight forward and continuous. But you should constantly question attitude, behaviour, eye contact, – why are they being aggressive, evasive, shall I challenge that now or later? Are they depressed, are they responding with a normal facial expression and body language? How are they responding to the person accompanying them? Why is THAT person accompanying them? Should I ask that person to go outside?

You can of course suspend the consultation at any time and go off on a therapeutic tangent, "I am just going to get a nebuliser, Venflon, can I check your pulse, blood pressure, chest while you are talking?" etc. No consultation should ever be set in stone. The whole point is that it wraps around the needs and presenting complaint of that patient at that time and adapts constantly as the information changes. And the only part of medical practice that is P.C. is the consultation. Patient centred. But doctor led.

Organising the consultation:

Before asking the patient directly, think like Sherlock Holmes or maybe more accurately that somewhat unsuccessful Southsea GP, Sir Arthur Conan Doyle. What can you see by looking?

How is the patient responding to others with them, children, newborn, spouse, boyfriend, partner? If there is someone else in the room you have an absolute right to question them – who they are and why they are there and if the patient wants them there? Teenagers with boyfriends, (or two teenage girls as often as not), if a young mother is tearful, should a nurse or receptionist look after her baby? If they are a teenager with a parent should you establish, diplomatically that you "always ask to see the patient alone for a few minutes, I hope no one minds" right at the start – you usually pick up on whether the consultation mood music is to do with sex, antisocial behaviour, depression, if you are being used as some sort of punishment, threat or back up (which occasionally you will be) or whether one or other protagonist is there under protest, within a few minutes of the start. You soon have a rough idea of who needs to stay and who needs to go. It is a small foible of mine but I always ask teenagers to switch off their phones and to spit chewing gum out into a bin before we start. I just say "mutual respect"-you wouldn't like me to be chewing gum would you?

Establish the reason:

This may seem easy and obvious. "Now what is the problem?", "What brings you here today?" or "What can I do for you?". It sounds straight forward but I can't count the number of patients who have then responded with a description of what appeared to be "the problem", I have taken a history, got them undressed, helped them onto the couch, examined them, got them dressed, discussed the diagnosis and treatment then written a prescription then I have stood up to say come back and see me if you are no better in a month, to which they have replied "Oh that isn't the reason I am here, It isn't my back, it's my diarrhoea."

Patients do not work on the same structured, organisational agenda that you have to. They don't work in 7 1/2 minute or 10 minute structured repeating cycles. If they take their jacket off before sitting down you know they are not self employed, they are in no rush, they do not respect your time pressure and you will have to manage the consultation actively or it will take 45 minutes. No generation of GPs, except perhaps those in the private sector has ever had enough time to manage their patients adequately or few enough patients to do a thorough job. We live with short cuts, follow ups, referrals and compromise.

Once you get to know which patients are less likely to have sorted their problems into a neat bundle for you, develop a phrase or technique that avoids this sort of frustration: "While we are here is there anything else I need to do?" "Is there anything else to discuss before I examine you?" I know perfectly reasonable GPs who will only see one patient problem per consultation and say "You will have to book another appointment for that". However frustrating it may be to have a biphasic consultation, I cannot see how they can justify this. The patient pays **them**, the patient paid for their training, (£500,000) – and what else has the GP to do? it is almost as if **that** GP is doing each patient a favour by letting himself be available. Our reason for existing is to consult and to be available for consulting, for everything and anything the great British public wants to ask. If you haven't realised that yet then you are in the wrong branch of medicine.

Take a good history:

It sounds obvious again but how poorly we do it. Take a common problem like back pain. Think of the common potential causes: Musculoskeletal pain from joints, muscles, ligaments, osteoporotic fracture, spinal pathology, abscess, tumour, disc, bony pain, trauma, secondaries, infection, renal pain, stones, infarct, tumour, infection, aortic dissection, bowel pathology, stress, shingles etc, etc. Ask about all the potential possible causes not just the common ones. So many contemporary politically driven analyses of the consultation place the expectations and beliefs of the patient high up the consulting agenda. Why? Who decided on this political world view? I assume this is to make the doctor seem less inaccessible, less authoritarian. More PC. (In the politically correct not the patient centred sense). But this approach has many disadvantages as well as being wrong: Some who are your potential patients profoundly believe that perforating the skin with small needles, even perforating small models of their enemies with needles, examining the shape of the skull, massaging the scalp, observing the colour of the irises, pushing specific parts of the feet, applying rocks, crystals, vacuum cups or leeches to the skin, smelling different aromatic vapours, inducing a stupor while watching a regular moving object, eating all sorts of herbs and foods, cutting off the foreskin or parts of the female perineum, even being physically touched by someone with a religious belief can positively influence their physical health. They are all wrong and I refuse to collude with them and their health beliefs. But

1) Being approachable, open and willing to discuss the implications of the diagnosis **you** have come to rationally is a far more honest way of being accessible and open, 2) Unless the patient has your medical knowledge and experience they are not going to get

an accurate or realistic diagnosis by applying unproven or irrational personal or cultural health beliefs, 3) By sticking to sound medical and scientific principles, not bending them to fit the hundreds of subjective beliefs that patients hold about their bodies, you will save time and get them better quicker. 4) My experience is that you have to be honest to yourself and your own experience in the end or you start believing and tolerating all sorts of indefensible grey wishful thinking nonsense.

If you have the time it is often extremely helpful to glance through the notes for an idea of the patient's history (if you don't know them personally), medical summary, last consultation, last out-patient summary and their current drug regime. Do this while they are coming in, getting undressed, etc.

Don't forget that the patient won't make connections and will only give you history of relevance as they see it. They may not think their breathlessness is worth mentioning while discussing black stools, or that their pet parrot is ill, or that they work with asylum seekers at the airport or etc.

So get the information you need, the history of the presenting and related symptoms, past medical history, previous drug and surgical history, smoking, drinking and occupational history, all medication, both prescribed and OTC, (this nearly always has some bearing on the symptoms), family history and try and get an idea of HOW OFTEN the patient consults. This, like it or not, has a significant bearing on the likely seriousness of their complaint. Then try and make connections. The thicker the notes (unless they have proven separate serious conditions or a known chronic poorly controlled one) the less likely each consultation is to be for a serious complaint. By now you should have a rough idea about what is wrong.

and then:

Perform a good examination

An older American physician recently wrote: **"Modern autopsy-less physicians including pathologists are whizz bang at computers, imaging, lab test panels, microbiomes, electronic medical records and coding. They are maybe not so great at physical exams, taking a useful personal and family history or gross and microscopic pathology. This latter list is where physicians once got really good at understanding what was wrong with their patients."** I couldn't agree more. I wish I knew who he was (I remember seeing his photograph in a journal) as I would write to him and say he isn't alone.

Virtually every consultation justifies at least a rudimentary examination. Especially the routine throats and bad backs which occasionally show unexpected pathology. Then perhaps we wouldn't have our Scarlet Fever epidemic. Cancers can present with back pain, so can aortic dissection, renal and bowel pathology. Certainly no new prescription for an antibiotic, analgesic, anti inflammatory and no referral should be issued without a proper examination. No patient should be dismissed as having "just a virus" without being examined properly either. I recall a partner who prescribed a broad spectrum antibiotic for a woman who presented with breathlessness and cough without undressing her. She came to see me worse a few days later. I asked about other symptoms, noting her pleuritic pain, the swollen calf and then what was a solid upper lobe when I examined her. I admitted her, she was anticoagulated and for some reason I persuaded her not to take action against my partner. Ironically a different partner in another practice missed an axillary vein thrombosis and upper lobe pneumonia by not undressing or listening to the chest of a different breathless patient ten years earlier. Both had been prescribed antibiotics, both came back to see me a few days later. Both were anti-coagulated and both wanted to complain but I calmed them down and agreed to act as their GP subsequently. My sympathies were with them. How long does it take to listen, to get a dozen deep breaths or percuss a chest a dozen times? or to think laterally?

In an American primary care discussion about "touching patients" in 2014, failure to properly examine the patient was at the top of the list of reasons for patients leaving a doctor's list. One doctor said "Touch is a social expectation: it is an integral part of the patient physician relationship" Another said "This intimate sharing of interpersonal space in a safe environment does a lot to win trust".

Examining the patient often discloses new information, makes many diagnoses, confirms or excludes others, reassures the patient, establishes a bond of trust and reassurance between the doctor and patient. The laying on of hands connects you with the patient and seems to help nearly all illnesses improve quicker in my experience. It certainly establishes a degree of trust, confidence and respect in your thoroughness and interest.

The Baby P. case and others regarding non accidental injury which have been so badly handled by our profession were in major part because the A and E doctor (and probably the GP) didn't strip the child off to exclude bruising and other external signs of injury. I assume the current anxiety regarding false accusations against the doctor were the subconscious justification for this. A successful accusation of assault against a doctor performing a justifiable medical examination with or without a chaperone is virtually unheard of. A fear of complaint should never prevent good practice and is an unprofessional justification of lazy, poor practice. Or even worse, the pressure of work and the inevitable difficulty of stopping mid surgery to find a totally unnecessary chaperone can lead to the decision to cut corners and just not bother. As no doubt they do hundreds of times every day throughout the surgeries, casualty units and out patients departments throughout the land. The law of unforeseen circumstances – politicians and lawyers (or amateur politicians and lawyers in our Royal Colleges) read about a handful of abusive doctors and decide that no intimate examination should therefore be done without the protection of a third party present. Then without considering the reality of medical life, protocols are written, training is instigated, the ethos and teaching of young doctors are changed and no one actually thinks about how completely impractical the new system of chaperones is in busy general practices or casualty units. Result: Doctors can't spare the time to get the chaperones as and when they are needed and hundreds of patients suffer the consequences of poorer medical standards.

There may be one other unadmitted reason GPs and lone casualty officers do not fully examine children when non accidental injury as a diagnosis flits through their heads. It is how to manage a bruised child and a potentially aggressive parent who knows why you are referring him/her to hospital or admitting their child. After all, why else, these days would a doctor whose face and demeanour just changed from friendly to suspicious insist on a second opinion the minute they see a bruise on your child? It is obvious what is going through their mind as the consultation for the parent suddenly becomes one where police arriving and an arrest are very real possibilities. No doctor happily rushes into what can be a very threatening and unpleasant situation on their own and some may just not bother to look. As a GP I dealt with bruises by asking about falls, saying all children were covered in bruises, but there were some blood disorders that caused bruising and could lead to internal bleeding and so I needed to arrange a hospital blood test. At least in hospital the doctor on the ward after my phone call would be prepared, not be single handed and by the time any blood test came back normal they would be with the Social Worker and Police.

I want to make the point here that all children ARE covered in bruises from the moment they learn to crawl and the VAST majority are not deliberately inflicted maliciously by adults.

So; **Undress the patient.** In children who may have been injured, look over every square inch of skin, in hot children, expose the buttocks, explaining to the child and parent that some rashes (i.e. petechiae and purpura) can start there.

While you are examining the patient, think laterally. So, with hand pain, examine the neck, with foot pain, examine the back, with headache in children, look at the low back and the buttocks for rashes, think like a medical student in a finals examination. Always check the throat if the patient has a temperature. If the patient is breathless or tired and losing weight – check everything that you can think of – and so on and so on.

Don't forget that General Practice is the management of sameness and repetition while trying to keep a high index of suspicion for rare serious underlying pathology. Sheep and goats.

I fully accept that timed appointments (mine are 7 1/2 minutes now), the patient as consumer, (the right to see the doctor within 48 hours as it was a few years ago), the burgeoning needs of QuoF, NICE guidance, new attitudes to good practice (following up of depressed and chronically ill patients regularly) and the increased number of consultations per patient per year have put extra pressure on the length of time we have with each patient. These are all things that have elbowed their way into the consultation within the last 20 years. They have affected the attitude we have had to develop and the thoroughness we allow ourselves in the consultation. We see far more patients for reasons we didn't used to. I worked as a locum private GP for 6 months thirty years ago and had half hour appointments. I currently do private GP sessions in a private hospital with the same length appointments. I did and do "proper" examinations as part of the consultation including full neurological examinations, go over the results of each blood test and its significance with the patient, perform Epley manoeuvres, inject joints during the consultation, manipulate displaced facet joints, demonstrate exercises and get a lot more fun out of each consultation. I actually refer far fewer patients too. Ironically it is probably more cost effective as well. But even in normal practice I could book double appointments and get patients I was worried about to come back.

When I first went in to practice, by luck I had a surgery with a spare examination room where I could put patients to change or get ready for my examination while I talked to the next patient. It meant I was far more efficient and thorough. So the current standard one room only surgery with the examination couch in the consulting room, no spare side room, lay-out of GP surgeries contributes, just like the chaperone ethos, to skimpy examinations and incomplete diagnoses and in the end, poor medicine.

By now you should have a good idea of whether

You should be dialling 999 already and whether the patient needs the emergency administration of drugs or treatment,

or if the patient needs to be admitted to hospital immediately,

or the patient needs to be admitted sometime soon,

or the patient is unwell but can be managed by you at home with medication and supervision by himself or family.

or if you need to call in and see them or call them by phone later, or tell them to phone the OOH service if (give clear instructions) they are not better,

or there is little that needs to be done except give reassurance.

or they have wasted your time completely.

Tell the patient what is wrong and be confident. Don't ask them what they think is wrong unless it is clearly only as part of information gathering as in order to reassure them. Many consultation models place a high value on the patient's own health beliefs. Does this have to stretch to the transfusion or transplant exclusions of some religions, male and female "circumcisions", (there are 120-170,000 young girls (different sources) in Britain who's parents' health beliefs included performing the butchery of female genital mutilation over just the one decade preceding 2014), voodoo, homeopathy, faith healing, or the belief widely held in parts of Nigeria and elsewhere that polio vaccine is contaminated by HIV or causes sterilisation etc? There is only one health model of value and that is the empirical, trial based, rational, research born, proven, double blind, conventional medicine practiced in the west by traditional GPs, hospital and other conventional doctors. On the other hand, the patient may have an idea or an underlying fear about what might be causing their mysterious symptoms. Often something serious. You should explain the rational cause of their illness and symptoms that you have formulated from their history and examination, using phrases like "usually this turns out to be due to" and "I would expect this to take.... weeks to improve", or "this is very common and most people are a lot better by...." and so on. Do this simply but not condescendingly, giving the treatment and the time span involved. This may entail simple, unprotracted explanations, diagrams, references to books (the most thumbed pages on my shelves are those with pictures of large bowel diverticulae, benign testicular lumps – Grants Atlas has a very good pictures of a lumpy epididymis and also a xiphoid process, (which patients are often discovering for the first time, decades after it actually appeared), the bones of the wrist and the foot, pictures of Molluscum Contagiosum, Pityriasis Rosea, Perioral Dermatitis, Slapped Cheek, what tonsils look like in "real" purulent tonsillitis, a picture of a Halo Naevus and melanomata. All useful adjuncts to have at hand in daily General Practice.

So listen and explain, say what is wrong and formulate a plan. The compliance of the patient is assumed. Again, many models of the consultation suggest doing all this in discussion, negotiation and with the cooperation of the patient. (Concordance is the term we sometimes use these days unless this discussion is being had in America where good old Compliance still has currency) –

Concordance: Agreement or harmony in relations between persons, musical notes or nations. A chord which is in itself satisfying to the ear and does not require resolution. Unanimous.

Compliance: Agreement, accord, complying with a request, the property of a body of undergoing plastic deformation, yielding to physical pressure.

What if the patient cannot or will not understand or accept the diagnosis or the cause? How often have you told a patient that their bad knee or back pain or diabetes is due to the 18 stone they carry around every day and the bottom line is that the anti inflammatory, the physiotherapy appointments or the antidiabetic medication are only a stop gap until they themselves do something about serious weight loss. Regular exercise (eg 20 minutes a day on a treadmill) and weight loss of a few Kg are more effective than any oral antidiabetic medication (viz bariatric surgery) and infinitely cheaper at getting HBA1C levels down. Regular exercise improves the outcome in most diseases including many cancers, depression, hypertension, cardiovascular disease etc. But how often is the result a blank refusal to accept the simple truth of the problem? I think that stating the facts and asking for agreement and acceptance of the facts (compliance) is often more likely to result in the patient getting better than a comfortable agreed understanding that accepts the patient's own health beliefs (concordance). Assuming of course that your formulation is accurate and the patient complies!

Any other business:

We are supposed to squeeze in all sorts of opportunistic things here.

Was there anything else you were worried about that we need to sort out while you are here?

Red or yellow flags come up on the computer – blood test due, blood pressure, missed check up with the nurse.

Screening of particular patient groups,

Opportunistic enquiries from your own knowledge of the patient's family – how is your mother, are you still the sole carer?

Alcohol or lifestyle advice,

The truth is you basically just don't have the time in most consultations for a lot of this other business. Unless you have half hour appointments of course.

Agree that you are now finished and arrange follow up:

No patient willingly leaves the consulting room unless the relationship with the doctor has been dreadful, the patient dysfunctionally aggressive or the relationship has really broken down. Indeed if they are keen to get out through the door after seeing you, you can assume the consultation was not a successful one. So you have to continue positive active management of the consultation (you have been totally accessible personally but in control of the process) by making it clear you have finished.

I have a series of terminating phrases. I never ask "What will you tell your wife we have discussed today?" (I try not to patronise the patient) or if "Was all that OK?" – I feel too much like I am asking to be graded on my performance. I may ask if they followed the explanation and then go over it again if they didn't. I would never show frustration or impatience at repeating a description and I will write the name of the diagnosis if they ask (with a warning about how unreliable and distorted the Internet and friends can be on medical topics) or give them the diagrams or the written explanations we have been over together to take away.

I will make it clear that we have finished by getting up and offering my hand and by one of a series of stock phrases: "OK, shall we compare notes in one month?, It's been nice seeing you. I would expect you to see an improvement in... definite time scale, but if you get... specific symptoms..... come and see me again in...... specific time frame". Do not be afraid to give a specific offer of follow up, if certain things do or don't happen because otherwise patients don't know whether to come back in a few days or not at all.

Then make sure you have kept proper notes about the consultation:

Which many of us are still poor at doing and which will be our only defence against future complaint, No Notes, No Defence. The notes, however brief, should cover and should remind the future doctor reading it (us and others) not just about the symptoms, history, findings and advice, but what we were thinking. So this includes potential management and treatment planning, as well as alternative diagnoses if it turns out we were wrong! The notes might also outline a brief plan for the next consultation, especially if the patient isn't better and if we have the time, what we said to the patient. If we record our thoughts in this way the notes will help us not to contradict ourselves and confuse the patient or duplicate investigations. It is most important for someone like me with a relatively poor memory for most of my 10,000 patient interactions a year, to have a rough outline of a reserve plan written down just in case an unexpected outcome happens in the interval between appointments. Also when they come back in a month you are back up to speed with the right questions and the right mindset straight away. The patient is also impressed that you recall their complaint and that have been mulling over their problem ever since you last saw them.

If you want a snappy mnemonic for the consultation:
AEIOU
Accessibility (Appointment, Access)
English Language Skills, (Engagement, Empathy).
Introduction (Invitation, Investigation, Inquisition)
Observation, (On Examination)
Understanding (Undertaking, Upshot, follow-**Up**)

Personality and Intelligence:
Your personality is of course, more important in the interaction between you and your patient than some learnt consultation technique of how to professionally interact, sympathise and support your fellow human being. There is of course no attempt at any stage in any training for any speciality to select candidates emotionally or individually best suited to their proposed job. To look at their personality.

IQ-yes. Who you are, what you are like – no. Where in the UKCAT, the personal statement, standard interview questions and the average work experience produced at medical school interview is the evidence base for the detection of kindness and empathy? Given the odd race and sex bias of medical school selection committees currently, where is their evidence that they are choosing the most suitable material to mould into future doctors? But then no grade is given for good listeners in psychiatry, good recollectors of minutiae or lateral thinkers in General Medicine, for people who genuinely relate well to and like children in paediatrics, (something I find to be a rare and special skill). Conversely there is no negative assessment at job interview or appraisal for the tremulous surgeons, stand-offish child specialists and GPs and specialists with an inflated sense of self importance, psychiatrists with no genuine human concern for their patients, mild Asperger's, poor empathy or lack of warmth. We are not even TRYING to fit the right people into the profession let alone the specialities and, like me, you must have met many colleagues who seem to be depressed having realised that they are not in the right career.

General Practice is the most personal, personally intrusive and vulnerable of all medical specialities from the doctor's perspective. In a real sense you are selling your own personality and opening **yourself** up to examination. If you do the job properly anyway. You are likely to see any number of your patients again and have a follow up consultation at no notice as you go shopping, pick up your children from school, go to the cinema or gym or at any time. It seems to me that more than ever before there are disproportionate numbers of doctors with the wrong personalities for genuine sympathetic consulting and empathising. Whether it is on the ward, in the surgery or on the high street.

As I have mentioned before, Atul Gawande, that insightful surgeon, Reith lecturer and commentator on professional behaviour quotes Schneider as saying that what patients want most from doctors "Isn't autonomy, it's competence and kindness."(Atul Gawande "Complications".) This is absolutely right but completely ignored by medical school selection committees, Royal Colleges and nearly everyone who currently teaches and trains in medicine. After all it isn't easy to score and grade a candidate's empathy or personal effectiveness is it?

Medical schools base their selections on A Level grades, unreliable personal statements, usually not written by the student, work experience and UKCAT assessments. These are often practiced and coached. So this is the ability to pass exams and present yourself positively and has nothing to do with "emotional intelligence" or empathy. Indeed, given the introversion, focus, self centredness and the obsessional traits that academic and highly intelligent individuals often demonstrate, the ability to feel and show warmth to patient after patient may be excluded by the very medical selection process itself. What results is an over intellectualised sometimes introverted work force, increasingly distant from the thoughts and feelings of their patients.

At some point in every trainer's progress they will undergo a largely pointless personality assessment so it might be worth mentioning this here:

There are various official ways of looking at and analysing personality:

The Belbin Self Perception Inventory of 9 team roles

A Plant,

A Resource investigator,

A Coordinator,

A Shaper,

A Monitor Evaluator,

A Team worker,

An Implementer,

A Finisher,

A Specialist.

and then we have:

Myers Briggs which has 16 personality types (4 dichotomies, 16 combinations).

Extraversion/Introversion,

Sensing/Intuition,

Thinking/Feeling,

Judging/Perception.

For instance: ESFP.

Conflict between the personalities of doctors within practices can make or break them with the frequent tendency of GPs to be non team players, to resent organisation (often the very reason many leave hospitals and enter General Practice in the first place) and to form cliques, particularly in practices of more than 6 partners. Part timers and full timers, doctors who have other roles and so see fewer patients, trainers and non trainers etc are often in conflict. The pooling of seniority, training and other income and how that is balanced by reduced patient commitment are constant bones of contention as is the inevitable sense of unfairness in workload. Doctors who take time off for illnesses perceived by others to be less than serious, intrusive family commitments, (especially sick children at short notice) and mutual unwillingness to cross cover are common issues raised at appraisal where partners' personalities are often the major stressors in a GP's professional life.

Audit:

The DOH defines audit as The systematic critical analysis of the quality of medical care including diagnosis, treatment, outcome, use of resources, and effects on quality of life for the patient.

Audit doesn't often turn out much like that and has unfortunately become almost an absolute requirement of appraisal, a marker of "good practice", part of the training curriculum and is beloved of medical academics everywhere. It was a compulsory part of the appraisal 5 year cycle until 2017. Yet it rarely discloses information of real clinical interest, is usually soft targeted at simple areas of data collection and is often actually carried out by practice administrators or an enthusiastic registrar. It is a product of the mass computerisation of practices. After all, we have all this data at the push of a computer key, we might as well analyse it. Audit (which actually means an ale formerly brewed in English colleges on the day of an official examination of the accounts) is usually done for convenience on the minimum number of patients and often on something simple like blood tests on Lithium or Methotrexate taking patients. It is yet another box we tick.

Wouldn't it be interesting to do a genuinely useful audit – like: Would male patients with personal medical problems actually prefer to consult male GPs in an all female practice? or How do patients rate the empathy levels of their doctors?, or do patients who are registered with full time partners have a more rewarding and consistent clinical experience than those who see part time or job sharing doctors over a long time period? Real problems that real patients care about that are never the subject of audit for some reason. To audit you need to collect numbers which you can then adjust and re-audit later. The number of manic depressives who had thyroid or Lithium bloods done in a defined time scale, the number of patients with diabetes who have had a cholesterol done. It is bean counting and then recounting. It can't contribute much to the really important questions, the ones which are analogue, subjective and can't be counted: Was the doctor competent, did they find out why you really went to see them, did you feel you were understood/ sympathised with, really helped by the doctor, did they actually listen, do you like them? etc etc.

The audit section of appraisal CAN be substituted for (hurrah) by two case reviews which demonstrate quality improvement and changed behaviour in the same way as an 8 stage audit. Or some other "Quality Improvement Activity (2017) which demonstrates changed behaviour or a better service.

This is how audits in exams and assessments are themselves assessed:

8 CRITERIA AUDIT MARKING SCHEDULE

Assessor's Name:	Date Sent for marking:	Date to be returned by assessor:
PG Certificate Student's Number:	Submission Date:	

ASSESSOR TO COMPLETE:

CRITERION	PRESENT	CRITERION PRESENT
Reason for choice of audit	Potential for change Relevant to the practice	
Criterion/Criteria Chosen	Relevant to audit subject and justifiable, e.g. Current literature	
Standards set	Targets towards a standard with a suitable timescale	
Preparation and Planning	Evidence of teamwork and adequate discussion where appropriate	
Data Collection (1)	Results compared against standard	
Change(s) to be evaluated	Actual example described	
Data Collection (2)	Comparison with data collection (1) and standard	

Conclusions	Summary of main issues learned	
A satisfactory audit should include all 8 criteria to be assessed as "Does meet criteria"		
This audit has been assessed as:	X Does not meet criteria	
Assessor Comments that will be used for feedback: Points for reflection:		

For instance:

Audit of Blood Test Monitoring for patients taking Methotrexate:

Thus:

Reason for choice of audit: I found one patient on Methotexate who hadn't had a blood test for several months. Methotrexate can cause blood dyscrasias and liver damage and current guidelines (referenced) are that FBC, renal and liver function be monitored before treatment, weekly until the dose is stable then every 12 weeks.

These patients should be made aware of and report the symptoms of potential side effects.

Criterion Chosen: Have a bold statement, in the title – you can say "All patients with X should have Y" – or "It is a marker of good care to increase/improve the number of patients taking methotrexate who have had appropriate bloods in the preceding 12 weeks."

All patients on a repeat prescription of methotrexate should have had their FBC, creatinine, U and Es and LFTs done in the last 12 weeks.

Standards Set: A standard of 90% was set. While in many circumstances a lower standard would be the norm, I felt a higher standard would be appropriate in view of the potential serious side effects of the medication. I felt we could achieve this within a 6 week time scale.

Method, Preparation and Planning: (Data collection)

I presented and discussed the topic with all the other doctors in the practice at our routine Monday Journal Club. They agreed: a) It was a clinically appropriate audit, b) It had not recently been assessed, c) It had clear potential patient benefits.

Then I made a computer search for all patients on Methotrexate medication for whatever reason. I pulled the notes and reviewed them to see if the above blood screens had been performed within the preceding 12 weeks.

Data Collection 1:(Be careful about exclusions and explain why these patients were excluded). Somewhere include a meeting with the partners if possible, don't mix criteria and standards. E.g. The initial search was on 1/1/14 finding all registered patients on that date taking Methotrexate on a repeat prescription. I checked all the notes (as well as up to date pathology results unfiled) to assess which patients had had their blood tests done within the preceding 12 weeks.

Number of patients on repeatMtx:	Number of patients with appropriate blood tests	with blood test results	Standard:
41	30	73.2%	90%

Change to be evaluated: On an 8 point audit (now mandatory in appraisal) start early in the year. I used a variety of means to improve the situation and improve the number of patients appropriately monitored. Each patient's electronic notes were flagged to prompt the next doctor or nurse seeing them to arrange a blood test and remind them of the importance of periodic screening. As patients are all on a 1 month repeat prescription, failure to comply would be identified at the next prescription request by administrative staff resulting in a personal conversation. This would be the time of the prescription request at the surgery, by E Mail or at the time of the phone call. The conversation would include the provision of a blood form and an explanation of the importance of future 3 monthly repeat testing. In addition a "Medication Review" Flag would be set up in each patient's notes at 3 monthly intervals to ensure the system was perpetuated.

Data collection 2: The second data search was performed from the patients' notes as above but on 1/3/14.

Number of patients with a repeat prescription for Methotrexate:	Number of patients with appropriately performed blood tests:	% with blood tests	Standard
41	38	92.7%	90%

Conclusions:

Our initial standard was significantly less than I had expected at 73% and meant that 11 patients were at risk. Even if the bloods were being done by, for instance a hospital Rheumatology department, good practice dictates that we should not, as responsible prescribers, issue a prescription in ignorance of the results. It took little effort to identify most of the patients who were not being monitored and to improve overall patient care and safety. The three patients yet to be tested will be phoned separately to bring them into the fold. If we still receive no response then we will write explaining our intention to remove them from repeat prescribing until either we have performed the blood testing or received results if done elsewhere.

Although we examined three monthly maintenance monitoring, the audit could easily have been adapted to examine the adequacy of initial monitoring which is more frequent and to see how closely this followed guidelines.

In the last Audit article I read, the authors recommended an annual meeting to audit the year's audits. But then I wondered, shouldn't they set up some sort of audit on the quality and outcomes of those meetings too just to ensure the auditing of the audits was audited appropriately??

Computerisation in general practice: (and distraction from the job in hand)

Is the process whereby consultations became focussed on the gathering of data and the recording of numbers. It was imposed on General Practice in the UK 20 or so years ago. Prior to that we had hand written notes in Lloyd George folders which permitted diagrams (of bruising and areas of tenderness, the site of scars, cutaneous abnormalities and injury), the addition of photographs, occasionally interesting and relevant evidence (I have seen foreign drug labels, some removed foreign bodies and dead dried insects in small specimen bottles) all impossible now. Prior to the symbolic and physical dominance of the display screen and keyboard, both of which take the doctors attention, gaze and concentration away from the patient, GPs spent far more of the consultation looking into the faces of their patient not at the backspace key and the delete buttons. The quality of the consultation, the role of the GP, the experience of the patient and the satisfaction of both have suffered. The more enthusiastic a practice is about data collection and about software, computers and new technology the less connected they become with their patients. This is a golden rule of General Practice.

You could almost argue the higher the QuoF and Audit numbers, the more IT Literate the partners, the more unhappy the patients. Well, almost.

Why did GPs have to accept the computer imposed and interposed literally between them and their patients?

Because Government via Health Authorities and PCTs wanted to exercise more control over the day to day behaviour of this effective, crucial but expensive part of the Health Service. – Why?

to facilitate data collection by government and official bodies

to monitor the activities of GPs to control and direct them

to enable GP's employers to pay them based on a throughput and item of service basis not on patient outcomes or satisfaction.

Most of the subsequent contracts were based, as well as QuoF payments etc on computerised data collection.

Computerisation of the consulting office is one of the commonest consistently harmful factors raised by American primary care physicians when asked about negative influences in the doctor patient relationship. It is an ongoing and vehement discussion amongst their primary healthcare doctors. In fact they have now had to be financially incentivised by healthcare insurers to use computers and record data "conveniently". By the end of 2014 however, the Medicare program was to penalise 257,000 American physicians and other "healthcare providers" 1% of their pay the following year for failing to "achieve meaningful use of electronic health record (EHR) technology in previous years." This number surprised the American Medical Association as it was more than 50% of eligible professionals. The AMA immediately adopted a resolution urging the centers for Medicare and Medicaid services to suspend all "meaningful use penalties" saying the requirements were too difficult for physicians to meet. Most American physicians clearly feel that the computer, whether financially incentivised or not, harms the rapport and interaction, indeed the very relationship between the doctor and the patient. A 2014 review found just 34% of American physicians were satisfied with their EHR system.

In an EHR review in August 2015, (Medscape) the more independent minded primary care physicians of the USA, not yet as brow beaten and demoralised as their UK GP counterparts reported as follows:

72% said EHRs made it difficult or very difficult to reduce their work load,

54% complained of higher operating costs,

43% had not yet returned to their pre EHR level of activity.

and I quote: These findings buttress numerous other reports of a backlash against EHRs, often said to reduce physicians to data entry clerks who are more preoccupied with satisfying federal meaningful use requirements than the patients they are treating. **So if we are honest, computerisation has cost us time, quality of consulting, extra work, extra money and reduced satisfaction. It has changed us to unskilled automatons. But also look at it from the patient's point of view (literally) and ask yourself whether computerisation has improved the patient's experience of seeing the doctor.**

Even worse, in a study published, ironically online, Jan 26, 2017 in JAMA Ophthalmology, Data in Electronic Health Records were shown not even to accurately record patient reported symptoms. So with the computer between us, we really aren't listening to the patient.

I believe the same is true of the patient experience in the UK and that of many doctors – at least those who care about doing their best for patients. Computerisation has partly ruined the doctor patient relationship, the quality of communication, involvement and connection between the doctor and the patient. Diagnoses are missed because the doctor is distracted by on screen tasks and not focussed on the patient. For many GPs, when PC should mean patient centred it too often means personal computer. How many illnesses are wrongly treated, signs and cues missed, early calls for help ignored because the screen and keyboard were in control of the doctor and he or she was preoccupied??

This was summed up by Dr John Mandrola speaking about "The worst mistakes in Medicine in 2015" regarding computerised medical notes (EHRs). He comments about computerisation in America but it is the same here:

"Policy makers including but not limited to President Obama, predicted that we could use the savings from digitising medical records to pay for extending insurance coverage. It is the worst prediction because what has resulted, the current day electronic health record, EHR, is an **unmitigated disaster**. EHRs not only remove humanity from the patient/doctor interaction, they distract care givers from what is most important. Distraction in my mind is our number one safety issue. EHRs make it worse."

This is basically saying that computers on our desks have damaged every consultation. Surely a statement of the blindingly obvious?

American doctors tend to be more forthright, vocal and independent than we are in Britain in openly and publically criticising the mistakes of modern medicine like computerisation but they also ask patients what they think a bit more than we do:

A study published in late 2015 confirmed that patients, particularly less sophisticated and less articulate patients think computerisation of consultations is a disaster too.

"Safety Net Hospitals" serve deprived communities in the US. A study (Nov 30 2015 JAMA Int Med. N. Ratanawongsa) of 71 videotaped consultations in these hospitals asked the patients to rate the care they were receiving. The videos were used to assess computer use by the physician, length of the visit, patient education level, clinical demographics, communication variables and so on.

You can guess, (– well if you are patient focussed, not a computer enthusiast, you can guess) what the patients thought of their doctors and their computer use. Less than half (48%) of the doctors with heavy computer use during the consultation had their care rated as excellent. Whereas 83% of patients with physicians "less engaged" with the computer thought their care was excellent.

High computer use was associated with observable "communication differences". Patients with doctors using the computer a lot engaged in more "chit chat" ("social rapport building"-presumably trying to engage with their doctor because they felt the doctor was not focussed enough on THEM). Those patients with doctors using computers less were observed to have a more positive demeanour. Physicians with high computer use engaged in more "negative rapport building" – making more statements to the patient involving criticism or disagreement. The authors commented:

"Concurrent computer use can inhibit authentic engagement and multitasking physicians may miss openings for deeper engagement. Negative rapport building may be an unintentional consequence of the Electronic Health Record". In an accompanying editorial, Richard Frankel from the Indiana University School of Medicine and Centre for Healthcare Information and Communication says "Our challenge is to find the best ways to incorporate computers in the examination room without losing the soul of medicine: the physician patient relationship". He suggested engaging in dialogue with the patient, without the computer then turning the screen toward the patient so he or she can see what is being written.

The alternative would be to turn the screen to the wall, call in the patient, consult, examine, prescribe and then write up once they have gone. Result: Everyone happy.

Useful Training/Learning/Reference Resources/Useful references:

Useful resources: Books, websites, apps, organisations etc etc

The single most useful book and resource to have on your desk and the thing you will use the most is a hard copy of an up to date MIMS. First published at a fraction of its current size in 1959, the Monthly Index of Medical Specialities is republished quarterly and free to all GPs. There is an online version at mims.co.uk and an app for your smart phone although this is nothing like as easy to use as the heavier original. MIMS contains information on most generic drugs, virtually all proprietary drugs as well as updated tables on antibiotic treatment in adults, withdrawing antidepressants, Calcium and Vitamin D preparations, contraceptives, diabetic medications and meters/test strips, ophthalmic treatments (including sensitising constituents), HRT, the routine childhood immunisation schedule, asthma treatments, topical steroids, smoking cessation treatments, vaccination and malaria guidance.

There are also the standard accepted clinical guidance algorithms for hypertension, preventing CVD, advice on fitness to drive, treatment of H. Pylori , IBS, Crohn's Disease, U.C., the management of asthma (BTS and SIGN),COPD, the menopause and a comparison of opioid potencies.

www.medilexicon.com A very useful and extensive list of medical acronyms and initials
www.bmj.learning.com
www.doctors.net ("The UK's largest professional network of doctors"?)
Doctor.net
SIGN Scottish Intercollegiate Guidelines Network. A useful collection of evidence based clinical guidelines.
IER Informatics Eden Resource – (BMJ) an education resource for health informatics
Patient advice leaflets (University Hospital Birmingham etc) – Good general Q and As
Frimley Green Medical Centre.
Filey Surgery
Bradford VTS Web pages – this is very well organised, includes "The Essential Handbook for GP Training and Education" etc. Very slick and accessible. I have used some

of their training information because I couldn't find it put or displayed better anywhere. Thank you to them.

http://www.gp-training.net/(protocol/protocol.htm)

eGuidelines Guidelines in practice (also an app)

Evidence based medicine www.herts.ac.uk/lis/subjects/health/ebm.htm

Bandolier http://www.medicine.ox.ac.uk/bandolier. (Evidence based medicine) A bandolier is a shoulder belt for bullets. I presume they thought that using it might give you ammunition for intellectual skirmishes and battles?

www.macmillan.org.uk Provides information on Macmillan nurses and the help they can provide for patients and their families.

Cochrane: http://cochrane.org/index.htm – The Cochrane library – "A collection of six databases of independent evidence to inform healthcare decisions" Systematic reviews of controlled trials etc.

GP Notebook: http://www.gpnotebook.co.uk Has a tracker recording what you have done.

GP-training.net

Onmedica.net CME courses PD tracker

eBNF

e textbooks: eMedicine (Medscape)

Merck Manual online

Bartleby.com-an electronic text archive including medical textbooks and a quotation database

The Genetics Home Reference website

Dermatlas.org Pictures of skin conditions

Safefetus.com (sorry about the spelling) Risks of various drugs to the developing foetus. It is American but very useful.

www.easyauscultation.com An excellent site with accessible descriptions of both adult and congenital heart murmurs.

Drugs.com For drug interactions and side effects etc

The Developmental Progress of infants and young Children Mary Sheridan (London Stationery Office) A book with illustrations. Your parents will tell you how to use one.

Aids to the Investigation of peripheral nerve injuries (HMSO) MRC No 7

Labtestsonline Although they are annoyingly reluctant to give normal levels.

The brilliant: Laboratory tests and Diagnostic Procedures by Chernecky and Berger which does give normal levels (W.B.Saunders) in old (American) and SI units and likely causes of abnormal results for every test you will ever want.

Science-Based Medicine website – evaluates medical (and alternative) treatments objectively.

Prodigy Clarity Informatics. Evidence summaries for NICE "CKS"-NICE Clinical knowledge summaries.

Arthritis Research UK: A great source of information and exercise/rehabilitation sheets for patients.-In fact nearly every disease has a dedicated charity which provides information and help to patients free of charge and can be accessed from your computer.

TOXBASE (you need to have a password).

The National Poisons Information Service 0870 600 6266

Global RPh: For normal drug levels

Web MD: General medical information, not particularly detailed.
Other information for patients:
www.nhschoices.nhs.uk
www.patient.co.uk
Http://sdm.rightcare.nhs.uk/
www.evidence.nhs.uk/
Http://guidance.nice.org.uk/
The National Cancer Institute Website for cancer facts, treatments, epidemiology but the statistics are American.
Breastcancer.org and
"Imaginis" are good breast cancer resource websites
Aftercure is an online support group for childhood cancer survivors.
    i Want Great Care www.iwgc.org   www.iwantgreatcare.org "The trusted site for healthcare reviews" from patients, about hospitals, surgeries, dentists, physios, nursing homes etc.
    www.healthmap.org shows world maps with the areas of outbreaks of:
Vectorborn, Gastrointestinal, Respiratory, Animal, Skin and Rash, Other Alerts, Neuro, Fever/Febrile, STD, Environmental, Haemorrhagic and MRSA/Hospital based infections worldwide.
    E Mail medadviser@dvla.gsi.gov.uk for all driving related questions.
    Therapeutic and toxic drug levels are available online from many sources including the very useful: http://www.globalrph.com/labs_drugs_levels.htm
    Please add other resources you like:

Training Theory:
(Which I have to admit all sounds a lot more useful than it actually is)

Maslow's Hierarchy:	Autonomy/Self factuation
Self Esteem	Esteem
Recognition	Learning
Confidence	Love and belonging
Safety	Safety
Survival	Physiological needs

The Inner Curriculum:

Autonomy
Self-Esteem
Recognition
Confidence
Safety
Survival

The inner curriculum is a "hierarchy of educational needs and achievements"

Teaching Styles:
Socratic
Didactic
Pedagogic
Andragogic

Learning Styles:	Learning Style Inventory:
Activist	Accommodator/Converger/Diverger/Assimilator
Reflector	
Theorist	
Pragmatist	
(Honey and Mumford)	

Some Learning Theory:

You may remember that the **Kolb Learning Cycle** Is: Active experimentation>Concrete experience>Reflective observation>Abstract conceptualisation and back to>Active experimentation.

Put more simply: Experience, reflection, conclusion, planning.

By the way, I hate the constant overuse by medical educators of the term **"Reflection"** – which we learnt at O Level (GCSE) physics means turning incoming data (e.g. light) back to front, inverted and reversed and meanwhile yourself, the reflector, (like a mirror) being completely unaffected by it. With learning we should be **"Diffracting"** (breaking into constituent parts – sieving, analysing and organising the incoming information logically) not Reflecting – That is if you really need to borrow a term for thinking about stuff from natural philosophy.

"Professional Boundaries":

Why are they important?: The conventional wisdom:

They help ensure the doctor will act in the best interest of the patient

They provide consistency, predictability and security in the doctor-patient relationship.

They help to promote transparency and clarity and to avoid ambiguity in the relationship.

They help the patient judge if the relationship is safe or not.

But why are they also subjective and dubious?

Clearly where a doctor lives in a community and is a parent, neighbour, co-worshipper, local councillor, community volunteer, recognised local resident and personality etc his (or her) relationship with his patients is more complex (and rewarding) than the urban doctor who's hours may be comparatively limited and who may live outside the practice area. The same rules cannot apply. Of course you make friends and develop relationships with people who happen to be your patients. Of course you celebrate and greave with them. Professionalism doesn't mean personal distance, coldness or lack of feeling.

How can the village doctor not celebrate the coming of age of a patient's disabled child, or attend the celebration of a patient's first year anniversary of remaining "dry" or go to dinner when invited by a family with similar attitudes and interests but who happen to be his or her patients? Should I have refused to go to the party of a long term heroin addict, wheel chair and house bound who I visited monthly for over a decade who through grim determination finally got herself off controlled drugs?

As so often in General Practice, there are actually no absolutes.

Appraisal and Revalidation:

The purpose of appraisal (for revalidation): The official definition goes something like:

To enable doctors to discuss practice and performance with the appraiser, to demonstrate they are up to "Good Medical Practice" and to "inform the "Responsible Officer's" revalidation recommendation to the GMC. Also to "Help GPs to consider and to plan professional development needs and to give doctors a chance to think if they are working productively and "in line" with the organisation in which they work. "

In practice: five acceptable annual appraisal folders = one Revalidation.

I have been an appraiser since the start of Revalidation (2002/3) and Relicensing (2009). I signed up with the very first group to do what I could to ensure that appraisal didn't get out of touch with the reality and the difficulties of doing what I call "real" General Practice. So that it didn't become another millstone around a good GP's neck. I feared appraisal could quickly become controlled by the expanding grasp of an organisation like the Royal College of GPs and its local deanery empires. Up until then The RCGP trained the trainers of aspiring GPs and set GP professional coming of age exams. The vast majority of GPs, even those with the exam qualification subsequently had little to do with what was seen as an unworldly and out of touch organisation. It might be hard to believe now but when appraisal started, the Royal College didn't own it or dictate its shape. Once it became part of the College's remit, the future funding of the College was assured. Also, they and the deaneries could justify their sizes, staff and costs. Indeed, they would be part of a regular compulsory legal process for all GPs and therefore part of the statutory establishment. But instead, many of us felt it needed down to earth, practical GPs not class room doctors out there appraising their colleagues. This is because the quality of a doctor's practice has little to do with educational theory, audits, selectively flattering feedback from colleagues, how many educational events you have attended or done on line and so on – and anyway you know what they say about teachers.

Unfortunately since then appraisal **has** become an academic exercise supervised by the College with standardised and largely pointless audits, significant events-which can be only be constructive as long as you make real changes to avoid the same mistakes again – and genuinely change yourself as part of the process, almost meaningless (and sometimes damaging) 360 degree feedback, an accountant's paradise of adding up the negotiated hours of impact and challenge of meetings and bartering the highly subjective value of learning (?!). It now (2016) appears that the age of the appraiser influences the "lenience" or strictness of the appraisal interaction as well (the older the more generous and forgiving) so it is hardly an objective process. Also there is patient feedback which can occasionally be almost 100% positive (as with my own patients latterly – and how does that help me to improve? – In fact it actually possibly caused resentment amongst my partners) or nit picking and sometimes mischievous criticism of doctors by difficult or manipulative patients. And there are plenty around of **them.**

If the patients hoped that the politicians and educators would use the Shipman horror to introduce a system to root out further murdering psychopaths or dangerous and uncaring doctors and improve the consulting, clinical and personal skills of the profession, forget it. Unfortunately this is not remotely what appraisal does. This is not surprising since the RCGP and their agents, the deaneries, are educators not critical assessors, not policemen, not staff sergeants, not prefects. Now we have an expensive bureaucratic and increasingly proscriptive examination of a doctor's willingness to engage with a standardised academia: nothing more. Does this make him a better GP? I doubt it. A safer GP? Probably not. A nicer GP, a more understanding or approachable GP? Of course not. And the most recent audit of GP opinion (GP magazine Aug 2017) was that 67% thought it had no beneficial effect on their practice at all.

But give me total control over the GMC, the Royal Colleges, the deaneries, the medical schools, the Department of Health and I would invent a much better, patient focussed and patient protecting way of assessing my colleagues fairly and honestly. It would root out any new Shipmans, improve standards and it would be a system that most doctors would respect and respond to.

It would not be under the control of those unelected, unrepresentative and unresponsive bodies, the RCGP and the GMC. It might involve feedback from undertakers and from relatives of the last five dead patients on the doctor's list. It wouldn't be annually either because it would take a lot longer than 2 hours face to face contact to get through. It would involve sitting in on surgeries, reading notes, interviewing real patients and partners in confidence. It would involve going over every complaint, formal and informal (with an open mind because not every complaint is FAIR) from the preceding 2-3 years. And each appraiser would have access to all preceding appraisal summaries (which we don't at present). It would put the patient's experience and outcome at the centre stage. Not the process – for what else other than "process" is the quality of an audit, the subjective impression of a colleague, the number of hours of personal or group study or the fatuous nonsense the "celebration of excellence"?

I used to go on appraiser update courses regularly and am stunned by what appraisal currently **excludes:**

These are some authoritative instructions from regional conferences run by our Deanery over the last few years:

I quote:

It is **"Not our responsibility to pursue health issues of the appraisee** if none are presented at appraisal" (including mental health issues). I have appraised doctors who had extreme OCD, depression, anxiety, even extremely poor hearing and communication skills all of which might have prevented them being effective doctors. None of this "is the concern of appraisal".

The appraiser should spend 20 minutes on the revalidation check list, then **the rest of the time (2-3hours) "celebrating the doctor's personal development".** *"Celebrating"* an interesting term if your real purpose is or should be investigating and improving standards and putting the patient's needs first.

"We are only there to assess "Up to date and safe practice" (not the patient's experience or the doctor's interpersonal skills) and that the doctor "Seems safe to practice" i.e. if "There is an absence of evidence of danger".

An absence of evidence of danger! – So a car is safe to drive and carry passengers if there is no obvious pool of brake fluid, oil on the ground or flat tyres when you stand and look at it?

I specifically asked at one appraisal conference what we should do if we were given evidence by another partner in a practice during their own appraisal of a colleague's lack of safety. In answer, a Deanery Appraisal Supervisor made it clear it was "Not our job to deal with this at appraisal" (KSS Appraiser Conference March 2012) so presumably we should pretend we hadn't heard it.

So: I am afraid appraisal has now become a sort of annual 11-plus exam which does nothing to assess a doctor's real competence, their patient value or safety and nothing to improve clinical standards. It is a: "How many courses and meetings have you attended?, how many "show" audits and significant events can you or someone else write up for you and have you organised questionnaires for the people you work with and the patients you see?" Tell me how **that** actually assesses how good at doctoring and how safe a doctor you are?

We are all sick of ticking boxes, of the clip board standardisation of the modern NHS so criticised by Robert Francis. It seems that no one trusts us to get on with our jobs without check lists, algorithms, reports or protocols anymore – except perhaps the patients. Even they, because we now concentrate so much on administration and the screen, worry that we no longer see their well being as the prime reason we come to work.

All appraisals are now done on computer, something that always slows down and interferes with the smooth running of the process. Just like the American Primary Care Physicians commenting on Electronic Health Notes, "Computerisation has cost us time, quality of consulting, extra work, extra money and reduced satisfaction" the same is true of appraisal and wherever computers poke their standardising, turgid, inflexible, soul destroying, disciplinarian heads in.

I was aware today while appraising a colleague and being constantly stopped from finishing by the computer "Toolkit" software that the format was quite literally a box ticking process. A whole list of boxes (actually circles) had to be ticked (the mouse pressed and the circles highlighted) after the completion of the appraisal but the answer to each was obvious from the preceding appraisal section and therefore actually superfluous. I had just written a report saying that I had no concerns about the probity, safety, competence etc of the doctor but I still had to tick all the boxes saying the same things again to satisfy the Toolkit and sign the thing off. Just ticking boxes. Doctors shouldn't have to act like simpletons in this way. You complete the various sections of the appraisal, sign them off, then tell the computer you have signed them off, then tell it you are happy the appraisal is complete and sign it off again. Usually you then find you haven't properly signed off one of the preceding sections and have to go back. Aaarrrgggghhhhhh.

The status of the profession by the start of 2017 was: Revalidation which takes place 5 yearly had been undergone by 205,000 of the 230,000 doctors on the medical register. A decision on whether or not to allow a doctor to continue is based on annual appraisals and feedback from patients and colleagues. It is up to Responsible Officers in each organi-sation- normally Medical Directors to make the recommendations. Minor issues lead to the deferral of revalidation for a short period while the problems are addressed. 40,000 doctors were in this position. Serious concerns lead to a referral to the GMC's disciplinary process. If the doctor does not engage with the process they lose their licence. This has happened to 3,500 doctors.

The "Forms": (Now on the Toolkits)

There are sections each appraisee has to personally complete on
knowledge, skills and performance,
safety and quality,
communication, partnership and teamwork and
maintaining trust.
Every individual interprets these headings differently and personally.
TRUST:
For instance: How do you summarise your ability to maintain trust and how can you objectively prove that your patients do actually trust you? What have you done to improve the trust your patients have in you? – Something like trust really only comes from famili-arity and repeated positive contact with you and your medical decisions over a long period of time. Trust is earned, it takes a long time and much of modern General Practice with sessional, locum and part time doctors, very large industrial practices where continuity of

care is the exception mitigate against trust EVER developing between patient and doctor. So the very idea of **Trust** demonstrates the problem of Appraisal as currently formulated and the sort of people who designed it. Indeed, if trust is important and of course it is, shouldn't continuity of care be considered the bedrock of good Primary Care just as it always used to be and something Royal College Presidents and The GMC should be campaigning for energetically?

Trust is a profound and significant word. It means a firm belief in the reliability, truth or ability of someone. A patient may not trust a part time doctor they rarely see or a new doctor as much as a full time or well established doctor. A patient must have had numerous subjectively successful interactions with positive outcomes to develop their own "Trust" in a doctor. It will depend for most people on familiarity. On the other hand some patients may trust some doctors by reputation or recommendation without any previous experience of them. A patient may not trust a doctor who made a wrong diagnosis once or who previously refused a treatment for good reasons that the patient thought they needed. Every patient and doctor will have a different definition of it. Some patients may never trust any doctor no matter what their experience of them because they have been previously disenchanted by medical failure or betrayal. Some may have blind and unjustified trust in the medical profession.

Trust sounds good but a little analysis exemplifies the unworldliness and irrelevance of it as a philosophical concept in this context and likewise many of the chapter headings of appraisal. How can real trust be earned, proven, demonstrated and how does it relate to competence, sympathy, caring, availability, actually being a good doctor?

This is all designed to **sound** good. The headings are worthy and honourable desires but the appraisal has no demonstrable purpose or objective focus. There is absolutely no common sense or rigour related to how *the patient* would view the job actually done by the GP. Most of the MSF questions are meaningless and you are prevented by the format from answering in any useful or constructive way. Even the patient feedback is notoriously manipulative, inconsistent, sample dependent and what do you do with it anyway? It's like this is all a philosophical assessment and not a rational investigation of clinical ability, safety, skill or competence at all.

A moment's thought about these subject headings and you realise that a committee must have thought them up and the members of that committee had their heads in books, wish fulfilment theory, how it would all sound later over supper and their feet were anywhere but on the hard ground of General Practice. The very idea that I could come into a stranger's surgery and assess something as nebulous as "Trust" having read a highly selected and edited summary of work items and feedback without the ability to interview anybody else is quite frankly, puerile. I have seen and appraised many doctors with excellent appraisal folders, well written and summarised, PDPs and audits according to the rules, good feedback, wordy summaries of clinical meetings and lots of "education". AND I have known through friends who are their patients how distant, disinterested, uncommunicative or self satisfied they are in their role as a doctor and wished that I were able to use appraisal to actually improve their performance.

Yes and sometimes to prick their bubble of complacency and pomposity.

So appraisal has become exactly what those of us outside the medical teaching establishment wanted it not to. A standardised, time consuming performance that we have to do annually and which is another depressing challenge to add to the list that GPs face every year.

By the way, appraisers were constantly told that appraisal should not be a "cosy fireside chat". In my opinion appraisal actually partially comes into its own when the appraiser is a GP of some experience and advises and supports the appraisee who is in a difficult practice situation, (partnership dysfunction, patient complaints, staff disharmony, substance abuse issues etc) and can act as a mentor and "friend" who has been through it and survived. I see no problem doing this next to a fire sitting down in a comfortable chair.

Regarding the fifty hours of Learning Activity: (– well, fifty credits rather than actual hours, some until 2016 made up from the combination of the *challenge* and the *impact* of the learning activity on, respectively, you and "your practice"): This is what Ben Goldacre, who writes about Bad Science and Bad Pharmacology in the Guardian (etc) says: "This is about the need to attend drug company sponsored educational events as a consequence of the educational points counting of appraisal:

In a rather odd game of consequences, this means that a set of new regulations, brought in to prevent doctors from murdering people, in reality has simply shepherded them even more into the hands of expensive industry sponsored promotional activity where they are misled about the benefits of expensive medicines, and so harm patients."

You need 250 one hour learning credits in a 5 year cycle. 50 hours per year. One hour of learning a week. If the one hour of learning has significant "patient impact" you can claim another credit for the impact. The same for the "challenge" or how hard it was to actually do the "learning". Reading a book, no challenge, getting to a distant lecture in a snowstorm or a flood, lots of challenge. That is how silly it is. There is a move in 2016 to end the dynamising of credits and hence end haggling at the appraisal itself.

CPD Continuous professional development, is based on the TIME spent on the activity. Personal reading can generally only be used for up to 10 credits. You can't say that you don't like going out to meetings, (as one of my appraisees did), or have a phobia of meeting other doctors or going out at night so all you ever do is read some journal or other for an hour a week. That would rather miss the point of the thing. Anyway most people think you learn as much from networking over coffee as you do from the actual meetings themselves. You shouldn't just use the one hour a week practice Journal Club as your only source of education either. I have learnt that most doctors attending post graduate meetings are part time female GPs who are desperate to talk to the other part time female GPs about

1) Their baby (ies)

2) How they resent having to go back to work and leave their baby in the hands of someone else after 6 months, 9 months etc.

3) How working three to four half days a week and clocking off at 12.00 o'clock is really hard work.

4) How they object to not having their voices heard and opinions taken note of by the other partners just because they never manage to attend practice meetings which are in the evening.

5) How their practice nice partners aren't so nice anymore and aren't happy about covering without notice when the baby is ill and aren't babies ill a lot?

6) Don't the other partners realise that they can't cover at short notice for the other

partners, they have a family now and their husband works etc etc.?

Back to credits:

There should be a good demonstration of a wide range of learning and a variety of types/sources. Practice organisational or management meetings without genuine educational or professional developmental content do not count. There MUST be reasonable REFLECTION (meaning personal consideration of the value of the activity and whether it will change or improve your practice, thought out, written down and discussed). Put to one side that the real meaning of reflection is: getting things back to front and being entirely unaffected by the incoming (light) information yourself – as in a mirror.

You need to do 1 MSF, from at least 10 colleagues, at least 5 of whom should be clinical, (Multi Source Feedback in this instance not Medicine Sans Frontieres) – this is colleague feedback, – however pointless, potentially harmful or cautiously over diplomatic the colleagues may be **in 5 years and**

1 patient survey (PSQ) Patient satisfaction questionnaire (slightly less pointless perhaps) in the same time. Generally speaking, the longer your patient list has known you and the more personal your list system is, the kinder the feedback becomes.

You also need to do ten significant event audits (or "clinical incidents", "significant untoward incidents" or "significant event analyses") although many appraisers are a bit confused about this, as the GMC does not require a minimum number of SEAs to be brought to appraisal for revalidation (2012 GMC doc pp 9) however the RCGP (RCGP doc pp 9 and 10) issued guidance in 2011 that a minimum of 2 SEAs should be brought to each appraisal. If there were no S.E. presented then case reviews would do (with a "learning outcome" good or bad) or reviews of "clinical outcomes", case review or discussion: The bottom line: It seems that most appraisers don't expect 2 significant event analyses a year – *but some do.* The cases don't have to be those you have personally been involved in or even cases your practice has been involved in.

and one eight phase clinical audit in five years – or two cases reviewed with an unproscriptive "it could have been done better if" summary included – hopefully showing quality improvement and change in behaviour.

Reviews of Quality Improvement activity (a highly subjective and flexible term) – **QIA.**

Our local deanery has put out the instruction that there should be "one substantial QIA" per 5 years (audit or similar) with smaller personal SEAs or case reviews in the other years of the 5 years cycle. The GMC says quality improvement activities "take many forms" but include clinical audit, review of clinical outcomes, case review or discussion, auditing or monitoring a teaching program or the very nebulous "evaluating the impact of a piece of health policy or management practice". See below**. Do you see now how this is an academic GP's dream and has nothing whatsoever to do with competent, safe or patient centred General Practice?

Discussion of Complaints and Compliments. We are British for goodness sake, we don't discuss compliments. BUT can I be honest? I have had a loyal and stable list for a third of a century. I have been devoted to them and most of them are pretty loyal to me. I go out at night and do my own terminal care, I attend their funerals if I can, I do my own post natal visits, I take the job home with me and worry about my decisions and treatment. I am angry about the failings of the NHS on their behalf and am personally upset if anyone writes a letter of complaint about me. The feedback is nearly all very nice so basically, I don't think a criticism in an MSF would make me change the way I do things now. Now that was a bit un-British wasn't it?

Professional Development Plans: Last and next year (at least three aims in each).

The development plan each year should have at least three "doable" intentions. These goals must be specific, measurable, achievable, relevant, time bounded – and with the constant love academics have for catchy acronyms this spells **SMART** which sounds American or TRAMS which sounds old fashioned and English or M, RATS which is meaningless.

There is also the **5p paradigm** which is often mentioned at this point in appraisal: person, practice, patient, population, politics. – you are supposed to ask how does the PDP connect with these various areas?

Nothing if not ambitious (or they could make it the 6 p paradigm with **pretentious!**)

Also you have to comment on Health and Probity. I have never had anyone raise anything vaguely questionable at appraisal regarding their own probity although I know practices that have advertisements on posters in waiting rooms, expensive delays on phone systems paid for by unsuspecting patients, first wave fund holders who invested in privately owned surgery premises with their fund holding profits, cost rent returns that far exceed mortgages, private cash in hand medicals, certificates and minor ops which go through no books, doctors on Local Commissioning Groups who have family businesses tendering for contracts and board members themselves directors of provider companies and so on. So what is the point of even asking about probity?

A record of other annual appraisals and old and current PDPs.

STOP PRESS:

At the turn of 2016/7 the rules on appraisal changed slightly: Perhaps because of another winter of unprecedented bed paucity, ambulance queues and this year, even cancer surgery cancellations due to lack of beds. All this was added to one month waits to see GPs and a "Humanitarian Crisis" (said the Red Cross) in hospitals and had resulted in numerous calls to end the distracting administrative millstones on GPs of appraisal, QuoF and CQC inspections.

The new appraisal changes were supposed to reflect the lamentable trend towards portfolio and sessional careers. These changes apply to England only. Scotland, Wales and Ulster were awaiting changes as of early 2017:

An end to the silly automatic doubling of credits for "impact" -which was always very subjective and open to haggling. Credits can be claimed for related proven activity such as giving your colleagues a teaching session on novel anticoagulants or long acting insulins after attending a half day course to learn about them. You can claim for your preparation and giving the talk. That is fairer than the old system of claiming for some nebulous effect that knowing about a new treatment was going to have on your "practice".

To claim a CPD point you now have to record a "reflection" on that learning- for instance if the specific new knowledge has made any difference to the way you will work. The reflection may be on teaching sessions, Significant Events, MSF, complaints (record these as a Serious Untoward Incidents) and compliments etc.

Reflection can be short winded and (hurray) negative. Towards the end of one's career an increasing number of meetings do seem repetitive and fairly pointless- and it has to be said, do not change the way one practices. I particularly refer to child protection, resuscitation, "dealing with change" and "the consultation", type meetings. Also a lot of hospital doctors haven't the faintest idea about the medicine of General Practice, our patients, their diseases, treatments and our working lives so they can sometimes seem irrelevant or patronising.

You only need to reflect on 50 credits/year.

No more Audits!! Instead various "Quality Improvement Activities" on all your various GP roles.

No more need to record two Significant Events a year. Appraisal now requires S.E. meetings and you can record them in your CPD with reflection and credits claimed if you wish.

You have to show one "Quality Improvement Activity" a year. This is self explanatory but could be an audit as before, a data search, SEA, case reviews, review of your referral or outcomes and reflecting on your various roles.

Serious Untoward Incidents are significant events that cause patient harm or significant risk of harm. There is a standard "Root Cause Analysis" proforma.

There should be a CPD, QIA, and some feedback for all GP roles outside the practice. NHS England will produce a suggested template although for the portfolio GP it is easy to see how time consuming this varied data collection will quickly become.

An MSF every 5 years with at least 35 patients feeding back, independently collated.

I don't know how long appraisal, adding as it does, a disproportionate load of work to the average GP and not really being fit for the purpose of weeding out dangerous and incompetent doctors, will survive. As I say elsewhere, the process should be more focused, more personal, more patient -experience based, more intense and a lot less frequent.

While we are on the subject of catchy acronyms, the appraiser still has a few more up his or her sleeve:

There is Excelllence for instance: (yes, three Ls)

When reviewing the appraiser's statements in the "output document", has Each role been considered? Have you excluded any prejudice? Challenged, supported and encouraged? Explained any reasons why any statements have not been signed off? Looked at supporting information regarding the GMC four domains? Looked at supporting information lessons learned and changes made? Last year's PDP? Encouraged excellence etc Noted any areas not covered in the revalidation requirements and how they will be addressed? Contains SMART PDP objectives? Explain the new PDP items?

OK this must be the worst aid memoire ever invented, stretching, padding and misspelling all in one largely unnecessary politically correct reminder. Sorry I even mentioned it.

Revalidation

Revalidation is to "assure patients and public that doctors are up to date and fit to practice". Basically it is standardised and based on 5 satisfactory annual appraisals.

Officially, appraisal is to enable discussion of the appraisee's practice and performance and to compare these with the "Good Medical Practice" publication from the GMC thus allowing the "Responsible Officer" to make a revalidation recommendation to the GMC. It is also "to enable doctors to plan their professional development".

So each year all appraisees submit a "Standard Portfolio" which is reviewed before appraisal by the appraiser, then discussed and completed by both at appraisal. Usually this is done on a "toolkit" – electronically these days. The available toolkits are all different, idiosyncratic and complicated.

The contents of "Good Medical Practice" are supposed to be used as evidence at appraisal. Then after the appraisal has been done, the boxes ticked and the appraisal office informed that all has been completed, the revalidation decision box is ticked by the R.O. (The local Responsible Officer). Then the GP is left alone for a year.

The Good Medical Practice Four Domains:

The "Good Medical Practice" booklet from the GMC:

The new edition was published in March 2013. It has on its cover a pretty smiling Asian female doctor who wears round her neck the now ubiquitous Trust I.D. card and is wearing a light blue dress or surgical scrubs.

The message the picture conveys is of a pleasant, welcoming, open minded, tolerant health service and you can stop worrying now. The image is aimed at the urban hospital doctor. The publication was no doubt designed by a PR firm with an inherently inclusive, everything is going to be all right if we work together brief. Ignoring the fact that two thirds of medical students are now women and a quarter are from ethnic minority groups, – in other words, medical school selection committees are racist and sexist against white males, who make up 43% of the population. They were probably unaware of the public's recent and apparently growing concerns about the quality and competence of some medical practitioners trained abroad. Indeed complaints and register suspensions are up to ten times more likely from some countries than for doctors trained in the UK. Most PR design team "creatives" are nice tolerant open minded people and they certainly wouldn't want a white, grey haired middle aged male doctor on the cover of "Good Medical Practice". So you can imagine the conversations about that sort of conservative cliché around the doughnuts, coffee and jelly beans at the East London design team table.

You may not think these things are relevant and I doubt whether the team who designed the final "Good Medical Practice" publication were aware that the GMC itself disciplines twice as many foreign trained graduates after complaints from the public regarding standards and behaviour as they do British graduates. I doubt whether they knew that only 20% of foreign trained doctors were at the median British medical school trained level – see page 40. You could argue that the pretty doctor on the cover could be a British graduate but usually it is a one glance visual image on a book cover that is designed to give its message in five seconds and not make you go away and ponder the hidden meaning. Possibly the cover carries a double irony and the final approval was very Machiavellian indeed – a kind of in-joke. Perhaps it just means that publicity and design companies, like medical supervisory and disciplinary bodies and the GMC itself are urban, London or big city based and have a clear political agenda in their attitudes, culture and opinions. They don't understand people who live in places smaller than Manchester-and are therefore somewhat out of contact with the general public. But more on that later.

London is as they say, a different country.

Anyway, to move back to Appraisal: The Attributes and Evidence:

Knowledge Skills and Performance: The so called "Attributes" are: Maintaining professional performance, applying knowledge and experience to practice, ensuring all records are clear accurate and legible.

Possible evidence would include: CPD and a reflective log, QuoF, PACT, case reviews etc.

Safety and quality: "Attributes" are: contributing to and complying with systems to protect patients, responding to safety risks, protecting colleagues and patients from risks posed by your own health.

Possible evidence: SEA, a health statement, complaints, child protection activity, CPR, audit, case/outcome reviews etc.

Communication, partnership and teamwork: "Attributes" are communicating effectively, working constructively and delegating effectively, establishing and maintaining partnerships with patients.

Possible evidence: Patient participation groups, patient feedback, colleague feedback, practice meetings, teaching, case discussion etc.

Maintaining Trust: (Perhaps the most nebulous, indefinable and subjective of all – see above:) "Attributes" are showing respect for patients, treating patients and colleagues fairly and without discrimination, acting with honesty and integrity.

Possible evidence: Complaints, probity statements, interaction with professional support groups, appraisals etc. None of which shows that your list genuinely **trusts** you because very little apart from the complaints has real currency.

All this sounds so reasonable and fair that it is the proverbial motherhood and apple pie, but when you begin to think about the reality of these "attributes" you realise yet again that they are far less helpful than they look– for instance: What if years of experience tells you that if you give every child with a temperature a big dose of broad spectrum antibiotic for at least a week then you avoid the need to see them with otitis, mastoiditis or secondary chest infections later and it does little REAL harm and occasionally you save a life. Or that it is better to give all women with dysuria expensive but effective antibiotics like Cefadroxil or Co Amoxiclav first line, in order to avoid Trimethoprim and Amoxicillin resistance and complications. Or people trying to stop smoking don't need to waste time with NRT but go straight on to Champix with or without vapourisors because traditional NRT works so rarely? That would be YOUR experience and you would be right as far as you are concerned. Risks to your own health? Since the 48 hour Working Time Directive, junior doctors have increased their sickness absence 300% compared with 30 years ago. They aren't any sicker but they are more willing to ask their tired hard pressed colleagues to cover for them. Is this ethical or fair? Are the risks to their own health actually greater than they were? Female doctors take more time off with emotional and physical ill health than male doctors – why?

There has been (2013) the new but unsurprising tabloid revelation that if you have an operation on a Friday you are between 40 and 50% more likely to die than if you have it on a Monday. This became a *cause celebre* subsequently. I don't know whether this was the case when we did twice to three times the current working week, knew our patients better, weekends on call in hospitals began on Friday morning and continued without a minute's pause until Monday evening, when we got a more intense (and stressful) apprenticeship and were therefore more competent much quicker. But it is possible that weekend continuity and quality was better under the doctor-unfriendly systems of the past. So there may be an inverse relationship between the risk to our health and that of our patients. The more hours we do, the greater our experience, the better the continuity, the fewer the handovers, the worse our work/life balance, the safer and better we are as doctors and the healthier the prognosis of our patients. But it is rather odd that we took less time off when we worked so much harder.

Delegating effectively? But what if I know I am the only person my own patients really want to see or maybe I am the best person at getting blood samples from neonates on the team or putting IUCDs in painlessly in the practice? Wouldn't it be unethical to delegate to someone else then? Partnerships with patients? I am all in favour of a friendly, informal, even affectionate (with some patients who in other situations might be my friends) relationship with patients but the very GMC who drew up these highly subjective "Attributes" will be a ton of bricks on my head if that partnership with any given patient overstepped their vague, undefined and very subjective "boundaries". Are the terms **affectionate or "close"** even allowed today between doctor and patient? I am absolutely sure the doctors of the past in reality as well as in history and literature had caring, affectionate, constructive, even loving relationships with patients (in a non sexual context) which were beneficial to both but would be completely misunderstood and rejected by today's professional (GMC) thought police. Think of Joel Fleischman in Northern Exposure, Dr Finlay, Doug Ross in ER, Drake Ramoray (Friends) Doogie Howser, Marcus Welby, Doc Martin, Gregory House, Hawkeye, Trapper, Beverley Crusher, Leonard McCoy, Stephen Maturin (Master and Commander), Dr Zhivago, Dr Kildare, the doctors of St Elsewhere's, Grey's Anatomy, Holby City, Out of Practice, ER, Scrubs and the thousands of fictional doctors we are fascinated by and admire. Were all these people emotional snow men and women or did they allow human feelings to creep into the professional arena occasionally? The films and books and story lines would have been pretty boring otherwise.

Honesty and integrity are the life blood of decent doctors but that isn't the same as blind acceptance of varied standards amongst our colleagues for the sake of some concept of "diversity". Don't confuse integrity with tolerance. Discriminating is what we are trained to do day in and day out. To discriminate the sick child from the well with almost similar signs, the suicidal from the only moderately depressed, the asthmatic who is "decompensating" from the asthmatic who is on the turn to getting better. I believe it is my professional and ethical duty to discriminate the good doctors I have worked with over the years from the bad and to take in to consideration a multitude of factors in that decision. Those factors may well include their training, cultural affinity with the average patient, ability to communicate colloquially and respond to subtle social and personal cues. If that means that some doctors who were trained abroad are not as safe and effective as some doctors born and bred and trained in the UK (of whatever cultural background) then it would be wrong to ignore that surely? If it means that some British born and trained doctors who have three digit IQs but no emotional intelligence or genuine empathy for their patients, then in my opinion they too should fail appraisal.

So discrimination in the interest of the patient is sometimes essential and Big Brother with his Equality and Diversity propaganda, which is forced on appraisers and trainers by the educational establishment has really lost the plot. – at least if the patient's needs trump the doctor's and health priorities trump politics.

So in summary:
Supporting Information for appraisal:
Six types: Information regarding:
Continuing professional development,
Quality improvement activity,
Significant events if any,
Colleague feedback,
Patient feedback,

Review of compliments and complaints.

The GMC had informed all GPs of the date of their first Revalidation by April 13 2013.

Also In the Portfolio should be other Statements relating to:

All professional roles and any contextual information,

Any exceptional circumstances,

Relevant appraisal summaries,

Past and present PDPs,

Statements relating to health, probity, adherence to GMP and authenticity of portfolio content,

Supporting evidence,

Any complaints and issues that you have been asked to raise by the PCO (Primary care organisation)/GMC,

Any additional information for the RO if appropriate.

All the appraisee's jobs must be included in the statement with evidence of competence and ongoing development, CPD, quality improvement and specific details of separate appraisals in other roles (ie GPSI).

Declarations:

There must be acceptance of the obligations in GMP (Good Medical Practice) relating to probity, health, confidentiality and personal responsibility for the accuracy of the portfolio.

The Appraisal **IS** now a pass or fail situation and you can fail just by not engaging adequately with it. "Engagement" is a highly subjective judgement which the appraiser will make based on the quality of the Toolkit, personal availability and the appraisee's willingness to make a proper and constructive effort. I think I would describe it as the appraisee's half of the mutual professional courtesy equation. I have had appraisees offer illegible written folders, folders without a single original thought or comment on their own professional life or way of working. Others with fifty X one sentence summaries of one hour practice journal clubs on a Monday lunchtime or fifty hours of journal reading at home. I have had others say that the way they practice has served them well for twenty five years so why should they change it and who else has a right to tell them what to do? (They could be right but they should at least be willing to prove it!) Revalidation and thus reli-censing will eventually depend on whether you "engage" with the process and the quality of the resultant Toolkit you present. If appraisal is worth anything, that is it. Whether the system is geared up to manage a significant proportion (let's say 5%) of "failures", I don't know. It is in everyone's interests to keep the bar fairly low. Except of course, the patient's.

The final statement is: "No information has been presented or discussed in the appraisal that raises concern about the doctor's fitness to practice"

As has been said many times by many people. This system, set up because of political anger over Harold Shipman is actually designed to pass people like him. He would no doubt have been very good at it.

Finally:

The Responsible Officer after considering the appraisal documentation (Toolkit) and other clinical governance data, can then affirm, defer, or refer to the GMC.

What is Quality Improvement Activity?:**

For doctors of my age, who managed to provide what seems in retrospect a much better, safer, health service with fewer doctors and no appraisals of any kind, even the concept that we should have to prove that we do – with "Quality Improvement Activity" or show others that we do relevant study, or rather pointless and highly standardised auditing of quantifiable data, or ask others we work with, who may have personal axes to grind, what they think of our abilities, is patronising and a sign of the progressive emasculation of our profession. Isn't continual self improvement, keeping up to date, trying to sharpen and modernise our performance the definition of a professional? Will this process make the patients safer and better looked after? I doubt it.

And **who are** all the Appraisal Leads, Clinical Governance Heads, Medical Directors, Responsible officers who have just sprung up out of nowhere and the self appointed administrative staff of this new multi million pound industry anyway? Have they been democratically elected into their positions of influence and power by their peers? Have they in some way proved their right to sit in judgement on us? Are they definitively better GPs? I had never heard of our region's Responsible Officer before he was appointed. And who chose him?! Are they well known by their colleagues for their long and successful GP careers which they have left at their peak in order to champion the side of the patient and the dedicated and hard working GP? Are they admired for the cleverness, dedication, skill and love of their patients, are they deeply missed by their partners and lists?

Of course not. I think you all know the answer to these questions..

The General Medical Council: The G.M.C.

Their Colleague Feedback Form:

The GMC Colleague Sample Questionnaire (should you need one) asks your colleagues to rate you as poor, less than satisfactory, satisfactory, good, very good or don't know on:

Clinical knowledge, diagnosis, clinical decision making, treatment (including practical procedures), prescribing, medical record keeping, recognising and working within limitations, keeping knowledge and skills up to date, reviewing and reflecting on own performance, teaching, supervising colleagues, commitment to the care and wellbeing of patients, communication with patients and relatives, working effectively with colleagues, effective time management, respecting patient confidentiality, honesty and trustworthiness, performance affected by ill health and the final question is: Is the doctor fit to practice medicine? Then the form asks for details about you and your actual contact with the doctor in question, your ethnic group but interestingly, not theirs.

To be honest, even with doctors I had worked with for 15 years I wouldn't be able to reliably answer half of those questions for half of my partners because General Practice is still a place where individuals work separately and not as part of a team. If one partner finds out that his or her diagnoses or clinical decision making aren't up to scratch from the universal feedback of their partners, what does the GMC suggest? They go back to medical school?

This is what the GMC says are the Duties of a doctor registered with them:

Make the care of your patient your first concern.

Treat each patient politely and considerately.

Respect each patient's dignity and privacy.

Listen to patients and respect their views.

Give patients information in a way they can understand.

Respect the rights of patients to be fully involved in decisions about their care.

Keep your professional knowledge and skills up to date.

Recognise the limits of your professional competence.

Be honest and trustworthy.

Respect and protect confidential information.

Make sure your personal beliefs do not prejudice your patients' care.

Act quickly to protect patients from risk if you have good reason to believe that you or a colleague may not be fit to practice.

Avoid abusing your position as a doctor.

Work with colleagues in the ways that best serve patients' interests.

Many of these statements are simply obvious platitudes that should not require stating at all and remind me of the hand washing sessions at infection-control courses. We make constant serious life and death decisions, we have years or decades of experience, we do a complicated and intellectually demanding job – so isn't this all a bit obvious?

Something has gone wrong in medical regulation and someone is missing the point. Harold Shipman murdered over 200 patients so we responded by introducing a system of expensive nationwide educational supervision with a bit of peremptory audit, all the wrong questions asked as well as some superficial feedback from colleagues and patients thrown in. That was our profession's and politician's response to one psychopathic mass murderer masquerading as a caring GP. In general, appraisal adds to the bureaucratic burden on doctors and is specifically **not** designed to detect the next Harold Shipman. That is what you get when you hand the job to the wrong people. People with spare time, who are currently at a loose end and volunteer rather than people who are chosen for their qualities and abilities, patient skills and track record.

Mid Staffs, Cardiff, Shipman, the soaring number of GMC complaints, the Heart Hospitals, the out of hours chaos have all come, one after another over the last few decades and destroyed the public's faith in the inherent service ethos and care of the NHS and its staff.

The profession's response is: Audits, 50 credits of learning, various dubious academic exercises, superficial and mostly pointless questions for people who come in contact with us and celebrating personal development and compliments.

Why?

Well look at the list of disasters above:

I am an experienced GP and NHS doctor who has had, as a patient or relative to see various doctors in the last few years, both for myself and close family members. I have also had feed-back on the experiences of my own grown up family who have visited their own GPs and various other NHS doctors recently. They and I are intelligent, reasonable, non confrontational and polite people. But I have been saddened by the poor quality of care and attitude of perhaps a third of their NHS nurses and doctors. Perhaps, for those living in London it has been an even higher percentage of their GPs. A few people close to me have had very serious illnesses and have experienced poor hospital ward in patient treatment and outpatients care too. There have been excellent and friendly nurses and doctors from many backgrounds but the professional and accessible doctor or nursing sister who can, through natural personality, a friendly attitude, medical knowledge, communication skills and language ability, relate well to a worried patient or relative is, these days, how can I put it?-far from ubiquitous. Simple administrative tasks like staffing an out patients or surgical list so that it runs on time or runs at all, or one hospital transferring a test or scan result or getting notes to another a few miles away is seemingly often impossible. The NHS of Radio 4 interviews and parliamentary questions is not the NHS of district general hospitals, casualty units, wards and outpatients in the real world.

I think it has been a serious mistake to select the most academic A star students for medical school. The most gifted academic applicants will pass the exams, jump the fences and present themselves advantageously but are almost guaranteed to be the least gifted in empathy, people handling, negotiation, managing difficult or worried patients and at communicating. Also, the huge influx of foreign trained doctors, so popular amongst politicians may have plugged manpower gaps in some areas of our NHS. The government may be depending on them to do this in the future – especially in female unfriendly specialities like A and E. It may have partly compensated for the disastrous 48 hour working time directive and the part-timism of the female dominated new NHS but many foreign doctors find conversational English, accents and forms of colloquial expression difficult. How could it be otherwise? To most doctors (other than anaesthetists or some surgeons) language is everything and even they, hopefully, need to explain what they are going to do before they do it. The huge number of foreign doctors and the free movement of workers within the EU who have had no official language requirements until recently, has almost guaranteed medical misunderstanding, mistakes and in the case of some (eg Ubani), deaths. It was only in June 2014 and after a number of high profile disasters that this particular example of politics trumping patients' rights was addressed and the GMC was handed powers to ban EU doctors with poor English skills. This was hailed as a "milestone in patient safety". Ubani was, by the way, fined E7,000 by a German regional administrative court for killing a British patient with a Heroin overdose and allowed to continue working.

The almost 70% graduates from most medical schools who are now female, has guaranteed part time working and discontinuity, a staffing crisis in the more family unfriendly (and harder) specialities such as A and E, orthopaedics and most surgery as well as the female popular speciality of Paediatrics. Here the problem is that the staff are off having their own babies so much of the time, that units cannot afford the locum cover. Female graduates show a lack of interest in proper GP partnerships, a disinclination to commit to full time jobs throughout the NHS, greater time off sick from every type of illness and this makes a long term doctor/patient relationship, – something the patient treasures above all else in General Practice, impossible to achieve. It also contributes to the staffing crisis throughout the NHS as three female doctors will work the same or fewer career hours as two male doctors but, obviously, take 50% more resources to train.

How can you have continuity if your doctor is off on maternity leave half of her first five years and then works part time or job shares with someone you, the patient, don't like?

Recognising limits: Well, no one taught me to inject finger joints but I have now done hundreds (my feedback says successfully), the same for ankle joints and toe joints. I was never told formally how to counsel suicidal patients or how to help drug addicts and alcoholics, I was certainly never given a minute's training in family therapy but I have spent most of the last thirty years doing all these things. If every doctor truly recognised their limits, we really would never do anything new or different. Does the GMC really know how real medical training works? In General Practice for my generation it wasn't "See one, do one, teach one", it was "Patient needs something, look it up, have a go at it, get better at it, teach it".

What about the constant complaint of my patients that they couldn't understand a word the outpatient doctor had said, could I interpret? Are these GMC "limits" or wasn't that the sort of thing they meant?

Confidentiality is a relative term within the bounds of family practice. A parent asks you if their teenage child who you have been looking after is taking drugs or is suicidal or pregnant and you have known them for 30 years. They are at their wits end with worry. Are you going to stone wall them or try to get them together and resolve the situation? I phoned my daughter's abysmal new GP in South London a few years ago to give him a quick summary about her longstanding difficult eczema just after she registered and before her notes arrived and he refused to take the call – even as I put it "as a professional courtesy". He told the receptionist to say he didn't talk to relatives because of "Data Protection". He was clearly intellectually inaccurate, legally wrong and professionally lazy.

I do not believe that voodoo is a valid faith system or that female circumcision (or male circumcision on religious grounds for that matter) is ever justified, or that blood transfusions are against God's will and so on. These are some of my beliefs that will influence how I treat patients and whether I respect their views. Oh and by the way, in the 40 years I have been in medicine about 20-25% of the doctors I have worked with have been out of date, pompous and self absorbed to the point of being inaccessible and dangerous, unwilling to change or listen, opinionated, inarticulate, incomprehensible through culture, background or intellect, or just thoroughly unpleasant people. They would all have been pretty close to missing the GMC good doctor guidelines in various aspects.

The GMC is much like the European Court of Human Rights. It has great power to dominate and control, to legislate and dictate rules and punishments but it seems to exercise that power in isolation from the views, opinions or feedback of those who it claims to represent.

What is worse it doesn't have any democratic validity since it isn't representative of or chosen by the profession.

It exists in splendid isolation from most doctors – except when it demands its annual subscription. It is undemocratic, never consults the opinion of the profession and does not seem to reflect the attitudes of the working doctor. Its ethics, attitudes, rules, professional guidelines and regulations are, like normal cholesterols and BMIs plucked out of the ether by a circle of the self appointed and faceless. Its rulings are slow, urban biased and for an NHS clinically overwhelmingly General Practice it is dominated by hospital and non clinical members and, of course, very expensive. It neither serves patients or doctors fairly or well. It describes best practice but I wonder how many of its paying members think this list comes close to reality.

I have been a doctor in the NHS for over 40 years but I have never been asked for an opinion on what constitutes good medical practice or ethics, I have never to my knowledge been asked to vote on the fitness for purpose of the "Chair" or members of the Council of the GMC. I have never met anyone else who has been asked either. Until recently when I did the research I had no idea who the members were, what their politics or careers had been and whether they were any good at being doctors themselves. Perhaps, like many doctors I have known, they were born to be teachers and politicians, destined for

Deaneries, Royal Colleges and Administrative Councils like the GMC but wholly incompetent as real doctors.

For instance: Have **you** ever been consulted whether it is always wrong for a doctor to treat his or her own family? Have you ever wondered why real doctors should never be judgemental or confrontational with patients (in other words have no feelings?) Have you ever wondered whether the committees who write the guidelines that we are supposed to abide by are truly experienced enough in the full scope of medicine, fully representative of all types of practice, have done it long enough, seen enough varied patients and represent a genuinely broad church, in other words, democratic?

The latest Handbook upon which we base appraisal and the way we are supposed to practice our medical craft is again called **"Good Medical Practice"**, although I have heard of no one who was consulted in its writing. It came out in April 2013 and as I mention elsewhere, it has a smiling Asian lady doctor on its cover. Whether she is to reassure the reader that medicine is an inclusive culture where trainers and appraisers are forced to attend annual equality and diversity training or a recognition that foreign trained doctors are three times more likely to come before the GMC I don't know. As I also mention elsewhere I suspect the creative design team was based in London and were displaying either their cool liberal credentials or making a rather naughty joke.

So who are the GMC members?

There are (2013/4) 12 members of the GMC Council, – at least 6 are not active doctors, 7 are women. Do they represent or reflect the profession? Are any of them aware of how General Practice (which constitutes most of British Medicine and 90% of the doctor/patient interactions) works?:

They are currently listed as (oddly they add up to 13)

A Professor of Therapeutics

A female Locum Consultant in Obs and Gynae,

A female lay member who has been involved in a great deal of community and voluntary work,

A consultant Gastroenterologist,

A female cross bench peer,

A Professor of Surgery,

A female Paediatric Hepatologist,

A female lay member with various previous jobs in the public sector,

A Professor of Medicine,

Another female lay member who has held various public positions,

Another female lay member who has held various public positions,

A doctor who is actually a career medical administrator and another lay member.

Until mid 2017 no GMC Council member had any direct experience of what 90% of NHS interactions consist:- Family Medicine, the General Practice interaction, how they are conducted, our way of life. Shocking isn't it? Even now (Autumn 2017) there is only one GMC Council member with any GP experience. These are the people who not only sit in judgement on and discipline us, their "Peers" but actually write our ethical rules and guidelines. Does it make you feel like you are in the trenches mid way through the Somme and the faceless unelected GMC is the top brass ensconced at the chateau miles away?

I recently read the GMC's publication on **The "Licence to Practise."**

This is the legal authority that permits us to be an NHS or private doctor, to sign death certificates, cremation forms and do all the other things in the UK that are restricted to registered and licensed doctors. But you can be or remain registered without a licence if you want. This allows you to show a third party that you are in "Good Standing" with the GMC and demonstrates your medical qualification. I am not quite sure what good this does you as you cannot prescribe or treat people. If you let your registration (and GMC subscription payment) end, for instance in a career break or retirement you cannot even call yourself a doctor (although I refuse to cow tow to this particular piece of bureaucratic infantilism). I will have Doctor carved on my gravestone and my heart long after I have stopped treating patients.

Registration with a licence to practise means you have to be revalidated annually. Registration without a licence means you cannot practice medicine, do not have to be revalidated, you can help the injured and sick in an emergency (but only as a "Good Samaritan" –) and enables you to sign passport photos – but that's about it.

Gone are the days when being a doctor was a vocation, a calling, a way of life. Now it is just a job, a temporary occupation, in the gift of the GMC. I thought that when I qualified I would never stop being a doctor. A doctor was what I was – not what I did. But apparently not now. That was a Victorian idea that no longer existed. If you are unregistered and unlicensed, it doesn't matter how long you have been looking after the sick, how many years and how much of your life you have devoted to medicine, the GMC says you can't call yourself a doctor anymore.

So add up this devaluing of the vocation of medicine, the undemocratic nature of its council, the emotional torture of its glacial and unsympathetic investigations, the absence of the majority of doctors – GPs, from its decision making processes, the often out of contact with reality rules and publications it promulgates and its clear urban bias and is it any wonder that many regard the GMC as out of touch, culturally alien, faceless and unfit for purpose? The number of suicides amongst doctors being investigated by the GMC seemed to come as a shock to its governing body in 2015/6. Various doctors' national representative bodies described the GMC complaints process as "Guilty until proven innocent", endless, unsupportive, victimising the doctor, despite the fact that nine tenths of doctors investigated had no action taken against them. The GMC's response: "Medical schools need to teach Emotional Resilience".

Good medical Practice:

Actually the booklet is not quite as bland and naive as it might have been: It is marked out in the famous FOUR DOMAINS:

Knowledge, Skills and Performance:
Make the care of the patient your first concern, keep up to date and don't exceed your competence.

Safety and Quality:
Take prompt action to protect the safety, dignity or comfort of the patient.

Communication, Partnership and Teamwork:
Treat patients politely and considerately, respect confidentiality. Work in partnership with patients, listen to and respond to their concerns, give information in a way they can understand, respect their right to reach decisions with you, help them to care for themselves, help colleagues to help patients.

Maintaining Trust:

Be honest and open, act with integrity, don't discriminate, don't abuse the trust in you or the profession.

The most important part though and the bit that bears repeating over and over is:

You are personally accountable for your professional practice and must always be prepared to justify your decisions and actions.

These 19 words are all we really need. They should be on the wall of every consulting room and out patients department, should be the new "Hippocratic Oath" and should have been used in evidence against Shipman, the doctors and nurses of Mid Staffs, Cardiff and everywhere else that professionals forgot who we are paid to serve and to whom we are accountable.

This is the best bit of the booklet and the only really memorable section. Much of the rest of it is naive committee generated stuff. Well meaning but imprecise, full of bland generalisations which mean little or nothing to the working doctor. If only they could have used a few full time apolitical undecorated real doctors with guidelines based on reality and honesty not the young socialist's guide book to a better society.

Some of the Metropolitan liberalisms that pepper the "Good Medical Practice"

The platitudes that fill out the bulk of the Good Medical practice Booklet –

You must be competent, you must keep up to date, you must provide a good standard of care are surely part of the definition of being in a "profession" and acting like a "professional". You can't imagine an architect ignoring new developments in materials technology or a barrister ignoring high court precedents. Do we really have to be told the absolutely obvious?

But there are a few points that I would take issue with:

for instance:

You must take account of spiritual, social and cultural factors. We are all human beings with human bodies prone to the same illnesses and cures. There is however a world of bizarre and conflicting cultures and beliefs out there held by millions, without a shred of proof. Just believing something or having a tradition doesn't make it right. I do not accept the cultural norms of male and female circumcision. These are cruel, damaging and harmful to otherwise healthy individuals and cannot be accepted or tolerated by any doctor. Neither can any irrational or improvable belief that harms someone or their children – voodoo, homeopathy, faith healing, witchcraft, the occult or a ban on transfusions (etc).

There is No Reason to accept the patient's harmful irrational medical beliefs and take them seriously. You must confront them and explain that western structured objective medicine slayed those dragons centuries ago.

You must assess the patient's conditions and "If necessary" examine the patient. I have been on the receiving end of a number of consultations in various situations over the last few years and I abhor the reluctance of many doctors to properly lay on hands for reassurance and for extra facts. I would say that at every consultation, a physical examination, however brief, should be **the norm** and there should be a good reason for you **not** to touch the patient. The formal, analytical, appropriately done laying on of firm hands inspires confidence, trust, familiarity and can often throw up unexpected extra information. Time and time again I have heard patients describe doctors as thorough, trustworthy and conscientious simply because they always offer the simplest examination as part of most consultations. So many new GPs seem to think their job is an office based one where they sit at a computer and give advice. How wrong they are. So often I have found something useful and unexpected by getting up out of my chair, going to the patient on the couch or asking them to lift up their shirt and just putting a stethoscope on skin or laying a hand on their abdomen. And getting off your backside regularly is in your own metabolic and circulatory best interests as well.

Respect a patient's right to seek a second opinion: Does that mean always refer them for a second opinion, or a third, or more – even if you believe it to be a waste of resources and a reinforcement of harmful and self destructive behaviour? What does that do to your own self worth and self confidence? Someone with medically unexplained symptoms and mild depression for instance. In the long run you can keep finding nothing wrong and be lead by the patient down endless diagnostic dead ends. "Just one more test and we will crack it doctor." The most honest and most difficult thing to do is to have the courage of your convictions and refuse further opinions. Accepting a patient's request and appearing unsure is the best way of losing the confidence and trust of the patient forever. And reinforcing mistaken self diagnoses. Why then would you not give in to a third or fourth opinion?

Wherever possible avoid providing medical care to yourself or anyone with whom you have a close personal relationship. Clearly the august GMC committee is thinking of the metropolitan drug addicts of London and the cities and the distressed minority of doctors who appear before them abusing prescription drugs. Only one new member of the GMC has any urban General Practice experience let alone rural GP experience. How on earth can they apply these rules about prescribing to one's own family when they don't have any idea what family medicine or family life in General practice is like? I go back to my point about democracy. These rules and attitudes are out of touch with primary care reality. They are based on the contact the committee has with the drug addicted doctors in severe trouble who appear before them. In my opinion it is **absolutely ethical** for a GP to prescribe appropriate drugs for him or herself and for members of their own families on some occasions. Elsewhere I describe the excellent country GP suspended for a year for prescribing two Fentanyl patches to her sister dying of breast cancer, visiting one weekend from France. This was an ethical and humane act and one for which she sacrificed a year of income, her reputation, a year's sanity, her partnership, her reputation and her hard won respect within her community. The committee who suspended her were simply not fit for purpose. I have discussed this case anonymously with colleagues since and each one seemed to know of a similar sorry story. Stories of the GMC's barrister based, confrontational, legalistic, glacial, inhumane, out of touch and bizarre procedures. These seem to be incomprehensibly reinstating dangerous and incompetent doctors just as often as suspending good doctors for trivial misdemeanours.

You must be satisfied you have consent before you carry out any examination or investigation. Again, the committee is assuming there are lecherous sexually perverted and repressed predators in all of us because of the despicable doctors who come before them, having abused their position of trust. Those men should be behind bars. They are very few and far between but the present obsession amongst registrars and newly qualified doctors for chaperones only serves to add suspicion and anxiety to their consultations. – Why is he asking if I need someone to keep an eye on him? What has he been up to? If you act in a friendly natural, informal way – " I'm afraid I just need to check, do you mind?" and you examine gently and professionally, i.e. quickly and efficiently and without unnatural eye contact, there should be few problems. I have performed tens of thousands of intimate examinations amongst my 1/3-1/2 million consultations over the last 40 years and I have on 2 or 3 occasions asked for a chaperone. This was when I knew of the patient's previous history of false accusations against other doctors or I felt threatened by an overly attentive lady patient. It was to protect me. There are other genuine reasons for not wanting chaperones as a standard accompaniment to intimate examinations: For instance: the tendency NOT to examine or to over refer when there is no female member of staff available to act as a chaperone. Both these alternatives put the patient at risk when sometimes a quick check that a fallopian tube or ovary is not tender can be very reassuring diagnostically. Also a third person in the consulting room always inhibits an honest exchange of information especially if the patient is young, worried, shy or embarrassed.

You must take part in regular reviews and audits: Be honest, most audits are done under protest on the simplest most unhelpful topics and by the registrar or administrative staff. They are popular because data collection is easy thanks to computerisation but they rarely have a *significant* clinical purpose, elicit change *which you shouldn't already have been aware of* and they have become a box we tick at appraisal and in training. They are almost never very interesting or productive.

I have never seen an interesting audit question:

(Do patients in this practice dislike being cared for by part time/job share doctors? Do the patients accept or resent prescribing incentive changes to their old familiar medication? Are patients happy that their doctors' attitudes are friendly and approachable? Have there been communication/language/attitude problems to do with sex/cultural/age differences that could be addressed? How do the patients regard the mode of dress or personal hygiene of their doctor? etc).

Reviewing patient feedback where it is available. I wonder how useful this is. I don't say this because mine was poor, but because it was uniformly good. Effusively good. I am sorry to blow my own trumpet and you will have to believe me when I say this and I didn't go round telling everyone my results but most years I was the most popular partner, against all parameters, in the practices I worked. The questions are subjective and of dubious real value. Like do you feel better able to cope with your illness after seeing the doctor? How well did the doctor put you at your ease?, How much did the doctor involve you in decisions about your care?, Rate the doctor's caring and concern for you, etc. Some are slightly more valuable and rational, like: How thoroughly did the doctor listen to what you had to say? How well did he explain your problems and treatment? What did you think of the time spent with you? and so on. Obviously these are highly subjective parameters and may depend upon one consultation, the patient's mood, previous experience of the doctor, how mean spirited or generous they happened to feel at the time, all sorts of variables unrelated to the quality of the doctor (even if that were something quantifiable!).

I have just partly retired but I had known most of the patients on my list for over 30 years. They collar me on the street now and berate me for leaving them and I do somehow feel a little guilty. They say they doubt whether anyone can look after them with the same commitment as me. I had known many since they were babies. I liked nearly all of them and so much of the prognosis and the satisfaction involved in any consultation actually depends upon whether the patient thinks YOU LIKE THEM, to some extent whether you **are** actually LIKE THEM, socially, culturally, personally and how much of their past history you share. Having the best practice feedback year after year was also in some ways a very negative factor as far as my partners were concerned. They worked hard too so why should I get so much positive feedback compared with them?

If you have concerns that a colleague may not be fit to practise you must ask for advice... I am the veteran of 3 partnerships in General Practice. Only one of my previous partners has been struck off – this was for inappropriate conduct with women. I knew he was a bad GP from his self important and pompous attitude to patients, partners and staff. He was one of a number of bad doctors I have worked with but I know that appraisal is not the way to find them. Within those partnerships there were probably three or four doctors I would not have wanted to see my family under any circumstances and amongst the registrars I come in contact with these days, I would say the majority are not fit to see patients independently by half way through their registrar year, long after they are seeing and prescribing alone. Are we really supposed to express concern about what in my opinion would be at least 10-20% of qualified doctors who are not good enough to see someone I care about at any time in their career? And how high are we setting the bar here?

You must listen to patients and take account of their views..unless those views include not exchange transfusing neonates on religious grounds, male and female circumcisions, Homeopathy, Spiritualism (and dare I say it: Prayer?) etc etc. I am a doctor, I practice medicine because conventional western medicine, double blind evidence based, empirical medicine is the only thing that makes people better reliably and the only thing I am willing to "take account of".

I suppose it does depend on what you mean by "take account of" – this is another committeeism. You **can** take an account of something (like the weather or the risk of war) and then totally ignore it, of course.

You must be considerate to those close to the patient and be sensitive and responsive in giving them information and support. I agree. So many doctors hide behind "patient confidentiality" or "Data Protection" excuses and refuse even to reassure desperately worried relatives about their loved ones. This is an abuse of power and position. It is often sheer cowardice or laziness. I phoned a London GP a couple of years ago to give him some information about the past history of my newly registered daughter (out of "professional courtesy") explaining to the receptionist who I was and why I was calling. My daughter had a complicated history with which I was very familiar. The receptionist said "He won't talk to you, he never talks to other people about his patients". I explained again why I was ringing, to **give him** information but she quoted "Data Protection", that meaningless catchall excuse, as his reason for not taking any call from any relatives and I never heard from him even after I phoned a second time. This was inappropriate and unethical. If a worried mum phones me about a teenager who I have seen and she thinks is suicidal, I will at least reassure her about drug abuse, prognosis, pregnancy, safety issues and all the things parents can be desperate about without giving away too many confidences. GP is complicated. You have many allegiances and responsibilities and you have to care for and about the Family. Confidentiality is relative. You are a Family Doctor. Your patient **is** the Family.

You must be polite and considerate: You must treat patients as individuals and respect their dignity and privacy. You must treat patients fairly and with respect whatever their life choices and beliefs. This is clearly wrong. For instance: A belief in the evil of a life saving transfusion, or of the rightness of circumcision or homeopathy or of a life style that involves promiscuity, obesity, drug taking, even voluntary benefits dependency etc etc. **The doctor is allowed feelings.** If you show you are involved enough to get angry, you show you care. All these GMC rules forget that we are not ciphers, not rubber stamps. Indeed the best doctors are those who are committed and involved enough with their patients to tell them they **are** wrong, they need to change that they are harming themselves and that we care enough to be annoyed and want them to change. This works and has been shown to work in a variety of acute and chronic diseases so you must forget the "Don't express or imply disapproval of beliefs and lifestyle" nonsense –, that is just liberal, intellectual, inexperienced, metropolitan, Islington dinner party, PC, non GP, GMC theory, hypothesising. It sounds right in the committee rooms of Harman Street, Manchester Or Euston Rd. London but it is rubbish in the sweaty, noisy, messy, primary care, face to face with the patient real world.

The investigations and treatment you provide must be based on the assessment you and your patient make of their needs and priorities etc. Really? when did the patient take a medical degree and acquire 30 or 40 years of medical experience to equate his assessment with mine? When did the GMC lose its common sense and decide that student attitudes towards politics and goodwill to all mankind actually invests a plumber or a street sweeper with the knowledge, wisdom and experience to match that of his doctor? I remember listening to a Radio 4 programme where a landscape gardener was given equal air time with the country's foremost epidemiologist during the MMR debate and whose argument was "I won't take the risk, there's no smoke without fire". You can only feel sympathy for his poor child and anger at the BBC and a country that allows a parent to act like this. Isn't this subliminal messaging exactly why we have measles and Whooping Cough epidemics now? The BBC subsequently apologised saying its charter obliged it to give equal air time to both sides of any argument. Andrew Wakefield was subsequently struck off and a national panic amongst parents to immunise their unimmunised teenagers followed. Wasn't it the same with Whooping cough damaged children – in the 70's because we allowed patients to believe their whims were on a par with medical fact and evidence? We don't have the resources to indulge everyone with every test they have read about on the Internet or fancy having because a friend might have mentioned it. That is why we doctors are here, with our experience, responsibility, our gate keeper role, knowledge, and hopefully our WISDOM.

So NO you don't allow the patient to make an assessment of priorities, you do that on their behalf.

You must respond promptly to complaints.. You must not allow a patient's complaint to adversely affect the care or treatment you provide. Rubbish. The doctor without feelings again. I have had a few informal complaints over the years and I always took them personally at some level or other. Whenever I talk to anyone in the real world about the benefits system or to employers about sickness absence they criticise the readiness of GPs to write certificates for trivial illnesses. I don't – and because I don't I have received a number of prolonged and personally vindictive complaints from patients. One of these was from a man who I knew was a busy black economy window cleaner I often saw out and about in local estates. He told me he was unfit to work. He and his wife confronted me together during one appointment and told me how he could not go back to driving buses and was often unable to leave the house. I had to renew his "sick note". I refused. His written complaint went as far as the Health Service Ombudsman and took 18 months before it was dismissed. There was no way I could have trusted him or continued friendly, personal General Practice care for him or his equally manipulative and mischievous wife thereafter. So I removed them from my list. I am entitled to my feelings and they had given me 18 months of relative misery. My attitude to other patients had became cynical, my morale was harmed, my sleep, my blood pressure, my mood and confidence suffered. Does the GMC think I am without any sensitivity, any feeling? I couldn't be objective with the couple afterwards and so I couldn't care for them properly and I suggest you use that defence if challenged. You have human rights too. No, you really do. – Freedom of thought, belief, expression, freedom from degrading treatment, the right to a family life. The Human Rights Act applies to doctors as well as the rest of the world and given the number who have ended their lives while being dealt with by the GMC I am surprised no case has been brought against them on behalf of an abused doctor using one or other clause of the act.

You should end a professional relationship with a patient only when the breakdown of trust means you cannot provide good clinical care....Again I think the GMC ignores the fact that many of us develop personal and friendly relationships with patients, as part of our professional interaction and that this is what makes us effective, useful and popular. We are not objective and distant, we are not ciphers, automatons, – we have feelings. We can be liked, needed and accessible, part of communities, we are Family Doctors. We use the trust and friendship, sometimes the affection, to the patient's advantage, – in a thera-peutic context, if you like. So the breakdown of trust happens in many subtle ways and it is not always an easy thing to explain to a committee – almost none of whom have ever done any General Practice and who sit in judgement in Manchester and London.

Honesty: You must not allow any interests you have to affect the way you prescribe, treat, refer or commission services... Absolutely. And to make sure that doesn't happen, no GP on a Commissioning Board should be allowed to have an interest or have a Family Member with a financial interest in any service bought by that board. Just to be on the safe side, no service provider should be allowed to purchase or commission services from any source where a GP or a GP's relative is on the board of the company or has any financial interest in it. On pain of imprisonment and removal from the medical list. This sort of family or personal financial relationship is corrupt or has the potential to be so. Too many GPs make too much money out of employing sessional doctors in their practices and offering various well reimbursed services to third parties (such as Prison Health, Occupational Health, Asylum and Immigration Health Services etc) and have made profits in the past from Fund Holding by getting in first and providing medical services of doubtful value which were temporarily well reimbursed. New research shows that Fund Holding failed to provide any sustained benefits for patients (See other sections). I hate to see the tax payer ripped off by entrepreneurial doctors even more than I do by corrupt politicians. On 11th November 2015, The Times lead on its front page was "GPs award £2.4Bn deals to their own companies" The story disclosed that PCGs had given more than 400 contracts to providers in which board members or their families had financial interests. In Birmingham "GP Leaders had awarded contracts worth £1.7m to a company in which three of them were share holders and one was a medical director. Of the 151 CCGs at least 50 had given at least one contract to enterprises in which members of their governing body had interests. 233 of these contracts saw GP surgeries being paid to provide extra services. This increases the partners' take home pay and the Patients Association representative said it would compromise trust between patient and doctor. An example of the Birmingham

South and Central CCG was given, awarding several contracts to "South Doc Services" in which three GPs were share holders, all on the CCG governing body and were earning hundreds of thousands of pounds outside their normal pay, the CCG paying the organisation £1m in 2014. Even the BMA criticised this arrangement as a "Conflict too far". The Times identified £16.6m being handed out in contracts to companies in which board members had interests. The BMA Chairman was quoted as saying no doctor who is a director in an organisation commissioned by a CCG should be a board member of the CCG. I **absolutely** agree and no member of his or her family either. On pain of striking off and prosecution. Surely this is the only way to guarantee probity given the temptations and the sums of money up for grabs. If doctors wash their hands so frequently why do so many of us have such sticky fingers? How will these doctors get through the probity section of appraisal and what I wonder will the Birmingham Responsible Officer do when their appraisals, probity: "no comment" sections come in? They all need an interview at least?

Even QuoF, as we all know, is and has always been milked by efficient practices who fund nurses to tick the boxes, see the patients and claim the money. Whether there have been long term, genuine patient health benefits of QuoF is open to debate too.

Clinical Governance:

If you qualified in the last 10-15 years you won't believe that we managed a (probably) better run, more humane, more caring and better loved health care system before concepts like Clinical Governance were invented. I suppose that we just thought what was best for the patient (or patients as a whole) and generally tried to do it. We governed *ourselves* clinically.

Then concepts such as clinical governance, honesty, integrity, probity, respect, human rights, trust, teamwork and so on, none of which mean anything if a patient isn't fed, watered, cleaned up or given pain relief on time, all started to be the academic currency of our profession. I don't know whether the tenets of clinical governance were being applied in Mid Staffs or at the Welsh hospital caring for Ann Clwyd's husband or in Morecambe Bay but I think for the patients involved, they would all have meant nothing compared with a caring member of staff just being willing to come to the bedside, feed, give water and to spend time doing some old fashioned nursing. Clinical governance is still for most of us a fairly meaningless concept that managers and educators like to use but this is the definition:

"An integrated approach that aims to ensure the continuous improvement of the quality of clinical services. The processes underpinning an integrated clinical governance approach require organisational analysis in order to understand the complex and dynamic methods of success."

Really? Isn't it actually far simpler than that and something that is learnt on wards with sleeves rolled up and not in class rooms with ring binders and laptop presentations? What all that means in real English is: Everyone do your job the best you can by putting the patient's interests first and let's try to do it together.

Our Local PCT put it this way in a handout:

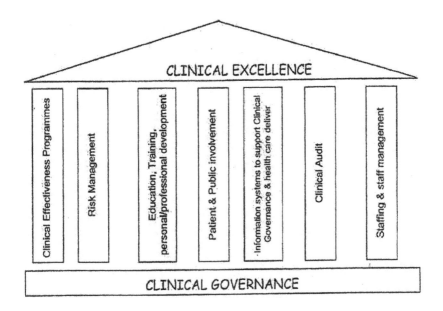

OUT OF HOURS

David Cameron was promising in October 2014 a return to 7 days a week GP services including GPs doing out of hours. He also, by the way, wanted a named doctor for us all (in other words a list system) and there was talk of scrapping appointments and having casualty style walk in and wait GP surgeries.

Many of us smiled wryly at these novel proposals and wondered: Why do politicians change everything if they are only going to swap it back, in due course to square one again later? All those things were in place when I started general practice 35 years ago.

It was one of the greatest primary care disasters in our history when the Blair/Brown government allowed the opt out of 24 hour care by GPs in 2004. This was great for we GPs who had seen patient demand out of hours grow from what were initially reasonable and usually justified visits and enquiries to frequent unjustified 24 hour calls for mostly trivia. This then became the consumer culture out of hours standard up to the early part of this century. Unfortunately for Cameron and his successors, the slaves had by now tasted freedom and the state couldn't afford to pay the going rate for adequate out of hours medical cover. Also of course, the newly 70% feminised GP work force just wouldn't work nights and weekends away from their families. At any rate. They had children to care for and a work life balance to think about. Further mass importation of foreign trained doctors is not, I hope, the answer either. I would also add that thousands of experienced retired doctors are positively discouraged from returning to work part time by nit picking appraisal rules and deadlines, the cost of insurance, the ease and seeming encouragement of trivial complaints, costly GMC registration and all the associated clinical governance, retraining, and Disclosure and Barring Investigations that have burgeoned in the last decade or so.

So what chance is there of returning to a proper, safe and effective, accessible, GP led OOH service?

By 2014/5 there was a crisis in GP out of hours cover, in the out of hours advice and triage system, the out of hours advice 111 phone number system and in A and E. – So that means all emergency care (other than day time General Practice, some walk in centres and what went on after patients had been admitted to hospitals). Indeed there was it seems, general confusion over what was available once the surgeries were closed and how to access it.

By 2014 a National Audit Office Census showed:

1 in 4 people had not even heard of OOH GP services.

1 in 5 were unaware of the new 111 urgent OOH phone number.

The numbers of patients using the OOH GP services by 2013-14 had fallen by a third in six years to 5.8 million. The report said this could be due to lack of awareness of the service or a lack of trust in it and as we know, visits to A and E had (have) risen significantly.

The report mentioned the 90% opt out of OOH services by GPs since being given the choice in 2004. It also described dissatisfaction with OOH services, patients struggling to access the services, 17% feeling the services were poor. The out of hours case type was said to have changed to "more complex cases" despite funding having dropped in real terms. The NAO said that funding had fallen by £75m in the last decade (OOH services cost £400m in the 2013/4 financial year). NHS England was said to have "Very limited over-sight" and was "Doing little to monitor performance." What a deterioration in ten years!

80% of casualty units did not have enough consultants for the 16 hours a day that is considered necessary for high quality care (Guardian 24 Jul 2013).

In the Autumn of 2015 the CQC reported that 3/4 of hospitals offered unacceptable standards of care. This was largely put down to low staffing levels. The figure for GP practices was that 31% were failing. Altogether: of 98 Hospital Trusts, 2 were outstanding, 22 good, 64 required improvement and 10 were found inadequate.

We know that in many hospitals mortality rates are up 30-40% at weekends and we should all know why this has happened. In 2015 representatives of the RCGP and BMA were confusingly saying either that we already had a 24/7 NHS or that it was unaffordable and unstaffable to provide one! The NHS was built up on and relied upon doctors working long hours. As I have often mentioned, 80 to 90 or more hours a week were normal when I qualified. On a 1 in 2 rota we did 136 hours a week. We, the doctors of the 70's 80's and 90's somehow accepted the chronic tiredness and low grade depression as our half of the contract. There are very few medical school places. It cost a fortune to educate each doctor. You felt privileged from the very start of the long process, it was a hard working apprenticeship and from the moment you qualified you knew you would earn a lot more than the average graduate. The average starting GP salary in 2015 without ANY out of hours is £90,000! The basic salary for junior doctors then was £23,000 and went up to £28,000 by the second year. (Pay for doctors-NHS careers). For doctors in specialist training jobs the basic salary is £30,000 – £47,000.

Undoubtedly there were times when you were dead on your feet a generation ago and I am not suggesting we should or could go back to such intense rotas. But you used to feel fortunate despite feeling constantly shattered in the mid 70's and my salary was a third or less of normal time for each hour of overtime then. The 2015 strike was about making

Saturday between 07.00 and 22.00 part of the normal working week and anti social hours only after ten O'Clock at night Monday to Friday. I think the "55,000 junior doctors in England" of 2015/6 were pushing their luck striking over their working conditions. They were being offered time and a half for Monday to Sunday 10pm to 7am and time and a third for 7pm-10 pm on Saturday and 7am to 10pm Sunday. Not one third time after 6pm every day, all night and all weekend like their seniors. Their working week is a half or a third of my generation's depending on whether we were on a 1 in 2 or 1 in 3 rota. (136 hours or 120 hours on a "duty week"). There must be thousands of potential applicants for medical school places who would happily sign the contract with the financial and social prospects of a doctor and what at 48 hours pro rata is still a relatively light duty rota. The average working week for **all workers** in London is 48 hours (Radio 4 August 2016).

I remember talking to an Inland Revenue inspector at a party a few years ago who said that apart from successful bankers and stock brokers, full time orthopaedic surgeons had the steepest income gradient of all professions after being appointed and there were many earning over a million pounds per year within 5 years of appointment. Incomes were guaranteed to rise in medicine if you could stick it and in some specialities, particularly some of the surgical ones, to rise exponentially.

Training to do medicine is a prized and rare goal for many ambitious young people but attitudes about their side of the bargain have changed drastically over the last couple of decades.

In my student year about 15% of the 90 students were women. By the present time (depending on the medical school) this has risen to 60-70%. Women give back about 60-65% of the career hours that men do and generally (not always, but generally) don't want to undertake the more grinding career pathways of Orthopaedics or most of the surgical specialities (8.7%), casualty, etc. They like portfolio careers, part time work, 9 to 5, they do sessions, want a work life balance, time off for pregnancy, bringing up children and increasingly, relatively minor illnesses (compared with their older female and current male counterparts). Few want to become full time partners in General Practice. There are staffing crises (2015) in A and E which women won't apply to do posts in and Paediatrics in which they fill 70% of the junior posts. Indeed, they were pregnant and taking maternity leave or working part time so much that 78% of children's units felt patient safety to be at danger in the Summer of 2015 (Telegraph Aug 2015). In a Woman's Hour programme on women in medicine in January 2015, involving four female Royal College presidents there was a comment that that 40% of Ophthalmic trainees were women and 69% of Pathology trainees were women. This was said to be entirely due to the easier on call rotas and later careers and when Jane Garvey asked why women didn't want to do the more difficult careers of casualty, surgery etc she "Couldn't describe the looks she was getting around the table!".

By 2014 one in eight medical graduates was seriously considering taking their skills and qualifications abroad in what I would regard as wholesale theft from the tax payer. They weren't off to help the starving and deprived by working in refugee camps in Syria or Palestine or in Zika or Ebola affected countries for MSF. During the strike as many as one in six said they were planning to work in either Australia or New Zealand "for a better quality of life".

By the Summer of 2013, the long evolving deterioration in emergency services came to a head. In the Today Programme expose that disclosed only 17% of A and E departments had full consultant cover during the week they also revealed that after the first three years of training 50% of emergency care doctors dropped out of the career due to the "demands of the rota". How many were female?

There have already been several media stories about the paucity of OOH GP doctors and the large areas covered by each in the community. We all know about the tendency for the out of hours 111 telephone and GP out of hours service triage protocols to default to "go to casualty". A far cry from my decades of being a one in three to a one in nine GP, covering seven to twenty thousand patients and personally visiting just about every one before admitting them. We are now familiar with ambulances queuing outside casualty departments so that waiting time figures can be fiddled and patients kept unsupervised on trolleys or having to nurse each other due to the shameful lack of beds and staff in many DGHs.

Casualty is a demanding but rewarding career choice. Varied and stimulating, it covers all medical areas and is like GP with surgery, drunks and trauma thrown in.

It isn't generally a career for a 9-5, female friendly profession. Newly qualified doctors do not expect a career of unsociable and excessive hours, anymore than a journeyman apprenticeship. Dare I say it, women try to avoid intoxicated, injured, aggressive and troublesome patients in understaffed casualty departments and anyway, there just isn't a sense of paying the tax payer back for your education anymore. The 48 hour Working Time Directive has caused many continuity and cover problems in and out of hours and has changed the mind set of young doctors as well. To put it bluntly they want their cake and eat it. A scarce, costly, privileged education, an undemanding, sympathetic and supportive training and a work life balance with the option of a part time and socially unchallenging job as well. How things have changed.

This is at least partly the result of the feminisation and socialisation of medicine.

Is all this true? – Are women avoiding full time, hard and demanding specialities because of biology? Well, many surgical jobs are just physically more demanding than many women can cope with. Take orthopaedics: In 2004, women made up 51 of 1776 consultants, just 2.9% ! They made up 8.7% of all Consultant Surgeons (2011). The highest proportion of surgeons was in paediatric surgery with 22% (RCS Surgical Careers, 2014) I suppose they just aren't prepared for the hours and the physical and emotional demands of the job especially if they are mothers. In GP, women now make up the majority of GPs, of part timers and job sharers and when patients complain that they can never see their doctor because they are "never there", the doctor is usually female. Women GPs tended to lead the move away from 24 hr personal responsibility 10-20 years ago, it was the women who often paid others to do their on-call in cooperatives and who are the group who tell me now when I discuss "Emergency General Practice" with colleagues that they "Don't deal with emergencies."

Practices are finding it harder to replace retiring partners with full time committed partners because so few full time male applicants are available to apply. There are already practices where male patients are unable to see a male doctor because there just isn't one. This, even though 90% men would rather see a male doctor for a genitourinary or personal sexual problem. This by the way is not true of women who tend to express no preference for similar personal conditions.

I can't remember a male doctor who was the delegated house husband in any couple I have ever worked with.

When female doctors do undertake traditionally demanding careers in medicine, say Anaesthetics – because it lends itself to sessional working, how prepared are they to adapt to patients' needs?

Let me quote from "Do no harm", a book by Henry Marsh – the Chief Neurosurgeon at Atkinson Morley/St George's Hospital who was doing his operating list one afternoon: "The next scheduled patient was a woman with a malignant brain tumour who had been put off once already: The nurse told him some unexpected news:

"The anaesthetist's turned up and said she'll have to be cancelled" "Oh for Christ's sake why?" I exploded. "Because she's on the end of the list and won't be finished by 5 O'clock" "Which bloody anaesthetist?" "The new locum, a slim blonde" I walked the few feet to the anaesthetic room and put my head through the door. The anaesthetist, Rachel, and her junior were leaning against the side of the worktop drinking coffee."What's all this about cancelling the last case?" I asked. "I'm not starting a meningioma at 4pm" she declared, turning towards me. "I've got no childcare this evening". "But we can't cancel it I protested, we have cancelled her once already" "Well I'm not doing it."

"Well I'll ask one of your colleagues then, " "I don't think they will – it's not an emergency."

For a few moments I was struck dumb. A few years ago this would never have happened. In the pre modern NHS consultants never counted their hours.......................

But the pre modern NHS wasn't in hock to a tidal wave of uncommitted and part time women doctors with a life/work balance definitely set in favour of life and against the needs of the patient.

We are now reaping the results: In January 2014 the Today Program on Radio 4 ran an interview with a voiced over female casualty SHO who said how hard it was working in casualty compared with other specialities. A representative (male) of the College of Emergency Medicine then brought up the subject of the problem of the number of female doctors and the difficulty of getting them to do the challenging work of casualty. 1:10 consultants and 1:6 junior staff in A and E were locums by then.

The government is promising to beef up staffing levels – presumably by importing doctors from abroad but this will cause its own problems. Some Indian applicants are being interviewed by Skype.

There is no short term solution. WE HAVE to increase the number of male medical students to at least 75% of the total.

We have to increase bed numbers in A and E units and DGHs by about 20%. We have to staff them with nurses, at least one nurse to 6-8 patients on each general ward, who are willing to nurse – not nurses who are graduates and just want to be executives and who feel they are above all the wet work. There has to be a real contract at medical school if medical students no longer accept an implicit one. In return for their expensive education they must agree to work full time, in the UK, for at least 5 years or ?75% of full time for 10 years after qualifying. They have to realise that you go into medicine for all sorts of reasons but a "work life balance" is not one of them. The career will reward you in all sorts of other ways in time but getting home ON TIME isn't one of them.

Also, no British medical graduate should be allowed to emigrate early without repaying at least half of their education costs. Fewer than half a dozen of my year of 90 graduates had gone to more lucrative or warmer countries within the first few years of qualifying but one in eight to one in six to GP trainees are said to be emigrating now. – But most of all, we MUST cut down the number of female medical students – we just can't afford their reduced, intermittent, restricted and selective careers. Oh, and end the 48 hour Working Time Directive. Obviously.

There: in less than a decade our staffing problems will be fixed.

In the Daily Mail, Oct 2014, the report on British doctors emigrating "to the sun" gave the disappointing news that 3,000 UK doctors are currently emigrating each year, primarily to Australia and New Zealand for a better "Work life balance". The NHS is replacing them with eastern European medical staff despite the fact that each British doctor costs £610,000-£850,000 to train. The other equally shocking statistic reported nationally in January 2017 is that only one in ten medical students plans to be a full time doctor. Despite full time being only 48 hours.

The cost of feminisation of medical schools:

Assume men work an arbitrary 100 career units and women 66% of the comparable career hours (assuming part time working, maternity leave, job sharing, late return to work, late in and early out, time off for ill children, picking up kids from school, higher sickness absence for emotional and physical illnesses etc, – this is an average from the various official estimates and articles I have read, it may well be less than this. Most of the female doctors I meet at medical lectures and courses work or plan to work less than 50% of available hours).

Medical schools vary but many seem to be selectively choosing the vast majority of their intake as female A Level entrants.

Apart from the effect on Surgical, Paediatric and Emergency specialities, forward planning and continuity in General Practice, how much more will this cost the tax payer, how many FEWER HOURS will an emasculated work force actually put in?

In the old days, probably up to 90% of graduates were male so they worked 90X100% of arbitrary male career equivalent hours and the 10% female graduates probably worked more than today's women doctors, let's say 70% of their comparable hours (from my contact with my 1975 year group) will do, so: The Class of '75 gave back 90x100% + 10x70% i.e. 97 Units of medical time.

Today 66% of graduates being female will give back 66% (or fewer) of their male colleague's hours so: The class of 2014 will give back 66 x66% + 33 x100% or 77 Units of medical time

In other words **productivity of the medical profession will drop by 20%** if it hasn't already, simply by the positive discrimination in favour of women going on all over British medical schools today.

The medical schools that answered my FOI enquiry (see Chapter 1) "Why are you so sexist against males?" said they simply chose on the basis of A Level results and the standard selection parameters and ignored the gender of the applicant. There is however a huge range from 25% to 58% in maleness between medical schools so clearly there is a great deal of individual choice being exercised by some selection committees. The social, financial, demographic, staffing, planning, management, indeed the actual structural ability to survive of the NHS as we know it is being ignored, indeed threatened by this sexism.

Administration:

Removing a patient from the list:

You cannot use race, sex, sexual orientation, disability, age, religion, a medical condition, need for specific treatments or a relationship to someone you have already removed from the list as a reason for removing a patient. You should not use a complaint as a reason either. (See "You must respond promptly to complaints")

If you do remove a patient, you have to notify the patient, giving reasons and also inform the NHS England Area Team (etc) of the removal.

You can remove the patient if the doctor patient relationship has irretrievably broken down.

But if a complaint is malicious, mischievous, manipulative, personal, hurtful or just plain unfair, as so many are these days, how can the relationship NOT have broken down? Usually you should have warned the patient in writing that they could be removed sometime within the previous 12 months.

You can also remove the patient if they have moved outside the practice area, (give them 30 days to make other arrangements – during which you are not responsible for their treatment).

You can remove them if you have reasonable grounds for thinking a warning might harm them or put you or your staff at risk and you have to be able to produce proof and dates for all of this.

Removal takes place 8 days after the NHS England Area Team receives the request. You are still responsible for them unless otherwise stated until then.

If the patient is violent or threatening, inform the police. The patient can be removed by informing the NHS England Area Team and the removal is immediate although it must be backed up in writing within 7 days. The patient still has to be informed why and a record made in the notes.

Death Certification (Coroner):

The GP must have seen the patient within 14 days to complete the death certificate.

Confirmation of death:

The doctor found, when she was dead, – her last disorder mortal.
Oliver Goldsmith.

There is no legal requirement for a death to be confirmed by a doctor but obviously a doctor is needed to certify a death. Where a patient dies outside the hospital the person discovering the body can confirm the patient is dead and summon the funeral directors. There is no need for the doctor to attend unless there is doubt about whether the patient is actually dead. GPs are required by statute to issue death certificates but this need not delay the removal of the body by the undertakers. It is incredibly rare for a live person to be carted off to the undertakers – although it has happened.

Unexpected Death of A Patient:

All unexpected deaths must be reported to the police (acting as Coroner's Officers) before a body can be moved.

An expected death where the patient has not been seen by his own GP for 14 days must also be reported to the police before the body can be removed. This is also a Coroner's case if you haven't seen him or her for >14 days. You can phone the Coroner or their officer to discuss if you did not find the death unexpected to discuss the likely cause of death from the past history and your knowledge of the patient.

Temporary Resident:

Must be resident in area >24 hrs, mustn't be registered with another local practice, up to 3 months.

Emergency Treatment:

<24 hours total stay, can be registered with another local GP. This is an emergency or accident situation.

Immediate Necessary Treatment:

Staying>24 hrs in your area, not registered with another local GP but you are not prepared to take them on as a patient. (You could have taken them onto your list or as a T/R) – if you believe that their condition cannot wait until they return to their own area. Responsible for them for 14 days.

Overseas visitors:

Overseas Visitors are entitled to free emergency treatment if they have a genuine emergency and go to casualty. Asylum seekers are all entitled to free NHS treatment.

Overseas visitors are entitled to free treatment if their medical condition has occurred or worsened since arriving and they are from:

The E.C.

Non E.C. countries including those that we have reciprocal arrangements with including most of the former Soviet Union and:

Anguilla,
New Zealand,
Australia,
Gibraltar,
British Virgin Islands,
St Helena,
Turks and Caicos Islands,
Falklands,
Hong Kong,
Iceland,
Malta,
Montserrat,
Norway,
Switzerland by special arrangement,
Barbados,
Channel Islands.

If the patient is not normally resident in the UK it doesn't matter what passport they hold (even a UK passport if they are ex-pats coming home on a visit), they have to pay. What is "Normally Resident"? This is a grey area and as you will have guessed, open to political, personal and human rights interference and interpretation. The legal definition includes terms such as "settled, living lawfully, voluntarily, for settled purposes, as part of the regular order of their life, for the time being, with an identifiable purpose for their residence here which has a sufficient degree of continuity to be properly described as settled". Go over those phrases again and think how unhelpful they are. The more legal definitions I read the more I realise how our august and respected Law Lords and senior judges almost never clarify anything after deliberating on it (see the Gillick Ruling, Legal Issues). What they do is restate the question in different terms and say: "Make up your own mind next time the problem reoccurs, Doc."

You can always phone the local NHS Fraud office and ask if in doubt.

Most people I have heard talking on the subject say that the patient either has to have been in the UK or is planning to stay in the UK for 6 months or preferably both.

A and E, walk in centre emergency treatment, compulsory psychiatric treatment and family planning are free. Likewise, emergency treatment by the GP, STD clinic treatment, notifiable/certain communicable disease treatment, are also all free.

Overseas Visitors: Who expect to move out of a practice area in 3 months can be registered as "Temporary Residents."

People eligible for NHS treatment are UK citizens,

"Ordinarily Resident" in the UK,

EEA nationals carrying form E128,

Other visitors are only entitled to "Immediate Necessary Treatment,"

The Form E112 entitles a visitor to seek treatment for a specific condition.

As I mentioned, the courts define someone "Ordinarily Resident" as: Lawfully, voluntarily, settled in the UK as part of the regular order of life, with an identifiable purpose for his or her residence and with sufficient continuity to describe the purpose as settled. Anyone intending to stay for less than 6 months will probably not qualify (the DOH suggests they should have an open ended passport allowing them to stay at least a year).

There is obviously a fair leeway for interpretation by the doctor and manipulation by patients who have been here less than 6 months I would say.

You can always offer to treat people privately if you are in doubt about their intentions or the regular conduct of their business.

So what is ordinarily resident? The usual legal fudge is to restate the obvious: "A sufficient degree of continuity to be properly described as settled." So would that be a travelling salesman who's home and family are in Tehran but who's main market and who's domicile for several months a year is in the UK but who flies all over the world at the drop of a hat and who pays no income tax here?

Termination of pregnancy: The Abortion Act 1967

Is legal up to 24 weeks despite this just about being a viable gestation in many premature baby units. 200,000 abortions are performed in the UK each year, largely on healthy fetuses and mothers. I remember the original debate in parliament on the Abortion Act well over 40 years ago and how it was promoted mainly to prevent back street abortions and save the tiny number of deaths each year caused by complications after these. There were arguments about multiple congenital abnormalities, the seriously ill mother and the case of the rape victim. I remember the emotional debate at the time. No one had any idea at the time that abortion would become an on demand, never seriously challenged or questioned, absolutely never refused, form of backstop birth control and in such huge numbers of healthy pregnancies.

How many lives of girls who might have been to back street abortionists did it actually save from perforated uteruses and puerperal sepsis etc? Judging by transcripts of the Commons Debate they thought the act would save large numbers of these hapless girls. The actual numbers are difficult to judge but the number of deaths before and after the Abortion Act in young women hardly changed from published mortality statistics. The best figures I can get from the statistics of deaths in young women in the UK pre and post the act are about five deaths a year.

Given the 200,000 normal babies per year currently denied the right to life and the huge change in personal sexual responsibility in society consequent to the awareness of free abortion for all comers, you can't help wondering if the nation should discuss this overused and potentially physically and emotionally damaging procedure again. After all, aborting on demand hundreds of thousands of healthy pregnant woman with normal babies wasn't exactly what they sold the bill to the nation as 40 years ago.

On the other hand, there is an interesting but slightly thought provoking fact that may also affect your attitude toward abortion. In the USA after a bitter (and still ongoing) debate about legalising abortion culminating in the "Roe vs Wade" decision in1973, huge numbers of unwanted babies could be aborted legally for the first time. In the first year 750,000 women had abortions and by 1980 1.6million abortions were taking place a year in the USA. Most of the women having abortions were teenage, poor, had restricted education and were single parents. All these factors are actually also predictors of their children subsequently becoming involved in crime. Sure enough, just at the time when the cohort of children would have become teenagers had they not been aborted, crime rates fell dramatically across America. Interestingly, the same fall occurred somewhat later in states that delayed the introduction of abortion. Unwanted babies lead to crime. I am not sure if the UK saw a similar benefit from about 1985 onwards.

Chiropody (Podiatry) Treatment:

1 in 3 older people cannot cut their own toenails. Of course that doesn't mean they can't get a relative to do it for them and every chiropody service seems to have its own rules regarding who they will see:

Locally my service is fairly typical and will see those
Of pensionable age,
Who are diabetic,
Pregnant.
Other services will see patients with severe mobility problems (ie hip OA) which prevent personal foot care,
People with Learning Disabilities,
Visual problems,
or those specifically referred by the GP.

Death Certificates:

It is not necessary (as some nursing homes claim) for a doctor to visit and confirm that a patient has died. Any member of the public may confirm a death, surprisingly. Doctors, of course, have to issue the death certificate as to the cause of death.

Rather prosaically, death is defined as the simultaneous and irreversible onset of apnoea and unconsciousness in the absence of the circulation. It is assumed that resuscitation is inappropriate, that this state has been observed for at least 5 minutes, (usually confirmed by the absence of a central pulse and heart sounds) and that after this period the pupils, motor responses to supra orbital pressure and corneal reflexes are found to be unreactive.

The time of death is recorded as the time at which these criteria are fulfilled. Unprofound and unpoetic in the extreme.

Caution should be exercised if the patient has been immersed in cold water, has taken alcohol or sedative drugs or is hypoglycaemic, hypothermic or in a coma. The patient may then not be beyond recovery though looking on first appearance dead.

If you did not expect the death, do not know the patient and you do attend, (I often do this out of courtesy unless the death was expected, inevitable and the patient's own doctor had been in regular attendance) check:

Major pulses,

Heart and breath sounds for one minute (and intermittently for up to five minutes),

Pupil and corneal reflexes.

Rigor starts to set in from 3 hours after circulation ceases.

So for practical purposes in General Practice, death may be said to have taken place in:

An unresponsive patient, temperature over 35°C who has not taken drugs or alcohol if:

There are no movements,

No respiratory effort over 1 minute of observation,

No heart sounds or palpable pulses over 1 minute of observing,

There are fixed dilated pupils and no corneal or other reflexes.

A quarter of deaths are certified by the Coroner, three quarters by other doctors.

You have to have been the attending doctor during the last illness to issue the medical certificate.

Coroners investigate violent, unnatural, unknown, sudden deaths, prison deaths and so on. These are about 12% of the total number of deaths.

A registrar will refer a death to the Coroner if:

the deceased was not attended during the last illness,

the deceased was not seen after death or 14 days before death,

the cause appears to be unknown,

the registrar has cause to believe the death was unnatural, suspicious, due to neglect, violence, abortion, during or shortly after an operation (anaesthetic related), or due to industrial disease or poisoning.

The Coroner: An independent judicial officer of the crown.

The Coroner has a statutory duty to investigate any death where he or she has reasonable cause to suspect a violent or unnatural death, the individual has died a sudden death – cause unknown, has died in prison or elsewhere which may require an inquest under any act of law. Coroners only hold inquests into 12% of the deaths certified. Three quarters of sudden deaths are due to circulatory diseases. 180,000 or so deaths are reported to coroners annually. 60% by doctors, 2% by registrars, 38% by others (mainly the police).

Causes of death in the UK: (Guardian Oct 2011)

There are 493,000 deaths in the UK annually:

Circulatory Diseases 160,000,

Cancer 140,000,

Respiratory Disease 67,000,

Digestive disease 26,000,
Mental/behavioural disorders 20,000,
Nervous system disease 18,000,
Death not caused by disease 17,000,
Genitourinary disease 12,000,
Other causes 9,800,
Endocrine, nutritional, metabolic 7,000,
Infectious, parasitic 5,000,
Musculoskeletal 4,000,
Congenital and chromosomal disorders 1,200,
Skin disease 2,000,
Blood and immune disease 1,000,
Babies dying around birth 224,
Pregnancy and childbirth 35,
Ears and mastoid diseases 20,
Eye diseases 11,

Death from injury or poisoning not known if deliberate 250,
Total accidents 6,400,
Transport accidents 1,453,
Falls 1,850,
Killed by falling object 30,
Bitten or struck by an animal 4,
Accidental drowning 170,
Drowning in bath 9,
Accidental hanging/strangulation 170,
Electric current/radiation/extreme temperature 35,
Smoke, fire and flames 123,
Wasps, hornets and bees 3,
Narcotics and hallucinogens 508,
Intentional self harm 2,600,
Assault 210,
Complications of medical or surgical care 220,
About 20 die each year in total from anaphylaxis.

So the **GP should refer the death to the Coroner** if he or she believes:
The cause of death is unknown,
If the certifying doctor did not see the deceased after death or within 14 days before death,
(ie the patient's attending doctor is away on holiday),
The death was violent, unnatural or suspicious,
The death was due to an accident,
The death was due to self neglect or neglect by others,
The death was due to industrial disease or related to the deceased's employment,
The death was due to an abortion (illegal),
The death occurred during an operation or before recovery from the anaesthetic,

The death was a suicide,

A "Doubtful stillbirth,"

The death took place during or shortly after police or prison custody,

Identity of the deceased unknown.

Even if you refer the death to the Coroner you can still complete a death certificate (after discussion with the Coroner or his officer and indicating on the death certificate that you have referred the death). The Coroner's officer is usually an incredibly helpful, understanding and sensible person, usually a police officer, who gives down to earth and practical advice about the process, forms, etc.

You should try and avoid vague terms on the death certificate; certainly "Old age" is inappropriate under 70. Avoid giving a mode of dying such as heart failure, shock, uraemia etc. unless you also give a background "causal sequence" – myocardial infarction, bleeding from perforated peptic ulcer etc.

So terms like Asphyxia, Asthenia, Cardiac arrest, Heart Failure, Liver or Renal Failure shock, Syncope, Uraemia, Ventricular Failure etc, need elaboration.

Sudden and unexpected deaths:

IHD 55%,

Other Heart Disease 9%,

PE 6%,

Ruptured Aortic Aneurysm 6%,

Acute Respiratory Disease 7%,

Acute Abdomen 2%,

Suicide 5%,

RTA 5%.

Virtually everyone dies of natural causes but at least once in a professional lifetime you will meet an unnatural death. One of mine was an elderly schizophrenic who murdered her husband with an axe, others were suicides by insulin overdose, hanging and exhaust gas.

Donating a patient's body to medicine

Is done via the Human Tissue Authority which has a website, phone numbers of medical schools and a pack to download. Consent and instructions have to be given before death in writing by the patient.

Post Mortems/Autopsies:

In hospital cases, PMs turn up a major ante mortem misdiagnosis in 40% cases. In a third of these patients, the patient would have lived had the diagnosis been made correctly. The rate of misdiagnosis (causing death) has not improved in 80 years despite all the imaging and pathology support that we have now. I assume the situation is about the same if not worse in GP given the paucity of diagnostic aids and facilities we have at our disposal.

Certificates:

How long should you give a medical certificate for?
Medical Certificates:

	Laparoscopic	Open
Abdominal/inguinal hernia:	1-2 weeks	2-3 weeks
Appendicectomy	1-2 weeks	2-3 weeks

I hate the term appendectomy which of course is the excision of an append and American.

	Laparoscopic	Open
Cholecystectomy	2-3 weeks	3-5 weeks

	Vaginal	Abdominal
Hysterectomy	3 weeks	7 weeks

Cardiac illness	
Angioplasty	0-4 weeks
Infarction	4-6 weeks
CABG	4-8 weeks

Medical Certificates and Reports: "Fit note."

Only a registered medical practitioner can issue official statements of a person's incapacity for work. Although osteopaths and occupational physicians etc may make a recommendation, it is you who decides, considering their opinion and you who carries the can.

The Old Med 3: Statement of incapacity for work: (used for Statutory sick pay and Social security) and Med 5 were replaced by a Statement of "Fitness to Work" in April 2010. The "Fit Note" is issued free of charge after 7 days off work as long as you believe the patient to have been unfit for their occupation.

The statement may be issued on the day the patient was assessed, after the assessment if you think it would have been reasonable to have issued a statement on the day of the assessment, after consideration of a written report by another doctor or "registered healthcare professional."

The changes in the new system are that the Med 3 and 5 are combined, phone consultations count as an assessment (strangely, – this must surely be open to huge manipulation, error and subjectivity), the "fit for work" option is removed and introduced is: "may be fit taking into account the following advice," there is more space for comments and the functional effects of the condition and tick boxes for altered hours and activity options.

To claim statutory sick pay for illness periods less than 7 days the patient may self certify (the SC2 or SC1 if self employed or unemployed are used to provide details of sickness absence of 4 or more days in a row) or they may ask for a private certificate. These are used to decide if the employee is entitled to Statutory Sick Pay.

ACAS has suggested standard disciplinary processes for employees frequently taking short periods off work and you can refuse to allow either the employee or employer to waste your time in this way.

The advice, as before, is not actually binding on employers and you do not need to see the employee at the end of the stated period.

You do not need to provide a patient with a sickness certificate until they have been off work 7 days. You can charge if their employer insists on one earlier, give a private certificate and a receipt. Some employers and some employees will always need proof that they have been ill.

The most frustrating and difficult situations and ones which seem to happen with the same difficult patients over and over again are for instance: Requests for retrospective certificates justifying a sick child's absence from school (with a background of regular non attendance and a "I didn't want to bring him down to the doctors or drag you out for a bad cold" scenario) Or "I need a certificate because I was too ill to attend community service/jury service/the case conference/my court appearance yesterday etc" (but I didn't bother to phone the doctor at the time) etc etc.

These are frustrating situations and I nearly always apologise as I refuse the certificate, with a "Sorry but this is practice policy and we can't retrospectively issue certificates" type of statement. I say this in a nice way and make sure there is a written statement somewhere in the practice handbook or in the waiting room which shows that regrettably I have no choice in the matter and next time if they ARE actually ill they will have to contact **me on the day** and do some negotiating, probably by **coming to see me**, not the other way round. I offer to see them in the surgery after a session has finished if they are worried about cross infection and reassure them that there is almost no condition that doesn't benefit from a trip outside in the fresh air.

Considering we spend 1/3 of our waking hours at work, that over half of all illnesses are work acquired, related or exacerbated and that medics are hopelessly naive about the daily world of work outside our own profession, it has always surprised me that we take so little interest in what our patients do for a living, who they are, what their work duties and worries, roles and responsibilities are and how little we contact their Occupational Health departments, Human Resources Teams or their managers or colleagues to intercede or enquire on their behalf. All these are normally very willing to report, advise or contribute information to the GP if asked.

DS 1500:

Is issued if the patient has a terminal illness, handed direct to the patient (or often via the D/N)

The DS1500 includes information on diagnosis, whether the patient is aware of the condition, current and proposed treatment and brief details of clinical findings.

For the purposes of this form, a terminal illness is one with a life expectancy of 6 months or less, they satisfy "Special Rules" and can claim Attendance Allowance, Incapacity Benefit (26 weeks off work instead of 52), Disability Living Allowance at the highest rate without waiting a qualifying period. The District Nurses tend to regard this as every terminally ill patient's right no matter what the personal or financial circumstances of the patient or family.

Dental Problems in General Practice and our Dental Colleagues:

Although dentists are obliged to arrange 24 hr emergency care for their patients, they can have on their answer machines advice to go straight to casualty if in severe pain, or there is bleeding, trauma or swelling. My last Saturday morning on call surgery commenced with three patients all suffering acute dental conditions who told my receptionist that their own dental practice either couldn't fit them in for a week or that the dental receptionist had advised them "just to get some antibiotics from the GP – it would be cheaper."

Our LMC suggested that some patients now play the system and know GPs will usually prescribe for dental infections, sometimes thus saving them time and money and that the patient isn't always completely honest in their dealing with GP receptionists. One of the patients I saw on this occasion was a PCT administrator! A dental "emergency" should receive a verbal response within a maximum of 6 hours with an average response time of 3 hours and a consultation within 24 hrs. Their "emergencies" are not the same as ours! Their answer machine message should be clear and up to date with information on the whereabouts of the local OOH Emergency Dental Service or the cover arrangements for their practice. One local emergency covering dental service refuses to see more than 12 patients a day at weekends!

Dentists can now prescribe Co Amoxiclav as well as Amoxicillin and Metronidazole, so they are more than capable of dealing with their own infections.

General topics:

Some Professional Structures, organisations and pressure groups you will encounter

Bandolier: An Independent evidence based health journal started in 1984 by two Oxford scientists now on line and free. I presume it is supposed to give you "ammunition" in any factual argument.

The Welcome Foundation: The Welcome Collection: Medical artifacts and works of Art.

The Welcome Trust: a global charitable foundation funding improvements in health care.

The King's Fund is a charity that defines its goal as analysing and improving the function of the NHS in England. They act as a pressure group to "Shape policy, transform services and bring about behavioral change." They undertake research and analysis in health matters and provide "Leadership development and service improvement." They also have a variety of resources to enable information gathering and sharing in health.

The Cochrane Collaboration: A global independent network of doctors, researchers and patient advocates who interpret medical research data.

Dr Foster: An organisation that "Works with healthcare organisations to achieve sustainable improvements in performance through better use of data." Slightly in the doghouse a few years ago because it gave a government department some negative comparative trust mortality data which didn't take into account the local deaths from a hospice.

MHRA (yellow card system). Drug side effect reporting system. The reports rise exponentially in the months after a new drug is released but once a common side effect is recognised nobody bothers to continue reporting it – the indomethacin or aspirin effect. Who bothers to send in a yellow card when a patient has a gastric bleed after taking these drugs these days?

But if the drug were brand new who wouldn't report it?

NHS Alliance: A group consisting of (at one time) for instance: PCTs, practices, some strategic health authorities and all sorts of patient and professional groups eg RCN, British Dental Association, National Associating of Non Principles and also *individuals* involved in health care. It calls itself the "Only voice to speak for the whole General Practice team" and its mission statement is to improve the NHS particularly via commissioning.

NICE; Now it is the National Institute for Health and Care Excellence. Which is actually NIFHACE – but this doesn't have the same ring as Nice does it? Their website says: NICE Guidance sets the standards for high quality healthcare and encourages healthy living. Their guidance can be used by the NHS, local authorities, employers, voluntary groups, and anyone else involved in delivering care or promoting wellbeing.

The NHS Confederation: Is the membership body for all organisations that commission and provide NHS services. "The only body to bring together and speak for the whole of the NHS."

Prodigy: Evidence summaries incorporated by NICE and now called Clinical Knowledge Summaries.

Criminal Records Bureau: Now the Disclosure and Barring Service (DBS, nothing to do with Aston Martins). The organisation that checks an applicant's past history with regard to safety of working with patients, children, with vulnerable patients/"clients" etc. Now using them may be called a Total Disclosure and Barring Service check rather than a "CRB check". There is a fee for this service which may be as much as £44.00 (2016).

The BMA: A trade union and professional association "for all UK doctors." It is involved in collective bargaining and national negotiation. I am not sure how it assesses the will of the profession except by rare attempts at national consultation. Still, that is much more often than either the GMC or RCGP. It has local and national forums and there is an annual representative meeting. I don't know anyone who has attended one of these. It has several committees, for consultants, GPs, junior doctors, ethics, etc. It suggests policies and the Head Office is in Tavistock Square, London but there are offices in each UK country. During the Junior doctors' strike its negotiating committee was said to include members active in extreme left wing politics. It has a reputation for negotiating intransigence and being politically far left and so is not exactly reflective of the politics of GPs as a whole.

Drug companies, Trials, Reps etc.

The NHS spends £9bn per year on drugs (about 8% of its budget) and drug companies spend 1/4 of the total cost of drugs on marketing. This is, surprisingly, twice as much as they spend on R and D.

Most new chemical entities that become prescribable drugs are produced by the R and D departments of pharmaceutical companies – not the NHS or university research departments. In other words the constantly criticised "Big Pharma". If we ever find new classes of resistance beating antibiotics, consistent treatments for drug resistant TB, antipsychotic drugs without side effects, new anti cancer drugs, the cure for Malaria or drugs that can repair arthritic joints or target faulty genes, it will be *probably* be private drug companies that manufacture them and market them. Pharmaceutical companies can make big profits but they are undoubtedly high risk businesses and not altruistic social services. Large numbers of drugs are discarded well into development because of side effects. Huge compensation claims are mounted and awarded against drug companies individually and as class actions. In the case of much needed new antibiotics which will be prescribed for courses of only a week and have the same limited licence period as drugs like antihypertensives that are prescribed continuously for years or anticancer drugs that command high prices, drug companies will have to be offered new financial incentives and possibly legal protection to develop them by governments. Otherwise they won't be financially worth researching and developing. Each drug that gets as far as receiving a license has cost more than £100m to develop, often a lot more. I remember being told that this was more than BMW spend on developing a whole new series of cars and since a significant proportion of drugs is withdrawn from the market early, it may often be a high profits but it is also a high risk business.

I don't tend to criticise the pharmaceutical industry as much as some doctors but then I don't usually see medical reps at the surgery either.

I used to count the Head Rep. of one drug company as a personal friend. My wife temporarily worked as a secretary in the same company while I was dragging her around the country on a series of SHO jobs thirty plus years ago. He became successful and popular by telling doctors he wasn't going to pretend the company's drug was exceptional, there were others like it, it wasn't the most expensive, it wasn't the most side effect laden but it might be worth giving it a try when the opportunity came up. He never called the drugs "products, " (something that instantly makes a doctor feel like a promoter of someone else's wares or a commercial salesman rather than a thoughtful professional). He never used misleading comparisons (for instance: his company's NSAID at a proper therapeutic dose compared with feeble Ibuprofen 200mg TDS), he never told you about more than one drug at each visit and he never took more than five minutes. Therefore, by going against all his rep-school training he became very successful.

I stopped seeing reps when my regular Thursday morning rep didn't turn up one day. As I usually saw them between morning surgery and my ante natal clinic, I thought I would do a quick visit in the half an hour that I now had spare.

The visit was to a fluey teenager, apparently too unwell to come to the surgery – I had no history other than that. When I got to the house, the boy's father called him to come downstairs to see me but there was no reply from the lad's bedroom. His dad was embarrassed, apologetic and annoyed but when I got upstairs and pulled back the covers from the silent boy, I saw the meningococcal purpura and an unresponsive septicaemic and unconscious young lad.

I don't know if my putting in an IV line, giving the Penicillin and Hydrocortisone and telling the father to go downstairs and dial 999 immediately saved the boy's life but I can't help thinking that my not seeing a rep that day and having the time to do the visit early might have done.

So I stopped seeing reps at that point, especially those who are out to encourage me to "promote products" for them, those who ask me directly if I am likely to prescribe **their own** product, telling me that their me – too or left handed molecule is a therapeutic milestone and on the way using highly selected or inherently biased trial data and unfair comparisons to exaggerate the benefits of their own drug.

Reps do provide some useful medical education and not all sponsored speakers have been "bought." They also, of course, feed us at most educational meetings but nice and personable though many of them are, their job is simple. To give doctors a one-sided view of their company's drugs leaving out all unflattering data and the evidence (at least from America) is that they are highly cost effective. With our PACT data, prescribing committees, budgets and limited prescribing freedom these days I doubt that they are quite so cost effective here.

Drugs: Development:

The search for new molecules for therapeutic use in man begins with the lab testing on target enzymes, proteins, bacteria etc, then:

Animal testing of the active agent to assess tolerability, toxicity and therapeutic indices.

Then testing on humans:

Phase 1, Human volunteers, low dose, gradually increasing,

Phase 2, A few to a hundred or so patients to determine short term outcomes, side effects and dose regimes,

Phase 3, Bigger groups of patients, perhaps thousands, randomised controlled trials (where neither the tester nor the tested knows whether an active or control substance is being given). Sometimes these tests are handed over to Clinical Research Organisations, – private companies who may compare the drug against placebo rather than the best drug available in its class currently so the trials often have to be examined at a bit more than their face value when presented to you.

New drugs are rarely completely new, of course. Once the first Beta Blocker, Statin, or Artan were produced, five to ten others followed over the following years (as "me-too" drugs) and these days drug companies even market left or right handed versions – (different chirality) of the original molecules (Escitalopram, Esomeprazole, Levocetirizine – called "me again" drugs) which extend the income stream from the original pool of R and D but make you wonder why any ethical manufacturer wouldn't have marketed the more effective enantiomer first. The answer is obvious really. By the way, just to demonstrate how differently these mirror molecules affect our bodies, thalidomide was a racemic mixture of the molecule (equal numbers of L and R handed forms). It was the L handed molecule that caused the phocomelia in exposed babies. The same sort of handedness occurs in nature: Caraway and spearmint are the same molecule, just mirror images of each other.

Trials:

It would take a GP 600 hours a month just to read all the UK GP related academic data published. There are only 720 hours in an average month, including the nights.

I am assuming that most of us are vaguely able to look at a trial and see if the drugs compared would be reasonable in the real world, that the trial hasn't been stopped before the dangerous side effects have become apparent, to know that surrogate outcomes (lowered cholesterols, BPs or HbA1Cs) don't always mean better survival, that the difference in outcomes is indeed of some statistical significance, that the study has been done by genuinely independent researchers, not by drug company ghost writers or stooges, etc.

We should all be aware of the useful concept of "Number needed to treat" (the number of patients over a predetermined time who need to be on a drug for one death or acute episode of illness to be prevented). If it is 1/Absolute risk reduction – For instance if a drug is effective at lowering blood pressure but the numbers needed to take the drug before a stroke or heart attack is prevented are thousands over a five year period, you may not think it is worth prescribing. If it prevents a stroke in every other patient you give it to for one year then it is a wonder drug.

Some Random Medical acronyms/initials:

AKT Applied knowledge test (end of training assessment)
ACP Advance care plan
ALOBA Agenda led outcome based analysis
BARD Behaviour aims room dialogue
BMA British Medical Association
CBD Case based discussion
COGPED Committee of GP education directors

COT Case observational tool

CRB Criminal records bureau.

CSA Clinical skills assessment: – A bit like OSCEs (done at an examination centre). An end of training assessment.

DBS Disclosure and Barring Service. What was the CRB. The authority that now assesses an individual's safety to work with the vulnerable, based on officially recorded information.

DES Directed Enhanced Services. Additional services a practice may choose to provide usually linked to national priorities and agreements.

DDA Disability Discrimination Act. I have a slightly negative view of the application of this in some healthcare situations since talking to a consultant psychiatrist friend. He told me he was forced to interview a totally deaf CPN who needed the constant presence of an interpreter and therefore would cost the employing authority twice the usual sum. Not only could they not afford this but the situation gave him and his team enormous headaches regarding confidentiality and handling paranoid, challenging and difficult patients.

DOP Direct Observation of Procedural Skills

DRC Disability Rights Commission

EOLC End of life care

EPU Early pregnancy Unit

FDR First degree relative (Not Franklin D Roosevelt)

GPC General Practice Committee (of the BMA, a registered Trade Union and Professional Association)

GPSI A GP with a special interest. Usually a GP who has qualifications and experience in a specialist area – e.g. Dermatology or ENT.

HRG Healthcare resource group. Not an organisation but a grouping together of similar treatment episodes with the same resources and clinical outcome. A standard model to assist in analysis of clinical procedures.

ICT Intermediate Care Team

JCPTGP Joint Committee on post graduate training for general practice. (Ended 2005)

LES Local Enhanced Services. Schemes agreed by PCTs in response to local needs and priorities

LL Learning Log

Mini CEX is Clinical Evaluation Exercise (Part of the WPBA) Is this supposed to sound like mini sex?" Since it should be Mini CEE, aren't we taking these acronyms a little too far here?

MMC Modernising Medical Careers.

MMSE Mini Mental state Examination.

MRHA Medicines and Healthcare products regulation Agency. As you can see this is MHRA not MRHA. They regulate medicines, do Drug Safety Update, The Yellow Card scheme since Thalidomide (1964) etc

MSF Multisource Feedback, Medicine Sans Frontieres

ORIF Open Reduction, Internal Fixation.

PBR Payment by results

PCLC Primary Care Led Commissioning.

PCRN Primary Care Research Network.

PDP Either Professional or Personal Development Plan

PEP Post Exposure Prophylaxis

PMETB Post graduate Medical Education Training Board (Merged with the GMC 2010)

POO Patient Orientated Outcome!

PSQ : Patient Satisfaction Questionnaire

QIA: Quality Improvement Activity

QUIPP: Quality Innovation Productivity and Prevention

RICE: Rest, Immobilisation, Cold, Elevation.

SDR: Second Degree Relative

SOP: Scope of Practice. Standard Operating Procedure

WPBA: Workplace Based Assessment: 6 Case Based Discussions, 6 Clinical Observation Tools (Video/case discussion) End of training assessment.

PLEASE ADD YOUR OWN NEW ACRONYMS

How big should your partnership be?

I was attached to a single handed GP as part of my trainee year and would have found his on call, day in day out, seven days a week cover rota intolerable. This is because I can never relax on call no matter how quiet it is. In single handed practices now almost nonexistent, doctors have to be thick skinned, imperturbable and without guilt. In rural Hampshire where the practice was, a few patients used to bigger practices would often be offended by his refusal to visit them for migraine or to see their children with high temperatures. He would instead manage them by phone, telling them to come to his house or go to casualty thirty miles away if they deteriorated. Occasionally he would visit those he considered genuinely at risk or seriously ill. I don't think his patients had a higher mortality rate than those attached to bigger rota practices and once people realised he was on call 24 hours a day seven days a week they rarely bothered him unless they thought they were **really** ill. He offered superb home terminal care.

I have also appraised many doctors in practices of twenty or so partners and assistants. They always have large numbers of part time doctors, many partners involved in outside activities, usually training, appraising, GPSI work. They often suffer from organisational (rota, cover and duty) confusion, communication and responsibility drift as well as a tendency to form partnership factions. Practice decisions are hard to make, consensus impossible and there are nearly always conflicting personality issues between partners. The part timers often feel excluded from decision making, the full timers feel the part timers can't wait to get off home and prioritise their families over their practice activities. The non trainers think the trainers and appraisers aren't seeing enough patients to make up for their time off and the pooled income isn't enough either. The other partners think the GPSIs are avoiding real, acute, demanding general practice and playing at cushy secondary care. Their patients find it difficult to develop continuity of care, an ongoing relationship with one doctor or even find out who is responsible for them and there is a constant potential for communication breakdown. This is particularly true when passing on messages from patients, establishing who has clinical responsibility for a given patient, who should return the call or do the visit and even who is on call. In big practices the on call demand becomes an impersonal white noise often offloaded to the part timers, registrars and least experienced doctors. The patients never see the same doctor at home twice with same acute illness.

The ideal size of a practice depends on what its main working parameters are. Are they patient continuity and accessibility, reliable absence cover for partners or ability to allow and encourage outside professional activities and "career development" for the partners? Are they partnership cohesion and informal relationships, good communication, a pool of flexible clinical (internal opinion and referrals) talent or administrative skills – what else that is important to the practice? These factors can sometimes become mutually exclusive: A larger variety of partner specialist skills means more partners and less cohesion in decision making and communication.

Put bluntly, patients feel alienated by big and therefore inherently impersonal practices but many doctors find smaller practices restrict income generation, variety of professional experience and confine practice planning.

I believe the ideal practice is 5-8 partners in size, administratively, cohesively and from the point of view of communication and continuity of care. This seems from American studies to be the most popular size from the patient's point of view. At this size however, most if not all partners need to be full time and not have **significant** outside commitments. A GP who works for the Deanery three sessions a week or teaches at the local Medical School or has a Community Health or GPSI commitment may be fulfilling a personal career plan but can put their partners under intolerable strain by doing so. This is something that often comes up at the other partners' appraisals if not at his or her practice meetings.

A recent American (2014) study showed that small practices reduced hospital admissions. 1-2 physicians had 33% fewer preventable hospital admissions per partner than practices with 10-19 physicians. Practices with 3-9 physicians had 27% fewer admissions. This was the first American study of its kind. This study also showed the interesting finding that if the physicians owned their own premises they made fewer unnecessary admissions (Health Affairs Aug 2014). Perhaps this gives a sense of belonging, of community, of commitment to the enterprise, of family almost.

The comments made by the authors were that smaller practices offered advantages such as more immediate appointments, easier telephone access to physicians, closer ties among patients, physicians and staff which lead to better outcomes. Those qualities should be considered in an environment that encourages and rewards consolidation, they said.

In America 83.2% of office based physicians are in practices of 10 or fewer, 38.6% in 1-2 physicians, 26.4% 3-5 physicians 18.2% have 6-10 physicians. It is interesting that there is currently a move towards GP factories with large numbers of doctors in each establishment here in the UK. Clearly this is not at the behest of the involved doctors' patients.

Complaints:

47,000 were made about General Practice in 2013/14. (HSCIC) of these 24,000 related to medical services (doctor and nurse services) and 22,600 were about administration.

Clinical issues were the most common cause for complaint (36%). 20% were related to "communication issues" which include the "the attitude" of staff.

Between 2012/13 and 13/14 hospital and community care complaints rose 4.6% from 109,316 to 114,308. Considering that 90% of patient consultations are in General Practice you could argue that GPs are doing pretty well compared with other health care "providers" in the NHS.

Altogether the NHS received 480 written complaints a day in 2013-14.

The Practice Team:

Second only to the practice nurse, the attached District Nurse is weight for weight the most valued member of the primary health care team from the GP's perspective. If your D/N is attached to your practice and better still, has a room in your surgery, then you are a communicative, tight and organised team. The patients are looked after better, decisions are communicated clearly and agreed. Generally, people in co-habiting teams work better with each other, know each other's faults better and work around them to the patient's advantage.

These days that particular model of practice organisation has been decimated by "virtual wards", sectorisation (areas of a town or city that have just one D/N team rather than individual practices each having their own D/N) and in my experience, the result has been low morale, a poorer service to the patient and poorer job satisfaction all round. All this has led in my area to a 40% loss in trained D/Ns over the last few years.

So yet again, a reorganisation in the primary care team that followed a failure to consult GPs, but looked good on paper has led to a worsening of services and the question, so often asked: "Why did they have to fix (and ruin) what was working well already?" The nurses, the G.P.s but particularly the patients these days all look back fondly to the time when each practice worked as a close knit and communicative professional family.

Essays:

Infection Control: The Sterile Environment: (An essay)

So here we are. Half a dozen GPs, a bacteriologist, a prescribing adviser and a nurse or two. All together in a stuffy upstairs room, giving up an afternoon of our working week and all learning about **Community Acquired Infection**.

Swine Flu, C.Diff, MRSA, drug resistant TB, these are the massed ranks of the 21st century's equivalent of the Black Death.

I calculate that the GPs here have about 220 year's clinical experience in total. So I may be wrong but I reckon this bunch of doctors will have consulted and treated 2.3 million patients between them. – No wonder they look tired.

We learn about C. Difficile, MRSA, the slippery Staphylococcus and how to prescribe "first line" antibiotics (– these are antibiotics that won't reliably do the job but **are** cheap).

We find out when the lab **wants** us to send a sample (usually after their recommended antibiotic has failed and the patient has got worse).

I have sat around tables listening to different doctors talking about infections and antibiotics ever since I started my love affair with medicine in 1970. I was a student then and I wondered what doctoring would be like when I was close to retiring, forty years later.

Stem Cell Organ Replacement? Gene Therapy? Magic Bullets of various kinds? The cure for cancer?

No. What we are now learning about today is how to wash our hands.

There is an "Infection Control nurse" here with a Power Point presentation and an ultraviolet light box telling us how to wash our hands.

I naively think that **all** nurses used to be infection control nurses. Didn't we learn that from Lister and Nightingale?

Here is a slide showing how to scrub, how to rub, how to rinse. Next we are told that touching people spreads disease. That we should have plastic covers over our keyboards, that we must remove all toys, ornaments and superfluous objects from the consulting area and that physical contact with the patient is a risky luxury we should try to avoid.

My mind fleetingly goes to Norman Rockwell's painting of the family doctor consulting a worried looking young couple. His gun hangs over the fireplace and his pipe rack is on top of the desk. Look closely and there is a border collie on a chair next to the fireplace.

But that was then and we have moved on now. This is the era of evidence based medicine.

So I ask if there is any evidence that any patient has contracted a serious disease just from touching his GP. Apparently that is not the point. The nurse replies: "Is there any evidence that patients **haven't** contracted infections from seeing their GP?"

I will let you take that in. It is a sign of the new weakness of we GPs as a profession that the assembled group didn't just all get up and walk out. I wonder whether it is worth asking for the evidence that turning hospital doctors into party goers with rolled up sleeves and without ties reduces cross infection. But I actually know there is no evidence for that so I don't bother.

How did we let it all get this far? Politicians and administrators, none of whom have the vaguest idea of what we do for a living, what medicine is or what patients value, are disseminating this patronising and irrelevant nonsense and we sit here and politely listen to it.

We are still the most accessible, valued and respected group of professionals that an average person ever consults. We exercise our day to day duties by applying science and art and assessing risks with common sense and reason. Something that most people think of as **wisdom** and most cultures still value highly.

But we now tolerate junk such as this because we are too tired or polite or punch drunk to resist the endless flow of politics and window dressing that now regulates us.

Don't they realise that we try to develop a "relationship" with each patient? That this is very often more than words. That **touching** in a proper, professional and purposeful way is a major and essential part of the consultation? That after seeing us, the patient will leave the surgery and touch thousands of objects that have touched the skin of thousands of other people?

Do they really think that we should take away toys, books, ornaments from the consulting room and make it emotionally (if not bacteriologically) sterile?

Don't they realise that patients **should** have their hands shaken, their chests listened to, their tummies examined. That proper professional, ethical, decent treatment **demands** that skin touches skin. That you can't do the job if you don't examine the patient.

I dare not mention the fact that some old ladies like a peck on the cheek and some old patient-friends an occasional reassuring hug.

I don't know whether she has heard of Microbiomes and the many trillions of bacteria they contain. And they are inside all of us. Has she heard how many mothers protect their Caesarian delivered children by rubbing their faces with swabs from their own VAGINAS! – and how those babies thrive compared with the cleaner babies! She would probably have apoplexy.

The infection control nurse is yet another disguised way of regulating the profession, of trying to distance us from the independence, the informal friendliness, common sense and trust inherent in good general practice.

General practice is not a sterile environment. Most of our patients are immunologically sound and are surrounded by endless other potential contaminants. They don't live in bubbles and nor do we.

Babies and bathwater are being thrown out. The consulting room must not become a sterile ITU. Informality, common sense and trust are going down the same drain as the miniscule and theoretical risk of infection.

Reflections in a cracked mirror

How I hate the modern obsession with "Reflection".

After every talk and lecture, at almost every trainers and appraisers meeting for the last few years and in everything associated with the medical learning industry I am encouraged to "reflect". To reflect on what I have learned and to shine that second hand light on how my new knowledge will change the way I practice.

There are now Structured Reflective Templates as part of our annual appraisals. A contradiction in terms if ever there was one.

I have been a doctor for forty years. Seeing, thinking, absorbing, accommodating and altering the way I work. Daily, hourly, constantly. I see what makes sense, what works better and I automatically adapt. Without thinking.

After all, isn't that what professional do?

Usually this is a natural and subliminal process without recourse to protected time, a formal thought pattern or that self conscious, unnecessary and artificial self analysis of reflection. We don't need to be told to do the obvious.

It works like this: Someone with more experience tells you what works for them and you try it out yourself next time an appropriate situation arises. Thus it has always been.

Or you do something that doesn't work and you don't do it that way again. In life as in medicine.

But for the last 5 to 10 years we have been encouraged **to reflect** on new information and how it will change us. This is like a photographer delaying the taking of a picture long enough to analyse why he is taking that particular picture. Or wondering how that picture will influence the viewer once he has taken it – rather than being spontaneous, instinctive, natural.

But it is worse than that. It isn't just that the whole process of being asked to reflect is artificial, pointless and patronising, reflection isn't even a correct use of the word.

I mean.. if they can get the concept so wrong, how can we trust anything they ask us to do?

You see the problem is this:

Reflecting is what mirrors and burnished surfaces do. They bounce incoming energy, i.e. light, off their surfaces. The light doesn't penetrate their smooth skins and in the process the light is turned upside down. They are blissfully unaffected by it. Lateral inversion, left to right, back to front.

So reflection is a process whereby the reflector is uninfluenced by the reflecting, the incoming energy is turned upside down and reality is distorted.

So next time you are asked to reflect on a piece of information or an experience just bear in mind the fact that doing so won't change you. The minute you start you will instantly get it all back to front, the wrong way round and anyway isn't it faintly narcissistic to keep reflecting like that?

Surely if we are talking about the physics of processing information, what we should be doing is **Refracting.** You shouldn't reflect on your experiences but refract them.

You see refraction is a process whereby a prism, lens or other **penetrable** transparent surface **absorbs** new information in the form of light, **separates** and defines the important constituents, changes them, interprets them in a new way and helps **tease out and clarify their secrets.**

It is an even more appropriate term when you find out that the refractive index is related to the denseness of the medium.

Also the process is often startlingly pretty and always a pleasant surprise.

Now Diffraction... that is something else again..

The MRCGP Video:

(These competencies and marking guidelines applied a few short years ago)

I was browsing through a copy of the B.M.J. looking for topics to discuss with my registrar in our next tutorial when I read a letter from Adrian Fogarty, a consultant in A and E of a year ago.

He complained about the current political correctness of so much teaching from the academic establishment. He exemplified this by quoting an article "Career Focus" that had suggested key competencies for G.P. registrars.

Of the 11 key competencies quoted, **only one related to clinical skills.** The rest were all management related. They included professional integrity, empathy, coping with pressure, sensitivity, organising and planning skills, legal and political awareness, conceptual thinking, etc.

He was worried that "clinical acumen" – something that patients rate above all else (Is this mole a cancer? Is my headache a brain tumour? Why am I so tired doctor?) had become so undervalued in our rush to make us patient friendly and politically correct that the next generation of G.P.s will be empathetic duffers. The doctors you go to see to be referred to the chap who **can** make the diagnosis and treat you.

I have to say that my experience of the new trainers induction year and most trainers' education sessions bear out this misplaced obsession with non clinical skills completely.

Then, in one of those odd moments of Déjà vu, I found myself looking at the M.R.C.G.P. examination, "consulting skills" component:

What are the competencies that the video judges value and score highly?

It won't surprise you to find they are similar to those decried by Dr. Fogarty and all doctors who care about the clinical competence of their trainees take note and despair...

The following are the criteria judged important in passing the Membership exam video:

1) **Encouraging the patient's contribution**. Why? In reality, you and I at the sharp end know we often have to **limit** the patient's contribution to relevant and constructive details, we cut them short because we have to actively manage every consultation and that patients contribute so much wood you often can't see the trees.

We have (in my case) seven and a half minutes to get to the nub of the consultation so it has to be guided.

2) **Responding to Cues**. This has now become an obsession amongst registrars who feel that every cue holds the hidden key to opening the door to patient Nirvana. In fact, like Agatha Christie's **clues,** most so-called cues are red herrings and you hardly ever open the secret door with a key question. Far more often, the receptionists are calling us on the intercom and asking that we respond to the **queues** that our sympathetic ear has caused to build up in the waiting room.

3) **Eliciting details to place the complaint in a social and psychological context**. Why? – There is frequently nothing we can do about a social context such as awful estates or neighbours from hell. –Isn't one reason that we are facing a recruitment crisis and what seem to be endless "non-medical" consultations precisely because too much social work is expected of G.P.s and because we have become society's emotional and social whipping boys? I know that isn't a popular view in some quarters but I AM a medic and I went to medical school to learn the art and science of medicine. What I do, want to do, do best and like doing is there in those words.

4) **Exploring Health Understanding**. Depressingly, this was a **MERIT CRITERION and It doesn't say explore their understanding and set them straight.** The implication is that we should show empathy and interest in the patient's beliefs even if the patient's health understanding, like their views on smoking and obesity, the risk of MMR and steroid inhalers, their views on circumcision, the benefits of homeopathy or reflexology,

are based on an irrational, personal or cultural bias and are wrong. To accept this at face value is to say that voodoo and circumcision are reasonable perspectives to incorporate in your management plan. Two millennia of rational western scientific evidence based medicine and all health beliefs are worth exploring and by implication valid? Follow this to its rational conclusion and the august Royal College of General Practitioners is going to award you a merit for colluding with homeopathy and reflexology.

5) Hooray, at last: "**The doctor obtains sufficient information for no serious condition to be missed**". At long last, something that will significantly affect the patient's life, which only *we, acting as doctors* can do and which the patient actually rates highly. Something, which, dare I say it, is harder than the rest of the list and comes from experience, training, skill and conscientiousness.

6) **The doctor chooses an appropriate examination**. Oddly enough, this is the only one of the fifteen criteria that involves **touching** the patient. Physical contact in an appropriate manner is part of the Doctor patient relationship and so important to the bond of trust and confidence that the consultation is built on. Patients get better quicker if they are examined. Why are we so frightened of it? Patients seek out reflexologists, faith healers, osteopaths, chiropracters, masseurs, sports physios. The power of touch is very basic and therapeutic.

My registrar once told me he had qualms asking to see a child's bottom as part of a full examination. This, in these days of doctor paranoia and "Doctor misses sepsis again" front page headlines is a natural anxiety but it is far more important to make sure that you are not missing the first purpuric spot.

(Or are we just supposed to be counsellors and advisers now, not healers?)

7) **The doctor makes an appropriate working diagnosis:** Although the frequency of "non specific abdominal pain", "stress", "benign paroxysmal vertigo", "dermatitis", "I.B.S.", "non ulcer dyspepsia", fibromyalgia and all the other vague and descriptive handles we give to problems attests to the relative rarity and luxury of a definite diagnosis in real family medicine.

8) **The doctor explains the diagnosis:** Yes, all well and good, but do **you** genuinely understand what fibromyalgia, C.F.S., chest pain for the umpteenth time in an anxious smoker, non specific abdominal pain or IBS, a raised P.S.A. in a 70 year old actually *mean*? There are almost too many variables to get it right in terms of implications, interpretation and how much the patient needs to know all the time. In any case our unbiased explanation will be coloured by our subjective anecdotal experience (The one nasty immunisation reaction we have seen), the cost of our prescribing budget, how we might be perceived by lawyers, our own moral and personal codes, religion, politics etc. What price an objective explanation when both the patient and we are so patently non standard and when "Gut Feelings" of experienced doctors have now been shown to be reliable clinical warning signs.

9) **The doctor uses appropriate language:** How patronising. Many patients feel treated like children if their problem is over simplified by a single syllable explanation. How do you explain genetic abnormalities, prions or serotonin deficiency to a cleaning lady with a vocabulary of 1000 words? What language do you use to explain the implications of multiple sclerosis for the first time? How will "depression" be perceived by an ex commando? How about dysmotility? What about the many patients who would be happier **without** the "truth" and deserve **more** than a 100% accurate diagnosis and prognosis?

Who decides what is appropriate? "You are making too much acid", "We need to reduce the inflammation", "Yes it is cancer but its only mild and the treatment is improving all the time"-Either you oversimplify and distort the truth or you need to spend the consultation giving a basic grounding in anatomy, physiology, biochemistry and so on. I think we denigrate ourselves and our role by oversimplifying what we do for purely political reasons. The husband and wife in a couple will frequently want different explanations of serious diagnosis or in the case of close relatives of mine a different approach to explaining. So be accurate, direct, honest, sympathetic and open. The worst thing that you can do is withhold information and have the "Why didn't you tell me this could happen?" conversation later.

10) **The doctor takes account of patient's beliefs:** This is the same as the "Health Understanding" section. How depressing that this, like 4) and 11) are merit criteria. Who decides all this? By now I am beginning to wonder whether the designers of training schedules and G.P. teaching manuals are undemocratic and out of touch with grass roots General Practice. Where is the professional consensus, the legitimacy?

The patient's beliefs: what about my lady who has been told that bottle feeding is safer than breast feeding and wrote a formal complaint about my correcting her? Is hers a valid belief? What about Jehovah's Witnesses, male and female circumcisions, what about our local homeopath who's baby with Pertussis nearly died due to his failure to seek conventional medical help, what about the baby with pyloric stenosis whose mother had her treated with cranial osteopathy until she was moribund ? **Sorry, but these are not valid health beliefs** and should not be accepted by real doctors who care about real patients.

11) **The doctor confirms the patient's understanding:** Which as we know, rarely lasts as far as the door and which varies with the patient's own intellectual abilities, language, education, culture and the patient's desire to please. It is much more important that the patient is clear about what they have to do to get better and what you are going to do to help them.

The fact that this is the third Merit Criterion confirms the vast distance of these rules from the reality of practice life.

12) **The Doctor uses an appropriate management plan.** The significant phrase is **"Management Plan"** – You will know, if you frequent deaneries and such centres of General Practice teaching that the doctors who work there regard themselves as executives in business organisations these days. Many have stopped being practising doctors. They have secretaries and assistants not receptionists or nurses. They are executives, administrators. That is why they have **Management Plans,** not "courses of treatment" or "therapy" and that is why number 13 is:

13) **The Doctor shares management options:** You and I Treat and we might suggest therapeutic alternatives. Administrators have management options.

14) **The Doctor Uses Appropriate prescribing behaviour:** No one in their right mind would argue for inappropriate prescribing behaviour, but we all know that placebos can be effective, that patient expectations, non licensed indications and personal experience may influence effective personal prescribing. Anyway, who decides what **is** appropriate, the local prescribing committee, the practice formulary, NICE? We are all aware of the unexpected negative effects that some "rational" prescribing trends have had in recent years. – The almost blanket withdrawal by GPs of antibiotics whatever the state of their patients throats was followed by a Scarlet Fever epidemic and, I assume, possible future Glomerulonephritis and Rheumatic Fever epidemics too?

15) **Doctor and patient appear to have established a rapport**. Which is more than some medical educators have done with grass roots G.P.s to judge by how they assess a good consultation!

As far as the consultation is concerned, these criteria are ignoring the basic fact that the whole process is based on experience and TRUST, not management options or exploring health understanding. This is not something that is fashionable at the moment even if it has always been the Holy Grail to most patients and their doctors.

What I am really trying to say is that educators must be more representative, more realistic and practical. More democratic, more in touch with real G.P.s and patients. They must reflect the real problems and practicalities of treating patients in the surgery.

It is time the profession stopped paying lip service to the political ideas exemplified by these criteria and a host of other guidelines and got back to a practical **medical** agenda.

By the way, while you are reflecting* on the somewhat cynical assessment of training attitudes I portray above, ask **yourself** if you think the next generation of G.P.s **will** be well prepared for the real job society expects them to do based on the competencies outlined and the drastically reduced training hours they will have experienced. If you think the answer is no, then someone somewhere is spending too much time philosophising with the other educational staff and needs to get out a bit more.

* For the real definition of this see above:

The thing the patients hate the most about modern registrars is how they sit quietly while the patient tells their symptoms, there is a long pause and then, as if from the Deanery Guide to "How not to inspire respect and confidence during the consultation" they ask the patient "Well what do YOU think might be going on?"

A few laws we could add to Number Ten's bonfire. No 2 (written in about 2012)

With the change of government, Ten Downing Street has set up an interesting new web site. This is intended to encourage the overregulated people of Britain to suggest laws that could be dumped on "Number Ten's Bonfire".

Think of the changes that have been imposed on we GPs over the last few years and I am pretty sure you will come up with several that could easily be dispensed with.

We GPs have, of course, benefitted from some changes to the law. The loss of 24 hr responsibility has given us our lives, sanity and health back. Though no daytime GP I know would tolerate the return of 24 hr responsibility, what sits in its place is a travesty of General Practice.

Why doesn't today's OOH care work? It is because of the sense of entitlement that many governments have given the people of Britain. Rights without responsibilities just don't work.

I don't see how we can resolve this without removing the right of patients to demand a free 24 hr consultation for all minor ailments – but that isn't going to happen.

If David Cameron wants GPs to restore 24 hour GP cover again (and how likely is that?) he is going to have to insist that patients either have a disincentive – like the need to pay up front to be seen out of hours or some sanction if they insist on a consultation not subsequently deemed serious by a panel of independent assessors: After all, the average patient has between one and two *real* emergencies in a lifetime but up to a dozen unpleasant and worryingly benign conditions.

But what other recent changes to the law can and should be removed? The endless screening and recording imposed by the new contract has turned us into clerks, administrative assistants and the evidence is that all the screening health checks we now have to do are, well basically, a waste of everybody's time. They make us more interested in the computer screen than the patient. So I say dump Quof.

The appraisal process can sometimes be productive, mentoring and informative for the appraisee but it is definitely NOT a way of rooting out the sort of psychopath whose serial murders prompted it. It costs a fortune and is largely superfluous. So dump Appraisal.

But the MOST harmful regulations that we must remove have come in almost unnoticed and have the potential to cause huge suffering. I mean those new laws covering the use of controlled drugs by GPs.

I was shocked to discover one unexpected effect of these burdensome regulations: I have believed for 30 years that one of the most useful and important drugs I had at my disposal was Diamorphine. It relieves pain, distress, dyspnoea, it is the treatment of choice in several clinical situations and is the cancer sufferer's friend. I hope to God my GP has it if and when I am dying of cancer, respiratory failure, motor neurone disease and a dozen other despicable natural causes. Yes it can be abused – and lawyers constantly threaten us with the consequences of its inappropriate use. But Diamorphine and Pethidine injections were always the drugs that I felt I could do the most good with – if potentially also the most harm.

The most tragic unforeseen result of the new regulations regarding the supervision of controlled drugs is that fewer than a third of my partners now carry these strong pain killers in their bags. They have decided that severe pain, renal and biliary colic, broken bones, traumatic accidents, the pain of terminal illness and myocardial pain are rare enough for them not to be bothered with the bureaucracy and inconvenience involved in carrying genuinely effective analgesics. They will just let the patient suffer while they wait for an ambulance.

This is the Law of Unforeseen Consequences. A political and legal solution to a vanishingly rare danger-that of *one medical psychopath*, has led to potential harm on a grand scale harming the very people that the new laws were designed to protect.

Before an evening meeting at a local post graduate centre I asked all the other GPs how many of them carried Pethidine or Diamorphine? I was shocked that I was the **only** doctor in the room still carrying these drugs. What a disastrous change in so short a time.

I believe that all those doctors (and most of my partners at the time) are now seriously letting their patients down. They have become moral cowards and made themselves unprepared for a life in real General Medical Practice.

Their justification is that they can call the ambulance rather than deal with these situations personally. They think they don't need to carry strong painkillers.

This is make-believe. The ambulance service is currently overwhelmed and you can't walk away from a patient in pain. I had a man in his 40's consult during afternoon surgery 3 weeks ago. He had chest pain and it was clear he was having a myocardial infarction. I phoned for a blue light ambulance while I did the ECG and it took 30 minutes to come. Thank God I had the drugs to relieve his pain and distress. It appears most of my colleagues would only have been able to wring their hands and offer sympathy. They are fearful that patients and relatives are now suspicious of their doctors and that all PCT administrators and compensation lawyers are falling over themselves to pillory GPs who are just trying to do a decent job. A few weeks later, I was summoned by a neighbour to a friend, a woman in her 60's who had fallen off a step ladder in the garden and had fractured her wrist. She was pale, shocked, tachycardic and in severe pain. Some IM Diamorphine and Cyclizine gave her the relief she needed and we chatted as the ambulance took its time to turn up. She has been "eternally grateful for my kindness" ever since.

Where is our professional courage? Where is the ethos that the patient's needs are paramount?

I am ashamed. Professional paranoia has led to collective moral cowardice. It is clear that the new and cumbersome regulations have resulted in a profound change in the role of family doctors and an abrogation of what every patient has the right to expect from us. – The treatment of what we all fear most, severe pain.

Why must we all be tarred with the same brush as Shipman? He was a psychopath and Daniel Ubani was incompetent. The rest of us aren't.

If Shipman had been a carpenter who stabbed to death a series of his customers, would the Government introduce new laws to regiment the obtaining, owning, storage, use, supervision and disposal of screwdrivers or chisels?

I know I am stretching the analogy a bit far, but strong pain killers ARE the tools of our trade. Used for centuries responsibly by the majority of us and without which we cannot do the job we are paid for.

We are all desperately sorry for the victims of Shipman and their relatives. We are shocked that one of our number cruelly abused the trust of his patients and the expectations of his colleagues in this way. But it is clear that the onerous new rules concerning controlled drugs and other recent legal changes – the expensive system of appraisal, the new intrusive and harmful requirements of the part 2 cremation form etc – all of which are laws made in reaction to Shipman, would simply not have detected or prevented him from committing his serial murders.

-And what is worse, these new laws just make it harder for the rest of us to care for patients properly.

Surely these above all are new laws that need to be incinerated on "Number Ten's Bonfire"?

THE MORNING AFTER PILL

There are two main frustrations in my life as a G.P.

-Being taken for granted and being expected to be all things to all people.

It is odd that it is these personal things that affront your sense of fairness and self esteem and wear you out so much, – not all the sick and suffering people.

Jaded and tired at the end of a frenetic surgery, I have to admit I was not my normal smiling self when the practice nurse bustled in waving a temporary resident form.

"Just need a prescription for the morning after pill, – a fourteen year old, the condom split".

This seemed to be enough explanation as far as the world was concerned, no need for any further complications. My nurse had become the local representative of the anonymous great unwashed, unthinking masses.

So much of this job has become morally and emotionally depressing. The loss of control, the expectations of unreasonable people. The time pressure, the lawyers on your back and the potential blame, the insistence that you go with the flow. The pervasive "Just stamp this for me, write me a note, give me the scrip, don't think about it, just do it" attitude.

It is summed up by a poster on our practice loo door that says: "Here to listen, not to tell"-

Well yes, but just look where the all listening and not telling of the last 2-3 decades has got society and this particular 14 year old "service user".

When I ponder about the complaints culture and the resulting liberal politics that have taken over our moral and medical codes of practice, our advisory committees and guidelines I really wonder who has dictated that agenda. No one I have ever worked with. Don't confront people, or correct them, or tell them they are wrong, just let them make their own mistakes. Ruin their lives, their health. It is easier just to give in to consumer attitudes, the depersonalisation of family medicine, the loss of the real family itself. I sometimes wonder if I am the only one in the world who sees the harm that all this hopeful, unquestioning indulgence has done.

I hate having to accept all lifestyles and behaviour without having an opinion, – all personal and other beliefs are OK. Why **should** I be un-judgemental? How can you be human and **not** have a valued opinion about how other people behave? Are we supposed to demure to anything and everything that people do to one another or to themselves? To always keep our own counsel? Is nothing right or wrong? Are doctors not allowed to have feelings and opinions?

I was, I admit a bit punch drunk that afternoon, with partners away, a coop session looming and a 16 hour day half way through.

I took the proffered T/R form half-heartedly only to find that the offending (or offended against) minor was actually registered with the practice up the road.

Why can't she see her own doctor? I asked. "She's shy" was the reply.

Well if she were so shy why did she need the morning after pill? I thought. The two hardly go together do they? It was as if a family doctor system based on personal lists and built up and worked at for decades by thousands of dedicated doctors was an inconvenience that should be thrown away without a thought to save an irresponsible child's embarrassment. Here to listen not to tell – Forget the personal service, the doctor patient relationship, the "FAMILY DOCTOR", – this is no longer a profession, this is a demand led service industry now. With fourteen year olds demanding to ruin their own lives.

Bold enough for sex, too shy to see her doctor to discuss the consequences. And my nurse asking me to condone the whole distorted, immoral, wrong, screwed up mess.

My resentment must have seemed genuine to my nurse because she gave up and just said "OK", leaving with the form in her hand.

The usual confusion, anger and guilt, a combination with which most GPs will be familiar, filled and frustrated me.

I wanted to help the nurse, the child, the child's family, I felt for the reputation of the profession and I wanted to be a good doctor. I wanted to be a warm approachable person coming to the aid of the vulnerable patient at a time of crisis, I wanted to make a difference-but this situation was soul destroying, confusing. Not what I signed up for when I applied to medical school. A whole cascade of thoughts went through my head.

Why do so many of our children and adolescents seem to have no sense of personal responsibility or morality? No behavioural grounding.

Do too many adults just listen and not tell?

Why was this child having sex at 14 anyway? She was not old enough to vote, to hold a credit card, to drink, to drive, to watch sex at the cinema but she was able to indulge in something potentially more serious, more responsible, potentially far more harmful than any of those things.

Would I be an accessory to this felony by condoning, abetting, aiding and encouraging this illegal underage copulation? On the other hand, should I be obliged to lecture the child and the no doubt surly baseball capped and inarticulate boy friend? If I just signed the prescription, could I justify my action to the parents if they found out? Aren't I obliged to investigate more of the child's background, to ensure her education, sexual and moral safety, to try to prevent a life of herpes, warts, chlamydia, infertility, early parenthood, delinquent, probably offending offspring and failed ambitions?

Let's face it, the only moral message of the last 20 years has been simple: Do what you want, – Just use a condom. And if you don't there is always abortion on demand, 200,000 a year, never refused. You have a human right to snuff out the life within you. The politicians voted on it and the judges say it applies to children too.

This may be the nexus, the crux point in her life where I could prevent her spiralling off into chaos, – I could be the support and direction she will remember all her life, mentioned on Desert Island Discs, and in her auto biography. I could really make a difference – as they say in the films.

But then again, I could just phone the police and social services. If I really had the interests of the moral majority, the child's future and the concept of a caring family at heart, the backbone upon which all societies rest, I should rail against this abomination. Shouldn't the condom forgetter or splitter be arrested? Shouldn't the girl be taken into protective custody and her parents (probably parent) enrolled on a compulsory parenting course?

And why do this couple expect me to believe that the condom split anyway? Do condoms split? Aren't they "electronically tested" for safety? Wasn't that phrase on a naughty album cover in the sixties, the Rolling Stones or Who or someone? Don't they have a Pearl Index of about 20 years? – the condoms I mean, not the Rolling Stones.

Is this just a code for "I have been stupid and now I want you to bail me out".

How old was the condom, what were they doing with it, why can't people read the instructions on the packet and delay their gratification by five minutes? If the damn things are on every corner shop counter and toilet wall why don't people use them according to the manufacturer's instructions?

You can bet she knows how to text funny faces and play games on her Nokia. How to sext.

Were they just counting on free morning after contraception when they planned their sexual escapade(s) ? Does the ready availability of a failsafe, a let-out, encourage people in risk – taking behaviour? Like people with cycle helmets actually get into more accidents. Is that why we have all the pregnancies, the STDs, the ruined lives? Because post coital contraception and abortion are accepted as part of normal life for teenagers and if you've got a seat belt and airbag why not drive a little faster?

This was clearly not going to be a two minute consultation for any doctor with a conscience.

Today, I wasn't in the mood to be a copulation condoner, a health professional for a service user, a passive listener. I would really get involved. I was resentful. Resentful of this silly child, her mindless self gratifying boy friend, liberal politics, soap operas, adult films, short term self indulgence, the messages that pour out of teenage magazines, TVs, videos, pop songs. The idea that sex without love is the norm.

I was going to tell her that sex should come as part of a maturing and evolving relationship between two people who care about one another and think they might have a future together. I was going to say don't be intimidated by fear of being laughed at, or being dumped, – you can say no. Wait till you feel comfortable and stable, wait, dare I say it, until there is love between you (whatever that may mean) – Men don't respect you if you give yourself too cheaply. You become a thing not a person. This is a fact of life.

But mainly, I wanted to shout at her, you are too young. Don't throw your life away. I want to tell you something and it may just be very important if **you** listen.

Well that was what I wanted to say.

But would she listen to me, would she care what I said, would she assume I just didn't know what sex and relationships can be like? Would she assume I didn't know about lust, intensity, desire?

Would she or her parent(s) make a complaint about my unsympathetic attitude, would they dismiss the good and ethical reasons for telling her to see her own doctor, someone who could see her more than just this once? Or if I told her to come back when I had more time, would everyone assume I was passing the buck, making life hard when it needn't be? Where would I stand, legally, ethically? – I had absolutely no idea.

Would some lawyer and amateur politician turn me into the wrong doer for exercising my own right to choose? Was I a cliché, a dinosaur just like the ones on the child friendly tie I happened to be wearing?

Is society's definition of a doctor nowadays so stretched and politicised by liberal attitudes that it means that I am allowed to make no valued judgements at all? Do I have to let everyone dig their own grave without sounding a warning? Doesn't the fact that we see lots of lives and lots of lives ruined give us the right and responsibility to say when someone is just plain stupid, or just plain wrong?

I half wanted to be Dr Finlay, – sensible, authoritarian, respected, always reliable and steady. No tacit encouragement to self destruction by him. I half wanted to be the Neighbours or E.R. doctors, – cool, phased by nothing, informal, on first name terms, everyone's friend.

There is no happy ending to this story. By the time I had called the girl on the tannoy, she had collected her scrip from a partner and was already on the way to an anonymous chemist. Blissfully unaware of the angst and self questioning that her split condom had caused. A shame it hadn't been her that felt it.

Uncertainty:

It has been said that General Practice involves the management of boredom, repetition and uncertainty.

Uncertainty in this context relates to the willingness of a doctor to make diagnosis and management decisions based on assumptions, subjective conclusions and his own experience. Without a strong evidence base or reasonable objective proof and by using subjective rather than objective influences. Uncertainty is something medical science has previously sought to exclude from the medical model, not to accept or embrace.

To some degree the combination of these unquantifiable factors can lead to increased rates of burn out, fear of litigation as well professional and personal insecurity. Uncertainty is the only constant feature of a life in General Practice and the natural GP is someone at home with it.

Confidence (though definitely not self satisfaction or self importance) is part of a good GP's character.

One could argue that the whole of human progress, experience, relationships, learning and so on has been gained by accepting uncertainty and learning from it. But this is anathema to the standard scientific model of medicine.

Contemporary medical training does not prepare new doctors for risk taking or vagueness of diagnosis or managed inadequate supervision of the progress of disease or an encouragement of educated guesswork in our professional lives.

The uncertainty that is part of consultations is many fold:

Let us start with factors that involve the doctor:

GPs are the only true generalists in medical practice these days. Physicians now all sub specialise and in any case, even **they** don't see the variety of surgical, paediatric, psychiatric, psychosocial and all the varied socio-medical presentations of modern general practice. It is impossible to be completely familiar with or be prepared for everything that might present on every average day to a family doctor. GPs have no filter to triage or prioritise the different types of patients, complaints and presenting formats (-while I am here, would you look at the baby, my husband won't come to see you but I am very worried, I know you are not on duty but would you pop in if you aren't too busy? etc) that can present without warning to the family doctor in or out of the surgery.

GPs **are** the triage, the gatekeepers, the initial assessors. GPs therefore, very early in every consultation have to decide on the potential or actual medical significance of each presenting problem. Not just accepting the raw symptoms at face value. They discard and ignore much that is presented for consideration in each consultation through a process of learnt valued judgment. This is the art of General Practice. (In a world where relatives, lawyers and colleagues assume it is usually a science). This involves risk assessment based on knowledge of the patient's previous help seeking behaviour, a knowledge of that patient's help seeking threshold, their stoicism, their reliability, their own experience of ill health and so on. So first time mothers, a friend who has just had a coronary, their family's sickness history (another child with a history of meningitis?) their personality and anxiety and so on may all be factored in. The so-called personal "health beliefs" may be part of this assessment.

The GP must also add to this risk assessment a knowledge of prevailing illness patterns (Is there meningitis, "flu", etc in the locality?) and a host of other factors.

In previous years, the GP would be familiar with the individuals themselves, their families, history and background of all his "list". There would have been the cushion of extended families, the reassurance of a stable culture and tradition within his community. The consistent and self confident patient. Add to this the bonding factor and uniformity of the list system (or panel) and familiarity and mutual trust tended to be the norm.

Today, populations are transient, mobile and of mixed culture. The demography of the standard nuclear family has changed and the overwhelming trend is to loosen the bond between individual patients and a specific individual doctor. Patients now register with a practice not an individual with whom they might develop familiarity, mutual memory and confidence over a period of time. Though the Government seems recently to have seen sense on this and may be restoring a list system again (Oct 2014).

This leads to either uncertainty in diagnosis and management or a safety culture of over treatment and over admission.

Medical training begins within a hospital and thus is a diagnosis based structure,

– the management of illness and disease, which is sometimes partially and half-heartedly adapted to include social, cultural and psychological modifiers. Health beliefs, expectations and other social issues are then tacked on to this standard (and very successful) evidence based approach.

It has been at the developing heart of western medicine since the discovery of circulation, microbes, effective drugs and treatments –in other words–for centuries.

It is based on observation; asking questions, evidence gathering and getting information – upon which a reasonable diagnosis and course of treatment can be based. –Ask, observe, examine, conclude, agree and prescribe. Above all, be objective. The heart of all medical consultations. It has been so successful that it has been universally adopted by all medical cultures and traditions.

Some of the uncertainty of General Practice is that so much of the proffered information is inaccurate, biased, subjective or wrong. Personal feelings, experience and interpretation of the "presenting complaint" in the doctor also dictate the emphasis which will be placed on the "raw data." In the real world of General Practice subjective as much as objective factors are of crucial importance. There are no golden rules.

Personality and confidence, age, experience of risk taking and litigation, psychological and personal factors are far more important to the general practice assessment than that of a hospital in patient or outpatient consultation.

The absence of attached staff, regular objective monitoring, accessible biometric data, or even of a reliable 4hrly pulse and temperature dictates that prognoses and diagnoses will always be a "best guess" in primary care.

This is why we must always have a clear idea of follow up and clear instructions regarding when and what-if, for the sick patient and relatives.

The patient presenting to a GP doesn't come with a referral letter. He or she has not been seen, assessed, triaged and referred appropriately by another professional. The initial assessment in general practice includes factors unknown to hospital colleagues: How ill (or otherwise) is the patient, why have they presented in this way, here and now, even factors such as do they actually need to be seen, why are they actually asking for help?

This is compounded by "Tesco" attitudes of consumerism in the supply and availability of medicine and of modern political attitudes. Patients' charters, the entitled demander and so on.

The net result is that there is no longer a mutual assumption of reasonable consulting behaviour between doctor and patient. The tacit understandings of the early NHS have gone.

The patient has been trained to consult early "just in case", to regard the doctor as like any other supplier of goods and services. The media exaggerate the risks of self-diagnosis and treatment. But also the risks of missing early symptoms of illness. The ever-present fear of rare serious illness combined with the ease of modern consulting has led to much inappropriate and early contact. We have all seen the 3 hour backache and sore throat. The free at the point of access, you can't be too careful generation. Mutual consideration of the roles and responsibilities of doctor and patient seem to have become a thing of the past. In the doctor's mind the reasonableness of the consulting situation is now as never before an issue in determining the outcome. So there is uncertainty in presentation, content and reasonableness.

Transience: Even in relatively stable social environments, families are now temporary and uncommitted to their locality and their environment. In many situations where stable family groups are the norm modern work practices and temporary relationships militate against social stability. The average GP loses and gains 10% or more of his list per year. Patients often don't know how best to use local medical services, are unfamiliar with a respected doctor and most individuals simply do not have the tradition of trust and familiarity with the existing family practice structure. They consult readily and this can lead to a sense of uncertainty and inconsistency between doctor and patient.

Accessibility: GPs have been encouraged to offer ready appointments to all patients – registered or not, who feel they need to be seen. As soon as possible. This has now ironically led to delays in seeing the doctor, unfriendly triage systems and surgeries that are booked up (with trivia) days or weeks ahead. We now have what the RCGP called a post code lottery for GP access. In June 2014 they published an analysis which showed in North, East and West Devon there are 60 GPs/100,000 patients. In Slough there are 22. In Bradford 22% of patients had "Problems" getting appointments but it was 5% in Bath and North East Somerset. 8/10 areas with longer waiting times had moderate or high levels of deprivation. None of this can be a surprise, surely. It used to be solved with financial incentives. Perhaps these just aren't high enough now. GPs do not pass all those exams, work hard for 30 years, exemplify classic professional upper middle class aspirations and attributes to seek out socially, culturally and for them emotionally deprived and unfamiliar city areas to work.

The ever-present worry of litigation can lead to GPs over treating and over investigating to remove uncertainty. The long-term result of this is an expensive second rate service for the patient and further anxiety for the doctor. The doctor is overwhelmed with unnecessary consultations and the patient can't get an appointment even if they feel they may be genuinely ill.

Uncertainty and the management of risk occur at every out of hours consultation now that emergency general practice is done by a different population of doctors with no knowledge of the patients that they might see. Often with little or no contact with the GPs either.

There is, of course, a huge cost issue in the increasing reluctance of patients and doctors to accept the management of uncertainty.

General practice remains an area where the management of the unknown is based upon knowledge, experience and familiarity. The GP must be given the authority and trust to make informed guesses and when mistakes occur to be forgiven – in the interests of the Health Service and of us all. Uncertainty cannot be factored out of the GP consultation without destroying its very identity or making it unaffordable.

GOOD PRACTICE:
LECTURE NOTES

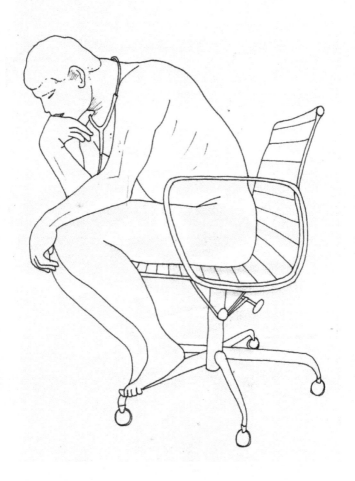

PART TWO

3: BASIC BIOLOGY:

Body surface area, adults and children. Height and Weight conversion charts.

ADULT HEIGHT CONVERSION

Feet and Inches	Cms	Metres
4'8"	142.2	1.422
4'9"	144.8	1.448
4'10"	147.3	1.473
4'11"	149.9	1.499
5'0"	152.4	1.524
5'1"	154.9	1.549
5'2"	157.5	1.575
5'3"	160.0	1.600
5'4"	162.6	1.626
5'5"	165.1	1.651
5'6"	167.6	1.676
5'7"	170.2	1.702
5'8"	172.7	1.727
5'9"	175.3	1.753
5'10"	177.8	1.778
5'11"	180.3	1.803
6'0"	182.9	1.829
6'1"	185.4	1.854
6'2"	188.0	1.880
6'3"	190.5	1.905
6'4"	193.0	1.930

	ADULT WEIGHTS in Kg				ADULT WEIGHTS in Kg					ADULT WEIGHTS in Kg				
7lb	84	98	112	126	140	154	168	182	196	210	224	238	252	266
5st	6	7	8	9	10	11	12	13	14	15	16	17	18	19
0lb	31.750	38.100	44.450	50.800	57.150	63.500	69.850	76.200	82.550	88.900	95.254	101.60	107.95	114.31	120.69
1lb	32.204	38.554	44.904	51.254	57.604	63.954	70.304	76.654	83.354	89.354	95.708	102.06	108.41	114.78	121.11
2lb	32.668	39.008	45.358	51.708	58.058	64.408	70.758	77.108	83.458	89.808	96.162	102.51	108.86	115.21	121.55
3lb	33.112	39.482	45.812	52.162	58.512	64.862	71.212	77.562	83.912	90.262	96.615	102.97	109.32	115.67	122.00
4lb	33.566	39.816	46.266	52.616	58.866	65.316	71.668	78.016	84.366	90.716	97.069	103.42	109.77	116.12	122.47
5lb	34.020	40.770	46.720	53.070	59.420	65.770	72.120	78.470	84.820	91.170	97.522	103.87	110.22	116.57	122.92
6lb	34.414	40.824	47.174	53.524	59.874	66.224	72.574	78.924	85.274	91.624	97.976	104.33	110.68	117.03	123.38
7lb	34.928	41.278	47.528	53.978	60.328	66.678	73.028	79.378	85.728	92.078	98.430	104.78	111.13	117.48	123.83
8lb	36.381	41.732	48.081	54.431	60.781	67.131	73.481	79.832	86.181	92.531	98.863	105.23	111.58	117.93	124.28
9lb	35.834	42.185	48.534	54.884	61.234	67.584	73.934	80.285	86.634	92.984	99.337	105.69	112.04	118.39	124.74
10lb	36.287	42.638	48.987	55.337	61.687	68.037	74.387	80.738	87.087	93.437	99.790	106.14	112.49	118.84	125.19
11lb	36.740	43.091	49.440	55.790	62.140	68.490	74.840	81.191	87.540	93.898	100.24	106.59	112.94	119.29	125.65
12lb	37.193	43.544	49.893	56.243	62.593	68.843	75.293	81.644	87.993	94.343	100.70	107.05	113.40	119.75	126.10
13lb	37.646	43.997	50.346	56.696	63.046	69.396	75.746	82.097	88.446	94.796	101.15	107.50	113.85	120.20	126.55

	BABY WEIGHTS in gm and Kg				BABY WEIGHTS in gm and Kg					BABY WEIGHTS in gm and Kg				
OUNCES	POUNDS				POUNDS					POUNDS				
	0	1	2	3	4	5	6	7	8	9	10	11	12	13
0	—	453.6gm	907.2gm	1.361	1.814	2.268	2.722	3.175	3,629	4.082	4.536	4.990	5.443	5.897
1	28.4gm	481.9	935.5	1.389	1.843	2.296	2.750	3.203	3.657	4.111	4.564	5.018	5.471	5.925
2	56.7	510.3	963.9	1.418	1.871	2.325	2.778	3.230	3.685	4.139	4.593	5.046	5.500	5.953
3	85.0	538.6	992.2	1.446	1.899	2.353	2.807	3.260	3.714	4.167	4.621	5.075	5.528	5.982
4	113.4	567.0	1.021 Kg	1.474	1.928	2.381	2.835	3.289	3.742	4.196	4.649	5.103	5.557	6.010
5	141.8	595.3	1.049	1.503	1.966	2.410	2.863	3.317	3.770	4.224	4.678	5.131	5.585	6.038
6	170.1	623.7	1.077	1.531	1.985	2.438	2.892	3.346	3.799	4.252	4.706	5.180	5.613	6.067
7	198.5	652.0	1.106	1.560	2.013	2.466	2.920	3.374	3.827	4.281	4.734	5.188	5.642	6.095
8	226.8	680.4	1.134	1.588	2.041	2.495	2.948	3.402	3.856	4.309	4.763	5.216	5.670	6.124
9	255.2	708.7	1.162	1.616	2.070	2.523	2.977	3.430	3.884	4.337	4.791	5.245	5.698	6.152
10	283.5	737.1	1.191	1.644	2.098	2.552	3.005	3.459	3.912	4.366	4.819	5.273	5.727	6.180
11	311.8	765.4	1.219	1.673	2.126	2.580	3.033	3.487	3.941	4.394	4.848	5.301	5.755	6.209
12	340.2	793.8	1.247	1.701	2.155	2.608	3.062	3.515	3.969	4.423	4.876	5.330	5.783	6.237
13	368.5	822.1	1.276	1.729	2.183	2.637	3.090	3.544	3.997	4.451	4.904	5.358	5.812	6.265
14	396.9	850.5	1.304	1.758	2.211	2.665	3.118	3.572	4.026	4.479	4.933	5.386	5.840	6.294
15	425.2	878.8	1.332	1.786	2.240	2.693	3.147	3.600	4.064	4.508	4.961	5.415	5.868	6.322

Body Surface Area of Children:

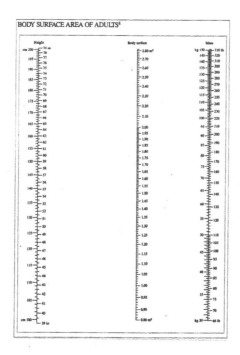

BODY SURFACE AREA OF ADULTS[8]

There are 13 organ systems in the body and according to Atul Gawande, 60,000 medical conditions that can go wrong with them. (Complications, the Reith Lectures, Being Mortal etc.) If you have a working knowledge of 60 of them and know where and how to access information on the rest, you will be a useful doctor.

Current life expectancy in the UK:
Male 79 years. Female 82 years – giving us joint 27th world ranking (Japan is first, the U.S. 33rd)
Zambia, Malawi, Angola, Mozambique, are all roughly equal at the bottom.

Calorific value of food:
Protein: 4.1Cal/Gr
Carbohydrates: 4.1Cal/Gr
Fat: 9.2 Cal/Gr
Note: 1Kg Adipose tissue= 7000KCals fat.

Exercise and calories:
Brisk uphill walking, swimming, cycling, racquet sports will burn 4-7 cals/min.
If you jog at 6mph (a mile in 10 minutes) for one hour and you weigh 10st. you will burn 600cals. You will have to jog for 11.7 hours to burn off 1KG of your weight.

Stuff you may have forgotten:

Life: These are the basic characteristics:
Movement
Respiration
Sensitivity
Growth
Reproduction
Excretion
Nutrition
Although some of my patients do seem to have evolved a way of compensating for atrophy of some characteristics, – movement and sensitivity, by hypertrophy in others – growth and reproduction.

Genetics, Evolution and Inheritance
The universe is thought to have started with a big bang 15-16 billion years ago when all our space and time began.
I have no idea why. Or how. Or *if*, even this is what happened.
What was occupying this space before the big bang? Most cosmologists would say that space itself started with the big bang so there was nothing before it. We are organisms that like to have rational explanations for the changes and events that happen around us so the paroxysmal coming into existence of *Everything – by chance* is a bit weird if you think about it. There wasn't even a where? before the Big Bang. A bit unlikely isn't it? On the otherhand there could have been an infinite number of *"wheres"* as in the Multiverse Theory where parallel universes exist but by definition can't be detected or proven. This is where Physics becomes Philosophy and thankfully has no parallel in medicine. (other than Homeopathy).
The origin of life on earth was 4 billion years ago, shortly after the planet earth

solidified. All the heavier elements necessary for life, including carbon and the luckily very stable iron atom were made in first or second generation stars and every star since by nuclear fusion and not the initial big bang. Hence Joni Mitchell's and Rush's "We are stardust". (Actually supernova dust.) Carbon is crucial for long chained molecules that make our DNA, proteins and connective tissue, iron for Haemoglobin etc. 2.7Bn years ago stromatolite bacteria began oxygenating the atmosphere long before photosynthesis in green plants subsequently took over. This oxygen eventually permitted animal life to develop. Oxygen is very toxic at higher concentrations than our atmosphere's 21% and not just to the premature baby's retina. 90% of the atmosphere is now of biological origin.

There are many amazing coincidences that allowed life to evolve up as far as we conscious, clever, self aware, space travelling beings and these all came together before and during the history of our planet and our own evolutionary biology. (The Goldilocks Enigma, everything "Just Right" for life) For instance:

We have just the right sized star to orbit around, not burning out and exploding before life could evolve, we are the right distance from that star so that liquid water can remain on the planet's surface-you need water for chemistry. The planet has a molten iron core to provide a magnetic field to shield us from the worst of the Sun's radiation and to regulate the climate. We have the presence of the moon, the correct tilt of the earth to provide planetary stability and seasons, the right distance from the Galaxy's core so that there isn't too much cosmic ray pressure but not so far out that we are flung out due to lack of gravitational pull, several large outlying planets to Hoover up most of the space debris that might cause another large extinction event like the one that wiped out the dinosaurs and (another serendipity) allowed us mammals our turn at evolving. Even the quantum world seems designed to encourage life: the size of the electron, the chemical properties of Carbon and Iron, the exact strength of the Nuclear Forces and Gravity, – The so called Goldilocks effect permits complex molecules to form, to remain stable and to make organic chemistry on which life is premised. On the other hand (The strong and weak Anthropic Principles), if we lived in one of the many multiverses where any of these variables were not quite right we wouldn't be here to write, read, think and talk about such erudite things in the first place. One alternative explanation, of course is that a sentient being made everything just right for us. So that we could have free will and the potential to improve things or mess them up.

So what about Life?

Organic compounds have been found in space, made in laboratories from primordial gases and electric sparks and seem to have a propensity for self assembly into complicated self replicating structures. All they need is time and luck. So that is basically a lot of time. RNA, DNA and cell membranes are self assembling molecules. Put them together and you have the basis of simple, unicellular, self copying "life."

One theory is that unicellular organisms became multicellular once they developed or acquired mitochondria. Mitochondrial DNA is like bacterial DNA and it is possible that our cells incorporated bacteria to generate the ATP they needed for energy. A genuine symbiotic relationship, perhaps accidental at first. Sex as a means of reproduction and institutionalising variation began 2Bn years ago. Evolution works through the magic of the self replication of DNA and mutant selection. Death and time. Thus biology is due to chemistry – as any chemist will tell you (and chemistry of course is due to physics as – any physicist will tell you).

We all know about the double Helix, an old fashioned telephone flex twisted around itself. I won't go over the medical school classic detective story of Watson, Crick and Rosalind Franklin's discoveries that disclosed the secret. Poor Rosalind Franklin died of ovarian cancer having taken the X Ray diffraction photographs of the DNA molecule, the cancer probably, like Marie Curie's, brought on by radiation. All amino Acids used in our bodies are L Amino Acids (by chance) and all sugars are D sugars.

The human Genome is 3.1 billion letters (base pairs) of DNA on 22 pairs of chromosomes plus an X and a Y. – Two meters (6'6") of DNA in each cell nucleus. 12Bn miles of DNA in your body. 6,000 genes per chromosome, two copies of each of the 150,000 genes in all. That is 3,100,000,000 A's, T's, G's and C's. Each person carries 2 genomes – one from each parent. There are only 3 genes identified so far that are unique to humans. Maize by comparison has 2.5-3Bn. separate letters. There are 4.6m bases in the genome of E Coli. Why a gram negative rod should need more base pair genetic information than one of us is a total mystery but clearly genome length has little to do with evolutionary development. Also the number of chromosomes of an organism is not a good guide to complexity – some plants can have thousands.

There are only 20,000-25,000 actual human protein coding genes, the same number as many plants, worms and flies. Mustard plants have 27,000 genes, ferns have 160,000m, amoebae for some reason, have 670,000m. Although we have 23 thousand "straight forward" genes and 10 trillion cells, (some references say 37.2 trillion human cells, some 50 trillion in an adult! – excluding bacteria) our WHOLE human organism ACTUALLY has up to 100 trillion cells and 100,000 – 3 million genes (different sources) if you include all the bacteria and other organisms inside us contributing symbiotically to our metabolism, digestion and existence. Where would our Vitamin K, B12, Folic Acid, Biotin, Niacin etc be without the help that bacteria give in absorbing them? We have ten times the number of bacteria in us that we that we have of our own cells.

The adult male makes 10Bn. sperm a month and these are the smallest cells, the ova being the largest although the long tract spinal neurones are the longest. Women are born with all their eggs in place. If it weren't for the chemical structure, the 3D shape of amino acids and proteins and their propensity to form long chains, none of this life would be possible.

All of life depends upon proteins. Proteins for structure, catalysts, manufactories, enzymes, hormones and body tissues from corneas and bone to teeth and brain cells. All are strings of amino acids making a variety of complex and simple proteins in a variety of 3D shapes.

Life on earth may have begun de novo from a primordial soup via methane, ammonia and lightning or near hydrothermal vents on ocean floors or even within submerged *Aero* like rocks, the bubbles providing a protected environment within. It may have been seeded by the process of "Pan spermia", – DNA or RNA having evolved elsewhere in the universe and being deposited from space. RNA based life may have existed before DNA based life evolved. But self copying molecules of RNA or DNA appeared on our planet about 4 billion years ago and have been replicating themselves in, on, above and under the surface of planet earth ever since.

As is now universally known, the rungs of the DNA ladder are bases (Adenine, Guanine, Thymine and Cytosine. In RNA, Thymine is substituted for by Uracil with A connected to T, C to G.) The double helix unravels, with each sequence of 3 bases, – a codon, a triplet, catching hold of an amino acid (this is in the ribosome), then these amino acids are strung together and thus new al la carte proteins are made. Many triplets can code for the same amino acid and the DNA blue print includes on/off, stop/go, start a new protein etc. instructions as well as the actual amino acid sequence list. ATG always starts a gene and "end a gene" is either TGA, TAG or TAA. All human amino acids are laevo rotatory, left handed, as it happens. There are only 23 universal proteins.

Our "*useful*" genome is only as little as 1.5% of our total DNA. Many of the other genes were thought until recently to be "Junk Genes" or "Introns" left over from our evolutionary past and redundant but it now appears that they have many roles including switching on and off the protein genes. Many of these act through a whole hierarchy of RNA programming rather than DNA and the importance and function of this system is only just beginning to be appreciated. All of this makes total sense when you think about it. Except, like the NHS, the genetic code does seem to be rather administratively heavy.

We have approximately 60 mutations each that our parents did not have. 70Bn of our cells die every day and are usually replaced.

Evolution:
All species evolved from a single cell 3.5Bn years ago, – our "Universal Common Ancestor", U.C.A. The three "domains of life all originated from this one life form. These domains are bacteria, bacteria-like microbes known as Archaea (single celled, no nucleus) and Eukaryotes (plants and multicellular species like us.)

Animals developed 700m years ago

Mammals developed 245m years ago,

Primates 70m years ago.

Apes and humans split from a common ancestor 7m yrs ago and "Humans" 3m years ago – you will have heard of "The African Lucy ", (or "Mitochodrial Eve") described in 1974 who was supposed to be our last common ancestor. We evolved down a complicated route Via Ardepithecus 4.4m yrs ago, Australopithecus (tools and a big brain) – 4m years ago, Homo Habilis 2.5m years ago, Homo Erectus 1.6m years ago, Homo Heidelbergensis, Homo Neanderthalensis (130,000 – 30,000 years ago, flint tools but no projectiles), Homo Sapiens 120,000+ years ago, Cro-Magnon Man (40,000 years ago). Africans and Aborigines diverged from Europeans 40,000 years ago.

The human race, now numbering 6Bn people, descended from approximately 10,000 individuals 100,000 – 150,000 years ago. The last single female ancestor of all living humans is thought to have existed 143,000 years ago.

We separated from the chimpanzees 250,000 generations ago and it is said that there have been 40,000 generations of men and women before us who "think like us".

Language as far as we can tell started 100,000 years ago.

Civilisation – the art of living within environments designed by humans rather than nature is 10,000 years old.

Human colonisation dates based on mitochondrial DNA:

Africa 130-170,000 years

W.Europe far East and India 39-51,000 years

Australia, 70,000 years

North and South America 12,000 years.

What about genetics?

Things you may have forgotten:

Diploid cells are most specialised bodily cells – liver, muscle, skin etc, and contain two complete sets of chromosomes. They reproduce by mitosis to make exact replicas of themselves. Haploid cells have half the diploid number of chromosomes and are the result of meiosis, the formation of a germ cell. At fertilisation two haploid gamete cells (sperm and ova cells) will merge to form a diploid zygote. Human cells have 23 pairs of chromosomes, 46 in all in normal diploid cells. 22 pairs, autosomes are the same in males and females, the other two are the X and Y.

The female is the default form of we human beings. The SRY gene on the Y chromosome switches on maleness.

In terms of **Personality,** people get most of their personality from their genes and their peer group (said to be 40%, 40%) – not their parents' influence (said to be 20%) – although abusing parents do give abusing genes to their children. Abused step children do not usually perpetuate the cycle.

Some **disadvantageous genes** may not have died out because they were geographically close to crucially important genes or because they were not as wholeheartedly negative in the past: For instance: As well as the different blood groups offering resistance to various infections, the Haemoglobinopathies (Sickle Cell Trait and Thalassaemia) also confer some malaria resistance and the heterozygous Cystic Fibrosis gene confers some resistance to Typhoid.

Do we know where the genes for various illnesses are? Since the human genome project was completed, we do have a good idea of where many diseases have their genetic basis – for instance: Asthma and Hay Fever genes are on chromosome 11 and are active if they are inherited from the mother. There hasn't been the expected (and Blair/Clinton promised) breakthrough in medicine since the first genome was mapped. What may be more productive is the UK's 100,000 genomes project (since 2012.) This consists of the mapping of 100,000 individual's genomes and then following them up for life to correlate their DNA to their subsequent medical history.

Handedness:

10% of the population are L handed. 25% of children of one left and one right handed parent are L handed. Flint tools which are both L and R handed appeared 1.8m years ago in our evolution.

Allergy:

Males develop allergy younger and they are more likely to grow out of it than females. You inherit asthma from allergic mothers not fathers.

Race:

All sorts of therapeutic and clinical differences (Haemoglobinopathies, storage diseases, risks of cardiovascular disease etc etc) are racially inherited. Afro-Caribbeans have twice the stroke rate, 50% increased risk of diabetes, increased prostatic cancer, respond better to CCBs and diuretics, than to BBs and ACEIs etc. Pancreatic cancer is much commoner in Ashkenazi (European) Jewish people, as are some storage diseases. 1% of Ashkenazi Jews have a defective copy of one of their BRCA2 genes and this increases the risk not just of pancreatic but breast and ovarian cancers. This risk comes from one individual 3000 years ago. 1.5% of European Jews also have the BRCA1 mutation which increases the risk of breast, ovarian, uterine, cervical, pancreatic and prostatic cancers (The Johns Hopkins Sol Goldman Pancreatic Cancer Research Centre.) In writing this book I have found references to high incidences of all sorts of inherited conditions in genetically restricted groups of people due to their cultural or religious constraints. The Muslim community in Bradford now has double the national incidence of some congenital abnormalities, the Ashkenazi Jewish community has high incidences of the above cancers and some storage diseases. Also Fanconi Syndrome, Gaucher's Disease, Kaposi's sarcoma and Tay Sachs Disease are more common in this group. These are diverse conditions – a renal tubular disorder, a sphingolipidosis, a genetic viral susceptibility and a gangliosidosis. A variety of physical disorders in a restricted gene pool. All evidence of the need for population freedom, diversity and genetic variation in order for human development and evolution to work properly.

Genetics:

A Gene:

Is a region of DNA that is transcribed as a single unit and carries information for a discrete hereditary characteristic, usually corresponding to:

(1) A single protein (or set of related proteins) or

(2) A single RNA (or set of closely related RNAs.)

'Gene Therapy' is a work in progress and, it has to be said has not lived up to its expectations after the excitement of the mapping of the genome. It can be defined as: the introduction of a new gene (or section of DNA) into the genome of an organism, with the aim of producing a new protein when the gene is transcribed – and thus an altered phenotype in the organism. Gene therapy need not introduce the new material into all the organism's cells – just the ones where the alternate phenotype is required. For example a gene therapy for cystic fibrosis need only affect lung cells and possibly the pancreas as they are the most significant of the cells in the body affected by the defective cystic fibrosis gene.

There are few practical examples of successful research applications of gene therapy for real illness. Gene therapy is notoriously hard to get to work to the extent where you get enough 'uptake' of the new gene – the rate of transformation of cells has always been historically very poor – meaning the new gene got into and was expressed by a very small proportion of the desired cells. Viral delivery vectors may have improved since I last looked into it, however.

There have been some successes in retinal disease, leukodystrophy, CLL, ALL, MM, lung cancer and Parkinson's disease but the treatments are by no means widespread, consistently reliable or readily available yet.

In January 2014 a promising viral mediated gene therapy which delivered a missing gene to the retina of almost blind sufferers of choroideremia was announced. The damaged gene and the substitute gene put into a virus and injected into the eye makes REP-1a. This is protein which keeps pigment retinal cells healthy. The researchers at Oxford University commented that ARMD and Retinitis Pigmentosa were conditions which might also benefit from this specific viral gene insertion therapy.

In cancer therapy, predictive biomarker studies are being undertaken to determine which patients will be susceptible to which particular treatments. For example, the RAS gene mutation in metastatic colorectal cancer means that the patient will not respond to Cetuximab. This is a sort of genetic parallel to hormone receptor status, determining the treatment regime to be used. There is also, of course, the risk prediction value of a growing number of gene biomarkers such as BRCA1 and BRCA2 – increasing risk for breast and ovarian cancers etc.

A new treatment for Huntington's Disease was announced in 2015. This was ISIS-HTT, a "Gene silencer", a mirror image of the Messenger RNA which leaves the cell nucleus with the code to make Huntingtin. The RNA is thus stuck on to and neutralised before it can start the process that leads to the damage of nerve cells.

Gene "Cut and Pasting" has now (2015) become a possibility via a technique known as Crispr-Cas9. This is "clustered regularly interspaced short palindromic repeats" Crisprs are sections of DNA and Cas9 is an enzyme which cuts DNA apart. They are used together by bacteria to prevent viral attacks. The Crispr examines the genome for the right section and the Cas9 cuts out that part of the DNA. Used clinically it would be possible to "edit" human genes and reprogram an individual's phenotype. Great excitement was generated by this technique amongst the sufferers of CF and Huntington's Disease and amongst many other sufferers of genetic disorders. But worries were expressed also about "Designer, made to order" babies.

There are also three areas of gene therapy which may be of use in cancer treatment: Immunotherapy, (genetically modified cells and viral particles which stimulate the immune system), Oncolytic Virotherapy (viral particles replicate within cancer cells killing them) and Gene Transfer (introduction of new genes into cancer cells to alter their growth, increasing apoptosis and rejection).

In June 2016 it was announced with the predictable mixed response that pig organs might be genetically cut and pasted to act as replacement donor organs for humans. The idea was to use human stem cells, pig DNA and gene editing to produce a human organ growing inside a pig host. The US authorities did not back this "Chimera" research. It would be interesting to see if the various religious groups that view pig meat with distaste would regard genetically human tissue grown inside a pig host acceptable or not.

Refer to a genetic clinic:

Colonic Cancer:
A FDR with onset <40 years.
2 FDRs both <70,
3 close relatives average age <60 or with one relative <50.
Familial Adenomatosis Polyposis.
Hereditary Non-Polyposis Colorectal Cancer Family: At least 3 relatives with large bowel cancer or an "HNPCC" related cancer (endometrial, ovarian, stomach, small bowel, ureter, renal pelvis.) One should be a FDR of the other 2 affected relatives. At least two successive generations should be affected. In one person the diagnosis should have been made <50.

Upper G.I. Cancer:
Consider referral in any FDR with age at onset <40 and in multiple first or second degree patients with upper GIT cancer (including pancreas.)

Breast Cancer:
Refer if your patient has 1 FDR and 1 SDR with breast cancer,
2 FDRs with breast cancer,
3 or more FDRs or SDRs with breast cancer,
1 FDR with breast cancer under 40,
1 FDR who is Jewish with breast cancer,

1 FDR who is male with breast cancer,
1 FDR with bilateral breast cancer,
1 FDR/SDR with breast cancer and 1 FDR/SDR with ovarian cancer,
1 FDR with breast cancer and ovarian cancer who is Jewish.
Ovarian Cancer:
Refer if your patient has
2 FDRs with ovarian cancer,
1 FDR with ovarian cancer and 1 FDR with breast cancer,
1 FDR with ovarian cancer and 2 SDRs with breast cancer,
1 FDR, male with breast cancer.

Other familial cancers include:
Familial Melanoma (CDK2NA.)
Refer patients with
Primary Melanoma and a F/H of 3 members with melanoma or 2 FDRs with melanoma, Primary Melanoma and associated pancreatic cancer and/or a neural tumour in a FDR,
Multiple Primary Melanomata.
Genetic Tests available (2013):
CDKN2A (Increased risk of various cancers including melanoma),
PTCH (BCCs etc),
Mismatch repair genes,
PTEN (Glioblastoma, endometrial cancer, prostate, lung and breast cancer etc),
Tuberous Sclerosis,
Fibrofolliculin (Papular skin lesions),
APC (Adenomatous Polyposis Coli),
NF1/2 (Neurofibromatosis),
These are mostly autosomal dominant.

Cystic Fibrosis and Autosomal Recessive Inheritance:

The commonest serious Autosomal Recessive disease. The world's highest incidence is actually in Ireland. It is possible that CF provided a "Heterozygote advantage" against such life threatening gut infections as Typhoid and Cholera, even against the pulmonary complications of TB or the diarrhoea of Lactose Intolerance after mankind took to drinking cows' milk – and therefore the mutation didn't die out. After all for every child with CF who would die, you would have 2 carriers:

Parents both carriers   cN x cN
Children: 1 affected, 2 carriers, 1 normal   cc   cN cN NN

4% population are carriers, incidence therefore $1/25 \times 1/25 \times 1/4$ = (Roughly!) 1:2000-3000. Less in non Caucasians.

4: Acute Medicine in General Practice:

Casualty:

Casualty units are busy and often unpleasant places to visit and to work in. They have always been so, especially on public holidays, Friday and Saturday evenings. This is clearly getting worse with the OOH confusion, the office hours and the difficulty in getting appointments of today's General practice. In an interview on Radio 4, March 2017, Simon Stevens, The NHS England Chief said that 300m patients saw GPs every year and 23m went to casualty. But 3m of these he added would be better dealt with in General Practice. How? Especially if GPs are going to be recruited to "Front of house" every casualty unit and therefore denude GP community numbers and at a time when GPs were calling for continental length appointments of 20-30 mins? In other words, expecting to see fewer patients for longer.

In one week before Christmas 2014, 44,000 people went to A and E, just under 90% of them being seen in four hours in England. That, of course, does not mean "treated" "diagnosed" or admitted", – just "seen". Not many countries actually publish the time people wait to be seen and England isn't the worst country in the UK for keeping people waiting – though it may be once the tidal wave of casualty phobic female doctors finishes washing over the beach of the NHS. If it ever does.

70% of casualty attendances are alcohol related at weekends in cities, 4-60% across weekdays. The commonest reasons for attending casualty: Trauma, followed by psychiatric conditions. (Parkinson et Al Emerg Med. J doi 10. 1136/emermed-2014-204581).

The magic four hour limit target changed from 98% to 95% in 2010 in England but despite this in 2015, 17 hospitals were declaring "Major Incidents" in order to trigger extra staff and resource deployment, the cancelling of routine surgery etc. due to unprecedented demand.

Indeed in the first week of 2015 I was struck by the irony of a Guardian article showing a half page photograph of city centre drunk mini skirted Liverpudlian girls staggering into an emergency ambulance. My reaction like, I imagine most people, was that these people were not emergency cases, they should not be treated free, that no one who is drunk should call an ambulance. Also shouldn't we have SOME mechanism for stopping this abuse of a system which can no longer assist the genuinely ill because its resources are funnelled off to help so many selfish, self indulgent, self destructive people?

The accompanying article "A and E Crisis: Experts explain the cause" stated that casualty units were under the greatest strain in living memory with elderly patients on trolleys for days, ambulances queuing for hours, staff under intolerable stress, patients aggressive and attending inappropriately.

The "Experts" included the following reasons for the crisis:

1) Attitudes. Younger people using the NHS far more than the older population. The younger generation has grown up with a free and universal service and a sense of entitlement to instant care. They have a "right now" society and this is a major problem for the NHS (Prof Keith Willett NHS England's Director of Acute Care).

2) The folly of reducing the number of District Nurses from 12,000 in 2003 to 5,500 had contributed said "Dr" Peter Carter Chief Executive of the R.C.N. (The "Doctor" title

is due to a PhD which was on the subject of "Why nurses abuse patients" – so he, according to my brother is a real doctor, not a quack like me. – My brother is a PhD in Chemistry). But then dentists call themselves doctors these days so maybe we REAL doctors should start calling ourselves professors.

He also said that dismantling NHS Direct and substituting (in 2013) NHS111 was a "huge mistake". Many of NHS Direct's staff were clinically trained with some nurses. They were more experienced, more likely to give experienced advice, take clinical responsibility and not just tell patients to go to casualty (a mixture of his words and mine but I agree completely).

3) We have too few beds: We need about 25% more beds in the NHS. We run the most "efficient" health service in the world with constant full bed occupancy, no flexibility and no ability to cope with even small fluctuations in demand for admission. Far too efficient (overwhelmed) to work effectively.

4) The growing population of the country means that casualty units and hospitals are just too small for the populations they serve particularly in some parts of the country and they can't recruit enough doctors and nurses. (Claire Murdoch Chief Exec of C and NW Lond. NHS Found Trust.) The UK population was expected to grow by 4.6m mainly due to EU migration and birth rates during the 2010s (Office of National Statistics) -the fastest growth in 50 years. The NHS has continued to shed beds and educate part time doctors for the last decade as if it lived in isolation from its potential pool of demand and its need to plan for the future.

5) No 24 hour Primary Care. I would add the fairly obvious factors of the sudden removal of a fully functioning primary care out of hours service within the last fifteen years. This is when problems really started to build up. The GP or his team took calls from all comers 24 hours day, triaged, negotiated with the patient and the hospital doctor, temporised, visited, treated, took clinical responsibility and all the risks. There is now almost no one in the system between patient and secondary care doing that. The out of hours GP was the bulwark who used to see and triage most sick patients at home, with GPs on call from their own home in rotas, then in cooperatives and he or she was the first port of call for most emergencies out of hours for five decades.

In a newspaper report (9/1/15) in the second week of 2015 the situation was said to be that 11% of patients were unable to get an appointment with their GP and 10% of these patients therefore went to casualty or their Walk-in Centre. David Cameron commented that this had contributed to an extra 1 million over 65s attending casualty "This year" compared with 4 years before.

You don't know what you've got til its gone (the on call GP, extended rotas then Cooperatives) – indeed.

6) The Feminisation of medicine:

There is now no chance of restoring a functioning primary care out of hours system unless the overwhelming number of female GPs (70% coming out of most medical schools) is vastly reduced or they are persuaded to increase the priority they put on their career as opposed to their family and home. Few will admit this in mixed groups but nearly all male doctors I know blame the feminisation of the medical schools of the last ten years for most of the staffing crises in the NHS. The greater sickness absence, depression and partimism, the maternity leave, their family priority and career selectivity of female doctors compared with men are at the root of most NHS medical staffing difficulties. We simply can't run a health service with this percentage of women doctors. Unless they are prepared to work the same hours as men. Female doctors neither want to do out of hours in General Practice or weekends or the more taxing training rotas in hospitals or work in the more challenging hospital specialities – especially casualty (see references elsewhere, including RCP census, the Representative of the College of Emergency medicine on the Today Programme 2014, or the Woman's Hour on Women in Medicine Jan 2015 etc). Where they do want to work (they are 70%+ of the junior staff of paediatric units) the crisis is because of excess time they take off in maternity leave and working part time.

As the function of the A and E department has had to change with the withdrawal of meaningful GP services at weekends and night and as the Health Secretary has commented, some casualty staff get to know some GP patients better than the GPs do themselves. Indeed, in a 2014 survey 1 in 4 patients had not "Heard of" out of hours GP services, one in five were unaware of the new 111 emergency number, the number of patients using OOH GP services had dropped by a third in six years and there had been a consequent rise in visits to the beleaguered A and E departments.

A survey done by Imperial College in 2014 showed a large drop in GP organised admissions and rise in admissions via Casualty. It found that 1.12m patients were admitted by GPs in England in 2001/2 compared with 0.93m in 2010/11. Over the same period hospital admissions through A and E had risen 72% from 2.1m to 3.6m. The researchers suggested a cause was "A failure of management in primary care and outpatient settings."

In a pre Christmas week 2014, The National Director of Commissioning Operations for NHS England Dr Barbara Hakin*, said: "This week saw over 110,100 emergency admissions to hospital and 436,229 attendances-up nearly 30,000 on the average for the same week over the past years".

Setting the (GP) slaves free was a huge mistake from the point of view of patient access to care, cost and safety. A majority female and part time work force neither wants to extend GP hours nor staff casualty departments so the prospect of restoring a quality primary care out of hours service or "manning" the overwhelmed casualty units is remote. Large numbers of British GP trainees are expressing the intention of leaving the UK once they have finished their rotation and working in Australia or New Zealand. This is for "Quality of Life" reasons. Even worse: a study was published in early 2017 which showed the results of the career intentions of today's cohort of medical students. A shocking nine tenths declared the intention to work part time on qualifying. So: An absence of meaningful out of hours GP services is just one aspect of the reduced holistic commitment of of today's doctors compared with their seniors.

This has led to a walk in Casualty Department ethos amongst patients and the interesting statistic that 40% of urgent treatment centre patients are now seen and sent home without any treatment at all. "Urgent" and "Emergency" are two of the most degraded words in English. Does this mean that the average patient has such little knowledge, confidence, common sense, is so risk averse or experience poor that the pursuit of reassurance has become a default essential in their life? The "you can't be too careful" culture? Is it time to consider putting the deterrent of an immediate financial charge into the calculation now?

Dr Cliff Mann of the College of Emergency Medicine was quoted in the first week of 2015 saying "The NHS non emergency line 111 was advising an increasing proportion of patients to seek emergency care." The implication was that 111 algorithms were risk averse, that the NHS was litigation driven, or the law biased towards a compensation culture. Primary care seemed to be non-existent for acute problems at inconvenient hours and the whole system was draining into casualty now. The problem, as always in a free system, is to separate out those that need care from those that just want attention and reassurance.

A research project in Ontario, quoted in Ben Goldacre's "I think you'll find it's a bit more complicated than that" looked at 22 million visits to casualty over five years. 14 million of these patients were sent home after being seen. The researchers then looked at the **average** waiting time in the A and E department (a proxy for the busyness of the department) when each discharged patient had arrived and whether the patient in question had subsequently died. It turned out that if a patient attended casualty when the average wait was 6 hours the death rate after being sent home was twice that of patients sent home if the average wait when they attended had been an hour. This was true for patients triaged as urgent or non urgent. Each increase in waiting time resulted in an increase in death and the statistically significant point was reached at three hours. What does this mean? Presumably that casualty staff sometimes get overworked, stressed, take short cuts and employ wishful thinking rather than good practice. All clinical work is the management of risk. If I had a ward full of empty beds, a quiet day as a Paediatric registrar and a *relatively* well new patient with an undiagnosed high temperature I would be more likely to admit the child for observation than send him home with instructions to return. If the beds were nearly full and the parents seemed competent, I might take a risk and trust them to keep a close eye on the child and come back if they were worried.

As you can tell, A and E departments can be hopelessly understaffed and unpleasantly crowded places. This, as is explained elsewhere was publicised by no less than the Representative of The College of Emergency Medicine. This was in no lesser forum than the *Today Programme* in January 2014 and is largely because women doctors dominate medical schools and the whole medical workforce now and don't want to work nights and weekends in A and E. Perhaps they prefer to become spokes people for Commissioning Organisations*. Casualties are the sumps that drain the misfits of every town and city as well as the sick and displaced. There is rarely any feeling of proper organisation or security or any sense that the really ill will get proper supervision or care in any reasonable time scale if you are waiting to be seen as a patient or even if you are a member of staff seeing the patients in casualty – at least in my experience.

The last time I accompanied a patient to casualty who I had intubated at home and hand ventilated in the back of an ambulance, we radioed ahead and were greeted by a single nursing auxiliary – the only member of staff in the unit at 8pm that evening. This was my local DGH.-Not exactly E.R.

That unit is now a walk in centre, no doubt a bit better staffed but consultants are still few and far between, about 3 times as many men as women, presumably because of the family unfriendly hours and demanding nature of some of the patients (figures for 2009 from NHS Medical Careers) and according to the red top headlines in September 2013, there were only 5 NHS casualty consultants covering their units in the whole of the UK during one night that month. To me, as far as quality of care is concerned, it is like most of medicine: there is not so much a north south divide or an urban rural divide but a: teaching hospital rotation and/out in the sticks divide.

25% of A and E patients at any time are children and they can get a particularly raw deal.

A recent headline (Sept 2013) told an unpalatable story which revealed several fault lines in the modern Health Service: Jeremy Hunt, the Secretary of State complained that casualty staff were more familiar with many GP's elderly patients than the GPs themselves and he suggested that GPs should re establish that lost relationship.

This sad situation is probably true now for the first time in the history of the NHS but is it one of many symptoms of the systematic break up of General Practice which used to form the back bone of the Health Service.

"It has been shown repeatedly that patients have the greatest confidence in their "Usual family doctor" and they will procrastinate if asked to see another unfamiliar doctor even if suffering quite serious symptoms. Wise clinicians confident in their own routes of access will provide a safety net for worried patients-none of this is available to patients or doctors in conveyor belt practices". (BMJ Oct 2008) Unfortunately many small scale practices are now banding together and gaining economies of scale and convenience while losing the core values of family medicine: a list system, accessibility, local roots, continuity, familiarity, an ongoing informal relationship, what I would call a "belonging" between doctors and patients. And the bigger the practice the more like a conveyer belt-particularly the new mega, factory practices which new (July 2016) research shows the patients hate and produce only income and rota benefits for doctors and "IT advantages."

Why have practices changed so much in the last decade or so? You can find out just by asking a few patients:

Elderly patients complain bitterly that they can't get appointments with their "own" doctor anymore because (and I hear this kind of conversation in Sainsbury's all the time).

1) "She is never there – She is on maternity leave/doesn't work alternate Wednesdays/is only part time, is a Clinical Assistant/portfolio GP/Registrar/Part Timer/Job Share/A Maternity or Sabbatical substitute. Why can't we just have a full time doctor like they used to have – someone we can get to know and he/she can get to know us?"

2) "She is always booked up because the phone is jammed from 8.30 every morning and when you can get through, all the on the day appointments are booked and the only ones left are in three weeks with her or with the training doctor who doesn't really seem to know very much, or you just get a telephone triage. But as you don't know them and they don't know you, how can they trust you or understand how bad you can actually get or know how ill you actually are?, I mean they can't see you can they?"

3) "She keeps taking time off at short notice because her child minder lets her down and her three children are always ill and then you have to see the Registrar who doesn't know very much and always asks you what is wrong."

4) " She is always training one of those registrars or off on a course somewhere so there is a locum I have to see who hasn't read the notes and who I will never see again and is often quite hard to understand as I am deaf."

5) "She works in a practice with 8, 9, or 10 partners and you never know who you are going to see and you aren't even registered with a person anymore are you? That awful Blaire/Brown government that paid the GPs so much and then let them stop coming out at night also said we had to be registered with a practice not a person. So now we never see one of our own doctors in an emergency AND we never get to be familiar with and trust an individual doctor at the surgery in the daytime either. It's the worst of all worlds". Practices used to be small and personal. You got to know the doctors and staff and they knew you. How can you have a professional relationship with a crowd? "You just don't

know who your doctor is anymore. How can you be registered with an organisation?" I have had all these conversations many times.

I was talking to a Practice Manager at a partnership I used to know very well about the recent personnel changes in her group. This was the practice in which my own Mother in Law had been unable to get her first appointment for two weeks after arriving and so registered elsewhere.

The manager mentioned in passing that one female partner had been off long term due to stress and in order to improve continuity they had taken on a new female assistant for a year. This new doctor then immediately announced her pregnancy and her intention to be absent on maternity leave for six months of that year. This was precisely what happened the last time I was working at the same practice as a partner and appointed a brand new practice nurse. We had discussed wanting her to start a much needed diabetic clinic, maybe a travel service, how we felt familiarity and continuity were key to good Family Medicine. She effusively agree at the interview. Then on the first working day, she arrived at work and made the announcement that she was pregnant. This ended any long term planning, there was a general sense of betrayal, then picking up the pieces and trying to book locums. After the birth of her child she decided (at short notice and again, after we had booked a week of clinics for her) not to return.

So what is ruining General Practice? Well, one of the things ruining the continuity, consistency, the long term relationship with a doctor you can get to know (– for most patients one of the most important aspects of medical care,) is the female bias of employment law, the feminisation of the medical work place and the ongoing 65-70% of female medical students now becoming established doctors. The patients have and are noticing the difference this has made. It is utterly dishonest that our profession is too cowardly to admit it, confront it and address the problems it is causing.

So Jeremy Hunt was partly right. Patients aren't registered with a doctor with whom they become familiar and develop trust anymore. This is **wrong** and that is why the List System is so much a key part of good General Practice and was so valued by patients and good GPs and why employment law that sanctifies a woman's choice to conceive whenever she wants and puts patients' rights at the bottom of the list is unfair. BUT the list system depends on most GPs being full time or nearly full time with limited non clinical outside commitments and therefore **available**. It also depends, of course, on having a sensible appointment system with reasonable numbers of on the day appointments.

The emasculation of medical schools over the last decade is sexist, short sighted and puts the patient's interests beneath soft politics again. The comparative paucity of male doctors means fewer general surgeons, fewer orthopaedic surgeons, fewer casualty consultants, chaotic A and E departments, paradoxically a feminised paediatric serviced manned (excuse the term) by expensive maternity cover locums, it means less availability of a GP you can get to know, fewer partners and full time GPs, less continuity in all areas of medicine. It obviously means more doctors off on maternity leave but it also means more doctors off sick with both physical and psychological ill health, more doctors part time, retiring early and being highly selective about their career options. Because all these are what women doctors do. Fewer career hours, less time commitment to the job.

Add it all up and I am sorry to say it but you **do** need a medical profession of mainly male doctors to give a service that puts patients first. The feminisation and part-timism of so many General Practices means it becomes very difficult to retain continuity, familiarity and trust, the three things of crucial importance to all patients, even (in my experience) children. Good General Practice is hard work; it **is** a commitment, a vocation, a way of life. It can't be done properly or with any degree of excellence a few sessions a week here and there. It means you have to make it your priority, your vocation. Perhaps even plan your pregnancy with some consideration to the needs of the practice and the patients. You never know when you will have to stay late so someone else will have look after YOUR children at short notice. Female doctors used to manage it. As if to pour salt into all the unsuccessful male medical school applicant's wounds, the Today Program ran an article on 12th June 2017 saying although girls did better at A Level, by the time it came to degrees they were lagging far behind boys academically.

So no wonder many patients turf up and see the casualty officer they saw last week and who knows and recognises them and gave them a same day appointment and remembers them from before. Who wouldn't?

Who should you tell to go straight to casualty or call an ambulance?

Significant overdose,

Uncontrolled epistaxis,

Genuine accident with significant residual injury,

Central chest pain,

Acute severe breathlessness,

An unconscious patient found at home and unrousable unless known to be diabetic on insulin or epileptic and you can get there soon,

Not breathing,

A sick child with a non blanching rash unless **you** can get there within a shorter time than an ambulance (and you probably **can**) to assess. All GPs will carry Benzyl Penicillin, an Injectable steroid and hopefully a blood culture bottle in date.

Death Rates and URTIs:

The riskiest weeks of the year in terms of mortality are the first couple of weeks of each New Year. This, especially the first week in January is when excess mortality usually peaks. Respiratory infections abound in winter especially RSV and flu and their bacterial community acquired secondary complications. The cause of "Colds", Rhinoviruses, are commoner in Autumn and Spring which I suppose is the reason we all say we need a "cold snap" to kill off the bugs. It doesn't kill them off but perhaps it reduces cross infection by keeping people inside. We associate unseasonal warmer temperatures with constant upper respiratory infections due to Rhinoviruses. There were 31,000 excess deaths in the UK winter of 2012-13 but counter intuitively these were spread across all income and social groups and were not concentrated in the deprived areas of big cities or the lower socio economic groups. Excess winter mortality is not related to income, one of many health political myths and indeed it isn't even worse in cold countries. We all know how better prepared Scandinavian transport systems are than ours for snow and ice but it turns out the highest winter mortalities are in the warmest (and presumably least prepared) southern European countries.

Discharge summaries: (Communication between primary and secondary care)

In these days of so called paperless medicine, one of our practice's audits in 2012 was of discharge summaries for patients admitted to our local District General Hospital (not just seen in casualty, these were even worse) and it showed:

20% were wholly or partly illegible,

17% had no diagnosis,

37% had no justification or reason for changes to pre existing drug treatments.

The patients themselves were, generally, completely unable to understand why treatments had been changed in hospital and what the new treatments were supposed to treat. They would subsequently bring in their bags of drugs to us, their GPs, with the summary as soon as they could get an appointment, asking for an explanation of what had happened to them over the last week. This applied to young and old and across all specialities.

It is hard to believe that communication skills are a huge part of medical student, GP, nurse and pharmacist training. It must all be negated by the preceding selection bias of three A stars at A level which produces academic, intense, introverted, often uncommunicative, unempathic and intellectual medical students. Intelligent but not necessarily emotionally intelligent. So the patient will often be at a loss as to why drugs have been changed and what their diagnosis was. The irony of course, as every GP will know is that most of the drugs that the SHO or registrar cleverly discontinued for the right theoretical reasons will have to be restarted by the GP in a few weeks. The patient's transient improvement in mood observed by the hospital doctor was due to all that excitement and entertainment on the ward but the isolation of home will soon restore the underlying depression. The nurses ensured that the patient kept to her prescribed diet and so her anti-diabetic medication was reduced as a consequence but as soon as she returned home and restarted the Kit Kats three times a day the Metformin would need to be increased by the GP again.

There has always been a schism between primary and secondary care but it is wider than ever today for a variety of reasons. This is a great shame and eventually to the patient's detriment.

One reason for this distance is because of the reorganisation of medical post-graduate training and the way education is funded. This has closed many local post graduate centres and ended routine weekly open meetings which were attended by GPs and hospital staff together.

Training now is less likely to be run by local consultants than by Commissioning Group Committees, Community Pharmacists, the various GP surgery inspection and Nursing Teams, Appraisal Groups, Drug companies, the local Hospice Team and so on and many of these are new arrivals in the community.

The schism is partly because of such initiatives as Choose and Book: (The Law of Unforeseen Consequences again:) GPs no longer need to be familiar with the local hospital consultants and have sent referral letters to "Dear Colleague" for several years not to "Dear John". So GPs and consultants are less likely to be familiar with each other, friends even, – and often no longer know each other personally. They meet socially less often and can no longer use that social contact to the advantage of their patients. Everywhere in my description of what has gone wrong with the NHS in the last 10-20 years there is the Law of Unforeseen Consequences. – If only we had thought a bit harder about the disadvantages of computerisation, standardisation, QuoF, Choose and Book, feminisation, slovenly dress standards, mass screening, giving up named lists and out of hours, the end of personal responsibility, or the way that Data Protection, Human Rights, Disability Rights, even Equality and Diversity Laws have been applied and would adversely affect patient care we might still have a functioning, personal and valued service and not one that has lost touch with its prime purpose.

Also the vast increase in part time doctors and those with other less committed careers in General Practice, including assistants and sessional doctors have caused a drifting away from the old informal hospital meetings for lunch and open MDT meetings that I and my contemporaries would often drop in on. Part timers have other things to do and other places to go.

The almost complete and much lamented loss of GP hospital beds means GPs are rarely wandering the wards or the canteen these days to say hello or to join a familiar group for coffee. How different this all was 20 years ago. And of course, the patient, not the doctor is the loser.

Acute Life Support:

Causes of collapse (Unresponsive, no pulse or respiration:)

Cardiac: Vascular occlusion, tamponade electric shock, drug effect, volume depletion, trauma, electrolyte imbalance, pneumothorax, arrhythmia.

Respiratory: Pulmonary embolism, respiratory obstruction, pneumo/haemothorax, drowning, pulmonary damage: (Infection, trauma, disease etc).

Central: Cerebral depression, overdose, drug effects, hypo/hyperthermia, trauma, shock, inflammation, infection, trauma, cerebral damage etc.

Assess situation/risk/summon help.

Assess and maintain airway >? Recovery, L Lateral position, neck extended.

If spinal injury is suspected use chin lift or jaw thrust without extending neck (if possible).

If apnoeic but pulse present: Give 2 Slow effective breaths 2 seconds each. Wait 10 seconds feeling for a carotid pulse. Repeat mouth to mouth inflation and check pulse after each inflation.

If the patient starts to breath, turn to L lat recovery position.

Cardiac arrest:

Give 2 slow effective breaths at the start (the importance of these is sometimes debated but I think they are useful as they initiate oxygenation, confirm a patent airway, exclude some potential diagnoses, can dislodge foreign bodies, it takes very little time and so on), check the pulse, then apply 30 compressions (5-6cms amplitude) to two inflations and repeat **30:2** until circulation returns or help arrives.

Some sources say give resus. for 1 minute then summon assistance. I think this depends on you, your experience and the situation.

When do you go for help if you are alone? The standard wisdom is to rush off and summon help or use your mobile before you start resuscitation UNLESS you think the victim is unconscious due to drowning or trauma (-in which case try resuscitation for a minute first). I have never been able to leave a newly collapsed and pulseless patient without having a go at recovering them straight away, believing those frontal cortical cells are disappearing in their millions every second and you might as well get a little oxygen into the local circulation. You can call for help in a few minutes; once the brain cells are dead you can't call them back.

Acute Coronary Syndromes:

For instance: 20 minutes or more of rest chest pain compatible with cardiac pain, recent onset of cardiac pain with minimal exertion or pre existing anginal type pain which has suddenly deteriorated. These patients should be seen by you and or referred to hospital straight away. Patients with these symptoms who have improved and are symptom free for 2 days when you see them need to be fully assessed and still referred – to be seen, if possible in O/P within 2 weeks.

Don't do what the GP of a friend recently did: The patient, a friend, was clearly suffering deteriorating effort associated chest pain and was seen on a Friday afternoon. Neither wanted the hassle of an ECG (no nurse available) and ambulance (no current pain) or an admission (a busy social weekend coming up) so they persuaded each other that she had reflux. It is easy enough to do with the wrong leading questions, omission of normal lines of enquiry and enough suggestion. A dishonest diagnosis was the mutually satisfactory but dangerous conclusion. This then prevented the administration even of aspirin which the GP knew might at least have been constructive, even life saving. You can imagine the outcome.

The acute coronary patient should be visited and the ambulance called. You will usually get there first, give important treatment and restore some faith in the GP as a real doctor.

Give Sublingual GTN, Aspirin (chewed, 300mg) oxygen if you have it (-I have to admit, I was wary of keeping this in a super heated car boot in the summer so it is the one emergency drug I keep at the surgery), get a Venflon or even a Butterfly into a vein (the ambulance crew will smile a bit at the retro amateurishness of the latter) and give Diamorphine.

ALL GPs SHOULD CARRY DIAMORPHINE. The arguments in favour of this anxiety, pain, dyspnoea and distress relieving analgesic, so irreplaceable in myocardial pain are unanswerable. It reduces circulatory load, catecholamine myocardial stress and relieves anxiety and pain. Your fears about car break-ins, worries about accusations of being a Shipman mark 2, accidental respiratory depression (-have in date Naloxone as well), the associated nausea, your pretence that ambulances always come quickly, that GPs are not an "Acute Service" and other *non controlled* drugs working just as well are simple fabrications to avoid having to keep and justify all the complex documentation now attached to controlled drugs.

The ratio of **Adult CPR** (See algorithms) is **30:2** Compressions: inflations.

Drug Treatment:

Diamorphine:
The dose is 5mg slowly IV (2.5mg in the elderly) at 1mg/min. I give it with Cyclizine 50mg but you can use:
Metoclopramide 10mg. (I have seen oculogyric crises with this but never with the former and this is treated with
Procyclidine 5-10mg IM repeated in 20 mins PRN) – which all GPs should carry too.
Other Drugs:
Atropine 300ug-1mg IV for bradycardia and hypotension.

Babies and Children:

Cardiac arrest is usually secondary to respiratory arrest, Apply CPR at **30:2** (larger children) for at least 1 minute before summoning help. In babies use one hand, two fingers, or squeeze the chest between forefinger and thumbs. Compress 1/3 the diameter of the chest. The ratio is **15:2** in babies and smaller children.

Resuscitation and urgent treatment algorithms:

(RCUK ETA 1-12) Resuscitation Council Guidelines. (My thanks to the Resuscitation Council for their permission to reproduce these)

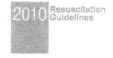 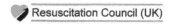

Adult Basic Life Support

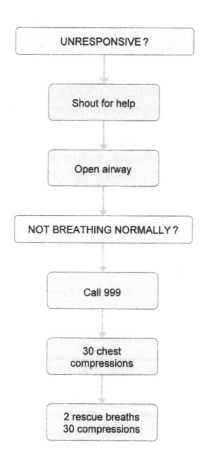

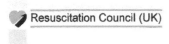

Resuscitation Council (UK)

Anaphylactic reactions – Initial treatment

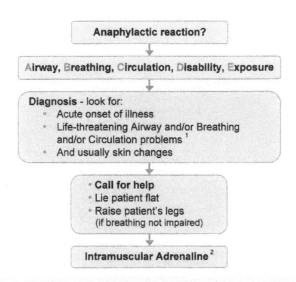

Anaphylactic reaction?

↓

Airway, Breathing, Circulation, Disability, Exposure

↓

Diagnosis - look for:
* Acute onset of illness
* Life-threatening Airway and/or Breathing and/or Circulation problems [1]
* And usually skin changes

↓

* **Call for help**
* Lie patient flat
* Raise patient's legs
  (if breathing not impaired)

↓

Intramuscular Adrenaline [2]

---

[1] **Life-threatening problems:**

Airway:	swelling, hoarseness, stridor
Breathing:	rapid breathing, wheeze, fatigue, cyanosis, SpO_2 < 92%, confusion
Circulation:	pale, clammy, low blood pressure, faintness, drowsy/coma

[2] **Intramuscular Adrenaline**

IM doses of 1:1000 adrenaline (repeat after 5 min if no better)

* Adult   500 micrograms IM (0.5 mL)
* Child more than 12 years: 500 micrograms IM (0.5 mL)
* Child 6 -12 years: 300 micrograms IM (0.3 mL)
* Child less than 6 years: 150 micrograms IM (0.15 mL)

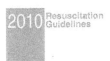

2010 Resuscitation Guidelines

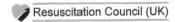

Resuscitation Council (UK)

Adult Advanced Life Support

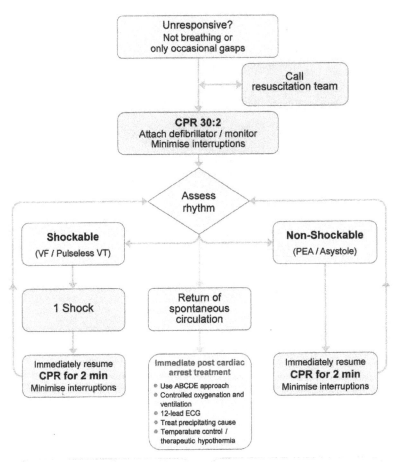

Unresponsive?
Not breathing or
only occasional gasps

Call resuscitation team

CPR 30:2
Attach defibrillator / monitor
Minimise interruptions

Assess rhythm

Shockable
(VF / Pulseless VT)

Non-Shockable
(PEA / Asystole)

1 Shock

Return of spontaneous circulation

Immediately resume
CPR for 2 min
Minimise interruptions

Immediate post cardiac arrest treatment
- Use ABCDE approach
- Controlled oxygenation and ventilation
- 12-lead ECG
- Treat precipitating cause
- Temperature control / therapeutic hypothermia

Immediately resume
CPR for 2 min
Minimise interruptions

During CPR
- Ensure high-quality CPR: rate, depth, recoil
- Plan actions before interrupting CPR
- Give oxygen
- Consider advanced airway and capnography
- Continuous chest compressions when advanced airway in place
- Vascular access (intravenous, intraosseous)
- Give adrenaline every 3-5 min
- Correct reversible causes

Reversible Causes
- Hypoxia
- Hypovolaemia
- Hypo- / hyperkalaemia / metabolic
- Hypothermia

- Thrombosis - coronary or pulmonary
- Tamponade - cardiac
- Toxins
- Tension pneumothorax

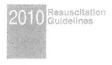 Resuscitation Guidelines

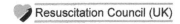

Adult Choking Treatment Algorithm

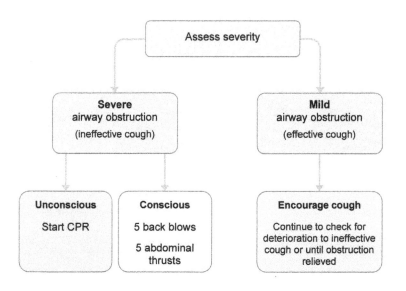

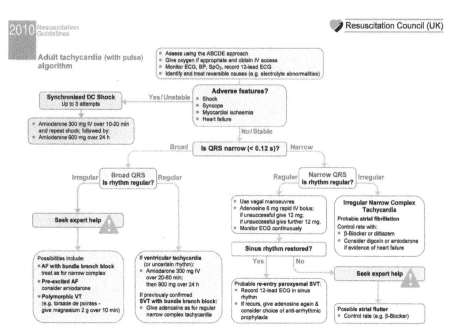

Adult tachycardia (with pulse) algorithm — 2010 Resuscitation Guidelines, Resuscitation Council (UK)

- Assess using the ABCDE approach
- Give oxygen if appropriate and obtain IV access
- Monitor ECG, BP, SpO$_2$, record 12-lead ECG
- Identify and treat reversible causes (e.g. electrolyte abnormalities)

Adverse features?
- Shock
- Syncope
- Myocardial ischaemia
- Heart failure

Yes / Unstable → **Synchronised DC Shock** Up to 3 attempts

- Amiodarone 300 mg IV over 10-20 min and repeat shock; followed by:
- Amiodarone 900 mg over 24 h

No / Stable → **Is QRS narrow (< 0.12 s)?**

Broad → **Broad QRS Is rhythm regular?**

Narrow → **Narrow QRS Is rhythm regular?**

Broad — Irregular → **Seek expert help**

Possibilities include:
- **AF with bundle branch block** treat as for narrow complex
- **Pre-excited AF** consider amiodarone
- **Polymorphic VT** (e.g. torsade de pointes – give magnesium 2 g over 10 min)

Broad — Regular:
If ventricular tachycardia (or uncertain rhythm):
- Amiodarone 300 mg IV over 20-60 min; then 900 mg over 24 h

If previously confirmed **SVT with bundle branch block:**
- Give adenosine as for regular narrow complex tachycardia

Narrow — Regular:
- Use vagal manoeuvres
- Adenosine 6 mg rapid IV bolus; if unsuccessful give 12 mg; if unsuccessful give further 12 mg.
- Monitor ECG continuously

Sinus rhythm restored?

Yes → Probable re-entry paroxysmal SVT:
- Record 12-lead ECG in sinus rhythm
- If recurs, give adenosine again & consider choice of anti-arrhythmic prophylaxis

No → **Seek expert help**

Possible atrial flutter
- Control rate (e.g. β-Blocker)

Narrow — Irregular → **Irregular Narrow Complex Tachycardia**
Probable atrial fibrillation
Control rate with:
- β-Blocker or diltiazem
- Consider digoxin or amiodarone if evidence of heart failure

[284]

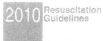 **Resuscitation Guidelines**

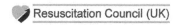 Resuscitation Council (UK)

Adult bradycardia algorithm

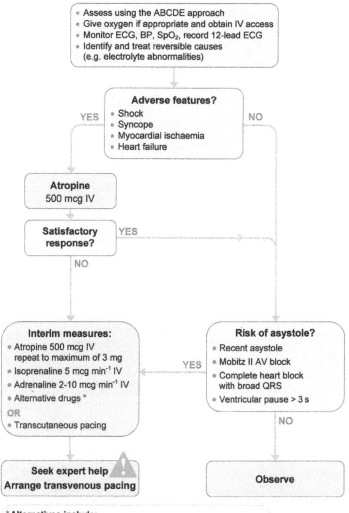

- Assess using the ABCDE approach
- Give oxygen if appropriate and obtain IV access
- Monitor ECG, BP, SpO$_2$, record 12-lead ECG
- Identify and treat reversible causes
  (e.g. electrolyte abnormalities)

Adverse features?
- Shock
- Syncope
- Myocardial ischaemia
- Heart failure

YES / NO

Atropine
500 mcg IV

Satisfactory response? — YES

NO

Interim measures:
- Atropine 500 mcg IV
  repeat to maximum of 3 mg
- Isoprenaline 5 mcg min^{-1} IV
- Adrenaline 2-10 mcg min^{-1} IV
- Alternative drugs *

OR
- Transcutaneous pacing

Risk of asystole?
- Recent asystole
- Mobitz II AV block
- Complete heart block
  with broad QRS
- Ventricular pause > 3 s

YES / NO

Seek expert help
Arrange transvenous pacing

Observe

*Alternatives include:
- Aminophylline
- Dopamine
- Glucagon (if beta-blocker or calcium channel blocker overdose)
- Glycopyrrolate can be used instead of atropine

ANAPHYLACTIC REACTIONS FOR ADULTS
Treatment by First Medical Responders

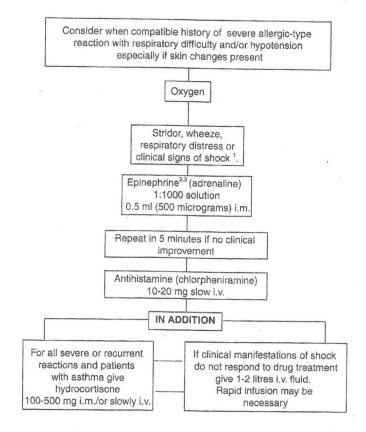

Consider when compatible history of severe allergic-type reaction with respiratory difficulty and/or hypotension especially if skin changes present

Oxygen

Stridor, wheeze, respiratory distress or clinical signs of shock [1].

Epinephrine[2,3] (adrenaline) 1:1000 solution 0.5 ml (500 micrograms) i.m.

Repeat in 5 minutes if no clinical improvement

Antihistamine (chlorpheniramine) 10-20 mg slow i.v.

IN ADDITION

For all severe or recurrent reactions and patients with asthma give hydrocortisone 100-500 mg i.m./or slowly i.v.

If clinical manifestations of shock do not respond to drug treatment give 1-2 litres i.v. fluid. Rapid infusion may be necessary

1. An inhaled β_2-agonist such as salbutamol may be used as an adjunctive measure if bronchospasm is severe and does not respond rapidly to other treatment.
2. If profound shock is judged immediately life threatening, give CPR/ALS if necessary. Consider slow i.v. epinephrine (adrenaline) 1:10,000 solution. This is hazardous and is recommended only for an experienced practitioner who can obtain i.v. access without delay.
Note the different strength of epinephrine (adrenaline) that may be required for i.v. use.
3. If adults are treated with an Epipen, then 300 micrograms will usually be sufficient. A second dose may be required.

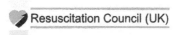 Resuscitation Council (UK)

Anaphylaxis algorithm

Anaphylactic reaction?

Airway, **B**reathing, **C**irculation, **D**isability, **E**xposure

Diagnosis - look for:
* Acute onset of illness
* Life-threatening Airway and/or Breathing and/or Circulation problems [1]
* And usually skin changes

* **Call for help**
* Lie patient flat
* Raise patient's legs

Adrenaline [2]

When skills and equipment available:
* Establish airway
* High flow oxygen
* IV fluid challenge [3]
* Chlorphenamine [4]
* Hydrocortisone [5]

Monitor:
* Pulse oximetry
* ECG
* Blood pressure

[1] **Life-threatening problems:**
Airway: swelling, hoarseness, stridor
Breathing: rapid breathing, wheeze, fatigue, cyanosis, SpO_2 < 92%, confusion
Circulation: pale, clammy, low blood pressure, faintness, drowsy/coma

[2] Adrenaline *(give IM unless experienced with IV adrenaline)*
IM doses of 1:1000 adrenaline (repeat after 5 min if no better)
* Adult   500 micrograms IM (0.5 mL)
* Child more than 12 years: 500 micrograms IM (0.5 mL)
* Child 6 -12 years: 300 micrograms IM (0.3 mL)
* Child less than 6 years: 150 micrograms IM (0.15 mL)

Adrenaline IV to be given **only by experienced specialists**
Titrate: Adults 50 micrograms; Children 1 microgram/kg

[3] IV fluid challenge:
Adult - 500 – 1000 mL
Child - crystalloid 20 mL/kg

Stop IV colloid
if this might be the cause
of anaphylaxis

	[4] Chlorphenamine (IM or slow IV)	[5] Hydrocortisone (IM or slow IV)
Adult or child more than 12 years	10 mg	200 mg
Child 6 - 12 years	5 mg	100 mg
Child 6 months to 6 years	2.5 mg	50 mg
Child less than 6 months	250 micrograms/kg	25 mg

See also: ▶ Anaphylactic reactions – Initial treatment

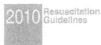 Resuscitation Guidelines

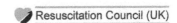 Resuscitation Council (UK)

Newborn Life Support

Dry the baby
Remove any wet towels and cover
Start the clock or note the time

Birth

↓

Assess (tone), breathing and heart rate

30 s

↓

If gasping or not breathing:
Open the airway
Give 5 inflation breaths
Consider SpO₂ monitoring

60 s

↓

Re-assess
If no increase in heart rate
look for chest movement

↓

If chest not moving:
Recheck head position
Consider 2-person airway control
and other airway manoeuvres
Repeat inflation breaths
Consider SpO₂ monitoring
Look for a response

Acceptable
pre-ductal SpO₂

2 min	60%
3 min	70%
4 min	80%
5 min	85%
10 min	90%

↑↓

If no increase in heart rate
look for chest movement

↓

When the chest is moving:
If heart rate is not detectable
or slow (< 60 min⁻¹)
Start chest compressions
3 compressions to each breath

↓

Reassess heart rate every 30 s
If heart rate is not detectable
or slow (<60 min⁻¹)
consider venous access and drugs

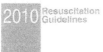

2010 Resuscitation Guidelines

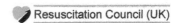 Resuscitation Council (UK)

Paediatric Basic Life Support
(Healthcare professionals with a duty to respond)

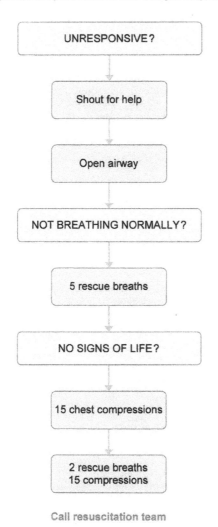

UNRESPONSIVE?

Shout for help

Open airway

NOT BREATHING NORMALLY?

5 rescue breaths

NO SIGNS OF LIFE?

15 chest compressions

2 rescue breaths
15 compressions

Call resuscitation team

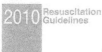 Resuscitation Guidelines

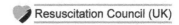 Resuscitation Council (UK)

Paediatric Advanced Life Support

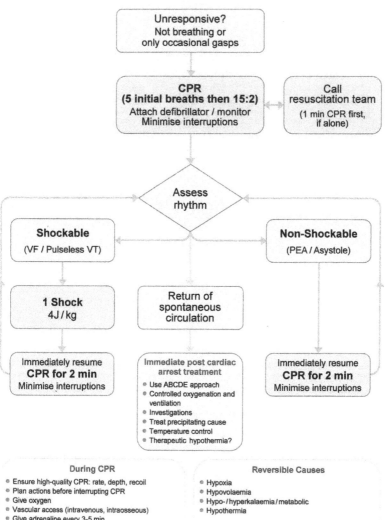

Unresponsive?
Not breathing or
only occasional gasps

CPR
(5 initial breaths then 15:2)
Attach defibrillator / monitor
Minimise interruptions

Call
resuscitation team
(1 min CPR first,
if alone)

Assess rhythm

Shockable
(VF / Pulseless VT)

Non-Shockable
(PEA / Asystole)

1 Shock
4 J / kg

Return of spontaneous circulation

Immediately resume
CPR for 2 min
Minimise interruptions

Immediate post cardiac arrest treatment
- Use ABCDE approach
- Controlled oxygenation and ventilation
- Investigations
- Treat precipitating cause
- Temperature control
- Therapeutic hypothermia?

Immediately resume
CPR for 2 min
Minimise interruptions

During CPR
- Ensure high-quality CPR: rate, depth, recoil
- Plan actions before interrupting CPR
- Give oxygen
- Vascular access (intravenous, intraosseous)
- Give adrenaline every 3-5 min
- Consider advanced airway and capnography
- Continuous chest compressions when advanced airway in place
- Correct reversible causes

Reversible Causes
- Hypoxia
- Hypovolaemia
- Hypo-/hyperkalaemia/metabolic
- Hypothermia
- Tension pneumothorax
- Toxins
- Tamponade - cardiac
- Thromboembolism

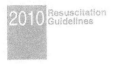

Resuscitation
Guidelines

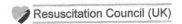

Resuscitation Council (UK)

Paediatric Choking Treatment Algorithm

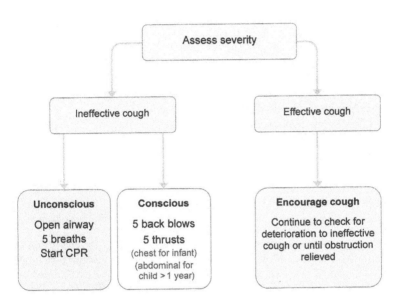

C.P.R.

Recent changes:

Hands only now and ok to start off with 100-120/min, 3 inch amplitude compression.

Early defibrillation in Children (do start with 5 breaths). Remember: airway: **30:2 In adults, in children 15:2.**

In adults the cardiac stimulation consists of (in order:) a precordial thump (if appropriate) and then two DC shocks of 200J followed thereafter by shocks of 360J.

CPR should be continued out of hospital for at least 35 minutes (Kanazawa Univ. Study European Soc Cardiology Congress 2015). 99% of both survivors and survivors with favourable neurological outcomes got their own circulation back within 35 minutes of the start of CPR. **No patients with a CPR duration longer than 53 minutes survived longer than one month after cardiac arrest.** There is no benefit of continuing after this time limit.

Severe Hypertension:

Measure with the patient seated and the arm supported at heart level.

Refer to hospital if: Systolic >220 or Diastolic >120mm Hg

Papilloedema/retinal haemorrhages

Encephalopathy, cerebral oedema,

LVF, dissecting aneurysm.

Some authorities suggest hospital referral if the BP is>140/90 with mild heart failure or renal impairment, age<30yrs, if there is a primary cause for the hypertension (Conn's, Renovascular disease etc) or failure to respond to GP treatment.

Acute Left ventricular Failure/Pulmonary Oedema:

Sudden onset of dyspnoea, sometimes wheezing, always sweating. They have basal creps, a third heart sound and a raised JVP.

Give:

Furosemide 10mg/ml, 40-80mg IV.

Diamorphine 5-10mg slowly IV (1mg/min) with Cyclizine/Metoclopramide which relieves back pressure, any pain and distress.

Sublingual GTN spray reduces pulmonary oedema.

High concentration of Oxygen.

Repeat the Furosemide and Diamorphine if no improvement after 20 mins.

Again, have Naloxone (0.8 – 2mg iv every 2-3 mins, Max 10mg) and Procyclidine (5-10mg IM, repeat after 20 mins PRN) available in case the Diamorphine or Metoclopramide cause respiratory depression or oculogyric crisis.

Pain relief:

Every GP worthy of the name should be able and willing to administer proper pain relief at short notice. They should never think, – as many of many colleagues incomprehensibly and inadequately say these days, that they are not an "acute medical service".

This is a consequence of the part-timism of our new General Practice and the foolhardy belief that what you will find during house calls is predictable, you won't pass any road accidents and your neighbours won't call on you at weekends when they fall off ladders.

Acute pain:

Diamorphine 5-10mg IM/IV slowly with 50mg Cyclizine.

Morphine is a slightly less soluble alternative.

Pethidine injection 100mg IV/IM – which has some specific advantages in migraine.

Tramadol injection/tablets 50mg/ml 50-100mg IM/IV this either works or has no analgesic effect whatsoever.

Meptazinol (Meptid) 100mg/ml 50-100mg IV/IM, Tabs 200mg.

If you carry opioids always also have in date:

Naloxone 400ug/ml, 0.4-2mg IV, repeated as and when necessary.

Diclofenac (25mg/ml) injection 75mg IM is useful for some pain, incl. migraine (you can give this to the regular migraineur rather than opioids to avoid habituation) and biliary/renal colic pain. A second dose can be given in a different site 30 mins later.

Dihydrocodeine, 30mg tabs. Good in diarrhoea too.

Diclofenac suppositories (25/50mg/100mg) are a useful alternative. Theoretical maximum daily dose is 150mg Diclofenac. Make sure that migraineurs have a supply and use them rather than home visits from you each time they get an attack. The absorption of suppositories can be somewhat unpredictable and remember the pain of migraine CAN be intolerable. 150mg is only the theoretical maximum dose per day.

Other NSAIDs:

Ibuprofen 400mg, Naproxen 250-500mg, or Diclofenac 50mg, or Etoricoxib 30, 60, 90mg tabs, (120mg tab for gout).

Nausea/Vomiting:

Cyclizine 50mg IM.

Domperidone (10mg tabs, 30mg supps). Prokinetic/centrally acting but now some concern regarding cardiac side effects in susceptible patients. I have never seen this.

Metoclopramide 10mg/2ml inj. Risk of dyskinesia especially in the young.

Promethazine (Phenergan) 10, 25mg tabs.

Prochloperazine (Stemetil) 12.5mg/ml inj.

Asthma:

Assess the severity from the patient's ability to complete sentences, the degree of anxiety – although regular sufferers often become blasé. Observe respiratory rate, accessory muscle use, recession, in-drawing, peak flow (<50% expected). Reliable signs of severity may be RR >25, Pulse >110, but transcutaneous oxygen monitors and your clinical assessment of central cyanosis (tongue) are notoriously dependent on other factors and unreliable. So is the subjective assessment of the chronic asthmatic who may have a peak flow virtually unrecordable and yet seem unbothered. You will have to make your assessment based on your knowledge of how the patient responded last time and how good a witness they are, how trustworthy the attendants are and what time of day it is as much as the blunt clinical signs.

Treatment:

Salbutamol MDI via a spacer device, 4-6 puffs each inhaled separately. It is almost impossible to

cause a significant overdose with more and more puffs in this way. So repeat every few minutes until a good response.

Terbutaline MDI can be given in the same way.

Prednisolone tablets. I always use the EC version, with some form of gastric protection*, 40-50mg daily, with no need to tail off if given for up to a week.

*PPI or H2 antagonist

Hydrocortisone 100mg IV can be given as an adjunct as the oral steroids. Orally, steroids will take several hours to kick in and even the IV steroids will take a few hours to have an effect.

Nebulised:

Salbutamol 2.5-5mg nebulised over 5-10 minutes. Make sure your nebuliser works efficiently. The patient's may not.

And Ipratropium 250-500ug should be given instead of the MDI and spacer if the patient is significantly unwell. Don't forget that the effect of inhaled drugs can be as short as an hour or two and have no concerns about increasing the frequency of the patient's regular inhaled medication to hourly or more initially – as long as you can trust them to recognise when things are going wrong.

Aminophylline. Still a useful, last try IV treatment in severe asthma (If the patient not taking oral theophylline) 5mg/kg (all ages) to a max 250-500mg over 20 mins +.

Oxygen, 40-60% by mask.

Life threatening asthma is indicated by a silent chest, cyanosis, poor respiratory effort, exhaustion, bradycardia and hypotension, PEFR <33% expected. Dial 999 and then give the nebuliser, oxygen, adrenaline and if you can, be prepared to intubate the patient (these chests feel rigid to the ambubag and mask or to your cuffed tube if the patient collapses and you have to intubate them).

Pneumothorax:

Most pneumothoraces are benign and resolve on their own (Primary spontaneous pneumothorax) and whether you send these patients to hospital depends on the state of the patient and the likely cause. It is the **tension** pneumothorax that becomes life threatening.

Usually in my experience, the patient is a tall male though not necessarily suffering from Marfan's Syndrome, often a smoker. There are tachycardia and tachypnoea, reduced breath sounds on the affected side as well as a resonant percussion note over the affected side of the chest and on the sternum – and possibly a visibly deviated trachea and apex beat. There can be hypoxia and cyanosis. These patients need X Rays and referral.

A secondary spontaneous pneumothorax occurs in a number of conditions, COPD, cystic fibrosis, asthma, infections, Marfan's, rheumatoid, sarcoid, A.S., cancer etc.

The diagnosis and extent are usually confirmed by X Ray if available and there is time. Then a wide bore needle inserted (above the rib below, the 2nd IC space above the 3rd rib in the mid clavicular line) or (4th-6th space in the midaxillary line). This applies to larger pnemothoraces and to the **tension pneumothorax** with the a chest drain then attached to a valve.

Infection:

Benzyl Penicillin 600mg IV for any suspicion of Meningococcal infection (with IV Hydrocortisone,

after a venous sample has been aspirated for culture and sent in a syringe

with the patient). Under 1 year 300mg.

Cefotaxime 1Gr IV/IM is an alternative (if allergic to penicillin). Children up to 12yrs 50mg/kg or even

Chloramphenicol 12.5-25mg/kg IV (Adults and children).

Diabetes:

Hypoglycaemia, (is usually defined as a BG<4mmol/li)

you can try hypostop or other forms of glucose including honey but

Intravenous Glucose 50mls IV of 20%

or 25mls IV of 50%

are always effective,

and in children: 10% 5 mls/kg IV

as is

Glucagon 1mg SC IM or IV in an adult if there is glycogen in the liver to be broken down and released

and in children 0-1m 20ug/kg IM

1m-2yrs 500ug IV

2-18 yrs <20kg Rx 500ug, >20Kg Rx 1mg

Ketoacidosis (Glucose and ketones in the urine) BG usually but not always >25mmol/li. In insulin dependent patients.

Usually the patient smells ketotic and has polydipsia, polyuria, is weak and has nausea and vomiting. There can be confusion, abdominal pain and failing consciousness.

These patients need to be admitted, preferably with some Normal saline running IV if you carry it.

Hyperglycaemic hyperosmolar non ketotic coma occurs in non insulin dependent diabetics with a coexistent illness, infection, MI or CVA. It can develop slowly. There is dehydration, coma and hyperglycaemia and may be the first sign in that patient of developing diabetes. Some drug treatments make the risk of coma worse and these include phenytoin, propranolol, cimetidine, various diuretics, steroids and chlorpromazine.

Psychiatric Emergencies:

If you are worried about personal risk when requested to visit a disturbed psychiatric patient you can always ask for police escort although this has to be finely judged and can inflame some situations. A few years ago I was accompanied by two police officers to the home of a psychotic patient after a report of bizarre nocturnal behaviour from a neighbour. We discovered her dead and decomposing husband in the living room but it was me who noticed the hatchet at her filthy bedside and within arm's reach as I was examining her.

Given the sparse and inaccessible out of hours psychiatry in the modern NHS, pharmaceutical emergency psychiatry is essential.

Haloperidol Tablets 1.5mg up to 5mg orally or 2-10mg of injection (5mg/ml) for severe anxiety and distress or for malignant vomiting.

Lorazepam 1mg 1-2 tabs orally or 1-2mg injection (4mg/ml) IM for the same indications.

Agitated, disturbed or violent patients:
Diazepam 10mg slowly IV.
Midazolam 2.5-10mg IV.
Chlorpromazine 25-50mg deep IM.

Benzodiazepine respiratory depression is reversed by
Flumazenil 200ug IV over 15 secs, then repeated as necessary.

Dystonic reactions/oculogyric crises etc to any of these drugs can be reversed by Procyclidine 5-10mg IM repeat dose after 20 minutes (Children 2-12 years 2-5mg, <2 years 0.5-2mg).

Convulsions:

Lorazepam injection 4mg/ml. 4mg IV for status epilepticus or
Diazepam IV or rectally 500ug/kg up to 30mg.
Midazolam 5mg/ml. 2mls buccally.

Bleeding:

N Saline (0.9%) and a set of Venflons/cannulae with a giving set is a good start.

Syntometrine (Ergometrine and Oxytocin) 1ml IM not IV can stop gynaecological bleeding but is more heat sensitive than most emergency drugs and the car boot is a highly labile thermal environment.

Anaphylaxis:

After food the reaction is usually 30-35 minutes, after a sting 10-15 minutes, after

IV drugs, about 5 minutes.

Again this is an example where the GP most definitely **is** an emergency service and can get to the patient and save a life waiting for the ambulance to arrive. All the following drugs should be in all our bags on every visit and IN DATE. But if they are out of date give them anyway. What have you got to lose?, drug expiry dates are notoriously conservative.

Elevate the feet.

Adrenaline 1mg/ml 1:1,000 IM or SC ½-1ml. (It can be diluted and given very slowly IV) Repeat at 5 minute intervals depending on BP response.

Child: <6m Adrenaline 1:1000 0.05mls (50ug) IM (or 0.5ml of 1:10,000)

6m-6yrs   0.12mls (120ug) IM

6-12 yrs   0.25mls (250ug) IM

All can be repeated at 5 minute intervals, ideally starting IV fluids if this is necessary.

If the patient is shocked then **IV** Adrenaline should be given as the muscles will not be properly perfused.

The doses of Adrenaline IV are: Adult: 100ug/min for 5mins (1ml of 1:10,000/min IV)

Child: 10ug/kg over several minutes (0.1ml/kg of 1:10,000 IV)

Oxygen (If you have it)

Chlorpheniramine 10mg/ml 10-20mg IM/SC/IV. Children <12 yrs 250ug/kg up to 10mg IM or slow IV

Hydrocortisone 100mg – 500mg IM or IV in an adult

Child: <1yr 2-4mg/kg)

1-6yrs 50mg)

6-12yrs 100mg) all IM or slow IV

Nebulised Salbutamol

IV Fluids if necessary

Death is almost never later than 6 hours after exposure so observe for this long in adults but for 24 hours in children.

Of the 20 deaths a year, the majority have Asthma.

Shock: Treatment:

Give 20mls Sodium Chloride/Kg over 5-10 minutes, can repeat twice with Albumen 4.5% Soln.

Toxic Shock;

Is caused by the Staphylococcus Aureus or Streptococcus Pyogenes toxins. The symptoms mimic many other conditions and are fever, malaise, diarrhoea and vomiting, myalgia, confusion and erythema of mucous membranes. There is a rapid deterioration to shock and organ failure (renal, hepatic and also thrombocytopoenia). There is an erythematous "sunburn" rash which much later desquamates.

If suspected, the patient must be admitted and given broad spectrum antibiotics before the ambulance arrives, IV. You obviously carry Benzyl Penicillin but you should also carry an injectable broad spectrum non penicillin antibiotic for the penicillin allergic patient you may suspect has meningitis. I carry Cefuroxime. The hospital treatment will involve a combination of various antibiotics: cephalosporins, penicillins, vancomycin, clindamycin, or gentamicin. I have often wondered whether the latter might be a better alternative to a broad spectrum penicillin for my bag and why it is spelt differently to the others.

Poisoning (Toxbase website or National Poisons Information Service, 0870 600 6266)
Remove yourself and the patient from noxious gas etc.

Treat shock, assess the need for resuscitation, give Oxygen if available, assess blood sugar, if opiates are suspected try Naloxone.

Coma:

Possible causes:
Drugs/toxins/poisons: From CO to controlled drugs, hypnotics and sedatives.

Metabolic/Endocrine: Hypo/hyperglycaemia, hypothyroidism, hypothermia, hepatic, renal, pituitary failure.

CNS pressure: Cerebral oedema, hydrocephalus, encephalitis, meningitis etc.

CNS injury: Concussion, fractures, haematomata.

Vascular: CVA including SAH, cardiac failure, shock.

Epilepsy: Including post ictal state.

Infection: Meningitis, encephalitis, septicaemia, infection elsewhere (pneumonia etc).

Respiratory failure.

The investigations and treatment need to be hospital based provided you have enough knowledge of the patient and the prognosis that this is in their best interests. While waiting you should perform a basic examination (exclude purpuric rash, hypoglycaemia, high or low temperature, assess BP and CVS, RS, pupils, reflexes, plantars etc). The Glasgow Coma Score is:

Glasgow Coma Score: GCS
(Max 15 is healthy)
Eye opening:
Spontaneously 4
To speech 3
To pain 2
None 1
Verbal response:
Orientated 5
Confused 4
Inappropriate 3
Incomprehensible 2
None 1
Motor Response:
Obeys commands 6
Localises to pain 5
Withdraws from pain 4
Flexion to pain 3
Extension to pain 2
None 1

PAEDIATRIC NORMAL VALUES

PEAK EXPIRATORY FLOW RATE

For use with EU / EN13826 scale PEF meters only

Height (m)	Height (ft)	Predicted EU PEFR (L/min)	Height (m)	Height (ft)	Predicted EU PEFR (L/min)
0.85	2'9"	87	1.30	4'3"	212
0.90	2'11"	95	1.35	4'5"	233
0.95	3'1"	104	1.40	4'7"	254
1.00	3'3"	115	1.45	4'9"	276
1.05	3'5"	127	1.50	4'11	299
1.10	3'7"	141	1.55	5'1	323
1.15	3'9"	157	1.60	5'3"	346
1.20	3'11"	174	1.65	5'5"	370
1.25	4'1"	192	1.70	5'7"	393

Normal PEF values in children correlate best with height; with increasing age, larger differences occur between the sexes. These predicted values are based on the formulae given in Lung Function by J.E. Cotes (Fourth Edition), adapted for EU scale Mini-Wright peak flow meters by Clement Clarke. Date of preparation – 7th October 2004

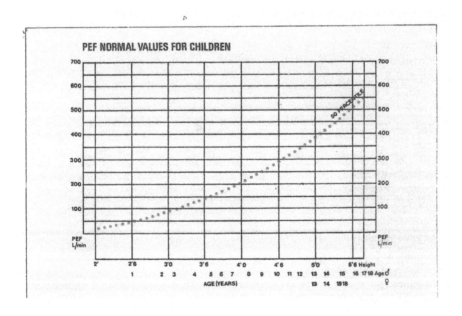

My thanks to Clement Clarke and Allen and Hanburys.

PEAK EXPIRATORY FLOW RATE - NORMAL VALUES
For use with EU/EN13826 scale PEF meters only

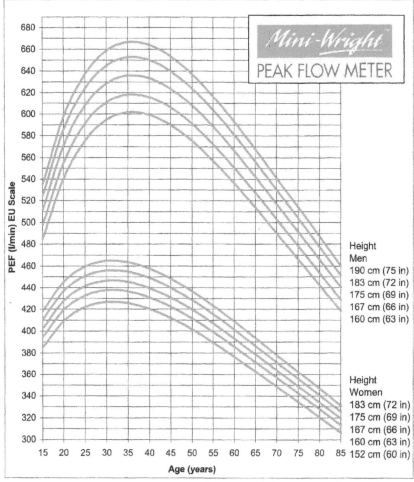

Adapted by Clement Clarke for use with EN13826 / EU scale peak flow meters from Nunn AJ Gregg I, Br Med J 1989:298;1068-70

DIAGRAM (PFV 1, PFV 2, PFV3) (includes adults)

Diagram X3 PFV2 and PFV1, PFV3

Children:

Asthma:

A sick child with asthma will have: A RR>40/min (>50/min if under 5 years of age), be too wheezy to complete sentences or feed, if older, have a PEFR <50% expected. They will be distressed or the opposite (floppy, weak, quiet and hypotonic) and have a hierarchy of recession and accessory muscles in use. There may be some intercostal and supraclavicular recession to start with and sternomastoids working hard, tripod posture or see saw respiration finally.

Treatment:

Salbutamol or Terbutaline MDI via a spacer device one puff breathed every 30 seconds X 10 puffs.

Repeat this every 20-30 minutes. Or

Nebulised Salbutamol 2.5mg or Terbutaline 5mg plus

Nebulised Ipratropium 125-250ug.

It is hard to imagine you can do any significant harm to a very sick asthmatic child by giving more than the above number of nebulised doses.

Prednisolone orally 5mg Sol tabs (disguise in juice) 1-2mg/kg or

IV hydrocortisone 4mg/kg (over at least a minute) – even the IV hydrocortisone will take an hour or two to work and the mainstay of the initial relief is frequent repeated nebulised medication.

Give oxygen, aiming for better than 92% saturation.

Croup:

Prednisolone 1-2mg/kg or

Dexamethasone 2mg/5mls oral soln, 150ug/kg.

Nebulised Adrenaline 1 in 1000 (1mg/ml) (400ug/kg, max 5mg.) Dilute in sterile saline and remember the effects only last 3 hours.

Even nebulised nasal decongestant drops (Xylometazoline, etc.) can work if you find you have run out of adrenaline and the ambulance hasn't arrived.

Infection:

Benzyl Penicillin in serious infections and where meningococcal infections are suspected: IV preferably,

<1yr 300mg

1-9 yrs 600mg

>10 years 1.2gr

Cefotaxime is an alternative

50mg/kg up to 12 yrs

1gr >12yrs as is

Chloramphenicol 12.5-25mg/kg

Diabetes: Hypoglycaemia

10-20gr glucose orally (a teaspoon of sugar is 5gr), hypostop/glucogel orally or

Glucagon 1mg/ml

<1m 20ug/kg

1m-2yrs 500ug

2-18yrs 0.5-1mg SC IM or IV plus or minus

Glucose 2-5mls/kg 10% I.V.

Convulsions:

Diazepam rectally <1m 1.25-2.5mg

1m-2yrs 5mg

2-12 yrs 5-10mg

12-18 yrs 10mg repeated after 5mins if necessary
Midazolam 5mg/ml 2mls can be given sublingually
<6m 300ug/kg
6m-1yr 2.5mg
1-5yrs 5mg
5-10yrs 7.5mg
10-18yrs 10mg

Analgesia:

The parents will presumably have given paracetamol and or ibuprofen (one hopes) to children. There is good evidence that doctors in the community and in hospitals under treat severe pain in childhood. I have used all strengths of soluble Co Codamol as well as codeine in children. (Don't forget to give lactulose or similar) as well as controlled drugs for more severe pain.

Morphine Injection 10mg/ml or oral solution 10mg/5ml can be used for severe pain
1-12m 200ug/kg 6hrly
1-5 yrs 2.5-5mg 4hrly
5-12 yrs 5-10mg
12-18yrs 10mg
as can
Diamorphine injection 10mg
1-3m 20ug/kg
3-6m 25-50ug/kg (both 6 hrly)
6-12m 75ug/kg
1-12yrs 75-100ug/kg
12-18yrs 2.5-5mg-10mg 4hrly
Naloxone 400ug/ml is used to antagonise opioid overdose,

1m-12yrs 10ug/kg then 100ug/kg if there is no response up to at 12-18 yrs 2mg repeated every 2-3 minutes. I don't know any GP who carries enough Naloxone to keep this going for long so be prepared to support the child's respiration and get it to hospital quickly if you have to use significant amounts of Naloxone in anger.

Nausea and vomiting:

Used as a last resort in children where fluid replacement is more important.

Domperidone tabs, liquid and supps cause less dystonia than Metoclopramide and Prochlorperazine
Prochlorperazine 12.5mg/ml, 5mg and 25mg supps, 5mg tabs
2-5 yrs 1.25-2.5mg
5-12yrs 5 – 6.25mg
12-18yrs 12.5mg
Cyclizine 50mg/ml,
1m-18yrs 0.5-1mg/kg (though not actually licensed in children)

Dystonic reactions (oculogyric crises etc) can be treated with
Procyclidine 5mg/ml IM or IV
<2 yrs 0.5-2mg
2-10yrs 2-5mg
10-18yrs 5-10mg

Other Paediatric Emergencies:

Acute Meningitis:

Meningococcal Meningitis:

Rx: 50mg/kg Penicillin G (Benzyl Penicillin)
Immediate Rx >10yrs 1.2Gr Penicillin
1-10yrs 600mg
Infant 300mg Stat. IV if possible, deep IM if not.

If genuinely allergic to penicillin, IV Chloramphenicol can be given. I carry Cefuroxime as the wait to get a purpuric child to hospital for IV second line antibiotics is worth the miniscule risk of cross allergy to cephalosporins. Of people who think they are allergic to penicillin only 10% actually are and of these, only 5-10% have a cross-reaction to cephalosporins. Meningococcal meningitis kills within minutes and whenever I have seen a drowsy or febrile child with a purpuric rash I have taken blood into a syringe, put the Penicillin back through the same needle followed by a bolus of Hydrocortisone. If they die, they die of septicaemia and adrenal shock. The Paediatric SHO will put the blood sample in a blood culture bottle if he knows what he is doing or a sharps bin if he doesn't. Dial 999 first, don't bother waiting for the interminable switchboard and registrar to answer the phone and bleep before you have transport organised. Make sure ambulance control knows it is a blue light call out.

That was Acute Medicine. What are the main Chronic Conditions in the NHS?

Cancer, heart disease, strokes, diabetes, dementia, obesity, arthritis, COPD, hypertension, mental ill health, epilepsy, asthma and substance abuse. 15 million patients in England have a chronic condition and this number will double in the next 20 years (Government statement 2016). 50% of GP appointments, 64% of OP appointments and 70% of in-patient beds are already taken up by patients with these chronic conditions.

5: ALCOHOL: (SEE PSYCHIATRY AND SLEEP SECTION)

Note: 8 grms alcohol (actually 7.9 grms) = 1U= 10mls.
A 750ml bottle of wine contains 736 grapes, about 750 calories 2.6lbs of fruit (1.18kg).
1ml of wine = 1 calorie !
85% of us drink alcohol at least occasionally. On average, 11.6 Li of pure alcohol a year. Alcohol is said to cost £21Bn a year in alcohol related crime, policing, NHS costs and lost productivity. At least £3.5Bn is NHS cost. 70% of casualty attendances are alcohol related at weekends.

3m people are said to die prematurely globally due to alcohol consumption and it is a leading cause of death in 16-50 year old males in the UK.

Recent "sensible" drinking limits for years were:
<21Us/week men,
<14us/week women.

But these have been revised and adjusted so often that few people take much notice of them.

These safe drinking limits were introduced in 1987, revised in 1995 and again by different agencies at various times, most recently by the government in 2016. The current "**Low risk daily guidelines**" were, until 2016 that men shouldn't exceed a daily intake of 3-4 units and women 2-3 units. These have been widely criticised and also, it has to be said, ignored.

The newest revised guidelines (Jan 2016) were that neither men nor women drink more than 3 us daily and that each have two days a week alcohol free. I wonder whether expectation of compliance with these guidelines is just as overoptimistic as with the guidelines of the past. They are sure to be just as ignored by large numbers of our younger fellow citizens.

It was announced in March 2016 that 9% of our community, mainly young men, drink their week's allowance in one day, – Actually I would think on **each** of **two** evenings a week. That is only about 7 pints after all. Given the revelation at almost the same time that most weekend A and E attendances are "alcohol related" these sort of guidelines seem destined to be ignored by 18-30 year olds.

It is quite fiddly working out how many units are present in drinks:
This is from the **Change for Life website (DoH):** (with thanks)

Glass of red, white or rose wine **(ABV 13%)**

Small 125ml

1.6 units

Standard 175ml

2.3 units

Large 250ml

3.3 units

750ml bottle of red, white or rose wine **(ABV 13.5%)**

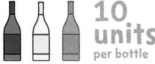

10 **units** per bottle

Beer, lager and cider
Regular (ABV 4%)

1.8 units   2.3 units

Strong (ABV 5.2%)

2.2 units   3 units

Extra strong (ABV 8%)

3.5 units   4.5 units

Other drinks (ABV varies)
25ml single spirit and mixer
(ABV 40%)
1 unit

275ml bottle of alcopop
(ABV 5.5%)
1.5 units

Beer is 3.5%-5% generally, spirits 40%, wine 11-13% alcohol but there are stronger examples of all of them.

For example:

A bottle of Sainsbury's House Montepulciano d'Abruzzo is only 12.5% vol. alcohol – a relatively weak red wine. Each 125ml glass is 92kcal and 1.6us alcohol. There being 6 glasses and 9.4 us per 750ml bottle.

Driving:

In most of the UK the legal alcohol limit for drivers is 80mg alcohol/100mls blood, 35ug/100mls breath or 107mg/100mls urine. It is less in most other European countries.

Scotland changed its legal alcohol driving level from 80mg % to 50mg % in 2014 and there is some debate about the rest of the kingdom following. This means that in "some circumstances" you would be over the limit after one pint of beer.

So, Current UK government consumption recommendations: (2015/16)

	Female	Male
Low risk	New 14 Old 15 Us	New 14 Old<20 Us/week
Old Moderate Risk	16-35 Us	21-50 Us
Old High Risk	>35 Us	>50 Us

Your advice on drinking will depend partly on what **you** believe to be safe given the constantly conflicting epidemiological evidence on alcohol. Also whether you think that your patient is likely to dismiss the very low guidelines as unrealistic and therefore just drink whatever he or she wants.

In the review of the previous year's drinking habits published in 2013 as part of the Opinions and Lifestyle Survey there were some slightly surprising findings: It is the young and smokers who drink heavily but the old drink frequently and consistently. Perhaps it is worth remembering this when an elderly patient complains of waking in the early hours (alcohol is a short acting sedative) or daytime somnolence. The social gatherings of the well off elderly seem to revolve around the consumption of significant amounts of alcohol but then again at their age, as long as their LFTs are normal, they are not driving or behaving antisocially, what other pleasures do they have?

Anyway, 58% of adults (people aged 16 and over) living in private households in Great Britain drank alcohol at least once in the week before being interviewed. This proportion has been declining both for men and women. Between 2005 and 2012 the proportion of men who drank alcohol in the week before being interviewed fell from 72% to 64%, and the proportion of women fell from 57% to 52%.

The proportion of adults who drank frequently (those who drank alcohol on at least five days in the week before being interviewed) has also been declining. Between 2005 and 2012 there was a fall from 22% to 14% in the proportion of men who were frequent drinkers – and from 13% to 9% in the proportion of women. In 2012 people aged 65 and over were most likely to have drunk frequently, both for men (23%) and women (14%).

Young people (those aged 16-24) were more likely to have drunk very heavily (more than 12 units for men and 9 units for women) at least once during the week (27%), with similar proportions for men (26%) and women (28%). Only 3% of those aged 65 and over were very heavy drinkers.

Smokers (25%) were more than twice as likely as non-smokers (11%) to have drunk very heavily at least once during the week.

On an average list, 200 patients are at intermediate risk, 55 patients are at high risk.

Blood Tests: GGT and MCV: – if both are raised they show you 62% of your alcoholics -also check the AST.

Although the Mediterranean paradox of long life despite an excess of saturated fat and smoking was said to be in part due to red wine, newer research suggests that moderate amounts of white wine are good for your general health as well but only if regular aerobic exercise is also part of the lifestyle. White wine does not contain the same high levels of antioxidants that most reds do and would therefore not be expected to protect against cancer. Procyanidins and Resveratrol in red wine have beneficial effects in a variety of ways, inducing cancer cell apoptosis, mitochondrial protection, "free radical chain reactions" and promoting resistance to radiation injury etc. Many of these protective properties are shared by red and blue coloured fruits and vegetables.

If there is severe dependency or biochemical damage there is no alternative to complete alcohol abstinence.

There are various detoxification regimes (see psychiatry section), the most traditional consists of high dose vitamins with Chlordiazepoxide or Carbamazepine or Clomethiazole (Heminevrin). Haloperidol or Olanzapine can be used as an add-on to the foregoing.

Alcohol withdrawal:

Diazepam, Lorazepam, Chlordiazepoxide, can be used at home in a slowly reducing regime. Plus or minus anti psychotics such as Haloperidol or Olanzapine if necessary. Sometimes you can be reluctantly forced into supervising an alcohol withdrawal at home as the least worst option in someone who convinces you they are now motivated to change, refuses to engage with secondary care and (most importantly) has a sensible and caring person living at home with them. Chloral Hydrate reduces some life threatening side effects, Carbamazepine or Topiramate can be used as anti convulsants. Clomethiazole, Heminevrin is still helpful as an adjunct sedative with or instead of benzodiazepines.

Other alternatives are Gabapentin and Baclofen (the latter in a highly variable dosage regime with very variable side effects and response rates).

I use Chlorpromazine or Chlordiazepoxide over 7-10 days. Stop all alcohol on the first day.

Thus:

Chlordiazepoxide 5-10mg (up to 15-20mg) 3-4X daily, slowly reducing.

Community detoxification should last 7-10 days and preferably be supervised by a motivated friend, partner, loved one, as well as you. You don't have to visit them every day but they do need someone else in attendance or close at hand who is sober of habit as well as sober – and you should probably phone daily at first and see them again at least on the last day (and a few weeks after at the surgery).

There is, of course, a small risk of Wernicke's Encephalopathy (the triad of opthalmoplegia, ataxia, and confusion and usually asthenia as well) (+/-Korsakoff psychosis) which can be prevented by supplementing Vitamin B1. Oral absorption is unpredictable so give big doses of B1 systemically, other B vitamins and Vitamin C, preferably a few days before detox begins. **Ideally** the B1 should be given **IM 250mg** Thiamine daily 3-5 days before or during the process.

Treat other symptoms of withdrawal, anxiety, hallucinations, confusion, diarrhoea, hyperthermia, nausea, headache, palpitations, tachycardia, tremors, paranoia, with Haloperidol, Heminevrin, Lomotil, beta blockers, increased doses of benzodiazepines etc.

Wernicke's Encephalopathy may prompt Korsakoff's Syndrome: poor memory, confabulation, confusion and change in personality. Wernicke's Encephalopathy may also follow Bariatric surgery.

Maintaining abstinence:

Antabuse: Disulfiram 200mg tabs. Initially 4 stat, then 3 on second day, 2, 2, then 1 daily, review regularly especially after 6 months. Any alcohol drunk is metabolised to acetaldehyde which causes the unpleasant symptoms. Avoid in pregnancy and avoid with Metronidazole. Up to 50% users remain abstinent.

Topiramate

Up to 75mg/day after detox.

Naltrexone

Opioid blocker (stops pain killers working) 6 month course. (Interestingly Low dose Naltrexone is an active anti cancer treatment used to treat various cancers by legitimate alternative cancer therapists – and does seem to work).

Acamprosate, Campral A Centrally acting stimulator of GABA receptors and a modifier of Glutamate levels, (which surge in concentration within the brain on alcohol withdrawal) this reduces the adverse effects of alcohol withdrawal and abstinence.

Nalmefene, Selincro. Has gained NICE approval (Oct 2014) "In conjunction with continuous psychosocial support" (whatever that is) for patients considered to have mild alcohol dependence and a high drinking level. This drug is intended for high risk patients (Daily consumption >60gr or 7.5Us for men or 40gr, 5Us for women). Overall, the drug, plus the support, adds up to a daily reduction of consumption of only 1.8Us per day.

There are various excellent community support agencies which include Alcoholics anonymous, Al Anon (friends and families of problem drinkers), Al Ateen (young Al Anon members, usually teenagers), Turning point (a national Charity with various support services).

Benefits of alcohol:

Combined with the CETP genome, alcohol beneficially affects HDL and if it also contains antioxidants such as those in red wine (etc) it may contribute to the Mediterranean paradox. A study was published in July 2017 (Diabetalogica J Tolstrup et Al) that showed a lower risk of diabetes (27% lower in men and 32% lower in women) in drinkers compared with abstainers. Wine was most beneficial and gin may have had the reverse effect. This was up to a weekly limit of 14Us in men and 9Us in women.

Carcinogenicity:

There is epidemiological evidence that alcohol contributes to cancer of the oropharynx, larynx, oesophagus, liver, colon, rectum and female breast.

6: ALLERGY:

What you may have forgotten:

Types of Allergic (Hypersensitivity) Reactions:

Type 1: Immediate or anaphylactic, includes contact urticaria, asthma, acute gut reactions etc. IgE. Within a few minutes, the anaphylactic response can be food (etc) related, histamine and mast cells involved.

Type 2: "Cytotoxic hypersensitivity". Also immediate, limited to cell membrane. Results in local damage, follows binding of IgG, IgM and complement activation. eg Drug induced haemolytic anaemia.

Type 3: "Immune complex hypersensitivity" Late reactions, immune complexes, IgG, IgM, complement system, involves skin and bronchi. eg Rh A, Serum Sickness, PAN etc.

Type 4: Allergic contact dermatitis, cell mediated 24-48 hrs after exposure. Delayed hypersensitivity. eg Tuberculin reaction. T lymphocytes in the atopic. Immune system memory, chronic inflammatory reaction and tissue damage.

T cells provide cellular immunity, antibodies attaching to the cells, (activated T cells).

B cells provide humoral immunity, producing the circulating antibodies.

The HLA system is genetically controlled by the 6th chromosome.

Asthma and hay fever are "on" chromosome 11 and active if inherited from the mother rather than the father.

Children who suck their thumbs and bite their nails are less likely to suffer sensitisation to common allergens as teenagers and adults than their peers. Asthma and hay fever are unaffected.

More evidence that cleanliness most definitely is not next to Godliness and for the hygiene hypothesis.

Useful Drugs:

Topical: Nose:

Antihistamine: Azelastine. Rhinolast nasal spray.
Mast Cell Stabiliser: Sodium cromoglicate, Rynacrom spray.
Anticholinergics. Ipratropium, Rinatec spray.
Steroids: Beconase, Rhinacort, Syntaris, Flixonase, Avamys, Nasonex, Nasacort,

Eyes:

Antihistamine: Azelastine, Optilast. Emedastine, Emadine.
Mast Cell stabilisers (etc) Ketotifen, Zaditen. Lodoxamide, Alomide. Nedocromil, Rapitil. Olopatadine, Opatanol. – and good old Sodium Cromoglicate, Opticrom.

Anaphylaxis:

Symptoms: Urticaria, pruritus, flushing, angio-oedema, dyspnoea, wheezing, stridor, hoarseness, dysphagia, dyspnoea, tachycardia, hypotension, sometimes coronary ischemia, shock, abdominal pain, anxiety etc.

There are said to be 20-30 deaths a year from anaphylaxis in the UK – that is roughly one every GP every 1000 years this includes about ten of these from peanuts. I would imagine, having given adrenaline for severe allergic symptoms a dozen or more times in the last thirty years, I have either been over diagnosing and treating anaphylaxis or have been heroically contributing to the remarkable low risk of dying of allergy in this country. Half of anaphylactic deaths are iatrogenic and a quarter each due to food or insect venom. This is obviously where GPs ARE an emergency service and you need to have some proper drugs with you at all times-in real anaphylaxis you will usually be able to get to the patient before the ambulance and that *might* be a matter of life and death.

Treatment:

Adrenaline: Adults: 0.3 – 1.0ml 1:1000 soln.
Children: 0.01ml/kg.
ie: I. M. Adrenaline 1 in 1000, adult and child >12 yrs 0.5mls, child 6-12 yrs 0.3mls and child <6 yrs 0.15ml
Auto devices:
Epipen Adults (>30kg) 300ug children 150ug
Jext: Adults (>30kg) 300ug children 150ug
For all: Give IM into antero-lateral thigh, repeat after 5-15mins if necessary. The effect of Epipens is said to last only 20 minutes.

A dose of Adrenaline can be given I.V. if shocked or if treatment is significantly delayed (3-5ml of 1:10,000 solution) If you know the patient is on a Tricyclic antidepressant, reduce the dose to one sixth. I always give IV Chlorpheniramine 10mg and Hydrocortisone 100mg at the same time. These are all drugs every GP worth the name with have, IN DATE, in his/her bag. 10% patients require a second dose of Adrenaline. You can give Glucagon as an inotropic to patients on Beta Blockers. Of the children who die of anaphylaxis up to 90% have a history of asthma.

Antihistamines:

Things you might have forgotten:

Histamine is secreted by all sorts of tissues, especially lung, skin and gut. Often the mechanism is that IgE binds to mast cells and the cell then releases histamine. Histamine thus plays a role in acute and delayed hypersensitivity reactions. We are all familiar with the flare and wheal skin reaction, angio – neurotic oedema and at the other extreme, anaphylaxis. Histamine causes some of these via vasodilatation and increased vascular permeability but other symptoms include itching, sweating, diarrhoea, headache, wheeze, flushing and vomiting.

Histamine is a also CNS neurotransmitter, it stimulates gastric acid secretion, it affects smooth muscle – it bronchoconstricts and vasodilates as well.

Histamine Receptors:

H1 Smooth muscle, endothelial cells	Acute allergic responses,
H2 Gastric parietal cells	Secretion of gastric acid,
H3 CNS	Neurotransmission,
H4 Mast cells, eosinophils, T cells, dendritic cells	Immune response.

So now you can see why Chlorpheniramine makes you tired, over the counter sleeping pills are antihistamines and why patients with severe itching and urticaria often do better on Cetirizine and Ranitidine together.

Antihistamines:

Sedative:

Hydroxyzine, Atarax 25mg nocte initially increasing to qds for acute and chronic dermatoses.

Cyproheptadine, Periactin 4mg tds initially. Clemastine, Tavegil. Ketotifen, Zaditen 1mg BD.

Alimemazine (Trimeprazine, which we all used to know as **Vallergan***).

Chlorpheniramine, (Piriton), Promethazine – **Phenergan***.

*These are the tradition treatments – or Chloral, for the endlessly nocturnally unsettled and screaming BUT WELL baby and the desperate mother. Use common sense, regular supervision, a Health Visitor if you have one and a defined time limit. But never say never to prescribing them.

"Non sedative":

Loratadine, Clarityn 10mg od. But sometimes you need a temporary bigger dose, (adults). OK for children>2yrs.

Desloratadine. The predictably named Neoclarityn. Adult dose 5mg, OK for children>2yrs. A "me as well" drug.

Cetirizine 10mg, Zirtek OK for children >2yrs.

Levocetirizine, Xyzal, (you'd have thought Neozirtek) 5mg OK for children >2yrs A "me as well" drug, as well.

Fexofenadine, Telfast. 120mg and 180mg (for chronic idiopathic urticaria).

Also Mizolastine, Mizollen 10mg and Rupatadine Rupafin 10mg (which will both no doubt appear in a Levo or Des form at a 5mg dose once the initial patent expires).

The latter is advocated for chronic idiopathic urticaria and allergic rhinitis – avoid with grapefruit juice, or you can try Ranitidine and the higher dose of Fexofenadine (Telfast 180) in the daytime plus Hydroxyzine (Atarax) at night.

Also Nalcrom which is Sodium Cromoglicate, the mast cell stabiliser 100mg 2 qds for food allergies.

Sledgehammer:

Systemic Steroids: such as:

Triamcinolone, Kenalog 40-100mg (deep) IM (40mg/ml) Gives relief from most symptoms of hay fever for 6-12 weeks and usually actually has few side effects.

Peanut Allergy:

One of the commonest allergies in childhood. Some allergy specialists recommend that pregnant mothers avoid eating peanut containing products during pregnancy to reduce the risk of sensitising their baby in highly atopic families and atopic children avoid them until age 3. Conversely "Level 1 scientific evidence from the LEAP trial" showed that we should recommend the introduction of peanut containing foods into the diet of high risk children between 4 and 11 months in countries with prevalent peanut allergy. Delaying the introduction "can be associated with and increased risk of peanut allergy". The ubiquitous refined peanut oil (arachis oil) was not thought to be generally allergenic because the protein was denatured by heating. That was until the Cambridge Team who are now desensitising children successfully suggested sensitisation takes place not in the mother's pregnancy but through the eczema damaged skin of babies via arachis and soya oils used in eczema creams. Gradually increasing doses of peanut flour did desensitise children from age 7-16 in one Cambridge paper (Lancet 30/1/14). Further research (Feb 2015) has suggested that the "1:50 children in the UK with a peanut allergy" can reduce the incidence 80% by regular consumption of peanut products before the age of 5 years. They suggest a peanut skin prick test be performed in the presence of eczema. If there is early reactivity then you have missed the boat and the oral desensitisation will not work.

Oral Allergy Syndrome:

The most common form of food allergy in adults.

The usual symptoms are swelling of the mouth, lips, throat and tongue after eating certain foods. This is in patients who suffer hay fever and their allergy to pollen cross reacts with certain food proteins as well.

Cooking or heating the foods reduces the reaction as the proteins are denatured somewhat.

The commonest primary allergen is birch pollen but grass and mugwort pollen as well as an allergy to latex can be amongst the underlying sensitivities. The symptoms are a redness, swelling and itching of the mouth and occasionally a rash on the lips and mouth, sometimes heartburn after eating certain (mainly raw) fruits and vegetables. Generalised symptoms are less common. RAST and skin prick tests are unhelpful but you can try a home-made skin prick battery using juices from uncooked fruits and vegetables. Almonds, walnuts and hazel nuts are the commonest nuts reacted to, not peanuts.

Severe reactions are very rare and O.A.S. is not generally associated with anaphylaxis or severe systemic reactions. Desensitisation does not work as yet and you may feel you need to give antihistamines for the patient to take PRN and occasionally an Adrenaline pen for reassurance. It is very unlikely to be needed.

A birch pollen reactor can suffer OAS with almond, apple, apricots, cherry, kiwi, nectarine, peaches, pear, carrot, parsley, parsnip, peppers and celery, coriander, fennel, hazelnuts. A rye pollen reactor can suffer O.A.S. with melon, tomato, peanuts. Someone who is allergic to latex can cross react and develop O.A.S. symptoms to apple, apricot, banana, cherry, figs, kiwi, mango, melon, papaya, passion fruit, peach, pear and plum. Also to almonds, chestnut, avocado, dill, ginger, sage, tomato and raw potato!

Salicylates in food:

Can contribute to acute and chronic urticaria, oral allergy, ADHD and behavioural problems in children.

The highest hidden levels are probably in asparagus, raisins, prunes, currants, dates, blueberries, raspberries, cherries, orange, curry spices, paprika, Worcestershire Sauce.

There are also high levels in:

Asparagus, currants, dates, raisins, prunes, blueberries, raspberries, oranges, cherries, aniseed, cayenne pepper, celery powder, curry powder, cinnamon, dill powder, five spice, garum m'sala, mace, mixed dried herbs, mustard, oregano powder, paprika, rosemary powder, dried sage and tarragon, turmeric, powdered thyme, Worcester sauce.

Fairly high levels in tea, coffee, apples (particularly the bitter ones like Granny Smith) other berries and citrus fruits, nectarines, dried fruits, figs, guava, grapes, kiwi, pineapple, peaches, plums, broccoli, chicory, endive, gherkins, mushroom, peppers, radish, watercress, bay leaf, chilli, cloves, ginger, mint, nutmeg, pepper, pickles, almonds, pistachios, peanuts, macadamia nuts, pine nuts, honey, liquorice, peppermint, chewing gum, wine, rum, port, cola, various liqueurs.

Somewhat less so but still present in apricot, lychees, melon, avocado, cucumber, cauliflower, onion, tinned tomato, tomato sauce, brazil nuts, walnuts, corn flour, beer, cider, sherry, preserves etc.

The Feingold Diet was an exclusion diet used for hyperactive children for decades after the war. It excluded Salicylate containing foods, foods with artificial colouring and flavouring, particularly Tartrazine, Saffron, Annato, BHT, MSG, Vanillin, barbecued food and indeed most bought and packet food. It was difficult to stick to but sometimes had dramatic positive effects.

Advice to patients allergic to house dust/mites:

House dust mites are ubiquitous in modern homes. They are 0.4mm long and live on shed epithelial cells. They produce faeces which contain an allergen called DerP1. Up to 80% of patients with severe asthma have a positive skin test to HDM allergen.

Avoid feather pillows, duvets and eiderdowns, replace them with synthetic fillings. Tell the patient to remove their under blanket (?)

Regularly vacuum the floor, the mattress, pillows, the base of the bed and divan, air the bedding and mattress. Shake the bedclothes outside every day. Bright sunshine (and microwaves) kill HDMs.

You can use a plastic cover for the top and sides of the mattress and damp dust it daily.

Once a week wash the pillow cases, sheets and under blanket, vacuum the bed base, carpet and covered mattress. Turn the mattress once a week.

Damp dust all the room surfaces at least weekly and include window sills, cupboard tops, pelmets etc. Keep the bedroom as dry as possible.

Replace woollen blankets with cotton or synthetic fibres.

Wash the curtains every so often.

Hospitals do not have carpets. Their shiny surfaces, vinyl, plastic and linoleum are easier to clean and harbour less dust.

All beds in a shared bedroom must be treated in the same way, the general house furniture should be vacuumed as well.

This may not be as clear cut as it all sounds though. There are studies that show Volatile Organic Compounds in foam and other synthetic fillings may worsen severe asthma and elsewhere I comment on the possible VOC contribution to cancer over a long period of time. Also some research has shown that feather pillows harbour no more house dust than synthetic fibres. Up to 10% of **any** pillow by weight can be HDM faeces after prolonged use!

General advice on patients with allergies:

1) Do not do allergy testing unless there is a clear trigger. The tests confirm a sensitisation and not an allergy.

2) Indication for auto-injector: Absolute is asthma or anaphylaxis, relative is nut allergy or living far away from a hospital A and E.

3) Egg allergy: MMR NOT contraindicated but should be given in hospital if anaphylactic. Can reintroduce egg at 24m. Skin prick remains positive so of no value in assessing.

4) Angioedema can affect anywhere in the patient's body. For instance, some patients may present only with abdominal pain due to oedema of the bowel. As well as allergens, trauma and infection can be triggers.

5) Rhinitis: Start treatment 2 weeks before the appropriate pollen season. Can use Kenalog or alternatively prednisolone 30mg for 1-3d to cover important events or very severe symptoms. Saline douching can work very well.

4) Urticaria: Start with non sedating antihistamine daily.

Step 2 – increase to qds if not working eg loratidine qds (try for 4-6wks before next step).
Step 3-add in leukotriene antagonist eg montelukast 10mg ON (again, try for 4-6wks).
Step 4-add in oral steroids for 1-3d.

The next step might be to refer for immunotherapy if it is available. Some of this is using the treatment off licence and this will need to be explained to the patient.
5) Document occupational allergens well, as the patient may be involved in seeking compensation.

Hay Fever: (Airborne allergens)
Early Tree Pollen: Jan/Feb/Mar: Alder, Hazel.
Mid/Late Tree Pollen: Mar/April Silver Birch
Grasses: May/Jul
Nettles and other weeds: July/Sep
Moulds persistent or intermittent, can be most of the Autumn, Winter and Spring.
More precisely: The **Pollen Callendar:**

	Jan Feb Mar Apr May Jun Jul Aug Sep Oct Nov Dec
Alder	xxxxxxxxxxxxxxxx Jan – Apr
Birch	xxxxxxxxxxxxxxx Mar-Jun
Oak	xxxxxxxxxxxxxxx Mar-Jun
Ash	xxxxxxxxxxxx Mar-May
Elm	xxxxxxxxxxx Feb-Apr
Poplar	xxxxxxx Mar-Apr
Mugwort	xxxxxxxxxxxx Jun-Sep
Grass	xxxxxxxxxxxxxxx May-Sep
Hazel	xxxxxxxxxxxxxxx Jan-Apr
Yew	xxxxxxxxxxxxxxx Jan-Apr
Willow	xxxxxxxxxxxxxx Feb-May
Oil seed rape	xxxxxxxxxxxxxxxx Mar-Jul
Pine	xxxxxxxxxxxxx Apr-Jul
Nettle	xxxxxxxxxxxxxx May-Sep

Food allergy Investigations: Exclusion Diet:

5 days of lamb (grilled, roast or cold), pears (not tinned), still spring water. Pear juice can be made with fresh pears, any salt must be pure sea salt.

Stop smoking.

On the first day a mild aperient can be taken (in the old days it was "Epsom salts" – magnesium sulphate).

Most tablets and medications include food products and should, if possible, be avoided. Don't even lick stamps or envelopes!

Teeth should be brushed with sodium bicarbonate solution.

Foods are tested in sequence, adding them in one at a time and assessing the response. Thus:

First test day: broccoli.
Second test day: plaice, fresh pineapple and turkey.
Third day: fresh tomatoes, fresh melon, grilled or roasted beef (own fat).
Fourth day: tap water, rice, cod.
Fifth day: banana, soy beans – soaked and boiled.
Sixth day: cow's milk, cabbage, chicken.

Seventh day: Indian tea, apple, yeast tablets (brewer's yeast, no vitamins).

Eighth day: butter, leeks, pork.

The more common allergens follow:

Eggs, wholemeal bread, percolated coffee, mushrooms, cane sugar (Demerara), oranges, grapes, beet sugar (packet sugar, "Silver spoon") lettuce, corn on the cob/glucose powder from maize, onion, fresh peanuts, cheddar cheese, spinach and so on. Following this list: white bread, coconut, garlic, plain chocolate (unless allergic to wheat/corn/sugars), grape-fruit, dates, courgettes or marrow, French beans, cauliflower, rye bread (may take 2 days for symptoms), black pepper, rhubarb, honey, instant coffee, (not if allergic to fresh coffee), asparagus, lemon, olive oil, parsnips, tinned carrots, (a test for allergy to the resin or these days plastic lining the tin), porridge oats, monosodium glutamate, – can be obtained in a pure form as a flavour enhancer from various supermarkets. Prawns/shrimps, Brussels sprouts, artificial sweeteners, herring, almonds, malt extract (from Boots), avocado, red/green peppers, raisins, etc.

Reactions may vary from headache to drowsiness, nausea to diarrhoea. Some people may get a tachycardia, some reactions (eg wheat) may develop a day after exposure. You can see how complicated the whole thing is and how motivated the patient has to be. Thankfully most patients, even those who are convinced they have a "food allergy" are not genuinely allergic to any food, even if they have some symptoms after eating certain foods. Serious food allergy is extremely rare (– I have never lost a patient from nut or **any** other food allergy in 40 years) and nearly all patients just eat what they find their guts and their sensitivities can tolerate.

Dirtiness in next to Godliness: The Hygiene Hypothesis

In the asthma section I mention how East German children without the benefits of Western immunisation schedules and freely available antibiotics and subject to smog and dirt had far less asthma than the pampered West Germans when the wall came down. Children who bite their nails and suck their thumbs are known to have fewer allergies.

There is a "Hygiene Hypothesis" (Strachan 1989) rooted in the finding that children brought up on farms or with pets tend to have fewer allergies and that early life exposure to bacterial lipopolysaccharide (microbial exposure beyond viruses) reduces the rate of subsequent allergic disease.

A study performed in Detroit, the Childhood Allergy Study, showed a similar effect in the urban US environment. The more dogs or cats a child had while growing up, the fewer allergies. The GABRIELA study showed less allergy with a more diverse microbiome due to greater exposures to a variety of bacteria in early life. The original hypothesis was based on the finding that the risk of hay fever diminished with more older siblings (and thus more dirt and infection at home-presumably). Children in double glazed homes have more asthma and babies who are born by Caesarean section have fewer illnesses if their faces are inoculated with their mother's vaginal secretions immediately after birth. All in all it is clear that a certain amount of dirt and infection is healthy in the development of a normal immune system, a normal microbiome and that too much cleanliness can be harmful. Western homes are much cleaner than ever before and the hypothesis is now used to explain not only the high levels of allergy but the increasing levels of disease with a possible immune component (Type 2DM, MS, IBD even Alzheimer's Disease, etc). Allergic illnesses are now being associated not only with cleanliness but double glazing, household heat efficiency and the possession of a dishwasher as well.

7: ANALGESICS:

The desire to take medicine is perhaps the greatest feature that distinguishes man from animals.

William Osler.

The clinical use of Controlled Drugs:

Terminal Care Analgesic Ladder:

Non opioids	>Weak opioids	>Strong opioids
(Usually an NSAID)	Codeine, Dipipanone, Co Proxamol,	Morphine
Paracetamol	Buprenorphine,	Diamorphine
	Diconal (Dipipanone and cyclizine)	
	Oxycodone with or w/o Naloxone (Targinact)	
	(also Oxycontin etc, Oxynorm etc)	

Terminal Care Opioid Equivalents:

Methadone Oral 20mg

Dipipanone Oral 60mg

Morphine Oral 30mg

Morphine IM 15mg

Diamorphine 10mg IM/SC

The equivalency of Morphine and extended release Oxycodone is said to be 2:1 although the latter often does not seem to be **this** potent clinically.

Interactions in solution

Diamorphine and:

High concentrations of both Cyclizine and Haloperidol may precipitate,

Hyoscine, metoclopramide, prochlorperazine (which may cause irritation given SC), are compatible,

as is the mixture with Methotrimeprazine.

Equivalent Doses: Mg

Oral Morphine		Sub Cut Morphine	Sub Cut Diamorphine		Oral Oxycodone		Sub Cut Oxycodone	
24hrs	4hrs	24hrs	24hrs	4hrs	24hrs	4hrs	24hrs	4hrs
30	5	15	10	2.5	15	2.5	7.5-10	1.25-2.5

Conversion Factors:

Oral Codeine to oral Morphine Divide by 10

Oral DHC to Oral Morphine Divide by 10

Oral Tramadol to oral Morphine Divide by 10

Oral Morphine to SC Diamorphine divide by 3

Oral Morphine to oral Oxycodone divide by 2

Oral Morphine to oral Hydromorphone divide by 7.5

Oral Morphine to SC Morphine divide by 2

Fentanyl Patches and oral Morphine Equivalents

24 Hr Oral Morphine	Fentanyl Patch (mcg/hr)
<90	25
90-134	37
135-189	50
225-314	75

315-404	100
495-584	150
675-764	200
1035-1124	300

Morphine or Diamorphine?

(Opium contains Morphine, Codeine, Dihydrocodeine, Narcotine and Papaverine btw).

Morphine

Causes more dysphoria and less euphoria (probably) than Diamorphine. It causes CNS depression, analgesia, cough suppression, vomiting and nausea, pupillary constriction, GI smooth muscle spasm, biliary spasm, bronchospasm, increased intraluminal gut pressure, constipation, dilatation of arterioles and veins, reduced sympathetic drive (as in PND and MI). It delays labour (unlike Pethidine) it is easier to titrate orally than Diamorphine as it is less water soluble. It is also less lipid soluble so has a slower onset of action systemically.

Diamorphine (Heroin, legal use is banned in the USA)

Is converted to Morphine in the body, more rapid onset by any route than Morphine, is more water and lipid soluble than Morphine, reduces pain (via pain sensation as well as ability to tolerate pain). Reduces cough (it was actually first marketed to combat the cough of TB). Causes respiratory depression through reduced sensitivity to CO_2 then to Hypoxia. Causes vasodilatation (an advantage in some clinical situations – acute LVF etc) causes convulsions in high doses. Reduces gastric motility, reduces gastric and biliary secretions, increased Sphincter of Oddi tone. Increases tone and reduces peristalsis of small and large bowel, constipates.

Less depression, less nausea, more pleasant psychic effect, fewer cardiovascular effects, twice the potency, more rapid onset than Morphine but probable effect only 3 hours IM. (25% shorter duration of effect). BUT peak levels depend a great deal on circulation, degree of shock and after an IM dose peak can be between as little as 20 to 100 minutes.

Despite it's addictive potential it does not cause addiction in acute pain situations or physical or mental decline in terminal care. No doctor should worry about abuse or habituation in cancer care.

Pethidine

Much weaker opioid receptor agonist than Morphine/Diamorphine. Causes respiratory depression and **some** smooth muscle spasm. But does not cause constipation significantly or suppress labour or cough. It IS antagonised by Naloxone. It can suppress newborn respiration. It does not increase Sphincter of Oddi contraction compared with Morphine and its relatives and is preferred for biliary and renal colic for its relatively benign smooth muscle effect.

Beneficial effects in migraine.

Naloxone

Reverses all the pharmacological effects, good and bad of Pethidine, Diamorphine and Morphine. So analgesia has to be via NSAIDs and non opiates while Naloxone still active. But Naloxone has a much shorter half life than either so another dose may be necessary *at least* an hour or two after the first in serious overdose situations. Thus reversal of severe opioid respiratory depression: Dose: 100-200mcg IV followed by 100mcg *up to every few minutes* if necessary IV until the patient is "reversed". Due to the short half life of Naloxone compared with opiates, even less severe cases may need a further dose 2hrs later. In children 10-20ug/kg IV every 2-3 mins initially. Repeat doses every hour if necessary. (But you **are** unlikely to be delivering a drug addict's baby at home).

Oxycodone and Naloxone (Targinact) Is a combination that is said to reduce constipation by a local gut activity of Naloxone. Some patients absorb Naloxone orally better than others though.

Other useful analgesics:

Paracetamol:(Acetaminophen in the US)

Analgesic, antipyretic but not anti-inflammatory.

Suppositories: Alvedon, 60mg, 125mg, 250mg.

Dose: Post immunisation pyrexia, at 2m 60mg Stat, 3-6m 60mg, 6m-2yrs 120mg, 2-4yrs 180mg, 4-6yrs 240mg, 6-8yrs 250mg, 8-10yrs 375mg, 10-12yrs 500mg, all qds.

Paracetamol has a low Therapeutic Index and is dangerous in overdose. It does have a specific antidote however. Metabolites of Paracetamol deplete the liver's Glutathione, an anti oxidant and death is from liver failure. The treatment of overdose can include activated charcoal, Acetylcysteine which is a Glutathione precursor and what treatment is used and what the outcome is depends on the speed of the presentation and the initial blood level of Paracetamol.

A toxic adult dose can be 8 tablets or as low as 4 gm, though some references do say 24 tabs is the limit and in children an acute dose >200mg/kg can lead to toxicity. To some extent this will depend on other factors, alcohol, liver disease, nutrition etc. The antidotes should be given in <15 hrs.

Paracetamol alone was the universal first analgesic recommendation for such situations as low back pain for years by groups such as NICE. Recently however it has slipped back to being considered little better than placebo. This is clearly not true, especially for the elderly, the relatively drug naive and for the many paracetamol/analgesic combinations. Let us hope that Co Proxamol will one day be reinstated to the ranks of prescribable mid range combination analgesics (See below).

After Paracetamol and Ibuprofen/Naproxen/Diclofenac:

Ketorolac, Toradol Tabs 10mg, Injection 30mg/ml. An NSAID. Short term management of moderate to severe pain.

Co Codamol comes in 3 strengths: Paracetamol/Codeine 500/8mg, 500/15mg and 500mg/30mg.

Co Dydramol is Paracetamol 500mg plus Dihydrocodeine 10mg. Note: Remedeine is Paracetamol 500mg and 20mg Dihydrocodeine. Remedeine Forte has 30mg Dihydrocodeine.

Dihydrocodeine is available on its own: DF 118, 40mg tabs and DHC Continus 60, 90, 120mg tabs BD.

Also as an injection, 50mg/ml.

These are notoriously constipating, sedative and often cause confusion. Far fewer side effects however follow the use of:

Co Proxamol, – the licences for which were cancelled by the MHRA in 2007 after advice from the CSM. The concerns were regarding overdose deaths, especially when taken with alcohol.

I think this decision was wrong. I believe Co proxamol was and is a very useful mid range analgesic with fewer side effects than Codeine and Dihydrocodeine containing analgesics. Anyone who seriously believes that it is no more effective than paracetamol alone has never treated patients in pain or taken a couple of Co proxamol themselves when **they** were in pain. Fewer manufacturers made it and it became much more expensive. So when our local PCT started threatening the GPs of patients taking this drug with its imminent withdrawal simply on the basis of cost, I felt angry and protective of them and many (usually sensible elderly patients) felt a sense of disbelief and betrayal. All were stable long term or intermittent short term analgesic users with no risk of abuse or overdose and all suffered unacceptable side effects on the alternative cheaper medication. They were usually arthritis sufferers who took two or three doses a day depending on what they planned to do. This complete withdrawal of Co Proxamol is one of many examples of the "Ignorance of power" demonstrated by many regulating decision makers over the last few decades. – Ignorance in the sense of the regulating and decision making authorities being out of touch with the patients they serve. Surely it is the job of the GP, once informed of a relative new risk of a drug (and Co Proxamol posed no risk to the vast majority of its takers) to assess and discuss the risk with each patient? I wouldn't blithely prescribe benzodiazepines to all my patients or dihydrocodeine or pethidine. I hope I would assess the suitability of each treatment for each individual patient at that time. When are representatives of the profession (or patients' informed representative groups) ever consulted on these far reaching undemocratic decisions?

While we are on the subject of unrepresentative decisions affecting the wellbeing of thousands:

I would include changes to cremation bureaucracy, controlled drug management (which have resulted in 90% of GPs simply not carrying controlled drugs at all), the disastrous time consuming change in the way oxygen is now supplied to General Practice patients, the imposition of dictation, correspondence and pathology software on every GP, the compulsory but clunky NHS net, appraisal and all the trivia associated with it, even the management decisions that have forced the computer keyboard and monitor to dominate every consultation-still such a hot topic in American primary care but a battle lost this side of the Atlantic. WE find General Practice in a crisis of overwork in 2016/7 and half the extra work is all these long winded administrative chores which used to be so easy, quick and simple. When it was paper based and we were trusted.

Anyway, Co Proxamol IS still available and IS a useful mid range analgesic drug with few side effects.

Tramadol: Zydol, is a weak opioid receptor agonist which also releases Serotonin and blocks the reuptake of Nor Adrenaline. Interestingly, the Dextropropoxyphene in Co Proxamol has some similar activities to Tramadol (SNRI) and the molecule of Tramadol is structurally like Venlafaxine, the antidepressant.

Dependence, constipation and lowering of the seizure threshold are side effects and patients either seem to gain *some* relief from Tramadol or none. It can be used with all the mid range Paracetamol combination analgesics and NSAIDs.

Oxycodone. Oxycontin Tablets, 5, 10, 15, 20, 30, 40, 60, 80, 120mg Sustained release, given BD

Oxynorm, 5, 10, 20mg Capsules, also Liquid (two strengths) and Injection 10mg/ml and 50mg/ml.

Combined with Naloxone in Targinact.

Diconal, Dipipanone 10mg and Cyclizine 30mg old fashioned but effective.

M.S.T. (Morphine sulphate tablets) continus. Colour Coded: 5mg white, 10mg brown, 15mg green, 30mg purple, 60mg orange, 100mg orange, 200mg green (again). The suspension comes in sachets.

Nepenthe is a mixture of anhydrous morphine 8.4mg/ml and "Disprin and Nepenthe" (Aspirin and Morphine in a palatable suspension) was an effective analgesic in bone pain. Probably no longer available. Nepenthe now seems to be used as a term to mean any drug or therapy that relieves pain and sorrow and helps you forget!

Pentazocine, Fortral, 25mg tabs, 50mg Caps 30mg/ml injection. Dysphoria, disorientation and nausea the common side effects.

Acupan Nefopam. 30-60mg TDS. Centrally acting non opioid analgesic that stops shivering.

Oramorph, Morphine sulphate soln 10mg/5mls (i.e. 2mg/ml) Oramorph concentrate 20mg/ml.

Buprenorphine, Temgesic 200ug and 400ug Sublingual tablet (nauseating) and BuTrans patches 5, 10, 20ug/hr. These last 7 days. Transtec patches 35, 52.5 and 70ug/hr need to be replaced twice weekly. Also Temgesic injection, 300ug/ml.

Meptazinol Meptid 200mg Tabs, Injection 100mg in 1ml. An opioid receptor mixed agonist/antagonist. Short onset, short duration.

Dexibuprofen, Seractil 400mg BD/TDS

Patches: include

Buprenorphine is BuTrans (Lower dose) 5ug/hr 10ug and 20ug/hr and also Transtec 35ug/hr, 52.5 and 70ug/hr

Fentanyl is Durogesic 12ug/hr, 25, 50, 75, 100ug/hr

8: Anticoagulants, Clotting, Thrombolysis, Blood etc:

Things you may have forgotten:

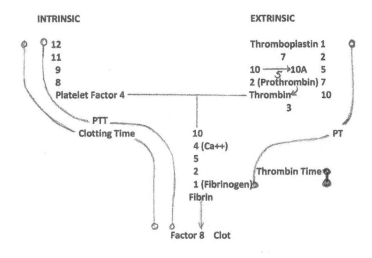

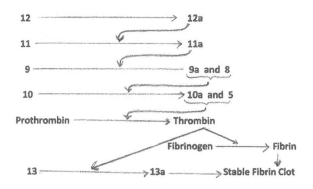

Diagram: The Clotting Cascade: (TCC1).

Blood Groups:

Blood Group:	Antigen on RBCs:	Antibody in plasma:	Can give blood to:	Can accept blood from:
A	A	Anti-B	A and AB	A and O
B	B	Anti-A	B and AB	B and O
AB	A and B	Neither	AB	All groups
O	Neither	Anti-A and Anti-B	All groups	O

Europeans:

40% are O

40% are A

15% are B

5% are AB

Why are there eight different groups? – Differences may have offered some survival advantages during our evolution:

Group AB is relatively immune to cholera.

Group O is susceptible to cholera but resistant to malaria and overall those with Group O have fewer cancers and are relatively resistant to Syphilis.

1/5 of the population do not secrete water soluble ABO proteins in saliva. They are more likely to succumb to meningitis and UTIs, but less likely to develop RSV and Flu.

Haemoglobinopathies (Sickle Cell trait and Thalassaemia) also confer some malaria resistance by the way.

Warfarin:

Prevents arterial and venous thrombosis and is useful in the primary and secondary prevention of stroke in non rheumatic atrial fibrillation. AF is found in about 15% of all stroke patients and up to 5% of AF patients have a stroke each year. 30% of AF patients are untreated at any given time and only 20% are on therapeutic doses of anticoagulant. It is surprising how many elderly patients have AF on one examination but not the next time you see them. Should you anticoagulate them on sight? Offer aspirin and a PPI and just say come back in a week after an ECG? – at least until you are sure they don't have a single episode of Paroxysmal AF? If it resolves, how can you be sure it is a single episode? Many cardiologists say it is better not to treat at all than to under anticoagulate a patient with AF. Presumably this is because of the bleeding risks but logically this doesn't make much sense. Is it better to ignore a raised cholesterol than to get it half way down towards the normal range? Surely a slightly lowered blood pressure constitutes less of a stroke risk than an untreated one? And anyway anticoagulation is and always has been a difficult decision which balances the real risk of bleeding to death (I have lost two patients on Warfarin to G. I. bleeds) against embolic catastrophe. My mother died of a stroke from sudden onset of AF in her eighties.

Dental Advice: No interruption of Warfarin continuity but dental procedure only to go ahead when INR<3.5 . Test within 72 hours or less of procedure. Maximum of 3 extractions at one time, sockets packed and sutured.

Interactions: Warfarin potentiates: Aspirin, NSAIDs, Amiodarone, Propafenone, Ciprofloxacin, Erythromycin, Aminoglycosides, Fibrates, Simvastatin, Thyroxine etc.

It should be avoided in pregnancy, especially during organogenesis (weeks 6-12).

Standard Warfarin treatment is associated with an annual risk of major haemorrhage of 1-9% (depending on the source you read) intracranial bleed about 0.5% and risk of death 0.2%.

Half life 48 hours.

Patients on Warfarin should have a detailed knowledge of the many interactions as well as the dietary sources of Vitamin K (a Warfarin antagonist and "antidote").

Thus: Vitamin K levels in various foods: (Various sources):

Low levels in green beans, cauliflower, celery, mushrooms, onions, green peppers, potato, tomatoes, most fruits including apples, blueberries, lemons, oranges, peaches, most meats, including beef, chicken, ham, pork, turkey, also fish, including mackerel, shrimp, tuna, in most vegetable oils, butter, most cheeses, eggs, yogurt, coffee, tea, milk etc.

Moderate Levels: asparagus, avocado, red cabbage, green peas, iceberg lettuce, margarine, olive oil, gherkins.

High Levels: broccoli, Brussels sprouts, cabbage, raw endive, kale, lettuce, mustard and cress, parsley, spinach, watercress, chard, mayonnaise, canola and soybean oil, cranberry juice, green tea and of course, Vitamin K tablets.

I have never heard of any Warfarinised patient being told to restrict any of these foods but if it is difficult to get your patient stable on a regular dose of Warfarin, ask if they eat large amounts of any of the above or take a vitamin supplement.

Coumarin treatment leads to soft tissue calcification (in blood vessels, cartilage etc) and this can be counteracted by giving a regular dose of Vitamin K2 with the Warfarin and stabilising the anticoagulant treatment on both.

Phenindione: Prophylaxis of embolisation in A.F., DVT, P.E.

Sinthrome (Acenocoumerol) is in the same group of oral anticoagulants.

Clopidogrel: (See below)

Note: beneficial effect reduced by Omeprazole and Lanzoprazole but not by Pantoprazole, Rabeprazole or Ezomeprazole.

Indications:

Prevention of atherothrombotic Events	within 35 days of M.I.
,, ,,	within 6m of Ischaemic Stroke,
Given with Aspirin to prevent	in Acute Coronary Syndrome
atherothrombotic events	without ST elevation,
Given with Aspirin	in Acute MI with ST elevation,

(300mg non EC aspirin and 300mg or 4X clopidogrel stat).

Given with Aspirin to prevent atherothrombotic and thromboembolic events in A.F.

How long?

Clopidogrel: 75mg

1m PCI with bare metal stent, post CABG surgery, after STEMI.

6m PFO closure.

1yr Acute coronary syndromes (ACS/NSTEMI) with PCI (Except STEMI).

Acute coronary syndromes (ACS/NSTEMI) without PCI (except STEMI).

Any PCI with drug eluting stent (DES).

Lifelong in established aspirin allergy.

After finishing Clopidogrel, Aspirin (75mg) continues for life (apart from PFO Closure, – D/W consultant).

FIBRINOLYTIC Treatment:

Alteplase, (Actilyse) Tissue Plasminogen Activator. tPA, PLAT

This catalyses plasminogen to plasmin the major enzyme responsible for clot breakdown.

Used in acute ischaemic stroke (after intracranial haemorrhage has been excluded, treatment should be started within 3 hours of onset of symptoms), acute M.I., acute pulmonary embolus.

Others include Tenecteplase, Urokinase, Reteplase, Streptokinase.

Low Molecular Weight Heparins/Heparin: Hyperkalaemia and thrombocytopenia are effects. Safe in pregnancy and breast feeding but Rx needs to be stopped before labour. Prolonged use can cause osteoporosis.

Doses:

Treatment of DVT, Unstable Angina, P.E., Peripheral Arterial Occlusion:

Heparin: 5000us I.V. Loading dose (10,000 us in "Severe P.E.") then 15,000us S.C. 12 hourly (do regular clotting studies).

Thromboprophylaxis in medical patients: 5000us (10,000us in pregnancy thrombo-prophylaxis) S.C. every 8-12 hrs.

Dalteparin: Fragmin 12,500us/ml (2500 us in 0.2ml) and 25,000us/ml (5,000us 7,500us, 10,000us, 12,5000us, 15,000us, 18,000us (in 0.2-0.72mls))

Doses:

Medical DVT Prophylaxis: 5000us every 24 hrs

Treatment of DVT/PE 7,500us-18,000us/day until oral anticoagulation effective.

Also:

Enoxaparin: Clexane 100mg/ml is 10,000us.

Tinzaparin: Innohep 10,000us/ml eg: A single daily dose for 6 days until Warfarinisation is established:

or

This was suggested to me by a haematologist:

One dose daily can be given as a **"Half way house to anticoagulation"** in a patient with a history of previous DVT if that patient has to fly long haul and is at risk of further DVT. Adult dose is 175 iu/kg. Advise a self administered dose the day before, the day of the flight and if possible the day after arriving??-(Likewise on the return journey) or you could start them on Warfarin a few weeks before and try to get the INR sorted out – but how impractical is that to get stable and then for the patient to monitor it abroad?

Novel Oral Anticoagulants NOACs, Non Vitamin K oral anticoagulants:

Target Thrombin (Dabigatran), Factor Xa (Rivaroxaban, Apixaban, Edoxaban). Lower rates of bleeding and fewer drug and food interactions than Warfarin. They also have a more predictable anticoagulant effect than Warfarin.

Dabigatran: Pradaxa A novel oral anticoagulant NOAC that "does not require moni-toring". (In fact you can't **practically** monitor it anyway). A direct thrombin inhibitor, there was no current specific antagonist**, unlike Warfarin and Heparin. Fewer significant bleed side effects than patients on Warfarin but more G.I. bleeds. If the patient is on Warfarin, stop it until INR <2. New patient: start Dabigatran, – maximum effect in 2-3 hours, half life approx 12 hours. If the patient is on Aspirin, either stop aspirin or can continue at <100mg aspirin and 110mg BD Dabigatran. Can be used in recurrent DVT and PE in adults. At 150mg BD reduces ischaemic and haemorrhagic stroke as well as systemic embolism. The general dose is 150mg BD or if >80 yrs 110mg BD. Measure effect with aPTT as INR is unreliable – stop treatment if aPTT>80 secs. Peak and trough levels are 2 hrs and 10-16 hrs. Prophylaxis in A.F. 150mg daily unless >80yrs, or on Verapamil or at high risk of bleeding then 110mg BD.

Rivaroxaban (Xarelto), Apixaban (Eliquis): Direct factor Xa inhibitors. These are other oral anticoagulants for AF, post DVT and for the prevention of VTE after hip or knee surgery. 15-20mg/day. Once daily NOAC (Novel oral anti coagulant).

Antidotes:

The Antidote for Heparin is Protamine Sulphate: Roughly speaking, 1mg neutralises 80-100us Heparin if given within 15mins of the Heparin.

The antidote to Warfarin is Vitamin K, (takes 4-6 hours), fresh frozen plasma or prothrombin complex concentrate if available.

The antidote to NOACs is prothrombin complex concentrate and soon specific antidotes will be available (2015).

Note: new ANTAGONIST** for Pradaxa, Dabigatran.

New clinical testing suggests Idarucizumab safely and effectively reverses the anticoagulant effect of Dabigatran (June 2015). Praxbind is given intravenously, the commonest S/Es being headache, hypokalaemia, confusion, fever. The anticoagulant effect of Dabigatran is effectively reversed within 4 hours of the administration of Idarucizumab (I think most doctors WILL just call it Praxbind).

Andexanet alfa, Ciraparantag also available (2016).

Warfarin Monitoring: I.N.R. International Normalised Ratio is basically the ratio of the patient's Prothrombin Time compared with a control.

A Normal Prothrombin Time is	10-14 seconds making the
Normal INR	0.8-1.2
DVT prophylaxis for general surgery:	2-2.5
Prophylaxis after hip surgery, M.I.	2-3
P.E., T.I.A.	2-3
Treatment of venous thrombo-embolism, DVT:	2-3
In VTE the lowest VTE and bleeding rates are at:	2.5
In PE with a mechanical heart valve:	3-4.5
In non-rheumatic A.F.:	2.0 may suffice
(but most authorities say non valvular AF, to reduce stroke:	>2)
A.F. If previous cerebral ischaemia:	2-3.9

Dentistry is OK if INR 2.0 or less. Warfarin is teratogenic: Causing Nasal hypoplasia, stippled epiphyses, foetal haemorrhage in the third trimester.

If in doubt, most indicated conditions warrant an INR of 2.5 or thereabouts.

Duration:

British Society for Haematology:

Calf vein thrombosis in non surgical low risk	3m
First PE or proximal DVT	6m
Post op calf DVT without risk factors	6wks

If "unprovoked", reassess after 3m and decide.
If two episodes of DVT or PE, "long term" treatment is advised.

American College of Chest Physicians recommend:

Symptomatic calf DVT (CVT)	6-12 weeks
Proximal DVT	at least 3 months
Acute PE	at least 6 months
One idiopathic proximal DVT or PE	Indefinite

So there seems to be a degree of consensus there anyway.

Atrial Fibrillation:

Non valvular:

If the AF Is persistent or paroxysmal or high risk (previous ischaemic stroke, TIA, systemic embolism, or 1 or 2 of: >75 yrs age, impaired L ventricular systolic function or heart failure, history of hypertension, diabetes), then long term anticoagulation is advisable.

Valvular:

For AF and patients with mitral stenosis long term anticoagulation is advisable, likewise in patients with AF and prosthetic valves (some need a higher INR and aspirin). Mechanical and bioprosthetic valves need INRs 2.5-3.5.

Myocardial infarction (with complications, i.e. large anterior infarcts, heart failure, intracardiac thrombus, A.F. or a thrombo-embolic event), need an INR of 2-3 plus aspirin for at least 3m.

Other risk factors:

Antiphospholipid Syndrome: Target INR 2.5, – lifetime. APS with recurrent thromboembolism, target INR 3, lifetime.

In acute A.F. anticoagulate if you cannot DC convert within 36 hours. If the L atrial diameter is >5.5cm (**N is 4cm**). Defibrillation tends not to work. A trans-oesophageal echo can exclude an atrial thrombosis.

The Sentinel Stroke National Audit Programme (SSNAP) (snappy title?) found that of AF patients admitted to hospital, in April to June 2015, 45.6% were taking anticoagulants. In July – September 2014 it was 41.2%. This prompted a debate about whether GPs should be more aggressive in anticoagulating all patients with AF or whether it was right to sometimes ignore NICE guidelines after discussion with the patient. Clearly the latter is often the case as long as the patient or the relatives are informed and aware of the risks (and possible benefits). Also it assumes that GPs know every patient on their list with AF at any given time. This of course is not possible.

Alternative approach to A.F. and anticoagulation (different source)
Anticoagulate all elderly with A.F.
A.F. if 60-80 years and no C.I.s.
    but>80 years use aspirin alone.
A.F. with mitral stenosis.
A.F. with cardiomegaly.
A.F. with previous thromboembolism.
A.F. with T.I.A.
Not young with A.F. alone??? – though 7% have a C.V.A. in the first year after onset.
Relationships between INR and risk of bleeding: (again)

INR 2 annual risk of bleeding %	0.3
3	1
4	3

Non Rheumatic A.F.: The benefits from Warfarin (DATB Factfile 94 32 57-60) **exceed the risks**. BUT under age 75, no diabetes, hypertension or cardiac disease, Aspirin 300mg a day (with PPI) is as effective.

Condition	Prothrombin time	Partial thromboplastin time	Bleeding time	Platelet count
Vitamin K deficiency or Warfarin	Prolonged	Normal or mildly prolonged	Unaffected	Unaffected
Disseminated intravascular coagulation	Prolonged	Prolonged	Prolonged	Decreased
Von Willebrand disease	Unaffected	Prolonged	Prolonged	Decreased or Normal or rejected
Haemophilia	Unaffected	Prolonged	Unaffected	Unaffected
Aspirin	Unaffected	Unaffected	Prolonged	Unaffected
Thrombocytopenia	Unaffected	Unaffected	Prolonged	Decreased
Liver failure, early	Prolonged	Unaffected	Unaffected	Unaffected
Liver failure, end-stage	Prolonged	Prolonged	Prolonged	Decreased
Uraemia	Unaffected	Unaffected	Prolonged	Unaffected
Congenital afibrinogenaemia	Prolonged	Prolonged	Prolonged	Unaffected
Factor V deficiency	Prolonged	Prolonged	Unaffected	Unaffected
Factor X deficiency as seen in amyloid purpura	Prolonged	Prolonged	Unaffected	Unaffected
Glanzmann's thrombasthenia	Unaffected	Unaffected	Prolonged	Unaffected
Bernard-Soulier syndrome	Unaffected	Unaffected	Prolonged	Decreased or unaffected
Factor XII deficiency	Unaffected	Prolonged	Unaffected	Unaffected

(My Thanks to Wikipedia)

	Cerebrovascular Disease:		Cardiovascular Dis:		Peripheral Art Dis.
	Acute Stroke:	2ndary Prev.	Acute M.I.	2ndary Prev.	
Aspirin:	300mg	75-150mg/d	150-300mg	75-150mg/d	

	Ischaemic Stroke	Unstable angina or non STEMI if 6m mort >1.5% with aspirin -treat until 1 year after last attack.
Clopidogrel:	from day 7-6m	Acute MI from a few days to 35 days with aspirin
(Plavix)		Also in patients undergoing stents after PCI* with aspirin
	75mg daily	Loading dose 300mg then 75mg daily 75mg/day
		Can be used alone in MI If Aspirin not tolerated

Dipyridamole TIA and Ischaemic Stroke
(Persantin) Alone or with aspirin depending on C/Is
200mg BD 2 years
*Percutaneous Coronary Intervention

A bit more on Aspirin:

In stroke, Aspirin benefits 4/5 patients with ischaemic stroke (most strokes are ischaemic – a secondary thrombosis on top of an atheroma). It isn't worth giving aspirin as prophylaxis (primary prevention) in healthy people as it increases the risk of haemorrhagic stroke and GI bleeds etc. – But give prophylactic aspirin to healthy patients with BP and previous TIAs, strokes.

Secondary prevention of stroke: Dipyridamole-persantin retard 200mg BD and aspirin gives 37% reduction in risk. (This also comes as Asasantin Retard).

Only 15% strokes are due to haemorrhage. Aspirin within 48 hours does not increase the risk of haemorrhage but you need a CT before thrombolysis (t-PA, Tissue Plasminogen Activator) gives much better reduction in incapacity.

Aspirin has long been known to have anticancer effects. A paper in Aug 2014 (Annals of Oncology) declared that the advantages of aspirin prophylaxis was third in line to stopping smoking and not being obese in preventing cancer. The authors showed that if patients between 50 and 65 years of age took daily aspirin for 10 years, there would be a 9% reduction in the number of cancers, strokes and heart attacks overall in men and 7% in women. The total number of deaths from any cause would be 4% lower over 20 years.

Long term aspirin reduces gastro intestinal cancers. We have known about polyposis cancer risk and aspirin for decades but – colorectal, oesophageal and gastric cancers as well as ?pancreatic, ovarian, lung and breast are reduced by aspirin prophylaxis too. An increasing number of well read cancer survivors are taking low dose aspirin to reduce metastases.

It takes 5 years of 75mg of daily aspirin to cut down cancer occurrence by 25%. (20% fewer ovarian cancers). Presumably this is partly because so many cancers are post inflammatory or because of the effects of aspirin on reducing angiogenesis of new cancers.

Controversially the US Preventative Services Task Force (USPSTF) suggested that all adults, men and women, aged 50-69 should take daily low dose aspirin for at least 10 years to reduce their risk of cardiovascular disease and colorectal cancer in the Autumn of 2015/Spring 2016. The caveats were: If they were in their 50's with a 10% or greater 10 year CVD risk, did not have bleeding risk and were willing to take the aspirin for 10 years. Patients in their 60's do have a higher bleeding risk. They had not enough information to extend the advice to the less than 50's or >69 year olds. This is the first time that primary prevention in otherwise healthy people at normal risk has been proposed using aspirin.

Not every medical agency in the US or elsewhere agreed. Also although aspirin reduces future risk of cancer and cardiovascular disease, one source said it doesn't appear to reduce the number of deaths from them. (This is contradicted by other sources, see below)

Still more on Aspirin:

The overall figures for aspirin and cancer (etc mortality, various sources) are:
5 years of daily aspirin use reduces colorectal cancer incidence by 37% and colorectal mortality by 52%. The risk of oesophageal cancer is reduced 58% by daily aspirin in clinical trials and 44% in cohort studies. Aspirin reduces stomach cancer mortality by from 31% to 41%. There is a negligible effect on pancreatic cancer. Aspirin reduces incident breast cancer by 18%. Cohort studies show a reduction in breast cancer of 8% in regular aspirin users. (There was no effect seen in the WHS). Aspirin has little effect on prostate cancer, it may slightly reduce lung cancer mortality but not incident lung cancer. Generally aspirin needs 3 years to reduce incidence and 5 years to reduce mortality. Any dose above 75mg is effective at preventing cancer. It reduces the rate of non fatal MIs, but primary prevention with aspirin does not reduce cardiovascular mortality. Aspirin increases the risk for haemorrhagic stroke by 32-36%. It also increases the risk of major extracranial bleeding by 30-70%. Overall by taking aspirin for 10 years between the ages of 50 and 65, the 15 year risk of MI, cancer or stroke is reduced by 9% among men and 7% among women (mainly through the effect on colorectal cancer). The NNT with aspirin for 10 years to prevent a major event is between 33 and 127. Aspirin should reduce the risk for death by 4% at 20 years (all through cancer mortality).

Anticoagulants and pregnancy:

Use Heparin in the first 6-9 weeks then oral anticoagulants 16th-36th week then heparin again. Heparin throughout can cause osteoporosis. Anticoagulation in some studies caused (in 7%) congenital abnormalities, S.B. or abortion, in 16% if the oral treatment were continued throughout pregnancy.

Warfarin if given perinatally can cause CNS defects, spontaneous abortion, SB, prematurity and haemorrhage. Ocular defects may occur if given anytime during pregnancy. There is a foetal Warfarin syndrome if given in the first trimester. (Nasal hypoplasia, hypoplasia of the extremities, developmental retardation). Most of these effects are dose dependent, especially >5mg/day. Epiphyseal stippling is seen on X Ray. 2/3 of foetuses exposed to Warfarin in pregnancy are born normal and breast fed babies of mothers taking Warfarin are generally considered safe. (Drugs. com)

D.V.T.

Risks:
Cancer, Trauma, Anti phospholipid syndrome, Previous DVT, Old Age, Surgery, Immobility, Contraceptives, Pregnancy, HRT, Post natal period, Obesity, HIV, Nephrotic syndrome, Central venous catheters, Polycythemia Vera, Chemotherapy, Blood factors – Non O blood group (double risk). (AND NOTE: protein C, protein S and anti thrombin prevent clotting so their absence increase the risk of DVT as does Factor V Leiden).

Half to 85% of DVTs are asymptomatic and only 25% of referrals with suspected DVTs actually have a DVT confirmed. Likewise only 25% of clinically suspected P.E.s are confirmed.

If the D Dimer is <220 there is only a 5% chance of a DVT.

A patient who has had an unprovoked DVT should have lifelong anti coagulation. The Probability is assessed by applying the Two-level DVT Wells score:

Clinical feature	Points	Patient score
Active cancer (treatment ongoing, within 6 months, or palliative)	1	
Paralysis, paresis or recent plaster immobilisation of the lower extremities	1	
Recently bedridden for 3 days or more or major surgery within 12 weeks requiring general or regional anaesthesia	1	
Localised tenderness along the distribution of the deep venous system	1	
Entire leg swollen	1	
Calf swelling at least 3 cm larger than asymptomatic side	1	
Pitting oedema confined to the symptomatic leg	1	
Collateral superficial veins (non-varicose)	1	
Previously documented DVT	1	
An alternative diagnosis is at least as likely as DVT	-2	
Clinical probability simplified score		
DVT *likely*	2 points or more	
DVT *unlikely*	1 point or less	

Likewise a tool for Pulmonary Emboli is the:

Two-level PE Wells score

Clinical feature	Points	Patient score		
Clinical signs and symptoms of DVT (minimum of leg swelling and pain with palpation of the deep veins)	3			
An alternative diagnosis is less likely than PE	3			
Heart rate > 100 beats per minute	1.5			
Immobilisation for more than 3 days or surgery in the previous 4 weeks	1.5			

Previous DVT/PE	1.5			
Haemoptysis	1			
Malignancy (on treatment, treated in the last 6 months, or palliative)	1			
Clinical probability simplified scores				
PE *likely*		More than 4 points		
PE *unlikely*		4 points or fewer		

Thank you to Dr Wells for his kind permission to use this calculator.

Atrial Fibrillation and the CHADS VASC Score:

CHADS2 Score:

Congestive heart failure	1 point
Hypertension >either 160?/90 (Some say 140/90)	1 point
Age>75	1 point
Diabetes	1 point
Prior stroke or TIA or thromboembolism	2 points
Consider Warfarin if = >2	

CHADS 2 Score: Stroke annual risk:

0	1.9%
1	2.8%
2	4.0%
3	5.9%
4	8.5%
5	12.5%
6	18.2%

So a good start in acute **Atrial Fibrillation** would be:
Give Digoxin first and add Bisoprolol (1.25mg for 2 weeks then 2.5mg a day) and start Warfarin thus:
One day of each of:
10mg
10mg then one day of
5mg then urgent INR after informing the lab.

Remember:

INR and Annual Risk Of Bleeding:

2	**0.3%**
3	**1%**
4	**3%**

Under 75 years without diabetes, hypertension, cardiac disease, then Aspirin 300mg/day is as effective at reducing embolic risk.

Dental Extraction and anticoagulation:
Stop treatment 2 days before or INR<2

Von Willebrand Disease:
Aut. Dom. (but some types are Aut. Rec). 1:100 in Italy, 3:1000 in UK. Mucocutaneous bleeding. Prolonged primary haemorrhage after trauma. Prolonged APTT due to an absent factor 8 carrier protein. Prolonged haemorrhages result if severely affected. Treatment includes cryo-precipitate and factor 8 with Von Willebrands factor concentrates which can be infused. Desmopressin releases Von Willebrand factor from endothelial cells and this as well as the oestrogen containing COCP and the anti fibrinolytic Tranexamic Acid, Cyklokapron can be also used in treatment. Von Willebrand factor is a carrier protein for factor 8, also prompting adhesion of platelets as its part in the clotting cascade.

Severe cases are rare and there are various types, most are inherited, some acquired – as in association with aortic stenosis, Wilm's tumour, hypothyroidism etc

Clotting Studies:

Prothrombin time	Partial thromboplastin time	Bleeding time	Platelets
Normal	Prolonged	Prolonged	Normal

Rapid Warfarinisation a reminder:
10mg 10mg 5mg on successive days and the fourth day request an INR with urgent result (Warfarin 3-9mg/day usually maintains the INR in the desired range)

Thrombophilia: (hypercoagulability)
This is the increased risk of clotting in some (about 5%) of patients. DVT and pulmonary emboli are common complications, as are thromboses in other venous sites, the arm veins and other deep veins, intra-cerebral, renal, hepatic (Budd-Chiari) etc.

Thrombophilia can cause recurrent miscarriage, pre-eclampsia, stillbirth and other pregnancy complications.

Investigations: **Thrombophilia screen:** FBC, homocysteine level, prothrombin time, partial thromboplastin time, thrombin time, protein C, protein S, thrombin 3, factor V Leiden and prothrombin gene variant, Lupus (anti) coagulant, anti cardiolipin antibodies, anti B2 glycoprotein1 antibody, activated protein C resistance, fibrinogen tests, etc.

Hypercoagulable states can be acquired: antiphospholipid antibodies, pregnancy, cancer, oestrogens, immobility, (plus or minus surgery), nephrotic syndrome, smoking, myeloproliferative diseases, obesity.

Or congenital: Factor V Leiden, prothrombin mutations, high homocysteine, sickle cell, protein C and protein S deficiencies, antithrombin deficiencies, vitamin deficiencies, etc.

9: THE BREAST:

Mastalgia/Breast Pain

Typical treatment options:

Pyridoxine 100mg OD.

Oil of Evening Primrose 160mg BD (Efamol) with or without Vitamin C.

Danazol 300mg reducing to 100mg over 3 months. Multiple side effects that limit its usefulness including amenorrhoea and weight gain.

Bromocriptine 1mg OD to 2.5mg BD. Suppression of lactation 2.5mg OD then BD for 2 weeks.

Cabergoline Used in hyperprolactinaemia. A dopamine receptor agonist.

Tamoxifen 10mg OD/BD for 3m. Mention that it is "sometimes used in breast cancer" but if taken long term reduces breast cancer. Otherwise a friend is bound to frighten them by saying "that's the cancer drug".

Goserelin (Zoladex)

Ibuprofen gel topically!

Fibrocystic disease of the breast:

Approximately half of all women in their child bearing years have lumpy breasts. Also called Diffuse Cystic Mastopathy. The breasts can ache, the upper outer breast margins are uncomfortable, particularly premenstrually.

Ultrasound and mammography can confirm the clinical impression of fibrocystic disease and help exclude an occult malignancy which is no more common than in a normal breast (unless there are "proliferative lesions" found on biopsy.)

Treatment is rarely necessary but the mastalgia treatments, the COCP and progestogens are amongst the alternatives. Fibrocystic cysts may be up to 2" across, the bigger ones can be aspirated in the surgery (send the fluid for cytology) and the condition does not adversely affect breast feeding.

Mammography:**

3 yearly from age of 47-72 now, – the UK programme having been gradually extended over recent years. The extension being completed by 2016. The extension to a lower age range is controversial. According to the publicity, the screening programme saves 2 – 2.5 lives for every "over-diagnosed case". The latest UK figures I have are: 1:20 are recalled for a second screen, the majority being normal.

However, mammography **is** controversial. In 2001 The Lancet published a paper (Gotzsche and Olsen) analysing the seven major studies upon which the National Mammography screening system had been based. The conclusion was that screening women (asymptomatic women at specific age groups) to improve health did not work and was actually harmful. "The test is largely ineffective as a screening tool for detecting cancer in sufficient time to influence survivability". There has been an active controversy with strong feelings on both sides ever since.

According to Toronto's Deputy Director of The Canadian National Breast Screening Study, Cornelia Baines, (regarding a younger age group) "For up to 11 years after the initiation of breast cancer screening in women aged 40-49, the screened women face a higher death rate from breast cancer than unscreened control women, although that is contrary to what one would expect..... three years after screening starts, their chance of death from breast cancer is more than double."

This is all every confusing and is exactly like the increase in deaths from screening asymptomatic younger men by doing PSA. More of them die.

The increase in the incidence of breast cancer in mammography screened pre meno-pausal women may be due to the effect of surgery on the breast primary which is thought to directly stimulate silent distant metastases, as do the effect of growth factors produced by the body following surgery as part of the healing process, the immune system may be suppressed following the trauma of surgery and of course mammography does use ionising radiation.

For every 10,000 women who have 3 yearly mammograms from 47-73 yrs there are 3-6 extra radiation caused cancers (Cancer Research UK.)

The benefits of screening start to become apparent over the age of 50.

In the three state study, USA, 96-03, the worst radiologists missed 40% of tumours and gave false positives in 8.3%. The very best radiologists missed 20% and had a false positives of 2.6%.

In 2000, a paper published the finding that by analysing 2,230 records of women screened between ages 40 and 69, after an average of 9 mammograms there was a false positive pick up rate of 43%.

In a more recent Canadian study (2014), annual mammograms failed to reduce breast cancer mortality in women (aged 40-59) compared with physical examination or routine care, according to a 25 year follow up. One haematologist at a national meeting in the US said that if mammographic screening were a drug and it had the same effects: cutting off breasts, courses of chemotherapy, hormones, life changing side effects and anxiety – while saving possibly only a few lives, it wouldn't get a licence: "The only reason mammography continues is that it isn't a medicine and subject to the same rigorous review" (Miller, Wall, Baines et al BMJ 2014 348 g 366.) quoted in Medscape March 2014.

In "I think you'll find it's a bit more complicated than that", Ben Goldacre, the medical statistician put it like this: screening patients every two years saves 2 deaths per thousand, aged 50-59 over 10 years. But achieving this requires those thousand women to have five thousand screenings resulting in 242 recalls and 64 women having at least one biopsy. Five women will have cancer detected and treated. In Jan 2017 A new Danish study (Ann Int Med) added weight to the anti screening argument. One in three women aged 50-69 who were diagnosed with breast cancer did not have a significant tumour. Neither did mammography reduce the number of advanced breast cancers found in women in the study. The author, Dr Jorgensen said "Breast screening was unlikely to improve breast cancer survival or reduce the use of invasive surgery. It also leads to unnecessary detection and treatment of many breast cancers".

I think there may be another obfuscating issue and one that frustratingly ignores rational argument when this subject is discussed these days. And that is of a strong feminist entitlement to spending on women's health. This often transcends rational discussion and is expressed frequently when I listen to debates on cervical smears, mammography, osteoporosis, HRT or any other purely female service. It is where politics transcends evidence in medicine, as it so often does these days. It is obvious at medical meetings on all the above topics where the status quo is now set in stone in the medical mind set. Suggest that worried teenagers or out of sequence women who have irregular bleeding should have smears on request or that mammogram money should be spent on cancer research or that calcium treatment and bisphosphonates are harmful treatments for most women with thin bones or that HRT should be actively discouraged for more than a brief period in the vast majority of patients and speakers are speechless with surprise and indignation.

Breast Cancer:

25,000 new cases a year in the UK. 11, 600 die a year (some sources say 15,000). 2/3 sufferers die of it. Only 1% breast cancer deaths were men in 2010. One of the cruellest things about breast cancer is that it seems to be able to recur very late – over ten to twelve years after the primary and long after the patient heaves a sigh of relief and has almost forgotten they ever had cancer. I know of no other common cancer that waits so long for its secondaries to make themselves noticed. There are all sorts of ways of cutting down the risk of this – from the menstrual timing of surgery to taking prophylactic aspirin and a handful of alternative treatments that mitigate against metastases (see cancer section).

Apparently (2014) the UK's survival in Breast Cancer is now better than it has been, deaths having dropped by 40% in the last 20 years due to better medical care.

The national screening campaign "saves one life for every £50,000" (800 lives saved a year in total). In the UK currently it is three yearly from age 50-70. Obesity is a huge cause of breast cancer compared with HRT, causing 50,000 cases in the last 10 years and survival being inversely proportional to BMI. Adipose tissue is, of course an endocrine organ and weight gain from 18 to the age of between 50 and 60 has consistently been associated with post menopausal breast cancer (as well as endometrial cancer – which is independent of menopausal status).

HRT does increase breast cancer, all routes and all types. The risk is increased for instance by 1.35X after 5 years with combined HRT. This is thought to be due to the synthetic progesterone. Unopposed HRT supplementation is a similar risk to not having "the menopause", a 2.3% increase in risk/year – still a slight increase in risk. There is less of a breast cancer risk if HRT is begun after a reasonable time into the menopause – a period of oestrogen deprivation. For instance if unopposed oestrogen is commenced 5 years after the LMP or combined HRT 3 years after the LMP there does not seem to be an increased risk. Tibolone probably has a risk in between opposed and unopposed HRT.

HRT is safe in oestrogen receptor negative breast cancer and probably safe in oestrogen receptor positive breast cancer if the patient is taking Tamoxifen but it may reduce the effectiveness of aromatase inhibitors.

Women who had taken antibiotics for 500 total days over a 17 year period were found to have double the breast cancer risk of women who had taken none in one study. Presumable via yet another obscure effect of the microbiome.

Personally I have never had a patient with breast cancer who wanted to take the risk of starting or continuing HRT and there are alternative treatments for most of the symptoms of the climacteric.

HRT polarises doctors' and patients' views more than most topics. I find whether they prescribe or take HRT as much a reflection of their politics and attitudes to soft feminism and women's rights as it is to actual safety. I have certainly attended courses on HRT where diametrically opposite views on HRT risk were promulgated by successive speakers quoting the same research! Elsewhere I compare HRT risks to drinking alcohol or being overweight. All these things increase a woman's breast cancer risk but just to put a critical view, here is Dr Walter Willett, Chair of Public Health at Harvard Medical School: "The downplaying of risk from HRT is even more despicable. The spin doctors calmly stated that for every 10,000 women on HRT during one year, only 8 more will have invasive breast cancer, seven more will have a heart attack, only 8 more will have a stroke, and only 18 more will have blood clots. Sounds benign doesn't it? Until you do the math.

There are (in the USA) 8-10 million women currently using HRT. Using conservative numbers, that adds up to 6, 400 cases of invasive breast cancer, 5,600 heart attacks, 6,400 strokes and 14,400 blood clots to organs like the lungs. That adds up to 32,800 cases of drug induced morbidity a year!"

There is a background 1 in 9 women lifetime risk (some authors say 1:12?), Peak age at diagnosis 60-64.

Survival figures up to 2003: 1 year 96%
5 years 85%
10 years 77%
20 years 65%
Some cases recur very late compared with other cancers.

National screening: 50-70 year olds. Highest incidence USA and the Netherlands, Lowest China.

Significant features: (other than any new breast lump), change in skin contour, – peau d'orange, skin tethering, bloody nipple discharge, retraction, distortion or nipple eczema. Diffuse breast pain is not usually a serious symptom, in fact *most* cancer generally isn't painful when it presents.

It takes a malignant cell approximately 4 years to become palpable in the breast.

There is a variety of recognised potential causes. Excess weight:

Obesity is a potent cause of breast cancer causing >50,000 deaths in the last 10 years (a huge risk compared with HRT.) Survival from breast cancer is inversely proportional to BMI.

A high number of periods: (Few pregnancies, early menarche, late menopause), HRT, alcohol consumption, exposure to oestrogen, radiation and now some suggestion that high stress occupations MAY increase the risk of breast cancer (possibly up to 1.7X) and genes of course. Ironically some caring occupations can reduce oestrogen levels and the risk of breast cancer. Unless they involve night shifts: artificial light reduces your endogenous anticancer Melatonin and increases the risk of breast cancer.

1/3 of secondaries are hormone sensitive. Aromatase inhibitors (Anastrozole (Non steroidal), Exemestane (Steroidal), Letrozole (Non steroidal)) stop endogenous androgens being converted to oestrogen.

Traditionally treatment was Tamoxifen>Megestrol>Aminoglutethimide.

The standard regime now is often 2 years Tamoxifen followed by 3 years of one of the Aromatase inhibitors.

Oestrogen or progesterone positive breast cancers can be treated with hormone therapies such as Tamoxifen. Herceptin works on tumours which are HER2-positive but 20% of breast cancers are "Triple negative" meaning chemotherapy, radiotherapy and surgery are the only options.

Typical Chemotherapy in HER2-Pos breast cancer is Herceptin – Trastuzamab. A monoclonal antibody that interferes with the HER2/neu receptor. These are cell membrane receptors that control cell reproduction. It is given at 3 weekly intervals for 1 year.

More on Mammography screening:**

Debate continues about the benefits and disadvantages of this (see above) and about the number and type of tumours detected (and what might have happened to the patients had they not been detected)

but one other British study showed these figures:

Total patients invited for screening: 23,164
Total screened: 16,951 (73%)
Referred for assessment: 1,417 (8%)
Biopsies 205 (1.2%)
Malignant 97 (0.6%)

The national screening campaign costs £40m/year and saves 800 lives (£50,000/life) Only 70% women take up the offer to be screened.

The Million women study:

Is flawed as it is based only on most recent HRT use, extrapolated and previous HRT history was ignored. (40% women change their HRT)

HRT is less of a breast cancer risk than being overweight or 1 glass of wine a day.

Risks:

Menarche <11 years X3
1st pregnancy >35 years X3
Menopause >50 X2
Weight >30 kg/SqM X2
2Us alcohol/day X2

The Major Studies:

HRT use WHI E+P X1.09 (Women's Health Initiative)
         E X0.99
Million women E+P X2 ?
         E X1.3 ?

E is American for Oestrogen
P is Progestogen

It used to be thought that in hormonal terms the breast cancer risk was simply related to the number of periods (the lifetime total oestrogen exposure) that a breast had undergone. If this is all there is to it, why is the age of the first pregnancy important? If you get pregnant at the age of 18 and you breast feed and (say for the sake of argument) you subtract 15 periods from your lifetime total, why is it better to have done this aged 18 than aged 38? Is the breast more vulnerable to the carcinogenic effects of hormones at certain ages than others?

10: Cancer and Terminal Care: (Also see Breast, Paediatrics)

If a lot of cures are suggested for a disease it means that the disease is incurable.

Anton Chekhov

Suffering is only intolerable when nobody cares.
Cicely Saunders, the founder of the modern hospice movement.

The global picture is this: In the next 60 seconds 15 people will die of cancer. One every 4 seconds, some 8m/year. Some current estimates are as high as 14 million. Statistics like this are frustratingly inconsistent in nearly every area I have researched and quote in this book. They are very different depending on the official source you access. I apologise for this. Despite the fact that if you cured all cancers you would only add on average 4 years to human life.

Cancer is however definitely on the increase in all developed nations, worldwide. WHO announced in 2014 that restrictions should be placed on smoking, obesity and alcohol to reduce cancer deaths. Good luck with that, WHO. Sometimes the advice we as doctors give about avoiding cancer (for instance avoiding sunshine) has the opposite effect. WHO said the number of cases would reach 24m a year by 2035. It is 8-14m/year now, predicted to rise to 19m/year by 2025, 22m/year by 2030.

More than half of all people born in 1960 will develop cancer at some point in their lives according to a 2015 report from Cancer Research UK. The previously generally accepted figure was one in three. This increase was originally explained by increasing longevity (Brit J Cancer Feb 2015).

The figures for those born in 1960 are 53.5% for men and 47.5% for women (compared with those born in 1930 that is an increase of 15% and 11% respectively). More than half of the cancers in the life time risk are diagnosed over the age of 70. Indeed, more than 60% of all cancers are diagnosed in people over the age of 65. Clearly a significant number of these are secondary to life and behavioural choices that patients make early on in their lives and those choices finally "catching up on them".

Major factors world-wide include HPV, late pregnancies, smoking, infections, alcohol, obesity and inactivity, radiation from the sun (though newer studies suggest avoiding radiation from the sun is an even bigger health risk), therapeutic radiation and air pollution. Only 10% of cancers are thought to have a genetic basis, 20% have an infectious aetiology. Recently however, such unexpected factors as tallness, stressful jobs, personality type, night work and low HDL (previously a wholeheartedly positive finding) have been found to be separate cancer promoting – or cancer associated factors.

In terms of the international incidence, tobacco has a lot to answer for. Smoking causes a quarter of cancer deaths. It increases cancer of the mouth, nose and sinuses, larynx, oesophagus, stomach, pancreas, bladder, liver, cervix, kidney, AML, ovary and bowel.

But surely it must be possible to genetically engineer a tobacco leaf that burns producing Nicotine and a tobacco taste with fewer hydrocarbon toxins and carcinogens? Wouldn't this be a public health and social boon? And wouldn't it make some innovative company a fortune?

People enjoy smoking for the pharmacological effect of Nicotine not the taste of smoke and tar and the sad truth is none of the alternative forms of self administration have the same cachet, social associations or instant pharmacological buzz. The jury is out on the e-cigarette although it is the closest of the NRTs to the real thing in performance, social ritual and pharmacology.

Lung cancer is the most common cancer worldwide, accounting for 1.2 million new cases annually; that is a new case every thirty seconds. This is followed by cancer of the breast, just over 1 million cases; colorectal, 940,000; stomach, 870,000; liver, 560,000; cervical, 470,000; oesophageal, 410,000; head and neck, 390,000; bladder, 330,000; malignant non-Hodgkin lymphomas, 290,000; leukaemia, 250,000; prostate and testicular, 250,000; pancreatic, 216,000; ovarian, 190,000; kidney, 190,000; endometrial, 188,000; nervous system, 175,000; melanoma, 133,000; thyroid, 123,000; pharynx, 65,000; and Hodgkin's Disease, 62,000 cases.

The three leading cancer killers are slightly different from the three most common forms, with lung cancer responsible for 17.8 per cent of all cancer deaths, stomach, 10.4 per cent and liver, 8.8 per cent.

Industrial nations with the highest overall cancer rates include: U.S.A, Italy, Australia, Germany, The Netherlands, Canada and France. Developing countries (areas) with the lowest cancer are in Northern Africa, Southern and Eastern Asia.

In the UK there are about 331,000 new cancer cases a year.

In 2015 processed meat – that is bacon, cured hams, salami, some of the nation's favourite foods were accused by the WHO of being carcinogenic. The nation started to wonder whether anything was safe to eat or conversely, whether any new food revelation was safe to believe. The actual facts are more digestible when put in context: WHO says of the 7,600,000 who die a year of cancer (Press release world cancer day):

34,000 cancer deaths worldwide per year are caused by processed meat,

50,000 cancer deaths may be caused worldwide by red meat,

200,000 deaths per year are due to air pollution,

600,000 deaths are due to alcohol consumption and

1,000,000 deaths a year are due to tobacco consumption.

The average GP loses 20 patients a year. 1/4 to cancer, 1/12 are sudden deaths, 1/3 "organ failure", and 1/3 "frailty or dementia"

Cancer management is improving in the UK with more effective treatment and a better prognoses for nearly all cancers over the last 20 years. The two week rule for suspected cancer cases has helped, but a quarter of cancers are still only detected as they present late in casualty units, many patients having previously been dismissed or reassured by their GPs. One thinks of the poor young women who die of aggressive cervical cancer. Some having previously presented with irregular PV bleeding requesting a smear and these are frequently refused because they are "too young". Or the multitude of women who present with non specific abdominal pain and whose ovarian cancers could have been picked up by an ultrasound. The figures are likewise bad for pancreatic cancer and CNS cancer (half and two thirds respectively are missed by primary care and diagnosed in casualty). There is a doubling of the death rate in the first year for these A and E cancer presentations compared with GP urgent referrals to secondary care cancer specialists.(Macmillan Cancer Support report April 2014)

In late 2014 NICE publicised the fairly obvious possible early warning signs of occult cancer. Two female members of my extended family, a fifty year old who presented with iron deficiency anaemia and a sixty year old with new onset recurrent abdominal pain were victims of this lack of GP focus. Both had been reassured and sent away without examination or investigation in the last few years by their day dreaming GPs. One was prescribed iron, the other, reassurance. If either GP had known the standard clinical guidance for either of these situations they would have investigated them fully. Even worse, a relative aged 70 presented a month ago with episodes of red rectal bleeding and was sent for a blood test without being examined. Now how hard is it to do a rectal examination? Sometimes I despair.

Casualty units diagnose 39% of all lung cancer and 32% of ovarian cancer. The problem here is at the stage of GPs and early diagnosis, the investigation of non specific symptoms. We in the UK do worse than most other developed countries. Why do GPs so frequently fail to pick up on vague but significant symptoms amongst the daily "background static"? Why do we fail to properly assess patients with what in retrospect were clearly worrying symptoms which should have prompted investigation? It seems GPs have become brow beaten into avoiding investigations, treatment and spending just like we are now avoiding prescribing antibiotics unless we have a blindingly obvious indication for them. Why have we become in twenty short years a profession of obedient sheep? Why are we no longer as bloody minded and determined to fight even for our patients' marginal interests? If you have read this book cover to cover you will know one of my answers at least – and blame medical school selection committees.

This situation and mind set is because of a perfect storm of:

1) Decades of pressure from administrators and supervisory GP groups emphasising cost of treatment as the prime management consideration rather than the patient's needs.

2) The training of GPs and registrars to be inflexible in the application of treatment protocols and management guidelines designed for populations not individuals. How often I hear this from patients presenting with significant symptoms only to be dismissed by doctors on the basis of "national guidelines", "protocols" and "probabilities" as if the GP had no choice or flexibility in the matter. Look at the current blanket reluctance to prescribe antibiotics for fear of being criticised by the CCG superbug police and the consequent rise of Scarlet Fever and deaths from paediatric "sepsis". Are my colleagues just saying "No" without fully assessing febrile patients?

3) This sense of continual external constraint has led to a change in the very personality of GPs and General Practice itself over the decades that I have known it. Or more likely, selection procedures as far back as medical school are excluding individuals who have the confidence, individuality and awkwardness to go against the crowd. WE ALL used to be misfits and characters – where have they all gone? We now seem to have lost the professional sense of purpose, the self confidence, the bloody mindedness we used to have on behalf of the patient. Gone are the prescribing and management freedom, the personal choice in decision making – all have been discouraged and even occasionally punished. In other words we now have standardisation and even uniformity of mind set based largely on the statistics of the health of populations, national guidelines and of cost. The individuality of Family Medicine, the GP doing what he or she thinks is best for the individual patient is now often shamelessly trumped by external sanctions and controls.

4) The absence of quick and accessible objective reassurance for the doctor and patient because of inaccessible investigations is also a block to diagnosis and reassurance: cervical smears at **any age,** blood tumour markers, ultrasound scans on demand, chest, other X rays, MRIs and CT scans, especially head CTs for GPs who are concerned about CNS symptoms: All these should be available without secondary care referral. How else can a

GP do his or her job properly?

In late 2014 a review showed that 27% of GPs were barred from non obstetric USS (how can we exclude early or even advanced ovarian cancer without referring tens of thousands of women with vague abdominal pain to outpatients for an opinion then? The 2012 "Direct Access to Diagnostic Tests for Cancer" report recommended a 2 week referral for investigation if the GP finds ascites and a pelvic mass. Great, the horse has bolted and what was that noise? the GP closing the stable door?

25% of GPs were not even able to order a chest X Ray – a shocking statistic in a country where TB is one of the three main public health infections and vague chest pain or a prolonged cough demands a CXR even in a non smoker. In fact a low dose CT is a better investigation to exclude lung cancer as CXR misses up to 25% of lung cancers but then if we cannot get access to a CXR, reliably reported, how many of us can order chest CTs?

50% of GPs could not refer directly for a flexible sigmoidoscopy the last time it was assessed – think of all those patients with IBS who have irregular bowel habits and who have to reach a certain threshold of their doctor's anxiety to be referred to a consultant. Patients with lifelong IBS do die of bowel cancer with depressing frequency never having reached their GP's level of **referral anxiety**.

Brain MRI: 50% of GPs do not have open access for the morning headache and nausea patients that abound and again have to persist with symptoms long enough or generate sufficient concern in the GP to break the threshold into a two week rule referral to a neurologist. We all know how few neurologists there are. So for most patients it is: Pay for the CT or referral yourself, wait for your headache to get worse or keep your fingers crossed your headache is benign. The CCGs control access to these routine investigations now and only 30% allowed their GPs access to all four basic tests in late 2014. Just imagine what would happen to the two week rule system if GPs referred all patients with what they thought could be a 10% chance of cancer?

The large number of patients presenting in this group with possible cancer symptoms, ignorance of guidelines, the implications of vague persisting symptoms and the fear of embarrassment are reasons GPs often don't refer. But as I have said elsewhere, too many women with abdominal pain and ovarian cancer are labelled as having IBS. Too many people with morning headache are being fobbed off as sinus pressure or stress. A rapid access USS and tumour marker blood test would help solve the problem or an open access head CT scan – (after the proper examinations have been performed) – or a quick out of protocol cervical smear in the irregular bleeding young patient. Why can't we have universal access to these? All GPs are working in the dark, flying by the seat of their pants. Compared with the cost of medical negligence claims they would all add up to but a drop in the ocean.

Tell each doctor to remember that protocols apply to POPULATIONS not INDIVIDUALS. Remind GPs that primary care only works from the patient's perspective if the GP is responsive to an individual's needs and FLEXIBLE. Also if they come back twice or three times with an improperly explained symptom that you have not effectively managed the patient and you are obliged to take it further.

The same Macmillan report I mentioned above complains about the lack of compassion shown to terminally ill patients and the diminishing chances of a pain free death. These too are directly due to the inflexible application of "Gold Standard Terminal Care Protocols", the inadequate number of hospices, the diminishing number of full time GPs who carry and are familiar with the use of Diamorphine, syringe drivers and controlled drugs, all due to the post Shipman rules. Thank you politicians. Add to these the poor out of hours care, in part because we have so many part time GPs. Very few of them are willing to be on call at night even for the few weeks it takes for their one or two terminal patients a year to undergo a dignified death at home. This is exacerbated by the part-timism and work/life/ family and child care preoccupations of the growing number of female doctors. Also by the fact that few practices have a proper list system for partners who can offer out of hours care to their own patients in exceptional circumstances. You do feel different about *your own patients* and only GPs with a personal list ever get to have **them**.

While we are discussing modern GP 's rationing out a short list of restricted services via external guidelines and denying access to any personally tailored service, this clearly hugely diminishes the quality of care that the patient receives. If the patient is old enough to remember the complete professional freedom, individuality, even quirkiness of the GP 20-30 years ago, the sense of loss is severe. This outside interference is bad enough from the patient's point of view but it also destroys any sense of professional pride, personal involvement and satisfaction that the GP will get from their work. What thought has the GP been called upon to give in the consultation? What choices, input, what decisions, what control ? How much involvement? How much personal interest and care ? What personal difference has he or she made? How much of them self has been shared when the doctor is simply applying a protocol?

As one particularly thoughtful observer put it to me in a discussion on the default consulting approach of young GPs, "You will get what you are training them for: No one who can think outside the box, no individuals, no one who can make a decision for themselves, no one who will discover or invent anything new, all probably depressed, anyone could do that job"

Again, I can't help feeling that this is at least partly because of the diminishing role of the full time (usually male) GP partner with a personal, professional, emotional, financial and historical commitment to his practice, partners and patient list – and young, part time, increasingly female GPs don't mind being rubber stamps, administrators of decisions made elsewhere because they have other priorities in their lives. Commitment, personal involvement and fulfilment three sides of the same coin.

So perhaps the late diagnosis of cancer in this country has many causes ranging from the white noise of the unrestricted access of 300 million mostly trivial primary care consultations per year, to the restricted access of most of us in primary care to various helpful differentiating investigations, to a restricted therapeutic freedom mindset in the new doctors, to restricted knowledge of some basic medicine amongst many of my colleagues old and young, to daily boredom and a poor therapeutic index of suspicion.

One source says 7% of the population have a truly genetic form of cancer, independent of other factors. For up to half of cancers, dietary, environmental and other influences are far more powerful determinants.

It seems that cancer levels in developed countries have doubled or tripled, depending on the cancer, since the second world war. There are many reasons for this. Better diagnosis, better recording and an older population play a part but many cancers are undoubtedly increasing in incidence and affecting younger age groups.

In America between grandmothers in the 1960s and their granddaughters, breast cancer has increased from 1:20 to 1:8. From 1985 to 1996 prostate cancer has increased from 85,000 to 317,000 and NHL has doubled since the early 70s.

There is evidence linking various cancers to environmental factors, breast and prostate to pesticide use (which is said to be oestrogenic), NHL to herbicide use. Breast, ovarian and uterine to hormone treatment and environmental oestrogens including those in plastics and various cancers to weight, diet and chemical pollutants. The effect of tobacco on the lung has been known since the 50's but now we know it contributes to multiple cancers of different systems.

Exercise reduces the incidence, even the recurrence rate and mortality of a variety of cancers. 30 minutes a day is enough, it doesn't have to be strenuous and breast and colonic cancers are amongst many that have been shown to respond.

Many would blame our alien diet in the developed world, with refined and processed sources of fat, carbohydrates and protein, industrial farming and the paucity of dietary vegetables, natural Omega 3 fats and fruits. There are however approximately 500,000 environmental chemicals, new since 1945, the long term effects of which are unknown, from oestrogens in the water supply to petrochemical fumes, plastic wrappers, bottles, can linings and vapours, (BPS and BPA), volatile organic (new carpet and new car) smells, dioxins, PCBs, phthalates, food additives and preservatives, solvents, paints, domestic and industrial insecticides and herbicides etc. The list is endless and none of these compounds have long term human safety data.

It is remarkable how every gynaecologist begins every talk on HRT with a safety broadcast on oestrogens. This is based on highly conflicting data and ignores environmental effects (feminisation of fish and fresh water reptiles due to high levels of oestrogen in fresh water and also in drinking water supplies) and the known effect of oestrogenic compounds on the growth of stem and cancer cells.

You can't help believing that oral contraceptives and HRT are no longer within the realm of rational debate amongst some doctors or journalists. You are with us or you are a dinosaur. Oestrogens and other female hormones are now a basic human right for all women and all risks to health and safety must just be accepted and ignored.

Lung cancer kills more in the UK than breast, bowel or prostate cancer. One recent set of comparative figures quoted: Prostate 15,000 new cases/year, breast 30,000 and cervix 3,000. Lung cancer 34,860.

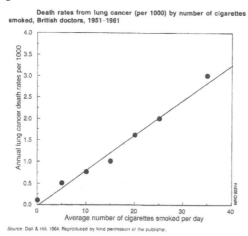

Death rates from lung cancer (per 1000) by number of cigarettes smoked, British doctors, 1951-1961

Source: Doll & Hill, 1964. Reproduced by kind permission of the publisher.

The **two week rule** system was set up in part to improve the UK's cancer outcomes. A recent study questioned its value as a rapid detection and life saving system. Only 1:10 referrals using strict criteria and a dedicated proforma actually proved to be upper GI cancers. The same was true for lower GI cancers. You may think that isn't bad but the point is that curative surgery was possible in less than 2% referrals.

I think that it all depends on what symptoms prompt the 2WR referral. If you refer a 50 year old male with iron deficiency and he turns out to have a R sided bowel cancer, the cure rate today is far higher than that.

Screening:

Patients are subjected to numerous screening tests throughout life, not just for the detection of cancer.

Screening begins in pregnancy with tests for nasal and nuchal U/S for Down's syndrome, then

blood tests for FBC and group, Rubella, Syphilis, Hepatitis B and C and HIV serology. Then the TORCH blood tests (Toxoplasma, Other {Coxsackie, Syphilis, VZV, and Parvovirus B19 serology} Rubella, CMV, Herpes Simplex Virus. After birth there is the heel prick test which is usually done between day 5 and 8, it includes tests for:

Phenyketonuria, Myxoedema, Sickle Cell Haemoglobinopathy, Cystic Fibrosis (Trypsin), MCAD (Medium chain Acyl CoA dehydrogenase), from May 2014 these were added:

Maple Syrup Urine Disease, Homocystinuria, Glutaric Acidaemia type 1, Isovaleric Acidaemia.

Occasionally these are performed too:

Galactosaemia, Biotinidase deficiency and CAH, depending on where you are.

also other inborn errors: including

Long chain Hydroxyacyl-CoA dehydrogenase deficiency (LCHADD).

Then the growth, hearing and development screening of the young takes place in the surgery or community.

Routine blood pressure, weight, diabetes and other screening tests are now part of a GP's "standard duties" sometimes attracting payment as part of QuoF or another contractual incentive.

Screening also exists for

Abdominal aortic aneurysm, Diabetic retinopathy, Raised intra ocular pressure, Breast cancer, Cervical cancer, Bowel cancer, Prostate cancer and various other conditions.

The risks of all this screening is of over-diagnosis, causing large numbers of worried well and treating patients for benign conditions which might never have done them harm. Then there are the risks of the screening itself (such as irradiation and unnecessary biopsy or surgery) and false reassurance if the screening actually doesn't save any lives. Indeed the Government's Science and Technology Committee criticised the NHS in October 2014 for its poor communication of the risks of screening to patients.

Breast cancer screening for instance became the subject of fierce controversy in 2012. An independent review showed that for every life saved by mammography, three women had treatment for a cancer that would never have been fatal. The figures for PSA and prostate cancer treatments were once thought far worse (but actually arent). Now mammogram leaflets are said to include more information, allowing an informed choice. (See above).

I wonder if informed consent really exists. Doesn't it depend upon an individual's ability to weigh up and accept personal risk? If YOU are the one who will get hurt, decisions are not usually very rational. Large numbers of men on "Active surveillance" seem to lose their nerve and have some sort of (probably) unnecessary prostate surgery sooner or later.

In 2015 the NEJM published data comparing metastatic breast and prostatic cancer. PSA and mammography screening had come into widespread use at roughly the same time in the US. 16 million women over 40 years were screened in the US in 2000. A total of 53,200 were diagnosed with breast cancer and followed 10 years. The screening increased cancer diagnoses by 16% but the death rate from the cancers didn't change. 25% more small tumours were detected and 7% more large tumours but this made no impact on mortality.

The trend in the data comparing prostate screening was startlingly different. The incidence of metastatic prostate cancer fell by approximately 50% within 7 years of the start of the widespread use of PSA in 1990. However, rates of metastatic breast cancer have remained remarkably stable since 1985 when widespread mammography was introduced. So despite the huge number of "false positives" treated, many men with prostate cancer had actually and surprisingly been saved by PSA testing. The far more expensive, often criticised but politically untouchable mammography screening campaign appears to have achieve nothing in comparison.

Finally, in a balanced Medscape review in Feb 2015, Dr S. Jha says that in America the US Preventative Services Task Force suggests breast screening should start age 50, their College of Radiology at 40 and The American Cancer Society at age 45! Major screening examples are given such as the Swedish Two County study in which mammograms reduced deaths by 30% and a Canadian study which showed no benefit (Miller, Wall, Baines: a 25 years FU study BMJ 2014 348 g 366). Over-diagnoses range from 0 to 30%. Whether screening is beneficial or not seems to depend on the background rate of breast cancer. Higher rates benefit the case for mammogram supporters as they limit over diagnoses. Lower background rates support the anti screening argument as these show the harms of over diagnosis and screening. Mammograms have never been shown to reduce all cause mortality, only deaths from breast cancer (Prasad, Lenzer, Newman BMJ 2016 352: h6080).

Any study on the benefits of screening must go on for at least 35 years and progress in techniques of screening will make the study redundant during that time. The conclusion of the article is that mammograms do save lives AND over-diagnose cancer. In America, false positive mammograms cost $4Bn a year. 3D mammograms and molecular breast imaging will save more lives at greater cost. The question no one is asking is: How much is a saved life worth?

End of life care:

Dying for human beings in a western civilised country can be a protracted miserable, painful process.

Only a third of dying patients have a conversation with their medical attendants about their own personal priorities, care preferences and wishes anytime before death.

Discussing issues around death is often seen as a failure by practitioners in a health care system which from medical school is focussed on diagnosis, treatment and CURE.

Atul Gawande discussed this issue in the Reith Lectures in 2014 when he suggested that a discussion about the reality of the situation should be made at the right moment and would be a relief to most patients. It might cover an understanding of "where they are" in terms of their illness, their fears and worries for the future, their goals for the future if time is running short (and what would be unacceptable to them) in an open, practical and frank way. Often hospice type care at home with maximum attention to pain and symptom control is what the patient wants when it is obvious there is no real hope of a cure. Sometimes individuals might prefer some pain to the drowsiness of strong opiates if the trade off were some meaningful last interaction with grandchildren or other members of the family or being able to paint, read, write, play an instrument or sort out their affairs.

He suggests five questions at this point:

What is your current understanding of your current health or condition?
If your current condition worsens, what are your goals?
What are your fears?
Are there any trade-offs you are willing to make or not?
and later: What would a good day be like?

This is clearly a time for the GP to stop in his or her tracks and connect with the patient in a quiet and personal way. To share medical decisions with an open mind, putting the patient's wishes and needs first and jettisoning personal bias, inappropriate protocols and outside influences-including those sometimes, of relatives.

Gawande also makes some other points which I allude to elsewhere in this book. The very brightest A – Level students get to be selected for medical school. They generally have little life experience, low levels of emotional maturity and in my experience, their intellectual excess implies limited empathy for the patients they deal with. It is very rare to see the sharp and the warm co exist in the same skull. The training of medical students values their intellect and technical skills far above their ability to show friendship, ability to connect or have empathy with the patient. This continues despite what I am told is endless role play (which, by the way has now been labelled as useless as a behaviour modifier and learning tool by one of its original proponents Prof Liz Stokoe (The Life Scientific 2014)). These lessons include for instance how to empathise and break bad news etc. at medical school. Students are bright but distant. Lighthouse doctors – not warm and close campfire doctors. To me this is why the doctor of today thrives on protocols, proforma and guidelines whereas the doctor of the 60's and 70's had the way to behave and relate to patients programmed as part of their life experience and personality. There are protocols for managing acute asthma and croup but for acute bereavement, the mother of a new stillbirth, the patient who is frightened of dying? What use is a proforma?

According to Gawande's "Being Mortal", in America, terminally ill patients are regularly intubated, defibrillated and ventilated, given combination chemotherapies or antibiotics even when their medical attendants know that their survival and more importantly their quality of life will not be improved but could be harmed. This is because the conversation about the patient's real priorities given the reality of limited time left to them has not been had, – the diagnosis of "dying" has never been discussed by their doctor. To me this is the job of the patient's GP. It is surprising how many patients in extreme old age and riddled with cancer, exhausted by heart failure or paralysed by Motor Neurone Disease can be on death's door but are not aware that their time and therapeutic options are limited or almost gone. At this point, or before it we should sit down with the family and the patient and talk and ask questions. What do you know about your illness? What would be the most important thing to you now? Freedom from pain, from breathlessness, being able to talk but maybe having some pain and so on. We should explain that active treatment has nothing more to offer and our goal should be to make what time is left as comfortable, as happy, content and if possible purposeful as we can. We should answer questions honestly because you will be surprised at the misconceptions about chances of survival and the process of dying that people have. We should ask the patient what to do if they get a chest infection or stop breathing, who they would like to see, where they would like to go, what they would like to do if at all possible. We should tell them that the palliative care drugs do work.

In a "Coping with Cancer" study performed in 2008 in the US, where these conversations weren't had with the patients, some dying patients were resuscitated, treated on ITU, given antibiotics and so on. (– Yes I don't know why things were allowed to go that far either).Not surprisingly in the last week of life the patients were assessed as having a substantially worse quality of life than those left without active intervention. AND Six months later the care givers (the family and friends) were 3X more likely to suffer major depression.

If you ask large numbers of patients who have been allowed to know that they are dying, what their priorities are, they aren't always keen that every small chance of extending their life a few days be taken. Their wishes are often to say: "I am sorry", or "I wish I had done this better", or "I love you", or to say "good bye" to their loved ones. Their priorities are to avoid suffering and fear, to strengthen relationships with family and friends to not be a burden and to achieve a sense for themselves that their life is complete.

How often does our interventionist, technical, don't mention the dying word approach achieve those goals? And when can we decide that people ARE dying anyway? When do we make that diagnosis given our ability to treat pneumonia, heart failure, ascites, cerebral oedema and so many other terminal events temporarily. The hard part of managing a dying patient isn't prescribing or diagnosing complications, it is helping the patient and in my experience, the relatives and loved ones accept that they have to confront the reality of the situation. Interventionist approaches to terminal illness do not, by the way, extend the life of the patient. There were found to be no significant differences in groups of U.S. dying patients who had intensive hospital care compared with symptomatic hospice care. Except for those with critical heart failure and they lasted up to 3 months longer with **non interventional** hospice care.

Prognoses:

When doctors are asked to estimate how long a patient has left, the better the doctor knows the patient, the longer the estimate. But the average estimate is 530% too long with 17% of guesses an under estimate and 63% being an over estimate. Only 20% are about right.

Currently (2014) around 500,000 people die each year in England and Wales. Of these, the figures in brackets are the 2014 figures from Medscape, the others were official figures from 2-3 years before – about 58% (53% 2014) patients die in hospital, 12% (5%) in a hospice and 30% (21%) at home (18% in care homes) (3% elsewhere). If there are supportive carers at home 73% die at home. Only 25% die at home if the carers say they are "unsure" about looking after the patient when asked beforehand. In America 50% of terminally ill patients die at home and 45% die in a hospice now (Atul Gawunde 2014). This is a rapid, recent, relative increase in this percentage.

In the UK (2014) two thirds of people say they would prefer to die at home and 29% in a hospice.

Goodness knows what the end of the Liverpool Pathway, the part-timism and emasculation of General Practice and the pseudo criminalisation of the use of (Dia) morphine by GPs will do to all our chances of dying at home. The majority of GPs are now women and very few female part time GPs are willing to visit terminally ill patients at night or even carry controlled drugs (own research). Most young female GPs I talk to about this subject say they are uncomfortable going out at night alone with controlled drugs. This, however, used to be accepted as what the job frequently entailed. There are notable exceptions, lauded in medical magazines but these are rare. Shipman and the politico-legal reaction to his murderous career have led to paranoia on the one hand and a suspicion on the other. This all relates to the assessment of appropriate pain relief and has caused immense harm to the only person that should matter here. The patient. To quote Wilkie Collins' Moonstone, regarding the doctor, Mr Candy: "Every medical man commits that act of treachery, Mr Blake, in the course of his practice. The ignorant distrust of opium (in England) is by no means confined to the lower and less cultivated classes. (Hear Hear!) Every doctor in large practice finds himself every now and then obliged to deceive his patients as Mr Candy deceived you".

When it comes down to the actual care of dying patients at home by GPs, once a syringe driver has been initiated and if the GP knows the family and patient well, many relatives and patients will try (counter intuitively) to expedite the process of dying, not to resist it. Giving drugs that will by their very nature, hasten death is the whole culture of medicine turned on its head of course for some doctors and nurses. This is a difficult situation ethically, culturally, personally, pharmacologically, emotionally and organisationally for all doctors and one where most of us are desperate to do well. Even though it is the only situation where the patient is the only person who cannot thank you for a good death.

The medical management of dying is today becoming less of a clinical pathway run by and focussed on doctors and nurses and their standard procedures but more of what it should be, something aimed at the patient's wants, needs and wishes. But this situation is a major culture shock for medics who spend the rest of their careers *treating* and preventing illnesses. Doing that job is how they are usually defined. Suddenly the sequence of treatable scenarios associated with cancer or Motor Neurone Disease or terminal heart failure, all of which usually have a clear therapeutic pathway, slip into symptom control with the purpose no longer being survival but patient comfort. Not really clearly measurable, definable or predictable and a realm where protocols fear to tread. In America (2016) 37% of cancer units have "Mind body and soul" in their mission statements. Many have "Complimentary Integrative Programs." As far as I am aware in 2016 the UK so far has none.

And everyone knows the prognosis and survival outcomes of each of these units, however caring.

Occasionally a patient you know well and who may have many weeks or months of poor quality opiate addled life left and who is in perpetual pain will ask you to precipitate their death. This has often happened to me and a discussion of aims, wishes, loose ends, family, saying goodbye, beliefs, regrets and fears should follow when you can come back and spare a quiet hour together. This may not change their mind. Their decision may be a rational one to you both. In this situation I am afraid that the humane injection of the British vet or the terminal drugs of Dignitas are not available to us and a rapid progressive increase in dose of the (for the family) distressing syringe driver is all that is legal.

In all honesty, most of the time the syringe driver is not used as a way of symptom response in the majority of desperately ill and deteriorating patients but a way of inducing coma and forcing the patient to die from the secondary complications of dehydration, starvation, stasis, postural pulmonary fluid retention, respiratory failure and occasionally from the direct complications of their primary illness. (See below).

A fifth of GPs said in an online poll (GP Online) in September 2016 that they would help a patient to end their life if the law allowed it. That is relatively *well* patients with a terminal illness who want to die before they had reached the syringe driver stage.

This is what the GMC says in its publications to doctors:

Patients wanting advice on ending their lives:

Our new guidance will help doctors to act within the law when a patient asks for advice on how to end their life. **Assisted suicide is illegal in the UK.**

Dignitas in Switzerland charges up to £6,000 depending on how much of the administration the patient wants them to undertake. It happens also to be legal in The Netherlands, Belgium, Oregon, Washington State and Vermont (2015).

The law in the UK is clear: providing information that could encourage or help someone to kill themselves is a criminal offence. However, doctors must listen to their patients, treat them with respect and compassion and be prepared to discuss the patient's reasons for wanting to end their life. The GMC says this can be a difficult balance to achieve.

You can say that again.

Like all GPs I have looked after dozens of my patients who had become friends and who at the end of their lives died at home.

Many times in this situation I have heard relatives say "you wouldn't let a dog suffer like that" – this is regarding a patient starving, dehydrating and dying in pain, slowly from prolonged opiate poisoning and starvation, dehydration and organ failure. These are often the real causes of death, but which don't go on the death certificate. The death is indirectly from an incurable cancer or wasting disease and I as the physician would be trying to relieve suffering but **already** worried about the rate at which I was increasing the speed of syringe driver. Often I would be looking over my therapeutic shoulder and wondering whether I was being thought of by nurses or relatives as another Harold Shipman.

The truth is that the most humane deaths I have seen have been sudden and unexpected or from the effects of clinically administered drugs in deliberately large doses. Natural deaths from wasting diseases never are. Doctors all know this and patients and relatives usually welcome our help even if High Court judges and politicians seem to forget it from time to time. We will all die and suffer death but we need not all die and meet death suffering.

My dog, a loved member of the family for the dog equivalent of 90 years developed pancreatic cancer a few years ago and this presented with deteriorating episodes of abdominal pain which brought me to tears. My caring and humane vet (humane to both me and the dog) after various treatments, saw him at no notice on a Saturday morning on the final occasion, explaining that he could only relieve my dog's suffering by painlessly ending his life. We both knew there was by now no more palliative or curative treatment. We then wrapped the dog in sheep skin and gave him a premed. injection. My dog became relaxed and drowsy, I was able to talk to him, hold his paw and stroke his head and 15 minutes later the Vet gave him an IM injection which put him calmly, contentedly, with my wife and myself holding him, to sleep. The bemused dog was staring puzzled into my tear stained eyes no doubt wondering what was wrong with me as he drifted off. This was one of the most thoughtful, caring, calm, peaceful deaths I had witnessed amongst the hundreds I had been involved with, in my life. Sometimes I come close to it if I am allowed full control of the terminal care of my patients at home. Sometimes, I am sorry to say, Hospice and GP care at home can result in a conflict of authority and responsibility. Sometimes relatives have impossible and unnatural expectations of what medicine can achieve in terminal situations. The GP should always be the arbiter of care for his or her patient but should in return be prepared to be available out of hours as terminal care is not a 9 to 5 job. I am available 24 hours a day for my dying patients and generally, I know them and the family well. It is ironic that our vetinary colleagues are now the rightful owners of the term Humane.

The Liverpool Pathway, of which we reached version 12, went the way of so many protocols – inflexible to the point of cruelty with some patients denied water and in some inexplicable cases, pain relief. I find it difficult to understand how any *humane* doctor or nurse so readily dispensed with the basic vocation of our professions – to care for the suffering and sick, to show compassion, to treat and cure when we can and to relieve suffering when we cannot. But always to do no harm. At the time, our own practice had meetings with the primary health care team and discussed the new **diagnosis of dying**. We included the Advanced Statement of Wishes under the Mental Capacity Act to make an advanced refusal to have treatment in specific circumstances and the "**Gold Standard Framework**" but it always struck me that formalising and standardising a process as unpredictable and individual as death was a bit like telling pregnant mothers exactly how their delivery would be "allowed to progress" in advance. To me this was all made worse by the financial rewards paid by the NHS for the use of the pathway. This always felt wrong- especially when a process, ideally taking place in the home and supervised by the patient's GP and district nursing team was designed and structured on a proforma by an Academic Hospital department of medicine and a hospice. Then, of course becoming carved in stone and becoming holy writ as far as some nurses and doctors were concerned.

The distressing stories from relatives about how some of these deaths were managed focus on how simple needs like pain relief and thirst were ignored because of a previously agreed protocol. It is odd that under advanced statements, patients can be encouraged to decline life prolonging treatment in advance should they be in no fit state to make a contemporary decision but they aren't allowed make an advanced decision to insist on four hourly morphine or water.

The Liverpool Pathway has been replaced by five new Priorities of Care (June 2014) placing greater emphasis on the wishes of the patient and on communication with their family. These priorities, which seem blindingly obvious, were created by The Leadership Alliance for the Care of Dying People in "One chance to get it right" and accept a named GP taking overall responsibility for the care of the patient. Baroness Julia Neuberger's report on The Liverpool Pathway had highlighted the rigid, impersonal and inhumane way that some of our colleagues had withdrawn drugs, fluids and empathy from their patients in the last few days and weeks of life. The New priorities emphasise communi- cation with the patient and relatives, responding to the patient's needs and wishes, regular reviews, involving the patient and relatives **to the extent that the dying patient wants**, consideration of the needs of families and an individual personalised compassionate care plan. This is exactly what full time GPs who care about their patients have always offered in an informal way and continued to offer despite the Liverpool Pathway and sometimes despite interference from hospice and other "experts".

I can only offer a rousing cheer for this common sense and say yet again as so many times in this book, that the GP is the pivot and secret of all good patient-centred care in the community. My worry (yet again) is that poor out of hours services including end of life care is due to the rarity of new full time GPs. This lack of traditional commitment to real General Practice by so many young doctors may well mean that old fashioned GPs who routinely care for their dying patients 24 hours a day may soon be extinct.

NICE put forward its "new proposals" – draft guidance for care of the dying in July 2015. These "encourage staff to communicate well and involve patients and relatives in decisions." They said many of the Liverpool Pathway's failings were due to how it was implemented: Described as an "Industrialised approach to managing dying people" by Professor Rob George, President of the Association of Palliative Medicine, "by inexperienced and box ticking staff." The new guidance focuses instead on personalised care, good communication and shared decisions between staff, relatives and patients where appropriate. "Staff" are encouraged to make daily reviews of medication, hydration and nutrition. That is a description of a good Family Doctor embedded in the community, available at night and well known to the patient's family – working with and communicating with the patient, D/N teams, relatives, the hospice teams and others. The sort of doctor who gives his mobile phone number to the relatives, is still prepared to go out at night, is familiar with end of life treatment and carries Diamorphine in his bag.

There are many times in this book that I wonder why and whether organisations like the GMC and other professional bodies, the RCGP, BMA, – our opinionated but often unrepresentative members of parliament and judiciary and so on have the right to say that they govern by representing the people of this country or the profession of medicine. Most people want to die at home. The person who should be able to care for them best in this is their GP. The GMC has currently only one doctor with previous GP experience amongst its council, so they have absolutely no understanding, experience of, or sympathy with the risks, challenges or benefits of home terminal care. Who do they actually represent? Where is their knowledge base? I know in my 40 years in medicine, no communication from any of these organisations has ever asked my opinion on a matter of ethics or medical politics so where do they get their laws, rules, guidelines, *legitimacy* from?

Let's *just suppose that* 90% of the profession felt that it was entirely reasonable for a dying and suffering patient of sound mind and in intractable pain to agree with his GP a rapidly increasing cocktail of sedatives and Morphine designed to render him unconscious and apnoeic? A quick, humane, consensual death. After all, we ARE supposed to have a "What are your priorities?" type conversation when this point is reached and some patients will say "A quick and painless death please doctor." Say they both agreed that the fairest and most humane way of achieving that would be over a timescale of, – say a couple of days. Well that **is** actually what does occasionally happen without it being stated out loud and has happened in secret since long before the days of Laudanum. At least that happens IF the family doctor is compassionate and cares about his patient. Suppose that most of the public (and I am sure they do) felt that this was an entirely reasonable thing for a doctor and his patient to do together?? Parliament voted against an assisted dying bill in 2015. They were afraid that sick patients who were not "on the verge of death" would be forced into ending their lives precipitously. So yet again, we have politicians involved in medical policy making: an unrepresentative and inexperienced group of the life-naive in Westminster, almost never canvassing their constituents on a matter of "conscience" making the majority of us suffer for fear of harming a tiny minority. To quote the GMC: It certainly IS a difficult balance to achieve -without offending someone. But why, as now, by perpetuating confusion and inhumanity do our legislators seem to offend nearly everyone?

Cancer and Food:

The anti cancer diet (see section on diet and nutrition) consists of avoiding refined white sugar and flour, avoiding Omega 6 in favour of Omega 3 oils, reducing saturated fats (there is evidence that high fat dairy consumption increases the risk of breast cancer), reducing salt intake (which in all western countries is consumed in multiples of our true requirement – around 1.25 gr/day, high intake can cause stomach cancer as well as cardio-vascular injury), supplementing the diet with anti oxidants, including Lycopene, Selenium, Vitamin D3, C and probably E, drinking green tea (Polyphenols and Catechins), red wine (Polyphenols including Resveratrol), supplementing the spice Turmeric (especially with black pepper), eating a great variety of fresh (organically growing does seem to increase the beneficial content) fruit and vegetables, especially the brightly coloured ones, especially blueberries, blackberries, raspberries, cherries, strawberries, pomegranate, (although recent research suggests these latter are not quite so good for prostates as originally suggested), eating tomatoes (slightly cooked or as sauce), cruciate vegetables, cabbage, Brussels sprouts, cauliflower, most herbs, olive oil, flax seed and canola oil, whole grain cereals, peas, lentils, muesli, garlic, onions, shallots, chives, mushrooms, especially the unpronounceable Japanese sounding ones, carrots, peppers, yams, broccoli, Bok Choy, sweet potatoes, beetroot, hazelnuts, pecans, walnuts, brazil nuts. Avoid all antiperspirants containing aluminium, scratched Teflon saucepans, dry cleaning smells, new paint, inhaling solvents, carpet and that lovely new car smell, herbicides, insecticides, eating and drinking from hot plastic containers, tins which are lined with plastic, microwaving food in plastic, bottled water that has been in plastic in hot shop windows active and passive smoking or inhaling any smoke from anything burning and so on.

Although this all sounds a bit new agey and alternative, most if not all the above has a real and growing research basis and is a response to the doubling of all cancers since the second world war in the developed world.

There are said to be 25 bioactive "epigenetic" compounds that help reduce cancer incidence and severity:

Vitamin D, Curcumin (Turmeric), Resveratrol, Omega 3 in fish and krill oils, Catechins (EGCG), Conjugated linoleic Acid, Coenzyme Q10, Indole 3 Carbinole/DIM, Sulphoraphanes, Quercetin, Grape seed extract, Modified citrus pectin, Anthocyanins (the blue/purple colour of plums, beetroot, , aubergines etc), Melatonin, Pomegranate, Soy/Genistein, Lycopene, Pterostilbene, Coffee Diterpines, Apigenin, Silibinin, N-acetylcysteine, Vitamin E, Coline, Piperine, and some minerals which are said to have a beneficial effect, including calcium, selenium and zinc. On the other hand, cadmium and mercury have harmful effects. (Canceractive, C Woolams Oct 2014).

The Liverpool Care Pathway:

Was introduced in the early years of the millennium and phased out just over ten years later. It gained a controversial and unsavoury reputation. This was because it was been seen as a way that medical and nursing staff prematurely and high handedly put a stop, simply for management convenience to the previously humane personal and **individual** terminal care generally offered to patients. It started to be seen as a rapid one way system to death. A system that consulted neither patient nor relatives. This wasn't the intention of the designers of the pathway of course. The Pathway's idea was to standardise good quality care and apply it everywhere. I don't know why, but almost all national protocols and guidelines which are promoted as "Gold Standard" or incentivised and generally adopted have a tendency to be applied rigidly like this. When this happens the individual patient's actual needs and wishes are submerged and lost in the pursuit of specious spreadsheet, tablets of stone rigidity. There should never be a protocol, a guideline or a gold standard so inflexible that it can't be bent, changed, ignored or suspended to fit a patient's contemporary needs. This is what worries me about the independent responsibilities given to so many nurse practitioners in many new nursing roles and the protocol and rules-driven approaches of new doctors. No doctor or nurse should ever be so resolute that they will not accept a colleague's experience might trump their algorithm or forget that all rules can be broken on behalf of the patient. Unfortunately, neither senior nurses or newly qualified doctors are known for their plasticity, broad mindedness or their adaptability.

The LCP summary from our local "facilitator" was full of the most atrocious newspeak that the immediate impression when I was first introduced to it was of the process being the whole point and not the outcome. Nothing new there. Read it and see whether it constantly refers you back to the patient or to the "system".

So they said: "The LCP is a multi-professional integrated care pathway (ICP) that provides a template of care for a person in the last few days of life. It facilities the use of local guidelines, promotes education and provides demonstrable outcomes to support clinical governance (Ellershaw and Wilkinson 2003). ICPs are flow sheets which outline the expected and realistic course of a patient's care. Deviations from the plan care are recorded as variances. Each part of the pathway can be tracked and monitored to ensure that the outcomes are within an accepted range of quality. ICPs are an agreed plan of care by a multi-professional team. The LCP replaces all other documentation".

That gives you a flavour of the sort of message we at the sharp end had to decode and how much a priority the patient's wellbeing had in it. It is typical of the modern NHS and shows how divorced much academia has become from the front end of General Practice.

No wonder it didn't work. The whole thing could have been written by George Orwell or J.G.Ballard.

The LCP was devised in 1977 at the Royal Liverpool University Hospital as a way of transferring the philosophy of care for dying patients from the hospice to other health care settings. It is a multi-disciplinary document for the last few days of life.

The LCP was divided into three parts:

Initial assessment

Ongoing assessment

Care after death.

The inflexibility of this attitude is not, I am sure, what was intended in the attempt to mimic hospice care by the doctors at The Royal Liverpool University Hospital. Indeed British hospice care has been rated as amongst the best in the world by an international survey published on World Hospice and Palliative Care Day 2015. This is all the more remarkable as £1bn is funded per year by public donations and £300m by Government contribution (2016). Hospice care should be and usually is at heart personal, flexible and patient focussed. How on earth can something designed and planned and about which the "multi-professional team" is instructed in advance, be flexible and respond to a constantly changing and entirely unpredictable situation? You can't draw up a fixed protocol for a situation which is different for each patient.

Anyway, the Liverpool Pathway Involved what should be a holistic assessment and review of the patient's end of life medical and personal needs to reduce unnecessary interference and make their passing as comfortable, dignified and peaceful as possible.

It should have included a review by the medical staff of:

- Whether any further medications and tests (such as taking the patient's temperature or blood pressure) are actually necessary,
- How to keep the patient as comfortable as possible, for example, by adjusting their position in bed or providing regular mouth care,
- Whether fluids should be given when a patient has stopped being able to eat or drink,
- The patient's spiritual or religious needs,
- Any other personal care needs of the patient and their own carers that are important.

Obviously this approach should only be used in consultation with the relatives/carers as it can involve an end to feeding and fluids and should only be considered when there is definitely no hope of survival.

At the time of writing and revising (July 2013 to late 2017) the Liverpool Pathway was in the process of being dropped. This is because it was used (or was seen as being used) to hasten the dying process and thus clearing hospital beds for the next occupant. People perceived it as another way that nurses and doctors could stop hands-on, personal involvement caring, some ward staff denying water to thirsty patients. Some, apparently, failing in the doctor and nurse's most important role, that of relieving pain or even *caring* at all.

It is ironic that our Prime Minister asked President Obama's ex health advisor, Professor Don Berwick, to investigate what went wrong with so many NHS initiatives and reorganisations of care. He has said staffing levels were inadequate (he suggested at least 1 nurse to 8 patients – which I think is correct) and that there should be a crime of "Wilful and reckless negligence" for which staff should be prosecuted. Predictably, the RCN's response was to criticise the possible downgrading of specialist nurses. Their concern was regarding a potential reduction in numbers of academic nurses in clinical decision making roles. But it is the very distancing of many nurses from basic caring through their focus on higher qualifications and pseudo doctoring that *is* the problem. Healthcare Assistants then take over their real job and this is exactly what many think has caused the general reduction in empathy and standards on the wards in the first place. It is depressing that The RCN should express such concern about *nurses' status* in a discussion solely about serious and cruel abuse of dying patients. Why does it take an American to tell us all this? And why are the Royal Colleges of Nursing and General Practice not only often wrong but DEAD WRONG, ABSOLUTELY and COMPLETELY WRONG, in fact the DEAD OPPOSITE OF RIGHT about so many important aspects of care like this? A degree can't teach you how to empathise with a dying patient.

So: He says that we now can't trust a nurse's or doctor's intrinsic vocation or kindness to ensure that they treat patients ethically anymore and we need to restore caring by making it mandatory. On pain of prosecution. What a sad reflection on our nursing and medical professions and their current ethics. So now we have to teach doctors to have emotional resilience according to the GMC and punish nurses for nor caring. Doctors are too emotionally soft and nurses too empathetically hard, – what an NHS.

There is a whole set of reasons why many NHS good intentions initiated through soft politics never work and often harm the patient. These apply to nursing, medical education, financial oversight, staffing and professional relationships and interfere with what was previously a good, functioning basic system. These affect terminal care, the post Shipman furore on controlled drugs and the consequent introduction of appraisal, drug auditing and prescribing limitations, inhumane local geriatric units and dysfunctional delivery units, nation-wide. Add to this the facts that there are not enough beds in any of our acute hospitals nowadays compared with 20 years ago, that there are too few nurses to cover them, too many of whom aren't able or willing to nurse humanely, that nurses are encouraged to focus on all the wrong things and are too busy to stop and attend to the patient and you begin to see the NHS' problem. There has been an over medicalisation and intellectualisation of the nursing profession in an attempt to turn nursing, which was an honourable and much loved way of life into pseudo medicine but without the practitioners having the full intellectual freedom, mind set, knowledge and training necessary to make independent medical decisions. There is also a constant drive for efficiency but where efficiency on the ward past a certain point nearly always means nurses having to ignore and therefore harm the patients. But politicians and managers who have no experience of medicine think they can make things ever more cost effective by interfering. Every change made in the day to day organisation of the Health Service over the last 30 years, almost without exception, has made things worse for the patients. Greater efficiency on the ward and in the surgery generally means worse care.

The days of the Quality Outcomes Framework may be numbered in each part of the UK and various historical incentives shown to be pointless but part of it was the **"Gold Standard Framework"** in cancer care: this was:

Palliative care indicators and other indicators relating to the GSF

PC 1 The practice has a complete register available of all patients in need of palliative care/support

PC 2 The practice has regular (at least 3-monthly) multidisciplinary case review meetings where all patients on the palliative care register are discussed

Other indicators:

CANCER 1 The practice can produce a register of all cancer patients defined as a register of patients with a diagnosis of cancer excluding non- melanotic skin cancers from 1 April 2003.

CANCER 3 The % of patients with cancer, diagnosed within the past 18 months who have a patient review recorded as occurring within 6 months of the practice receiving confirmation of the diagnosis.

EDUCATION 7 The practice has undertaken a minimum of 12 significant event reviews in the past 3 years which could include:
– any death occurring in the practice premises,
– new cancer diagnoses,

– deaths where terminal care has taken place at home,
– any suicides,
– admission under the Mental Health Act,
– child protection cases,
– medication errors.

EDUCATION 10 The practice has undertaken a minimum of 3 significant event reviews, within the past year.

RECORDS 13 There is a system to alert the out of hours service or duty doctor to patients dying at home.

Does all this look like it will improve the **actual care** that a dying individual experiences from a doctor or nurse or is it all Liverpool Pathway-looks-good-on-paper-stuff?

Chemotherapy:

Each new chemotherapeutic agent costs £500m to bring to clinical availability and as cytotoxic drugs are supposed to be toxic they pose a particular problem in terms of side effect reporting, yellow cards, what side effects are therapeutically predictable, expected, unpredicted, long term, indeed catered for as part of a treatment regime. After all what other course of treatment includes "toxic" in the title?

When do you withdraw a cytotoxic drug because it is too toxic or for instance how do you balance the benefits of a drug that puts most patients with a serious untreatable cancer into remission only to cause leukaemia two years later, or infertility?

Chemotherapy with any agent is labour intensive with monitoring, frequent dosing and supervision of the response, admission for complications. Then there is the cost of the drugs involved.

Pressure groups, the media and manufacturers all push for the rapid and often inappropriate adoption of new treatments but how much is an extra year or few months of life worth if the patient is seventy ? (-is it worth more than an extra year for a teenager who hasn't contributed anything to the exchequer – since the old patient has paid a great deal in tax?) Is this monetary value less if the side effects of treatment itself affect the "quality" of life?

All chemotherapeutic agents are either toxic, immunosuppressive or carcinogenic (Dr D Burke, Chief Chemist at The National cancer Institute 1974). Carcinogens include doxorubicin, streptozocin, BCNU, various hormonal treatments, melphalan, cyclophosphamide, chlorambucil, busulphan, cisplatin, etoposide, adriamycin, daunorubicin and others in the same groups.

Tumours curable in advanced stages by chemotherapy:
Choriocarcinoma, A.L.L. in adults and children, Hodgkin's, Differentiated Large Cell Lymphoma, Lymphoblastic Lymphoma, adults and children, Follicular Mixed Lymphoma, Testicular Cancer, Peripheral Neuroepithelioma, Acute Myelogenous Leukaemia, Wilm's Tumour (Kidney Nephroblastoma), Burkitt's Lymphoma, Neuroblastoma, Small Cell Lung Cancer, Embryonic Rhabdomyosarcoma, Ewings Sarcoma, Ovarian Cancer.

Tumours curable in the adjuvant setting: (An agent that stimulates immunity but is not itself anticancer).
Breast Cancer, Osteogenic Sarcoma, Soft Tissue Sarcoma, Colorectal Cancer.

Tumours responsive in an advanced stage but not yet curable:
Bladder Cancer, Chronic Myeloid Leukaemia, Chronic Lymphatic Leukaemia, Hairy Cell Leukaemia, Multiple Myeloma, Follicular Small Cleaved Cell Lymphoma, Gastric

Cancer, Adrenocortical Cancer, Medulloblastoma, P.R.V., Prostatic Cancer, Insulinoma, Breast Cancer, Cervical Cancer, Soft Tissue Sarcoma, Head and Neck Cancer, Endometrial Cancer, Carcinoid Tumours.

Tumours poorly responsive to conventional treatments in advanced stages: Pancreatic Carcinoma, Osteogenic Sarcoma, Renal Carcinoma, Thyroid Carcinoma, Carcinoma of Penis, Colorectal Carcinoma, Vulval Carcinoma, Melanoma, Non Small Cell Lung Carcinoma, Hepatocellular Carcinoma.

Staging of cancers:

Generally now done as: The TNM System.

Tumour (T) usually based on the size of the primary and its local spread. (1-4). Tx the main tumour cannot be measured. T0 main tumour not discovered. (Stage 0: Carcinoma in situ, no local spread).

Nodes (N) (0-3)

Metastases (M) (0 or 1, – meaning metastases). In lung cancer M1a means spread to the other lung, M1b means spread to the rest of the body.

Breast cancer: (see Breastcancer.org) and "Imaginis" (Good breast cancer resource websites). Also see Hormone section and Screening above.

Breast cancer management has improved in the UK over the last 20 years such that the death rate has dropped 40%. This is said to be due to better UK cancer medical care.

Breast cancer causes/risk factors: Age, being female, BRCA1 and BRCA2 genes, family history, breast cancer in the opposite breast previously, dense breast tissue on USS, lobular CIS, a prolonged menstrual life, having children late, exposure to various hormones – medroxyprogesterone, post menopausal oestrogens and progestogens, not breast feeding, being obese or overweight, alcohol, breast radiation while young, exposure to stilboestrol while in utero, exposure to oestrogenic environmental compounds/plastics/parabens in creams, hormones, shift work, and so on.

Lowering Hb A1C by not eating at night for at least 13 hours reduces the risk of breast cancer recurrence. A raised HbA1C actually increases the risk of every cancer except liver cancer.

Ibuprofen, aspirin and metformin reduce breast cancer incidence. Bisphosphonates reduce boney metastases.

Prognosis is based on the tumour size and histology. Tubular structures, pleomorphism, mitosis count, differentiation, lymph node status and degree of vascular invasion are all taken into account. Hormone receptor status, (– oestrogen and progesterone receptor) – patients who are ER and PR positive have a better prognosis. The HER2 (Human Epidermal Growth Receptor 2) may be over expressed in some tumours resulting in excessive growth and a poorer prognosis. This may respond to Herceptin – or Trastuzamab – humanised monoclonal anti-HER2 antibody.

There are other factors: DNA cytometry and DNA ploidy measure aggressiveness of cancer cells and so on.

There is some evidence that beta blockers may reduce metastasisation of breast cancer cells and improve breast cancer prognosis. (D. Powe, Nottingham Univ. etc). Cancer Research UK was backing a study with 30,000 patients in 2014 but given that some reports say that BBs halve secondary spread if given pre-surgery, what would you say to a patient if she came to you a week before her biopsy/lumpectomy/mastectomy and asked for 80mg of propranolol daily? I for one wouldn't be able to refuse as long as she didn't have asthma.

There are several studies that show that the consumption of walnuts (?) due to omega 3 fatty acids and vitamin E as well as polyphenols etc may reduce the incidence and growth of breast cancer, (American Institute for Cancer Research website), bowel cancer (Journal of Nutritional Biochemistry May 2015) as well as prostate cancers.

Other dietary strategies to protect against breast cancer would include the consumption of supplementary iodine, nocturnal melatonin, green tea, Vitamin D3 to raise blood levels to 65-75 ng/ml (usually 5000IU/day), if over the age of 45 years ?Progesterone cream? and plenty of cruciferous vegetables (cauliflower, cabbage, broccoli, Brussels sprouts, kale, bok choy etc).

Also if you have your breast surgery in the second half of the menstrual cycle some studies say you double your survival. (?Due to an increased progesterone level) (Mohr Br J Cancer 1996).

Supplementary iron MAY increase the risk of breast cancer.

The incidence of breast cancer is clearly increasing. In the 1960's in America 1:20 women presented with the disease. By 2005 it was 1:8. This is only from the Grandmothers' generation to the granddaughters'.

There is a 1 in 9 women lifetime risk (some authors say 1:12), we have national screening of: 50-70 year olds. Worldwide the highest incidence is in the USA and the Netherlands and the lowest in China.

There are roughly 22,000-25,000 patients/year in the UK (different sources), 25% are dead at 4 years, 50% dead at 12 years although this mortality rate gets better every year and may already (2017) be out of date. 11,600 die a year. Only 1% breast cancer deaths were men in 2010. In Lobular carcinoma in situ, LCIS, there is a >7% risk of cancer after 10 years and the breast cancer risk is >1% of recurrence on the contra-lateral side of a previous cancer, per year.

Significant features: (other than any new breast lump) change in skin contour, skin tethering, bloody nipple discharge, retraction, distortion or nipple eczema. Diffuse breast pain is not usually a serious symptom, in fact cancer generally isn't painful when it presents.

Treatment:

1/3 of secondaries are hormone sensitive. Aromatase inhibitors (Anastrozole (non steroidal), Exemestane (steroidal), Letrozole (non steroidal) stop endogenous androgens being converted to oestrogen.

Traditionally treatment is excision, local or mastectomy, axillary clearance with or without DXT, Tamoxifen>Megestrol>Aminoglutethimide.

The standard regime now is often 2 years Tamoxifen followed by 3 years of one of the Aromatase inhibitors.

Typical Chemotherapy in HER2-Pos breast cancer is Herceptin – Trastuzamab. A monoclonal antibody that interferes with the HER2/neu receptor. These are cell membrane receptors that control cell reproduction. It is given at 3 weekly intervals for 1 year.

Breast Cancer can be graded under the T, N M system or:

Stages: **Stage 0**   Non invasive tumour ie DCIS.

  Stage 1A   **Invasive** tumour up to 2 cms diameter, no spread, no nodes.

  1B   Invasive tumour is only found in nodes, not the breast and are 0.2-2 mms diameter or Invasive tumour in the breast <2cms diameter and the nodes affected 0.2-2mm diameter. Microscopic invasion is possible in Stage 1 but is <1mm.

  Stage 2A   No tumour found in breast but >2mm cancer found in 1-3 axillary or other local nodes. The tumour is <2cms diameter and has spread to axillary nodes or the breast tumour is 2-5 cms diameter without axillary spread.

  2B   The breast tumour is 2-5 cms diameter and 0.2-2mm cancer is found in lymph nodes or 2-5 cms diameter and 1-3 axillary or other local nodes. The breast tumour is 5cms diameter without nodal spread.

  Stage 3A   No breast tumour or the tumour can be any size, with 4-9 axillary or other nodes. The tumour is >5cms with 0.2-2mm diameter secondary spread in the nodes or the tumour is >5cms and spread to 1-3 axillary or other nodes.

  3B   The tumour is any size and has spread to the chest wall and or skin of the breast and may have spread to 9 axillary nodes or to other nodes. **Inflammatory breast cancer** is stage 3B or worse – Reddened or swollen skin, tumour in nodes and may be found in the skin.

  3C   Any sized or no detectable breast tumour, but if there is a tumour it may have spread to the chest wall/skin, and spread to 10 or more axillary or supra and infraclavicular nodes or axillary and sternal nodes.

  4   Invasive cancer that has spread beyond the breast and regional nodes to distant nodes and organs.

ER and PR positive denotes (o) estrogen or progesterone receptor positive tumour cells and therefore the tumour is likely to respond to hormonal manipulation. (Tamoxifen, Exemestane).

The HER2/neu marker on the tumour cells indicates aggressiveness but "Herceptin" (Trastuzumab) is used in this type of tumour, – an antibody to the receptor.

Triple negative cancer (15-25% of the total) is ER, PR and HER2/neu negative and has no selective treatment but standard chemotherapy/radiotherapy are used. The risk of relapse is higher than for hormone positive breast cancers in the first 3-5 years but becomes relatively much less after that.

Mastectomy vs. Lumpectomy:

Lumpectomy is less traumatic, there is a quicker recovery, BUT the post op radiation therapy is longer (5-7 weeks). This affects breast reconstruction and there is a higher risk of local recurrence. It is not possible to re-irradiate the area if there is a local recurrence in future. Further local surgery may be needed if the margins are not clear.

Mastectomy is more likely to remove the whole tumour at one go but requires a longer recovery, more extensive reconstruction and if axillary nodes are removed (and as in radiotherapy to the area), there may be arm lymphoedema.

Sentinel node biopsy is the removal of a limited number of axillary nodes and causes less oedema risk.

Radiotherapy can be used to the breast after lumpectomy ("breast preservation surgery"), if the tumour is early stage, <4cms, in one site and excised with clear margins.

Radiotherapy is given to the remaining breast tissue after mastectomy especially if the tumour is >5cms, there is lymph or vascular invasion, 1 node (premenopausal) or >4 nodes (postmenopausal) involved, there are positive margins of resection or there is skin invasion.

Screening: 1:9 women (or thereabouts) will get breast cancer at sometime in their lives. They are screened by mammogram in the UK 3 yearly from the age of 50 to 70.

4% will be asked to go back and of those 1 in 8 turn out to have cancer.

Family History of Breast cancer: Lifetime risk

1 relative >40 years	1:8
2 relatives 50-60 yrs	1:8
2 relatives 40-50	1:4 – 1:6
2 relatives 30-40	1:3 – 1:4
3 relatives average age 40-50	1:3

The BRCA1 and BRCA2 genes: The Angelina Jolie effect:

Breast cancer: 12% of the general female population will get breast cancer in their lifetime.(One source). 55-65% of women with the BRCA1 mutation and 45% of women with the BRCA2 mutation will have breast cancer by the age of 70. In terms of ovarian cancer these risks are 1.3% for the general population during their lifetime, 39% for women with BRCA1 and 11-17% of women with the BRCA2 mutation will get ovarian cancer by the age of 70.

Angelina Jolie had a bilateral mastectomy followed by bilateral oophorectomy and salpingectomy saying she had the BRCA1 gene which gave her an "87% risk of breast cancer and a 50% risk of ovarian cancer" quoted in Mail Online March 2015. Perhaps she has the right to some hyperbole given her profession and the emotion that comes with this sort of assault on who you are and how you perceive yourself.

Bowel Cancer: Lifetime risk

General population	1:35
More than 2 first degree relatives affected (suggests dominant pedigree)	1:3
Two first degree relatives	1:6
One first degree relative <45 years	1:10
One first degree and one second degree relative	1:12
One first degree relative >45 yrs	1:17

Familial adenomatous polyposis (1:4 are spontaneous mutations, almost all will develop cancer).

Hereditary non polyposis colorectal cancer (Lynch syndrome) increases various intra abdominal cancers. Causes 40% of bowel cancer in patients under 30. 90% men and 70% women with this mutation develop bowel cancer by 70.

Colorectal Cancer:

Dukes Staging – Largely superseded by the T, N, M. (Tumour, Nodes, Metastases) system.

Frequency at diagnosis and 5 year survival (now slightly out of date and pessimistic)

A	Localised in bowel wall	11%	83%
B	Penetrates the bowel	35%	64%
C	Spread to lymph glands	26%	38%
D	Distant metastases	29%	3%

15,000 deaths in 1996 in England and Wales, 68% Colon, 32% Rectal.

Causes:

Risks are doubled by a close relative who has had the disease, previous IBS (never just assume an exacerbation of symptoms is benign especially in an older patient), too much salt, pickles, animal fat, (trans fats can increase polyps), processed meat, alcohol, smoking, laziness. Diabetics have 3X the risk of colorectal cancer.

COX – 2 activity which is thought to be behind bowel tumour formation can be lowered by regular low doses of aspirin, ibuprofen, other COX 2 inhibitors, fish oils, Turmeric, (Circumin, Curcumin), garlic and ginger. Bowel cancer is rarer in India.

Aspirin also prevents established bowel cancer metastasising as does Cimetidine (but none of the other H2 antagonists). (Gut 1994, 35:1632-1636, Lancet 24/12/94 Vol 344 1768-1769 Warwick Adams Morris etc).

Aspirin has long been known to have anticancer effects. A paper in Aug 2014 (Annals of Oncology) declared that the advantages of aspirin prophylaxis was third in line to stopping smoking and not being obese in preventing cancer. Nowadays you can add not avoiding sunshine to that list if you are discussing "Cancer prevention". The authors showed that if patients between 50 and 65 years of age took daily aspirin for 10 years, there would be a 9% reduction in the number of cancers, strokes and heart attacks overall in men and 7% in women. The total number of deaths from any cause would be 4% lower over 20 years. Long term aspirin reduces various gastro intestinal cancers. – colorectal, oesophageal and gastric cancers and an increasing number of well read cancer survivors are taking low dose aspirin to reduce metastases unbeknown to their oncologists.(See anticoagulant section). More recently, (Sept 2015) the American US preventive Services Task Force has suggested that all adults aged 50-69 should all take aspirin daily for at least 10 years to reduce their risk from CVD and colorectal cancer. At the time, the American Cancer Society recommended against aspirin prophylaxis as a prevention strategy for colorectal cancer. The Task Force contradicting this, said that there was evidence of benefit between these ages but insufficient evidence to recommend prophylactic aspirin outside the 50-70 year group. Low dose aspirin taken in conjunction with active cancer treatment is associated with a 15-20% mortality reduction in a range of cancers. The reductions are (from a review in PLoS One in 2016) respectively: 24% in colonic cancer, breast cancer 13% and 11% in prostate cancer. It may be that the benefit is limited to cancers with the mutation PIK3CA, HLA class1 Ag, or over expression of COX2. Overall the reduction in mortality was found to be 17%. There was a 23% reduction in relative risk of metastatic spread. Long term Metformin seems to reduce the rate of various cancers – including pancreas, colon and hepatocellular carcinoma.

So the overall figures for aspirin and cancer (etc mortality) are:

5 years of daily aspirin use reduces colorectal cancer incidence by 37% and colorectal mortality by 52%.

The risk of oesophageal cancer is reduced 58% by daily aspirin in clinical trials and 44% in cohort studies.

Aspirin reduces stomach cancer mortality by from 31% to 41%.

There is a negligible effect on pancreatic cancer.

Aspirin reduces incident breast cancer by 18%.

Cohort studies show a reduction in breast cancer of 8% in regular aspirin users. Oddly there was no effect seen in the WHS-This isn't W H Smiths, this is the Women's Health Study, 1993-2004 (Brigham and Women's Hospital and Harvard) to look at low dose aspirin and vitamin E regarding primary prevention of cardiovascular disease and cancer. In all, it spawned 400 published research reports directly and indirectly related to general population cardiovascular issues.

Aspirin has little effect on prostate cancer. It may slightly reduce lung cancer mortality but not incident lung cancer.

Generally Aspirin needs 3 years to reduce incidence and 5 years to reduce mortality.

Any dose above 75mg is effective at preventing the cancers it prevents.

It reduces the rate of non fatal MIs but primary prevention with aspirin does not reduce cardiovascular mortality.

Aspirin increases the risk of haemorrhagic stroke by 32-36%.

It also increases the risk of major extracranial bleeding by 30-70%.

Overall by taking aspirin for 10 years between the ages of 50 and 65, the 15 year risk of MI, cancer or stroke is reduced by 9% among men and 7% among women (mainly through the effect on colorectal cancer).

The NNT with aspirin for 10 years to prevent a major event is between 33 and 127.

Aspirin should reduce the risk for death by 4% at 20 years (all through cancer mortality). Vitamin D significantly reduces incidence and apparently Vitamin E and Magnesium supplementation lower the risk of gut cancer too – though surprisingly, a high fibre diet is now **not** thought to reduce the risk. How attitudes change. Low levels of Vitamin B12, Folic Acid and Biotin may increase risk through a negative effect on gut micro flora. Previous suspicions relating bowel cancer to red meat and coffee consumption are still debated. Folic Acid supplementation reduces colorectal adenoma (Cancer Prevention Research 16/05/2013).

So if a patient with bowel cancer comes to you and asks what you would think about prescribing them aspirin, Cimetidine, Bisphosphonates and Vitamin D, it is quite possible that, according to some studies you would be reducing the risk of recurrence by at least half. I believe it would be unethical to refuse.

Higher doses of Metformin are associated with increased survival in colorectal cancer patients (Cancer epidemiology, biomarkers and prevention 10/6/2013) and Metformin reduces the risk of non smokers developing lung cancer (Kaiser Permanente, Oakland, Jan 2015) by half over 5 years of use. Oddly though it seems to increase the risk for smokers.

Screening: The national occult blood stool screening campaign detects 2 cancer patients per 1000 samples. It started by testing 60-69 year olds but will be extended to 74.

Bowel cancer screening:

Faecal occult Blood and M2-PK (an enzyme biomarker) screening reduces the risk of dying of bowel cancer by 16%. The NHS screening is done 2 yearly from 60 to 69 and is being extended to 74 yrs. The patient is posted a card with six areas upon which to smear a sample of stool using cardboard spatulae. The result comes back in two weeks.

The local "Programme hub" is contactable on 0800 707 6060 in the UK.

The incidence and mortality of bowel cancer have been declining in the USA over recent years, presumably due to their extensive screening of the over 50's. However a paper from Texas (JAMA Surgery Nov 5 2014) highlighted the rising incidence in younger, unscreened adults. The biggest increase being in those between 20 and 34, in colon and rectal cancer at all stages. The authors predicted a doubling in incidence in the younger population within 15 years so that 1 in 6 of colon cancers and 1 in 4 of rectal cancers will be in the under 50 year olds. Never assume a change in bowel habit or persistent rectal bleeding even in a teenager is benign. The young patient tends to have a left sided tumour and amongst the current theories regarding the increased incidence are dietary changes, reduction in milk (calcium is protective), increase in sugar intake and diabetes, processed foods, obesity, sedentary lifestyle, antibiotics and changes in the microbiome, etc.

A study published in 2015 (Nature Medicine) looked at genetic markers of bowel cancer in order to link clinical behaviour and response to treatment to molecular subtype. It found that nearly all tumours fell into four groups: CMS1 CMS2 CMS3 and CMS4.

Subtype CMS4 had the worst prognosis and needed the most extensive treatment while CMS2 had better survival rates even on recurrence of the cancer.

If these tests become generally available, they should allow oncologists to grade the treatment appropriately for the cancer risk.

Pancreatic Cancer:

8,000/year, one of the commonest 10 cancers.

75%>65 yrs age,

1 yr survival 10-20%,

Symptoms depend upon location.

50% are head of pancreas (some present with jaundice, some with back or abdominal pain).

Jaundice and rapid weight loss indicate a worse prognosis.

Diabetes may be a clue.

Family history, personal past history of pancreatitis, diabetes, obesity and smoking and being an Ashkenazi Jew are all risk factors.

Urgent upper abdominal USS or CT are mandatory in recent onset upper abdominal pain in an older patient with weight loss with or without back pain, diabetes etc.

High levels of enzymes LYVE1, REG1A and TFF1 are present in the urine of patients with pancreatic cancer compared with chronic pancreatitis and normal controls. The combination of all three allows for a 90% accurate stage 1 or 2 diagnosis. (Queen Mary Un. Lond. 2015)

Lung cancer:

The second commonest UK cancer and the biggest cause of death from cancer. Although smoking is the major aetiological factor, many new lung cancer patients have either never smoked (less than 100 cigarettes in their life) or have given up. Apparently 80,000 UK citizens still die every year directly from smoking. Despite moves to prevent all smoking on hospital property in 2013, aimed at patients and staff (Isn't "Hospital property" public property and don't smokers pay more in taxes for a shorter life expectancy than non smokers and thus become less of a drain on NHS resources in retirement than non smokers?) 20% of adult patients still smoke (2015). If you look at psychiatric patients it is actually 70%. As with many other cancers, some foods and regular exercise seem to protect against lung cancer even in smokers. A study in 2014 found that the higher you live above sea level, the lower your lung cancer risk. For every 1000m higher you are, lung cancer decreases by 7.23/100,000 – a 13% drop.

There is a linear relationship between number of cigarettes smoked and the risk of getting lung cancer (Doll, Hill etc 1964 who studied what killed 40,000 British doctors). If you doubled the number of cigarettes you smoked, you doubled your risk. 40 a day was twice the risk of 20, 20 a day twice the risk of 10 etc. This is probably the most famous epidemiological study of all time. Electronic cigarettes, e-cigarettes, which vapourise Nicotine without the other noxious constituents of tobacco, are currently causing some controversy. They figure in pop videos and some have flavourings such as cherry, bubble gum, spearmint, etc, attractive to teenagers. Public Health commentators fear they may be a gateway to real smoking for the young. They do however offer a real way of stopping smoking and are at least as effective as old style Nicotine replacement patches. Sadly, in the first published trial comparing the two, fewer than 10% gave up smoking (e-cigarettes 7.3%, Nicotine patches 5.8%, placebo e-cigarettes 4.1%). Hardly impressive for any substitute.

Non small cell lung cancer has increased in America from 12% to 40% of the total in the last 20 years. It is not smoking related but is like many cancers, oestrogen sensitive: (Breast, colon, some brain tumours, prostate, testicular and ovarian cancers). This is thought to be secondary to the increase in environmental oestrogens – presumably excreted waste products as well as the oestrogenic chemicals in urine, food, plastics, pollutants and so on. After a patient has given up smoking, his or her risk of lung cancer is higher the older they were when they gave up and the longer they smoked before they gave up. It is less if they exercise regularly after stopping smoking.

The never smoked lung cancer sufferers vary tremendously depending on the source you read, – from 10% in some American texts to the 60% quoted above. In non smokers, recognised risk factors include second hand smoke, natural radon exposure, asbestos, arsenic and silica. Tumour suppressor genes and proto-oncogenes have different mutational profiles in the smoker and non smoker cancer populations (namely TP53, KRAS and EGFR). Gefitinib and Erlotinib work better in the non smoker cancers.

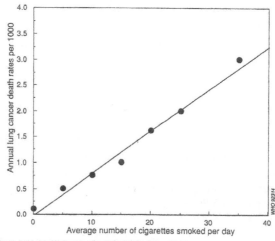

Death rates from lung cancer (per 1000) by number of cigarettes smoked, British doctors, 1951–1961

Source: Doll & Hill, 1964. Reproduced by kind permission of the publisher.

Death Rates From lung cancer per 1000 (DRLC) by number of cigarettes smoked. Reproduced by kind permission of the publisher.

Roy Castle, the singer and trumpeter, died of lung cancer in 1994 never having smoked but, presumably having passively smoked in pubs and clubs a great deal.

Lung cancers are: Non small cell lung cancers including oat cell which are adenocarcinomata (40% total lung cancers but the commonest in non smokers), squamous cell carcinoma (30% total lung cancers, smoking related), large cell carcinoma (9% of total lung cancers) and small cell lung cancer (usually smoking related). Small cell cancers metastasise early, are smoking associated and can produce endocrine symptoms. Carcinoids can develop in the lungs.

A large number of other cancers spread to the filter that is the lung vascular bed.

The majority of lung cancers are related to smoking (85%), the other known factors being radon, asbestos (which also causes pleural cancer, mesothelioma), genetic factors, pollution and passive smoking.

Overall there is only a 15% 5 year survival and symptoms depend on where and how big the tumour is. Cough, haemoptysis, weight loss, dyspnoea, audible wheeze, clubbing, dysphagia, venous obstruction, Horner's Syndrome etc. are the commoner presenting features.

Lung cancers have a variety of systemic "paraneoplastic" presentations: These include myasthenia, inappropriate ADH, hypercalcaemia, etc.

Spread is to brain, bone, adrenals, local spread, kidneys, pericardium and the opposite lung.

Treatment is excision, radiotherapy and chemotherapy with a platinum drug plus etoposide, or a variety of other agents.

A good explanation of staging of lung cancer is in the NICE "Diagnosis and Treatment of Lung cancer" (Feb 2005).

But in summary:
The primary tumour:
Tx cannot be assessed.
T0 No evidence of primary tumour.
T1 <3cm.
T2>3cm, involving main bronchus, >2cm distal to carina etc.
T3 Any size invading chest wall, diaphragm, pericardium etc.
T4 Any size invading mediastinum, heart, great vessels etc.
Regional Nodes:
Nx Can't be assessed.
N0 No regional node metastases.
N1 Metastases to ipsilateral peribronchial or hilar nodes etc.
N2 Metastases to ipsilateral mediastinal or subcarinal nodes.
N3 Metastases to contralateral mediastinal, hilar, ipsilateral scalene or supraclavicular nodes etc.
Distant Metastases:
Mx Cannot be assessed.
M0 No distant metastases.
M1 Distant metastases present.

Oesophageal cancer:
Is usually squamous (usually tobacco and alcohol related, mostly in the upper 2/3) or adenocarcinoma (usually reflux related, via a transition of Barrett's oesophagus and usually in the lower 1/3). 2M:1F. Dysphagia, weight loss, odynophagia, (pain on swallowing), heartburn, food sticking, regurgitation, occasionally nausea and or vomiting are the usual presenting symptoms. There may also be hoarseness (recurrent LN palsy) or haemoptysis/ haematemesis.

Causes of gullet cancer include the afore mentioned smoking and heavy alcohol consumption, bisphosphonates (which double the risk), chronic reflux, often silent but via Barrett's oesophagus, obesity-which quadruples oesophageal cancer and may act via reflux, (being overweight causes 1:4 of all cases in the UK), HPV, Plummer Vinson Syndrome, (oesophageal web due to iron deficiency), Coeliac Disease (which increases the risk of squamous carcinoma) and achalasia.

Small doses of aspirin reduce the risk (as with other GI neoplasms) and cruciferous vegetables and highly coloured fruit and vegetables are protective – as they are against virtually all cancers – see diet section. Bizarrely, Helicobacter gastric infection may be slightly protective. Roasted, fried and barbequed meat is thought to increase the risk, so does exposure to soot and the manufacture of rubber.

Diagnosis is generally done via upper GI endoscopy. Staging is by CT or PET scanning,

Treatment includes stenting, resection, radiotherapy and chemotherapy.

The 5 year survival is about 15%, Staging is the usual T N M system.

Prostate cancer: (See Urology and PCA3/PSA in pathology and screening above:)
The second most common male cancer cause of death (to lung cancer) and the most commonly diagnosed cancer in men (next in order are: Lung, bowel, bladder, NHL, MM,

kidney, oesophagus, leukaemia and stomach). 10,800 men die annually in the UK from the disease, 41,700 new cases being diagnosed.

The average age of diagnosis is 70-74 years and average age of death 80-84. (NHS Prostate Cancer Risk Management Programme booklet 2009). This is slightly confusing as some life expectancy statistics (Office of National Statistics 2006-8) put male life expectancy in the South East of England at 79.2 years, Scotland 75 years. I cannot believe a diagnosis of prostate cancer is good for you. By the age of 80, 80% of men will have positive biopsies for prostate cancer. Only 1:26 men die of the disease though – so a lot of men die with the histology still in their prostates but not *of the "disease"*. 1:2 men will die of cardiovascular disease of course.

Genes:

The BRCA1 gene confers 2X the risk and BRCA2 up to 8X the risk of prostate cancer (ie a positive family history of prostate or breast cancer). New research is directed at finding a gene marker for the proportion of men with a raised PSA who have the rare potentially aggressive prostatic cancer rather than those with indolent cancers that can safely be left and watched. There are five separate subset types of prostate cancer genetically with 100 individual genes linked to the development of prostatic cancer.

Age and family history are risk factors. Race: Being black is a 3X risk factor, with South Asian men having a lower incidence than white men. Diet, chronic inflammation, the HPC1 HPC2 HPCX and CAPB genes and exposure to the defoliant, agent orange are other contributory factors. Living near or working on golf courses increases prostate cancer incidence and is thought to be due to toxic pesticide sprays.

Gleason Scoring:

A biopsy of the prostate is done and the two most common histological types looked for and graded. The most common tissue in the microscope field is listed first. These two tissues are graded from 1 to 5, 1 being the most benign (normal prostate), 5 the most aggressive (poorly differentiated tumour). This is the Gleason Grading.

Then the two scores are given in the report – for instance "3+4"

A "Gleason Score" of 3+4 (total 7) Is not as bad as 4+3 as the commonest tissue (4) in the latter is more aggressive then the commonest tissue (3) in the former.

PIN, Prostatic Intraepithelial Neoplasia, needs follow up. ASAP, (not as soon as possible but "Atypical Small Acinar Proliferation") suggests possible cancer and the need (unfortunately) for another biopsy.

So the higher the **Gleason Score** the worse the prognosis.

Thus: Gleason score and survival:

4-5 mean survival	20 years
6	16
7	10
8-10	5 although these are roughly millenium figures and prognosis is getting better all the time.

20% tumours are missed at biopsy as they tend to be at the front of the gland, the biopsy usually being done transrectally, from behind. (Unless the 30 needles technique of the perineal TEMPLATE BIOPSY is used – this approach being from below through the perineal skin). The transrectal approach is why DRE misses many tumours as well. This is leading to a call for routine prostate MRI scans for men with raised PSAs (MPMRI – the multiparametric MRI). Most prostate tumours especially in older men are fairly indolent and new research is directed towards finding the genetic keys in the 100 genes linked to prostate cancer to identify the smallish percentage of aggressive tumours. There are 5 basic genetic types of tumour and few of them are particularly likely to become highly malignant.

Staging:

T1 in the prostate gland

T2 still in gland T2a only in 1/2 of 1 lobe

T2b >1/2 of 1 lobe

T2c in both lobes

T3a through capsule

T3b into seminal vesicles

T4 local spread e.g. to rectum or bladder or pelvic muscles-locally advanced.

Nodes:	Metastases:
Nx Nodes not checked	M0 No cancer outside the pelvis
N0 No local nodes affected	M1 Cancer outside pelvis
N1 Tumour in nodes	M1A Cancer in nodes outside pelvis
M1B Cancer in bone	
M1C Cancer elsewhere.	

1/4 – 1/3 of men present with metastases. A surprising analysis of data published in Nov 2015 in the NEJM showed that since the widespread introduction of PSA testing (admittedly there is a large number of tumours treated that would never have killed their owners), the incidence of metastatic prostate cancer has dropped 50%. So PSA is not a brilliant specific screening test but apparently it does save lives overall. Early cancers are usually peripheral within the gland and asymptomatic.

The section on diet gives a lot of information about why prostate cancer has become a bit of an epidemic since the second world war. An ageing population, better cancer registration, better detection and diagnosis are all part of this increase but there does also seem to be a genuine increase in incidence too.

Food plays a significant negative and positive effect in the prostate cancer story with obesity, red meat and dairy products (a straight line correlation) probably all increasing risk, omega three fatty acids, Resveratrol, Turmeric, Saw Palmetto, even Broccoli, various nuts and mushrooms possibly reducing the risk.

It appears that various pesticides increase the risk of prostate cancer (Am J Epidemiology, 2013), Fonofos, Malathion, Terbufos and Aldrin all increase the risk of aggressive prostate cancer in farmers and agricultural workers. It may be worth mentioning that Malathion is used as a conventional treatment for head lice, crab lice and scabies as well as wood worming treatment for lofts and old buildings. Oestrogenic compounds including various "plastic" residues, (Bisphenol A, BPA from bottles and the plastic lining of drinks cans) are also thought to cause increase rates of prostatic malignancy.

13 Xeno-oestrogens are now linked to prostate cancer.

There is now some evidence that statins may reduce the progress of prostate cancer (April 2014).

Conventional cancer treatment largely and strangely ignores the powerful effect of diet in causing and treating cancer. There is now a huge conventional and persuasive literature on the subject. As well as lycopene, (tomatoes), pomegranate, broccoli, grape seed, selenium and various antioxidants in red fruit, vegetables and drink it seems that metformin reduces the death rate from prostate cancer recurrence by a up to quarter for each 6 months "treatment". It does something similar in bowel, lung and other cancers. This is something as surprising as it is unexpected and as unknown and unbroadcast as it is underutilised. You could also advise your patients to eat lightly cooked tomatoes and broccoli as both have specific anti prostate cancer properties. Indeed a diet with relatively increased vegetable fat reduces the death rate from established prostatic cancer (JAMA Internal Medicine 10/06/2013). A low vitamin D level worsens the prognosis in prostatic cancer as it seems to in many conditions.

Vasectomy has been under suspicion as a potential cause of prostate cancer for many years. I have always reassured my patients that there was no link but a study in J Clin oncology Jul 2014 showed a 20% increased risk of the most aggressive, most lethal prostate cancers in vasectomised men. The American Urological Association, spurred in to action by this report performed a meta analysis of evidence incorporating 8 cohort studies and came to the conclusion that there was no clinically or statistically significant association. Phew.

In other words, if there is an association, it is very small.

Fish oil consumption reduces the incidence of prostate cancer – the seemingly universally beneficial marine Omega 3 oils contribute here but there is some evidence that the few patients who over supplement their diet with fish oils may slightly increase their risk. Strange.

Ejaculating frequently reduces the rate of prostate cancer: It being 20% lower in men who ejaculate 21 times a month compared with those who ejaculate 4-7 times a month. This 20% reduction applies to age groups 20-29 and 40-49 – and for the lifetime average.

The main problem with screening and the most difficult treatment issue for GPs is that neoplasia is common but prostate cancer death is rare. Morbidity from investigation (biopsies) and treatment (radiation and surgery) is significant and most cancers are indolent but **some** are very aggressive and it is difficult to differentiate the two in advance. That is the PSA dilemma in a walnut sized nutshell.

Walnuts, by the way, reduce the incidence of various cancers, containing as they do omega 3 fatty acids and twice as many antioxidants as any other commonly eaten nut. Gamma tocopherol, a form of Vitamin E in walnuts helps reduce incidence of breast, prostate and lung cancer. They also reduce endothelin, a substance associated with blood vessel inflammation and found raised in prostate cancer patients. They reduce bowel cancer via miRNA expression (which affects inflammation, vascularity and proliferation in bowel cancer) – at least in mice bowel tumours.

So specifically (all the following have been the results of a number of controlled studies at reputable centres by the way):

Dairy products increase the rate of prostate, breast, ovarian and colorectal cancers.

Broccoli and tomatoes (Lycopene) decrease prostate cancer risk.

Various nuts reduce all sorts of cancers (pecans – breast and prostate, walnuts – breast, prostate, ?bowel and lung).

Turmeric (Cu/ircumin) reduces bowel cancer.

Red grape polyphenols reduce many cancers.

Vitamin D reduces cancer of the colon, prostate and breast and probably various other cancers.

Vitamin K reduces metastasisation from colonic cancer.

Colon cancer is increased by salt, red meat, being sedentary, possibly by low fibre in the diet.

Beta carotene reduces the incidence of a number of cancers – including colonic, as do

The anti oxidants Selenium, Zinc, Vitamin C as well as

Some forms of Vitamin E (but not Alpha Tocopherol).

Vitamin K.

Vitamin A.

Niacin,

Biotin,

Co Enzyme Q10 (which also helps reduce some statin side effects) all non specifically reduce cancer risks.

But back to prostates and diet:

The American Society of Clinical Oncology 2013 was presented a placebo controlled double blind study on treatment refractory prostate cancer patients. The study related to the effect of a combination of nutrients on PSA levels. There was a 64% reduction in PSA when patients took pomegranate seed, broccoli, green tea and turmeric. Very few conventional treatments are as effective as this.

So in summary: **Supplementary treatments**, any of which you could advise your prostate cancer patients to take which all seem to have at least some scientific basis:

Flaxseed, Boron, Cruciferous vegetables, (incl: Broccoli) Vitamin D (Big doses) – 4000Us a day, Soy Isoflavones, Green tea, Omega 3 Fatty Acids, Circumin (Turmeric), Co Enzyme Q10, Gamma Tocopherol Vitamin E, Lycopene, Selenium, Zinc, Milk Thistle, Gamma Linoleic Acid, Zeaxanthin, Pomegranate, Saw Palmetto, Resveratrol, Lignans, Vitamin K, Beta-Sitosterol, Apigenin, Ginger, Inositol, N-Acetylcysteine, Quercetin, Reishi, 5-Loxin, Watercress, Grapeseed, Glycyrrhizin, Modified Citrus Pectin, (Life Extension Dec 2013).

Ovarian Cancer:

Risk factors:

A family history of cancer, being infertile or having fertility treatment, using an intra uterine device, using hormone replacement therapy, being overweight or tall, having endometriosis, using talcum powder, smoking, dietary factors, having breast cancer.

The main histotypes are epithelial in origin and include high-grade serous carcinoma, clear cell carcinoma, endometrioid carcinoma, low-grade serous carcinoma and mucinous carcinoma. There are many other rare types that are non-epithelial in origin. Each varies in aggressiveness and response to treatment. High grade serous carcinoma is the most malignant form and is up to 70% of the total. Most actually come from the fallopian tube rather than the ovary and often present already having spread into the abdomen. Up to 25% of sufferers have the BRCA 1/2 mutation.

Clear cell carcinoma, the second commonest type makes up just over 10% and may be associated with pre existing endometriosis. These patients respond poorly to chemotherapy, better to standard radiotherapy.

Endometroid carcinoma again arises from endometriosis and requires surgical rather than chemotherapy treatment.

Mucinous cacinoma makes up about 4% and has a poor response rate to chemotherapy.

Some express the HER2 oncogene.

Low grade serous carcinomas have a poor prognosis but are rare.

Non epithelial tumours include:

Germ cell tumours, Stromal Tumours.

In 2004 Shih and Kurman divided ovarian tumours into Types I (associated with BRAF and KRAS alterations, the least malignant) and II (associated with p53 alterations and includes the most malignant serous carcinomata). Recent published data has shown fallopian epithelium can seed and encyst the adjacent ovary initiating an ovarian cancer. It is postulated that prior salpingectomy would prevent most serous ovarian cancers. Hence Angelina Jolie's bilateral Salpingo – oophorectomy.

Death rates from ovarian cancer have not changed much in 50 years.

There is a lifetime risk of 1:80 of ovarian cancer for UK women. The risk is doubled by a glass of milk a day (American Journal of Clinical Nutrition, The Rainbow Diet, pp113).

The main worrying symptoms are pelvic or abdominal pain, loss of appetite, urinary frequency or urgency, early fullness or distension, bloating, weight loss, fatigue, change of bowel habit. You should never diagnose new onset of IBS in anyone over 50 – and while we are on the subject, never assume iron deficiency is benign in anyone of the same age either. The first is ovarian cancer and the second bowel cancer until proven otherwise.

Check CA125, plus do an USS if in doubt. A large scale study in 2015 (the UK Collaborative Trial of Ovarian Cancer Screening) performed annual Ca125s on post menopausal women in over 13 NHS trusts and found that screening Ca125 for changing levels may be a more reliable way of early detection over time than the absolute level. If levels became relatively elevated the patient was given an USS. 86% of cancers were detected.

The COCP slightly reduces the risk of ovarian cancer, the benefit lasting up to 30 years. The COCP slightly increases the risk of cervical cancer. HRT increases the risk of ovarian cancer.

8% women with ovarian cancer will have a family history, increasing the risk 3X. With 2 affected relatives the risk goes up 10X. The genes include the BRCA genes involved with hereditary ovarian and breast cancer (BRCA1 and BRCA2, both Aut. Dom. and inherited via either parent) as well as the mismatch repair genes of hereditary non polyposis colon cancer-HNPCC.

BRCA1 is a gene on Chromosome 17 and should produce a DNA repair protein. Mutations of this gene cause most (75%) of inherited ovarian cancers. The frequency of this gene is about 0.1% in the general population but higher in certain gene pools (eg Ashkenazi Jews). It causes inherited breast cancer as well as ovarian cancer.

BRCA2 is on chromosome 13 and should also encode a DNA repair protein. This defect causes 10% of inherited ovarian cancers. This is also commoner in Ashkenazi Jews. It also contributes towards inherited breast cancers too.

BRCA1 may increase the risk for prostate cancer and BRCA2 for pancreatic cancer as well as for the female cancers. Fallopian tube cancer risk is higher in BRCA carriers as is peritoneal carcinoma which originates from the same embryological tissue as ovarian tissue.

HNPCC (Hereditary nonpolyposis colorectal cancer, Lynch syndrome) families have an increased risk of colorectal cancer, as well as endometrial, ovarian, stomach, urothelial and pancreatic cancers. The culprit genes are: MLH1 and MSH2 and both are Aut. Dom.

These families have strong and multiple family histories of bowel cancer.

Screening is by colonoscopy, ovarian and endometrial screening (etc) where appropriate.

Beta blockers increase patient survival in ovarian cancer, Beta 2 and 3 adrenergic receptors being on various ovarian cancer cell surfaces and contributing to their own (cell) survival. In May 2017 a paper showed a pooled analysis that a comorbid condition of hypertension was associated with a 46% lower risk of ovarian cancer progression.

Endometrial cancer:

Risk factors

Early menarche, late menopause, nulliparity, PCO, obesity, unopposed oestrogen regimes or HRT with inadequate progestogen, Tamoxifen, family history.

Post menopausal bleeding is due to endometrial cancer in 9% of women in their 50s, 16% in their 60s, 28% in their 70s and 60% in their 80s.

Cervical Cancer:

The common symptoms/signs are: Post coital PV bleeding, persistent intermenstrual bleeding, persistent PV discharge, an abnormal looking and feeling cervix.

Cervical cancer screening:

Nationally is currently performed between 25 and 50 years of age 3 yearly and between 51 and 64 years 5 yearly. The advice is that over 65 years of age, only screen those who haven't been screened since 50 or those with one of the last three tests abnormal – ie if three tests are normal, no further F/U. You can smear mid trimester in pregnancy if necessary. There is a current (2015) debate about extending the age limit for smears as half of cervical cancer deaths occur >65years and 25% present >65 years.

My advice is to do a smear and look at the cervix on any woman of any age who requests a smear for any gynaecological symptom of significance or if she has irregular bleeding or spotting before during or after the cervical screening age range. There are many who have died, younger and older than the screening guidelines by simply being refused smears by their GPs. This is simply bad medicine.

Brain Tumours:

Kill more people under 40 than any cancer. There are 120 types in all, primary and secondary.

The main primary brain tumours are: Gliomas: More than half of the total. Astrocytomas and glioblastomas, oligodendrogliomas, ependymomas. Meningiomas: 25% of the total. Pituitary Adenomas: Usually benign, 10% of the total. Medulloblastomas: A paediatric cerebellar tumour.

The common secondaries are: Cancer of the bladder, breast, some sarcomas, germ cell tumours, renal cancer, leukaemia, lung cancer, lymphoma and melanoma (which metastasises to the brain more commonly in men). Occasionally colonic or prostatic cancer can metastasise to the brain too. Fewer than 10% of brain secondaries are found before the primary. Metastatic brain tumours are the commonest adult brain tumours. >80% are multiple.

Symptoms include morning and nocturnal headache, nausea and vomiting, fits, weakness or numbness, ataxia, hearing loss, various visual disturbances, dysphasia or dysarthria, poor concentration and memory, disorientation, drowsiness etc.

Investigations: MRI with gadolinium enhancement, CT (though less resolution and less good at soft tissue generally speaking than MRI), EEG, angiogram, biopsy etc.

Treatments include excision, radiotherapy, chemotherapy, proton therapy, some gene therapies, anti angiogenesis therapy.

Hodgkin's Disease – Hodgkin's Lymphoma.

More common after EB Virus infection. Classically the types are:

Lymphocyte Predominant: Young men, good prognosis, often isolated high neck lesions.

Nodular Sclerotic: Young women, a bit more aggressive, the commonest type.

Mixed Cellularity: Men, systemic symptoms, moderately aggressive.

Lymphocyte Depleted: Older patients, more aggressive.

Staging: I: Single node region or a single extra lymph node site.

II: Two contiguous node sites on the same side of the diaphragm or one nodal region and one extra nodal site.

III: Nodes on both sides of the diaphragm which may include the spleen or a limited extralymphatic site.

IV: Disseminated involvement of one or more extralymphatic organs.

Add "B" if systemic symptoms. Itching, night sweats, lymphadenopathy, weight loss, hepatosplenomegaly, cyclical fever etc.

In all types there is a T Cell mediated immune defect. There are various immune dysfunctions including haemolytic anaemia, thrombocytopenia. Other systemic symptoms: fever, sweats, weight loss, alcohol related node pain, Pel Ebstein fever (one to two week cycles). Infections are the cause of 50% deaths.

Chemotherapy may involve: Doxorubicin/Bleomycin/Vincristine/Vinblastine?Cyclophosphamide/Etoposide/Prednisolone etc.

TERMINAL CARE:

Dry Mouth:

Glandosane spray, Carboxymethyl Cellulose in natural, lemon, mint flavours. Salivix pastilles, Aquoral etc.

Mucositis:

Mugard – Carbomer, Difflam-Benzydamine.

Chemotherapy Stomatitis/Oral ulcers.

Difflam rinse, Corsodyl Mouth wash, Sucralfate (Antepsin) Susp. 1g in 5mls QDS. Duraphat 2800ppm fluoride toothpaste and 5000ppm mouth wash (private prescription).

Antiemetics:

Stuff you might have forgotten:

The vomit centre (American: vomiting center) in the medulla coordinates incoming messages from the chemoreceptor trigger zone next door (on the floor of the 4th ventricle) and other sources. The Area Postrema nearby is outside the Blood Brain Barrier and therefore I suppose best able to detect noxious non lipid soluble plasma contaminants. It detects toxins in the blood and irritants in the upper GI tract and initiates vomiting. The vomit centre's receptors include H1 histaminic and muscarinic cholinergic receptors as well as dopamine receptors. That must cover most noxious things. So drugs as varied as Anticholinergics (Hyoscine, Cyclizine, Promethazine, Dimenhydrinate), Dopamine antagonists, (Antidopaminergics-Domperidone, Metoclopramide, Haloperidol, Droperidol, Phenothiazines, etc) and Steroids (Dexamethasone/Methylprednisolone in cytotoxic vomiting), Cannabinoids (Nabilone) and Benzodiazepines (Diazepam etc) are effective anti emetics in specific situations, eg: Cyclizine 50mg 4 hrly injection and tablets, Domperidone (Motilium) tabs and suppositories 30mg, Promethazine (Phenergan) elix, tabs 10/25mg, Prochlorperazine (Stemetil) injection 12.5mg/ml and tablets 5mg and syrup, Nabilone, Cesamet 1mg 1-2, starting the night before chemotherapy. This is a cannabinoid. Ondansetron (Zofran) and related drugs are 5HT3 antagonists, 4mg, 8mg and are very expensive but usually effective at stopping this miserable side effect of certain chemotherapy regimes.

All the 5HT3 antagonists end in "setron": Palonosetron, Granisetron, Ondansetron.

The antihistamines are: Cinnarizine, Dimenhydrinate, Promethazine, Cyclizine, Promethazine.

The Neurokinin NK1 antagonists are: Aprepitant Fosapreptitant (For Cisplatin and other chemotherapy).

and the age old Phenothiazines, Prochlorperazine (Stemetil), Trifluoperazine (Stelazine) etc.

For PAIN RELIEF, dyspnoea and agitation:

Oral:

Oramorph Morphine Sulph soln, 10mg/5mls, Oramorph conc 100mg/5ml.

MST, 10mg (brown), 30mg (purple), 60mg (orange), 100mg (grey), 200mg (turquoise). MST suspension (sachets).

Sevredol (Morphine Sulph) tabs, 10mg, 20mg, 50mg tabs and solution.

MXL Controlled release Morphine caps (30-200mg caps) i od.

Palladone Hydromorphone caps 1.3mg, 2.6mg. Fewer S/Es than Morphine.

Zomorph, Morphine Sulph caps, cheaper than MST.

Oxycodone, Oxycontin Tabs, 5mg, 10mg, 20mg, 40mg, 80mg, 120mg Tabs (120mg tabs are approx £6 each).

Oxycodone combined with naloxone (which reduces constipation) is Targinact, 5mg/2.5mg (blue) 10mg/5mg (white) 20mg/10mg (pink) and 40mg/20mg (yellow) (these are almost £3 a tablet).

Fentanyl Lozenges (very expensive and very bad for the teeth). Actiq 200, 400, 600, 800, 1600mcg (30 of the latter are £210) !

Fentanyl comes in various other forms including a sublingual tablet (Abstral) but note that 10 of the cheapest tablets (400ug) are £50.

Clearly synthetic controlled drugs are very expensive.

Patches:

Transdermal Fentanyl Durogesic patches 25, 50, 75, 100mcg/hr. Change every 72hrs, (£28-£92 for 5 patches)

(25ug/hr Fentanyl is equivalent to a 4 hrly. Morphine dose of 5-20mg,

50ug =25-35mg
75ug=40-50mg
100ug=55-65mg
125ug=70-80mg
150ug=85-95mg
175ug=100-110mg
200ug=115-125mg
225ug=130-140mg

250ug=145-155mg

275ug=160-175mg etc.

Buprenorphine, Transtec 35ug, 52.5ug, 70ug every 3 days/Butrans patches 5ug, 10ug, 20ug/hr every 7days.

Rectally:

NSAIDS (particularly useful in bone pain:) Flurbiprofen and Indomet(h) acin supps.

Systemic:

Diamorphine injection 10-20mg initially 4 hrly for an average adult IM/SC or by syringe driver.

or Morphine sulphate 40-80mg over 24 hrs based on Oramorph dose of 80-160mg in 24 hrs.

Morphine and Diamorphine are covered under "Controlled Drugs" but as a rough guide, Injected Diamorphine (more soluble than Morphine) is twice to three times the potency of oral Morphine and three times the potency of MST for the purposes of initiating the syringe driver.

3mg oral Morphine=2mg oral Diamorphine=1mg parenteral Diamorphine.

A subcutaneous loading dose equivalent to the previous four hour oral dose may be required.

See "The Clinical Use of Controlled Drugs" below:

SEDATIVES/Tranquillisers:

Methotrimeprazine, Levomepromazine, Nozinan, is extremely useful and should be in every GP's bag. It is an anti psychotic, anti emetic, sedative AND analgesic. 25mg Tabs, the inj. is 25mg/ml.

Midazolam, Hypnovel is a muscle relaxant, pre med and also an anticonvulsant, 10mg/2ml inj. and is used as a sedative. A sub lingual form is used to terminate convulsions (Buccolam).

Haloperidol is antiemetic as well as anxiolytic 1.5mg 4-6hrly orally or 5mg/ml, 20mg/ml inj.

SECRETIONS: (Anticholinergic)

Hyoscine (also antispasmodic) 400mcg and 600mcg/ml inj. dries pulmonary secretions, terminal cough, chestiness which are usually probably more distressing to relatives than to the patient. Short acting.

Glycopyrronium bromide, Robinul 1200-1800ug (1.2-1.8mg)/24 hrs similar action.

NAUSEA/Vomiting:

Haloperidol 1-2mg IM, Metoclopramide 10mg IM, Cyclizine 50mg IM, Levomepromazine 12.5-25mg IM, Domperidone 10mg IM, Hyoscine 200-600ug IM, Granisetron (1mg, 2mg tabs oral).

Syringe driver:

Can be mixed over a 24-30 hour period:

Diamorphine, Cyclizine, Haloperidol, Metoclopramide, Methotrimeprazine (Levomepromazine), Midazolam (Hypnovel), Hyoscine (Buscopan).

Morphine is **less soluble** in small volumes than Diamorphine which is preferred.

Some terminal care drugs may cause severe **subcutaneous reactions: (ie avoid in syringe drivers)** – Diazepam, Chlorpromazine, Prochlorperazine.

A Good starting combination is:

Diamorphine 5-10mg 4hrly,

Midazolam (Hypnovel) 10mg in 2mls/4hrly OR
Levomepromazine (Nozinan) 25mg in 1ml, 1-2mls 4hrly,
Glycopyrronium (Robinul) 0.2mg/ml, 1ml 4hrly,
Plus water for injections to make up the syringe driver volume.

Cyclizine 50mg is a good injectable antiemetic if needed and Haloperidol is a good PRN sedative, anxiolytic and antipsychotic.

Levomepromazine, (Methotrimeprazine, Nozinan) is a sedative antiemetic, Midazolam (Hypnovel) is an anxiolytic antiepileptic, Hyoscine (Buscopan) an antispasmodic that dries mucous and salivary secretions, Metoclopramide a prokinetic anti emetic, Diamorphine a powerful sedative analgesic, and Ketoralac injection Toradol 30mg/ml is an NSAID, – **ALL CAN SAFELY BE MIXED IN A SYRINGE DRIVER FOR A 30 HOUR PERIOD.**

The following either **cannot be mixed** or irritate subcutaneously so must be administered by a separate syringe driver:

Diazepam, Chlorpromazine, Stemetil, Dexamethasone, Phenobarbitone.

Don't forget to keep your own record of any stat doses of controlled drugs you need to give. I do not need to tell you how unreasonably interfering and suspicious the big brothers at the PCT/Health Authority, (now presumably the Clinical Commissioning Group) have become since Shipman and how much harder it has become to administer humane pain relief with them and their clip boards auditing every ampoule of controlled drug. Also despite the generally good relationship GPs have with hospice doctors and nurses it is important to realise that you have invited them to advise and assist in the management of YOUR patient. Overall care and control, management of the drug regime and terminal care supervision is your responsibility. They are there to help you not the other way round.

You will also, of course, need to inform the OOH organisation that you have a terminally ill patient at home unless you give the carers your home number and to have discussed with the relatives and signed a DNR form to be left at the home. The last thing you and the relatives want is an ambulance crew resuscitating your patient who is dying with carcinomatosis. There are many examples of this disaster having happened through poor communication. It can be incredibly distressing for everyone.

CONSTIPATION:

Lactulose, Movicol Sachets (Polyeth Glycol, Sod Bicarb) 1-8 sachets/day, Sodium picosulphate (Laxoberal), Picolax sachets, Dioctyl Docusate caps 100-500mg/day. Stool softener. Macrogol (Idrolax) sachets, Co Danthrusate (Normax), Co Danthramer (which **is** restricted to the terminally Ill now), Bisacodyl, Liqu. paraffin and Mg OH Emulsion.

Chemotherapy for different cancers: With common abbreviation.

Name	Components	Example of uses, and other notes
ABVD	Adriamycin (doxorubicin), bleomycin, vinblastine, dacarbazine	Hodgkin's lymphoma
AC	Adriamycin (doxorubicin), cyclophosphamide	Breast cancer
BEACOPP	Bleomycin, etoposide, adriamycin (doxorubicin), cyclophosphamide, Oncovin (vincristine), procarbazine, prednisone	Hodgkin's lymphoma
BEP	Bleomycin, etoposide, platinum agent (cisplatin (Platinol))	Testicular cancer, germ cell tumours
CA	Cyclophosphamide, adriamycin (doxorubicin) (same as AC)	Breast cancer
CAF	Cyclophosphamide, adriamycin (doxorubicin), fluorouracil (5-FU)	Breast cancer
CAV	Cyclophosphamide, adriamycin (doxorubicin), vincristine	Lung cancer
CBV	Cyclophosphamide, BCNU (carmustine), VP-16 (etoposide)	Lymphoma
ChlVPP/EVA	Chlorambucil, vincristine (Oncovin), procarbazine, prednisone, etoposide, vinblastine, adriamycin (doxorubicin)	Hodgkin's lymphoma
CHOP	Cyclophosphamide, hydroxydaunorubicin (doxorubicin), vincristine (Oncovin), prednisone	Non-Hodgkin lymphoma
CHOP-R or R-CHOP	CHOP + rituximab	B Cell Non-Hodgkin lymphoma
COP or CVP	Cyclophosphamide, Oncovin (vincristine), prednisone	Non-Hodgkin lymphoma in patients with history of cardiovascular disease
CMF	Cyclophosphamide, methotrexate, fluorouracil (5-FU)	Breast cancer
COPP	Cyclophosphamide, Oncovin (vincristine), procarbazine, prednisone	Non-Hodgkin lymphoma
CVAD/HyperCVAD	Cyclophosphamide, vincristine, adriamycin (doxorubicin), dexamethasone	Aggressive non-Hodgkin lymphoma, lymphoblastic lymphoma, some forms of leukaemia
DT-PACE	Dexamethasone, Thalidomide, cisplatin or Platinol, adriamycin or doxorubicin, cyclophosphamide, etoposide	Multiple myeloma
EC	Epirubicin, cyclophosphamide	Breast cancer
ECF	Epirubicin, cisplatin, fluorouracil (5-FU)	Gastric cancer and oesophageal cancer

EP	Etoposide, platinum agent (cisplatin (Platinol))	Testicular cancer, germ cell tumours
EPOCH	Etoposide, prednisone, Oncovin, cyclophosphamide, and hydroxydaunorubicin	Lymphomas
FEC	Fluorouracil (5-FU), epirubicin, cyclophosphamide	Breast cancer
FL (Also known as Mayo)	Fluorouracil (5-FU), leucovorin (folinic acid)	Colorectal cancer
FOLFOX	Fluorouracil (5-FU), leucovorin (folinic acid), oxaliplatin	Colorectal cancer
FOLFIRI	Fluorouracil (5-FU), leucovorin (folinic acid), irinotecan	Colorectal cancer
ICE	Ifosfamide, carboplatin, etoposide (VP-16)	Aggressive lymphomas, progressive neuroblastoma
ICE-R	ICE + rituximab	High-risk progressive or recurrent lymphomas
m-BACOD	Methotrexate, bleomycin, adriamycin (doxorubicin), cyclophosphamide, Oncovin (vincristine), dexamethasone	Non-Hodgkin lymphoma
MACOP-B	Methotrexate, leucovorin (folinic acid), adriamycin (doxorubicin), cyclophosphamide, Oncovin (vincristine), prednisone, bleomycin	Non-Hodgkin lymphoma
MOPP	Mechlorethamine, Oncovin (vincristine), procarbazine, prednisone	Hodgkin's lymphoma
MVAC	Methotrexate, vinblastine, adriamycin, cisplatin	Advanced bladder cancer[4]
PCV	Procarbazine, CCNU (lomustine), vincristine	Brain tumours
POMP	6-mercaptopurine (Purinethol), vincristine (Oncovin), methotrexate, and prednisone	Acute adult leukaemia[5]
ProMACE-MOPP	Methotrexate, adriamycin (doxorubicin), cyclophosphamide, etoposide + MOPP	Non-Hodgkin lymphoma
ProMACE-CytaBOM	Prednisone, doxorubicin (adriamycin), Cyclophosphamide, etoposide, cytarabine, bleomycin, Oncovin (vincristine), methotrexate, leucovorin	Non-Hodgkin lymphoma
R-FCM	Rituximab, fludarabine, cyclophosphamide, mitoxantrone	B cell Non-Hodgkin lymphoma
Stanford V	Doxorubicin, mechlorethamine, bleomycin, vinblastine, vincristine, etoposide, prednisone	Hodgkin lymphoma

Thal/Dex	Thalidomide, dexamethasone	Multiple myeloma
TIP	Paclitaxel, ifosfamide, platinum agent cisplatin (Platinol)	Testicular cancer, germ cell tumours in salvage therapy
EE-4A	Vincristine, actinomycin[6]	**Wilms' Tumour**
DD-4A	Vincristine, actinomycin, doxorubicin[6]	WIlms' Tumour
VAC	Vincristine, actinomycin, Cyclophosphamide	Rhabdomyosarcoma
VAD	Vincristine, adriamycin (doxorubicin), dexamethasone	Multiple myeloma
VAMP	One of 3 combinations of Vincristine and others	Hodgkin's lymphoma, leukaemia, multiple myeloma
Regimen I	Vincristine, adriamycin (doxorubicin), etoposide, cyclophosphamide	Wilms'Tumour
VAPEC-B	Vincristine, adriamycin (doxorubicin), prednisone, etoposide, cyclophosphamide, bleomycin	Hodgkin's lymphoma
VIP	Vinblastin, ifosfamide, platinum agent cisplatin (Platinol)	Testicular cancer, germ cell tumours

Others: Oxaliplatin (IV infusion) and Capecitabine (oral) in bowel cancer (two weeks treatment in total every three weeks, repeated) (CAPOX)

Why chemotherapy often fails:

CHEMORESISTANCE

When a cell undergoes a series of successive mutations, it can acquire the ability to multiply unrestricted by the body's normal regulatory mechanisms, becoming cancerous and forming a tumour. Because tumour cells already contain a number of mutations, the barriers to their further mutation are lower than those for healthy cells. Thus with every successive mutation, the chance of a further one increases. When natural selection is added to this increasingly frequent mutational change, it is easy to see how those tumour cells which are best adapted to survive will do so. These cells will out-compete their less well-adapted kin and go on to propagate the tumour.

While chemotherapy is toxic to cells and especially to rapidly dividing cells, this toxicity provides another selective pressure to drive further tumour evolution: in the presence of the harsh environment of toxic chemotherapy, the most resilient tumour cells will stand the best chance of surviving and go on to propagate further tumour growth. Thus if a tumour survives after a course of chemotherapy, it is likely to be more virulent than before the treatment began. Tumours that metastasise have already demonstrated an aptitude for survival in foreign environments and are therefore likely to be even better placed to mutate further and resist chemotherapy. A simple evolutionary process therefore drives chemoresistance in tumours over time.

In addition, recent research [Ref 1] has shown that the cytotoxic effects of chemotherapy can drive changes in non-tumour cells located in the immediate vicinity of tumours, altering their levels of cell signalling and having a direct impact on the growth of the tumour. Sun et al found in vivo evidence that prostate cancer chemotherapy using mitoxantrone and docetaxel damaged fibroblasts in the prostate stroma to the extent where gene expression changes took place and these cells secreted elevated levels of the signalling protein WNT16B. This drove **enhanced** tumour growth. They observed similar results in breast and ovarian cancers in vitro.

[Ref 1] *Nat. Med. 2012 Sep;18(9): 1359-68. Treatment-induced damage to the tumor microenvironment promotes prostate cancer therapy resistance through WNT16B. Sun Y, Campisi J, Higano C, Beer TM, Porter P, Coleman I, True L, Nelson PS.*

Alex Heath BSc MSc

Targeted anticancer therapy:

Most chemotherapy kills actively dividing cells at a rate proportional to their cell division and of their uptake of the drug. This is not specific and has many damaging short and long term side effects. Not least is the long term risk of chemotherapy generated cancer. Some chemotherapeutic regimes specifically target the abnormal metabolism of cancer cells and are aimed at tumour cell growth signalling and angiogenesis, causing apoptosis, stimulating the immune system to target cancer cells or at delivering toxic drugs direct to cancer cells.

Most targeted drugs are either small molecule drugs or monoclonal antibodies:

Selective "Estrogen" (Oestrogen) Receptor Modulators (SERMs) act as anti cancer drugs in ER positive breast cancer. Tamoxifen competes at the oestrogen cellular receptor, Fulvestrant destroys it.

Aromatase inhibitors act in the metabolic pathway producing oestrogen, thus lowering body levels of the hormone. A.I.s include: Anastrozole (Arimidex), Exemestane (Aromasin) and Letrozole (Femara).

Other targeted therapies include:

Imatinib, Dasatinib, Nilotinib, Bosutinib, Trastuzumab (Herceptin, which works in some breast cancers and lower oesophageal tumours: It is a monoclonal antibody to the receptor 2 of human epidermal growth factor, inhibiting growth in the tumour and probably focussing immune attack on the cancer cells too). Pertuzumab, Lapatinib, Gefitinib, Eriotinib, Cetuximab, Temsirolimus, Everolimus, Romidepsin, Bexarotene, Bevacizumab (Avastin which prevents new blood vessel growth). Likewise Sunitinib, (Sutent), Rituximab, etc. There are actually dozens of targeted anticancer therapies available for specific cancers now. Some more details at: http://www.cancer.gov/cancertopics/factsheet/Therapy/targeted

Food Supplements:

Many PCT Commissioning Groups are balking at the prescription of food supplements to cachectic and terminal patients when rich shop bought foods (creamy yogurts, puddings, biscuits, etc) are available "OTC". I think this is unreasonable and disloyal when these patients are elderly, vulnerable and have trusted and paid their taxes faithfully to the NHS for decades and now need some simple constructive help with their nutrition.

I am happy to prescribe a variety of supplements BUT some are very sweet and some are very sickly. I let the patient decide which he or she likes best:

For instance (most are ACBS):

Complan sachets.

Ensure. Carbohydrate and protein supplement, various flavours.

Ensure plus. Higher calorie content than Ensure. Milk shake style.

Fresubin 5kcal shot high fat. Incomplete.

Provide extra.

Fortimel. Carbohydrate and high protein.

Fortisip. Nutritionally complete, cow's milk based, various flavours.

Caloreen. Glucose polymer, low electrolyte, high carbohydrate.

Clinifeed. Mixed liquid feed, nutritionally complete.

Hycal. Carbohydrate only.

Maxijul. Glucose polymer carbohydrate supplement.

Formance Mousse.

Scandishake. Fat/protein/carbohydrate. Not complete.

Calshake. Fat/Carbohydrate supplement.

Calshake, Scandishake, Enshake 2 Kcal/ml – The 1.5KCal alternatives are Ensure Plus/Fresubin Energy.

If you have ever tasted either the syrupy sweet or sickly creamy food supplements listed here you will know how unappetising or queasily nauseating most of them are. You wouldn't normally have consumed manufactured bad tasting high calorie supplements before you had cancer and now that you have the chemo-nausea and other treatment side effects you shouldn't have to start. They are not what most GPs would call "healthy foods". Full of sugar and fat and generally without healthy anti oxidants, vitamins, minerals, an appetising taste or anything that comes under the heading of "a healthy supplement".

It is worth mentioning that high calorie foods so espoused by many NHS cancer units and usually promoted in their hand-outs for patients are very unhealthy diets in a number of ways. We would not normally recommend high sugar and fat diets for our normal, non cancer patients and simply preventing catabolism by overwhelming the body with excessive calories does not lead to healthy anabolic repair and growth of tissue. Extra fat and sugar encourage hyperglycaemia, hyperlipidaemia and unhealthy fat deposition in sick patients just as they do in healthy ones. Cancer cells do grow better in a high carbohydrate medium and by encouraging sugary foods you may help maintain a patient's weight but there is good evidence that you are feeding the cancer too. We should be encouraging what we all know to be a good diet (See "The Rainbow Diet" by Chris Woolams). A variety of bright coloured fresh fruits and vegetables, lean protein, fish, chicken, pulses, rice, beans, nuts and especially cruciferous vegetables are by far the healthier alternative. The colourful foods happen to have the healthiest natural anti cancer activity but fresh food, a wide variety, plenty of fibre, vitamins and trace minerals where there is an evidence base to support them, unprocessed food, not a high calorie sugar and fat based diet. This offers the best outcomes and survival statistics in virtually all cancers.

Other cancer topics:

Ascites/Oedema due to Liver Failure: Sometimes Dexamethasone 4mg daily and Spironolactone 100mg BD/TDS will buy some extra time and comfort when all else fails.

Bone Pain: Etidronate 800mg/day, plus steroids (especially in myeloma).

Sodium Clodronate, Bonefos controls pain and reduces hypercalcaemia in osteolytic breast secondaries, myeloma.

The Clinical Use of Controlled Drugs:

Terminal Care Analgesic Ladder:

Non opioids   **>Weak opioids**   **>Strong opioids**

(Usually an NSAID) Codeine, DHC, Dipipanone, Co Proxamol (etc), Buprenorphine, Morphine,
(Co Dydramol, Co Codamol 8mg, 15mg, 30mg)
Diconal (Dipipanone and Cyclizine)   Diamorphine

Terminal Care Opioid Equivalents:

Methadone Oral 20mg
Dipipanone Oral 60mg
Morphine Oral 30mg
Morphine IM 15mg
Diamorphine IM/SC 10mg

Interactions in solution (See above)

Diamorphine and:

High concentrations of both Cyclizine and Haloperidol may precipitate,
Hyoscine, Metoclopramide, Prochlorperazine (which may cause irritation given SC),
are compatible, as is the mixture with Methotrimeprazine.

Equivalent Doses: Mg

Oral Morphine		Sub Cut Morphine	Sub Cut Diamorphine		Oral Oxycodone		Sub Cut Oxycodone	
24hrs	4hrs	24hrs	24hrs	4hrs	24hrs	4hrs	24hrs	4hrs
30	5	15	10	2.5	15	2.5	7.5-10	1.25-2.5

Conversion Factors:

Oral Codeine to oral Morphine divide by 10,
Oral DHC to Oral Morphine divide by 10,
Oral Tramadol to oral Morphine divide by 10,
Oral Morphine to SC Diamorphine divide by 3,
Oral Morphine to oral Oxycodone divide by 2,
Oral Morphine to oral Hydromorphone divide by 7.5,
Oral Morphine to SC Morphine divide by 2.

Fentanyl Patches and oral Morphine Equivalents

24 Hr Oral Morphine mg	Fentanyl Patch (mcg/hr)
<90	25
90-134	37
135-189	50
225-314	75
315-404	100
495-584	150
675-764	200
1035-1124	300

CD analgesic equivalents: (different routes)
4hrly oral Morphine 5mg = 4hrly oral Oxycodone 2.5mg = 10mg SC Diamorphine in
24 hrs = 25mcg 72 hr Fentanyl patch.

Morphine, Diamorphine or Laudanum?

Note: Opium contains Morphine, Codeine, Dihydrocodeine, Narcotine and Papaverine.

Laudanum, the Victorian middle and upper class drug answer to all ills including baby colic, insomnia, Nicotine withdrawal, pain and anxiety was an 10% alcoholic solution of powdered opium. It was flavoured, often with cinnamon or saffron. It seems to have been used like paracetamol is used now. Its use was only prohibited in 1928 and you could get it until then without prescription OTC. Every notable poet and Victorian writer – Poe, Dickens, Carroll, Keats, Shelley, Coleridge and Byron took it. Lizzie Siddal, one of the pre Raphaelite "Stunners" and Ophelia in Millais' famous painting died of it.

Wilkie Collins' The Moonstone, the first ever detective novel, is based on its side effects when given to the dashing hero to alleviate Nicotine withdrawal.

We do not use Laudanum as such now and it and related drugs certainly aren't legally available without prescription. There are some differences between the various powerful opiates. Morphine itself causes more dysphoria and less euphoria (probably) than Diamorphine. It causes CNS depression, analgesia, cough suppression, vomiting and nausea, pupillary constriction, GI smooth muscle spasm, biliary spasm, bronchospasm, increased intraluminal gut pressure, constipation, dilatation of arterioles and veins, reduced sympathetic drive (as in PND and MI). It delays labour (unlike Pethidine) and it is easier to titrate orally than Diamorphine as it is less water soluble. It is also less lipid soluble so has a slower onset of action systemically.

Diamorphine (Heroin, legal use is banned in the USA), is converted to Morphine in the body, more rapid onset by any route than Morphine, is more water and lipid soluble than Morphine, reduces pain (via pain sensation as well as ability to tolerate pain). Reduces cough (it was actually first marketed to combat the cough of TB and still very useful in this regard). Causes respiratory depression through reduced sensitivity to CO_2 then to hypoxia. Causes vasodilatation (an advantage in some clinical situations – acute LVF etc) causes convulsions in high doses. Reduces gastric motility, reduces gastric and biliary secretions, increased Sphincter of Oddi tone. Increases tone and reduces peristalsis of small and large bowel, constipates. Less depression, less nausea, more pleasant psychic effects, fewer cardiovascular effects, twice the potency, more rapid onset than Morphine but probable effect lasts only 3 hours IM. (25% shorter duration of effect). BUT **peak levels** depend a great deal on circulation, shock and after an IM dose can be between 20 and 100 minutes. Does not cause addiction in acute pain situations or physical or mental decline in terminal care.

Naloxone Reverses all the pharmacological effects, good and bad of Diamorphine as well as Morphine. So analgesia has to be via NSAIDs and non opiates while Naloxone is still active. But Naloxone has a much shorter half life than either so another dose may be necessary an hour or two after the first in serious overdose situations. Thus reversal of opioid respiratory depression: Dose: 100-200mcg IV followed by 100mcg every few minutes initially if necessary IV until the patient is "reversed". Due to the short half life of Naloxone compared with opiates, may need further dose 2hrs later. In children 10-20mcg/kg IV every 2-3 mins. initially. Repeat doses every hour if necessary. (But you **are** unlikely to be delivering a drug addict's baby at home)

Oxycodone and Naloxone (Targinact) Is a combination that is said to reduce constipation by the local gut activity of Naloxone. Some patients absorb Naloxone orally better than others though.

Pethidine: Much weaker opioid receptor agonist than Morphine/Diamorphine. Causes respiratory depression and **some** smooth muscle spasm. But does not cause constipation significantly or suppress labour or cough. It IS antagonised by Naloxone. It can suppress newborn respiration. It does not increase Sphincter of Oddi contraction compared with Morphine and its relatives and is preferred for biliary and renal colic for its relatively benign smooth muscle effect.

Ritalin (Methyphenidate) can be co prescribed with Morphine and other strong opiates if the patient wants to remain less drowsy and more aware of their surroundings in their last weeks. Useful to know in terminal care situations if you want to try and achieve the best of both worlds.

CONTROLLED DRUGS AND PRESCRIPTIONS:

Diamorphine and other opioids come under The Misuse of Drugs Regulations 1973 and hence are denoted "Controlled Drugs" or CDs. This has nothing (directly) to do with the Corps Diplomatique or Compact Discs.

1) Prescriptions must be signed and dated by the prescriber with the prescriber's address and indelible.

2) They must, of course have the name and address of the patient.

3) and include the form and (where appropriate) the strength of the preparation eg [Diamorphine powder for injection ampoules (ten mg) 'CD', 10 (Ten) ampoules]

4) The total quantity of the drug or preparation or the number of dose units in words and figures (10 (Ten) Ampoules)

5) The dose: eg: 3-6 ampoules SC as instructed (Via syringe driver over 24 hours and when required one to two as a stat dose 3-4 hrly for pain)

The prescription for schedule 2, 3 or 4 CDs is valid for only 28 days. Computer generated CD scrips can now be issued. The hand writing requirement ended in 2005. A CD prescription may request that the prescription is dispensed in instalments, the amount at each instalment and the interval being specified. Schedule 4 and 5 drugs may be subject to repeat prescriptions.

The regulations also require the doctor to notify the Chief Medical Officer if he suspects a patient may be addicted to Diamorphine. Only licensed doctors may prescribe for addicts. The rest of us must refer them to treatment centres.

Scheduled Drugs:

Different drugs with abuse potential come under a number of legal restrictions and are categorised as being in various "Schedules" as follows: For instance:

Schedule 1) Ecstasy, Cannabis.

Schedule 2) Opiates, Diamorphine, Pethidine, Amphetamines, Barbiturates, Quinalbarbitone.

Schedule 3) Minor stimulants, Benzphetamine, Buprenorphine, Temazepam.

Schedule 4) Benzodiazepines, Anabolic, Androgenic Steroids.

Schedule 5) Low strength Codeine, Cocaine, Morphine, Pholcodeine.

Genetics and Cancer:

Between 5 and 10% of all cancers are inherited and the possible markers of genetic cancers are:

Many cases of a rare cancer in the family,

Cancers at a younger than normal age.

More than one cancer in one person (e.g. breast and ovary).

Cancers in both of a pair of organs (breasts, ovaries, retinas etc).

More than one childhood cancer in a set of siblings (e.g. a sarcoma in each of a brother and sister).

Breast cancer: 5% will be in women with a mutation in BRCA1 or BRCA2.

Bowel cancer: 5% will be due to inheritance of a mutation in BRCA1 or BRCA2.

Breast Cancer Screening:

From age 50 every 3 years to 70

AT LEAST 1:12 women develop breast cancer (This depends on the country and the source of information). 15,000 women die each year of it in the UK. 2/3 sufferers currently die of it.

These are some figures of one local screening project:

Total Invited: 23,160,

Screened: 17,000,

Referred for assessment: 1420,

Biopsied: 205,

Malignant: 97 or 0.6%

Refer to a family history clinic if:

1 FDR (parents, children, siblings) and 1 SDR (grandparents, grandchildren, aunts, uncles, nephews, nieces, half brother, half sister) with breast cancer.

2 FDR with breast cancer,

3 or more FDRs or SDRs with breast cancer.

1 FDR with breast cancer <40 years old.

1 FDR of Jewish extraction with breast cancer.

1 male FDR with breast cancer.

1 FDR with bilateral breast cancer.

1 FDR/SDR with breast cancer and 1 FDR/SDR with ovarian cancer.

1 FDR with breast cancer and ovarian cancer and who is Jewish.

One FDR male with breast cancer.

(FDR First degree relative, SDR Second degree relative (Uncle, aunt, nephew, niece, grandparent, grandchild, half sibling – someone who shares a quarter of their genes with the index person)).

Ovarian cancer screening:

Is done if 2 relatives on the same side of the family have been diagnosed with breast cancer or ovarian cancer before the age of 50. Screening is by annual USS and Ca 125. **But** 50% of early Ca ovary sufferers have N markers as do 15% of total ovarian cancer sufferers.

Screening is done from 35 years of age or from 5 years before the age of the relative at diagnosis.

Ovarian cancer risk in general population by age 70, 1%.

If first degree relative, 3%.

Families at high risk of ovarian cancer:

Families with two or more individuals with ovarian cancer at any age who are first degree relatives of each other.

One with ovarian cancer at any age and one breast cancer <50 years who are first degree relatives of each other.

One ovarian cancer at any age and 2 with breast cancer <60 years who are first degree relatives of each other.

One individual with known ovarian cancer genes.

Three individuals with colorectal cancer, at least one diagnosis <50 years and one ovarian cancer who are first degree relatives.

Genes that predispose to both breast and ovarian cancer are BRCA1 and BRCA2, Aut. Dom., maternal or paternal inheritance.

Screening by USS and CA125 from age 35 years.

Mutations in a gene on chromosome 17 increase the risk of prostate cancer and there is usually a positive family history but BRCA gene mutations increase breast and prostate cancer incidence in men too.

Gastro-intestinal Cancer:

Colonic carcinoma: refer to a family history clinic if the patient had

1 x FDR age at onset <40 yrs.

2 x FDRs both <70 yrs.

3 close relatives, average age <60 with one <50yrs.

Familial Adenomatosis Polyposis.

Hereditary Non-Polyposis Colorectal Cancer: At least 3 relatives should have large bowel cancer or and HNPCC related cancer (includes endometrial, ovarian, stomach, small bowel, ureter, renal pelvis etc). One should be a FDR of the other 2 affected relatives; at least 2 successive generations should be affected, in one person the cancer must be diagnosed below 50 yrs.

Upper GI cancer: Consider referral in any FDR, age at presentation <40 yrs, or multiple first or second degree relatives with upper GI cancer (includes pancreas.)

Genetic Testing for Cancers:

CDK2NA (Melanoma.)

PTCH.

Mismatch repair genes.

PTEN.

Tuberous Sclerosis.

Fibrofolliculin.

APC.

NF1/2.

Most of these are autosomal dominant.

Treatment of patients with complications on Chemotherapy:

Neutropenic Sepsis:

Usually occurs 7-14 days post chemotherapy. This is particularly true in the elderly, frail and in haematological malignancy. It can happen after chemotherapy has been completed so pyrexia and other signs of infection should be taken seriously even (sometimes) with a normal WBC (poor general immune response in some haematology patients).

Refer urgently to hospital (the specialist chemotherapy unit if you can but my experience is that they rarely if ever have beds and you are often referred to the medics on call at your DGH) if: Temp >38°c (Don't forget that steroids, NSAIDs and paracetamol may mask the febrile reaction to infection), there are rigors, unexplained hypotension or tachycardia and the patient is generally feeling unwell. All this is especially true if there is a central line, Hickman, Groshong, PICC, Portacath etc.

Central Lines: These avoid the need for recurrent re-cannulation of peripheral veins when recurrent sampling or IV drug administration are necessary. They allow dilution of often irritant chemotherapeutic agents in fast flowing vessels, avoiding endothelial irritation, reduce superficial infections but they also increase the risk of central sepsis.

The Hickman line is inserted under sedation and local anaesthetic with an incision over the jugular vein as well as an incision lower down the anterior chest wall. The central line itself is inserted down the jugular to the SVC just outside the RA, the other end being advanced subcutaneously to the exit site where it is held down with a cuff.

PICC lines are peripherally inserted central catheters. The tip is often in the SVC but the origin is in a peripheral (arm) vein. The lines may have multiple lumens (lumina) and stay in place for up to 6 months. They need to be covered in showers and are quite restricting (they need covering and protecting during vigorous activity, playing sports etc).

The Portacath is a subcutaneous port (reservoir) that is inserted under sedation and local anaesthetic, usually in the anterior upper chest with the tip in a deep central vein. Its lifespan is longer than the 6m or so of a PICC line and as it is completely covered by skin, the patient can undertake normal activities without extra precautions and it isn't supposed to need flushing as often as the PICC.

General Symptoms:

Nausea/Vomiting:

If the patient is having oral chemotherapy or recently completed IV treatment then some systemic treatment (Cyclizine/Metoclopramide/Domperidone etc) may be required. If they are febrile consider sepsis.

Diarrhoea/Constipation:

Capecitabine and 5FU, common cytotoxic agents are potential causes of severe diarrhoea. Up to 4 loose stools a day can be treated with extra fluids and loperamide. Nocturnal diarrhoea and 5-6 motions a day indicate the need for referral to review electrolyte loss and hydration. Diarrhoea is a symptom of neutropenic sepsis.

Constipation: Can be caused by the Vinca Alkaloids (Vincristine, Vinorelbine, Vinblastine) and by Granisetron, the anti emetic. Occasionally a stimulant and stool softener will be needed. Avoid enemas in neutropenic patients.

Stomatitis

Many regimes cause this, it occurring up to a week after chemotherapy and lasting up to 10 days.

Try Difflam mouthwash, Corsodyl Mouthwash, Sucralfate mouthwash (Antepsin suspension), Carbomer (Mugard mouthwash), Hyaluronate (Gelclair, Gengigel) and in my experience, with chemotherapy which incorporates Methotrexate, try Folinic Acid as a mouthwash.

Treat oral thrush with Daktarin oral gel and or Fluconazole capsules.

Grief:

There are various ways of analysing grief and describing the phases and emotions involved:

Shock and numbness (disbelief).

Yearning and searching, a period when the bereaved person can briefly forget the dead person has actually died.

Disorganisation and despair. Often with symptoms of depression, confused thinking, organisation, planning, poor sleep concentration, lowered mood and emotional lability.

Reorganisation. The beginning of recovery, resolution and adjustment.

Alternatively in grief – some describe stages of:

Denial and Isolation,

Anger,

Bargaining,

Depression,

Acceptance. MRI imaging shows grief emotions arise in primitive parts of the brain including the limbic system and these are present in animals. This seems to add support to copious observational evidence that animals from swans and dogs to elephants and primates experience emotions including grief.

From the doctor's point of view it is important to have shown involvement, concern and responsiveness to the family and relatives during a terminal illness or to have given unbiased sympathy to them during the sudden bereavement of an accident or a violent death. Regular visiting, an unquibbling attitude to pain relief and these days, to prescribing expensive dietary supplements and treatments will help establish you as on their side. – Whatever the preceding history between doctor and patient.

Many relatives will direct their own guilt or anger toward their GP – this for a late or missed diagnosis or sometimes a perceived lack of sympathy. So an attentive (but not servile) caring supervision at this time, especially if it includes out of hours visits or phone calls will be hugely appreciated.

Terminal care and the management of pain and other distressing symptoms and of the relatives' needs before during and after the actual death differentiate real GPs from those just playing at the job.

Free prescriptions and Cancer:

Free NHS prescriptions are now a bit of a sick joke. The young and the old get them, a whole list of illogical historical illnesses qualify you for them, if you are pregnant, can't go out without someone else, have a fistula, Addison's Disease, Hypopituitrism, Hypoparathyroidism, Diabetes apart from that treated solely by diet, Myasthenia Gravis, Epilepsy on prophylaxis, Myxoedema, if you are lucky enough to have Coeliac disease, (in which case the tax payer will pay for your meals (-there is **a free lunch** for **you**)). If you live in Wales (as I discovered on holiday) or Scotland or Northern Ireland *But not England* you can get all your Calpol, Brufen and everything else on the taxpayer and if you are on benefits, looking for work etc you get free prescriptions. 90% of the public get their drugs free in fact as long as they get the doctor to write an FP10. You don't get free prescriptions if you have Cushing's, hyperthyroidism, a prolactinoma or Muscular Dystrophy, or are just normal, live in England and work. The whole system is irrational and unfair. Pay your taxes, work hard and be honest and you get taken for a ride.

The retail cost of most OTC drugs is of course a scandal and so this makes it economically worthwhile if you have the time, to go to the surgery and get a scrip for even easily available OTC medications and it takes a stubborn and determined doctor to refuse.

Prescriptions cost 20p when I started medicine so they have gone up by a multiple of 42X since then. Even petrol has only increased 20X (– 7p/li >140p/li)) in the same 40 odd years and this occasionally comes down in price-unlike prescription charges. This is an exponential increase but what is worse is that **so few** people actually and unfairly pay for their prescriptions.

Since 2009, patients with cancer have been entitled to free prescriptions and no doubt, like you, I said a good thing too – at first. It seemed far more sensible than patients with mild myxoedema on a 6 month thyroxine prescription (which costs them and the NHS very little) getting everything else free too. But I have had patients claiming that their rodent ulcers and squamous cell carcinomas, even solar keratoses – all benign lesions really, were forms of cancer. Other patients thought their colposcopy polyps entitled them to free prescriptions, or needing a sunscreen to avoid developing cancer and even others who had been successfully treated for questionable cancers 20 years ago submitted their forms for free prescriptions. The largess of politicians pursuing popularity is just another factor in the slow progressive demise of the impossible "free everything for (nearly) everyone" Health Service.

Exemption certificates for cancer patients actually **last 5 years** and are valid for the whole of that time even if the cancer treatment finished 4 years and 11 months before.

The patient must have been **undergoing** treatment for cancer, the effects of cancer or the effects of cancer treatment. The small print, should you need to stand your ground, says that the exemption does not apply to patients who have **been treated** and are now apparently clear of cancer and where no further treatment is planned. It does not include patients having routine F/U appointments with no active treatments.

How do you solve the prescription problem?

Charge **everyone** an affordable sum for each prescription (say £2) with no exceptions. This must include children, the unemployed and all those with current exemptions – though possibly not the retired elderly. They have paid through the nose in taxation all their lives.

Force retailers to sell basic OTCs at affordable (NHS) prices.

Prevent GPs prescribing OTC medications on FP10s unless there are exceptional reasons for doing so.

Allow GPs to prescribe 6 months worth of long term maintenance therapies (like we used to) for patients with stable conditions.

Allow retail pharmacies to recycle unused drug returns if returned in original packaging, unopened and to pay the patient a nominal sum for returning unused drugs.

The current drugs system is designed to maximise costs and waste and patients are dumbstruck at the idiocy of some of the inexplicable institutional restrictions on sensible cost saving that exist in relation to drug prescribing and dispensing. I even had a partner who was sanctioned and threatened with a charge of professional misconduct for giving a patient on Telmisartan a packet of 3 months of the same dose of (in date) Telmisartan, returned by a relative of a dead patient. Sheer nonsense. He should have been given a commendation.

Alternative treatments:

There are many unconventional treatments for cancer (i.e. not the "conventional" big three: surgery, radiotherapy and chemotherapy – what are colloquially known as slash, burn and poison) and some of these treatments as well as being free of side effects do have impressive results. I mean documented improved outcomes in terms of survival, longevity, response and actual verifiable cures. These results have been demonstrated not just by people with axes to grind or a financial interest but by independent academic and research departments, over and over again.

If you are dyed in the wool standard medical material like me, you need a very open mind to accept even why cancer is happening at such an increased rate, (processed food, environmental pollutants, herbicides, pesticides, plastic residues, diesel fumes, solvents, dry cleaning fumes and flame retardants and so on) and much of that requires almost a betrayal of what you are supposed to stand for. But conventional medicine is not really doing very well at detecting cancer early and treating it safely, cleanly and effectively. The long term unselected cancer survival rates are poor and the short and long term morbidity, even mortality of conventional treatments is not impressive by the standards of the treatment of tuberculosis, a host of infectious diseases, diabetes, chronic kidney disease, vitamin deficiencies, myxoedema, epilepsy or many of the mystery killers of the past.

Alternative treatments do take a bit of a cultural shift and a broadening of the mind to accept.

We all make several cancers each week but our efficient immune systems destroy them naturally. A blood specimen taken at random will show half a dozen mixed histologically malignant cells in the peripheral blood at any time. DNA is after all a system that has random variation as its raison d'etre and part of its design. The immune system must recognise the abnormality the vast majority of times and trigger a destructive cellular/humoral response and this must happen over and over again in our lives. Indeed one of the prophylactic effects of aspirin in reducing the poor prognoses of many cancers is thought to be via its ability to uncover the cancer cell/metastasis cleverly hiding behind its cloak of camouflage platelets.

Many times in this book I have mentioned the adverse effect our modern refined, cleaned up and almost valueless diet is having on health. The processed colourless, white rice, white bread, white flour, white sugar diet. We recognise its effect on cancer development and progress, function of the heart, diabetes, blood pressure, stroke risk, its influence on the paediatric and adult gut, on allergy and immune function. Increasingly we know the importance of the commensal trillions of bacteria we harbour in our guts as the "Microbiome" and how they influence a myriad of bodily functions. I am sure the relatively recent loss of many trace elements and nutrients from soil, our farming methods and changes to food which our bodies had adapted to over millions of years are amongst the contributing factors of the cancer epidemic of the last 60 years as well.

I am also convinced that the right and (I am sorry but they probably have to be) organically grown mix of varied fresh fruit, vegetables, pulses, herbs and spices, unless you are iron deficient, green tea, red wine, dark chocolate, no antiperspirants, deodorants, non stick pans, (see the diet and other sections) and low sugar intake, will improve your chances of avoiding cancer and your recovery from it. There is a lot of controlled evidence and real proof related to that. You could call a diet and environment suited to our 3 million year adapted body "alternative" or you could call modern life and diet just idiotic.

Back to other alternative treatments:

Like you, I have to take a deep breath when I consider SOME alternative and so called natural therapies: Homeopathy, Iridology, Crystal Therapy, Faith Healing, Colour Therapy, Aromatherapy, Colonic Hydrotherapy and so on. – Where is the proof, the evidence? Therein lays the problem. Treatments are either conventional, state funded, widely accepted as the norm, the "side" to which all state educated doctors like me have to be loyal, – "The home team" or

"Fringe", private, fee paying, unregulated, provided by just anybody with an opinion, a front room and a persuasive personality – The opposition.

But as far as cancer therapy is concerned, it isn't quite that clear cut.

There is a famous therapy called The Gerson Therapy: This consists of a primarily dietary approach, with organic food, low protein and fat, no milk or soya, no pulses, filtered water for consumption as well as washing, plenty of fruit and vegetable juices, fruit and vegetables lightly cooked or raw, including some potatoes and oatmeal. There are specified essential foods or banned foods, the way the food is juiced is specifically laid out and there are regular coffee enemas. (Yes – this apparently raises levels of Glutathione S transferases, one of a group of liver detoxifying enzymes). Also included is Co Enzyme Q10, castor oil and pancreatic enzyme treatment. This may seem weird but apparently there are impressive responses to this kind of "toxin removal and elemental dietary approach" in some forms of cancer. There are lots of pros and cons on the Internet, as you would expect. The bottom line is that, against my preconceptions, this unconventional treatment seems to treat all kinds of cancer patients safely and effectively. For the alternative, rational view visit "We are MacMillan cancer support".

There is apparently a "conspiracy against formal public controlled trials" of its beneficial effect not by Gerson therapists (who are usually American MDs and willing to demonstrate its efficacy) but apparently by the American FDA. This is hearsay: there is a huge positive literature on the Internet. If you have a patient with severe cancer or chemotherapy side effects, you might want to find out a bit more about it and other alternatives with them. What have you both got to lose? Especially with the **Saatchi Law** (the Saatchi or Medical Innovation Bill) having been debated (2014, which would have indemnified doctors for trying alternative treatments "when there are no other treatment options and every option holds serious risks"). It does seem that public opinion about cancer and alternative treatments is slowly changing. What isn't changing is that politicians do not seem to canvass public opinion before making laws.

There was an editorial in The Lancet Oncology during the passage of the bill which said that Lord Saatchi was promoting "Precisely the type of response that evidence based practice seeks to avoid". This in my opinion misses several relevant points. Presumably the Lancet editorial was saying that progress in cancer treatment comes from large clinical trials and the random allocation of patients into trials which may well administer sick patients ineffective placebos, less effective treatments or doses. Indeed I did this for a living, to children, as a large part of my early career. I wholeheartedly agreed with the scientific, one step at a time approach while I was young. The editorial implies that huge numbers of cannon fodder patients are needed in this way, as this is the scientific method and the only way to detect small benefits between competing treatments. But if I were one of those patients or a relative of one (which I have been) I would want a treatment known to be at least *partially* effective at a dose known to be reasonable and when I was beyond conventional hope I would take my chances with *any* non poisonous therapy. Isn't randomisation of a sick patient into a non treatment or worse treatment group unethical? Do no harm? To hell with being one of a nameless number, unknowingly deprived of the best known treatment or treatment of any kind for the sake of a double blind controlled trial and future generations. Given the outcome of most chemotherapy treatment, those huge numbers of less well treated patients were sacrificing their lives for very little territorial gain. Can't we design computer programs to compare results from two groups of good active treatments, taking in all variables, both known to be or thought to be effective without deliberately and knowingly giving one group a much better treatment?

There is:

The Plaskett Therapy which is a vegan version of dietary therapy, similar in approach to the Gerson therapy, low protein, with various modifications and scientific adaptations.

Hoxsey Therapy: A mixture of herbal medicines with marked anti tumour effect.

Essiac herbal tea: An anti tumour effect.

Laetrile: Vitamin B17, Amygdalin (a cyanide containing molecule that is in many foods but has an anti cancer effect) It isn't really a vitamin and it is found naturally in bitter almonds, peach and apricot stones. The sale of Laetrile is banned by the FDA and EU.

Protocel: Is sold in the USA as a food supplement but was originally used with great success as a chemotherapeutic treatment for various cancers. The FDA seems to have prevented controlled trials on it and also prevented registered doctors from using it as a standard cancer treatment. Read about it from various legitimate sources however and it is hard not to be impressed by its results in cancer of all kinds. Unfortunately nearly every "alternative" cancer writer in the American literature is a conspiracy theorist with the FDA and "Big Pharma" as the main bogeymen and many alternative treatments are therefore characterised as victimised not by virtue of their risks, but because they threaten the medical establishment and other vested interests. So it is often hard to get an unbiased view of some non standard anticancer treatments – without a degree of persecution paranoia.

Many alternative anticancer theories assume cancer cells have abnormal lipid membranes and highly acidic, hypoxic (anaerobic) interiors. The acid interiors may be related to the associated fact that some cancer theories postulate different cellular metabolisms, including alternative energy generating mitochondrial pathways. Some say the evidence is that cancer is not just a genetic but a mitochondrial disease and that cancer cells ferment rather than respire to obtain energy. Thus carbohydrates and to a lesser extent some amino acids (such as glutamine) are the main sustenance of cancer cells. It is undoubtedly true that a diet high in vegetables, particularly colourful vegetables and fruit improves health and survival in cancer and cancer therapy. Conversely there is good reason to assume a carbohydrate, calorie rich diet, as suggested by the dieticians in so many NHS cancer units may well be feeding the cancer rather than the recovery.

For instance, Protocel is said to act on the ATP in cells reducing its activity. The theory is that cancer cells survive on an anaerobic glycolytic metabolism and by down regulating their oxidative metabolism still further push down the "Redox" pathway. Protocel thus causing lysis of acidotic cells. Non acidotic (non cancerous) cells are unaffected and so there are no side effects.

Flaxseed oil and cottage cheese. I know this sounds bizarre but if it were renamed Omega 3 and 6 essential fatty acids and sulphur based protein treatment to repair and replace damaged cancer cell membranes would it sound any less weird and new agey? Many of us are indeed omega 3 and 6 deficient and these EFAs make up part of the structure of cell membranes. Flaxseed (which is linseed oil) is particularly rich in these EFAs – 25% Linoleic Acid and 50-60% Alpha Linoleic Acid. Omega 3 EFAs not only make up cell membranes, they contribute towards oxygen transport in cells and prostaglandin synthesis. If there is inadequate appropriate membrane lipid, the membrane prevents proper cell division, the cell does not replicate properly, abnormal fats in the membrane (see elsewhere, saturated and hydrogenated fats affect cell membranes) affect oxygen diffusion and all this can trigger neoplastic change. The sulphur based proteins in cottage cheese render the EFAS in flaxseed water soluble and the cell membranes are restored and repaired. That is the theory and a brief Internet trawl will glean some interesting results and no adverse effects of the treatment.

The Rife Machine: Uses sound frequencies to destroy cancer forming organisms (theoretically).

Caesium treatment. Caesium chloride, one of the most alkaline metallic salts is given to the patient. The idea is that it then penetrates the intracellular environment of all cells and as cancer cells are acidic the treatment raises the intracellular pH and selectively kills cancer cells.

Palladium lipoic complex with vitamins and amino acids.

Low Dose Naltrexone (the opioid blocking drug) 3-5mg/day. The dose in MIMS for maintenance of abstinence in alcohol dependency is 50mg/day. It stimulates the immune system and as well as increasing endorphins, increases the number of NK, or Natural Killer cells. It affects opiate receptors on tumour cell membranes then endorphins cause apoptosis via these opiate receptors.

Pau D'arco (Napthaquinone in the bark is cytotoxic).

Ellagic Acid (In various fruits, especially raspberries and red berries).

Dr Kelley's enzyme theory: Is that trophoblastic cells are normal "healing" cells in adults. Trophoblastic and cancer cells are said to "share many common features", including a negative electrostatic charge (camouflage from immune recognition) and a lack of differentiation. When the healing process gets "out of control in a certain area, a cancer forms". Trophoblastic cells are normally under the control of humoral pancreatic enzymes and when these are inadequate, cancer is more likely. Cancer is three times more common in diabetics. A little far-fetched ? Yes I agree.

Burzynski antineoplastons. These are naturally occurring peptides which are said to activate tumour suppressor genes or switch off oncogenes causing cancer cells to revert to normal or die.

This is a brief summary of the main "evidence based" alternative cancer therapies which are used by hundreds of thousands of people in the UK, USA and Europe and which your patients may well ask you for and your opinion about. As you can see there is a lot of unconventional theory and strange concepts of how the body works at a micro level in some of these ideas. But isn't that what Pasteur's microbiological concept of infection must have sounded like in the 19th C? Or infections causing peptic ulcers, antibiotics affecting gut flora affecting the development of allergy and so on?

Having been on the receiving and giving ends, I know that virtually ALL of the specialists at the best UK cancer hospitals are currently unaware even of the name of the most popular and ?**effective** of these alternative therapies. Certainly, even traditional sources like the MacMillan website are basically negative about virtually any unconventional cancer treatment. Thus:

"We know that the scientific evidence base is growing for the use of some therapies in cancer care. However, we would like to see more high-quality research into complementary therapies in order to support patients, health professionals and commissioners to make informed decisions on the application of these therapies.

We make a clear distinction between supportive therapies used in conjunction with anti-cancer treatment and so-called alternative treatments, which are promoted as having an effect on the illness to be used instead of conventional treatment.

We do not advocate the use of alternative therapies. "

I was no better when I worked as a registrar at the Marsden in the early 80's; I would have seen the discussion of "alternative therapies" as an annoying distraction from the reality of surgery, chemotherapy and radiotherapy. But I sometimes felt slightly unreasonable as the NHS doctor – was the role ethically conflicting? Was it always in the patient's best interests to be in a large multicentre chemotherapy trial when the outcomes for most drug treatments were so bad? These trials are designed for large populations and basically compare different combinations of chemotherapy poisons against each other. The outcomes in most cancers and drug regimes are rarely impressive, so why should we be reluctant even to consider alternative therapies? – Can they be any worse than some of our traditional complications, side effects and outcomes? Some patients do call cancer treatments slash, burn and poison after all.

This is illustrated by the situation with intravenous Vitamin C, hyperthermia, hyperbaric oxygen. I had never heard of these treatments until recently and neither had the any of the oncology registrars looking after two close friends of mine when they asked. In fact the response was a predictably terse dismissal of these, as of all alternative treatment modalities.

So much so that even the inoffensive word "alternative" has taken on sinister, potentially dangerous, insulting and threatening connotations in the minds of some, more paranoid doctors.

It is however a newsworthy and current topic of conversation in many American cancer treatment centres. IV Ascorbic Acid reaches far higher serum levels than any oral dose can. The gut limits absorption and systemic administration is therefore used in a number of US and a few non NHS UK centres treating cancer patients in order to reach the high levels necessary.

Ascorbic Acid is both an antioxidant and a pro-oxidant. It converts free radicals to Hydrogen Peroxide in the presence of metallic elements. Tumour cells concentrate this effect, the result being damage to their DNA and mitochondria. Its supporters, and there are many amongst conventional oncologists, (in the USA) say this can be effective and non toxic in cancer of the lung, brain, colon, ovary, breast and pancreas. Vitamin C (and other anti-oxidant) treatments coincident with conventional chemotherapy CAN block some chemotherapy activity but presumably, given separately it could be additive via the localised oxidative cell damage. It does illustrate how poorly most doctors (and I would include myself in the early part of my career) respond to genuine questions on unconventional treatments from patients. We make the mistake of assuming all traditional medicine is evidence based, respectable and legitimate and all alternative treatments not worth investigating or even discussing. This may be true of Homeopathy, Iridology, Phrenology etc-which could not work in any rational world but why do we doctors fail to even show curiosity about other treatment modalities? We should be well informed about all treatments available to our patients especially those which have the *possibility* of a scientific basis. I don't understand the irrational rules of quantum mechanics, Heisenberg uncertainty, Schrödinger's Cat or Relativity but SAT Navs seem to work. Surely we shouldn't judge a question or a potential treatment purely on its provenance but on 1) How well knowing about it equips us to counsel and empathise with our patients.

2) Whether we have actually considered if it could be effective after all.

3) And anyway, are you sure that every drug and treatment modality that we currently support has quite the evidence base we think it does? Most negative trials are not available or publicised (as with some very popular, over prescribed seasonal anti-virals and other drugs) and there are several popular drug and surgical treatments which became conventional for decades and now we wouldn't recommend to our patients. I am sure you can think of various types of hip replacements, tonsillectomies, neonatal heart operations, total meniscectomies, numerous late drug withdrawals due to serious side effects and so on. These were treatments which you and I were keen on and promoted at one time or other because they were "conventional medicine" and now would rather forget. Why do we therefore so readily dismiss other treatments about which our patients want our unbiased advice, have been used, often extensively, elsewhere in the world and may turn out to be just as – or even more effective?

Retasking of old drugs as an adjunct to cancer therapy:
Loratadine/desloratadine in breast cancer, reducing metastases.
Mebendazole, which blocks cell division in lung, brain and colorectal cancer.
Metformin which has similar anti cancer effects to long term calorie restriction.
Statins lower the risk of colorectal and skin cancers.
Doxycycline works against bone secondaries for instance from breast cancer.
Cimetidine which reduces metastases from colorectal and gastric cancers.
Dutasteride reduces prostatic cancer progression and incidence.
Low dose Naltrexone (see above) used in alcohol and opioid addiction which has an effect on a number of cancers.
Clomipramine and
Aspirin which reduces recurrence of GI cancers including oesophageal cancers (but not pancreatic).
Bisphosphonates reduces skeletal metastatic spread of breast cancer.
Vitamin K2 prevents hepatic metastatic spread of breast cancer.

Irrespective of traditional or alternative therapies, survival in virtually all cancers is improved in patients who;
Take regular exercise,
Take Fish Oils and Curcumin supplements,
Have a "good sex life", (3 orgasms a week),
and believe in God (may improve survival up to 700%!).
Just being married improves your prognosis after cancer treatment 20% (JCO 2013) -27% (Cancer 2016).

Do not attempt Cardiopulmonary Resuscitation: DNACPR

Adults aged 16 years or older. This form to be retained by the patient or with the patient at his/her home.

Name
Address
DOB
NHS/Hospital No.

In the event of a cardiac or respiratory arrest, no attempt at life saving resuscitation should be made. All other treatment and care should continue as appropriate.

Does the patient have the mental and physical capacity to make and communicate this decision freely? If yes skip the rest of this section:
If No, are you aware of a valid advance decision refusing CPR relevant to the current condition?
Has the patient appointed a Welfare Attorney on their behalf- if yes, that person must be consulted.
All decisions must be made in the patient's best interests.

Summary of main clinical (and other relevant) problems why CPR would be inappropriate, unsuccessful or not in the patient's best interests:

Summary of communication with patient or Welfare Attorney or if not discussed with either, the reason why:

Summary of discussions with patient's relatives and friends: (with names and dates if possible)

Names of the MDT members contributing to the decision:

Healthcare professional completing or endorsing the DNACPR order:
Name
Position
Organisation
Date

Review date or No review date:

Do not attempt Cardiopulmonary Resuscitation Form

11: CARDIOLOGY:

Things you may have forgotten:

The ECG

Intervals, rates etc: 1 small sq= 0.04 sec.

Multiply the small squares on the ECG tracing by 0.04 to get the time interval in fractions of a second.

To get the rate per minute, divide 300 by the number of large squares between the complexes.

P is 2-3mm tall, 3 small squares wide, 3mm, 120 msec, notched in p mitrale, peaked in p pulmonale.

PR 120-210msec, (3.5-4 small sq). In paediatrics: <1yr 0.07-0.12 sec >1 yr 0.09-0.16 sec.

ST should be on the baseline, raised with exercise, ischaemia, acute infarction.

T is <5mm tall in standard leads <10mm tall in chest leads. Taller in infarction and ischaemia, ventricular strain, hyper kalaemia, CVA. Smaller in emphysema, thick chest wall, pericardial effusion, myxoedema, ischaemia, cardiomyopathy.

QT 10 small squares <420msec. is <half of preceding RR. Longer in CCF, MI, low Ca++, myocarditis. Short with digoxin, high Ca++, high K+.

U (best seen in V3) high with low K+, digoxin, high Ca++, exercise.

QRS Duration 0.05-0.10sec 2.5 small sq. in standard limb leads. Long in BBB or ventricular arrythmias.

Amplitude: If <5mm in 3 standard leads, coronary A disease, CCF, pericardial effusion, myxoedema, amyloid, obesity, emphysema.

Q: Amplitude: 1mm is N in AVL, AVF, V5, V6. Deep Qs N in AVR.

QT Interval drugs: (See SADS – Sudden Arrhythmic Death Syndrome on the internet):

In the normal adult it should be 0.33-0.44 secs. If >0.44 secs, it is a marker of myocardial electrical instability – prolongation of the QT is associated with possible ventricular arrhythmia, syncope and sudden death.

A huge number of drugs affect the cardiac QT interval, increasing the risk of arrhythmia and sudden death in susceptible patients. In fact it would be easier to consider those drugs that don't affect QT.

Those that **do** include:

Adrenaline
Alfuzosin
Amantidine
Amiodarone
Amitriptyline and other TCADs
Amoxapine
Astemizole, Terfenadine

Azithromycin, Clarithromycin, Erythromycin
Chloral

Haloperidol
Indapamide
Lithium
Methadone
Methylphenidate
Moexipril/Hydrochlorthiazide
Naratriptan, Sumatriptan, Zolmitriptan
Nicardipine
Ocreotide

Chloroquine
Ofloxacin
Chlorpromazine
Ciprofloxacin etc
Cisapride
Citalopram
Co Trimoxazole
d-Sotalol Sotalol

Diphenylhydramine
Disopyramide
Domperidone
Flecainide
Fluconazole, Itraconazole, Ketoconazole, etc
Fluoxetine, Sertraline, Trazadone, Venlafaxine
Granisetron, Ondansetron

Paroxetine
Prochlorperazine, Trifluoperazine
Quetiapine, Risperidone
Quinine/Quinidine
Ritodrine
Salbutamol, Salmeterol,
Terbutyline
Solifenacin
Tacrolimus
Tamoxifen
Thioridazine
Tolterodine
Vasopressin
and many others.

Cardiology: Things you may have forgotten:

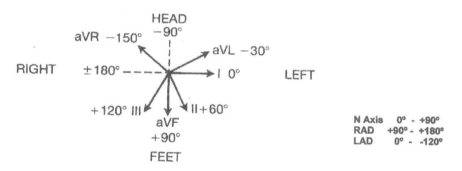

Diagram of Cardiac Axis (CA 1).

Classic ECG changes:

Myocardial Infarction:

ST elevation can occur within minutes, Q waves occur within days, then ST depression, T wave inversion within hours. A Q in III or AVF must be accompanied by a Q in II before making a diagnosis of MI.

Anterior: Small: V3-V4 Extensive V2-V5
Anteroseptal: I, AVL, V1-4
Anterolateral: I, AVL, V4-6
Lateral: I, II, AVL
Inferior: II, III, AVF
True posterior: Tall R waves in V1 V2 (reciprocal)
Sub endocardial: ST depression and T wave inversion in overlying leads with reciprocal

elevation of ST and upright Ts in leads from opposite surface and in cavity leads. Any lead.

Pulmonary Embolus:

S1, Q3, T3. Wide QRS in R Leads, rSR V1.

LVH:

R in AVL>13mm or

R in V5 or V6 >27mm or

S in V1 +R in V5 or V6 >35mm.

Largest R and S >40 small squares.

RVH:

Rs or qR in V1 or V3r with R ventricular activation time >0.03 sec,

QRS <0.12 sec +RAD. Tall R in V1,

R>S in V1. T wave inversion in V1-3. Deep S in V6 usually accompanied by RAD.

Cor Pulmonale:

RAD i.e. dominant S in I, R in III, P Pulmonale (best in II and>2.5mm). RVH with prominent R and T wave inversion in V1-3 partial or complete RBBB.

Digoxin Toxicity:

Bradycardia, coupling, reversed tick ST depression, shortening of QT, AF, VF, prolonged QRS, delayed conduction.

Calcium: HyperCa++ shortens, HypoCa++ lengthens QT.

Heart Sounds and Murmurs:

Things you may have forgotten:

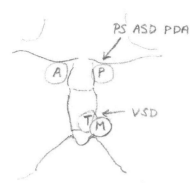

HEART SOUNDS

CLOSURE SOUNDS (First and Second Heart Sounds)

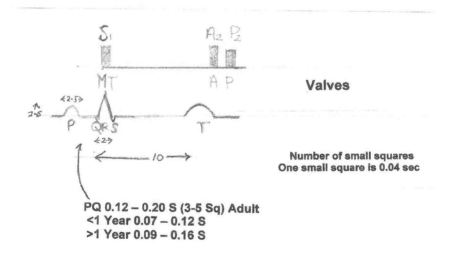

Valves

Number of small squares
One small square is 0.04 sec

PQ 0.12 – 0.20 S (3-5 Sq) Adult
<1 Year 0.07 – 0.12 S
>1 Year 0.09 – 0.16 S

Aortic area

--------->Neck in (A)S P2 May be single or reversed

Ejection click if valvular

Pulmonary Area

Second sound split in (P)S
Best area for pulmonary second sound
Loud 2nd sound in pulmonary hypertension
Fixed splitting in ASD, paradoxical in LBBB

(P)S ASD

(P) Apex

(T)Murmur

Fixed split second sound, ASD
An Ostium Primum (low) may involve T and M valves
with an apical pan systolic (M)incomp murmur (rare)

PDA (P)area c thrill. Pulm P2 may be absent

------VSD Small

Maladie de Roger Tricuspd posn. 4LIS c thrill

---- Large

P2 Sound may be single   3 Apex (M)flow
in pulmonary area

Tricuspid Area (L sternal edge)

------ (T)R

------- VSD

(A)R Austin Flint. Lean forward, hold breath in expiration

(T)S ASD Fixed splitting

Mitral Area

(M)R ----------> Axilla

(M)S Carey Coombes-Increased M flow in Rh F. Pre
OS   systolic accentuation unless in AF.

Graham Steell. Early diastolic pulm regurgitant murmur due to pulmonary hypertension (cor pulmonale)

A2

Ejection sound Single P2 ---------- Fallots Heard in Tricuspid position

VSD Ⓟ S

Coarctation Often loudest at back, absent femoral pulses, associated c PDA, A valve lesions.

Diagram of murmurs/heart sounds (MHS 1, 2 and 3).

Hypertension:

As you will see, this is a moving target. Not only do the national standards as to what levels we should aim for change depending on new survival data, but as we all know, definitions and targets constantly move and we can take the blood pressure one minute and it has changed by the time the patient is in the car park. What's worse, the law of thirds means that most patients aren't even taking their tablets properly all the time and you may take the blood pressure at one of those times, overdosing them with the next prescription in compensation.

What is blood pressure anyway? Best practice suggests that the patient is seated and rested for at least 5 minutes before recording the level. I think I did that a few times during half hour medicals on stressed patients a few years ago. Most of us however just don't have the time to spare to wait 5 minutes and how often will the patient actually be rested and relaxed like this in "real life". How relevant IS that reading anyway?

Home BP and ambulatory BP readings are better at predicting end organ damage and incident cardiovascular disease than surgery readings. Ambulatory readings are better than separate home readings.

To diagnose "hypertension" there have to be three separate readings of >140/90 and despite the obvious caveats on the anxiety of having your blood pressure done in the stressful environment of the surgery (have you ever sat in a doctor's waiting room?) it may not be quite such an artificial environment to have it checked as I used to think. Life is one long string of stressful events, – frustrations in the car, in the queue at the bank, at work, arguments at home, worries about the children and neighbours, a saw tooth of blood pressure one after another and one day one of them is going to be the straw that ruptures an endothelial plaque in your anterior descending or your middle meningeal artery. So you might as well calibrate your drug treatment to the elevated blood pressure of the waiting room in anticipation of life's slings and arrows.-Is this right? I often go to lectures where they say that everyone, no matter what age or condition should have their blood pressure dragged down to 120/70. Perhaps they don't see the postural hypotension, the fractured hips, the syncope, the loss of vasomotor tone that causes the falls and the faints when the patient is more relaxed at home. Is survival to 100 worth it if we faint every time we stand up or if we need support stockings in bed? Falling in the elderly is the most common symptom causing admission to a nursing home or care home. Most people want to avoid this loss of independence in old age like the plague.

New research shows that actual *fluctuations* in both systolic and diastolic BP increase fatal CHD, stroke and heart failure, not just the absolute levels themselves.

Indeed the *very newest* evidence (Imp Coll. August 2016) suggests that with existing coronary artery disease, the doctor dragging blood pressure down to "normal" ("120/70") increases the risk of MI if not stroke. So over treating blood pressure clearly has its risks too. NO blood pressure treatment guarantees a consistent safe reduction in blood pressure and no blood pressure measurement tells you what the patient's blood pressure will continue to be for any length of time after you have measured it.

Hypertension: WHO definition:

160/95 but the treatment target now generally considered to be 130/85 and

Normal is	<130/<85
High normal	130-139/85-89 (i.e. no higher than 140/90)
Mild Hypertension	140-159/90-99

Isolated Systolic Hypertension is generally defined as >160

Since 2006: The NICE Hypertension recommendations were:

Thresholds for treatment:

Without diabetes:	>140/90 treat if 10 yr CVD risk>20% or existing CVD or TOD.
	>160/100 treat all.
Type 2 diabetes:	>140/80 treat if 10 year CVD risk >20% or history of CVD or microalbuminuria or proteinuria.
Type 1 diabetes:	>135/85 treat all.
	>130/80 treat if abn. albumin excretion or 2+ features of metabolic syndrome.

Targets for treatment:

Without diabetes:	140/90,
Type 2 diabetes:	140/80 (135/75 if microalbuminuria or proteinuria),
Type 1 diabetes:	135/85 (130/80 if nephropathy).

(TOD Target organ damage)

NICE 2015

Offer ambulatory monitoring, annual cardiovascular risk monitoring, testing for target organ damage.

Treated hypertension	<80 yrs 140/90,
	>80 yrs 150/90,

For a clinic BP of 140/90 the ABPM daytime average (home monitoring average) is
135/85,
160/100   150/95.

Note: Targets: (BHS 1999)

Hypertension	<140/85,
Hypertension with diabetes	<140/80,
Hypertension with diabetes and nephropathy	<130/80,

| Hypertension in the elderly | <140/85, |
| Hypertension with other CHD risks | <140/85. |

In America the 2014 JNC 8 recommendations were:

- In patients 60 years or over, start treatment in blood pressures >150mm Hg systolic or >90mm Hg diastolic and treat to under those thresholds.
- In patients <60 years, treatment initiation and goals should be 140/90mm Hg, the same threshold used in patients >18 years with either chronic kidney disease (CKD) or diabetes.
- In nonblack patients with hypertension, initial treatment can be a thiazide-type diuretic, CCB, ACE inhibitor, or ARB, while in the general black population, initial therapy should be a thiazide-type diuretic or CCB.
- In patients >18 years with CKD, initial or add-on therapy should be an ACE inhibitor or ARB, regardless of race or diabetes status.

JNC 8 is mostly in line with the **European Society of Hypertension** (ESH) guidelines also released in 2014 which suggested a target of <140mm Hg systolic BP for all patients, with some caveats. In patients with diabetes, the ESH guidelines suggest a diastolic BP of <85mm Hg, and for patients under 80 years. They suggest a target systolic of between 140 and 150, going lower only if the patient is fit and in good health.

Then there is the 9000 **Heartwire trial** (– actually "SPRINT", – Systolic BP Intervention Trial – OK I know it spells SBPIT which sounds like "spit" but sprint does sound cooler than spit doesn't it?) of hypertensive patients at risk, which showed that a systolic target of less than 120mm Hg (!!) was associated with lower risks of MI, ACS, Stroke, Acute HF, CV death, all cause mortality. As you might expect however, there were higher rates of hypotension, syncope and AKI. I assume higher rates of hip fracture, compulsory nursing home admission, falls, dependency and a poorer quality of whatever life they had. Later (different) research also showed more MI in patients with existing CVS disease dragged down to very low blood pressures on treatment.

In Atul Gawunde's Book "Being Mortal" he makes the point that the frequent and banal situation of recurrent falling at home is one of the commonest reasons for older patients being forced against their will into living in supervised accommodation or a nursing home. Here they can lose not just their independence but morale, spirit, interests, friends, outlook and hope. So if you treat their blood pressure down to the ground when you are taking it (presumably even lower in the peace and quiet of home when the patient leaves the surgery) then you vastly increase their chances of postural hypotension, injury, loss of independent living and loss of...............everything they live for.

So although we have had effective treatment for raised blood pressure and cholesterol for thirty years, we are still a bit unsure about what the targets for both treatments should be!

Note: The correct diastolic is taken as the Karotkoff Phase V – the loss of all sound. I suspect most doctors DO NOT use this as the diastolic level, but erroneously use the change **in** sound.

What Drugs to use?

Treatment:

Current UK Guidelines:

Step	Less than 55 years.	Over 55yrs or Black, any age.
1	ACEI (or BB*)	CCB or Thiazide
2 If still hypertensive:	ACEI (or BB*) plus CCB OR ACEI plus Thiazide to either group	
3 If still hypertensive:	ACEI (or BB*) plus CCB plus Thiazide to both groups	

Then add further diuretic, (**Spironolactone) Amiloride, Alpha blocker, or Beta blocker,

possibly refer. ACEIs and BBs are ineffective in black people as monotherapy.

*Guidance at various times, I find works well. **This is more likely to work with a raised Renin (random 0.5-3.1pg/ml/hr)

Step 6 is Alpha blocker, moxonidine, or alpha and B blocker.

Thus: Ramipril, Bendrofluazide and Amlodipine are the current cheap and cheerful evidence-based first line drugs for straight forward uncomplicated hypertension.

You might want to try the slightly stronger diuretics Hydrochlorthiazide or Chlort(h)alidone in the elderly, (>80 yrs), those at risk of heart failure or with oedema.

Hypertension in diabetic patients:

Drug of choice a Thiazide (Bendroflumethazide) and/or ACEI (Ramipril, with second line Lisinopril based on cost). Try to avoid Beta Blockers, CCBs are not first line and although diabetogenic, Thiazides still improve outcomes.

A few points: A 24 hour BP monitor is extremely helpful in assessing the significance of a patient's raised readings. I find sitting in G.P.'s waiting room one of the most frustrating and annoying experiences I can have and it must take 10-15 minutes for my BP to settle after I enter the haven of peace and tranquillity which is my doctor's consulting room. As a G.P. I find Beta Blockers far more useful at an early stage in many patients than the above chart suggests. The clue is in the patient's "You're running late" comment, or "You're busy again today" after only a 10-20 minute wait. The patient is usually male, middle age or young, self employed and in a suit. If they are headache prone then prescribe a slow release or long half life, non selective BB, starting at a low dose, provided they are not asthmatic and do not get too many side effects. I would start this between stage 1 and 2.

A BP is only a "still photo" from a long running film and we all know that it will be completely different in an hour, 3 hours, 24 hours. What we are looking for is an overall trend and unless the levels are very high – 220/120 or there are other symptoms (or the patient is pregnant), I do not overreact to one reading. The guidance always tells us to take the blood pressure three times and we know we should treat the patient not the blood pressure. There is the famous law of thirds, the fact that if the patient feels tired or drained they will soon stop taking their medication and that every day is full of an infinite number of blood pressure influencing variables so trying to apply precision to blood pressure recording and management is a bit like trying to control a kite on a windy day with an elastic string.

There are of course hundreds of iconic blood pressure trials with catchy acronyms: ACCORD (Action to control cardiovascular risk in diabetes), SHEP (Systolic hypertension in the elderly), HOT (Hypertension optimal treatment), AASK (African American study of kidney disease and hypertension) and so on. ALLHAT, the Antihypertensive and lipid lowering treatment to prevent heart attack study began in 1994 with 33,000 patients and monitored the lowering of BP and lipids to see the cardiovascular benefits. Surprisingly perhaps, it found old fashioned Chlort(h) alidone (nowadays spelt without the h) was safer than the (then) newer CCB Amlodipine (BadPharma. Ben Goldacre). Also that CCBs and thiazides were better than Lisinopril at reducing Coronary artery disease and stroke. The study also came up with the fact that ACEIs reduce CCF with diuretics, protect against CVS morbidity and also prevent stroke.

We know that reducing cholesterol in co morbid situations and getting significantly raised blood pressure down saves lives. There is of course a plethora of clinical trials constantly going on to compare the various anti hypertensives amongst themselves. The last time I checked MIMS there were 160 antihypertensive preparations for us to chose from.

Spironolactone is often a last ditch but very effective add on antihypertensive when all else fails despite seeming old fashioned. Presumably the patients who respond have high Renin levels so you should start treatment very slowly, titrate and watch electrolytes closely.

Grip strength is related to coronary risk (Leong, Lancet May 2015) The average male adult grip strength is 38.1kg, female is 26.6kg. For each 5kg decline in grip strength there was found to be a 17% increased cardiovascular death rate, a 9% higher stroke risk and a 7% higher MI risk. The reason for the connection between forearm weakness and circulatory health is unknown and what's more important, it is not known whether building up grip strength reduces your systemic circulatory risk. It seems unlikely though.

Cardiovascular 10 year risk charts:

Cardiovascular 10 year risk charts: Non Diabetic Men/Women. Non Smoker/Smoker. (Thanks to Professor Paul Durrington of Manchester University for his kind permission to reproduce these.) Don't forget they are only guides and the risks are higher in the overweight, Asians, patients with co existing other risk factors and illnesses, in women with premature menopauses, in the presence of strong family histories etc.

Nondiabetic Men

CVD risk < 10% over next 10 years
CVD risk 10-20% over next 10 years
CVD risk > 20% over next 10 years

CVD risk over next 10 years 30%

10% 20%

SBP = systolic blood pressure mmHg
TC : HDL = serum total cholesterol to HDL cholesterol ratio

| Non - smoker | Smoker |

Age under 50 years

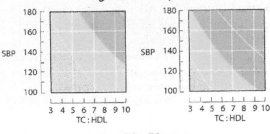

Age 50 - 59 years

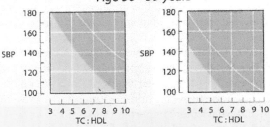

Age 60 years and over

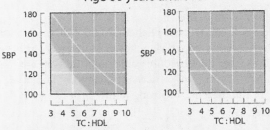

Copyright University of Manchester

Note 1:
These charts are for estimating cardiovascular disease (CVD) risk – non-fatal myocardial infarction (MI) and stroke, coronary and stroke death and new angina pectoris – *for individuals who have not already developed coronary heart disease (CHD) or other major atherosclerotic disease*. They are an aid to making clinical decisions about how intensively to intervene in lifestyle and whether to use antihypertensive medication, lipid-lowering medication and/or aspirin.

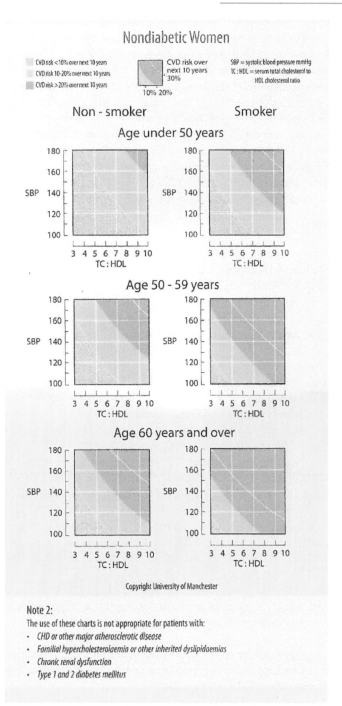

Nondiabetic Women

CVD risk <10% over next 10 years
CVD risk 10-20% over next 10 years
CVD risk >20% over next 10 years

CVD risk over next 10 years 30%

10% 20%

SBP = systolic blood pressure mmHg
TC : HDL = serum total cholesterol to HDL cholesterol ratio

Non - smoker   **Smoker**

Age under 50 years

Age 50 - 59 years

Age 60 years and over

Copyright University of Manchester

Note 2:

The use of these charts is not appropriate for patients with:

- CHD or other major atherosclerotic disease
- Familial hypercholesterolaemia or other inherited dyslipidaemias
- Chronic renal dysfunction
- Type 1 and 2 diabetes mellitus

Non Diabetic Men, Non Diabetic Women, CVD risk charts.

The NHS Routine Health Check: (introduced in 2009)

Thought by many of us to be a waste of time from the start – another almost pointless burden to add to our work load. More questions to ask and tasks to perform before the patient is allowed to get to their own agenda in the consultation. More a political show-piece than a cost effective use of resources and it turned out to be just that, pretty much a waste of time. Research done at ICL funded and commissioned by the DH in 2016 found that the checks reduce 10 year cardiovascular risk by 0.21%. That is one cardiovascular event (MI or stroke) every 4,762 screened patients. The study (Chang, Canadian Med Assocn. J) followed 139,000 patients between 2009 and 2013 and looked at them again 2 years later. The checks increased the number of detected hypertensives by a meagre 3% and diabetics by 1.3%. Their weight dropped 0.27kg/Sq M and Tot Chol 0.15mmol/li. Only 21% of eligible people even attended their appointment which gives the patient's verdict on the checks too.

ACEIs:

Before starting treatment with ACEIs and ARBs I always check for renal bruits but I have only heard a handful in thirty years (-In which case I do an USS and then refer, treating hypertension with something other than ACEIs, ARBs, Eplerenone or Spironolactone etc). So significant **renal artery stenosis** in GP is rare even though 1 in 5 adults between 65 and 75 is said to have some degree of RAS and 42%>75 years! Presumably most of these are not functionally significant. It is said that if the creatinine increases >15% over pre-treatment levels on an ACEI, then RAS may be present. The recommended ACEI regime is therefore:

Check K and creatinine, start Rx, recheck K and creatinine after 1 week, watch for hyperkalaemia and raised creatinine, titrate to an effective dose and if no change in renal function then do annual creatinine and electrolytes.

ACEIs are more likely to adversely affect renal function in arteriopaths (claudication, aneurysm etc.).

Despite the official figures, I suspect 25-30% of patients on ACEIs develop a **dry cough**. Try a topical nasal steroid spray as a first approach – as even patients on ACEIs get post nasal drip. Then try a Cromoglicate MDI (Intal)) or Nedocromil (Tilade). ACEIs increase serum bradykinin (which is normally metabolised by ACE) and the inhalers counteract this, amongst other actions. Alternatively try ARBs or a different anti hyper-tensive. Ramipril is supposed to cause more cough than any other ACEI so you could also try another ACEI if you are dead set on avoiding the cost of an Artan. If you are, shame on you.

There is a risk of first dose hypotension on any ACEI but this is rare unless the patient is in heart failure or on a biggish dose of a loop diuretic (eg Furosemide 80mg). I have never seen it despite the dire warnings.

So: **A.C.E.I.s:**

Help reduce progression of renal disease in diabetes and CKD of various causes. But avoid in pregnancy and can cause angio-oedema and dry cough. **Risk of hyperkalaemia.**

Lisinopril Carace, Zestril, 2.5-40mg a day.

Captopril, Capoten, Acepril. (As most Aces have either ace or pril in the name, this is a clever combination of ACE and PRIL! I wonder if the creative team got an industry prize for that?) 12.5mg-50mg BD.

Enalapril, Innovace 2.5-20mg daily.
Fosinopril, Staril.
Cilazepril, Vascace.
Ramipril, Tritace 1.25mg initially-10mg daily. Good evidence of M.I and stroke reduction.
Perindopril, Coversyl. 24 hour control.
Quinapril, Accupro.
Trandolapril, Gopten "Longest half life"?

Stated Half Lives of ACEIs
Captopril 2 hrs,
Enalapril 11 hrs,
Lisinopril 12 hrs,
Quinapril 2-2.5, (25hrs elimination), Peak 2-6 hrs.
Ramipril 4, 10-18, >50hrs Triphasic,
Trandolapril 15-24hrs,
Fosinopril 12hrs.
These are the T 1/2 of the active drug in hours and don't necessarily equate to its clinical effect.
Ramipril and Perindopril are said to have particularly good CVS mortality profiles.

Stuff you may have forgotten:
Veins contain 70% of the circulating blood volume, arteries 17%, the remaining 13% is in the organs.

The Renin-Angiotensin system:
The Liver produces Angiotensinogen into the systemic circulation

v

Low BP>Kidney Juxta-glomerular apparatus secretes>Renin into the circulation>>>>>converts v

v

Angiotensinogen to Angiotensin 1

v

The lungs contain the enzyme: Angiotensin converting enzyme

v

which converts Angiotensin 1 to Angiotensin 2

Angiotensin 2 vasoconstricts, stimulates Aldosterone secretion (from the Adrenal cortex), which then increases renal tubular sodium and water reabsorbtion (and excretion of potassium) which increases blood pressure.
ACEIs, ARBs, Spironolactone, Eplerenone and Aliskiren all act along this pathway blocking various stages **(and so the potential risk of Hyperkalaemia).**
Epleronone does not cause gynaecomastia, Aldosterone often does.

Angotensin II Receptor Antagonists (The Artans):
Can increase K, so avoid with potassium sparing diuretics.
Losartan, Cozaar, Valsartan, Diovan, Irbesartan, Aprovel Long Half Life.
Candesartan, Amias, Olmesartan, Olmetec. The most effective anti hypertensive Artan?

Eprosartan, Teveten. Affects peripheral sympathetic tone, no drug interactions. Telmisartan, Micardis. Good 24 hour control. Long half life.

etc.

and don't forget the cholesterol. Lowering the cholesterol in a hypertensive reduces the cardiovascular risk more than lowering the blood pressure. Certainly this applies to diabetics.

Renin Inhibitors:

Aliskiren. Rasilez. Interactions, predictably, with ACEIs, Artans, Digoxin and K+ sparing drugs. Also Furosemide, grapefruit juice St John's Wort etc.

Newish warnings (April 2014) have been issued by the American FDA to be careful ("Must not prescribe") Aliskiren with other drugs acting along the RAS in patients with diabetes, with renal impairment (GFR <60mL/min) because of the risk of deterioration in renal function, hyperkalaemia, hypotension.

Potassium:

A systematic American review and meta analysis of 22 trials and 11 cohort studies published in 2015 examined the effect of potassium intake on blood pressure, kidney function, lipids, mortality, CVD, stroke and CHD. **The mortality rate dropped with increased potassium intake.** The highest intake of potassium (4700mg/day) gave the best SBP drop.

Potassium is in higher concentrations (see diet section) in:

Prunes, dates, most nuts, avocados, bran wheat germ, oranges, bananas, spinach, beetroot, steak, chips, figs, tomatoes, pineapple etc.

Most people consume far less than an optimum amount of potassium from a blood pressure point of view.

Renal Adverse reactions: AKI

In a 2015 article about "pernicious drug reactions" – the combination of a RAS inhibitor, diuretic, (especially a loop diuretic) and an oral aldosterone antagonist and diuretic were given as a common causes of acute kidney injury, particularly in the older patient. Those patients who developed a drug related acute kidney injury were 10X more likely to be admitted to hospital and 4-5X more likely to die. Adding an NSAID makes everything even worse. This bumps up the risk by a further 66%.

So when treating hypertension you should always avoid wherever possible having an older patient with reduced renal function taking the combination of: NSAID, RAS inhibitor, loop diuretic and an aldosterone antagonist. Other drugs that cause AKI include COX II Inhibitors, Aminoglycosides and Iodine contrast media.

Beta Blockers:

What you may have forgotten:

These are useful and currently a little out of fashion but with a plethora of uses and beneficial actions.

There are 3 types of B (catecholamine) receptors:

B1 are mainly cardiac and renal. They are selectively blocked by "Selective" Beta blockers.

B2 are in the lungs, G.I.T, liver, uterus, leukocyte, vascular smooth muscle and skeletal smooth muscle.

B3 are in fat cells.

(Note: Alpha 1 receptors are in blood vessels, Alpha 2 in the kidney, central nervous system (hypotensive), adipocytes and platelets).

Beta Blockers have a multiplicity of clinical uses including:

Rate limiting rapid AF, angina, some arrhythmias, some forms of headache, some types of CCF, tremor, glaucoma, hypertension, migraine prevention, arrhythmia suppression after MI, phaeochromocytoma, HOCM, hyperhydrosis, chronic and acute anxiety states (stage fright), etc.

Specific Beta blockers have different properties:

Those used in Heart Failure: (with an ACEI and diuretic)
Bisoprolol, Nebivolol, Carvedilol, SR Metoprolol.

Those with **Intrinsic Sympathomimetic Activity:** (Avoiding excess bradycardia through a partial AGONIST effect at the B receptor):-So best avoided after M.I., in angina, tachyarrhythmia.

Oxprenolol,
Pindolol,
Penbutolol,
Acebutolol.

Alpha 1 Blocking and Beta blocking Beta blockers: Causing arteriolar vasodilatation as well as cardiac slowing etc.
Labetalol, Carvedilol.

Selectivity:

Non selective B Blockers exacerbate asthma etc but are better in migraine and tremor. Alprenolol. Carteolol, ISA. Carvedilol, alpha blocking too. Labetalol, alpha blocking too. Nadolol, hydrophilic. Oxprenolol, ISA. Pindolol, ISA, membrane stabilising. Propranolol, membrane stabilising. Sotalol, hydrophilic. Timolol.

B1 Selective B Blockers: Less effect on Lipids, sexual function, glucose metabolism, peripheral circulation, COPD.

Acebutolol. ISA, membrane stabilising. Atenolol. Hydrophilic Betaxolol. Membrane stabilising. Bisoprolol. Celiprolol. ISA, hydrophilic, vasodilating partial B2 agonist activity, "no effect on lipids or glucose", Metoprolol, Nebivolol. Said to have no effect on diabetes or lipids.

I.S.A.:(Intrinsic Sympathomimetic Activity)

Acebutalol, Oxprenolol, Pindolol.

Beta Blockers and problem drug interactions:

Beta Blockers may cause bradycardia with rate limiting CCBs eg Diltiazem, Verapamil. Beta Blockers can cause bradycardia with Digoxin, Mefloquine.

Hypotension with Verapamil, Nifedipine, Nisoldipine and various other antihypertensives but there can be rebound hypertension on discontinuing Clonidine while taking a Beta Blocker.

Some antipsychotics interact with Beta Blockers increasing the risk of arrhythmias.

Use in Migraine:

Propranolol, Metoprolol, Nadolol, Timolol.

Specific clinical areas of hypertension:

Hypertension in Afro-Caribbean patients:
Thiazides, Calcium Channel Blockers and Alpha Blockers work but ACEIs and BBs are ineffective as monotherapy.

Hypertension in pregnancy:
Methyl Dopa, Labetalol, Amlodipine, Hydrallazine IV, Doxazosin. Also Aspirin/ Calcium.

Hypertensive Crisis: (or emergency if there is evidence of organ damage):
Systolic is = or >180/Diastolic is = or >120.
Severe hypertension with impairment of more than one organ systems.
Signs and symptoms include: Retinal haemorrhage or exudates, papilloedema, (sine qua non), RICP, HA, nausea, possible haematuria, proteinuria, sometimes arryhthmias, epistaxis, etc
Treatment:
Nifedipine 10mg 4-6hrly, Atenolol 25mg, Sodium Nitroprusside IV, Labetalol IV, Nitrates IV, Hydrallazine IV.

Other antihypertensives:
Indapamide: Natrilix. A thiazide, used in isolated systolic hypertension.
A Daily Mail wonder Drug of relatively limited effect on BP that your patients may ask you about.

Angina:
"Angine" is the French word for quinsy and sore throat – and indeed angina – an ischaemic myocardium can cause mouth pain, neck pain, throat pain, epigastric pain, inter scapular pain as well as retrosternal pain. It isn't always clearly exercise related. It can, for instance, be associated with anticipation of stressful situations or driving. It may only happen at night. Ischaemic heart pain is worth thinking of when anyone who might be an arteriopath, who has smoked or otherwise might have less than pristine coronary arteries looks pale and sweaty and feels ill with paroxysmal pain above the abdomen.

Angina generally: Treatment:
Aspirin 300mg stat then 75mg daily,
B Blocker, or
Verapamil, or
Diltiazem (Avoid B.B. with Verapamil and caution with Diltiazem because of bradycardia).
GTN,
Nicorandil can help as an add on,
Statin, aim for a cholesterol of <5.
And Nitrates:
ISDN – the Dinitrate, dosing a.m. and mid afternoon (the active moiety is NO) – has a short half life, or alternatively ISMN – the Mononitrate, much less first pass metabolism than the Dinitrate (but avoid with Viagra type drugs) – and it does have a longer half life.
Nifedipine can be used with a BB.
NOTE: Dihydropyridine CCBs are Amlodipine, Felodipine, Lacidipine, Nifedipine, Nicardipine etc,

Phenylalkylamines CCBs are Verapamil etc,
Benzothiazepine CCBs include Diltiazem,
Non selective CCBs include Mibefradil etc,
Ziconotide is an analgesic CCB.
See below:
You can try Ivabradine, Procoralan – a sinus node inhibitor 5mg BD, which acts at the S.A. node. Take care when co prescribing drugs that can cause bradycardia (BBs, Verapamil, Diltiazem) or monitor heart rate first.

Note: **The Bruce Protocol** is a standardised regime of graded exercise on a treadmill. The grade of this is increased every three minutes thus:

Stage	minutes	% Incline	Km/hr	MPH
1	up to 3	10	2.7	1.7
2	6	12	4.0	2.5
3	9	14	5.4	3.4
4	12	16	6.7	4.2
5	15	18	8.0	5.0
6	18	20	8.8	5.5
7	21	22	9.6	6.0

Coronary Syndrome X:

There is a variety of clinical situations called "Syndrome X": Coronary syndrome X, Metabolic Syndrome (central obesity, insulin resistance etc), Turner Syndrome XO (see eponyms) and so on.

Coronary syndrome X is exercise/stress chest pain (classic anginal type pain) with normal coronary arteries on angiogram. The patients may have ST depression on ETT or not. They can be helped by treatment with CCBs but have a very good prognosis. Although many cardiologists do not even accept that the condition actually exists, some believe the ischaemia is at a microvascular level rather than further upstream.

Calcium Score: (EBCT)

Electron beam computerised tomography: Equivalent to 30 CXRs in terms of radiation. Performs a rapid CT sweep of the heart in a fraction of a second by having an electronically generated X Ray source, rotating in a circle rapidly around the patient. The procedure takes half an hour or so in total and gives good quality pictures of the size, position and density of coronary calcification.

The EBCT detects coronary calcification and then using the Agatston scoring method a coronary calcium score is used to assess the subsequent cardiac risk.

Many units will offer this investigation *for a price*. Other than the radiation, it is non invasive, can be used to avoid an angiogram and its risks in a patient with chest pain – and as long as the score is low, can be very reassuring.

A Coronary artery calcium score
0 No significant plaque is likely
>100 Above average risk of a coronary event in 5 years
>1000 A high risk of a cardiac event

Myocardial Infarction:

Anatomy

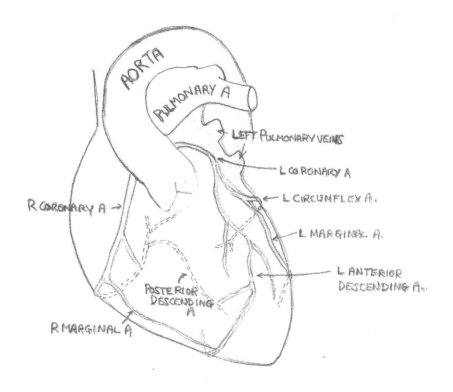

Diagram of Coronary Circulation (CC1)

Myocardial Infarction ECG Criteria:
Q>30ms in AVF
R<10ms and <0.1mv in V2
R>40ms in V1
ST Elevation >0.1mV in 2 leads or evolving Q waves.

Anatomy:

Infarct	Artery	Area	ECG
Anterior:	LAD	Ant.wall of LV	ST elevation in 1 aVL V1-6
		Intraventricular septum	ST depression in II III and aVF
Inferior:	R Circumflex	Inferior surface of L ventricle	ST elevation in II III aVF
		Sometimes R Ventricle	ST depression in I aVL
		and intraventricular septum	and precordial leads
Lateral	L Circumflex	Lat wall of L ventricle	ST elevation in I aVL V4-6

The ECG changes of:

Inferior infarction

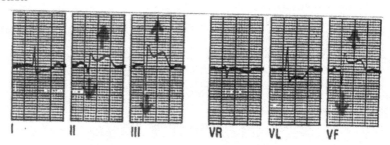

Anterior infarction

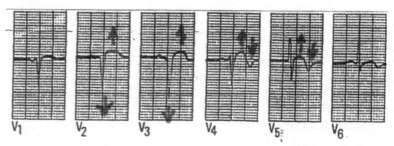

Subendocardial infarction

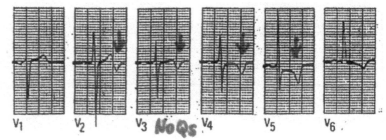

Ischaemia

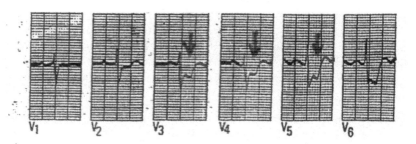

Diagram: Electrical changes of acute Myocardial infarction and ischaemia: (MIOECG) (MIOECG2)

Acute Myocardial Infarction: Treatment:
Sub Lingual GTN,
300mg Non enteric coated aspirin,
4x 75mg Clopidogrel,
I.V. Cannula.
=/– IM/IV Diamorphine 10mg
Cyclizine 50mg.
Oxygen.

Anti thrombosis agents and current recommendations:

	Cerebrovascular Disease:		Cardiovascular Dis:		Peripheral Art Dis.
	Acute Stroke:	2ndary Prev.	Acute M.I.	2ndary Prev.	
Aspirin:	300mg	75-150mg/d	150-300mg	75-150mg/d	
	Ischaemic Stroke		Unstable angina or non STEMI if 6m mort >1.5% with aspirin -treat until 1 year after last attack.		
Clopidogrel: (Plavix)	from day 7-6m		Acute MI from a few days to 35 days with aspirin Also in patients undergoing stents after PCI* with aspirin		
	75mg daily		Loading dose 300mg then 75mg daily Can be used alone in MI If Aspirin not tolerated		75mg/day
Dipyridamole (Persantin)	TIA and Ischaemic Stroke Alone or with aspirin depending on C/Is 200mg BD 2 years				

*Percutaneous Coronary Intervention

Unstable Angina and non ST segment elevation MI. Non STEMI: NICE 2010
Assess 6m mortality. Give 300mg stat aspirin, continue indefinitely or Clopidogrel monotherapy if allergic to aspirin.

If 6m mortality >1.5% give 300mg Clopidogrel with the aspirin.

Give 300mg Clopidogrel to patients about to undergo PCI.

Give Clopidogrel for 12m to patients with NSTEMI.

Consider stopping Clopidogrel 5 days before CABG.

Glycoprotein IIb and IIIa inhibitors:
Consider IV Eptifibatide or Tirofiban if 6m mortality >3% and scheduled for angiography within 96hrs of admission. Consider Abciximab as an adjunct to PCI.

Antithrombin therapy

Offer Fondaparinux unless angiography is planned within 24 hrs of admission, unfractionated Heparin if the angiography is within 24 hours

Do angiogram +/– PCI within 96 hrs of admission if 6m mortality >3%. Conservative management (no early angiogram) if risk <3%. Review if ischaemia is experienced or demonstrated by testing.

Assess LV function in all patients who have had an MI or who have unstable angina.

S T segment elevation myocardial infarction: STEMI. NICE 2015
This follows a complete coronary artery obstruction and although we are all familiar with the classic symptoms of chest heaviness or pain, sweating, dyspnoea, nausea and palpitations, occasionally diabetics, women and any patient in fact may not have typical symptoms.

A third die from ventricular arrhythmias early but the in-hospital mortality is now only 5%.

Primary Percutaneous Coronary Intervention, PPCI covers the techniques of stenting, coronary angioplasty and thrombus extraction via catheters. This is the preferred treatment as long as the patient has emergency access to a catheter lab. Otherwise it is fibrinolysis. PPCI is meant to be performed within the 2 hours that fibrinolysis would have been administered.

In Acute STEMI:

Offer coronary angiography if presentation is within 12 hours of symptom onset followed by PPCI

(If this can be done within 2 hours of the time fibrinolysis would have been given)

Give fibrinolysis if presenting within 12 hours of onset of symptoms if PPCI isn't available within 2hrs.

Give an antithrombin at same time as fibrinolysis, Give standard medical therapy to all including those not eligible for reperfusion therapy. Consider angiography +/– PPCI if ongoing ischaemia.

Avoid glycoprotein IIb IIIa inhibitors and fibrinolytics if PPCI is planned. Do an angiogram after recovered cardiogenic shock.

After fibrinolysis: do ECG 60-90 mins later, – if raised ST do angiogram with PCI if indicated. Consider an angiogram after fibrinolysis if further symptoms of ischaemia and even if clinically stable.

The antiplatelet agents prior to PPCI are Clopidogrel, Prasugrel and Ticagrelor with Heparin or Bivalirudin the anticoagulants after.

The obvious smoking, weight, statin, blood pressure and exercise advice and management come next.

Aspirin: its clinical uses:

Aspirin is indicated for secondary prevention in those who have already suffered a cardiovascular event (MI or CVA) but it hasn't convincingly been shown to improve cardiovascular mortality or all-cause mortality in patients at high risk without a previous event history (primary prevention). It is also not recommended for older healthy patients. This is all due to the risk of Intra cerebral and GI bleeding. Interestingly though, one official American medical group now (the US Preventative Services Task Force (USPSTF) (2015)) recommends primary use of aspirin in older healthy individuals but this is very controversial. The statistics are related to CVD and colorectal cancer benefit.

Only half of patients with ischaemic vascular disease and 1/6 of those who are at significant other preventable risk are on aspirin (2014). Aspirin reduces the incidence of various cancers as well as improving their outcomes. This latter is via an effect on "unmasking metastases" to the immune system.

Primary prevention trials contradict each other: men's hearts benefit more than their brains and in women it is the other way round. Other trials show a benefit in terms of cardiovascular events in both sexes but not on mortality. Diabetics may need a BD dose schedule to gain benefit from aspirin, by the way and are at higher risk of cardiovascular events so the threshold for treating them is lower.

Currently (2015) in America aspirin is recommended prophylactically if the male patient has a 10% and the female patient a 20% or greater 10 year risk CHD risk. The 10% figure of CHD risk also applies to diabetics.

In cancer, aspirin is protective in colorectal cancers and to a lesser degree in breast, oesophageal, biliary, lung, oral, prostate and stomach cancers. It probably takes 5-10 years to have a significant clinical benefit. It doesn't prevent pancreatic cancers.

Aspirin inhibits COX 2 which promotes cell proliferation, it initiates apoptosis, it inhibits NFk-B (which reduces neoplasia). Aspirin seems to reduce distant metastases rather than local spread. This action works on several different established forms of cancer and at different stages in the cancer life cycle.

Aspirin treatment constitutes a 54% increase risk in GI bleeding, (though this isn't "fatal" bleeding, oddly). This risk is worse in the first month, possibly returning to normal after 5 years. The concomitant use of CCBs and NSAIDs increases the risk.

The risk of haemorrhagic stroke is increased by aspirin but only if the blood pressure is raised.

NSAID cardiovascular risk: See Odd Drugs:

Post Infarct:

Current advice is:

NICE 2007: Secondary Prevention:

20-30mins exercise a day (to the point of slight dyspnoea).

Mediterranean Diet.

ACEI, aspirin, BB, statin.

If the patient has signs of heart failure then they should be on an aldosterone antagonist (after ACEI started) (or plus an ARB).

Aspirin is given to all MI patients indefinitely. In aspirin and Clopidogrel intolerance, warfarin may be substituted (INR 2-3) for 4 years. In some circumstances Warfarin and aspirin may be given together.

Clopidogrel with low dose aspirin for 12m after the last non ST elevation coronary episode. Thereafter aspirin alone.

After ST elevation MI, aspirin and Clopidogrel for the first 4 weeks then aspirin alone.

All patients should be assessed for the possibility of revascularisation.

They should be advised to take 7gr of Omega 3 fatty acids a week (usually oily fish though this isn't the only source). If they are not eating the fish then prescribe 1gr daily of Omega 3 for 4 years. Cut out butter and cheese. Only 21 us alcohol/week for men, 14 for women and at least 20-30minutes of exercise a day. Lose weight, stop smoking, cardiac rehabilitation programme, they can usually fly within 2-3 weeks, ED drugs are not advised less than 6m after an MI and then not with Nicorandil or Nitrates. Good luck with maintaining the exercise and healthy diet then.

New NICE recommendations (Aug 2016) are for heart or stroke patients to receive Ticagrelor for up to 3 years after their initial 12 month dose. This is given with low dose aspirin for a year in ST elevation MI treated by percutaneous coronary intervention, non ST segment MI, or when admitted with unstable angina.

Rehabilitation after an infarct:

The first two weeks at home: Advise the patient to get up late, go to bed early. Potter about at home, gradually increase physical activity, snooze in the afternoon. They will feel more tired than normal.

By the third week the patient should be getting up and down stairs freely, going out more.

By the fourth week doing light household activities, increasing walking distances.

Assuming no significant excess tiredness, chest pain, dyspnoea etc, younger patients should be up to 4-5 miles walking 8 weeks after an M.I.

Older patients and those limited by symptoms can modify their expectations and slow down their progress. Walking against cold wind, sudden strenuous or violent activity should be avoided.

If the patient played golf before their coronary, they should be up to 18 holes by 3 months.

Return to work depends on the patient's job, pre episode fitness, confidence and the severity of the episode itself. Part time or light full time work is usually possible 6-10 weeks after discharge. As in all conditions, the self employed and owners of their own businesses will be champing at the bit sooner than the salaried patient.

Excessively physical jobs may not be possible and the GP may need to make recommendations on the "Fitness Certificate" or write to the Occupational Health Department or even the local Disablement Resettlement Officer, National Careers Service (or equivalent) about this. Virtually all patients should be back at work by 10-12 weeks but they should have thought about their job and all other personal factors that led to the coronary – and modify their risks of having another through stress and lifestyle factors.

The patient should not drive for at least 1 month and not then if driving brings on cardiac symptoms – although they don't usually have to inform the DVLA of and uncomplicated infarct. All professional drivers must inform the DVLA however and they may need to undergo further specific tests before resuming professional driving.

Sex: Marriage, -that is the state of being married, improves survival rates after infarcts as it does in most illnesses. The ACALM study, a 16% benefit (Carter et Al 2017). Less than 1% of coronaries occur during sex. Of those dying during sex, 90% are men and 75% of those are having extramarital sex with a younger woman! There are no figures for extramarital sex with an older woman. The only patient of mine who I discovered had died while having sex was indeed having sex with another, younger, women, not his wife, he was hypertensive, though ostensibly well controlled and had bought Viagra from the Internet. We always got on very well, I knew his wife well and it was very difficult protecting her from the details on the hospital report.

It is probably sensible to leave gentle sex for the first time for at least 4 weeks and then to take it easy.

The old advice was to avoid flying for 10 weeks. Newer advice is: After a recent MI (within 21 days of an acute episode of ischaemia): Patients should be "Able to walk 80m and climb 10-12 stairs without symptoms. With Heart Failure, as a rough guide the patient should also "be able to walk 80m and climb 10-12 stairs without symptoms" before flying. – So flying depends on what the patient is capable of doing on the ground.

What are Oily Fish?

Sardines, Herring, Anchovies, Salmon, Trout, Mackerel, Tuna, Marlin, Swordfish, Shark. These fish do not live at the bottom of the sea but forage at various depths. Oily fish concentrate contaminants (eg mercury in Minamata was in Tuna) and fat soluble vitamins. They are good sources of Omega 3 fatty acids and the consumption of oily fish may reduce dementia, macular degeneration, as well as improving cardiovascular health. There is, however an upper recommended limit of 4 servings a week (2 for women of child bearing age) due to possible mercury contamination.

White fish tend to be bottom feeders and are not oily (having only oil in their livers eg Cod liver oil) for instance Cod, Haddock and Flatfish. Generally speaking the oilier the fish tastes, the better it is for you-unfortunately.

Antibiotic Prophylaxis in cardiac disorders:

Opinions still differ as to whether this is necessary but as SABE is almost impossible to diagnose clinically, can be devastating and antibiotics are amongst the safest drugs we prescribe, (In 40 years I have yet to lose a patient to a resistant infection, pseudo membranous colitis, severe Stevens Johnson syndrome, severe SLE like syndromes, dyscrasias, renal failure, or anaphylaxis etc due to an antibiotic I have prescribed). I still advise prophylaxis.

Amoxicillin 3gr 4 hours before or Clindamycin 600mg 1 hour before treatment.

Child<5yrs 1/4 Adult dose, 5-10 years 1/2 adult dose.

Advice to the patient: (!) Avoid body piercings and tattoos, maintain good dental hygiene etc

NICE recommended cessation of antibiotic prophylaxis in 2008 but the European Society of Cardiology and other expert groups take issue with this guidance. They say there should be a risk assessment based on previous cyanotic heart disease, a prosthetic heart valve or prosthetic repair material being present. I say just give it.

Heart Failure:

10% of >85 year olds as well as surprisingly large numbers of younger patients are affected. Average prognosis is only 3 years once diagnosed. Life expectancy is inversely proportional to the dose of diuretic that the patient regularly needs to alleviate dyspnoea. However most patients are stabilised on a third of the dose that it takes to correct the heart failure in the first place. Those that aren't are quickly stabilised by going back on the original bigger dose. The common causes of heart failure are ischaemic, valvular, myocardial or hypertensive heart disease. Various drugs can contribute toward CCF including NSAIDs, Diltiazem, cytotoxics, Cyclophosphamide, Paclitaxel, antiarrythmics, beta blockers (although low doses of some BBs are beneficial), NSAIDs – Prostaglandins are more important in water homeostasis in heart failure than in the normal individual, CCBs, anaesthetics, immune modulators, SSRIs, TCAs, and so on.

Investigations:

CXR, echo cardiogram: Left ventricular systolic function, N LVEF (Ejection Fraction) is >55%

BNP, -Brain Natriuretic Peptide (>400 is an abnormal NTproBNP).

B.N.P. Basic/Brain Natriuretic Peptide If>400pg/ml, (116 pmol/li) arrange an echo, if >2000 arrange an urgent echo. This is a marker of heart failure.

<100 makes CCF unlikely

>500 on treatment means a poor prognosis and unless you are confident in the treatment of heart failure, or there are good reasons not too, referral is needed soon.

BBs. ARBs and ACEIs reduce the level.

Generally the advice is for a specialist referral if the level is BNP>400pg/

ml (116pmol/li) or NTproBNP>2000pg/ml (236pmol/li) (N-Terminal prohormone of brain natriuretic peptide). See Pathology for details.

This used to be called Brain natriuretic peptide because it was found in pig brains. It is now called

Basic Natriuretic Peptide or B-Type Natriuretic Peptide. In humans is comes from heart muscle, in response to excessive stretching.

Heart Failure Treatment:

Digoxin:

Half life 36 hrs, take blood level 6 hrs after last dose. Improves symptoms in heart failure with or without AF.

Maintenance dose: Maximum range 62.5-750mcg/day, usually 125-250mcg/day, in the elderly: 62.5-250ug/day.

Rapid Digitalisation: 0.75mg-1.5mg over 24 hours.

Colour coding: 62.5ug Blue, 125ug yellow, 250ug white.

Other Heart Failure Treatment: Thiazides with ACEIs eg Ramipril 2.5 >5mg, ARBs, other Diuretics.

Once the patient is more stable and not acutely breathless: Some Beta Blockers can be added (Carvedilol, Bisoprolol 1.25mg, Slow release Metoprolol, Nebivolol) – Very slow titration.

For instance add Carvedilol to diuretic and ACEI at a dose of 3.125mg bd slowly increasing. Maximum 50mg bd.

Spironolactone (Can use with an ACEI but watch K+).

Alternatively in Heart Failure: Treatment may include:

Loop diuretics, Bumetanide, Furosemide, Torasemide,

Thiazides, Bendroflumathazide, Indapamide,

Metolazone,

Don't forget there is a synergistic effect between different acting diuretics – for instance Bendroflumethazide and Furosemide.

Potassium Sparing diuretics Amiloride, Triamterene, Spironolactone,

ACEIs OK if K<5.9.

Beta Blockers, Bisoprolol, Carvedilol. Reduce if pulse <50-don't stop suddenly.

Spironolactone 12.5-25mg/day. A specific aldosterone antagonist, do not use with a creatinine >200umol/li. Up titrate ACEI first and keep an eye on K+.

Do chemistry at 1, 4, 8, weeks and 6, 9, 12 months if the patient is still alive then 6 monthly thereafter.

Digoxin: Important use in A.F. patients but no effect on actual mortality. Reduces hospital admissions though.

A rise in creatinine is expected with diuretics and ACEIs. A 30% rise in creatinine is acceptable. Ignore relative hypotension if it is asymptomatic but if symptomatic it is "renal failure" and warrants referral to secondary care. In this situation stop hypotensive drugs and NSAIDs and stop spironolactone before ACEI.

Recommended exercise in heart failure:

Aerobic exercise to 60-80% **maximal heart rate (which is usually considered to be 220-age)** for 20 minutes, 3 times a week. – which is actually good advice whether you have heart failure or not.

Exotic treatments include biventricular pacing, +inotropic stimulation, ultrafiltration, intra aortic balloon counter pulsation, ventricular assist devices, transplantation.

Vasovagal Syncope:

Rx: Support stockings, some advise Beta Blockers though I cannot quite see how antag-onising catecholamines should be helpful and I would suggest great caution, Midodrine – an alpha agonist, fludrocortisone, SSRIs and graded exercise.

Syncope. Definition:

Transient LOC (transient global cerebral hypoperfusion), transient, rapid onset, short duration, complete recovery. The incidence peaks in small children then reflex syncope increases in teens then various more serious causes crop up in older patients.

Half of adults will have one episode in their life.

Reflex syncope constitutes the majority.

Orthostatic 10%,

Cardiac 5-10%,

Unexplained 15-20%.

3 main types of syncope:

Reflex syncope-(Neurally mediated) ;

Loss of upright vasoconstrictor tone, bradycardic, – or mixed.

Vasovagal, simple faint (fear, pain, orthostatic stress).

Situational (cough, post prandial, exercise, lifting).

Carotid sinus syndrome.

Atypical.

Orthostatic hypotension;

Primary autonomic failure-Parkinsons, Lewy body dementia,

Secondary autonomic failure DM, amyloid etc,

Drug induced,

Alcohol,

Volume depleted.

Cardiac syncope

Arrythmia-primary and secondary, WPW, ARVC.

Structural, valvular, HCM, IHD etc.

PE, pulmonary hypertension etc.

History is diagnostic in 50%.

Red flags: Any conduction abnormality, QT >450ms or <350ms, QTc, any abnormality of ST or T.

Assess Hb, biochemistry, blood glucose (if necessary fasting) etc, etc.

Faints are classic: Posture, provocation and or prodrome.

Orthostatic hypotension if no other significant features and do lying and standing BP then BP after 3 minutes standing.

Refer to a cardiologist unless you are sure the diagnosis is a simple faint, situational syncope, orthostatic hypotension or clear epilepsy.

Refer quickly if you find an abnormal ECG, heart failure, T-LOC during exertion, palpitations, breathlessness, FH of sudden death, murmur.

Treatment of reflex syncope: Fluids, tilt training, support stockings, occasionally Midodrine/pacing.

Classical Orthostatic Hypotension:

Decrease in systole 20mm/diastole 10mm Hg within 3 minutes of standing.

Treatment: 2-3 li fluid a day/10 gr salt a day. Sleep with head raised 10 degrees. Physical counter pressure manoeuvres, compression stockings. Midodrine (alpha agonist) 5-20mg TDS, Fludrocortisone 0.1-0.3mg/day, EPO, Desmopressin.

Midrodine (2.5mg, 5mg, peripheral alpha 1 adrenergic stimulator) Bramox

Driving:

Patients with Syncope should not drive while awaiting specialist assessment so nearly everyone who can afford it sees the cardiologist privately at first anyway.

DVLA Guidelines:

Solitary Loss of consciousness/loss of awareness

Likely to be unexplained syncope but with a high probability of reflex vagal syncope.

	Licence revoked	
Group 1	No restriction	
Group 2	Can drive after 3 months.	

Likely to be cardiovascular in origin:

	No cause licence revoked	Cause found and treated
Group 1	6 months	Can drive after 4 weeks
Group 2	12 months	Can drive after 3 months.

No clinical pointers; (expected to see a cardiologist AND neurologist):

Group 1	6 months
Group 2	12 months.

Calcium Channel Blockers:

There are three classes, all with different properties and uses:

Dihydropyridines: Nifedipine, Amlodipine, Felodipine (No effect on A/V conduction, no interactions with rate limiting drugs-Digoxin), Nicardipine – Increase the heart rate and are good combined with B.Bs etc

The most vascular selective group. Various interactions including Grapefruit Juice which effectively reduces the liver metabolism of the drug and increases its plasma level.

Lercanidipine, Zanidip is marketed as being particularly useful in isolated systolic hypertension.

This group can take a couple of months to start to work in hypertension.

Phenylalkylamines: Verapamil, – Rate limiting, good in A.F and migraine.

Benzothiazepines: Diltiazem, – Rate limiting, avoid with other rate limiting drugs like B.Bs and antiarrythmics.

On the other hand, you can combine Verapamil with Beta Blockers if you increase the dose slowly and watch the pulse, maximum dose (in Cluster Headache, migraine, etc) 240-400mg/day in 2-3 doses. Cordilox, Securon, Univer etc.

Diltiazem too can be used with caution with Beta Blockers, Adizem, Dilzem, etc 60-120mg TDS. But don't use in conduction disorders (heart block etc).

Avoid Nitrates with Dihydropyridines (tachycardia).

I find Felodipine to be the CCB with the fewest side effects (ankle oedema and itchy shins and feet is a major problem with Amlodipine), in hypertension and

Verapamil is effective in Migraine and Cluster headache provided you use a big enough dose. Often in long standing severe migraine, Verapamil works where nothing else has.

Alpha Blockers:

Doxazosin, Cardura 1mg-16mg. Prazosin 500ug – 20mg. Also Terazosin, Indoramin. Start low, titrate slowly and these drugs have a theoretical advantage in BPH, Beta Blocker cold hands and feet, as well as some symptoms of anxiety and post traumatic stress (for instance bad dreams!)

Note that alpha blockers and Viagra (Sildenafil) may cause hypotension together.

Statins: HMG Co reductase inhibitors/Cholesterol etc

Summary:

Until 2013 statins were advised if the cardiovascular risk in the following 10 years was: >20%. New guidelines introduced in 2014 lowered this to anything over a 10% risk. As of 2015 NICE has back tracked a bit, now piloting the 10% level to see if it is practical. 180,000 die of cardiovascular disease a year and the NHS spends £450m a year (pre review of recommendation) on statins.

Monitor LFTs before starting Rx, at 3m, (LFTs, CPK) and repeat lipids, LFTS and CPK 3months after dose changes. When clinically stable do annual bloods.

Whatever the initial level of cholesterol, statins are supposed to reduce coronary risk, but they aren't quite as innocent and wholeheartedly positive as some people paint them. As many as half of patients stop treatment because of side effects varying from vague muscle aches and tiredness to muzzy headedness, bad dreams and depression. Then there are the deranged liver function, the serious muscle and kidney side effects, an apparent increase in diabetes especially in women. Also a new study (2015, Diabetologica) reported that men on statins had a 46% higher chance of developing Type 2DM, the risk being dose dependent for Simvastatin and Atorvastatin. High dose Simvastatin showed a 44% increased risk and low dose Simvastatin a 28% increased risk. The obese and those with a family history of diabetes are at greater risk-and there are even long term effects on cataract development. Patients also tend to eat more and put on more weight when on statins. Whether this is because of a biochemical switch being flipped or a sense that they will be protected from the consequence of further dietary excess is not known. A recent (2014) study gave the benefits and risks like this: for every patient whose life is saved (primary prevention) statins cause 1 diabetic, prevent 2 MIs and half a CVA.

When statins are used in low risk patients without heart disease (primary prevention) there is no mortality benefit, irrespective of how much the statin lowers the cholesterol level. There is a small reduction in vascular events (stroke, heart attack) over 5-10 years. the risk reduction is around 7/1000. In other words you have to treat 140 patients with a statin for 5 years to prevent one event or for 99.3% of treated patients there is no benefit. The benefit is about the same as the increased risk of diabetes. (Medscan June 2014). So statins have been associated with diabetes, dementia, fatigue, weakness, muscle wasting, depression, congestive heart failure (?) and something called "mitochondrial toxicity". They inhibit selenium containing enzymes such as glutathione peroxidase. Inhibition of this and selenium activated protein synthesis may be contributory to heart failure.

It isn't quite such an easy decision in General Practice as it may be in a university research department. See below.

Although some studies have thrown up an association WITH dementia, there are also studies that link certain patient groups taking statins with a decrease in Alzheimer's dementia. (JAMA Neurology Dec 2016): thus:

Women, two year statin treatment, top 50% number of prescriptions, had a 15% lower risk
Men (non black)   "   had a 12% lower risk.

Different statins had different effects:

Atorvastatin lowered Alzheimer's risk in white and black women and in Hispanic men and women

Simvastatin was associated with a lower Alzheimer's risk in white men.

Pravastatin and rosuvastatin reduced Alzheimer's in white women.

So white women benefited from all statins but lipophilic statins were more beneficial than hydrophilic statins. -Another reason for not necessarily just following local prescribing guidelines and prescribing the cheapest statin. (See my comments elsewhere).

There are many drug interactions involving statins. The latest to come to attention involve Dabigatran and both Simvastatin and Lovastatin. The combination of this NOAC and these statins showed a significant increased stroke risk. (Canad Med Ass Journal Dec 2016).

Also, statins in a recent review were found to have saved the lives of only 14% of the 20,000 avoided CVS deaths in England between 2000 and 2007. These were deaths avoided by the patients getting their blood pressure and cholesterol levels down but the majority of lives saved were through weight lost and increased exercise.(University of Liverpool data 2014/5).

Data published in 2014/5 showed that 7 million people in the UK take statins. 750 lives a year are saved by this treatment. Lowering salt and increasing exercise however prevent 4,600 UK deaths a year (Telegraph 23/1/15).

Many websites suggest we are worrying about the wrong types of cholesterol in any case. Total cholesterol, LDL, ratios, – what really gives us accurate mortality data? One convincing source I read suggested it was oxidised LDL that was the "newest circulating fat" (in evolutionary terms) that our bodies were unable to cope with and the major vascular risk factor. Oxidised LDL is the result of super heated fat and meat in cooking (frying, roasting, barbequing) and therefore entirely unfamiliar to us in our body's genesis. The suggestion being that if we do not overcook meat and superheat cooking oil/fats we will avoid raising our levels of oxidised LDL. As you know, our profession has had an epiphany of sorts on saturated fat over the last decade, red meat, dairy products and even butter being partially rehabilitated. The only really harmful fats under all circumstances seem to be manufactured hydrogenated fats and burnt oil and meat.

Co Enzyme Q10

Many of your switched-on patients will be taking this common supplement without mentioning it to you.

Statins deplete cells of Co enzyme Q10. CoQ10 is an essential nutrient co enzyme for mitochondrial ATP production and is a fat soluble anti oxidant. It is present in the diet and is synthesized in cells. It diminishes in tissues and blood after age 30. Statins decrease CoQ10, and this correlates with decreased ATP production in the cell, increased ischaemia reperfusion injury, skeletal muscle injury and increased mortality in animal studies.

Studies in humans relate depletion of Co Q10 to treatment with statins, which has been shown to be associated with diminished L Ventricular function, an elevation of lactate to pyruvate ratio and other significant cellular metabolic changes.

These changes are worse in pre existing heart failure and in the elderly and can be avoided by CoQ10 supplementation (easily obtained from health food stores and the

Internet) without affecting the lipid lowering effect of the statin. You can't help wondering if statins despite their lipid benefits may be contributing to the seeming heart failure epidemic in this way.

Usual guideline: In patients with a confident diagnosis of ischaemic disease if cholesterol>5.0mmol and <70yrs.

Aim to keep Total cholesterol <5.0mmol, LDL C <3mmol, HDL>1.4MMOL, Tg <2.0.

and in Secondary prevention: Total <4mmol, LDL <2mmol

NICE Guideline 67 (2010) But remember "NICE guidance does not override the individual responsibility of healthcare professionals with regard to drugs they are considering and the circumstances of the individual patient" which as you know, takes into account a multiplicity of variables in coming to a decision about drug treatment. Like all guidance to GPs, legal or clinical it seems to come down to "It's up to you after considering all the alternatives". Indeed in 2015 Dr R Haslam was suggesting a committee of GP grandees be set up to consider whether NICE guidelines were reasonable, practical or realistic for most GPs to advise their patients to follow. Good for him. This is the first time I have heard the concepts of practicality or realism applied to NICE guideline advice. Given what has happened to so many gold standard frameworks, protocols and guidelines set free from academic departments and committees into the actual world of GP, then only to fall prey to *real life*, it's about time.

Check LFTs, renal function, fasting glucose, as well as fasting lipids. I always add CPK. Actually you only need to do Total Cholesterol and HDL nowadays and these are non fasting but if the patient is fasting for the glucose you might as well check the triglycerides as well. Obviously tell the patient to stop smoking and offer help towards this (it might work), to reduce alcohol consumption (it depends) and tell them to lose weight and take exercise (it won't).

There are now reports of renal damage occurring to patients on long term statins and the MRHA warned in 2008 that any statin could cause depression, sleep disturbance, memory loss, sexual dysfunction and rarely, interstitial lung disease. We are all aware of the muscle damage and diabetes risk.

Some believe that Co Enzyme Q10 can correct some of these (but not all) the side effects and it is taken as a supplement extensively for this purpose in America. (See above)

Statins are indeed a controversial and much argued about treatment. The American testing guidelines are that only non fasting total cholesterol and HDL need be measured now.

Primary prevention:

If according to the charts there is a >20% (since 2014, it is suggested we might consider a 10% risk and pilot studies to see if this is "practical in General Practice "were started in 2015) 10 year risk of cardiovascular disease, offer a statin. Which statin used to depend on cost and tolerance but NICE now suggests fixed doses of Atorvastatin – see below:

Obviously treat raised BP, any abnormal thyroid function etc. Once the patient has started the statin, NICE says don't worry about cholesterol measurements. I **would** however do bloods every so often – to check LFTs, to give you the opportunity to check compliance and side effects and look at CPK if necessary.

Ezetemibe is supposed to be reserved for "Primary Hypercholesterolaemia" but I think that is a somewhat narrow and restrictive use of this useful drug.

Secondary Prevention:

Assuming the "coronary event" has acted as a "wake up call", the patient is likely to be more receptive to your dietary and lifestyle advice. He or she may well be obsessional about blood pressure, you can increase the statin until the total Cholesterol is <4mmol/li and LDL<2mmol/li.

Again, NICE seems to suggest a big fixed dose of Atorvastatin (2014).

Use a fibrate if the patient is unable to tolerate a particular statin, this raises HDL, but doesn't do much for mortality (I would try a more expensive statin first). Then you can try Nicotinic Acid, resins, and you can use Ezetemibe in primary hypercholesterolaemia.

I would advise checking LFTs and CPK 3monthly or more often initially, settling to annually if the patient is well.

NICE says check LFTs before treatment, at 3m and 12m only, CPK if muscle pains occur, less than 3X ULN LFTs are OK and usually if CPK is<5X ULN that is considered OK too.

Stop statins if a peripheral neuropathy develops.

The NICE guidelines mention that various groups are at higher risk: South Asian Men, HIV patients, patients on antipsychotic medication, patients with CKD and patients with SLE and Rh.A etc.

The Guidelines also mention diet (increased vegetables, fruit and fish, reduced fat to <30% total calories, saturated fat <10% total calories, cholesterol <300mg/day etc) and exercise (at least 30 minutes of sweaty exercise a day five times a week). Are there any GPs on NICE advisory committees? This exercise level seems a pretty unobtainable counsel of perfection for the average coronary patient.

In 2014 the new NICE guidelines proposed reducing the 10 year threshold to 10%, something which proved controversial and difficult to promote (see above). So difficult in fact that NICE subsequently decided to pilot the idea first. It is doubtful whether there would be significant mortality benefit and there has been much simultaneous debate in medical and non medical literature about lipid side effects ("buried" by drug companies in published trials and perhaps more obvious to GPs who are at the daily sharp end of thera-peutics). The NNT to prevent one CVA or MI at this 10% level is apparently 140 patients over 5 years. Other new recommendations included statins for Type 1 Diabetes (not just the existing recommended Type 2), for CKD Stages 1-4 and the above mentioned fixed dose regimes of 20mg in primary prevention and 80mg of Atorvastatin in secondary prevention.

The blood tests recommended are not LDL cholesterol but "Non HDL cholesterol" – this does not have to be fasting. The Americans are suggesting at the same time that you don't need to fast and only need to measure Total and HDL Cholesterol.

In the largest study conducted on diet and risk, (De Souza, Aug 11, 2015 BMJ) an already confusing area wasn't helped much by the facts. The healthy dietary advice used to be: Avoid butter, cheese, dairy products, meat, eggs, frying, roasting, barbequing; instead have unsaturated fats, vegetables, fish oils and olive oil, fruit and vegetables and keep a healthy weight. We now know it is healthy to be slightly overweight, that the standard weight centiles, lipid and cholesterol norms were virtually random figures from the start. Added to all that, salt isn't really that bad, sugar is probably far worse than salt or fat in the long run and that much of the advice we gave and our patients largely ignored was wrong anyway. Something else that won't surprise GPs much is that patients don't take tablets that make them feel ill for some tiny potential future benefit: In a study published in Feb 2017 (Eu J Prev Card) it turned out that patients with side effects were more than three times more likely to miss their cholesterol target than those who were side effect free. This made them almost level with those not taking statins. It turned out that in a normal population 57% of the patients studied on statin treatment were "Not meeting their LDL target of 1.8mmol/l at F/U." Muscle pain and other side effects were the biggest cause of missed targets followed by the inevitable (and consequent) "not taking the tablets"! Well there's a surprise (I suspect to everyone except we cynical GPs.)

Eat butter and cheese but avoid margarine and crisps:
In the largest collective study on saturated fat consumption, it was found that saturated fat does not have an effect on all cause mortality, cardiovascular disease incidence, coronary heart disease incidence, ischaemic stroke or diabetes. There was a trend for a "borderline" association between saturated fat and CHD mortality. On the other hand, **trans fat** consumption (hydrogenated vegetable oils) **is** associated with all cause mortality, total coronary heart disease and CHD mortality. There are some natural trans fats in the diet but the majority are industrial and synthetic. Making trans fats is by a process of bubbling hydrogen gas through hot liquid fats. This solidifies them at lower temperatures so they can be spread – who wants liquid butter on their toast ?

Perhaps it might be just as easy to persuade the patient to take Folic Acid and related B vitamins which reduce homocysteine and reduce heart disease, ischaemic stroke and even some cancers(?) while encouraging non smoking and alcohol cessation/reduction.

Liver enzymes 3X the ULN are a good reason to postpone chemotherapy so it has always struck me as bizarre that statin treatment is the only clinical situation where it is reasonable to accept such abnormal liver function tests. – by which I mean transaminases up to 3x the ULN and CPK up to 5X (-10x?) ULN. These enzymes indicate hepatitis and myositis and would be of real concern in any other clinical situation, warranting investigation. So why are we prepared to accept potentially decades of inflammation with who knows what long term consequences (cancer is often a consequence of long term inflammation in any given tissue) just because the patient is on statin treatment?

There is an increased risk of myopathy with
Statin treatment, Hypothyroidism, Renal disease, Alcoholism, Other muscle diseases, Other lipid lowering drugs, P 450 Drugs (Erythromycin, conazoles, inavirs, etc).
It is possible that Co enzyme Q10 reduces the muscle side effects of statins.

There are Interactions between Statins and all sorts of drugs,
Digoxin, Warfarin, Other lipid lowering drugs, Erythromycin, Niacin, Verapamil, Amiodarone, Diltiazem, Oral Hypoglycaemics and so on.
Hydrophilic and Lipophilic Statins: (lipophilic means crosses the BBB and causes dreams).

Hydrophilic: Rosuvastatin and Pravastatin. The most lipophilic was Cerivastatin which was withdrawn because of rhabdomyolysis.

So MOST LIPOHILIC Ceriva (withdrawn) >Simva>Fluva>Atorva>Rosuva>Pravastatin>LEAST LIPOPHILIC.

Cerivastatin was the most lipophilic and had the most serious side effects.(Mainly

Rhabdomyolysis and other muscle problems for which it was withdrawn in 2001). GENERALLY speaking, the hydrophilic statins have the fewest side effects.

Statins have multiple interactions via the cytochrome P450 3A4 pathway. Rosuvastatin definitely has the fewest.

Statins and Grapefruit Juice:

Grapefruit juice contains Bergamottin which interferes with the Cytochrome P-450 enzyme which metabolises statins. Their serum levels can then become elevated if Grapefruit juice and the statin are taken simultaneously and hepatic and muscle damage can occur.

The statins which interact with grapefruit juice are:
Simvastatin,
Atorvastatin,
Lovastatin.

Statins with NO Grapefruit juice interaction are:
Rosuvastatin,
Pravastatin,
Fluvastatin,
Pitavastatin.

The least likely statin to cause muscle pain is probably Rosusvastatin, Crestor.

Fibrates:

Specifically raise HDL and lower Tgs. (Statins lower Chol and LDL).

A reduction of 10% total Cholesterol leads to a 20% drop in CHD death rate. 20% acute CHD events still occur <6mmol/li

So again the evidence on **targets for cholesterol** suggest LDL<3mmol/li and Tot <5mmol/li and secondary and high risk prevention levels of LDL <2 mmol/li and Tot <4mmol/li. Indeed, if you can achieve it, secondary protection even up to age 80 years, in diabetics post M.I. as well as angina patients is now supposed to be 3.5mmol/li. It is the HDLC that is beneficial, aim for and HDL>1.4.

CETP Inhibitors eg Torcetrapib, Dalcetrapib, raise HDL cholesterol levels. (Between 30 and 70%.) But this isolated rise in "Good Cholesterol" has not so far improved clinical outcomes. Indeed Torcetrapib increased death rates and CV events.

PCSK9 inhibitors are the latest treatment option for patients who are not at their LDL-C target but with a family history and CVD. Alirocumab can be used with other lipid drugs.

Ezetimibe, Ezetrol 10mg OD. Alone or with a statin: (Inegy).

Use in statin intolerance, Lowers cholesterol absorption 50%.Use if elevation of LDL despite statin treatment or in combination with statins in familial hypercholesterolaemia Lowers LDL. There are conflicting trial data about end results at the moment, although new information suggests (2015) a clinical benefit in adding Ezetimibe to a statin in post Acute Coronary Syndrome therapy (IMPROVE-IT Study).

Omacor Omega-3-Acid ethyl esters. (Eicosapentaenoic and docosahexaenoic acids-EPA, DHA.) Many benefits – lowers triglycerides, is antiplatelet, reduces post infarct mortality (?) increases bleeding etc. You will never see a patient who has too much Omega 3. But the FDA in America is now putting out alarm warnings not to take more than 3gr/

day in a diet of the EPA and DHA, the two Omega 3 fats in fish oils that are actually in fish as well as supplements. The risks of overdosing on Omega 3s are bleeding, stroke, raised LDL and poorer glycaemic control in diabetes. Apparently Omega 3 supplements are very popular in the USA.

Homocysteine and the heart:

Homocysteine is an Amino Acid, mostly protein bound in plasma which promotes atherosclerosis through endothelial damage and local clot formation. It causes vascular smooth muscle hypertrophy and prevents arteriolar vasodilatation. It also causes platelet aggregates, lipoproteins to precipitate and these effects are obviously contributory factors to coronary obstruction and infarction.

High levels of **Homocysteine** (>14umol/li) are associated with heart disease death.

There seems to be a linear relationship between the two. There is an inverse relationship however between Folic Acid intake (and its and plasma levels) and plasma Homocysteine. Generally speaking there is in fact an inverse correlation between Vitamin intake (especially B Vitamins like Folic Acid and Pyridoxine) and heart disease. This is another good reason for consuming green leafy vegetables, nuts, pulses, bright coloured fruits and even the occasional glass of beer in a varied mixed diet – or a vitamin supplement every day.

Exercise:

I am, as you may have gathered, a little cynical about how effectively we can promote one of the cheapest and most important therapeutic interventions that we doctors can make in cardiovascular and indeed many other diseases:

It has always entertained me that even people using a gym seem to park their cars as closely to the front door as possible to avoid any extra unplanned exercise and avoid having to walk from the far end of the car park. The average overweight man and woman in the street will do anything rather than use the stairs, buy a bicycle, or go for a brisk walk. As soon as they do, their over stressed joints, muscles and tendons hurt and get strained in any case as they are so unused to being used. Even people who recognise the value of exercise as having positive "payoffs" find it something they have to "do" rather than something that they incorporate into a normal part of existence. Much of our culture regards inessential movement as unpleasant or undignified. But we GPs should all encourage constant unnecessary movement. Especially since in August 2017 PHE announced that 45% of adults were not even having a 10 minute brisk walk a month.

Take-away meals are bad for you not only because they are usually unhealthy to eat but most of them are now delivered to your door. You don't even have the exercise of walking to the restaurant to collect them. The fairest way to charge a passenger on a bus or plane is to weigh them and their luggage together. The total is proportional to the fuel burnt getting them from A to B and if they have a tiny piece of hand luggage but weigh 20 stone, shouldn't they pay for two? Exercise has as much benefit as antidepressant treatment on the depressed, or anxiolytic treatment on the stressed, improves survival in most cancers, recovery from most orthopaedic procedures and is the only intervention known to reduce lung cancer in smokers who have given up smoking. Exercise and the resultant weight loss reduces HbA1C more than most anti diabetic drugs and of course, aerobic exercise improves lung function in asthma and COPD. Weight bearing exercise improves balance and reduces falls in the elderly as well as reducing osteoporosis and fractures. It improves all circulatory conditions, central and peripheral. There is no drug or class of drugs that has the same breadth or degree of benefits. But try to get your overweight, sedentary, elderly or just slothful patient to increase their regular daily exercise regime consistently – even a little and you might as well have asked them to fly.

Other Cardiovascular drugs:

Aspirin and Clopidogrel:
In Non STEMI Rx Aspirin 75mg for life,
Clopidogrel 75mg for 1 year.
In STEMI Rx Aspirin 75mg for life,
Clopidogrel 75mg 1 month if no intervention, 1m if stent.

Diuretics: Where they act:

Thiazides..**Distal convoluted tubule**
Bendroflumethiazide Aprinox,
Prestim,
Co-Tenidone, Atenolol and Chlort(h) alidone,
Hygroton, Tenoret 50,
Tenoretic,
Cyclopenthiazide Navidrex,
Hydrochlorothiazide,
Indapamide Coversyl Plus, Natrilix,
Metolazone Metenix 5,
Xipamide Diurexan,

Loop...**Loop of Henle**
Bumetanide Burinex 1mg Bumetanide is equivalent in diuresis terms to 40mg Frusemide.
Furosemide Lasix (Frusemide),
Torasemide Torem 5-40mg daily, better K+ control than Furosemide.
Ethacrynic Acid.

Potassium-sparing......................................**Cortical collecting tubule**
Eplerenone Inspra,
Spironolactone, Aldactone, Co-flumactone,
Lasilactone,
Spironolactone,
Triamterene, Frusene, Co-triamterzide,
Dyazide, Dytide, Kalspare,
Amiloride Amilamont,
Co-Amilofruse, Burinex,
Co-amilozide, Frumil,
Moduret 25,
Moduretic.

Osmotic...**Loop of Henle and Proximal tubule**
Mannitol.

Carbonic Anhydrase Inhibitors...............................**Proximal tubule**
Acetazolamide.

Diuretics are recommended as one of the first line blood pressure treatments but they are probably the cause of most cases of middle age and old age **gout** in General Practice. They are a good combination with Ccbs which often cause ankle swelling if given alone. Avoid the combination of ACEIs/ARBs and potassium sparing diuretics or watch the K+ closely.

Thiazides are more likely to cause hyponatraemia, hypomagnesaemia* and hypocalcaemia than loop diuretics.

Hypomagnesaemia is more likely with thiazides, particularly together with cortisone, loop diuretics, PPIs, aminoglycosides and excess sweating etc* (see Pathology Section)

Combination Diuretics: Co Amilofruse: Frusemide/Amiloride (Frumil etc)
Co Amilozide: Hydrochlorthiazide/Amiloride (Moduretic etc)
Co Triamterzide: Hydrochlorthiazide/Triamterine (Dyazide)
Cyclopenthiazide and Amiloride (Navispare)
Chlort(h) alidone and Triamterene (Kalspare)
Frusemide and Spironolactone (Lasilactone)
Frusemide and Triamterene (Frusene)
Note: Bumetanide 1mg with Amiloride 5mg (non prop) gives a prompt diuresis and is K sparing

Presumably this is Co Amilonide or Co Bumetoride or Co Bumetamiloridanide!.
Hydroflumethazide and Spironolactone (Aldactide)

Which first line Thiazide?

An observational study of 30,000 Canadian patients taking either Chlort(h) alidone or Hydrochlorthiazide was published in 2015 to assess which diuretic to start hypertensive patients on.

The risk of death or adverse CV events was similar in the two treatment groups. The Chlort(h) alidone group individuals were more likely to be admitted with hypokalaemia or hyponatraemia though.

So it looks like Hydrochlorthiazide is the first line mild thiazide diuretic for hypertension.

Atrial Fibrillation: (and the CHADSVASC risk score)

A half of all arrhythmias are AF. 10% of 80 year olds have AF and every GP has 20-25 patients with AF. One paper gave the lifetime risk as 1:4. (Based on Framingham and Rotterdam studies, Clin Med, 2016, V0l 16 P272 etc) The risk is, of course, left atrial embolism and stroke which is 5-6X increased and CVAs in AF have a worse prognosis than those in sinus rhythm. 90% of strokes in AF come from the left atrial appendage and as an alternative to long term anticoagulation or defibrillation, you can therapeutically occlude the LAA through the atrial septum using a "Watchman device". This is an umbrella shaped device introduced at cardiac catheterisation that "locks" into position at the neck of the LAA. 87% of patients can then come off Warfarin. Overall 1.2% of the population have AF. There will be between 14 and 17 million in Europe by 2030. Only 20% of these patients are currently properly anticoagulated. Heart Failure and AF frequently co exist and have a mutually deleterious effect on one another. AF is a marker of HF severity and an independent prognostic factor in HF.

Up to 40% of patients with AF develop HF and up to 40% of patients with HF develop AF.

Anything over 7 days is called persistent atrial fibrillation.

It can be secondary to or associated with:

Hyper/hypothyroidism, Mitral valve disease, CABG, COPD, Prosthetic heart valves, M.I./I.H.D, Pericarditis, Pulmonary embolism, Pneumonia, Alcohol etc.

Estimates vary but the "non valvular" risk of CVA/thromboembolism is 5-12%/year in AF. Alternative therapies include radiofrequency ablation or atrial pacing.

If you are sure the A.F. has been going <36 hours then it is safe to defibrillate, otherwise you will need to anticoagulate first.

A trans-oesophageal echo excludes a L atrial clot. Assess L atrial diameter (normal is 4 cms) if >5.5cms, then defibrillation will not work.

Anticoagulation:
Atrial Fibrillation and the CHADS VASC Score:
CHADS2 Score:

Congestive Heart Failure	1 point
Hypertension >160?/90	1 point
Age>75	1 point
Diabetes	1 point
Prior Stroke or TIA or thromboembolism	2 points
Consider Warfarin if	= >2

CHADS 2 Score: Stroke Annual Risk:

0	1.9%
1	2.8%
2	4.0%
3	5.9%
4	8.5%
5	12.5%
6	18.2%

and CHADS VASC adds in female sex as a risk factor as well as lower age group and vasculopathy.

	Risk Factor	Score
C	Congestive heart failure/Left ventricular dysfunction	1
H	Hypertension — high blood pressure	1
A_2	Age≥75	2
D	Diabetes mellitus	1
S_2	Stroke/TIA/TE (thromboembolism)	2
V	Vascular disease — coronary artery disease (CAD), myocardial infarction (heart attack), peripheral artery disease (PAD), or aortic plaque	1
A	Age 65-74	1
Sc	Sex category — Female gender	1

So a good start to treating acute **Atrial Fibrillation** would be:

Give Digoxin first (initially 125ug), and add Bisoprolol (1.25mg for 2 weeks then 2.5mg a day) and starting Warfarin thus:

One day of each of:

10mg

10mg

5mg – then urgent INR after informing the lab.

You might also need Ramipril (2.5mg initially) and Furosemide (20mg initially).

Other Oral Anticoagulants: Warfarin reduces stroke in AF by 2/3, Aspirin by 1/5.

Dabigatran (Pradaxa) (or other NOAC etc), 110mg or 150mg BD – renal failure extends the half life – the lower dose is as beneficial as warfarin with lower bleeding risk, the higher is said to be better with the same bleeding risk.

INR and Annual Risk Of Bleeding:

2   0.3%

3   1%

4   3%

Under 75 years without diabetes, hypertension, cardiac disease, then Aspirin 300mg/day is as effective at reducing embolic risk.

Put another way: The RCP Guidance on AF is:

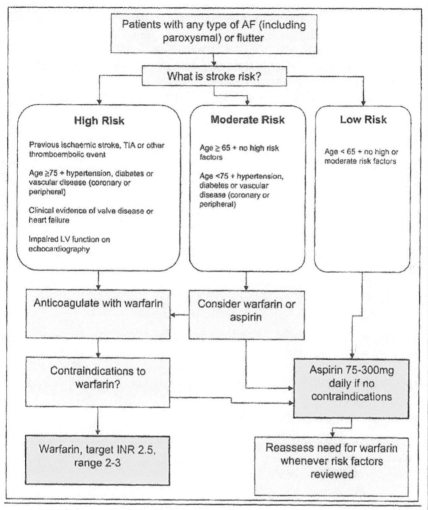

Patients with any type of AF (including paroxysmal) or flutter

What is stroke risk?

High Risk

Previous ischaemic stroke, TIA or other thromboembolic event

Age ≥75 + hypertension, diabetes or vascular disease (coronary or peripheral)

Clinical evidence of valve disease or heart failure

Impaired LV function on echocardiography

Moderate Risk

Age ≥ 65 + no high risk factors

Age <75 + hypertension, diabetes or vascular disease (coronary or peripheral)

Low Risk

Age < 65 + no high or moderate risk factors

Anticoagulate with warfarin

Consider warfarin or aspirin

Contraindications to warfarin?

Aspirin 75-300mg daily if no contraindications

Warfarin, target INR 2.5, range 2-3

Reassess need for warfarin whenever risk factors reviewed

Adapted from National Collaborating Centre for Chronic Conditions. *Atrial fibrillation: national clinical guideline for management in primary and secondary care.* London: Royal College of Physicians, 2006

(Diagram AFSR 1) What's the stroke risk?

Apart from **Warfarin (a Vitamin K antagonist, VKA) there are the other "NOACs or direct oral anticoagulants", Apixaban, (BD) Rivaroxaban, (OD) and Dabigatran (BD).** Dabigatran inhibits activated Factor II (or IIa or thrombin) The anti-Xa drugs are Rivaroxaban and Apixaban (also one called Edoxaban)

The commonest in use is the direct oral thrombin inhibitor:

Dabigatran (Pradaxa). This has been used since 2008 for post orthopaedic surgery

DVT prophylaxis. The RELY study compared Dabigatran at its two doses (110mg and 150mg bd) with Warfarin. Dabigtran had fewer haemorrhagic strokes and intracranial bleeds. Dabigatran 150mg bd had less stroke and systemic embolism but more GI bleeding than Warfarin and Dabigatran 110mg bd, a better net clinical benefit than Warfarin, similar major bleeding but less than the lower dose of Dabigatran. Dabigatran 110mg was similar to Warfarin for stroke and systemic embolism but less major bleeding than Warfarin. Those on Dabigatran had more dyspepsia than Warfarin and higher discontinuation rates. The advice was to use the lower dose of 110mg bd in the older, those at higher risk of stroke and if on Verapamil. New patients are in the therapeutic range within 30 minutes but Warfarin has to be discontinued until the INR is <2. NOTE: **INR does not monitor Dabigatran. Some authorities recommend the aPTT and if this is abnormal in an urgent situation Thrombin time or Ecarin Clotting Time if the results are needed to change the management (ie overdose). This given the relatively short half life of Dabigatran (Peak 2-4 hrs after administration and half life 12-14 hours).**

Rhythm control
There are various "Classes" of drugs used in the treatment of Rhythm Control of Atrial fibrillation:
Class 1 A B C Quinidine, Lidocaine, Flecainide.
Class 11 B Blockers (eg highly selective, Bisoprolol).
Class 111 Amiodarone, Bretylium, Sotalol (Also class 11).
Class IV Ca Channel Blockers including Verapamil – Dihydropyridines.

Paroxysmal Atrial Fibrillation: "Adrenergic or Vagal".
Vagal, avoid B Bs and Digoxin but use Quinidine, Disopyramide, Flecainide.
In "Adrenergic" type, treat underlying cardiac problem and use B Blockers – eg Sotalol, Atenolol, Amiodarone.
Various new agents Ibutilide, Azimilide etc
Avoid Digoxin in PAF – it makes PAF more likely.

Cardioversion if A.F.>48 Hours.
Pill in the pocket (Flecainide/Propafenone).

So: Atrial Fibrillation Treatment Put Simply:
Rate Control: BB, Atenolol, Bisoprolol, Metoprolol, or Rate limiting CCB, Verapamil, Diltiazem, either of these with Digoxin, >(?Via OPA) Amiodarone,
Rhythm Control: Standard BB, Sotalol, Amiodarone, Class 1C agent-Flecainide or Propafenone,
OR Anticoagulant: Warfarin, INR 2-2.5 Heparin, Pill in the pocket, BB, Amiodarone, Class 1c, Sotalol.
Note: **Warfarin Loading Dose** is 10mg, 10mg, 5mg on successive days then INR OR use NOAC*
Can use Sotalol, Bisoprolol, with Digoxin and anticoagulant.
Aspirin alone reduces stroke 22%.
or * eg **Dabigatran**: Standard dose, 110mg or 150mg depending on age (in AF 80 years is the dose cut off age).

Rate-control treatment algorithm for permanent (and some cases of persistent) AF

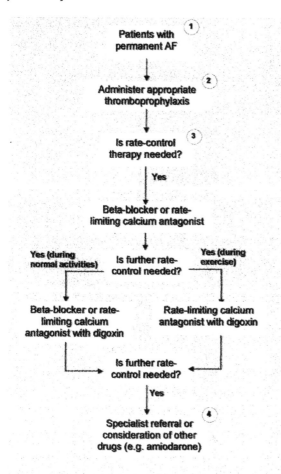

1. Patients with permanent AF includes those with persistent AF who have been selected for a rate-control treatment strategy.

2. Based on stroke risk stratification algorithm.

3. Target a resting heart rate of less than 90 bpm (110 bpm for those with recent-onset AF). Target an exercise heart rate of less than 110 bpm (inactive), 200 minus age (active).

4. Referral for further specialist investigation should be considered especially in those with lone AF or ECG evidence of an underlying electrophysiological disorder (e.g. WPW syndrome) or where pharmacological therapy has failed.

Rhythm-control treatment algorithm for paroxysmal AF

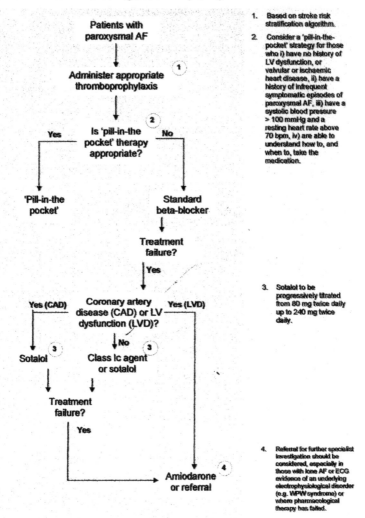

1. Based on stroke risk stratification algorithm.

2. Consider a 'pill-in-the-pocket' strategy for those who i) have no history of LV dysfunction, or valvular or ischaemic heart disease, ii) have a history of infrequent symptomatic episodes of paroxysmal AF, iii) have a systolic blood pressure > 100 mmHg and a resting heart rate above 70 bpm, iv) are able to understand how to, and when to, take the medication.

3. Sotalol to be progressively titrated from 80 mg twice daily up to 240 mg twice daily.

4. Referral for further specialist investigation should be considered, especially in those with lone AF or ECG evidence of an underlying electrophysiological disorder (e.g. WPW syndrome) or where pharmacological therapy has failed.

Stroke risk stratification algorithm

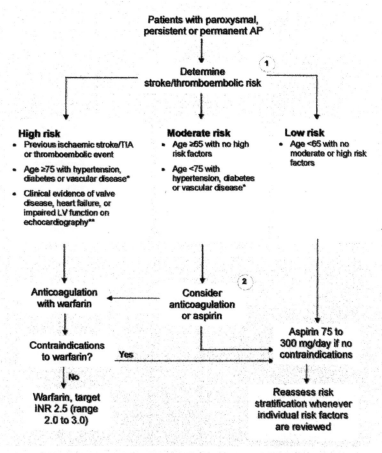

Patients with paroxysmal, persistent or permanent AF

↓

Determine stroke/thromboembolic risk (1)

High risk
- Previous ischaemic stroke/TIA or thromboembolic event
- Age ≥75 with hypertension, diabetes or vascular disease*
- Clinical evidence of valve disease, heart failure, or impaired LV function on echocardiography**

Moderate risk
- Age ≥65 with no high risk factors
- Age <75 with hypertension, diabetes or vascular disease*

Low risk
- Age <65 with no moderate or high risk factors

Anticoagulation with warfarin ← **Consider anticoagulation or aspirin** (2)

↓

Contraindications to warfarin? — Yes → **Aspirin 75 to 300 mg/day if no contraindications**

↓ No

Warfarin, target INR 2.5 (range 2.0 to 3.0)

Reassess risk stratification whenever individual risk factors are reviewed

1. Note that risk factors are not mutually exclusive, and are additive to each other in producing a composite risk. Since the incidence of stroke and thromboembolic events in patients with thyrotoxicosis appears similar to that in patients with other aetiologies of AF, antithrombotic treatments should be chosen based on the presence of validated stroke risk factors.
2. Owing to lack of sufficient clear-cut evidence, treatment may be decided on an individual basis, and the physician must balance the risk and benefits of warfarin versus aspirin. As stroke risk factors are cumulative, warfarin may, for example, be used in the presence of two or more moderate stroke risk factors. Referral and echocardiography may help in cases of uncertainty.

*Coronary artery disease or peripheral artery disease.

** An echocardiogram is not needed for routine assessment, but refines clinical risk stratification in the case of moderate or severe LV dysfunction and valve disease.

Cardioversion treatment algorithm

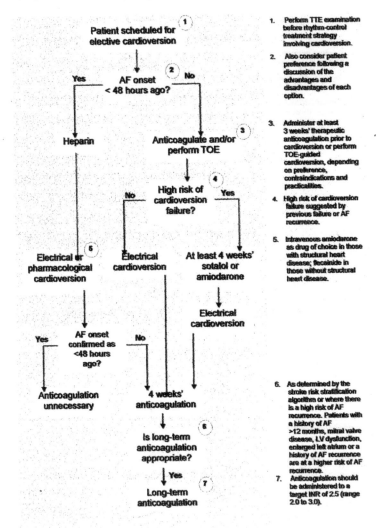

1. Perform TTE examination before rhythm-control treatment strategy involving cardioversion.

2. Also consider patient preference following a discussion of the advantages and disadvantages of each option.

3. Administer at least 3 weeks' therapeutic anticoagulation prior to cardioversion or perform TOE-guided cardioversion, depending on preference, contraindications and practicalities.

4. High risk of cardioversion failure suggested by previous failure or AF recurrence.

5. Intravenous amiodarone as drug of choice in those with structural heart disease; flecainide in those without structural heart disease.

6. As determined by the stroke risk stratification algorithm or where there is a high risk of AF recurrence. Patients with a history of AF >12 months, mitral valve disease, LV dysfunction, enlarged left atrium or a history of AF recurrence are at a higher risk of AF recurrence.

7. Anticoagulation should be administered to a target INR of 2.5 (range 2.0 to 3.0).

Rhythm-control treatment algorithm for persistent AF

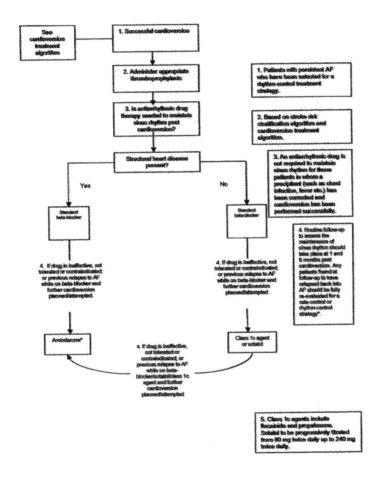

* If rhythm-control fails, consider the patient for rate-control strategy, or specialist referral for those with lone AF or ECG evidence of underlying electrophysiological disorder (e.g. Wolff–Parkinson–White [WPW] syndrome).

Sudden adult (arrhythmic) death syndrome S.A.D.S. (SADSUK, www.sads. org) and occult serious heart disease in the young:

This can be due to an arrhythmia or an unrecognised muscle or structural cardiac abnormality that can affect children and adults: Sudden cardiac death in young people is not as rare as you might think. There are 3,500/annum between 16 and 64 years. At PM of course, there is a coronary (ischaemic) cause found in the majority but 4.1% have innocent coronaries and no other indication of an aetiology. These are called sudden adult death syndrome or sudden unexpected death syndrome.

A brief list:

Genetic Conditions, HCM, Arrythmogenic R Ventricular Cardiomyopathy (A.R.V.C.), Long QT Syndrome, Brugada Syndrome (ECG looks like RBBB with ST elevation), Catecholaminergic Polymorphic Ventricular Tachycardia (C.P.V.T.), Progressive Cardiac Conduction Defect (P.C.C.D.), Idiopathic Ventricular Fibrillation (I.V.F.), Sodium Channel Disease, Conduction Disease, Structural Heart Disease (ARVC, DCM, HCM, Mitral Prolapse, WPW), WPW.

The British Heart Foundation does an excellent leaflet which can be downloaded summarising all this – "Sudden Cardiac Death in Young people".

The "Cardiac ion Channelopathies" are: Long QT, Brugada, Progressive Cardiac Conduction Disease and Catecholaminergic Polymorphic Ventricular Tachycardia.

They are potentially inherited and so relatives of any adult who suddenly and unexpectedly dies with a normal PM must be referred and assessed. They should at the very least have ECG, Echo, Holter monitor and an exercise ECG. Other genetic conditions which are missed at PM include Arrythmogenic Right Ventricular Cardiomyopathy, HOCM, Dilated Cardiomyopathy, Dystrophia Myotonica, WPW Syndrome and Mitral Valve Prolapse. None are detectable clinically except perhaps Mitral Valve Prolapse and so your ears should prick up when you hear a patient mention this kind of history. I have had two cases, – I don't include the regular seemingly healthy young people who are fit regular joggers or footballers who die on half marathons or the London to Brighton bike ride with unpredicted coronary narrowing. One was a brother of a patient who at 30 went to bed in the normal way and didn't wake up and the other a ten year old who I assume had a cardiomyopathy who collapsed in the playground one morning. Neither had shown any warning symptoms.

David Frost's son died while jogging at 31 from Hypertrophic Cardiomyopathy. This was also found at his father's PM (who died of a "heart attack" aged 74) but the family were not told or screened. There is a 1:2 chance that his children would inherit this cardiac condition

Other Arrythmias:

Premature Arial Contractions:
Benign and common, Nicotine, caffeine, alcohol. Treatment: BBs

Premature Ventricular Contractions:
Very common, optimise treatment of co existing cardiac and pulmonary conditions. Treatment: BBs, occasionally ablation.

Sinus Bradycardia:
HR <60/min. Every QRS Narrow, preceded by a "p". HR can be 45 or less in athletes and 30 bpm in sleep in normal adults with up to 2 second pauses.

Sinus Arrythmia:
Increase in rate with inspiration. Exaggerated in athletes, young adults and children. Is normal but can be due to disease or digoxin.

Sick Sinus Syndrome:
All these result in bradycardia. Often alternates with some form of atrial tachyardia (e.g. A.F.)

Supraventricular Tachycardias:

Sinus Tachycardia >100 BPM.

Paroxysmal Supraventricular Tachycardia: Sudden start and finish. Atrial rates 140-250, normal QRS, usually a re-entry mechanism. Carotid sinus massage, Adenosine, CCBs, BBs can terminate the arrhythmia. Various triggers: stress, caffeine, alcohol, pseudoephedrine etc.

The Valsalva manoeuvre can be tried and its success rate improved by lying the patient flat but with legs elevated after the "strain". The manoeuvre's success rate can be improved in this way from 5-20% to about 44%.

Multifocal Atrial Tachycardia: Usually if hypoxic (severe pulmonary disease etc) the ECG shows at least 3 p wave morphologies.

Atrial Flutter: Saw tooth ECG at 250-350 rate. Often degenerates to AF. Treatment is electrical cardioversion.

Pre excitation Syndrome (Wolff Parkinson White Syndrome): Various short circuit pathways but the Bundle of Kent is the commonest.

Atrial Fibrillation: See above but here is a SUMMARY: No p waves, narrow QRS. Rhythm control. TREATMENT: Cardioversion under heparin if onset within the last 24-48 hours (sometimes hard to tell though). Need a trans oesophageal echo (confusingly called a T.E.E. not a TOE) if valvular disease as a high risk of embolism. If >24-48 hours then must pre anticoagulate orally for 4-6 weeks and after conversion for a further 4-12 weeks. Complications: embolism, CVA, heart failure. Treatment: treat the various underlying causes (see above), ventricular rate control (BBs, CCBs, – Verapamil, Diltiazem, Digoxin, Amiodarone), anticoagulation, (INR 2.0-3.0, -use if CHADS score >2), antiarrythmics to try to restore sinus rhythm, cardioversion (results in SR in 90% but it remains in only 30-50% at 1 year. Class 1a, 1c, and III agents improve that chance to up to 70%), catheter ablation (success **up to** 70%).

Ventricular Arrythmias:

Ventricular Tachycardia: >30 seconds is "sustained" and <30 seconds is defined as "non-sustained VT". May cause LOC and hypotension.

Non sustained: Life threatening. Needs referral as the patient requires a fairly full work up: An echocardiogram and stress test to exclude a cardiac abnormality, Holter monitoring, treatment of existing arrhythmias and electrophysiology studies. Will need an indwelling cardiac defibrillator.

Torsade de Pointes: Variation in the QRS amplitude, a "polymorphic ventricular tachycardia". These episodes have a variety of causes, drop the blood pressure and cause syncope then return to normal but may degenerate to VF. The condition is associated with long QT (which causes R on T and this can trigger the Torsade chaos).

The ECG shows rotation of the axis, a long QT and a premature ventricular contraction preceding.

Although there is a risk of sudden death, most episodes do resolve spontaneously.

Torsade de Pointes can be triggered off by low Mg and K, even by severe episodes of diarrhoea and fluid loss in susceptible individuals. It is associated with alcoholism, various drug interactions and even drug grapefruit interactions can cause it (see Diet section).

Antiarrythmics:

Amiodarone: Must do LFTs, U and Es, TFTs and CXR before and the bloods every 6m on treatment. Eye checks every 6m, UVA and UVB screens. Can cause neonatal thyroid problems if given in pregnancy/breast feeding. The worst S/E is Amiodarone-Lung: Reduction in pulmonary gas transfer but also light sensitivity, thyroid disturbance, neuropathy and tremor etc.

Initially 200mg TDS reducing to OD. Interacts with Warfarin and Digoxin, potentiating both. Good at controlling PAF. Half Life >60 days.

Alternatively:

Dronedarone, Multaq for AF, PAF. Do ECG (QT) and U and Es, Mg before treatment, after 1 week then monthly to 6 months and then periodically.

Verapamil, Cordilox for SVTs 40-120mg TDS.

Disopyramide Rythmodan.

Procainamide.

Quinidine.

Drug induced arrhythmias:

Are common:

Antihistamines: Diphenhydramine, Chlorpheniramine, Hydroxyzine etc. Cetirizine, Terfenidine, Astemizole. Sympathomimetics: Dextroamphetamine, Methylphenidate, Fenfluramine, Ecstasy, (MDMA) Cocaine, Pseudoephedrine. Phenylpropanolamine. Beta stimulants: Salmeterol, Salbutamol etc. Phencyclidine (PCP). MAOIs. Methylxanthines: Theophylline, Aminophylline, Caffeine, TCAS, Scopolamine, Probantheline, Cisapride, Erythromycin, Pentamidine, Chloroquine, Amantadine, Antiarryhthmics: 1A Disopyramide, Quinidine, Procainamide, 1B Lidocaine, Tocainide, Mexiletine, 1C Propafenone, Flecainide, II Beta Blockers, Propranolol etc, II Sotalol, Amiodarone, Digoxin, Milrinone, Clonidine.

But a significant number of previously innocent drugs are now guilty of causing arrhythmias, from Azithromycin to Levofloxacin and Domperidone.

Takayasu's Arteritis: (Aortic Arch Syndrome)

An arteritis of the aorta and main branches, often detected by angiogram or by raised inflammatory markers. Rare. This is a progressive inflammatory disorder causing either occlusion or aneurysm of the various arteries and hence the various symptoms and upper limb asymmetry of blood pressure (>10mm).

Young women, (F9:M1) usually of oriental Asian descent, fever, fatigue, weight loss, tender arteries, claudication (jaw, etc) angina, T.I.A.s, BP different in the two arms, bruits, pulseless upper limbs.

The phases are usually described as Systemic (generalised symptoms plus arterial tenderness) then Occlusive with ischaemic symptoms (plus or minus ocular involvement), loss of various pulses, claudication, bruits (subclavians), hypertension, dizziness, headache, abdominal pain, haematuria, haemoptysis and so on. Raynaud's may be present, some aneurysms may rupture. Treatment is steroids/anticoagulants/steroid sparing Methotrexate, Azathioprine, Cyclophosphamide. Recently Anti-TNF. Cause unknown.

There is a tremendous variation in mortality (2-35% over 5 years). Up to 80% have one or more relapses, but over 90% can achieve long term remission.

Bundle Branch Block: (only present if QRS>0.12 secs, 3 sm squares)
LBBB:QS or rS in V1, monophasic R in I and V6, QRS>120ms
RBBB: Wide QRS >100ms, terminal R wave in V1
and slurred S in I and V6

LBBB: Wide QRS W in V1 M in V6
RBBB: M in V1 W in V6

LBBB Caused by A stenosis, dilated cardiomyopathy, IHD, hypertension, myocarditis, M.I. coronary A disease, dilated aortic root, etc **Patients need cardiac evaluation.**
RBBB Harmless especially in the young, RV strain (especially in P.E.), ASD, (Ostium Secundum), ischaemia, myocarditis.
The risk of developing heart failure is 3X higher in LBBB than in RBBB in middle aged men.

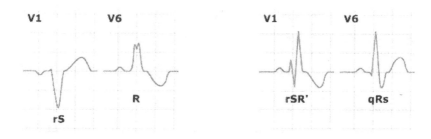

Diagram Left Bundle Branch Block and Right Bundle Branch Block

Heart Block:
1st degree: PR>200ms. Can be caused by a variety of drugs including CCBs, BBs, digoxin, etc. There is an increased risk of A.F. If accompanied by a wide QRS – refer to cardiologist as higher risk of progression to 2nd or 3rd degree block. Otherwise if asymptomatic is benign.

2nd degree: Type 1 is a progressive increase in PR subsequently leading to a dropped QRS (2-10% of long distance runners!) – can be secondary to drugs and most patients do not need pacing. Also called Mobitz type 1 or Wenckebach. This is usually a benign condition.

2nd degree Type 2 is a normal PR with a sudden failure of P to conduct – Mobitz type 2/Hay type. **This is a serious condition** which can lead to sudden unexpected death. The lesion is below the AV node and accompanied by RBBB or fascicular block. Often causes pre-syncope. Exercise exacerbates symptoms. Usually need pacing.

3rd degree Complete PR dissociation – always need a rapid referral and pacing, **This is a serious condition can degenerate to Ventricular tachycardia/fibrillation.**

Claudication: Peripheral Arterial Disease:

(Peripheral artery occlusive or peripheral vascular disease) is occlusion, acute or chronic of the large and medium sized vasculature, usually from atheroma but also from inflammation, embolism or thombosis etc.

It causes ischaemia downstream and its severity is often graded in "Fontaine stages":
Stage I Asymptomatic (subtle changes include colour and nail changes and hair loss),
Stage II Mild Claudication,
Stage IIa Claudication >200m walking distance,
Stage IIb Claudication <200m walking distance,
Stage III Rest pain,
Stage IV Necrosis or gangrene.

The risk factors for peripheral vascular disease are smoking, diabetes, hyperlipidaemia, hypertension, increasing age and rarer hypercoagulability states.

The severity of the obstruction is assessed (usually by referral to a vascular nurse or vascular surgeon) by measuring the ankle/brachial pressure index (assuming the brachial artery is reasonably patent).

Various treatments:

Cilastazol, Pletal is an arterial vasodilator and inhibitor of platelet aggregation (via phosphodiesterase inhibition). Aspirin and Clopidogrel. Naftidrofuryl, Praxilene. Inositol nicotinate, Hexopal. Pentoxifylline, Trental. Cilostazol. Statins.

Surgery via angioplasty, bypass grafting, occasionally sympathectomy.

This is clearly one situation where the outcome depends upon the patient stopping smoking and complying with medication.

Abdominal Aortic Aneurysm:

Risk of rupture:

Size on USS	Risk Of Rupture
<5.5cm	<1%/year
5.5-5.9cms	3.5% (1%F) (4%F)
6-6.9cms	15%
7-8cms	25%

Although these percentages do vary in different studies.

Can reduce risk of rupture by stopping smoking and by prescribing statins, antiplatelet treatment. Size>5.5cms or growth>1cm/year requires treatment. Mini laparotomy repair has <1% mortality. It used to be said that the "normal" rate of growth is 1mm/year.

One American study looking at when **thoracic aneurysms** ruptured, showed diameters of 5.9 cm for (ascending) and 7.2cm (descending) thoracic aneurysms as the (mean) size at rupture. They grew at 1mm a year, like the AAAs.

A "Cardiac" Diet:

should include oily fish, extra soluble fibre, 2 units of alcohol a day (especially red wine which increases HDL, lowers LDL), some garlic, (beneficial effect on coagulation). Possibly extra doses of Vitamin C, E, and A, ??

But less sugar and alcohol generally. A cardiovascular "Lifestyle" is, of course less flab, more exercise, better control of blood sugar in diabetics, a tight watch on renal function, thyroid supervision etc etc

E.C.Gs:

Myocardial Infarction ECG Criteria:
Q>30ms in AVF
R<10ms and <0.1mv in V2
R>40ms in V1
ST Elevation >0.1mV in 2 leads or evolving Q waves

Pulmonary Embolus ECG Criteria:
Tall R in V1 P Pulmonale (Peaked) in inferior leads, possible T inversion in V123. Possibly: R=S in V5 or 6.
S1 Q3 T3. (R Ventricular strain pattern) Incomplete or complete RBBB, T inversion in ant chest leads.

Drug Monitoring and ECGs
Verapamil: (especially high dose in cluster headache),
Aricept,
Lithium,
Quetiapine.

Cardiomyopathy:

Generally classified as extrinsic or Intrinsic to the muscle:
Intrinsic: Hypertrophic Cardiomyopathy HOCM/HCM, Arrhythmogenic RV Cardiomyopathy, Mitochondrial Cardiomyopathy, Dilated Cardiomyopathy, Restrictive Cardiomyopathy. Extrinsic: Amyloid Haemochromatosis, Diabetic Cardiomyopathy, Hyperthyroid Cardiomyopathy, Acromegalic Cardiomyopathy, Alcohol, Chemotherapy, Muscular Dystrophy, Obesity Associated, Coronary Artery Disease Ischaemic etc.

Can cause sudden death with a relatively normal post mortem. Familial Hypertrophic Cardiomyopathy F.H.C. Aut Dom, Prolonged QT on ECG.

Dilated Cardiomyopathy can be viral e.g. Coxsackie B, due to Chaga's Disease (Trypanosomiasis), Alcohol damage, auto immune, Adriamycin toxicity, due to thyroid disease. Men 2: Women1, Associated with HLA DQw4 and DR4, 20% inherited.

The patient may have 3rd and 4th heart sounds, mitral and tricuspid regurgitation (systolic murmurs) and tachycardia.

Treatment is diuretics, ACEIs, Digoxin, transplant, anticoagulation in AF.

Infective Endocarditis: SBE

25 cases/million. Mortality 20%. About a quarter follow dental treatment or disease. Other potential causes are drug abuse, surgery, cystoscopy etc but in half no preceding at risk activity is detected.

Signs are as follows:
Pyrexia 84%, Malaise 79%, Pallor 47%, Dyspnoea 42%, Weight loss 39%, Splinter Haemorrhages 26%, Splenomegaly 21%, Clubbing 9%, Ocular emboli 9%.
The mean duration of symptoms before diagnosis is 6+ weeks.

Diagnosis is by thinking about it in the first place, because the signs and symptoms are vague and difficult to detect. Tests: trans-oesophageal echo (for vegetations on the valve/s) and blood cultures.

One of the most occult and difficult diagnoses in medicine and one of the most damaging diseases. That is why I still stick to antibiotic prophylaxis with patients who have heart and valve lesions and dental or minor surgery.

12: Some useful clinical signs/tests/data:

Reflexes: Spinal levels
C5/6 Biceps, Musculocutaneous N, flexes elbow.
C5/6 Brachioradialis. Radial N, flexes, aids pronation/supination forearm.
C7/8 Radial N. Also C56, T1, Triceps, extension of elbow and extensor of wrist and hand. Sensation of back of hand.

L3/4 Knee jerk/Knee extension. Femoral N
L5 Lifts toes/Dorsiflexion of toes
S1/2 Ankle jerk. Sciatic N/Plantar flexion of ankle
Plantar response (Babinski) for UMNL. (This is pos until 6m of age.)

Useful Clinical Signs, Some common (ish) Eponymous Diseases and Interesting Conditions:

Apert Syndrome: Craniosynostosis and syndactyly. Odd facies and intellectual disability. FGFR2 gene abnormality.

Arnold-Chiari Syndrome: Downward herniation of the cerebellar tonsils through the foramen magnum with resultant neurological symptoms. F3:M1. Seen more readily in standing MRIs. Two types. In I, the cerebellum herniates, in II, the cerebellum and brain stem herniate downward.

Asperger Syndrome: Part of the autistic spectrum affecting social understanding and communication in relating to others. Read The Rosie Project, any Sherlock Holmes or the curious Incident of the dog in the night-time.

Barrett's Oesophagus: A precancerous oesophageal change related to recurrent and chronic acid reflux. 1:11 patients with chronic reflux develop Barrett's and one in 800 with Barrett's develop carcinoma of the oesophagus (NHS Choices).

Batten Disease: A rare liposomal storage disorder, begins in childhood, slow progressive neurological deterioration. Fatal. Usually aut rec. (occasionally dom).

Behcet's Diseases: Apthous and genital ulcers, uveitis. Sometimes aneurysms, E. Nodosum. Pyoderma Gangrenosum, arthralgia, CNS symptoms, multiple inflammatory symptoms in various systems. An autoimmune vasculitis. Treatment: Steroids, Anti-TNF, Interferon alpha 2, Azathioprine etc.

Bell's Palsy: Cranial N. 7 weakness, patients CANNOT MOVE UPPER FACE/FOREHEAD as it is a LMNL (differentiates it from a CVA). Occasionally bilateral, H. Zoster, EBV, pregnancy, DM, HIV. 70% complete recovery, can take many months. May recur in 15%. Look for blisters in outer ear (Facial N Zoster, the **Ramsay-Hunt Syndrome**). Loss of taste from ant 2/3 tongue. Facial palsy can occur in Lyme disease. Rx steroids, Aciclovir (etc).

Bornholm's Disease: Coxsackie B epidemic, pleurodynia. Severe pleuritic pain is characteristic. Echo viruses and Coxsackie A viruses can be the culprits. Can last 4-6 weeks, non specific treatment.

Brudzinski's Sign: There are several Brudzinski signs. The main one is flexing the head causes reflex hip flexion. It is positive in meningeal irritation (meningo-encephalitis, sub arachnoid bleed etc).

Budd Chiari Syndrome: Hepatic venous thrombosis, abdominal pain, ascites, hepatomegaly.

Burkitts Lymphoma: B cell NHL, fastest growing tumour. Specific gene mutations.

Calve Disease: of spine. Osteochondritis of a vertebral body.

Legg Calve Perthes' Disease: Ischaemic necrosis of the femoral head.

Caplans Syndrome: Pulmonary nodules, pulmonary fibrosis and Rheumatoid arthritis. A form of pneumoconiosis in people with Rheumatoid.

Charcot's Disease: Neuropathic (analgesic) arthropathy.

Charcot Marie Tooth Disease: Hereditary motor and sensory neuropathy. The most common inherited neurological disorder. Muscle wasting is characteristic – inverted champagne bottle legs. No treatment.

Conn's Syndrome: Primary hyperaldosteronism.

Cooley's Anaemia: Beta thalassaemia major. Both Hb beta chain genes have deletions. Aut Rec.

Cornelia De Lange Syndrome: Thick eyebrows, dev. delay, microcephaly, odd facies, CHD, autism etc.

Cri du Chat Syndrome: (Lejeune Syndrome) Partial deletion of short arm of chromosome 5. Affected babies have the charactarisitic cry. Severe mental retardation and speech, growth, motor and developmental delay. Behavioural features include repetitious movements, aggression, tantrums. Various other features: salivation, charactaristic facies, congenital heart lesions etc.

Crigler Najjar Syndrome: Types I (Severe) and II (Less severe). Congenital jaundice Aut Rec. Unconjugated hyperbilirubinaemia. An absence of Glucuronyl Transferase.

Crohn's Disease: Inflammatory bowel disease, fistulae, abscesses, systemic complications, uveitis, sacroileitis, E. nodosum. etc.

Crouzon Syndrome: Aut dom. 1st branchial arch Syndrome. Craniosynostosis, exopthalmos, concave facies.

Cushing's Disease: An ACTH secreting pituitary tumour. Cushing's Syndrome is the result of excess ACTH, cortisol secretion or steroid use. Weight gain, bruising, stretch marks, moon face, weakness etc.

Dandy Walker Syndrome: Congenital cerebral abnormalities, large 4th ventricle, absence of cerebral vermis, basal cyst, other cerebral abnormalities, motor delay and associated physical malformations. Can occasionally be caused by Warfarin taken in first trimester.

de Quervain Disease: Tenosynovitis (at radial side of wrist and base of thumb) Positive **Finkelstein** test.

de Quervain Thyroiditis: Giant cell thyroiditis.

Down('s) Syndrome: Trisomy 21. (Non disjunction or translocation) Charactaristic facies, intellectual disability, heart disease, umbilical hernia, increased nuchal thickness in 2nd trimester and increased neck skin (fold), hypotonia, large tongue etc.

Dubin Johnson Syndrome: Aut rec. Benign conjugated hyperbilirubinaemia.

Duchenne muscular dystrophy: Sex linked muscular dystrophy. Calf pseudo hypertrophy, wheelchair by teenage. Life expectancy mid 20's.

Dupuytren Contracture: Fibrotic flexion of fingers 4 and 5. M10:F1. Alcohol and rock climbers etc

Ebstein's Anomaly: Congenital tricuspid anomaly with apical displacement of the septal and posterior leaflets. Atrialisation of some of the RV.

Edwards Syndrome: Trisomy 18. 80% female. Congenital heart defects, mental retardation, multiple cong. abnormalities, muscle contractures, odd facies, etc

Ehlers Danlos Syndrome: A Collagen disorder, aut dom or recessive. Hyperelasticity, fragility, bruising. Joint dislocation. Ocular abnormalities including blue sclerae. Multiple systemic disorders including cardiac abnormalities. Six current sub types.

Eisenmenger Syndrome: A cyanotic heart condition caused by the reversal of a congenital R to L cardiac shunt after the development of pulmonary hypertension.

Erb's Palsy: (Erb Duchenne Palsy) C5 6 Brachial plexus injury. Waiter's tip position of affected arm.

Fabry Disease: An X linked alpha galactosidase-A deficiency. A sphingolipidosis.

Fallot's Tetralogy: The most common cyanotic congenital heart disease consisting of infundibular pulmonary stenosis, VSD, R ventricular hypertrophy and an overriding aorta with the aortic valve at least partially, sometimes mainly attached to the R ventricle.

Fanconi Anaemia: Aut recessive aplastic anaemia associated with various congenital abnormalities.

Fanconi Syndrome: Renal disorder with an incompetent proximal renal tubule.

Fish odour Syndrome: Trimethyaminuria. Most cases are autosomal recessive. The poor sufferer smells of fish as the enzyme Flavin is missing and Trimethylamine builds up and is excreted in sweat, urine and breath. The treatment is to avoid eggs, meats, beans and grains. Can try probiotics, charcoal, Riboflavin. There are specialists in various hospitals including Queens Square who collect cases.

Fragile X Syndrome: X linked

Well actually the inheritance is a bit more complicated than that: Parents can pass "premutations" of the fragile X gene, making the mutation more unstable each time a mother passes it to her child. When men pass on the premutation on their X chromosome, it doesn't become the full mutation. Men and women with the premutation are called carriers, women carrying it sometimes having a premature menopause. Some male carriers develop something like Parkinson's in later life but neither have the features of Fragile X itself.

1:4,000M 1:6,000F. Girls are less affected by Fragile X than boys, the normal X presumably opposing some of the effects of the damaged one. Intellectual disability for instance tends to be worse in boys. The basic problem is a failure to produce the FMR (Fragile X Mental Retardation) protein which facilitates neuronal connection as an essential part of learning and development. The result being developmental delay and mental retardation as well as a number of physical characteristics. The gene is FMR 1 on the long arm of the X chromosome.

Fragile X is the most common inherited cause of mental impairment/learning disability and the most common known cause of autism amongst boys so it is a major source of inherited mental disability.

Although early milestones may be on time, social, language, speech, (with various mannerisms) etc delays are almost universal.

The symptoms and signs include characteristic elongated facies, flat feet, hypotonia, double jointed fingers and thumbs, large ears, large testicles in the boys affected, variable, sometimes severe mental retardation, social awkwardness, autism and stereotypical movements. There are social anxiety, ADHD, sensory hypersensitivity, distractibility and a higher incidence of seizures.

There is no treatment of the root cause but various treatments for the symptoms and complications.

Freiberg Disease: Epiphysitis of head of 2nd metatarsal in the pubertal, especially girls.

Freidrich's Ataxia: Aut recessive progressive neurological condition. Begins in childhood, with ataxia, abnormal gait, heart disease and diabetes. Cognition intact.

Gaucher's Disease: Homozygous or compound heterozygous lysosomal storage disorder. Three types. GBA gene mutation.

Gilbert's Syndrome: At least 5% of population. Unconjugated hyperbilirubinaemia. Harmless. In one of my house jobs I was in a room with five junior doctors one Monday morning. Someone commented on my yellowish sclerae. Three of us, it turned out, had Gilbert's syndrome and went yellow after a weekend on call. Those were the days when a weekend on call was 80 hours of continuous duty of coffee and fluorescent lights. These were wedged in between two long weeks on call. When consultants knew the first names of the junior staff (See "Do No Harm, Henry Marsh) because they were on the wards long enough to be recognised. The days when the GMC didn't think we need extra toughening up, via extra teaching in "Emotional Resilience".

Goodpasture's Syndrome: Autoimmune damage of the basement membrane of lungs and kidneys resulting in haemoptysis, haematuria and renal failure.

Grave's Disease: Autoimmune hyperthyroidism and goitre (and Grave's ophthalmopathy).

Guillain Barre Syndrome: Post infection auto immune peripheral neuropathy. Follows various infections including respiratory and gastroenterological infection, Campylobacter, Cytomegalovirus, EBV, VZV, Flu and flu vaccination, Mycoplasma, Hep E and Dengue.

Hashimoto Thyroiditis: The first recognised auto immune disease, leads to myxoedema though periods of hyperthyroidism occur. 7F:1M.

Henoch-Schonlein (anaphylactoid) purpura: Petechial rash, on the legs and often starting on the buttocks, (in a child with abdominal pain, always check the buttocks however embarrassing and whether or not you have a chaperone), colicky abdominal pain, occasionally intussusception, blood in stool, arthralgia and arthritis, especially of lower limbs, proteinuria and haematuria. IgA vasculitis following URTI or other infections, various drugs etc. Some develop nephrotic syndrome or chronic kidney failure. Rx early steroids, anti immune treatments if kidney damage. Give the steroids in a decent dose, early.

L'Hermitte's Sign: An electric shock sensation in the limbs and body on neck flexion, or tingling down the back of the neck radiating into the legs, due to irritation of the cervical cord. This is also known as the barber's chair phenomenon and is said to be classic for MS (2/3 MS patients have it at sometime) but it can occur in all sorts of spinal cord conditions, B12 deficiency, cervical spondylosis, cord compression, the Arnold Chiari malformation etc. (my one case, missed by the casualty officer with disastrous results was of a previously normal young woman with a staphylococcal spinal abscess which she had developed for no apparent reason without warning. She is now partially paraplegic).

Hirschsprung(s) Disease: Congenital megacolon due to failure of intra uterine nerve cell migration to the myenteric and submucosal nerve plexuses and inability of the colon or part of it to relax. No perinatal meconium is passed. Abdominal distension and signs of obstruction often relieved by digital rectal examination if a low, short segment. There are many associated genes and syndromes and treatment is surgical.

Hodgkin(s) Disease: A form of lymphoma (cancer of lymphocytes). Four histological types: Nodular sclerosing, Mixed cellularity, Lymphocyte predominant, Lymphocyte depleted. Reed Sternberg cells are characteristic histologically. Treatment: Chemo, DXT, BMT. 80% + 5 years survival.

Horner Syndrome: Unilateral ptosis, constricted (miotic) pupil, anhydrosis as well as occasional unilateral facial flushing. Due to a sympathetic palsy in the neck and this may be secondary to; MS, cerebral, lung or thyroid tumour, cervical rib, brachial plexus injury, neck trauma, aneurysm, carotid A. dissection, cavernous sinus thrombosis, migraine or cluster HA, even local infection, including middle ear infection.

Holmes-Adie pupil: Large irregular pupil, poor constriction in response to light but good to accommodation and remains constricted for a prolonged interval – a tonic pupil. Usually this is a "normal" situation, rarely a parasympathetic efferent pathway lesion.

Holmes Adie Syndrome: is the Holmes Adie pupil plus absent deep tendon reflexes and sweating abnormalities. (Ciliary ganglion damage affecting parasympathetic control of the eye).

Hunter Syndrome: X linked. Mucopolysaccharidosis II. Mental retardation, hearing and visual handicap, hepatosplenomegaly, thickened heart valves, similar to Hurler's Syndrome but no corneal clouding.

Huntington's Disease: Aut dom. disorder affecting various parts of the brain including the basal ganglia, cortex, hippocampus, cerebellum etc. – resulting in chorea, dementia, punctuated by falls, behavioural problems and a life expectancy of 20 years from presentation. Some patients have seizures, most have psychiatric, memory and cognition problems leading to dementia. Usually presents in 30s or 40s. 50% of children of affected parents develop the disorder. One of the most unpleasant and cruellest familial conditions there is. A sword of Damocles for the young in the affected families.

Hurler Syndrome: Mucopolysaccharidosis 1, a lysosomal storage disease. Aut rec. Odd facies (Gargoylism), dwarfism, hepatosplenomegaly, hirsuitism, macroglossia, corneal clouding, cardiac valve thickening. Ante natal diagnosis is possible (CVS, amnio). Therapies are being tried with enzyme replacement therapy, bone marrow transplant and (soon) gene therapy.

Jakob Creutzfeldt disease: CJD. (Human mad cow disease). Prion mediated incurable CNS disease.

Kaposi's Sarcoma: Skin tumour(s) secondary to Herpes virus 8 infection, (STD and vertical transmission) associated with HIV Aids. Four different kinds depending on the clinical setting.

Kartagener Syndrome: Aut Rec. Primary ciliary dyskinesia, situs inversus, chronic sinus infection and bronchiectasis. Also involves sperm and oviductal immotility, glue ear, anosmia.

Kawasaki Disease (Syndrome): Mucocutaneous lymph node syndrome. Auto immune medium size vasculitis. A disease of children, fever, inflammation of conjunctivae, uveitis, iritis, oral membranes, strawberry tongue, cervical lymphadenopathy, skin and lymph nodes. Medium sized necrotising vasculitis, arthralgia, rash, multiple other symptoms. Cardiac involvement is the worry via myocarditis then vasculitis and coronary aneurysm causing MI. Various theories about cause. An odd association with high atmospheric wind patterns (presumably an infectious agent as yet unknown).
Diagnosis from 5 days of pyrexia then: oral redness, trunk rash, redness or swelling of hands or feet, conjunctival injection, cervical lymphadenopathy at least 15mm.

Treatment IV Immunog, Salicylate (vaccinate against VZV), steroids, Infliximab.

Kernigs test: Bend the hip to 90 deg with the knee bent at a right angle. Then straighten the knee. This is painful and resisted. It is a sign of meningism (infection or haemorrhage) or lumbar disc irritation.

Klinefelter Syndrome: 47XXY. Spontaneous mutation via non disjunction. Hypogonadism, delayed puberty, infertility, hypospadias, can be tall, little body hair and libido, same risk as that of women for breast cancer and SLE. Sometimes learning disabilities, reading and speech problems are common. More severe features with extra X's, -48, XXXY etc, less severe in mosaic 46, XY/47, XXY.

Korsakoff Syndrome/psychosis: Memory loss from thiamine (B1) deficiency usually secondary to alcoholism but can be caused by HIV Aids, starvation, dialysis, carcinomatosis, recurrent vomiting. Can follow acute Wernicke encephalopathy.

Lesch Nyhan Syndrome: Hyperuricaemia, secondary to absence of the enzyme HPRT. Dystonia, mental retardation, self injury. Sex linked.

Mallory-Weiss Syndrome: Gastro oesophageal tear and bleeding following forceful vomiting. Small haematemeses are common after repeated periods of vomiting in children and are virtually always benign.

Marfan Syndrome: Not a common condition, but a potentially devastating one – Sir John Tavener and Paganini suffered although it doesn't *always* confer musicality. Chromosome 15 Aut Dom. 1: 3,300 (regardless of sex or race) M:F 1:1, 25% new mutations, there is a "type 2" which is less severe. Average age at death is 44 years. The defect is in the connective tissue-Fibrillin 1 gene. Features: Tall (Abraham Lincoln was long thought to have had "Marfan's" but this is currently in doubt). Upward dislocated lenses, flat corneas, cataracts. Various cardiac abnormalities-aortic dilation and dissection, (may be antagonised by ARBs especially in pregnancy), aortic regurgitation, mitral regurgitation, dilation of pulmonary artery and thoracic and pulmonary aorta. Spontaneous pneumothoraces, apical blebs. Dural blebs, dysautonomia, vasovagal syncope, orthostastic hypotension, inappropriate sinus tachycardia, pectus excavatum.

High arched palate, crowded dentition, joint hyper mobility, positive thumb sign (the thumb extends beyond the palm when flexed over the palm). Arm span tends to be greater than height, scoliosis, arachnodactyly, hyper mobile joints, long limbs and high arched palate are characteristic. Dislocated lenses are present in over half of patients by 11 years of age. **All first degree relatives should be screened.**

Beta blocker treatment and Losartan delay aortic dilatation. The aortic root size should be (MRI or USS) monitored and replaced with or without the aortic valve once it reaches 5 cms. (from its normal 2.2-3.8cm diameter.)

Meniere's Disease (Syndrome): Episodes of tinnitus, pressure sensation in the ear(s), hearing loss and vertigo lasting half an hour to several hours. Commoner in women. Sometimes attacks occur in clusters. May be associated with migraine, drop attacks. Exclude migraine associated vertigo, familial benign recurrent vertigo (Rx Acetazolamide).

Munchausen Syndrome: A situation where an individual feigns illness (factitious disorder) to gain sympathy. Clues are inconsistent illogical, unwitnessed symptoms, over familiarity with hospitals and procedures, extensive medical knowledge, frequent or extensive previous medical contact, endless new symptoms. Lack of self esteem.

Munchausen Syndrome by proxy: The parent or carer of a child invents symptoms in the child or deliberately makes them ill. The parent, usually the mother, is often a health care professional or knows a good deal about medical care and medicine. Usually seen as hands-on and caring.

Noonan Syndrome: Aut dom "male Turner's Syndrome" or spontaneous mutation and can affect girls. Neck webbing, odd face, pulmonary stenosis, ASD, cardiomyopathy, short stature, can include learning difficulties, bleeding disorders. The damaged chromosome is 12. Various anaesthetic complications. 4 known abnormal genes. 50% of Noonans sufferers have PTPN11 gene mutations, 20% have mutations of SOS1. Up to a half of affected individuals have an affected parent.

Osgood Schlatter Disease: Apophysitis of the upper anterior tibial tubercle in athletic adolescents.

Paget's Disease of bone: Rapid localised bone turnover with risk of deformity, fracture, erythema, even high output CCF, neurological symptoms, pain, deafness etc. Detected by XR, Alk P'ase, bone scan. Treatment includes bisphosphonates, Calcitonin.

Paget's Disease of the breast (or nipple and areola): Can indicate ductal carcinoma in situ or invasive breast cancer within the affected breast. A quarter of breast cancer is said to involve Paget's Disease. The appearance is that of eczema: scalyness, itching, crusting, of the areola and nipple, flattening of the nipple with a discharge.

Also Paget's Disease of the penis and vulva as well as Paget Schroetter Disease!

Parkinson's Disease: Progressive damage to the basal ganglia (substantia nigra) causing tremor, rigidity, bradykinesia, gait disturbance, followed by thought and behaviour disruption, depression, dementia. Lewy Bodies are a pathological finding and dopamine is depleted. May be primary or secondary. Treatment (see neurology section) is diverse but not yet impressive.

Patau Syndrome: Trisomy 13. Increased risk with maternal age. Microcephaly, micropthalmia, hand, finger, spine and eye defects, genital, kidney and heart defects, abnormal facial appearance, rocker bottom feet, polydactyly. Non disjunction, translocation (inherited) or mosaic. 80% die in first year.

Perthes' Disease: (Legg-Calve-Perthes' disease). Avascular necrosis of the femoral head. Age 4-8, (or "5-10 years") commoner in short statured hyperactive caucasian boys with delayed bone age. The Ligamentum Teres artery fails before the medial femoral circumflex artery can take over. Treatment includes osteotomy, non weight bearing, avoidance of high impact sports, traction. The earlier the onset the better the prognosis for spontaneous remodelling of the femoral head.

Peutz Jeghers Syndrome: Aut Dom. Intestinal polyposis and melanin spots on lips, oral mucosa and fingers. 50-57% die of cancer, 15X the N incidence of GI cancer. 11% suffer pancreatic cancer. 50% suffer intussusception. Other associations are Addison's Disease, McCune Albright Syndrome (endocrine disorders, skin macules, fibrous dysplasia of bone). Cumulative risk of cancers by age 70 is 85%.

Phalen's Sign (test): Reversed praying: Numb central fingers in CTS.

Pick's Disease: Fronto temporal dementia. Personality, language and thinking symptoms. Personality changes predate memory symptoms unlike in Alzheimers.

Plummer Vinson Syndrome: Upper oesophageal web, iron deficiency, dysphagia, 90% women, now seems to be disappearing.

Phosphenes: Flashing lights in optic neuritis analagous to L'Hermitte's sign.

Prader Willi Syndrome: Abnormal chromosome 15, affects males and females. Hypotonia, short stature, delayed sexual development, later childhood obesity, learning difficulty, characteristic elongated face, behavioural problems, compulsive behaviour, anxiety, hallucinations, depression etc.

Prinzmetal angina: (Cardiac Syndrome X). Coronary artery spasm which can result in MI, commoner in female, aggressive, after certain drugs including illegal drugs, anti migraine, chemotherapy and some antibiotics. Dysfunctional endothelial NO release? Treatment: Nitrates and CCBs.

Ramsay Hunt Syndrome: Zoster of 7th (Facial) N. Rash on tympanic membrane, ear lobe, tongue, roof of mouth, facial weakness, unilateral hearing loss, vertigo.

Raynaud's Disease:(Primary Raynaud's phenomenon) which is idiopathic or Raynauds Syndrome (secondary Raynaud's phenomenon) due to: SLE and other connective tissue disorders, anorexia, Takayasu's, Lyme Disease, beta blockers, Bromocriptine, Ergotamine, Ciclosporin, Sulphasalazine etc. On cooling, the extremities go white, blue and on warming pink, throbbing and tingling. Smoking, caffeine and other vasoconstrictors worsen symptoms as does migraine and angina. Other causes include vibrating tools, malignancy, CFS, CTS, MS, Mg deficiency, hypothyroidism.

Reiter's Syndrome: Arthritis, conjunctivitis, uveitis, iritis, urethritis, penile ulceration, pustules and rash on palms and soles of feet. Associated with HLA-B27 and STI with Chlamydia or other infections with Salmonella, Shigella, Yersinia, Campylobacter organisms.

Reye's Syndrome: Encephalopathy and liver damage from the combination of a viral infection, Varicella or Influenza and Aspirin treatment in childhood.

Rinne Test: A tuning fork held against the mastoid until it goes quiet should still be audible via air conduction in front of the ear.

In conductive loss (middle ear disease) the patient cannot hear the tuning fork still vibrating in front of the ear).

In sensorineural loss both AC and BC are diminished but the patient usually hears the sound louder on bone.

Always do in combination with: Weber's Test (see below)

Romberg's Test: (Romberg's sign) This tests is for proprioception, middle ear disease or lower limb sensory ataxia.

Get the patient to stand with feet together, hands at their sides and eyes closed, then watch for swaying. Be prepared to catch them if they fall.

The test is positive if the patient falls when their eyes are closed.

Balancing with eyes closed depends on dorsal columns (Pyramidal tract) and proprioceptor input from joints. The test is positive in Tabes Dorsalis (neurosyphilis) and peripheral sensory neuropathies.

The test is not a test for cerebellar function as in this test the patient has to be able to balance with their eyes open before closing them. With Cerebellar Ataxia they are unsteady even with eyes open.

Rotor Syndrome: Aut Rec. Conjugated hyperbilirubinaemia. Common in Philippines. Benign.

Schamberg's Disease: Progressive Pigmentary Dermatosis (Purpura Pigmentosa Progressiva). Haemosiderin deposition as "Cayenne pepper" spots spread from feet to rest of body.

Scheuermann's Disease: Juvenile osteochondrosis of the spine resulting in marked kyphosis.

Schober's Test: A mark 10cms above L5 should stretch by 5cms on forward bending unless patient has AS.

Sever's Disease: Calcaneal apophysitis. Adolescents, overuse, benign. Squeeze test is positive.

Sheehan's Syndrome: Pituitary necrosis following intra or post partum haemorrhage. Results in no breast milk, amenorrhoea, tiredness, loss of body hair, hypotension.

Simmond's Disease: Pan hypopituitrism not due to intrapartum hypotension. Due to anterior pituitary lobe pituitary damage. Usually fatal.

Sjogren's Syndrome: Autoimmune condition resulting in destruction of tear, salivary and other exocrine glands. May include peripheral neuropathy and chronic bronchitis. May be primary or secondary to a connective tissue disorder. 9F:1M

Smith Lemli Opitz Syndrome: Aut rec. Microcephaly, odd facies, cerebral malformations, finger malformations, congenital heart abnormalities, genital, pulmonary, kidney, liver and ophthalmic abnormalities. Defect in cholesterol metabolism affecting the hedgehog signalling pathway. (An embryonic cell organising system).

Stevens Johnson Syndrome: A less severe form of Toxic Epidermal Necrolysis (up to 10% of body area in SJS, over 30% in TEN). The dermis and epidermis separate at a layer of necrosis due to what is believed to be a delayed hypersensitivity reaction. Various drugs and infections can trigger both. Fever, sore throat, orogenital ulcers, conjunctivitis and a generalised rash are the usual sequence of events and the list of drug triggers is long. Allopurinol, valproate, levofloxacin, diclofenac, azithromycin, sitagliptin, lamotrigine, ibuprofen, carbamazepine as well as sulphonamides, penicillins, anticonvulsants, etc. Also after URTIs and a variety of bacterial, mycoplasmal, fungal and viral infections. The mortality depends on the extent of the skin involvement.

Sturge Weber Syndrome: A visible facial (ophthalmic and trigeminal areas normally) port wine stain associated with an intracranial vascular anomaly, ipsilateral hemisphere hypo perfusion, plus or minus developmental delay, ADHD, learning difficulties, epilepsy, various visual symptoms and glaucoma. Severity varies a great deal.

Still's Disease: Juvenile Idiopathic Arthritis. Usually Rh F Neg. Morning stiffness, iridocyclitis, growth retardation. Three clinical sub types: Oligo/Polyarticular and Systemic. No characteristic blood result (Rh F not always pos). Treatment: Physio, Mtx, NSAIDs, TNF, biological agents, alpha blockers etc.

Takayasu's Arteritis: Pulseless disease. Inflammation of large arteries. 9F:1M. Flu, rash, tender carotids, vertigo, dyspnoea all can happen but the diagnosis is made on: 3 or more of: Age under or =40 yrs, claudication of an extremity, reduced brachial pulsation, difference of >10mm Hg systolic between the two arm BPs, aortic or subclavian bruit, abnormal angiography. Treatment: steroids, Mtx, Azathioprine, biologic therapies. etc. The disease is commonly relapsing/remitting but mortality is low.

Tay-Sach's Disease: Aut rec Lethal sphingolipidosis. Mutation on chromosome 15. Commoner in Ashkenazi Jews. Progressive neurological deterioration from 6m to death at around four.

Tietz Syndrome: Pain and swelling in one or some of the anterior costochondral or sterno clavicular joints. Pain is pleuritic, postural and movement related. This can be viral and must be differentiated from Coxsackie pleurodynia, Bornholm Disease. Treatment: NSAIDs, manipulation (osteopathy), steroid injection into or around the joint.

Tinel's Sign: Tapping the ventral surface of the wrist in CTS causes a sensation of electric shocks in the fingers. (There is a Tinel's Test at the knee for the Peroneal N. and in various other parts of the body where peripheral nerves are compromised).

Tourette Syndrome: An inherited condition characterised by multiple motor and at least one phonic "tic". ADHD and OCD may co exist. The most frequent tics are between ages 8 and 12. Most but not all improve as the patient gets older. Various treatments may be tried from CBT to Risperidone, Clonidine, Pimozide, Atomoxetine, SSRIs, TCADs and etc.

Treacher Collins Syndrome: Aut Dom. Facial abnormalities, micrognathia, hearing loss, malformed ears, droopy lower eye lids, cleft palate, normal intelligence.

Trendellenberg Test: Lie the patient down. Empty the leg veins by lifting the leg and then apply a tourniquet tight enough to occlude the superficial but not deep veins. Get the patient to stand.

Normally the superficial saphenous vein will fill from below in about 30secs (from capillaries) If it fills quicker than this there is deep or communicating vein valvular incompetence. After 20 seconds release the tourniquet and see if there is sudden filling. If there is, the deep and communicating veins are competent but the superficial veins are not.

Trendellenberg Sign: Is positive when the hip abductors (Gluteus medius and minimus) are weak or paralysed or when the leg the patient is standing on causes pain (eg hip joint pathology). This results in the unsupported side of the pelvis dropping. The hip supporting the weight is the affected hip – eg Gluteus Medius tear etc.

Tudor Hart's Inverse Care Law: Poorer people need more healthcare and yet get poorer healthcare. It is also true that poorer people and people who would gain most advantage from a change in lifestyle and who might benefit most from health education are the groups least likely to be accessible or respond to the health message.

Turner Syndrome: 45XO.Webbed neck, low ears and rear hair line, wide spaced nipples, aortic stenosis, bicuspid aortic valve, coarctation, short stature. Infertility, amenorrhoea, cong. heart dis. more common, as are DM and myxoedema. Visual and hearing disorders despite N. IQ, ADHD. Most affected foetuses are spontaneously aborted.

Trendelenberg Sign/Test: Stand patient on one leg and if the pelvis tips down on the opposite side, this is a positive Trendelenberg sign. This occurs when the hip abductors are weak on the weight bearing side or when that side is a painful hip. With congenital dislocation of the hip for instance, assuming the child is old enough to stand, when standing on both feet, the pelvis is level but when weight is borne by the affected side, the opposite pelvis drops due to weak hip abductors on the affected side.

The other Trendelenberg Test: is to demonstrate incompetent saphenous valves and is the saphenous and lower superficial veins of the leg filling despite a suitably tight upper thigh tourniquet. (After the leg has first been emptied of blood by elevation).

Unterberger's Test: Ask the patient to walk on the spot with their eyes closed. If they rotate they may have a labyrinthine disorder on that side.

Vincent's Angina: Pharyngitis and gingivitis caused by Borrelia Vincenti (spirochaete) and Fusiformis Fusiformis (Gr neg Bacillus). Necrotising ulcerative gingivitis, responds to dental hygiene and penicillin. Angine is the French for throat infection.

Von Recklinhausen's Disease: Neurofibromatosis 1 is characterised by skin macules, cafe au lait spots, nerve tumours, CNS and eye tumours, bony abnormalities, short stature, scoliosis, macrocephaly, learning difficulties, ADD, increased risk of various cancers. It presents in childhood.

Neurofibromatosis 2 presents a bit later than 1 and the main symptoms are due to nerve tumours which usually present in the patient's twenties with meningiomas, Schwannomas (eg cranial N 8), spinal tumours cause cord compression. Cataracts are common.

Von Willebrand Disease: The commonest inherited clotting disorder. An absence of Von Willebrand factor leading to haemorrhage, menorrhagia and easy bruising. Factor VIII and PTT are abnormal.

Waldenstrom's Macroglobulinaemia: A Non Hodgkins lymphoma, a cancer of B lymphocytes in bone marrow and these lymph cells generate excess monoclonal IgM which is the macroglobulin. This causes bruising, infections, night sweating, blurred vision, headaches, weight loss etc.

Waterhouse Friderichsen Syndrome: Adrenal haemorrhage and failure leading to septic shock during the course of septicaemia, often but not always due to meningococcal infection.

Weber Test:
The tuning fork is held on the apex of the head, centrally. A normal patient hears it equally in both ears. If it is heard louder on one side then compare the result with the Rinne test. This means either the louder side has a conductive deficit (-If it had shown a pos Rinnes on that side) or the other side has a sensorineural loss. (-If the Rinnes showed both AC and BC were reduced on the opposite side).

Wegener's Granulomatosis: (also called granulomatosis with polyangiitis). An auto immune vasculitis affecting the nose and URT as well as lungs and kidneys. Symptoms include PUO, tiredness, sweating, arthralgia, recurrent ear or sinus infections, epistaxes, chest symptoms, cough, dyspnoea, haemoptysis and haematuria. Treatment includes steroids, Mtx, Rituximab, plasma exchange.

Werdnig Hoffmann Disease: Aut rec. Spinal muscular atrophy (Type 1). Degeneration of ant. horn cells, second most common lethal Aut rec condition in white people after CF. The other SMAs are slower to progress and later onset. It is untreatable, progressive and presents with hypotonia. The babies affected are otherwise neurologically normal.

West Syndrome: Symptoms begin 3-6m. It is responsible for up to a quarter of first year epilepsies. **Infantile spasms** (Jack knife and other forms, up to 100 episodes in a row), EEG hypsarrythmia, mental retardation. A variety of cerebral insults can result in West Syndrome, these include Tuberous Sclerosis, perinatal asphyxia, etc. Treatment consists of steroids and anticonvulsants. The infantile spasms usually resolve by age 5 but half grow into other forms of epilepsy and some have permanent cerebral damage.

Wernicke's Encephalopathy: Alcohol related B vitamin deficiency (mainly Thiamine, B1). Can co exist with Korsakoff Syndrome. Ophthalmoplegia, ataxia and confusion are classic but hearing and vision loss, dysphagia, sleep apnoea, amnesia, psychosis, neuropathies etc can also occur.

Whipple's Disease: An infection with Tropheryma whippleyi causing weight loss joint pain steatorrhoea and malabsorption, CNS symptoms. The infecting organism is an Actinomycetes. Treatment is with the appropriate antibiotic for up to 2 years. Goodness knows what that does to your microbiome. No treatment means death through CNS involvement though.

Whipple's Procedure: for cancer of the pancreas involves removing the head of the pancreas, the duodenum, part of the stomach and other tissues.

Wilm's Tumour: Nephroblastoma. 90% five year survival.

Wolff Parkinson White Syndrome: A cardiac pre excitation phenomenon causing tachycardia via an accessory pathway – the Bundle of Kent. Short PR, Delta wave on the ECG. Treatment via AV nodal blocking drugs and catheter ablation.

Zollinger Ellison Syndrome: Over production of gastrin, usually by pancreatic gastrinoma, many being malignant. Causes bleeding from upper GI ulcers of stomach, duodenum, small bowel.

The Trisomies: (Meiotic non disjunction or translocation) All increase in incidence with maternal age.

Down's Syndrome: Trisomy 21, mental retardation, characteristic facies, hypotonia, congenital cardiac abnormalities, hearing problems, leukaemia, epilepsy, hypothyroidism, Coeliac Disease, obesity etc. Screened for via nuchal translucency 11-14 weeks and thickness at 18-22 weeks, (which is non specific and can disclose other Trisomies, Turner's, Cong Heart Dis, as well as various other congenital disorders), quadruple test 14-20/52, (detailed USS 19-20/52.) Occurs in 1:600-800 births. Most are spontaneous, 5% are inherited. Incidence is age related:

Age	Risk ratio:
<20	1:1600
20	1:1500
30	1:800
35	1:270
40	1:100
45	1:50

An invasive rapid antenatal investigation is the QF-PCR (aneuploidy) test, – the quantitative fluorescent polymerase chain reaction marker analysis (looks for Trisomy 21, 13 and 18).

Edward's Syndrome: Trisomy 18, 1:6000 live births but 1:2500 pregnancies. Higher fatality rate in boys than girls so 80% of affected babies are girls and only 50% full term affected infants are born alive. Congenital heart and renal abnormalities, exomphalos, gut atresia, growth and feeding disorders, arthrogryposis, microcephaly, abnormal facies. Rocker bottom feet, choroid plexus cysts etc. Median lifespan 5-15 days.

Patau Syndrome: Trisomy 13. 1 in 10,000-20,000 births. Microcephaly, failure of cerebral development, eye and spinal abnormalities, rocker bottom feet, exomphalos, cleft palate, overlapping digits, abnormal kidneys, genitals, various heart defects, single umbilical A. Most affected babies are stillborn or die soon after birth. 1:3 make it to 6m, 1:10 to 1 yr.

Autoimmune conditions:

S.L.E.

A Relapsing remitting illness of unknown cause but associated with autoimmunity.

Hair loss, fatigue/malaise, rashes (butterfly), scattered epithelial ulcers, recurrent glandular fever/ME, women aged 15-45 (9 W: 1 M), photosensitive rashes, aches and pains, especially arthralgia, headache, depression, pleurisy, multiple allergies, recurrent miscarriage, teenage migraines, teenage growing pains, peri, myo and endo carditis, P.E., renal damage, tests: ANA positive in 90%, (anti dsDNA), Anti ENA, DNA very specific anticardiolipin Ab. Associated with the antiphospholipid syndrome, etc. **Treatment:** NSAIDs, Hydroxychloroquine, steroids, immunosuppressives, treatment for cholesterol, BP, osteoporosis, sun protection etc.

Hughes Syndrome:
(Sticky blood, antiphospholipid syndrome).
Teenage migraine, tendency to thrombosis, TIAs, CVAS, memory loss, recurrent miscarriage, livedo-blotchy circulation, ataxia, giddiness, visual disturbance, "atypical MS", venous ulcers, occasionally low platelets, arterial and venous thromboses, occasional murmurs, thrombocytopoenia. **Treatment**: Aspirin, Heparin in pregnancy, Warfarin.

Sjogren's Syndrome:
Aches, joint swelling, fatigue, depression, scratchy dry eyes, dry mouth, previous "GF", fluctuating arthritis, raised ESR, Rh factor, often drug allergies (e.g. Septrin), food allergies, sun rash, often misdiagnosed as ME., vaginal dryness, interstitial cystitis, thyroid family history, ANA and ENA pos (especially anti RO). **Treatment**: Artificial tears, dental care, Hydroxychloroquine, steroids for flares.

Tuberous Sclerosis:
40% adult females with TS have Lymphangioleiomyomatosis of the lungs which gets worse with the COCP.

Add your own unusual conditions and eponyms:

13: DERMATOLOGY:

> I'd tried so, not to give in
> And I said to myself this affair it never will go so well
> But why should I try to resist when baby I know so well
> That I've got you under my skin
> — Cole Porter

Topical Local Anaesthetics:

EMLA Cream Lidocaine/Prilocaine. 5g, 30g and occlusive dressings. Apply 1-5 Hrs before painful procedure. Use cling film and any kind of adhesive tape to maintain occlusive contact. This speeds onset and prolongs duration of its action.

Taking Blood.

When taking blood in children, get the patient to apply topical local anaesthetic cream in various areas where veins might be found if they are difficult bleeders. Both antecubital fossae and backs of hands just in case.

Remember anxiety venoconstricts, but warmth, (putting the hand in hot water for 2-3 minutes), dependency (hanging the arm down a while) all help to vasodilate and a gentle tourniquet (between diastolic and systolic pressure) lets blood in but not out of the ligatured limb. On a cold winter's morning, make sure the child/baby has had a chance to warm up in the waiting room a while. For small babies use the broken needle dripping from the back of the hand in to a paediatric sample bottle technique. (Warn the parent it can be messy). Always go for the vein you can feel especially in the ante-cubital fossa (avoiding the brachial artery) rather than the one you can see especially in fat toddlers.

Don't forget that different phlebotomy techniques, including prolonged venous stasis can affect various results from clotting to electrolytes.

The mother will have spent time making herself and the child nervous by excessive and unnatural reassurance so there is often an atmosphere of tension when children or babies are brought in for blood samples. Sometimes it is a good idea to warn the mother that they might be asked to leave the room as soon as you suggest the blood test. You need a nurse who knows how to reassure mother and child but to hold the child still and you need a steady hand. A few millimetres of overshoot as you penetrate the skin can make the difference between a successful sample and a stressful morning and a haematoma in a chubby toddler.

Common Skin Lesions – A Brief Guide:

Viral Warts: Leave or treat topically.
Molluscum Contagiosum: Leave or if really necessary topical phenol (can scar).
Skin tags: Shave or excise. Cosmetic. Send for histology unless tiny.
Seborrhoeic Warts/Keratoses: Cryotherapy, curettage or cautery if a problem. Cosmetic. Could mask something else though?
Pyogenic Granulomata: Curettage and cautery (send for histology always).
Actinic (Solar) Keratoses: Solaraze (Diclofenac Gel) or Efudix (5-Fluorouracil Cr), Imiquimod Cr. (Aldara), cryotherapy, curettage, cautery.
Campbell de Morgan spots, Spider Naevi: "Cosmetic".
Bowen's Disease: Cryotherapy or curettage and cautery or Efudix.
Benign Naevi/moles: Shave and cautery. Usually cosmetic. Always send for histology if

any recent change in size or shape/irregular colour or edge/itching/bleeding etc.

Basal Cell Carcinoma: Refer

Squamous Cell Carcinoma: Refer.

Melanoma, sure or suspected: Refer 2WR.

Sebaceous Cysts/Lipomata: Minor op in house.

Dermatofibroma (Histiocytoma). Minor op, excision, curettage if really necessary. Cosmetic. Leaves a scar.

Keratin Horn: Curettage and cautery. Histology essential.

Kerato Acanthoma. Refer, 2WR if Squamous Cell Ca suspected (hard to differentiate).

Solar Comedones: Usually due to sun and smoking. Incision and contents expressed. If >5mm can excise. Cosmetic.

Solar Lentigines: Benign pigmented spots, the plural of solar lentigo. Cosmetic.

Sebaceous Naevus. Excise in adulthood. Refer. Risk of malignancy.

Congenital Naevi. Cosmetic.

Lentigo Maligna. Refer. The rate of melanoma transformation is proportional to the size.

Raynauds: Phenomenon/Disease/Syndrome: Up to 20% of adults are affected but it can be seen at any age from childhood on. Runs in families. The skin goes White>Blue >Red (with burning/tingling) as the vasodilatation restores the colour and life to the fingers/toes. The ears and nose can be affected.

Primary or secondary, it can be associated with connective tissue disorders (secondary) – Scleroderma, SLE, Rh.A, but the majority are benign and isolated.

Cold, stress, smoking, gripping and other factors make it worse, as do vibrating instruments and tools.

Treatments include Nifedipine, Amlodipine, ACEIs, Artans, SSRIs, Vit E 100-400iu/ day, Vit C 500-1000mg/day, Cinnarizine, Oil of Evening Primrose.

Obviously you will need to have checked an AIP before reassuring.

Dermatitis Herpetiformis:

Itchy blisters, knees elbows, scalp, Rx Dapsone, assoc c Coeliac Disease.

Molluscum Contagiosum:

Central punctum, supposed to look like little "molluscs". Nearly always gone within 18m, spread by rubbing but trauma hastens the immune response which sometimes gets rid of all lesions virtually overnight. Rx Podophyllotoxin, Condyline, try to avoid phenol as "leaving it to nature" leaves no scars. Phenol and curetting hurt and leave permanent white marks.

Bullous Pemphigoid:

Topical or Oral Steroids, Azathioprine, Tetracycline.

Milia:

Differin (Adapalene gel), Hyprefactor.

Angular Cheilitis:

Can be due to iron deficiency, thrush, H.Simplex or Staph Aureus infections, riboflavin deficiency, UC, Crohns, oral retinoids, Down's Syndrome, poorly fitting dentures etc.

Treatments include:

Short contact Lotriderm (Betnovate and Canestan), lots of Vaseline (or similar barrier especially at night), topical antiseptics, antifungals, oral antifungals, flucloxacillin, topical steroids, injected fillers, depending on the cause (swab) and "education".

Perioral Dermatitis:
Common in children (lip licking) and young women. Often secondary to the long term use of steroid creams on the face. Other causes may be fluoridated toothpastes, UV light, the OCP. Topical treatments containing antibiotics (Erythromycin, Metronidazole (Rozex)) or Pimecrolimus or Tacrolimus/Pimecrolimus or Oral antibiotics (Minocycline in adults) as if you were treating acne are usually effective. In lip licking children, plaster the perioral region with Vaseline every night.

Lumps on the pinna: are usually Chondrodermatitis Nodularis and are harmless. If you have to treat them, a short contact strongish steroid cream may soften them. They go eventually and are commoner after sun exposure.

Keratosis Pilaris:
Autosomal Dominant, a common cause for consultation and a blank response from the GP (or in the words of the GP in the Geoffrey Archer play "Can you hear me at the back" "It's a C.K. rash" – What is that? "Christ Knows")
But it is due to plugged hair follicles, of thighs, upper outer arms, face, eyebrows. They tend to look worse at puberty and can be slightly improved by salicylic acid or urea containing creams or by a vigorous rubbing with a dry towel after showers and baths.

Schamberg Disease:
Progressive pigmentary dermatosis. Rusty coloured spots, usually on the legs, especially the ankles, slowly extending over the body. More common in men. This is due to leaking capillaries which leave a haemosiderin stain but no symptoms. They look like "Cayenne pepper", can be slightly itchy (treat with topical steroids) but the lesions have no serious implications and no real treatment.

Dermatofibroma:
(Histiocytoma) These are common especially on the legs of young women (? due to shaving?) and may be initiated by a prick from a thorn, sting, or other F.B. They are harmless and often the treatment is to curette (though the usual pumice stone and emery board are uncomfortable and ineffectual) or excision – exchanging a benign lump for a scar.

Perianal Dermatitis:
Advise against too much cleanliness. Too much obsessional cleaning of the perianal area especially with wipes and deodorised cleansers removes the epidermal protective surface oils and damages epithelial continuity. This allows chapping, irritation and infection to persist. Cleanliness definitely is not next to Godliness – I assume Angels don't need to open their bowels.
Perianal dermatitis is often a stress or occupational condition and perpetuated by scratching especially at night. In all patients exclude thread worms, even in adults (actually it is probably just easier to treat the whole family on spec). Avoid frequent washing, avoid use of soap and advise loose underwear and no tights in women. Try Dermovate oint, (short term), aqueous cream for washing, Hydroxyzine, Atarax 10-20mg at night.

Vitiligo:
Associated with Diabetes, Thyroid Disease, Pernicious Anaemia. Exclude Pityriasis Versicolor, can try treatment with Pimecrolimus cream for 2 months. Some studies suggest 50-100% repigmentation!

Alopecia:
Less than 9 months usually needs no treatment. One or two persistent patches:

Intralesional Triamcinolone, Dithranol.

Patchy hair loss <30%: Try Betnovate (etc) scalp lotion for children, Dermovate for adults – daily for 3 months. >30% contact allergen (local irritant) therapy using Diphencyprone (Diphenylcyclopropenone) in Alopecia Areata and Totalis/Universalis.

There are also: Minoxidil (Regaine), Finasteride, (Propecia).

Erythema Nodosum:
Associated with the COCP,
Strep throat,
Cat scratch,
Fungal infections,
Glandular Fever,
Sarcoid,
Behcets,
Inflammatory Bowel Disease,
Pregnancy,
Treatment: Steroids, Colchicine.

Tinea Skin Infections:

Virtually any of the antifungal creams can work topically, Clotrimazole, Ketoconazole, Miconazole, Terbinafine etc. Even dabbing Selsun, the Selenium Sulphide containing antidandruff shampoo on the lesions each night for a month can get rid of them.

Treatment orally:
Terbinafine, Lamisil 250mg OD,
Adult Tinea Pedis 2-6 weeks,
Tinea Cruris 2-4 weeks,
Tinea Corporis 4 weeks,
Finger Nail infections 6-12 weeks (Tricophyton Microsporum and Epidermophyton).

Toe nails 3-6 months (review at 3 months and check the new nail growth is healthy and transparent),

or use "Sporanox Pulse" – Itraconazole 100mg 2 bd for 7 days then wait 3 weeks and repeat the cycle. They suggest 2 cycles for finger nails and three for toe nails.

Topical nail treatments include Amorolfine, Loceryl, applied Mondays and Thursdays (or whatever twice weekly regime the patient can remember) and Tioconazole, Trosyl, applied twice daily for up to year. Send off clippings for mycology as fungal infections are not the only things that turn nails white. (Liver disease, diabetes, CHF, hyperthyroidism, malnutrition, dysproteinaemia, psoriasis, trauma, iron deficiency, etc).

I find that the simple application of Terbinafine cream (Lamisil) to the affected nail fold in chronic fungal paronychia, massaged in to the freshly damp (and absorbent) nail after a bath (or before and after the gym) slowly clears fungal nail infections. It takes three or four months but it works as well as lotions or lacquers.

An alternative OTC treatment that seems to work is "Ozonated organic olive oil" which sounds a bit new agey, smells a bit sickly and looks like vaseline but does seem to eradicate fungal nail infections. This is applied to the nail fold at night with a cotton bud.

Cellulitis:
Amoxicillin and Flucloxacillin,
Co Amoxiclav or
Levofloxacin 500mg/day for 5 days which is said to have 98% overall success.

Hirsuitism:

Could try: Spironolactone, Dianette, Finasteride in appropriate patients.

Eczema:

Steroid Creams/Ointments:

If steroids are used topically you use an effective strength for the shortest effective duration. In the old days, endless and ineffective applications of weak steroids, usually 1/2% or 1% Hydrocortisone were used for weeks and months for fear of skin atrophy. Consequently itchy, miserable children lost sleep, got secondary infections and excoriated scarring of their skin. So use a moderately potent steroid on the body (Betnovate or equivalent) and Eumovate or similar on the face for short periods if the severity justifies it. Nocturnal sedative antihistamines (Alimemazine, Chlorphenamine, Promethazine) and occlusion using small plastic bags on hands and feet may be necessary. Always remember that Staph Aureus stops eczema getting better and that antibiotics effective against Staph may be needed over and over again. Do nasal and perianal swabs if this is the case and use Fucidin H, Fucibet, Naseptin, Mupiricin (Bactroban) where appropriate.

ALSO I suppose, given the modern world's obsession with Health and Safety, I ought to warn against the risk of suffocation when small children and plastic bags are in close proximity. I suppose you ought to make a few small holes in the bags to avoid the vanishingly small risk that this might happen.... but then again there is such a thing as being too careful.

Creams rather than ointments are more acceptable to most parents as they dry quicker on the skin, are not sticky and are water soluble when the applying hands are washed. They persist on the skin for a shorter period however and are less effective clinically.

If the patient has unilateral hand eczema always consider a fungal infection.

Hydrocortisone and urea: Urea is a hydrating agent and moistens dry skin. Alphaderm, Calmurid HC.

Children with severe atopic eczema can suffer extremely disturbed sleep. This is because of the vicious circle of itching, scratching, irritation and wakefulness which causes a miserable exhausted child (and parents), excoriated infected, scarred eczema and often a hospital admission. Sometimes strong sedative antihistamines or oral steroids are appropriate to stop the itching, also to aid sleep but that natural sleep regulator, Melatonin, has been shown to improve atopic eczema too. This is presumably by breaking the vicious circle by restoring deeper, restorative sleep and reducing scratching.

Topical Steroids:

Mild:

Hydrocortisone,

Canestan HC (fungal infections),

Daktacort (fungal and some bacterial infections),

Nystaform HC and Timodine. Mixed infection and inflammation (especially bad nappy rash).

Hydrocortisone and crotamiton. (Scabicidal and antipruritic). Eurax Hydrocortisone.

Hydrocortisone and Urea. Alphaderm, Calmurid HC. Dry skin.

Moderate:

Betnovate RD (0.025%) 100gr. Cr, oint.

Modrasone, Alclometasone.

Eumovate, Clobetasone.

Haelan, Fludroxycortide.
Synalar 1 in 4.(Fluocinolone)
Trimovate, (Eumovate with Nystatin and Oxytetracycline). Stains underwear.
Potent:
Betamethasone valerate,
Betnovate, oint and cream,
Betnovate C, with Clioquinol (active against candida and bacterial infection),
Betnovate N, with Neomycin (active against bacterial infection),
Betnovate with Canestan (Clotrimazole) is Lotriderm,
Fucibet with Fusidic acid (active against bacteria, especially Staph),
Diflucortolone, Nerisone cream, oily cream and oint.
Fluocinolone 0.025%. Synalar cream and oint. Gel for scalp and Synalar C and N for infections.
Fluocinolide, Metosyn cream and oint,
Fluticasone, Cutivate cream and oint,
Hydrocortisone butyrate, Locoid-various.
Betamethasone with Salicylic Acid, Diprosalic oint and scalp appl.
Lotriderm is half strength Betnovate with Canestan.
Very Potent:
Clobetasol, Dermovate. Cream, oint, scalp appl.
Diflucortolone, Nerisone Forte, oily cream and oint
Clobetasol/neomycin/nystatin cream and oint.

You can still get the pharmacist to make up an old fashioned cream or ointment to your own specification and feel like a real doctor: Thus for hyperkeratotic skin on the soles of the feet, 6% Coal Tar, 2% Salicylic Acid, 25% Dermovate oint.
Immunomodulators:
Pimecrolimus, Elidel 1% cream. Tacrolimus, Protopic 0.03% 0.1% oint, I find these effective and they are safe, in children where steroid creams have not worked at reasonable doses. The data sheets recommend time limited treatment and regular reviews and predictable caveats regarding infections and potential neoplasia.
Topical treatments for superficial infections, Impetigo, Staph, etc.
Bactroban, Mupirocin, oint and cream. Neomycin cream. Retapamulin, Altargo oint (Includes MRSA), Sodium Fusidate, Fucidin cream and oint.
Dermol lotion and cream both contain chlorhexidine. This is effective against Gram pos, Gram neg bacteria and some fungi and viruses. At the moment.
There is an increasing world-wide literature that the ubiquitous hand scrub dispensers in hospitals, the topical antiseptics for teenagers to rub on their acne covered faces, the antiseptic surface sprays sold to housewives for kitchens and loos, the daily use of agents that "kill all household germs", the disinfectant and antiseptic mouthwashes, medicated soaps, the pocket spirit gel dispensers and so on are simply creating super races of resistant bacteria immune to current disinfectants, antiseptics and antibiotics. That far from protecting us from C Difficile, MRSA and new strains of "superbugs", the constant use of environmental germ warfare is adversely affecting the microbiome upon which so many body systems depend as well as encouraging new resistant organisms. That IS how natural selection works isn't it?

There is interesting research that shows simple unmedicated soap and water is just as effective in preventing cross infection as antiseptics soaps and gels. What is actually needed is not bacteriocidal chemicals but proper hand washing rituals reliably and consistently performed between patients. Like so much of the polemic in this book, Lister, Pasteur and Nightingale knew this stuff in the 19th Century. Why are we so advanced that we have forgotten it? We don't need to dispense with ties and be bare below the elbows, we just need to relearn how to scrub our hands properly. And to keep doing it.

In 2015 a paper was published in Antimicrobial agents Chemoth (2015;60:1121-1128) disclosing that 45% of nosocomial Staph Aureus isolates in Texas Children's Hospital carried one or more genes associated with chlorhexidine tolerance. Strains carrying these tolerance genes were associated with reduced susceptibility to systemic antimicrobials and increased rates of septicaemia.

Emollients:

Urea: Cream (Aquadrate) with lactic acid (Calmurid cream).

WSP and Liquid Paraffin: Lotion (Aquamol) (Cetraben in pump dispensers, the bath additive is light liquid paraffin).

Aqueous Cream.

Colloidal Oatmeal: Bath and shower oil, cream (Aveeno).

Soya Oil: Cream, oil etc, (Balneum).

Liquid Paraffin (etc) with Chlorhexidine/Benzalkonium: Dermol lotion, cream, bath emollient.

Liquid Paraffin and WSP etc: Diprobase Cr, oint (pump dispenser) emulsion, Diprobath.

Liquid Paraffin, Isopropyl Myristate. Doublebase, gel, includes a pump dispenser, bath additive, shower gel etc.

WSP, Lanolin, Light Liquid Paraffin: E45 cream, pump, bath oil, wash cream, lotion, etc.

YSP, liquid Paraffin, emulsifying wax, Epaderm cream, Hydromol oint. etc.

Almond oil, Liquid Paraffin, Imuderm liquid.

Light liquid Paraffin, WSP: Oilatum cream, pump, emollient, gel etc.

WSP and liquid Paraffin: Emollient: Ultrabase.

Colloidal Anh Silica, Liqu Paraffin, WSP, Glycerol etc: Unguentum M: oint, dispenser etc.

After new evidence that creams containing arachis oil may be responsible for causing peanut sensitivity in very small children you may want to look closely at the constituents of the creams you prescribe to small children.

Dermatitis of the hands:

Almost any smelly or coloured agent used can cause hand dermatitis. Allowing the hands to be washed or wet a lot makes the skin vulnerable to sensitisation (nurses, young mums). Some professions are particularly susceptible: hair dressers, nurses, lab technicians (especially working with animals – rodent urine and epithelial cells are potent sensitizers), builders (chromium in cement etc), mechanics (oils and solvents) and so on.

To improve healing and reduce the risk of relapse, advise:

Hand washing with a soap substitute (aqueous cream, etc) and lukewarm water. Dry with a clean towel.

Avoid direct skin contact with detergents, washing up liquid, shampoo, (wear plastic gloves when washing hair), hair lotion, cream or dye etc. Avoid direct skin contact with all polishes and all cleaning agents. Avoid direct contact with all solvents, meths, turps, White Spirit, petrol and thinners, glues, sealants, paints etc.

Avoid peeling citrus fruit with bare hands, wear gloves in cold weather, don't wear rings while doing housework or when getting hands wet, when washing up use as much fresh running water as you dare and long handled brushes. Use PVC not rubber or latex gloves and don't get sweaty or allow water inside them (wear them for no more than 20 minutes). Wear gloves when preparing food and in contact with all fruits and vegetables.

Scalp dermatitis:

Seborrhoeic Dermatitis: "Scurf". Capasal Shampoo, Nizoral Shampoo, Selsun shampoo (Selenium Sulphide, OTC).

Leg Ulcers:

Venous Ulcers:

If infected, take swabs then Co Amoxiclav or Metronidazole (Often the nastier the smell the more sensitive to the latter). Flamazine (Silver Sulfadiazine) cream or even Povidone Iodine (Betadine) spray.

The key to a cure in my opinion is elevation and exposure. Not dressings and bandage techniques. Exercising the calf while the leg is horizontal or elevated makes logical sense. All the silver mesh, honey and systemic antibiotics seem to make very little difference once the ulcer is established and infection becomes chronic.

Varicose veins:

Cause a number of dermatological changes secondary to venous congestion, extravasation and oedema. One obvious visible change is the skin thickening of **lipodermatosclerosis**. The treatment which nearly always includes elevation and compression can sometimes include the anabolic steroid Stanozolol.

Silver Nitrate Solution 1.7% or 5% for Granulomata (umbilical)/warts etc. The Silver Nitrate (caustic) pencil contains Silver Nitrate and Potassium Nitrate. Protect surrounding normal skin with Vaseline.

Chilblains: Balmosa Cream, (Menthol, Camphor, Methyl Salicylate, Capsicum). Nicotinic Acid (Vitamin B3) 50mg BD.

Hyperhydrosis/Sweating:

Deeply embarrassing to many adolescents and young adults with soaking clothes and dripping hands. Try anything but be aware that Botox and surgery are the only really effective treatments. Also be aware that some reputable writers suspect aluminium containing antiperspirants are contributing to the doubling of cancer incidence in the west since the second world war.

Driclor: (etc) Aluminium Chloride antiperspirant. Apply at night, wash off the next morning.

Robinul 2mg BD (If the pharmacist can source it).

Probantheline, Beta Blockers, Clonidine.

Axillary Botox and the definitive cervical/lumbar sympathectomy, which are performed at a few specialist centres – (risk of pneumothorax with the former).

Pruritus/Itching:

Causes:

Hepatic: Obstructive Jaundice, pregnancy,

Blood: Reticuloses, Leukaemia, Polycythaemia, Iron Deficiency, Mastocytosis,

Carcinoma: especially lung, stomach, colon, breast, prostate,

Chronic Renal Disease (probably due to 2ndary Hyperparathyroidism),

Endocrine: Diabetes Mellitus, Insipidus, Myxoedema, Hyperthyroidism, Gout, Carcinoid,

Neurological, Tabes, G.P.I. Thalamic Tumour,

Drugs: Cocaine, Morphine, drug allergies,

Parasites: Roundworms, Trichiniasis, Onchocerciasis etc,

Psychogenic.

Skin Diseases: Mites, Scabies, Bites, Pediculoses, Eczema, Urticaria, Lichen Planus, D. Herpetiformis, Lichen Simplex Chronicus, Miliaria Rubra – Prickly Heat, Nodular Prurigo, pemphigoid.

Rx Doxepin, Xepin Cream. Hydroxyzine, Atarax Tabs, 10-100mg Nocte.

Patient advice regarding scabies:

The commonest sites for the burrows are the palms, fingers and wrists. There is an allergic generalised rash that takes a while to develop after catching the infection and the same time to settle even after the mite has been killed.

Transfer is by direct skin contact, not via cutlery, clothes, sheets, towels etc. Scabies is common and not related to standards of hygiene.

Cream and lotions need to be applied to all the skin especially between fingers and toes, even under nails and the soles of the feet. The head should be treated too, avoiding the eyes. Some medications need to be reapplied 3-7 days later.

All household and close contacts should be treated, even if asymptomatic.

The itching may take 2-3 weeks after treatment to improve. Anti pruritic creams can help during this time. Treatment failure can be due to inadequate application of the cream or re-infection. Retreatment may be required.

Chronic Idiopathic Urticaria:

Some 30-50% of these patients are genuinely autoimmune. They have antibodies against IgE or its high affinity receptor and some have thyroid antibodies. They suffer daily wheals and itching for at least 6 weeks. 90% also have angio oedema.

Try Rupatadine 10mg 1 od, antihistamines, low dose steroids, ciclosporin.

Male pattern baldness:

Finasteride, Propecia (3-6m Rx) is also Proscar, (1mg and 5mg respectively) – a 5 alpha reductase inhibitor used in BPH. It can cause impotence and gynaecomastia so the patient must really want the extra hair. Minoxidil, Regaine can be used in both sexes-a private prescription, keep trying for a year. Usually causes a fine downy growth that in my experience isn't really much like the real thing. Both work better at the crown than hair line.

Acne:

If a woman is on the pill, change from Levonorgestrel to Norethisterone as the progestogen, (i.e. Logynon to Binovum)

or to Desogestrel, Marvelon, Mercilon.

Dianette (Co-Cyprindiol), Cyproterone plus 35ug Ethinylo estrodiol is used in severe acne, idiopathic hirsuitism. Withdraw 3-4 cycles after condition resolved.

Oral antibiotics:

Minocycline 100mg od is one of the most effective but can cause Pulmonary Eosinophilia, photosensitivity, arthropathy, benign RICP, lupus, skin pigmentation and liver damage requiring LFTs so try

Cheap and cheerful Oxytetracycline 250-500mg BD or slightly more effective Lymecycline 300mg equiv. od first. Remember no antacids or milk and take on an empty stomach. Organising this into a teenager's early morning schedule can be problematic.

Topical treatments in Acne: Include:

Azelaic Acid, Skinoren, apply bd. (Inhibits Propionibacteria and reduces the number of keratinocytes).

Clindamycin, Dalacin T, apply bd.

Erythromycin with and without zinc, Stiemycin and Zineryt soln.(OK In pregnancy but acne often improves then anyway). Apply bd. There is also topical:

Metronidazole, Metrogel, Rozex, for **Rosacea**. Apply bd – also used in perioral dermatitis.

Ivermectin, Soolantra is used for papulo-pustular rosacea and is anti parasitic as well as anti inflammatory.

The Retinoids, Vitamin A analogues include topical Adapalene, Differin, which comes as a once daily cream and gel.

Isotretinoin gel 0.05% Isotrex.

Tretinoin Gel 0.01% and 0.025% Retin-A.

These are said to be better where comedones, papules and pustules predominate, in other words, non inflammatory acne.

As well as oral:

Roaccutane. 10mg, 20mg (Consultant supervision). Risk of depression, sometimes severe, inflammatory bowel disease. Now withdrawn in the USA.

There are various keratolytic and retinoid/antibiotic combinations, Adapalene and Benzoyl Peroxide, Epiduo, Clindamycin and Benzoyl Peroxide, Duac Gel, apply once in the evening. As well as

Erythromycin and Isotretinoin – Isotrexin gel, Aknemycin soln, apply once or twice a day.

The bleach/peeling agent:

Benzoyl Peroxide, Panoxyl, Brevoxl etc is a keratolytic which causes drying, scaling and redness of the top layer of the skin and bleaching of clothes and pillows. The idea is to start with the lowest strength and it strips off a thin layer of epidermis, unblocking the infected pores. Presumably

Salicylic Acid, Acnisal does much the same.

Nicotinamide, Nicam Gel, Vitamin B3, has an anti-inflammatory effect when applied to inflamed acne lesions.

So: Start with something topical like Duac for mild to moderate acne or Differin if comedones, papules and pustules predominate. Add an oral tetracycline (erythromycin if you are worried about teeth staining) and then:

If all else fails and severe acne looks like it is not responding or it may be scarring a young patient's face or confidence then refer for consideration of Roaccutane, Isotretinoin.

This nearly always works despite the dry mouth and eyes, risk of blood dyscrasias, the need to monitor LFTs and Tgs, risk of pancreatitis, possible haematuria and psychiatric reactions. – none of which I have ever seen in over 3 decades of General Practice.

Actinic (Solar) Keratoses:

Solareze (Diclofenac gel) bd for 60-90 days maximum effect may take until 30 days post treatment. Also Imiquimod, Aldara. Apply 3 times a week for 4 weeks, wash off the next morning, – can repeat course after 4 weeks. Fluorouracil cream, Efudix – a variety of treatment regimes. For a simple scalp A.K. try using daily for 10 days, stop, reassess and repeat if necessary.

Psoriasis:

There are many proprietary creams and ointments that work. If you want to try an older approach and if you have a chemist willing to go back to basics:

A) 6% Coal Tar soln.
2% Sal Acid.
25% Dermovate in YSP.
B) 5% Coal Tar Soln (or 10%).
2% Sal Acid in WSP.
C) 10% Coal Tar.
0.5% Sal Acid in 0.1% Halog Cr.

Then there is Dithranol, a derivative of anthracene which slows cell turn over and inhibits DNA synthesis, – in the form of Dithrocream 0.1 0.25 0.5 1 and 2%. Start weak and build up. Short contact is half to one hour then washing off or overnight contact then washing off. It is slow onset.

Psorin is coal tar, dithranol, and salicylic ac. oint.

Vitamin D and analogues:

It was found that patients with psoriasis improved while taking vitamin D for osteoporosis. Immune T cell receptors involved in psoriasis have some common features with Vitamin D receptors hence the small risk of hypercalcaemia with these drugs. Vitamin D (See section on vitamins) improves virtually every condition from Alzheimer's and Parkinson's to various cancers, asthma and hypertension. So there is probably no reason to withhold supplements of at least 5,000Us a day in your psoriasis patients. Oral and topical treatment together are recommended by various dermatological sources.

Calcipotriol oint, Dovonex. (Also comes as a scalp lotion and combined with betamethasone as Dovobet),

Tacalcitol, Curatoderm (oint and lotion) and

Calcitriol, Silkis (oint and lotion).

The Retinoids are related to Vitamin A:

Retinoids are used in inflammatory, rapid turn-over conditions, (acne, psoriasis, etc) as anti aging agents and in some skin cancers. Some are oral (Isotretioin, Roaccutane) and some topical.

Tazarotene, Zorac gel.

Acitretin, Neotigason.

Scalp psoriasis:

Responds well to Diprosalic (Betamethasone and Salicylic acid) and Capasal shampoo (Salicylic Acid, Coal Tar, Coconut Oil) but warn the patient their scalp will tingle.

Seborrhoeic Dermatitis:

Scaley, itchy and red scalp, nasolabial folds, sternum. It may be due to overproduction of sebum and a super infection with yeast. It is one of the common causes of a cradle cap type scalp rash in babies. Depending on the age, the site of the rash and the thickness of the scales, topical keratolytics and steroids (eg Diprosalic) and or anti fungals (Daktarin Cream, Miconazole, Nizoral cream, Ketoconazole), may work as may Selsun shampoo (Selenium Sulphide) left in situ as long as possible before washing off. Capasal Shampoo.

Pruritus:

For which no other treatable cause has been found:
Hydroxyzine, Atarax 25mg Nocte to qds. Can be used over 6m. Naltrexone, (Adepend, usually used in alcohol dependence, low dose used in cancer treatment), Buprenorphine, Paroxetine, Gabapentin.

Melasma, Pigmentation.

Azelaic Acid, Hydroxyquinone, Tretinoin. Sometimes Laser treatment.

Contact Dermatitis:

From Plants: Phytophotodermatitis-due to Psoralens (Just like those used in Psoriasis) which photosensitise the skin to UVA radiation. Sun block and topical steroids help and absolute avoidance in the future. Present in many plants including:
Hogweed, Cow Parsnip, Celery, Rue, Various weeds, Parsley, Daisy, Chrysanthemums, Dandelion, Lettuce, Colophony in Pine, Cypressus Leylandii, Angelica, Fennel, Dill, Anise, Lime, Lemon, Bergamot (as in Earl Grey Tea), Fig, Mustard, Wild Carrot etc.

Occupational causes of skin disease (80% of occupational skin disease is dermatitis)

are legion but include:
Chromates in cement, Cobalt, Nickel, Formaldehyde, Epoxy Resins, Engineering oils and greases, Cutting fluid, Plant psoralens, Coal tar distillation products (creosote, pitch etc), Chloronaphthalenes, chlorodi-phenyls, chlorotriphenyls, hexachlorodibenzo-p-dioxin, tetrachloroazoxybenzene and tetrachlorodibenzodioxin (TCDD), (acne).
Any occupation that causes sweating etc.

Malignant Melanoma:

UVB radiation from sunshine exposure, decades before, is the main aetiological factor. (it is UVA that is supposed to cause the skin changes of aging). This is not now thought to be due to simple exposure and "browning" of the skin (avoiding the sun is now listed with obesity, poor diet and smoking in terms of *absolute harms* to long term health) but due to previous burning episodes.

Major features: (Any one needs rapid referral):
Change in size or new growth of the skin lesion, Irregular shape, Irregular colour,
Minor features:
Largest diameter 7mm or >, Inflammation, Oozing, Crusting, Bleeding, Change in sensation.

If major feature =2 points and minor = 1 point then refer if the patient has one major feature or >3 points.

Breslow thickness is prognostic. This is the vertical height from top to bottom of the tumour from the biopsy specimen:

The prognosis is inversely proportional to this thickness (depth), thus:

less than 1mm: 5-year survival is 95% to 100%,

1 to 2mm: 5-year survival is 80% to 96%,

2.1 to 4mm: 5-year survival is 60% to 75%,

greater than 4mm: 5-year survival is 37% to 50%.

The Clarke grading system is based on the layer of the dermis that the melanoma has penetrated to:

Level I: confined to the epidermis (top-most layer of skin) ; – in situ melanoma; 100% cure rate,

Level II: invasion of the papillary (upper) dermis,

Level III: filling of the papillary dermis, but no extension in to the reticular (lower) dermis,

Level IV: invasion of the reticular dermis,

Level V: invasion of the deep, subcutaneous tissue,

Again prognosis is roughly related to these stages but Breslow staging is more generally reliable.

The Cancer Research Campaign suggested a 7 point code for Melanomata:

Major signs:

If an existing mole is getting bigger or a new one is growing,

If the mole has an irregular outline,

The colours are mixed shades of brown or black.

Minor Signs:

If the mole is bigger than the blunt end of a pencil,

It is inflamed or has a reddish edge,

It is bleeding, oozing or crusting,

If it starts to feel different to the patient – itching or pain,

Referral guidelines:

One or more major signs >consider rapid referral,

Additional presence of one or more minor signs – increasing possibility of melanoma,

3 or 4 minor signs without a major sign >consider referral.

Odds and ends:

Pitted keratolysis:

Of soles of feet (one cause of smelly feet): Can be due to a chronic Corynebacterium infection, Rx Fucidin.

Moh's Surgery:

This is piecemeal excision of superficial skin cancers – Rodent Ulcers, (Basal Cell Cancers) or Squamous Cell Cancers. It has been used for some Melanomata and other superficial skin pathology. Usually done under a local anaesthetic. Per op, the excised samples are frozen or fixed and examined microscopically to assess whether the excision is complete and when the borders are clear the lesion is repaired. The cure rates are virtually 100% for BCCs, slightly less for SCCs. The technique is usually used in areas of the body where tissue preservation is important – the face etc. It leaves less of a scar.

14: DIABETES: (See also page 514)

422 million people globally are "living with diabetes" (2016, WHO) with 4.9 million attributable deaths in 2014. So a very large number of people are clearly dying of diabetes too.

Global Prevalence: 2002 2.8% but by 2030 4.45%, and 90% will be type 2. This has increased 4X since 1980. The most rapid increases have been in some of the poorest countries but in Qatar and Kuwait 40% of older citizens have diabetes.

UK prevalence is 3.6% with Indians 3X more likely and Pakistani and Bangladeshi 6X more likely than average. In 2014 the UK had 2.7 million Muslims, 325,000 of whom had diabetes – a population at risk during long fasts. Approximately 2% of diabetics are "monogenic" with a single gene mutation at fault. For instance Maturity Onset Diabetes of the Young is usually caused by a mutation in the HNF1A or GCK genes. Neonatal diabetes is usually caused by a mutation in either of the KCNJ11, ABCC8 or INS genes.

In 2014 the news was that 1/3 of English adults had impaired glucose tolerance ("prediabetes") and the NHS was spending 1/10 of its whole budget on patients with diabetes and its complications. 5-10% of "pre-diabetics" develop diabetes each year. These levels of impaired glucose handling have increased dramatically from 11.6% of adults in 2003 to 35.3% by 2011 and can be attributed to increased weight and lack of exercise. Gluttony and sloth. Put another way, 740 Type 2 Diabetics are diagnosed in the UK each day, 280,000 a year. T2DM has increased 60% in the last decade (2015).

A poorly controlled diabetic potential mother, (in other words hyperglycaemia in pregnancy), produces overweight babies and those babies grow into overweight adults. We also know that the patient's weight, – lower birth weight, (starvation stress in utero), race, activity, genes and diet are important factors in the causation of diabetes. Certain specific dietary constituents may also influence diabetic risk. Also, taking two to five courses of penicillin in the preceding year increases the risk of developing type 2 DM by 8%. The risk is 23% for more than 5 courses. Other antibiotic groups, cephalosporins, macrolides and quinolones increase T2DM risk as well – the latter increasing the subsequent risk to 37%. These findings suggest a mechanism involving gut flora and internal biochemical mechanisms controlling glucose homeostasis. Either this,or as in some other cases, the infections themselves resulting in diabetes. It is currently fashionable to blame antibiotics for many bodily ills but we used to believe diabetes could result from a low grade viral pancreatitis. Perhaps this could be part of a nasty systemic viral infection for which the antibiotic was given?

But: The whole concept of the gut flora powerfully influencing so many disparate bodily systems would have been entirely alien to the profession only twenty years ago. It would certainly have been fanciful and laughable had it been suggested when I was training four decades ago. Indeed I do find some of the claims relating to the distant control exercised by our gut commensals a bit hard to swallow. It has now become part of the medical zeitgeist that by encouraging dirt and supporting our local microbiotic communities we can improve all sorts of health issues. So much so that The Times ran a spread against hand washing and caesarean sections and in favour of faecal transplants and smearing neonates with body fluids in Nov 2015. This was the same edition that ran the old news that children with pets or who lived on farms had less asthma. By the 21st Century, cleanliness has become next to sinfulness. I don't include simple hand washing with soap in between patients in this general enthusiasm for nature. Clearly, we need to scrub with more enthusiasm. However I wouldn't use *antiseptic* scrubs or gels given the Texas research 2016 finding that some hospital bacteria now have genes for chlorhexidine resistance and that these confer systemic antibiotic resistance. Also, in September 2016 the American FDA banned soaps and washes containing Triclosan and Triclocarban, "The two most common antibacterial ingredients". Triclosan was found to affect antibiotic resistance, affect the human microbiome and even affect developing foetuses. So is it really sensible to have antiseptic gels and scrubs on every hospital corridor and ward?

There are many conditions that require weeks, months or (for instance, Immune disorders, Cystic Fibrosis, COPD, Whipple's disease, HIV) sometimes years of broad spectrum antibiotic treatment. I am not aware that all these patients develop diabetes or serious systemic complications in some unrelated bodily system. So my own jury on the key and central role of the microbiota is still deliberating.

However, the research increasingly suggests that the "microbiota" *is* responsible for many previously unknown, seemingly unrelated disease processes. There seems to be no association between antibiotic use and Type 1 DM. Certain whole fruits, -blueberries, grapes and apple consumption all reduce diabetes risk but the consumption of fruit juices (presumably because of the amount of added sugar) increases the risk of developing diabetes as an adult. The consumption of sugar and sugary drinks generally is prospectively associated with Type2DM as well as adiposity – this was reported in a July 2015 paper in the BMJ. In normoglycaemic individuals the risk of T2DM developing is 4 fold higher if the patient has various raised fasting amino acids: isoleucine, phenylalanine and tyrosine – suggesting a link between amino acid and glucose metabolic dysfuncion.

Exposure to pesticides leads to a 60% increase in Type 2 DM risk (EASD 2015).

Pre-diabetes can be addressed by a permanent improvement (if you can achieve it) in levels of both exercise and weight. Indeed Type 2 diabetes is so closely related to BMI that in 2004 NICE suggested gastric banding in Type 2 diabetics with BMIs of only 30 and above. There is a dramatic improvement in all parameters of type 2 DM after surgical restriction of calorie intake by gastric banding or gastric bypass-including renal and CVS risk factors. Indeed at least a quarter to a third of obese type two diabetics are cured of their illness by the surgery and many of the rest are improved. The earlier the surgery the better the results. Newer results suggest however that even if the gastric bands or other weight loss treatments stay in situ, the weight loss may not be sustained after a period of two or three years. So I assume neither will a diabetes cure. Interestingly, self harm increases in the second and third year in women following bariatric surgery too. It is as if the body and mind start to resent the nonstop punishment of calorie restriction and fight against it after a couple of years like a child denied sweeties for being naughty. After all, from early child hood and probably for hundreds of years across many human cultures, sweet things have been a reward, a pleasure, a treat and not an intrinsic part of our regular diet. Denying this through an alien gastric stricture may be subconsciously interpreted as an ongoing punishment and an imposed harm.

In Type 1DM there is an association with HLA DR3 and DR4, also with Coxsackie and Rubella infection, low Vit D (but what isn't ?) and cow's milk consumption via an auto immune mechanism.

Symptoms: Polyuria, polydipsia, weight loss, tiredness, delayed healing, blurred vision, thrush etc are some of the common symptoms of T1 and T2DM.

Type I: is normally diagnosed from the pattern of symptoms at presentation, including hyperglycaemia, ketosis, rapid weight loss, age below 50, BMI <25kg/m2 and a personal or FH of auto immune disease. You could measure C-Peptide to confirm or diabetes specific autoantibody titres but these probably won't be necessary.

Diabetic ketosis is associated with blood glucose levels consistently >15mmol/li and causes the above plus:

Abdominal pain, air hunger or sighing respiration (secondary to metabolic acidosis), hyperventilation (Kussmaul respiration), confusion, nausea, vomiting, the foetor of ketosis as fatty acids are broken down as an energy source instead of glucose and sometimes coma. This usually indicates a relative lack of insulin. Ketosis may be secondary to infection, other illnesses, dehydration, vomiting or the way T1DM or occasionally T2DM presents.

Pathology: (See Pathology Section)

Random venous glucose >11.1mmol/li.

or Fasting plasma glucose (8hrs without calories) >7.0mmol/li (this should be 3.5-6mmol/li) OR do a

Glucose Tolerance Test: after 75gr glucose by mouth. (OGTT) or:

(The "Gold Standard" is 3 days normal exercise and diet, fast overnight for 12 hours, no smoking, use a small bottle of *Lucozade* from which the lid had been removed the day before (so it is "flat") it must be at room temperature. Then bloods are taken after fasting at 30 minutes and at 2 hours).

Abnormal is:

>9mmol at 30min.

2 hour plasma glucose >11.1 mmol/li ("New" 2000 criteria).

Non diabetics should be back to N at 2 hours.

"Pre-diabetes" is fasting plasma glucose 6.1-7.0 mmol/li (and OGTT 2 hour level <7.8mmol/li) Manage these patients with diet, weight reduction and close supervision. Risk of progression to actual diabetes is about 2%/annum (more if you believe Diabetes. co.uk).

"Impaired glucose tolerance" is fasting plasma glucose <7mmol/li. OGTT at 2 hours >7.8 but <11.1 mmol/li. The risk of diabetes here is nearly 5%/annum (one reference). There is a much higher cardiovascular risk in impaired glucose tolerance. If you are interested in alternative medicine, there is some evidence that increasing magnesium intake can lower Insulin resistance in Type 2 DM and also in areas where there is high black tea consumption there is a lower incidence of diabetes. Up to 3/4 of patients with impaired glucose tolerance develop diabetes within a decade (another reference: Diabetes.co.uk).

Recommended glucose targets: HbA1C <7%, Fasting glucose 4-7mmol/li. self monitoring before meals 4-7mmol/li.

Interpretation (WHO criteria) (Alternative Source)

Venous Plasma Glucose mmol/L

	Normal	Diabetes Mellitus	Diabetes Mellitus ("Provisional")	Impaired Glucose Tolerance	Impaired fasting glycaemia
Fasting	6.0 and below	7.0 and above	7.0 and above	Below 7.0	6.1 – 6.9
	and	and	or	and	and
2 hour	7.7 and below	11.1 and above	11.1 and above	7.8 – 11.0	7.7 and below
			Note: If at least one other abnormal level on another occasion, then diagnosis of DM can be made		

HbA1C: SEE PATHOLOGY (Glycated, Glycosylated haemoglobin): Glucose binds to the Beta chain of haemoglobin and remains irreversibly attached. The amount bound is proportional to the ambient blood glucose and the duration it has been raised over 1-3months. The reference units were changed in the UK at the end of 2012.

The normal range is 20-40 mmol/mol (4%-5.9%).

It used to be suggested that:

A well controlled diabetic would have a level of 48 mmol/mol (6.5%).

Recent research suggests 53mmol/mol (7%) is more appropriate – as aiming lower may introduce an unacceptable risk of hypos.

Indeed, it is a level about 7.5% in diabetic patients that is actually associated with the lowest all cause mortality (MeReC Extra 45). The Accord study showed an increased risk below an HbA1C of 6 and The ADVANCE study showed a target <6.5 had no beneficial effect on macrovascular events or all cause mortality.

This is all very strange as a brief trawl of the literature also gives the following information:

HbA1C Concentration:

Mortality	<5%	5-5.4%	5.5-6.9%	7% or >
All cause	1.0	1.41	2.07	2.64
CV	1.0	2.53	2.46	5.04
Ischaemic	1.0	2.74	2.77	5.20

Note: that Sickle Cell Anaemia (other haemoglobinopathies) and G6PD deficiency give a falsely low HbA1C but B12 and folate deficiency give falsely elevated levels. The Fructosamine level may be used when the patient has a haemoglobinopathy.

So roughly speaking,

A **HbA1C** of 5% (31 mmol/mol) suggests an average blood glucose around 5.5 mmol/li

HbA1C			
6%	42 mmol/mol		7 mol/li
7	53		8.5
8	64		10.2
9	75		12
10	86		13.5
11	97		15 etc

	HbA1C%	Fasting Pl Gluc mg/dl	OGTT mg/dl	mmol/L
Diabetes	6.5 or above	126 or above (7.0mmol)	200 or above	11.1 or above on GTT
Prediabetes	5.7-6.4	100-125 (5.6-6.9mmol)	140-199	7.8-11.1 on GTT
Normal	About 5	99 or less (5.5mmol)	139 or less	7.7 or less on GTT

The latest NICE guidance (2015) to reduce vascular complications in **Type 1DM** is a target HbA1C of 48mmol/mol (6.5%) or less (this is lower than the 2014 7.5% for the prevention of microvascular damage and 6.5% for those patients at increased risk of arterial disease).

A target of 48 mmol/mol (6.5%) is recommended in children and the younger patient In Type 1 and 2 DM (the previous target was 7.5%).

Plasma glucose targets should be around:

5-7mmol/L on waking

4-7mmol/L before meals

5-9 mmol/L 90 mins after eating.

All Type 1 patients should be offered a structured education programme (DAFNE – Dose adjustment for normal eating) and multiple daily injection basal-bolus insulin regimens should be the insulin regime of choice.

The Types:

- Type 1 diabetes mellitus 5-10% of the total.

- Type 2 diabetes mellitus 75% of the total.

- LADA 10% – Latent autoimmune diabetes of adults, thin patients who become insulin dependent.

- Maturity onset diabetes of the young* 2%.

- Gestational diabetes.

- Endocrine causes (1-5%) Polycystic Ovary Syndrome, Acromegaly, Cushing's Syndrome, Thyroid disease, Addisons, Somatostatinoma, Glucagonoma, Phaeochromocytoma.

- Genetic causes (1-5%) MODY* 1-6: Disorders of beta-cell function, Down's Syndrome, Friedreich's Ataxia, Haemochromatosis, Myotonic Dystrophy, Turner Syndrome, Kleinfelter's Syndrome.

In the presence of polyuria, weight loss, tiredness and a BG>11.1mmol/li Type 1DM is assumed and SC Insulin commenced.

In straight forward Type 2DM, 2 fasting BGs will be>7mmol/li (or HbA1C>6.5 on 2 separate days) or a 75gr OGTT if the 2 hour level is >11.1mmol.

Type 1 and Type 2

These are not quite as clear cut as they once were. Not all type 1s are diagnosed in childhood or youth. Not all type 2s are overweight, 20% of type 2 diabetics are of normal weight. Some Type 2s start needing insulin as part of their treatment and are insulin dependent Type 2s.

But Generally:

Type 1 Diabetes:	Type 2 Diabetes:
Often presents in childhood or youth	Usually presents over 30 years
Not usually overweight	Usually overweight
Often presents with ketosis	Presentation associated with raised BP and cholesterol
Treatment involves insulin	Initial treatment is either orally or without medication
Cannot be controlled without insulin	Sometimes possible to stop medication
There is an auto immunity to Beta cells.	There is insulin resistance.

Some patients with Type 2 diabetes may need insulin injections as well as their Type 2 medication if they develop either a low insulin output or a reduced insulin sensitivity.

Diabetes and the work place:

Those treated with diet alone can do virtually any job. If treated with oral hypoglycaemics, the patient cannot join the police, armed forces, fire brigade or fly a commercial aircraft.

Insulin dependent diabetics cannot fly aircraft, drive trains, work at sea or dive. It may be undesirable for them to work at heights or for them to do jobs requiring vigilance (ie Air Traffic Control) – Jobs that require vigilance? What about medicine? I have known many doctors with all forms of diabetes, who worked full time – but then I have known doctors who have fasted while on duty and became hypoglycaemic and confused, doctors with dyslexia who regularly wrote down doses and names of drugs that were wrong, doctors with recurrent severe depression, personality disorders, various forms of unpredictable epilepsy, doctors who worked at detailed operative surgery despite an incapacitating tremor, senior colleagues who continued cardiac catheterisation of children despite the after effects of a severe hemiplegia. No one stopped them, no one seemed entitled to stop them. I wonder how many of these doctors would have been honest enough to admit they were not fit to work (-or how many of their appraisers would be brave enough or been *allowed to stop them* from working?)

Driving and diabetes:

Group 2 vehicles

Since 2013 drivers on insulin or oral medication that can induce hypoglycaemia can drive a group 2 vehicle (bus and lorry) provided they:

Have had no episodes of hypoglycaemia requiring the assistance of another person in the past 12 months.

Have full hypoglycaemic awareness (that is, are able to avoid the onset of hypoglycaemia by taking action after warning symptoms).

Can demonstrate regular blood glucose monitoring at least twice daily with a meter with memory function.

Have no other debarring complications of diabetes, such as eye problems.

The DVLA will arrange annual review by an independent diabetic consultant, who must examine three months of blood sugar readings, which the patient collects on a blood glucose meter.

If patients change from oral hypoglycaemics to insulin, they must tell the DVLA and stop driving group 2 vehicles.

Group 1 vehicles

Drivers must inform the DVLA if they are taking insulin. Drivers of group 1 vehicles (cars and motorbikes) using insulin must have an awareness of hypoglycaemia, have adequate blood glucose monitoring, not be a danger to the public and meet eyesight standards.

Patients must inform the DVLA if they have had more than one episode of hypoglycaemia requiring assistance from another person in a year. You should advise patients not to drive if they have had an episode requiring admission to A&E, treatment by paramedics or assistance from a partner/friend who had to administer glucagon/glucose because the patient could not do this.

The patient does not have to report an episode of hypoglycaemia if they were conscious of it and able to take appropriate action independently.

Patients taking insulin temporarily (less than three months), for example due to gestational diabetes, need not inform the DVLA as long as they are under medical supervision and not at risk of disabling hypoglycaemia.

My own opinion is that the loosening of rules relating to large vehicles and hypoglycaemic diabetes treatments is utterly wrong. It exaggerates the right to drive a large, extremely dangerous weapon of potential mass destruction and diminishes the simple human right of all of us to go about our lives in as much safety as possible. We all know from what happened in December 2014 in Queen St Glasgow how many innocent people can be killed by a heavy vehicle with its driver unconscious at the wheel. In America, drivers who knowingly take risks and drive unsafely, killing others as a consequence are regularly imprisoned for life. Here they seem to be let off scot free. Diabetic patients who drive for a living can do other jobs. Who said that controlling a motor vehicle trumps the right to life, the right to walk the pavement with our children or stand at a bus queue without the added risk of being mown down by an out of control bus or HGV? The GMC revised its rules on confidentiality at last in May 2017 saying that the GP's responsibility to the potential victim of his patient who he (or she) had deemed medically unfit to drive outweighed his duty of confidentiality. I would hope you had already realised this.

Metabolic Syndrome* (see below) is a catchall phrase but in the context of Diabetes means central obesity (or a raised BMI) plus two of:

Raised Tgs
Raised BP
Raised Fasting BG
Low HDL (Nicotinic Acid can raise) (low HDL-C).

It is associated with or includes: Hypertension, microalbuminuria, fatty liver disease, steatohepatitis, PCO, ED, low total testosterone levels, hyperuricaemia, impaired fibrinolysis and affects (in some studies) up to a third of (for instance) the US adult population.

DESMOND is "Diabetes Education and Self Management for Ongoing and Newly Diagnosed Diabetics". It is a foundation training course and an ongoing education network. The DESMOND organisation provides information (eg the safer Ramadan Toolkit etc) and Training Courses (The lay educator study support days etc) as well as a support structure for diabetes education country wide.

DAFNE is "Dose Adjustment For Normal Eating".

Complications of diabetes are to small vessels, causing retinopathy, nephropathy, neuropathy, ED, and big vessel damage, CVD, CVAs, gangrene, ulcers, peripheral vascular disease, infections.

Diabetic Risks:

BUPA uses a Diabetic Risk Score questionnaire which goes as follows:

1) Age

Under 45 yrs	0 points
45-54 yrs	2
55-64 yrs	3
>64 yrs	4

2) BMI

<25Kg/M2	0
25-30	1
>30	2

3) Waist Circumference (between ribs and top of hip)

Men		Women	
<94 cm	0	<80 cm	0
94-102 cm	3	80-88 cm	3
>102 cm	4	>88 cm	4

4) Do you have at least 30 minutes of physical activity daily?

Yes	0
No	2

5) How often do you eat vegetables or fruit?

Every day	0
Not every day	1

6) Have you ever taken antihypertensive medication regularly?

No	0
Yes	3

7) Have you been found to have a raised blood glucose at any routine test?

No	0
Yes	2

8) Have any family members got any form of diabetes?

No	0
Yes but not FDR	3
FDR	5

Risk of developing Diabetes in 10 years is

Score <7	1:100
7-11	1:25
12-14	1:6
15-20	1:3
>20	1:2

I am grateful to BUPA for permission to reproduce this score chart.

Medico-legal issues:

The number of claims against doctors for failing to diagnose or manage diabetes properly have gone up by 28% in the 10 years up to 2015. The MDU said in September 2015 that the number of claims increased from 162 to 207 from 2003/7 to 2008/12. The charity Diabetes UK estimated that the number of adults with diabetes has gone up from 1.2m to 3.3m over the ten years to 2015. Clearly more patients are aware of the symptoms, investigations and treatment of diabetes these days. 75% of litigation involves GPs and the MDU recommends that we avoid this by:

Recording management and F/U plans,
Ensuring patients know what to do if symptoms persist,
Having a computer warning system to flag up patients "of concern",
Being familiar with management guidelines,
Ensuring regular monitoring and screening,
Chasing up DNA diabetic patients who default reviews,
Analysing medication errors and diagnostic delays (?SEAs),
And that we explain and apologise if things go wrong.

Retinopathy:

Background retinopathy is the commonest form of diabetic retinopathy. It consists of microaneurysms ("dots") and haemorrhages ("blots") – which are larger than "dots" and are deep haemorrhages within the retina. There are also hard exudates in a circinate pattern around damaged, leaky blood vessels – if near the retina this is exudative retinopathy and the patient needs referral. There are also cotton wool spots which are ill defined white lesions – retinal nerve fibre layer infarcts.

Maculopathy, of which there are four types – focal or exudative, cystoid, ischaemic and "mixed". In "focal" maculopathy, oedema and/or hard exudates encroach on the fovea and affect vision. The treatment is photocoagulation of the damaged leaky vessel.

Proliferative retinopathy affects 5% of diabetics and can be asymptomatic until sudden visual loss occurs. This is due to vitreous haemorrhage or retinal detachment. Neovascularisation is the growth of fine new blood vessels, the most harmful being near the disc. This is treated by photocoagulation.

Type 2 Treatments:

Metformin is the good old standby, a Biguanide, the first drug to use in almost all diabetics (non insulin dependent) especially the overweight, unless the patient has a low GFR. You are supposed to check renal function twice yearly because of the risk of lactic acidosis. If the patient develops a shock state from any cause, the Metformin should be suspended. OK in pregnancy and breast feeding, the commonest side effect is diarrhoea. It might be worth checking for Vitamin B12 deficiency annually as pernicious anaemia can be a long term side effect of Metformin.

It suppresses liver glucose production, increases Insulin sensitivity, reduces gut glucose absorption and increases peripheral glucose uptake. It lowers LDL and Tgs and reduces diabetic cardiovascular complications – strokes and heart attacks. It is also used in such conditions as PCO, non alcoholic fatty liver disease and premature puberty (Insulin resistance seems to be its forte).

Interestingly it has a non specific effect on suppressing proliferation of a number of cancer cell lines as well. It reduces the incidence of pancreatic cancer, breast, colon, ovary, lung and prostate cancer. Why this isn't recognised and used more by oncologists is a puzzle to me. Whereas diabetics generally suffer an above average level of cancers of most cell types, those on Metformin have half the number of the non diabetic public. The cancers suffered are less aggressive in patients taking Metformin as well. The one thing it doesn't do is reduce lung cancer in smoking diabetics-where it actually increases the risk (Kaiser Permanente, Oakland, Cal 2015, Medline) Diabetes Care 2009 Sep 32 (9) 1620-5.

Basically, after Metformin you seem to be able to add any other drug in combination with it.

The drug groups are: (See end of chapter)

Sulphonylureas: Increase insulin secretion from B cells. Gliclazide 40-320mg per day as a once or twice daily dose. Also Glipizide, Glimepiride etc.

Biguanides: Basically Metformin is the only one in clinical use now. Phenformin, available when I qualified, was withdrawn because of the side effect of higher levels of lethal lactic acidosis. Metformin reduces insulin resistance, reduces gluconeogenesis, (the release of glucose from non carbohydrate sources, usually causing ketosis) and reduces hepatic glucose output. Avoid if Creatinine>150umol/li. See above.

Prandial Glucose Regulators: Oral insulin secretion stimulator. Nateglinide, Starlix, 60mg 30mins or so before meals, titrate the dose up. Repaglinide, Prandin. 0.5mg 15mins before meals, titrate up.

Alpha-Glucosidase inhibitor: Acarbose, Glucobay. Chew with first mouthful of food. Start with 50mg with main meal and increase to 100mg TDS.

Glitazones: (Thiazolidinediones, TZDs.) Activate PPARs, nuclear receptors which have a variety of metabolic actions including decreasing insulin resistance, increased glucose uptake, reduction in circulating fatty acids and Tgs, they increase HDL-C and LDL-C. Tend not to cause hypos. Avoid in heart failure or if high risk of fracture.

Pioglitazone, Actos 15-45mg OD acts at the genome regulating insulin. It modulates the transcription of insulin sensitive genes reducing insulin resistance in the liver and peripheral tissues. Can be used in Type 2 DM as mono therapy particularly if the patient is overweight or with Metformin or a Sulphonyurea.

Various Glitazones have been withdrawn including Troglitazone, Romozin, Rosiglitazone, Avandia. (Cardiac side effects).

Can use Glitazones with Metformin and Sulphonylureas or with Insulin.

Incretins: are gastrointestinal hormones that stimulate insulin release. They reduce the rate of gastric emptying. They inhibit Glucagon release from the Alpha cells of the pancreas. Both GLP-1 and GIP are Incretins and are inactivated by the enzyme DPP-4. Therapeutically the analogues are currently (**GLP-1 agonists/analogues/Incretin mimetics**)

Exenatide, Byetta/Bydureon and

Liraglutide, Victoza, and

Lixisenatide, Lixumia and

Dulaglutide, Trulicity. These can be used with sulphonylureas and metformin.

In other words they are GLP-1 analogues (GLP-1 is an endogenous "Incretin" that potentiates B Cell insulin release, is natriuretic, lowers appetite, lowers glucagon, increases insulin and reduces progression of Type 2 Diabetes) which improve B cell function, lower the patient's weight and improve B Cell function.

So to summarise: GLP-1 (Glucagon like peptide, half life 2 minutes) analogues

– Exanatide, Byetta and Liraglutide, Victoza, etc are analogues of gut Incretins. DPP 4 (Dipeptyl peptidase) is an enzyme that metabolises Incretins – and the Gliptins inhibit DPP4. It all sounds more complicated than it is.

DPP-4 Inhibitors, Gliptins. These are weight neutral. Diabetics have high DPP-4 and low GLP-1.

DPP-4 inactivates GLP-1 and GLP-1 stimulates insulin release and inhibits glucagon release. Sitagliptin. Januvia, Vildagliptin, Galvus. Saxagliptin, Onglyza, Linagliptin, Trajenta.

Side effects include severe joint pains, heart failure.

SGLT-2 Inhibitors – The **Sodium glucose co-transporter 2 inhibitors** prevent active glucose reabsorption from the PCT. Weight loss is a side effect and these include: Empagliflozin (Jardiance) Dapagliflozin (Forxiga) and Canagliflozin (Invokana) which can also be used in combination with insulin and with or without other anti-diabetic drugs. In addition, they can be offered (orally) as triple therapy when taken with metformin and either a Sulfonylurea or a Thiazolidinedione.

This is the tenth NICE-approved treatment to reduce blood sugar levels in type 2 diabetes.

They work by blocking reabsorption of excess glucose in the kidneys, enabling it to pass into the urine.

There is a risk of ketoacidosis (with relatively low BG levels (eg <14mmol/li)) with SGLT2 inhibitors.

[(Typical symptoms of Ketoacidosis are: Nausea, vomiting, anorexia, abdominal pain, thirst, dyspnoea, confusion, fatigue, sleepiness). The treatment of DKA is IV fluid, potassium, Insulin 0.1U/kg/hr IV and monitoring fluid output/balance.]

Put another way:

Hypoglycaemic	No Hypos
Insulins	Metformin
Sulphonylureas	Acarbose
Meglitinides (glinides) Repaglinide, Nateglinide,	Pioglitazone
	GLP1 agonists/analogues (from L cells)
	– incretin mimetics
	injectable-Exanetide
	Liraglutide, Lixisenatide, Abiglutide etc
	DPP4 inhibitors gliptins-tabs. Lina, Sita, Vilda, Saxagliptin
	SGLT2 inhibs Forxiga, Dapagliflozin – tabs Invokana,
	Canagliflozin tabs.

So in Type 2DM, if monotherapy with Metformin does not achieve the appropriate HbA1, current guidelines in the USA and UK say you can add in:

an SU/glinide

TZD

DPP-4 Inhibitor (weight neutral)

GLP-1 RA

Basal Insulin.

All diabetics over 40 should have a statin as the cardiovascular risk is the main killer.

Insulin: (see the comparative table in MIMS and end of chapter)

When added as a third line treatment, insulin is better at improving glycaemic control than alternative oral treatments in T2DM especially in patients with an HbA1c of 9% or higher. The commonest side effects are hypoglycaemia and weight gain. 7-15% of patients with T2DM on insulin have at least 1 hypoglycaemic episode per year and 1% – 2% have a severe episode. In the UK Hypoglycaemia Study it was found that within the first two years of insulin therapy, the hypoglycaemic risk was no worse than with a sulfonylurea and it was lower than in type 1 diabetes patients during the first 5 years of treatment. (UKPDS, ADVANCE, ACCORD).

Basal/bolus insulin regimes aim to mimic physiological insulin secretion but Neutral Protamine Hagedorn (NPH) has a peak in profile after 4-8 hours and this can lead to hypoglycaemia.

Novel insulin analogues shorten its action – Aspart, Lispro, Glulisine or lengthen it, acting as basal insulins – Detemir, Glargine (action starts in 1-4 hours, duration up to 24 hours).

Degludec has a very long duration of action (>42 hrs, half life 25 hrs) with genuine once daily dosing.

Other new long acting insulins include: Insulin Glargine U300 and Peglispro.

The usual strategy for achieving glycaemic control is to target Fasting Plasma Glucose using basal insulin or other methods. If HbA1c remains elevated once the FPG has been optimized, the contribution of postprandial hyperglycaemia should be addressed (Post Prandial Glucose – PPG).

The International Diabetes Federation (IDF) recommends an HbA1c target of lower than 7% or even lower if it can be easily and safely achieved.

(Fasting plasma and post prandial glucose)

	FPG	PPG
IDF	6.5mmol/li	9.0mmol/li **Blood glucose levels.**

Insulin is ultimately needed in many T2DM patients and it is likely to be more effective than most other agents when used in triple therapy, especially if HbA1c levels are very high (≥9%). It can also be an effective first line agent or second line agent with Metformin. Patients who benefit most are generally those with an HbA1c higher than 8.0%, who are taking 2 or more oral antihyperglycemic agents or a GLP-1 receptor agonist and who have long-standing T2DM. Also likely to benefit most are those who have a greater increase in their FPG than their PPG, leaner patients (likely to be insulin deficient), patients on a GLP-1 RA who are obese on insulin or whose FPG stays high. A basal insulin is probably going to be the most effective next therapeutic move for these patients.

T2DM treatment, a reminder:

In the stepwise approach recommended by most guidelines, first-line therapy usually consists of metformin plus lifestyle changes, progressing to dual therapy if HbA1c targets are not met after 3 months, then advancing to triple therapy if targets are not met after a further 3 months.

For example, after 3 months of therapy with metformin and failure to reach an HbA1c target, either add a sulfonylurea, thiazolidinedione, glucagon-like peptide-1 (GLP-1) receptor agonist, dipeptidyl peptidase-4 (DPP-4) inhibitor, sodium glucose cotransporter 2 (SGLT2) inhibitor, or basal insulin to the patient's regimen. If HbA1c remains above target after a further 3 months, the guidelines recommend adding a third different glucose-lowering agent from this list. You get the idea.

Insulins duration of action:

Insulin type	Example	Onset (h)	Peak (h)	Duration (h)	Administration
Short-acting insulin	Soluble insulin, regular insulin	0.5	1-3	4-8	0.5h before a meal
Rapid-acting insulin analogue	Aspart, lispro, glulisine	0.25-0.50	0.5-1.0	2-5	Immediately before a meal
Intermediate-acting insulin	NPH	1-2	4-8	8-20	Between meals or twice daily (as basal insulin)
Premixed insulin	NPH (70%)/regular insulin (30%)	0.5-1.0	1-12	22	Once or twice daily before meals
	NPL (70%)/lispro (30%) or	0.25	2	22	
	NPL (50%)/lispro (50%)	0.25	1-4	24	
	NPA (70%)/aspart (30%)				
Basal insulin analogue	Glargine, detemir	0.5-1.0	Almost no peak	16- 24	Once or twice daily
Second-generation basal insulin analogues	Degludec	Steady state within 3 days	No peak	>42	Once daily
Coformulated basal insulin analogues	Degludec/aspart	As per individual components	As per individual components	As per individual components	Once or twice daily
	Degludec/liraglutide*	As per individual components	As per individual components	As per individual components	Once daily

Commonly used Insulins:

Short Acting: Lispro (Humalog short peak) 15mins – 2-5 hrs. Give before or soon after meals. Aspart, Novorapid immediately before or with a meal, 10mins to 3-5 hrs. Neutral, Soluble, Actrapid Up to 8 hrs.

Glulisine, Apidra.

Intermediate: Isophane, NPH. Humulin, Hypurin Porcine, Insulatard, up to approx 20-24 hours.

Long acting: Lente, IZS. Hypurin Bovine, Detemir (Levemir). Insulin Glargine (Lantus), 24 hrs + Smooth action, no peak. Insulin degludec Tresiba, the bioidentical Glargine, – Abasria

Various mixtures make up the biphasic Insulins: Novomix30 (Soluble insulin/ Protamine insulin 30/70%) Humalog Mix 25 and Mix 50: (Lispro insulin and Lispro protamine 25/75% and 50/50%). Humulin M3 (Soluble and Isophane insulin 30/70%) etc.

Various "Pens" to give small doses of insulin.

Insulin requirements are increased by:

OCPs, Thyroxine, Danazol, Steroids, Beta 2 stimulants.

Decreased by:

Oral hypoglycaemics, Salicylates, Sulphonamides, Some antidepressants, Some ACEIs, Beta Blockers, Alcohol, Ocreotide (used in Carcinoid etc).

Neuropathy:

65% diabetics develop neuropathy but intensive therapy can reduce it 70%. 7-8% diabetics present with the symptoms of neuropathy.

Risks include:

Duration, height, smoking, BP, being male, poor control etc.

It is a distal symmetrical neuropathy (vibration, pin prick, fine touch, temperature).

Painful neuropathy, leg ulcers, Charcot neuroarthropathy.

Exclude uraemia, B12, Pb, EtOh, HIV, malignancy, etc.

Other neuropathies include:

Proximal motor neuropathy, Diabetic amyotrophy: Males in 50s, Type 2 DM, must image L/S and exclude other causes.

TS/Mononeuropathies (thigh pain, severe). Common peroneal N, Lat Cut N entrapment,

Cranial Mononeuropathies, 3rd or 6th Cranial Ns.

Acute insulin neuritis –peripheral neuropathy after sudden improvements in BG.

Autonomic Neuropathy: Erectile dysfunction in 40%, but GI, bladder, postural hypotension, (>30mm Hg postural drop) etc involved Rx Fludrocortisone.

Diabetic Neuropathic Pain: Treatment:

Treatments include: Some recommend Duloxetine (Cymbalta), TCAs (Amitriptyline) as the first two to try. There are also: Gabapentin, 300mg on first day, increasing to maximum of 800mg TDS. Avoid sudden withdrawal. Pregabalin. Lacosamide, Vimpat. Also Clonazepam 0.5mg Nocte, increasing to 1mg BD if tolerated. Paroxetine, Citalopram, Carbamazepine, Phenytoin, Lamotrigine (very slow titration, as with all the anticonvulsants, 25mg alt days, increasing in 2 weeks to OD) Epilim, Venlafaxine, Topiramate, Mirtazapine, Topical Capsaicin, – Zacin cream, Axsain and lignocaine cream. The plethora of alternatives tells you that none of them work very well and/or that all have serious side effects. It may be worth mentioning that as well as damaging peripheral nerves, the persistently elevated blood glucose of Type 2 Diabetes increases the incidence of **Dementia** as well.

Diabetes and Kidney Disease:

A third of patients c T2D have CKD 2-5 (impaired kidney function) (<60 GFR). Diabetes is the commonest cause of end stage renal disease.

Annual Transition:

No nephropathy 1.4% Microalb 3.0% Macroalb 4.6% Elevated creatinine or renal replacement Rx 19%.

Proteinuria is an independent risk factor in DM 2. The CV event rate is increased both with diabetes and CKD

Metabolic Syndrome: *

Often called Metabolic Syndrome X, it can be confused with Fragile X – (which is long facies, learning difficulties, often autism etc) and with Cardiac Syndrome X (angina with no ischaemia) or with Turners Syndrome, (XO) So let's stick to Metabolic Syndrome which is:

Insulin resistance,

Glucose intolerance,

Hyperinsulinaemia,

Raised Triglycerides,

Low HDL,

Hypertension,

Central obesity.

The deadly combination of upper body central obesity, glucose intolerance, (hyper-insulinaemia and Insulin resistance), raised triglycerides, hypertension, hyperuricaemia, impaired fibrinolysis and endothelial dysfunction, is called "civilisation syndrome" although it is not an inevitable consequence of modern life.

The treatment is, of course to eat properly, lose weight and exercise more.

This comes under the heading of: TLC which in this case means therapeutic lifestyle changes – (Try to lose corpulence) but if necessary, added to this can be Metformin, lipid lowering and anti hypertensive drugs.

Up to 20% of the adult population has metabolic syndrome. We should aim for waists to be <100 cms for men and 90cms for women or 40" or 35". Marks and Spencer which stocked 30" waist trousers all my life no longer finds it cost effective to do so – Is the spread of visceral fat ubiquitous and relentless and affecting the middle classes as well as the lower social classes?

Gestational Diabetes is commoner in women with central obesity and excess visceral fat. 3% of British pregnancies are affected. In a 2016 study (Zhang, BMJ Jan 2016) following 22,000 pregnancies over 10 years, there was a 27% increase in GD in the (nurses) who ate 2-4 servings of potatoes a week. Over 5 portions a week and the risk went up 50%. Chips, boiled, mashed, any kind of potato exacerbated risk but other vegetables and whole grains reduced it. Much as you would expect. Gestational diabetes increases the risk of pre-eclampsia and hypertension during the pregnancy. After delivery there is a long term increased risk of Type 2 DM, CVD and Metabolic Syndrome (Waist circ is a surrogate for visceral fat – apple shaped people not pear shaped).

The Metabolic Syndrome WHO criteria are an increased waist circ and 2 of:

Tg>1.7,

HDL <1,

BP >130/85,

FBG>5.6mmol/li,

ACR>3.4 (Albumin/creatinine ratio).

Visceral fat is increased in women with GD but subcutaneous (metabolically inactive) fat isn't.

GDM in one pregnancy means it will almost certainly occur in the next. Metformin is safe in pregnancy, controls glucose and helps in the long term fat distribution of offspring (less visceral fat, more subcutaneous fat).

The Fat (Thrifty) Gene Theory (or myth)

-There may be a reason why so many of us have a propensity to hyperglycaemia, insulin resistance, raised triglycerides, excessive fat stores, NAFLD, raised blood pressure, central obesity and hyperuricaemia. This is what some have called "diabesity" and it is now thought to be due to a specific genetic mutation that saved our ape ancestors from starvation. At least, this is the "Thrifty Gene" or "Fat Gene" Hypothesis: That Insulin resistance and extra stores of body fat confer an advantage during times of famine despite the obvious disadvantage when food is plentiful.

The earliest apes diverged from a common ancestor with monkeys in East Africa 26m years ago. These apes lived primarily on a fructose rich fruit diet, slowly spreading north into Europe and elsewhere while the world climate remained mild. Then the planet cooled, food became scarcer and competition for sustenance increased. During the northern winters some apes starved but a fortuitous gene mutation occurred which blocked the enzyme for breaking down uric acid and this it turned out had some wide ranging metabolic and survival benefits during times of hardship. The European apes kept this new survival mutation and spread, some back in to Africa, eventually evolving in to humans.

The theory involves the fact that the gene for Uricase is blocked in modern great apes and humans. As we share the same mutation blocking the gene, this suggests a common ancestor 13-17m years ago – which is when famines and starvation started happening to our ape predecessors.

Uricase breaks down uric acid and so the mutation blocking it leads to hyperuricaemia. This is worse in obese patients eating a protein and sugar rich western diet. Hyperuricaemia raises BP via an action on the kidneys causing salt retention and also raises BP via vasoconstriction due to oxidative stress. Raised uric acid also causes raised fructose (fruit sugar) levels to be converted to fat and fructose itself is converted to uric acid in cells – this action being unlike other sugars. So a high fructose diet in the absence of uricase causes hyperuricaemia and various features of metabolic syndrome including adiposity. Each of these features happens to have improved the survival of great apes in times of starvation. Increased blood glucose, body fat, blood pressure and blood lipids. The European apes which returned to Africa with the disabled uricase gene were thus better able to survive famine than the indigenous African apes who still had uricase and presumably couldn't compete in times of hardship – thus becoming extinct. This effect would have taken many generations and individuals and many, many years.

Various commentators used the fat gene as an excuse for large numbers of us becoming overweight through no fault of their own. However a study in Arch Ped and Ad Med looked at the *actual* effect of the "obesity gene" on individuals. The actual effect of the fat gene on

BMI was only 0.65,

Waist circumference was 0.6cm,

and Body Fat was 0.04%.

So in population and genetic terms the fat gene might make a small survival difference over several generations but in the individual it is nothing compared with the weight gain of gluttony and sloth.

Lipid Targets:

60% of diabetic patients are failing to reach the NICE targets (2013):

"If a person is found to be at high risk of cardiovascular disease, they should be offered statins to achieve total cholesterol levels of less than 4.0 mmol/litre, HDL cholesterol not exceeding 1.4 mmol/litre, or total low-density cholesterol levels of less than 2.0 mmol/litre." (Usually Tgs <1.7mmol).

Measure the waist and advise to lose inches. Advise them to lose 5% or more of body weight. Increase activity – 30mins a day for 5 days each week. Decrease total fat intake to less (much less) than 30% total calories and increase fibre. 80% people with type 2 diabetes are overweight/obese.

Micro albumin screening – Type 1 diabetes for >5 yrs and >12 yrs old, Type 2 diabetes if presentation <60yrs:

	Normal	Microalbumin	Macroalbumin
Urine albumin	<20mg/li	20-200	>200
Albumin/creatinine ratio	<3mg/mmol	3-30	>30

Action: Up to 3X ULN retest in 1yr. 3-10X ULN retest on 2 or more occasions in 6m.

>10X ULN + Albustix positive)

Treatment: Normoalbuminuria: Treat any BP>130/80, Optimise BG.

Biannual albumen concentration. First voided specimen. Recheck if >20mg/li.

Microalbuminuria: Urinary albumin 2-3X/yr on a timed specimen. Optimise glucose control, treat BP>130/80. Consider ACEI, avoid excess protein diet.

Macroalbuminuria: (>200mg/li) – Dipstick positive proteinuria, tendency to increased Se creatinine,

do quantitative proteinuria 2-4X/yr, serum U and Es and creatinine 2-4X/yr,

Control BP, restrict protein to 0.7gr/kg body wt.

Refer to nephrologist when creatinine>200umol/li.

End stage renal failure >500umol/li. >Dialysis/Transplantation.

Blood pressure:	No diabetes	Diabetes
Optimal treated BP	<140/85	<130/80
Audit standard	<150/90	<140/80

British Hypertension Guidelines for patients with Diabetes:

Type 1 Diabetes:

No nephropathy: Treat >140/90 Aim for <130/<80 Audit standard: <140/<80

Nephropathy: (Proteinuria>1gr in 24hr) Target BP <130/80 or lower (<125/75)

ACEIs or ARBs reduce decline in renal function.

Type 2 Diabetes: (ISH common and difficult to control) (Isolated Systolic Hypertension)

No Nephropathy: Treat >140/90 aim for <130/<80

Nephropathy: Target is <130/80 or lower (<125/75) when there is >1g/24hr proteinuria. ACEIs and ARBs reduce the decline in renal function.

Statins should definitely be used in Type 2 Diabetics with hypertension and probably with Type 1 diabetics as well. Also consider aspirin over 50 yrs if 10 yrs CVD risk >20%.

NICE says: Do the BP annually, give lifestyle advice, review BP in 1m if >150/90, 2m if >140/80, 2m if >130/80 and there is vascular damage.

Start medication if **BP >140/80 or >130/80 with kidney, eye or cerebrovascular damage.**

Do BP 1-2 monthly and ramp up treatment until you get these levels.

The drugs suggested are ACEIs, unless the patient is black or could become pregnant (CCBs).

ARBs are suggested if the patient cannot tolerate ACEIs. Dual therapy: with CCBs or diuretics (eg Bendroflumethazide) or triple therapy with all three, then adding an alpha blocker, beta blocker, potassium sparing diuretic (watch K+) in sequence, watching the BP every 4-6m.

Guidelines for Type 2 Diabetes:

Lifestyle measures
HbA1C >/= 6.5%   Metformin (avoid if low GFR)
Then can try either of:
Adding a Sulphonyurea (unless weight gain or hypoglycaemia problematic)
a Thiazolidinedione (Glitazone) if hypoglycaemia a big risk or if patients have Metabolic Syndrome
or a Gliptin if hypoglycaemia or weight gain are concerns or to avoid #s and CHF with TZD.
Exenatide can be considered as second line to lose weight for instance in sleep apnoea.
If HbA1C >/= 7.5%
Third line therapy: Add a Gliptin, TZD, Exenatide, Insulin
HbA1C>/= 7.5%   Insulin plus or minus other agents.
Increased insulin regime.

Diabetes and Cardiovascular Disease:

Heart disease and stroke are increased by Diabetes by a factor of 2-4x. Better control of BP, cholesterol and blood glucose all reduce risk. Diabetics have strokes and heart attacks younger than non diabetics and a patient with T2DM in middle age is at the same risk of an MI as a non diabetic who has already had one MI. Sometimes the MI may be silent due to afferent neuropathy.

Diabetics' higher risks can be due to hypertension which is twice as common in diabetics, hyperlipidaemia, central obesity, accelerated arteriopathy and add on, of course, smoking.

In DM atherosclerosis is more likely and develops quicker than in non diabetics and heart attacks are more severe. Cerebrovascular disease is also worse in diabetes: With DM and raised BP, stroke is twice as likely as without DM. TIAs are 2-6X higher than non diabetics. Peripheral arterial disease and heart failure are both more common in diabetics. Intermittent claudication being 3X more common in male diabetics and 9X more common in female diabetics.

A recent study put the risk for Type 1 diabetics of being admitted with heart failure as 4X that of the matched non diabetic population.

Diabetes Therapies:

BLOOD GLUCOSE METERS

MANUFACTURER	METER	STRIP/ TEST CASSETTE REQUIRED	SAMPLE VOLUME	TIME FOR TEST (SECS)	BLOOD GLUCOSE RANGE (MMOL/L)
Abbot Diabetes Care	FreeStyle Freedom Life	FreeStyle Lite Test Strips	0.3	5 (average)	1.1-27.8
	FreeStyle InsuLinx	Freestyle Lite Test Strips	0.3	5 (average)	1.1-27.8

	FreeStyle Optium Neo	FreeStyle Optium Blood Glucose Test Strips	0.6	5	1.1-27.8
AgaMatrix Europe Ltd	WaveSense JAZZ	WaveSense JAZZ Test Strips WaveSense JAZZ DUO Test Strips	0.5	5 (minimum)	1.1-33.3
Arctic Medical	IME-DC	IME-DC Test Strips	2.0	10	1.1-33.3
Bayer Diabetes Care	CONTOUR XT	CONTOUR NEXT Test Strips	0.6	5	0.6-33.3
	CONTOUR NEXT	CONTOUR NEXT Test Strips	0.6	5	1.1-33.3
	CONTOUR NEXT Link	CONTOUR NEXT Test Strips	0.6	5	1.1-33.3
B Braun	Omni Test 3	Omnitest 3 Blood Glucose Test Strips	0.3	3	0.6-33.3
GlucoRx Ltd	GlucoRx Nexus TD-4277	GlucoRx Nexus Test Strips	0.5	5	1.1-33.3
	GlucoRx Nexus mini TD-4287	GlucoRx Nexus Test Strips	0.5	5	1.1-33.3
	GlucoRx Nexus Voice TD-4280	GlucoRx Nexus Test Strips	0.5	5	1.1-33.3
LifeScan	OneTouch Verio	OneTouch Verio Test Strips	0.4	5	1.1-33.3
	OneTouch VerioIQ	OneTouch Verio Test Strips	0.4	5	1.1-33.3
Menarini Diagnostics	GlucoMen GM	GlucoMen GM Sensors	0.5	7	0.6-33.3
	GlucoMen LX Plus	GlucoMen LX Sensors and GlucoMen LX Ketone Sensors	0.3	4	1.1-33.3

MANUFACTURER	METER	STRIP/ TEST CASSETTE REQUIRED	SAMPLE VOLUME	TIME FOR TEST (SECS)	BLOOD GLUCOSE RANGE (MMOL/L)
Mendor Ltd	Mendor Discreet	Mendor Discreet Test Strip Cartridge	0.5	5	1.1-33.3
Nipro Diagnostics UK Ltd	TRUEone	TRUEone Test Strips	1	5	1.1-33.3
	TRUEresult	TRUEresult Test Strips	0.5	4	1.1-33.3
	TRUEresult twist	TRUEresult Test Strips	0.5	4	1.1-33.3
	TRUEyou mini	TRUEyou Test Strips	0.5	4	1.1-33.3
	TRUEyou	TRUEyou Test Strips	0.5	4	1.1-33.3
Roche Diabetes Care	Accu-Chek Mobile	Mobile Test Cassette	0.3	5 (approx)	0.6-33.3
	Accu-Chek Aviva	Aviva Test Strips	0.6	5	0.6-33.3
	Accu-Chek Aviva Nano	Aviva Test Strips	0.6	5	0.6-33.3
	Accu-Chek Avivia Expert	Aviva Test Strips	0.6	5	0.6-33.3
	Accu-Chek Active	Active Test Strips	1-2	Approx 5 (test strip in meter) /8 (test strip outside meter)	0.6-33.3
Sanofi	iBGStar	BGStar Blood Glucose Test Strips	0.5	5 (average)	1.1-33.3
	BGStar	BGStar Blood Glucose Test Strips	0.5	5 (average)	1.1-33.3
	My Star Extra	BGStar Blood Glucose Test Strips	0.5	5 (average)	1.1-33.3
Spirit Healthcare	CareSens N	CareSens N Test Strips	0.5	5	1.1-33.3

	CareSens N POP	CareSens N Test Strips	0.5	5	1.1-33.3
	CareSens N Voice	CareSens N Test Strips	0.5	5	1.1-33.3
	TEE2	TEE2 Test Strips	0.5	5	1.1-33.3
Ypsomed Ltd	mylife Pura	Mylife Pura Test Strips	1	5	0.6-33.3
	mylife Unio	Mylife Unio Test Strips	0.7	5	0.6-33.3

INSULIN PENS

MANUFACTURER	NAME	DOSAGE (MIN-MAX)	INSULIN USED IN PENS	PEN NEEDLES COMPATIBLE
INJEX UK LTD	INJEX 30	5-30 units	All 10ml Insulin vials and cartridges	None. Insulin administered by needle-free jet injections using patient-activated spring-loaded mechanism through a micro-aperture
LILLY	Humalog HumaPen Savvio	1-60 units	Humalog, Humalog Mix 25, Humalog Mix 50, Humulin I, Humulin M3, Humulin S	BD Micro-Fine +
	Humalog Kwik-Pen Humalog Mix 25 Kwik-Pen Humalog Mix50 Kwik-Pen	1-60 units	Humalog, Humalog Mix 25, Humalog Mix 50	BD Micro-Fine +
	Humulin I Kwik-Pen, Humulin M3 Kwik-Pen	1-60 units	Humulin I, Humulin M3	BD Micro-Fine+
	HumaPen Luxura HD	0.5-30 units (half-unit increments)	Lilly 3ml cartridges from Humalog and Humulin ranges	BD Micro-Fine+

MANUFACTURER	NAME	DOSAGE (MIN-MAX)	INSULIN USED IN PENS	PEN NEEDLES COMPATIBLE
	Humalog 200 units/ml Kwik-Pen	1-60 units	Humalog 200 units/ml	BD Micro-Fine+
NOVO NORDISK	FlexPen	1-60 units	NovoRapid, Levemir, NovoMix 30	NovoFine, NovoFine Autocover, NovoTwist
	InnoLet	1-50 units	Insulatard, Levemir	NovoFine, NovoFine Autocover, NovoTwist
	NovoPen 4	1-60 units	All Novo Norsdiak 3ml penfill cartridges	NovoFine, NovoFine Autocover, NovoTwist
	PenMate	Automatically inserts needle when button is pushed. Fits NovoPen 3, NovoPen 3 Demi and NovoPen 3 Junior only		NovoFine, NovoFine Autocover, NovoTwist
	NovoPen Echo	0.5-30 units (1½ unit increments)	All NovoNordisk 3ml penfill cartridges	Novofine, Novofine Autocover, NovoTwist
	Tresiba FlexTouch	2-160 (2 unit increments)	Tresiba	Novofine, Novofine Autocover, NovoTwist
	Tresiba FlexTouch	1-80 units (1 unit increments)	Tresiba	Novofine, Novofine Autocover, NovoTwist
	NovoRapid FlexTouch	1-80 units (1 unit increments)	NovoRapid	Novofine, Novofine Autocover, NovoTwist
OWEN MUMFORD	Autopen Classic	1-21 units (green) 2-42 units (blue)	Lilly or Wockhardt UK 3ml insulin cartridges	Penfine universal click, Unifine Pentips, BD Micro-Fine+, NovoFine
	Autopen 24	1-21 units (green) 2-42 units (blue)	Sanofi 3ml insulin cartridges	Penfine universal click, Unifine Pentips, BD Micro-Fine+, NovoFine

SANOFI	SoloSTAR	1-80 units	Apidra, Lantus, Insuman Basal and Insuman Comb 25	BD Micro-Fine_, Penfine universal click, ultrafine Pentips, Unifine Pentips, Insupen
	ClikSTAR	1-80 units	Apidra, Lantus, Insuman (all presentations)	B D MicroFine+, Penfine universal click, ultrafine Pentips, Unifine Pentips, Insupen
	JuniorSTAR	1-30 units	Apidra, Lantus, Insuman (all presentations)	B D MicroFine+, Penfine universal click, ultrafine Pentips, Unifine Pentips
SPIRIT HEALTHCARE	Insujet	4-40 units	All 3ml and 10ml UK Insulin cartridges	None. Insulin administered by needle-free jet injections using compressed air through a precision nozzle

INSULIN PUMPS

Dana Diabecare R
Advanced Therapeutics (UK) Ltd

Animas Vibe
Animas Corporation

Paradigm Veo 554 & 754
Medtronic

Accu-Chek Combo
Roche Diabetes Care

Accu-Chek Insight
Roche Diabetes Care

Mylife OmniPod System
Ypsomed Ltd

INSULIN

NAME	MANUFACTURER	SOURCE	DELIVERY SYSTEM	TAKEN
Rapid-acting analogue				
NovoRapid	Novo Nordisk	Analogue	Vial, cartridge, Novo prefilled pens, 1.6ml PumpCart	Just before/with/just after food
Humalog	Lilly	Analogue	Vial, cartridge, prefilled pen	Just before/with/just after food
Apidra	Sanofi	Analogue	Vial, cartridge, prefilled pen	0-15 mins before, or soon after, a meal
Short-acting/neutral				
Actrapid	Novo Nordisk	Human	Vial	30 mins before food
Humulin S	Lilly	Human	Vial, cartridge	20-45 mins before food
Hypurin Bovine Neutral	Wockhardt UK	Bovine	Vial, cartridge	As advised by your doctor
Hypurin Porcine Neutral	Wockhardt UK	Porcine	Vial, cartridge	As advised by your doctor
Insuman Rapid	Sanofi	Human	Cartridge	15-20 mins before food
Medium and long-acting				
Insulatard	Novo Nordisk	Human	Vial, cartridge, prefilled insulin doser	As advised by your doctor
Humulin I	Lilly	Human	Vial, cartridge, prefilled pen	As advised by your doctor
Hypurin Bovine Isophane	Wockhardt UK	Bovine	Vial, cartridge	As advised by your doctor
Hypurin Porcine Isophane	Wockhardt UK	Porcine	Vial, cartridge	As advised by your doctor
Hypurin Bovine Protamine Zinc	Wockhardt UK	Bovine	Vial	As advised by your doctor
Hypurin Bovine Lente	Wockhardt UK	Bovine	Vial	As advised by your doctor
Insuman Basak	Sanofi	Human	Vial, cartridge, prefilled pen	45-60 mins before food
MIXED				
Humulin M3	Lilly	Human	Vial, cartridge, prefilled pen	20-45 mins before food

Hypurin Porcine 30/70 Mix	Wockhardt UK	Porcine	Vial, cartridge	As advised by your doctor
Insuman Comb 15	Sanofi	Human	Cartridge	30-45 mins before food
Insuman Comb 25	Sanofi	Human	Vial, cartridge, prefilled pen	30-45 mins before food
Insuman Comb 50	Sanofi	Human	Cartridge	20-30 mins before food
Humalog Mix 25	Lilly	Analogue	Vial, cartridge, prefilled pen	Just before/with/just after food
Humalog Mix 50	Lilly	Analogue	Cartridge, prefilled pen	Just before/with/just after food
NovoMix	Novo Nordisk	Analogue	Cartridge, prefilled pen	Just before/with/just after food
LONG-ACTING ANALOGUE				
Lantus	Sanofi	Analogue	Vial, cartridge, prefilled pen	Once a day, anytime (but at the same time each day)
Levemir	Novo Nordisk	Analogue	Cartridge, prefilled pen, prefilled insulin doser	Once or twice a day, anytime (at same time each day)
Tresiba	Novo Nordisk	Analogue	Tresiba Penfill 100 units/ml & prefilled Tresiba FlexTouch 100 units/ml & Tresiba FlexTouch 200 units/ml (NB the 3ml FlexTouch pen for 200units/ml contains 600 units)	Once a day, anytime (but preferably at the same time of the day

MEDICATIONS

GENERIC NAME	TRADE NAME	DOSAGE SIZE/ STRENGTH	MIN-MAX DAILY DOSE	WHEN TAKEN	TIMES PER DAY
BIGUANIDES					
Metformin	Glucophage	500mg, 850mg	500-3,000mg	With or after food	2-3 times
	Metformin Oral solution	500mg per 5ml	500-3,000mg	During or after meals	2-3 times
Metformin prolonged release	Glucophage SR	500mg, 750mg, 1,000mg	500-2,000mg	With, or after, evening meals if once. Breakfast and evening meal if twice. Swallow whole	Once (dose can be split if not tolerated or glycaemic control still inadequate)
SULPHONY-LUREAS					
Glibenclamide	Gliben-clamide	2.5mg, 5mg	2.5-15mg	With or immed after breakfast or first main meal of the day	Once
Gliclazide	Diamicron	80mg	40-320mg	Take with water before a meal. Swallow whole	1-2 times
	Diamicron MR	30mg	30-120mg	Take with water at breakfast. Swallow whole	Once
Glimepiride	Amaryl	1mg, 2mg, 3mg, 4mg	1-6mg	Shortly before or with first main meal	Once
Glipizide	Minodiab	5mg	5-20mg	Before food	1-2 times
Tolbutamide	Tolbutamide	500mg	500-2,000mg	With or immediately after food	1-3 times
PRANDIAL GLUCOSE REGULATORS					
Nateglinide	Starlix	60mg, 120mg, 180mg	60-540mg	Up to 30 minutes before meals	Up to 3 times

Repaglinide	Prandin	0.5mg, 1mg, 2mg	0.5-16mg	Usually within 15 minutes prior to main meals, but up to 30 minutes before	Up to 4 times
ALPHA-GLUCOSIDASE INHIBITORS					
Acarbose	Glucobay	50mg, 100mg	50-600mg	Chewed with first mouthful of food, or swallowed whole with water directly before	3 times
THIAZOLIDI-NEDIONE-S (GLITAZONES)					
Pioglitazone	Actos	15mg, 30mg, 45mg	15-45mg alone, or in dual or triple therapy or with insulin	With or without food	Once
INCRETIN MIMETICS					
Exenatide	Byetta	5mcg, 10mcg (injection pens)	10-20mcg	Within 60 minutes prior to the two main meals of the day, approx 6 hours apart	Twice
Liraglutide	Victoza	Injection pen: selection of 0.6mg, 1.2mg, 1.8mg	0.6mg starting dose, then 1.2mg, then 1.8mg	Once a day at any time, independent of meals, around same time of day	Once
Exenatide prolonged-release	Bydureon – Single Dose Kit	2mg powder and solvent to prolonged-release suspension for injection	2mg once weekly	Once weekly	Once weekly. The day of weekly administration can be changed if necessary as long as the next dose is administered at least one day (24 hours) later
Exenatide prolonged-release	Bydureon – Pre-Filled Pen	2mg powder and solvent for prolonged-release suspension for injection in pre-filled pen	2mg once weekly	Once weekly	As above

GENERIC NAME	TRADE NAME	DOSAGE SIZE/ STRENGTH	MIN-MAX DAILY DOSE	WHEN TAKEN	TIMES PER DAY
Lixisenatide	Lyxumia	10mcg, 20mcg (fixed dose injection)	10mcg once daily for 14 days, then 20mcg once daily maintenance dose from day 15 onwards	Administered once daily, within the hour prior to any meal of the day. It is preferable that the prandial injection of Lysumia is performed before the same meal every day when the most convenient meal has been chosen	Once
SGLT-2 INHIBITORS					
Canagliflozin	Invokana	100mg, 300mg	100mg monotherapy/ add on, increasing to 300mg for tighter glycaemic control. If eGFR drops below 60ml/min/1.73m2 use 100mg; discontinue if <45	Best taken before the first meal of the day	Once
Dapagliflozin	Forxiga	5mg, 10mg	10mg for monotherapy and add-on combination therapy with other glucose-lowering medicinal products. 5mg for people with severe hepatic impairment increasing to 10mg if well tolerated. Discontinue if eGFR<60ml/ min/1.73m2		

Empagliflozin	Jardiance	10mg, 25mg	Initiate with 10mg; titrate to 25mg. If tighter glycaemic control needed (and if eGFR is 60ml/min/1.73m2 or above). If eGFR<60, use 10mg, discontinue if <45. Monotherapy or add-on.	With or without food at any time of day	Once
DPP-4 INHIBITORS					
Saxagliptin	Onglyza	2.5mg, 5mg	5mg alone or in dual or triple therapy, or with insulin (reduce to 2.5mg in moderate or severe renal impairment)	With or without food at any time of day	Once
Alogliptin	Vipidia	6.25mg, 12.5mg, 25mg	25mg w.metformin/thiazolidinedione/sulphonylurea/insulin or triple therapy w.metformin & thiazolidinedione/sulphonylurea/insulin. 12.5/6.25mg in moderate/severe renal disease	Once daily with or without food	Once
Linagliptin	Trajenta	5mg	5mg alone, or with metformin, or with sulphonylurea and metformin, or with insulin. No dose adjustment needed in renal impairment	With or without food	Once
Sitagliptin	Januvia	100mg, 50m, 25mg	100mg alone, or in dual or triple therapy, or add on to insulin. Reduce to 50mg in moderate renal impairment (CrCl>/=30 to <50ml/min) Reduce to 25mg in severe renal impairment or with end-stage renal disease (dialysis)	With or without food	Once

GENERIC NAME	TRADE NAME	DOSAGE SIZE/ STRENGTH	MIN-MAX DAILY DOSE	WHEN TAKEN	TIMES PER DAY
Vildagliptin	Galvus	50mg	100mg as monotherapy, in combination with metformin, metformin and a sulphonylurea, thiazolidinedione, or with insulin (with or without metformin) ; 50mg with a sulphonylurea. If moderate or severe renal impairment or with end-stage renal disease (ESRD), recommended dose is 50mg once daily	With or without food	50mg in the morning, 50mg in the evening, except in dual combination with a sulphony-lureawhere administration is 50mg in the morning.
COMBINED FORMULATION MEDICATIONS					
Pioglitazone + metformin	Competact	15mg/850mg	One 15mg/850mg tablet	With or just after food	Twice
Vildaglipin + metformin	Eucreas	50mg/850mg, 50mg/1,000mg. Also licensed as triple therapy with a sulphonylurea or insulin	50mg/850mg-50mg/1,000mg twice	With or just after food	Twice
Sitagliptin + metformin	Janurnet	50mg/1,000mg	50mg/1,000mg	With food	Twice
Saxagliptin + metformin	Komboglyze	2.5mg/850mg, 2.5mg/1,000mg	5mg/1700mg – 5mg/2000mg	With meals	Twice
Alogliptin+ metformin	Vipdomet	12.5mg/1,000mg	12.5mg/1000mg	With meals	Twice
Linagliptin+ metformin	Jentadueto	2.5mg/850mg, 2.5mg/1,000mg	2.5mg/850mg – 2.5/1000mg	With meals	Twice

15: Diet, Diets, Nutrition, Vitamins etc:

The best doctors are Dr Diet, Dr Quiet and Dr Merryman.

Old English Proverb

Weight:

Based on the Body Mass Index: (BMI) a measure derived by dividing the weight in Kgs. by the square of the height in metres.

BMI	Kg/Sq M
Very severely underweight	BMI <15
Severely underweight	BMI 15-16
Underweight	BMI 16-18.5
Normal	**BMI 18.5-25**
Overweight	BMI 25-30
Moderately obese	BMI 30-35
Severely obese	BMI 35-40
Very severely obese	BMI >40

In July 2016 a Public Health England "Health Matters" report suggested that GPs should become "Health role models for physical health" to their patients. In this way we would be better able to discuss and promote physical activity with them. One in four patients would be more active if their GP advised them to do more exercise. This report followed The Chief Medical Officer Dame Sally Davies publically announcing in 2014 that no doctor should be overweight or obese. She was "perpetually surprised at how many nurses and doctors were overweight". I have worked with partners who smoked and whose rooms smelt of cigarette smoke while advising patients to give up and with morbidly obese doctors who were advising type 2 diabetics about calorie controlled diets. I can think of recent presidents of The RCGP who were, if not obese then pretty close to it. Perhaps their work colleagues should say something?

Weight and bedtime: Preschool children who go to bed after 9.00 pm are twice as likely to be obese in later life. (Journal of Ped. online, S Anderson et al, June 2016.) This holds true even when controlled for birth weight, mother's weight, ethnicity and income. About a quarter of the preschool aged study population went to bed after 9.00 pm. The study didn't explain why staying up late led to later weight gain. Perhaps allowing children to stay up late is a "surrogate" indicator of lack of supervision, lack of proper management or an over indulgent parental attitude. Perhaps that extends from bedtime to other aspects of behaviour like snacking. Perhaps just being up late gives children an opportunity to eat for an extended period. You don't eat when you are asleep.

Very obese

Obese

Overweight

Body Mass Index

Healthy

Underweight

HEIGHT (Feet and Inches)

	4'10"	5'0"	2"	4"	6"	8"	10"	6'0"	2"	4"	6"	
126	59 58 56 55 53 52 50 49 48 47 46 45 44 43 42 41 40 39 38 37 36 36 35 34 34 33 32 32											20st
124	58 57 55 54 52 51 50 48 47 46 45 44 43 42 41 40 39 38 37 37 36 35 34 34 33 32 32 31											7lb
122	57 56 54 53 51 50 49 48 47 46 44 43 42 41 40 39 38 38 37 36 35 35 34 33 32 32 31 30											
120	56 55 53 52 51 49 48 47 46 45 43 43 42 41 40 39 38 37 36 36 35 34 33 33 32 31 31 30											19st
118	55 54 52 51 50 49 47 46 45 44 43 42 41 40 39 38 37 36 36 35 34 33 33 32 31 31 30 30											7lb
116	54 52 52 50 49 48 46 45 44 43 41 40 39 38 37 37 36 35 34 34 33 32 31 31 30 30 29											
114	54 52 51 49 48 47 46 45 44 43 41 40 39 39 38 37 36 35 34 34 33 32 32 31 30 30 29 29											18st
112	53 51 50 48 47 46 45 44 43 42 41 40 39 38 37 36 35 35 34 33 32 32 31 30 30 29 29 28											
110	52 50 49 48 46 45 44 43 42 41 40 39 38 37 36 36 35 34 33 32 32 31 30 30 29 29 28 27											7lb
108	51 49 48 47 46 44 43 42 41 40 39 38 37 37 36 35 34 34 33 33 32 31 31 30 29 29 28 28 27											17st
106	50 48 47 46 45 44 42 41 40 39 38 38 37 36 35 34 33 33 32 31 31 30 29 29 28 28 27 26											
104	49 47 46 45 44 43 42 41 40 39 38 37 36 35 34 34 33 32 31 31 30 29 29 28 28 27 27 26											7lb
102	48 47 45 44 43 42 41 40 39 38 37 36 35 34 34 33 32 31 31 30 29 28 28 27 27 26 25											
100	47 46 44 43 42 41 40 39 38 37 36 35 35 34 33 32 32 31 30 30 29 28 28 27 27 26 26 25											16st
98	46 45 44 43 41 40 39 38 37 36 36 35 34 33 32 32 31 30 30 29 28 28 27 27 26 26 25 24											7lb
96	45 44 43 42 40 39 38 37 37 36 35 34 33 32 32 31 30 30 29 28 28 27 27 26 26 25 25 24											
94	44 43 42 41 40 39 38 37 36 35 34 33 33 32 31 30 30 29 28 28 27 27 26 25 25 24 24 23											15st
92	43 42 41 40 39 38 37 36 35 34 33 33 32 31 30 30 29 28 28 27 27 26 25 25 24 24 23 23											7lb
90	42 41 40 39 38 37 36 35 34 33 33 32 31 30 30 29 28 28 27 27 26 25 25 24 24 23 23 22											
88	41 40 39 38 37 36 35 34 34 33 32 31 30 30 29 28 28 27 27 26 25 25 24 24 23 23 22 22											14st
86	40 39 38 37 36 35 34 34 33 32 31 30 30 29 28 28 27 27 26 25 25 24 24 23 23 22 22 21											7lb
84	39 38 37 36 35 35 34 33 32 31 30 30 29 28 28 27 27 26 25 25 24 24 23 23 22 22 21 21											
82	38 37 36 35 35 34 33 32 31 30 30 29 28 28 27 26 26 25 25 24 24 23 23 22 22 21 21 20											13st
80	38 37 36 35 34 33 32 31 30 30 29 28 28 27 26 26 25 25 24 24 23 23 22 22 21 21 20 20											7lb
78	37 36 35 34 33 32 31 30 30 29 28 28 27 26 26 25 25 24 24 23 23 22 22 21 21 20 20 19											
76	36 35 34 33 32 31 30 30 29 28 28 27 26 26 25 25 24 23 23 22 22 21 21 20 20 19 19											12st
74	35 34 33 32 31 30 30 29 28 28 27 26 26 25 24 24 23 23 22 22 21 21 20 20 19 19 18											
72	34 33 32 31 30 30 29 28 27 27 26 26 25 24 24 23 23 22 22 21 21 20 20 19 19 18 18											7lb
70	33 32 31 30 30 29 28 27 27 26 25 25 24 24 23 23 22 22 21 21 20 19 19 19 18 18 18 17											
68	32 31 30 29 29 28 27 27 26 25 25 24 24 23 22 22 21 21 20 20 19 19 18 18 18 18 17 17											11st
66	31 30 29 29 28 27 26 26 25 24 24 23 23 22 22 21 21 20 20 19 19 19 18 18 18 17 17 16											7lb
64	30 29 28 28 27 26 26 25 24 24 23 23 22 22 21 21 20 20 19 19 18 18 18 17 17 17 16 16											
62	29 28 28 27 26 25 25 24 24 23 22 22 21 21 20 20 19 19 18 18 18 17 17 16 16 16 15											10st
60	28 27 27 26 25 25 24 23 23 22 22 21 21 20 20 19 19 19 18 18 17 17 17 16 16 16 15 15											7lb
58	27 26 26 25 24 24 23 23 22 22 21 21 20 20 19 19 18 18 18 17 17 17 16 16 16 15 15 15 14											
56	26 26 25 24 24 23 22 22 21 21 20 20 19 19 18 18 18 17 17 17 16 16 16 15 15 15 14 14											9st
54	25 25 24 23 23 22 22 21 21 20 20 19 19 18 18 18 17 17 17 16 16 16 15 15 15 14 14 14 13											7lb
52	24 24 23 23 22 21 21 20 20 19 19 18 18 18 17 17 16 16 16 15 15 15 14 14 14 14 13 13											
50	23 23 22 22 21 21 20 20 19 19 18 18 17 17 17 16 16 15 15 15 14 14 14 14 13 13 13 12											8st
	1.48	1.52	1.56	1.60	1.64	1.68	1.72	1.76	1.80	1.84	1.88	1.92 1.96 2.00	

HEIGHT (Metres)

WEIGHT (Kilograms) · WEIGHT (Stones and Pounds)

Diagram BMI (BMI1)

Calorie Intake:

Current advice:

Male: 2200-2800 KCals Female 1500-1800 KCals/day

11 million British citizens are on a diet at any given time (Sun Times 11/1/15)

A fifth of secondary school children are obese at school entry aged 12.

Cancers known to be weight associated include breast, (9kg excess weight increases risk 40%, 30 kg doubles the risk, BMIs >30 increase the risk 10 fold) prostate, ovary, oesophagus, pancreas, colon, rectum, endometrium, kidney, thyroid and gallbladder. In fact (Lancet 2014:10.1016/S0140-6736 etc) a high BMI was found to be associated with 17 of 22 common cancers, varying in degree. There was, in this research, a linear relationship between each 5kg/m2 increase in BMI and uterine, cervical, gall bladder, renal and thyroid cancers as well as leukaemia. There was also a relationship with liver, colon, ovary and post menopausal breast tumours, although other factors complicate the direct relationship.

In 2002 – and it has deteriorated since, 26% of the USA population were obese

21%   UK

6.8%   Swiss

2.9%   Japanese

Even more worrying, 1/3 boys in the UK <6years old are overweight or obese, rising to 50% by the age of 16.

In 2014 28% of UK adults were obese (BMI>30)

In 2014 62% were overweight with a BMI >25

The latest figures (2016) are that 64% of adults in the UK are overweight or obese (65% men and 58% women)

Globally the percentage of adults with a BMI>25 increased from 23% to 34% between 1980 and 2008.

Any statistic I quote that is a few years old will underestimate any obesity problem.

In Australia they suggest 2 portions of fruit and 5 of vegetables each day as being the healthy diet for all. Certainly vegetables have more useful anti oxidants, iron and more health giving vitamins than fruits per se. But 47% UK children eat no vegetables other than potato in a week and think chips are part of their 5 a day. 90% fail to eat the 5 a day. "Cruciferous" vegetables (green leafed vegetables, the brassicaceae-cauliflower, cabbage, cress, bok choi, broccoli, Brussels sprouts, etc) and vegetables which are red, purple or blue have an anticancer effect and have many health benefits other than weight control over a long period of regular consumption.

In fact 2/3 of British adults do not manage to eat 5 a day either let alone the new 7 or 10 helpings of fruits and vegetables a day we should be eating according to recent research (2014).

Calorie restriction and weight reduction increases longevity and reduces death rates from diabetes, circulatory diseases and cancer. A 10-30% reduction in calories doubles rat life spans although strangely, being slightly overweight increases life expectancy too. A study of 2.9m people published in JAMA, Jan 2013, seemed to show that people who were overweight but not obese were 6% less likely to die than normal weight people during the study period. Authors explained this by saying perhaps this was because they had a little more reserve to survive serious illness or perhaps by being overweight they attracted more attention from their medical attendants. Neither are very likely I would have thought.

Protein Intake:

The Institute of Medicine recommends a daily intake of:
56 Grams for men and
46 Grams for women with a 25% increase for
athletes, the elderly, those recovering from illness or injury and those who are pregnant or lactating.

Vitamins:

Vitamin A: Improves skin and mucous membranes. It is involved in the health of the immune system, also in night vision. Although the World War Two rumour that bomber and night fighter crew ate carrots to see in the dark was a ploy to keep radar a secret.

Beta Carotene (plant carotenoids are provitamin As) is an anti oxidant, mopping up free radicals. (Free radicals are any reactive oxygen species that cause damage to body macro-molecules, cell death and diseases of aging). Usually the yellow pigment in various fruits and vegetables, over consumption turning your skin yellow too. They reduce ARMD (age related macular degeneration) but high doses in smokers may increase lung cancer. There is some suspicion that high doses increase prostate cancer too. Said to reduce (in very high doses, – 50,000IU with Folic Acid) recurrence and incidence of colonic cancer. Toxicity can be treated by a warm bath with Vitamin C dissolved in it (2oz in a bath of warm water). Exposure to sunshine is now known to be beneficial in health terms, it may age you but it doesn't kill you. Indeed a large Swedish survey (J Int Med. March 16 2016.)showed that smoking and sun exposure gave the same life expectancy as avoiding the sun while not smoking. Indeed all the decades of slip, slop, slap may have been doing us far more harm than good. We certainly all need more Vitamin D but sunburn and significant skin cancers may be avoided by taking extra Vitamin A. The Swedish study reassuring us about sun exposure did not attribute the benefits solely to Vitamin D outright. Sun exposure generally doesn't cause dangerous skin cancer (melanoma), sunburn does. Also melanomas in patients not often exposed to the sun have a worse prognosis than those in tanned patients.

The current RDA for Vitamin A is 0.7mg a day for men and 0.6mg a day for women. (UK)

The Americans say the limits should be: 3,000mcg RAE (or 10,000 IU) of preformed Vit A from supplements, animal sources and fortified foods daily (Babycenter expertadvice)/100mcg in pregnancy, 350mcg in breast feeding (Aptaclub).

Vitamin A is in liver, fish oils, cheese, fortified spreads, yogurt, eggs, carrots, oranges, sweet potatoes, apricots etc.

More than 1.5mg regularly may make older bones brittle so supplements containing Vit A should be avoided in osteoporosis. This is in fact the absolute upper limit to take for any length of time (NHS Choices). This sort of "Overdose level" could be reached by having as little as two servings of liver or liver pate a week. Fish oils contain Vitamin A, and pregnant women should avoid these and vitamin A supplements. Too much vitamin A in pregnancy can be teratogenic and cause liver damage.

The Retinoids used in acne are Vitamin A analogues, Tretinoin being the carboxylic acid form of vitamin A.

Vitamin B1: Thiamine. Essential for CHO metabolism and neurological function. Supplemented in alcohol withdrawal regimes to prevent Wernicke's encephalopathy and Korsakov's Psychosis.

Vitamin B2: Riboflavin. Energy metabolism, skin and visual function.

Vitamin B3: Niacin, Niacinamide, Nicotinic Acid, Nicotinamide. Anti inflammatory, anti-cholesterol, anti acne (Nicam gel) and anxiolytic in its different forms. Has recently (2015) been found at a dose of 500mg BD for 1 year to reduce skin cancer (BCCs and SCCs) recurrence by 23%, reduces actinic keratoses, in Australians. Niacin causes flushing, niacinamide does not. It is found naturally in various foods and in high levels in "organ meats and brewer's yeast". In combination with fish oils has been used to reduce stroke damage- presumably via the effect both have on micro circulation.

Vitamin B4 is a former designation given to a number of compounds which are no longer considered essential vitamins. It includes Adenine, one of the key bases of nucleic acids RNA and DNA is a constituent of of ATP.

Vitamin B5: Pantothenic Acid: Involved in energy metabolism. Deficiency very rare.

Vitamin B6: Pyridoxine. Good at hormonal mood stabilisation. (ie PMT) >50mg/day is said to cause peripheral neuropathy, the general public can only buy 10mg. Depleted by long term NSAID use.

Vitamin B7: ("Vitamin H") Biotin. Involved in fatty acid synthesis, gluconeogenesis and the metabolism of amino acids. Produced by intestinal bacteria in abundance. Deficiency may be an issue in alcoholics, smokers, possibly in some pregnant women. Lack affects skin and hair initially.

Vitamin B9 Folic Acid: Important to DNA Metabolism, aids rapid cell division and growth (childhood and pregnancy), RBC metabolism. Found in green leaves, bread, fortified cereals. Deficiency causes neural tube defects in foetuses, macrocytic anaemia, glossitis, supplements decrease CVAs etc.

Folic Acid may improve fertility and sperm quality, it reduces Homocysteine levels and stroke risk. (Ischaemic but not haemorrhagic – check B12 first).

One study showed 300-400ug/day reduces CVA risk. The China Stroke Prevention Trial 2008-2013-showed 800ug was effective. Another showed combining 0.8mg Folic Acid with Enalapril reduced stroke risk by 21%.(Also helped specifically by thiazides). Its effect on different cancers at different stages varies. Generally Folic Acid and B vitamin supplementation is considered to be beneficial in heart disease (via lowered homocysteine) and anti cancer – but also a number of anticancer drugs are anti – folate. Oral Folinic acid as a mouthwash reduces chemotherapy glossitis and mouth ulceration.

Pregnancy and Folic Acid: Supplementation prior to conception and following stopping contraception is 0.4mg/day. This reduces the incidence of neural tube defects, (spina bifida, anencephaly), cleft lip, congenital heart disease, abortion, abruption and pre eclampsia as well as autism. Although Folic Acid supplementation has been recommended since 1992 only 28% of pregnant women take pregnancy supplements at the correct time (2016). In the US the incidence of Neural Tube defects has dropped 23% since they started supplementing bread and flour with Folic Acid. A similar policy in the UK would have prevented 1800 cases of NTD cases in the 14 years up to 2012. Supplementation is recommended in Crohn's Disease, Coeliac Disease, epilepsy.

The RDA for pregnant women is 600-800ug/day (twice the normal RDA).

Folic acid comes as 400mcg and 5mg tabs. The public can buy up to 500mcg/day. 5mg/day is needed to reduce the risk of recurrent neural tube defects and may reduce facial cleft defects.

0.4mg/day is the recommended daily dose before pregnancy and up to at least 12 weeks to reduce NTD but 4 or 5mg/day to reduce recurrence. Also 5mg a day if either parent has a NTD, or a FH of NTD, or previous affected pregnancy, or if the mother has malabsorption including Coeliac Disease, or DM, SCA or is taking an AED including Carbamazepine and prophylaxis against abruption. This is at least up to week 12.

Naturally occurring folates are in green vegetables, liver, breakfast cereals, kidneys, yeast, beef extracts, sprouts, cauliflower, green beans, spinach, orange juice, Bovril, milk, fortified Corn Flakes, and bread, most foods in small amounts. It is heat sensitive and soluble.

The highest levels are in lightly cooked sprouts, spinach, soft grain bread and corn-flakes (both fortified) and Bovril.

Doses >500ug/day need a prescription, doses of 5mg a day may cause SACD in the B12 deficient. (Sub Acute Combined Degeneration).

Preparations include 400ug, 5mg Tabs, 2.5mg/5ml susp. Lexpec. Folic Acid supplementation is said to reduce the rate of colonic cancer. See Pregnancy.

In 2016 Scotland decided to fortify its flour with Folic Acid joining the US and 77 other countries.

Folinic Acid is Leucovorin (Calcium Folinate) and is used as an adjuvant in chemotherapy with Methotrexate (as a "rescue") and 5 FU (as adjuvant therapy, making the 5FU more effective). It is a "vitaminer" for Folic Acid, having the full vitamin activity of Folic Acid. The vials of Folinic Acid can be used as a mouth wash in the oral ulceration and mucousitis of chemotherapy.

Vitamin B6 Pyridoxine. Essential in protein metabolism and CNS function. Used therapeutically (and it **does** work) for hormonal depression, mood swings and PMT. 50-100mg/day – but it may take several weeks to start working.

Vitamin B12. Helps maintain the structure of cells, RBCs and CNS function. Deficiency causes macrocytosis, pernicious anaemia, Sub Acute Combined Degeneration of the spinal cord.

60% of breast cancer sufferers are B12 deficient as are 3/4 of vegetarians. Deficiency is surprisingly common. It ranges from 3 to 15% in various adult studies.

Preparations:

Oral Cyanocobalamin (which needs Intrinsic Factor from the stomach to bind and be absorbed in the terminal Ileum, as does natural B12). So oral B12 won't work in the presence of gastric parietal antibodies or with inflammation of the terminal ileum.

Hydroxocobalamin is the injectable form and comes as 1mg/ml amps. – (and can also be used as an antidote in Cyanide poisoning). The dose in pernicious anaemia is: 500ug IM on alt days for 2 weeks, then 250ug weekly until normal FBC, then 1mg every 3m. In pernicious anaemia WITH "neurological involvement" the dose is: 1mg IM on alternate days while improvement is occurring, maintenance 1mg IM every 2m. Hopefully you will never see B12 deficiency reach that severity. The oral form (assuming the patient has some residual Intrinsic Factor) is Cyanocobalamin 50-150ug/day. (Endorse scrip "SLS").

It is hard to overdose on B12 as it is water soluble and just overflows into the urine.

The **Schilling Test** detects Pernicious Anaemia. This is done thus: First replace the deficient B12 stores before the test – this can take weeks. Then on the day of the test, give an oral radio labelled B12 dose, then 1 hour later an IM injection of unlabelled B12 to saturate liver and other body stores so that any absorbed B12 spills straight out into the urine. Then a 24 hr urine collection is performed. A normal result is at least 10% of the radiolabelled B12 found in the urine in 24 hrs. A second test after the co administration of

Intrinsic Factor and labelled B12 then demonstrates malabsorption due to terminal ileitis. Vegans are recommended to take regular B12 supplements by their Society.

Antidepressants are supposed to work better if B12 is given too. Apparently Hitler and many 1930s film stars had their weekly shots of B12 to keep their morale up.

B-17, Laetrile (synthetic) and Amygdalin (natural) may have some anti cancer effect. Found in apricot kernels. High doses of B vitamins (B6, B8 and B12) can reduce the symptoms of schizophrenia (Psychological Medicine).

Vitamin C: Aids connective tissue integrity, Iron absorption (non meat sources), healing, infection (WBC integrity), Biotin, protein and fat metabolism. An antioxidant. Intravenous Vitamin C improves the efficacy of various chemotherapy regimes and cancer survival and in high doses IV is effective against EB virus infections, reducing EB virus antibody levels during active infection.

Vitamin D: Regulates calcium absorption, growth of bones and teeth. Deficiency is associated with a large variety of cancers and medical conditions from prostate cancer to Alzheimers.(See elsewhere)

Vitamin E: Protects cell structure and lipids against oxygenation. An anti oxidant (is said to mop up "free radicals")

Vitamin K: Blood clotting.

Minerals:

Calcium: (Normal 2.2-2.6 mmol/li) is needed for the normal function, growth and structure of bones and teeth. Prescribed with Bisphosphonates, Vitamin D, HRT in osteoporosis/osteopoenia. Calcium is also essential to the normal function of nerves and muscle. Hypocalcaemia (Hypoparathyroidism, low vitamin D, CKD), causes tetany, ECG changes, seizures.

Hypercalcaemia can cause renal and biliary stones, bone pain, abdominal pain, polyuria, depression and cognitive dysfunction. Found in cheese dairy products, fish.

Red wine protects slightly against osteoporosis in men and probably women, yet another of its beneficial medicinal effects.

Calcium supplementation may adversely affect cholesterol and carotid intima-media thickness in post menopausal women (Am J Clin Nutr 2013). Many believe calcium supplementation in the asymptomatic elderly can lead to coronary artery disease and renal calculi without improving bone density (although the coronary artery harm is disputed: (World Congress on Osteoporosis, April 16, Abstract P311)) 2000-2500mg/day is said to be safe from a CVS point of view. The current consensus seems to be that the universal supplementation of Vitamin D and/or Calcium in normally active adequately nourished people of any age, who are not institutionalised or otherwise special cases, is unnecessary. It can be harmful.

Phosphorous is needed for skeletal function

Potassium: See below for foods rich in potassium – but most fruits and vegetables are actually fairly rich in this element. Potassium rich foods can lower blood pressure and reduce stroke risk (this in post menopausal women without hypertension). In women with hypertension, potassium supplements reduce death rates but oddly not stroke risk. (Stroke Sept 2014 10.1161.). More recent evidence seems to suggest that supplementing magnesium, potassium and calcium may lower stroke risk. The American Dept of Agriculture suggests a potassium intake (for women) of 4,700mg/day. WHO suggests 3,510mg.

Magnesium is needed for good skeletal, nerve and muscle function. It is important in energy metabolism and in cardiovascular function. As many as two thirds of teenagers and the elderly may be consuming two thirds of their daily needs or less. There was a lot of Internet chatter after the sudden unexpected cardiac death of Carrie Fisher that she may have died of Hypomagnesaemia. (G. Lundberg Feb 2017 Medscape). Magnesium protects against osteoporosis. Magnesium may be malabsorbed during PPI or lost in diuretic therapy. 30% of alcoholics are hypomagnesaemic. Other causes include antibiotic therapy, Digitalis, Cisplatin, Ciclosporin, Mycophenolate therapy. Lack of Vitamin D, B6 or selenium deficiency, various forms of diarrhoea, zinc supplementation, diabetes (glycosuria), acute MI, malabsorption, pancreatitis etc. Magnesium is found in soya beans, pasta, seafood, nuts (particularly almonds, peanuts and cashews), pulses, melons, mango, sweet corn, jacket potatoes, bananas, green leaves, particularly spinach, whole grains, oats, wheat germ, brown rice, black beans, kidney beans, whole wheat bread and salmon (Atlantic). High levels of dairy calcium in the diet depress serum magnesium and Vitamin D. Tea, coffee, alcohol, sugar, fat and physical activity lower magnesium levels. Magnesium supplementation reduces the incidence of colorectal cancer and migraine.

The commonest cause of raised magnesium seems to be iatrogenic. It may be a good idea to put everyone on a PPI on extra magnesium.

(Less than 0.7mmol/li is hypomagnesaemia)

40% adults are Magnesium deficient in the West. Low Magnesium reduces Vitamin D synthesis. Instead of giving our elderly patients calcium we should probably be giving them magnesium.

The adult supplementary dose of magnesium is 320mg (F) or 420mg (M)/day of the citrate or other salts.

Copper is, with Zinc and Magnesium part of an anti oxidant enzyme system. Used by the body in melanin, bone and iron metabolism. Found in meat, fish, pulses.

Zinc is involved in Vitamin C absorption, helps prevent prostate cancer and is prevented from being absorbed itself by fat. Zinc mainly comes from meat and is one of the dietary constituents that probably needs to be supplemented in vegetarians.

Zinc and Vitamin C really do prevent upper respiratory tract viral infections but the only forms of zinc that are active are Zinc Acetate and Gluconate (the former has been shown to cut the duration of colds in half). No other form of zinc has been shown to be effective (-so this excludes most effervescent Vitamin C and Zinc that I have looked at in pharmacies in the UK!) Zinc supplements increase the number and function of T Cells in older people. 30% of nursing home residents are deficient in Zinc and more likely to develop pneumonia infections. Apparently Zinc supplements taste much worse if your levels are replete.

As well as playing a role in immunity, zinc is important in wound healing, sexual function and in the proper function of sight, taste and smell.

Zinc decreases more than any other metallic mineral in milk as breast feeding continues and like most others, decreases slightly if breast milk is pasteurised. Its level in breast milk is not affected by maternal age or supplements. Regular supplementation should be between 7.5 and 15mg/day. (Shallenberger, Second Opinion Dec 2016).

Chromium Used in glucose and lipid metabolism. In wholegrain cereal.

Iodine: Thyroid metabolism and in regulating BMR. In seafood, dairy products, grain.

Iron. Part of Haemoglobin, the oxygen carrying red cell metalloprotein. Found in liver, red meat, cereals. Iron deficiency and the secondary hypochromic, microcytic anaemia are common. The various causes include menorrhagia, pregnancy, (haemodilution in pregnancy lowers maternal haemoglobin as well as the iron demands of the baby), blood loss elsewhere, especially gastro intestinal bleeding (see GI section). Iron deficiency with no obvious cause or which persists or in an older patient should always be assumed to be due to gastro intestinal bleeding and investigated. NSAID treatment is a frequent cause of upper GI blood loss, peptic ulcer and GI malignancy need to be excluded. Other causes include Angiodysplasia, CKD, IBD, oesophagitis. Epistaxes and the various causes of haematuria. Poor iron absorption, which includes poor diet, coeliac disease, vegetarianism and veganism of course.

Manganese: With copper and Zinc, part of an anti oxidant enzyme system. Used in the metabolism of bones, sex hormones, nerves and joints. In greens, nuts, whole cereals.

Molybdenum: Involved in Iron and Uric Acid metabolism. Needed for normal male sexual function. Found in vegetables, pulses, cereals.

Selenium: Antioxidant, involved in thyroid metabolism. Controversially, deficiency has been linked to some forms of cancer, -stomach and breast, exacerbations of prostate and melanoma, even infections with TB and HIV. Found in cereals, nuts (esp. fresh Brazil), kidney, liver, garlic, tuna, oily fish, onions, sunflower seeds, wheat germ, eggs, even chicken breast.

It is possible that more than 55mcg daily Selenium supplementation may increase the risk of developing diabetes. Free Radic Biol Med. 2013 Dec;65:1557-64. doi: 10.1016/j. freeradbiomed. 2013.04.003. Epub 2013 Apr 16. – although the relationship between Selenium and diabetes is complicated.

Also, although Selenium supplements used to be thought of as benefitting prostate tissue, one study, JNCI Feb 21 2014, demonstrated an increased risk of aggressive prostate cancer if the patient already has high (toe nail) body levels of Selenium. If the patient has low body levels of Selenium, Vitamin E supplements increase the risk of prostate cancer too.

Various studies have shown that Selenium supplementation slows disease progression in thyroiditis. (80-200ug/day). The FDA in America recommends at least 55ug/day of Selenium for adults up to "a tolerable upper intake level of" 400ug.

Zinc: Is involved in Vitamin A and C metabolism, immune function, tissue repair and for smell and taste function. Found in meat, eggs, some seeds, wheat germ, oysters, pork, greens. Supplementation reduces prostate cancer, deficiency showing as white finger nail flecks. Many people believe Zinc, especially with Vitamin C improves resistance to viral infections. In a meta analysis published in 2015 it was only Zinc Acetate and to a lesser extent Gluconate that were found to have a significant anti viral effect. This is postulated to be via its anti rhinoviral activity, the stimulation of interferon gamma and through its effect on a cell surface molecule ICAM-1. Ionic zinc also has an anti histaminic effect, reducing nasal congestion, rhinorrhoea etc. The dose is at least 75mg, best administered topically over a longish period as a lozenge. None of the OTC fizzy zinc and Vitamin C that I could find in UK retail stores had zinc in either the Acetate or Gluconate form.

Typical Multivitamins: Which I have prescribed for 25 years for post viral malaise, Glandular Fever and other forms of generalised tiredness, brief episodes of mild depression where physical symptoms predominate, especially where a healthy mixed diet is unlikely, include such preparations as Forceval. These are large capsules, quite hard to swallow and very much a reminder of the doctor in your pocket. I suggest that adults take 3 a day for 10 days then 1 a day for a couple of months. This nearly always improves wellbeing and energy levels and solves the acute problem. I would, of course, have examined, spoken to and talked up the effect to be gained from this treatment before writing the scrip-and this process is no doubt as much a part of the treatment as the Red/Brown Gelatine Capsule itself.

Forceval Caps (24 Vitamins and Trace Elements for adults, 22 for children). You could try any other multivitamin preparation, for instance Dalavit drops.etc instead.

Too many vitamins: It is obviously true that someone who is well and eating a proper mixed diet shouldn't need extra vitamin supplementation. You should certainly be a little careful about too much Vitamin A in pregnancy. It is equally true that many people take huge doses of vitamins and other supplements which may occasionally do them harm. There have been some associations between high dose Vitamin A and bone fractures, high dose vitamin E and lung cancer. Are many of our patients deficient in vitamins? Given the fact that most children eat such a vegetable poor diet and the vast majority of their vegetable intake is potato, it seems inevitable that subclinical vitamin C, Vitamin D, B vitamin and iron deficiency will be present in a significant number of patients. Many vegetarians are at least Zinc and B12 deficient. Possibly iron, vitamin D, Creatine and carnosine should be supplemented too. Most adults in the UK would benefit from taking Vitamin D supplements, not only by virtue of their bone metabolism but by the reduction of a large number of other illnesses and cancers. Rickets is increasingly common in certain subgroups and all adults seem to be chronically Vitamin D deficient with several diseases more frequent as a consequence. Many recommended daily allowances of vitamins are inadequate. The RDA for vitamin D can be made in the skin during less than one minute of bright sunlight exposure on a naked pink body.

Nutrition:(Calories)

Protein gives 4.1 KCal/gr.
Carbohydrate 4.1 KCal/gr.
Fats 9.2KCal/gr.
1Kg Adipose tissue =7000 Kcalories fat
1ml of wine gives 1 KCal.

GDA: (Guideline Daily Amounts)	Female	Child	Men
Energy	2000Kcal	1800	2,500
Protein	45gr	24	55
Carbohydrate	230gr	220	300
of which sugars	90gr	85	120
Fat	70gr	70	95
of which saturates	20gr	20	30
Fibre	24gr	15	24
Salt	6gr	4	6

Approximate Calorie expenditure per hour:	90kg	60kg
Average male sitting in a room	84	
Average male sitting in a sauna	120-150	
Average Dancing	340	210
Serious dancing	460	285
Golf	440	270
Riding a horse slowly	270	165

Trotting	550	338
Climbing a mountain	800	500
Rowing gently	400	250
Rowing machine 20/min	1100	680
Running 5.5mph	890	530
9mph 2.5% uphill	1500	900
Skiing downhill	790	480
Football	730	450
Squash	850	520
Breast stroke 20yds/min	390	240
Crawl 20yds/min	390	240
Tennis vigorous	800	490
Walking 2mph	290	176
Wrestling	1050	640

Source AAHPERD Virginia USA

Calories, sugar and cardiovascular risk:

The average Briton eats 30kg of sugar a year and if your diet consists of a significant amount of added sugar, your cardiovascular risk is greatly increased. Indeed, research published in 2014/5 suggested sugar was as bad or worse than salt as a cardiovascular risk factor. If a quarter of your daily calories are from added sugar then your risk of cardiovascular disease is 3X greater than someone who derives less than 10% of their calories from added sugar. In a paper published in JAMA Jan 2014, those who derived 17-21% of their calories from added sugar had a 38% higher risk of dying from cardiovascular disease. Over 21% of sugar calories and the CVS risk was more than doubled. Natural sugars in fruits do not have this effect but sucrose and fructose (corn syrup) are particularly implicated in hypertension. Most American adults consume the equivalent of 22 teaspoons full of sugar per day and I expect the UK isn't far behind. The American Heart Association recommends 6 teaspoons full of sugar or fewer for women (100Kcals) per day and 9 teaspoons full of sugar (150Kcals) or fewer for men.

A can of fizzy drink has 35 grm, 8.75 teaspoons of sugar, – 140 Kcals. (American Heart Association)

New food labelling is confusing as it may give the food as a percentage of "total sugar" rather than a percentage of the lower "added sugar" per day. For instance added ("free") sugar should be no more than 5% of energy intake. (30g/day for an adult) and it should form no more than a third of the total 90gr of all sugars in food. In which case a 330ml can of Coca cola has 35gr sugar (9 tsp). This is actually 117% of the recommended daily intake of sugar (added) though only 39% of total sugars. In other words one whole can of normal coke is too much **added sugar** for an adult to have in one day.

But fizzy drinks aren't the only sweet liquids we imbibe: A 250mls serving of:

Pure red grape juice has	41grm sugar!!
Coca Cola has	26.5grm sugar
Fresh squeezed orange juice has	24grm sugar!!
Milk	12.5grm
Double gin and normal tonic has	10grm (50mls gin 200mls tonic)
Tea with two sugars	8grm
Dry Chardonnay	1grm

Diet, food and antioxidants:

Anti oxidants and heart disease: Free radicals are associated with compromised anti oxidant protection which causes atherosclerosis via PUFAs in LDL. Anti oxidants in the diet thus prevent LDL oxidation by free radicals and reduce atherosclerosis. (LDLs are only atherogenic when oxidised). Antioxidants prevent this: eg Vitamin E, Beta Carotene, Vitamin C, Selenium, Flavonoids in red wine, Gluthathione. Mono-unsaturates and saturates are less vulnerable than polyunsaturates. Anti oxidants also protect against cancers.

Antioxidant nutrients involved in protection against oxygen free radicals include: Copper, Zinc, Manganese, Selenium, Vitamin E (may protect against cataracts too) specifically Alpha Tocopherol, Vitamin C, Beta carotene and other carotenoids, Vitamin A, Riboflavin, Vitamin B2 etc.

The dietary sources of the main anti oxidants: Vitamin E: Vegetable oils, nuts, whole grains, Tocopherols: seeds, sweet potatoes, margarine, liver, Tocotrienol (Vitamin E family): yolk, dark green vegetables, Carotenes (600 compounds): yellow, green and orange veg. and fruits, carrots, mangoes, apricots, spinach, kale, greens, watercress, broccoli, green beans, spinach, peppers etc. Vitamin C: Fruit and veg, kiwi, blackcurrants, strawberries, green peppers, bean sprouts, new potatoes. Flavonoids: – (3000 compounds), coloured fruit and veg. (skins), apples, onions, potatoes, tea, red wine. Ubiquinone-10: soya beans, sardines, mackerel, nuts, wheat germ, beans, garlic, spinach, other veg. Selenium: grains, fish, liver, pork, cheese, egg, walnuts, brazil nuts.

Electrolytes:

High **Potassium** Foods: (over 250mg/100gr):

Boiled Spinach*	Roast chicken (meat only) *
Raw celery	Lean grilled lamb chop*
Boiled parsnips	Lean grilled pork chop*
Boiled beetroot*	Lean grilled rump steak*
Boiled new potatoes*	Lean grilled bacon*
Chips**	Grilled pork sausage
Boiled haricot beans*	Cod in batter*
Canned beans in tomato sauce*	Fried haddock*
Dried dates** Figs**	Fried plaice
Dried raisins** Prunes**	Fried scampi*
Bananas*	
Raw tomatoes Lima beans**	
Fresh pineapple	
Molasses	
Seaweed**	
Tree nuts **	
Avocados**	
Bran**	
Wheat germ**	

*The highest levels of potassium. **The very highest

In this list the highest sodium levels are rather predictably: The canned and processed peas, the baked beans (presumably not the low salt version), the bacon, the pork sausage, the fried haddock and plaice. The lowest salt containing foods were the raw fruits, the runner beans, frozen peas, boiled sprouts, cabbage, cauliflower (not spinach and not raw celery).

Salt: (Sodium)

We should all know that salt is a contributor to many bodily ills. 5gr/day is the recommended intake. The body is 0.15% sodium and 0.15% chlorine by weight, a total of only 210 gms sodium chloride. In evolutionary terms our predecessors ate no more than 0.24 gm salt daily for millions of years. But as communities and societies developed we ate more fish, meat and preserved food and our sodium intake increased. Now most people ingest 9-12 gm salt/day. 80% is added by manufacturers, only 15% at the table.

Virtually every human on the planet ingests too much salt. Reducing salt intake positively improves the outlook in hypertension, cardiovascular and chronic renal disease.

Prepared bought food, tinned food, packet food, crisps, sauces and processed food are usually high in salt. Most cooks add salt during the cooking process to enhance flavour and our palates grow up used to this. Just look at the salt in some "big names" pasta sauces to see how much salt is being added to your family's diet without you knowing it. Salt and sugar are the new cholesterol.

Salt intake elevates population blood pressure, an increase of 6 gr/day raising SBP by 9mm Hg over 30 years. On the other hand, reducing dietary salt has a fairly brisk reverse effect. Reducing salt by 4.4 gr/day for 4 weeks lowers SBP by 4mm Hg. (and DBP by 2mm Hg)

Salt has a direct effect on arterial walls, causing them to be less elastic, it increases BP and counteracts the effects of antihypertensives working on the Renin-Angiotensin system.

In CKD sodium excretion is reduced and patients are even more sensitive to dietary sodium. Salt increases BP even more in CKD and it counteracts the effects of drugs acting on the Renin Angiotensin system even more in CKD than in patients with healthy kidneys. There is on average, 40% less salt in bread (2017) than there was 10 years ago (Today programme).

Salt content: (from my kitchen cupboard)

Heinz ketchup has	0.3 grm/serving
	1.8 grm/100 grm
Fruit and Fibre Cereal	1 grm/100 grm
Taste the Difference salted caramels	0.1 grm/chocolate
Panetone	0.23 grm/slice
Heinz Baked Beans	2.4 grm/can
Dolmio Bolognese Sauce	0.8 grm/100 grm
Gravy granules	0.8 grm/70mls serving
Newman's BBQ Sauce	Na 1.3 grm/100 grm
Sultana fingers	1 grm/100 grm
Sainsbury's Basic Salsa	0.43 grm/50 grm serving

Grapefruit Juice:

A CYP3A4 inhibitor (via Bergamottin)

Avoid with Cyclosporin, most Calcium Channel Blockers, incl. Verapamil, Dihydropyridines (Amlodipine, Felodipine etc), Terfenadine, Saquinavir (An Antiretroviral), Ritonavir, Cyclosporin, Tacrolimus, Omeprazole, Midazolam, Triazolam,

Zolpidem, Sertraline, Fluvoxamine, Trazadone, Buspirone, Quetiapine, statins except Pravastatin, benzodiazepines, Losartan, Dextromethorphan, Repaglinide, antiarrythmics, Amiodarone, Dronaderone, Quinidine, Propafenone, Carvedilol, all the Sildenafil Type drugs, Codeine, Tramadol, Methadone, Buprenorphine, Oxycodone (but not Morphine), Oral Marijuana, Carbamazepine, Mebendazole (Vermox).

The following list of Grapefruit Interactions is published by the Canceractive website which specialises in dietary advice on treating cancer. Grapefruit juice can affect cytotoxic therapy significantly and since it actually tastes fairly unpleasant why not suggest blueberry, raspberry or cherry juice each of which have anti cancer (anti oxidant) properties?

Crizotinib, cyclophosphamide, dasatinib, erlotinib, everolimus, imatinib, lapatinib, nilotinib, pazopanib, sorafenib, sunitinib, vandetanib, venurafenib, repaglinide, saxagliptin, albendazole, artemether, erythromycin, etravirine, halofantrine, maraviroc, praziquantel, primaquine, quinine, rilpivirine, saquinivir, budesonide-oral, colchicine, methylprednisolone-oral, atorvastatin, lovastatin, simvastatin, amiodarone, amlodipine, apixaban, cilostazol, clopidogrel, dronedarone, eplerenone, ergotamine, felodipine, losartan, manidipine, nicardipine, nifedipine, nimodipine, nisoldipine, nitrendipine, propafenone, quinidine, rivaroxaban, sibutramine, sildenafil, tadalafil, ticagrelor, vardenafil, aprepitant, alfentanil-oral, buspirone, carbamazepine, dextromethorphan, diazepam, fentanyl-oral, fluvoxamine, ketamine-oral, lurasidone, methadone, midazolam, -oral, oxycodone, pimozide, quazepam, quetiapine, sertraline, triazolam, ziprasidone, estradiol, ethinylestradiol, cisapride, domperidone, cyclosporine, everolimus, sirolimus, tacrolimus, darifenacin, festerodine, solifenacin, silodosin, tamsulosin.

Grapefruit juice does not affect systemically administered drugs but its affect on the above can last 24hrs. Not all these interactions are clinically noticeable of course.

Coffee:

Coffee, once considered a relative health disadvantage through its caffeine content and possible pancreatic cancer risk has now been medically rehabilitated. 2.25 billion cups are drunk worldwide each day. (7 million tons of coffee beans consumed a year). Contemporary studies now suggest various benefits including:

In Parkinson's Disease, diabetes mellitus, symptomatic gall bladder disease, CVA and in a variety of chronic liver diseases. These include in NAFLD (Non alcoholic fatty liver disease) alone, steatohepatitis in NAFLD, in raised GGT and raised levels of other LFTs, to slow progression of cirrhosis, mortality in cirrhosis, HCC development rates, (Hepato Cellular Carcinoma), improved antiviral response in hepatitis C etc. Coffee enemata were used (are used) as part of the Gerson anti cancer therapy to "detoxify" the liver – if you believe that sort of thing. (See Cancer section). A study in The NEJM in 2014 showed the overall death rate for coffee drinkers is 16% lower than non drinkers. Recent research has shown advantages in the areas of CVS disease (lower coronary calcium scores), Metabolic Syndrome, Type 2 Diabetes, neurodegeneration, (dementia), stroke, liver, kidney and other cancers and malignant melanoma. The dietary Guidelines Committee in the US said in 2015 that up to 5 cups a day (400mg caffeine) were not associated with long term health disadvantages. A 2012 study of 400,000 people (NEJM) demonstrated a 10% all cause reduction in mortality associated with 3-4 cups per day. The anti oxidants in coffee reduce oxidation of LDL and 2 cups a day mitigate against heart failure despite caffeine's temporary hypertensive affect. Despite decades of dogma it doesn't cause ectopics either (!). Various studies over the last decade have produced data showing 1-6 cups a day reduce stroke risk by up to 25%.

The highest coffee consumers have the lowest risk of diabetes. Three or more cups a day produce a 37% lower risk than one cup a day. One and a half cups a day give an 11% lower diabetes risk. Coffee also reduces insulin resistance and increases insulin secretion.

Caffeine reduces gout. Xanthine oxidase metabolises caffeine and makes uric acid. Drinking coffee preoccupies it and takes its mind off making gout crystals.

Cancer seems to be affected by coffee consumption too: Endometrial, prostate, head and neck, BCC, melanoma and breast cancer incidences are reduced by coffee consumption due to its anti mutagenic and antioxidant properties.

Coffee can inhibit dementia progression and depression. One recent study showed that caffeine enhances memory consolidation. It may also be beneficial in PD and MS.

A 2015 study showed, relative to no coffee, pooled mortality was
0.95 for 1 cup a day
0.91 for 1.1 – 3 cups a day
0.93 for 3.1 – 5 cups a day
1.02 for >5 cups a day
Caffeinated and decaffeinated coffee benefits were the same. Smoking however was a "strong confounder" of the benefits of coffee.

Among never smokers, coffee consumption was inversely associated with the mortality risk due to cardiovascular and neurological disease and suicide. For cardiovascular disease:
0.95 for 1 cup a day
0.94 for 1-3 cups a day
0.81 for 3-5 cups a day
0.91 for >5 cups a day
The benefits must come from something other than caffeine, presumably the anti oxidant content, – chlorogenic acid or the lignans etc or one of the thousand other unknown compounds it contains.

JAMA Internal Medicine Oct 2015

HOWEVER: Just before we all rush down to the hospital's branch of Costa or Starbucks, the very latest study of 18-45 year olds from Italy came like an double espresso blast from the past. In this age group with untreated mild hypertension, those who drank 1-3 espressos per day were found to be three times more likely to have a cardiovascular event (usually an MI) within a decade compared with non coffee drinkers. Moreover "heavy coffee drinkers, ie those drinking 4 or more expressos per day, were 4X as likely to have a cardiovascular event as abstainers. (European Soc of Cardiology Congress poster 2015) So there you are: the hypertensive effect of caffeine may be mild but you can become habituated to it and coffee can cause some organ damage along with multiple varied metabolic benefits. Ask a urologist and he or she will tell anyone with bladder symptoms to avoid all caffeine including coffee as abstaining does seem to help symptoms of irritable bladder. Coffee is also thought to contribute to glaucoma development.

While we are on the subject of coffee, Caffeine is in many compound drug preparations and foods:

Caffeine:

Caffeine is a stimulant, causing tachycardia, raising BP and antagonising fatigue and loss of alertness.

It is in coffee, tea, many fizzy drinks, especially the small volume "energy drinks" marketed as such, as well as chocolate, some herbal and over the counter preparations.

Individual sensitivity to caffeine's effects varies enormously. Generally caffeine can cause a physiological response from 15 minutes to up to 7 hours after consumption.

There are 135mg caffeine in an average cup of coffee and there are from 40-120mg in a cup of tea.

A can of fizzy drink may have 35-70mg.

Chocolate has 10-35mg depending on the size of the helping.

So called energy drinks may have up to 300mg in 20oz.

Pure drip coffee 151 mg/ 250mls

Brewed coffee 141 mg/ 250mls

Red Bull Energy 80 mg/ 250mls

Black Tea 5min Brew 77mg/250mls

„   3min Brew 70mg/250mls

„   1min Brew 47mg/250mls

Green Tea 5min Brew 52 mg/250mls

„   3min Brew 45 mg/250mls

„   1min Brew 23 mg/250mls

Coca Cola Classic 25 mg/250mls

(New Scientist March 2017)

Caffeine increases the rate of absorption of analgesics and is included in some compound pain killers.

What are Oily Fish?

Sardines, Herring, Anchovies, Salmon, Trout, Mackerel, Tuna, Marlin, Swordfish, Shark. These fish do not live at the bottom of the sea but forage at various depths. Oily fish concentrate contaminants (Mercury in Minamata disease was in Tuna) and fat soluble vitamins. They are good sources of Omega 3 fatty acids and the consumption of oily fish may reduce dementia, macular degeneration, as well as improving cardiovascular health. There is, however, an upper recommended limit of 4 servings a week (2 for women of child bearing age) due to possible mercury contamination.

White fish tend to be bottom feeders and are not oily (having only oil in their livers eg Cod liver oil) for instance Cod, Haddock and Flatfish. Generally speaking the oilier the fish tastes, the better it is for you-unfortunately.

Farmed salmon nowadays have half the Omega 3 that their wild cousins do. This is because they are not eating wild anchovies.

Oily fish: Reduce your cardiovascular risk and new evidence suggests fish oil supplementation has a protective effect on cognitive function and the maintenance of brain volume in older men and women. Omega 3 supplementation in the last three months of pregnancy also reduces asthma, wheeze and lower respiratory infection for six months in the baby.

The beneficial ones are: Mackerel, Pilchards, Herring, Sardines, Kippers, and Salmon

Less so is the much nicer tasting and less reflux inducing: Tuna.

Omega 3 oils: (Polyunsaturated fatty acids.)

Omega 6 fatty acids are generally found in nuts (walnuts) and seeds and Omega 3s in fish and some vegetable matter. Some research suggests the consumption of 7 grams of Omega 3 oils (EPA and DHA eicosapentaenoic acid and docosahexaenoic acid)

(preferably marine) per week after an MI reduces the risk of recurrence. Omacor was marketed for this. It has been suggested for some time that fish oils had various cardiovascular beneficial effects. 4 small portions or 2 large portions of the right fish a week provide 1 gram of Omega 3 a day.

Other benefits are the reduction of breast cancer (in mice) and reduction of flu (H1N1) infections. The latest research shows Omega 3s may reduce the extent of vascular damage after stroke.

Unfortunately some studies are now throwing up that high blood levels of Omega 3 are associated with high and low grade prostate cancer although this is not *generally* accepted as yet.

A large portion would be 5oz of salmon, mackerel or trout fillet, a 212gr tin of salmon. A small portion 125gr of sardines, 105gr salmon or 100gr smoked salmon.

Omega 3 oils are in high concentrations in:

Flax seeds and oil, Salmon fish oil, Chia seeds, Caviar, Sardine oil, Cod liver oil, Fish Roe, Mackerel, Sprouted Radish seeds, Butternuts, Atlantic Salmon, Walnuts, Fresh Basil, Oregano, Cloves, Marjoram, Walnut oil, Cooked Broccoli, Herring, Spinach, Canola oil, etc.

Generally speaking, animals fed outside before slaughter (organic or wild) and eating their "normal" diet of fresh green grass etc, have flesh, milk and eggs higher in Omega 3 oils than animals reared inside and fed concentrated or dried feed. Organic foods generally have a healthier ratio of omega 3 to 6. This applies to animal and vegetable sources of fatty acids. Over the last century the ratio of Omega 6 to Omega 3 fatty acids in the western diet has dramatically increased. Most people are getting 10-15 times as much Omega 6 as Omega 3. The ideal ratio is between 2 and 3. Organic milk has for instance 25% less Omega 6 and 62% more Omega 3 fatty acids. The ratio of these two types of fatty acid is key to a number of chronic health problems associated with civilisation, especially cardiovascular disease.

Cooking and oils: Avoid frying with sunflower and corn oil now.

Although frying and roasting undoubtedly add to the taste and texture of many foods, the high temperature involved denatures many proteins (roasted meats, egg white etc) carbohydrates and fats (crackling, crisps, roast potatoes and so on) and the oils themselves are chemically changed. The end result is that the oils can become carcinogenic in the long term and that certain oils are worse than others. Roasting and frying are certainly unnatural ways of preparing food but then so is cooking food at all. The least bad oils to cook with are coconut oil, macadamia nut oil, sesame and olive oils. The saturated fat in Palm Oil raises LDL and denatures when heated.

What happens is that when heated above a certain temperature, oils oxidise forming various carcinogenic substances which include aldehydes and lipid peroxides. This happens particularly at higher temperatures, when oil passes its "smoke point". Polyunsaturated oils make more aldehydes when heated and these include corn oil and sunflower oil. Aldehydes promote heart disease, dementia and cancers.

Olive oil, cold pressed rape seed oil, butter and goose fat produce fewer aldehydes when heated as they are richer in monounsaturated and saturated fats which are more stable at high temperatures. Lower levels of less toxic compounds are produced when these oils are heated.

So you and your patients should avoid fats that are polyunsaturated when frying and try to fry below the "smoke point" of the fat. Olive oil is the ideal compromise at 14% saturates, 10% polyunsaturates, extra virgin olive oil giving no extra benefit in cooking. Coconut oil is good too as it is also high in saturates. Keep oils out of sunlight and don't reuse oils you have cooked with as this will concentrate toxic aldehydes and other harmful compounds. Lard is better than polyunsaturates for cooking (who would ever have thought lard had a dietary advantage of any kind?!) though sunflower and vegetable oils are healthy consumed cold. Barbeques and woks rely on very high temperatures and both are likely to be unhealthy forms of food preparation.

Nuts:

The benefits of nuts are mentioned in various other sections. Some have been shown to have anticancer effects, (walnuts and breast, prostate, bowel and lung, pecans against breast and prostate). Most have high levels of trace elements and anti oxidants. Some do have high levels of salicylates and are allergenic. Arachis oil from peanuts is in many dermatological creams and skin preparations. Most are high in magnesium and vitamin E.

Brazil nuts, for instance, contain protein, fibre, selenium, healthy omega 3 oils, vitamin E, magnesium, zinc, and various B vitamins.

Walnuts are particularly high in omega 3 fats. (High ratio of omega 3 to omega 6 fatty acids and a good source of vitamin E). They are not only beneficial in terms of colonic and other cancers but in preventing CVD, DM and some neurological conditions.

Weight reducing and Anorectic Agents:

Dexfenfluramine, Adifax, (caused heart valve and pulmonary problems), Phenteramine, Duromine, Ionamin, Ponderax, Fenfluramine, Reductil, Sibutramine have all been withdrawn during my career due to toxic side effects.

They seemed to be related to amphetamines and worked while they were being taken, had cardiovascular side effects and caused rebound weight gain once you managed to get the patient off them. Then there was Rimonabant, Acomplia (an inverse agonist for a cannabinoid receptor), – withdrawn because of psychiatric reactions.We don't have that many to choose from now.

You can try filling the stomach up with Sterculia (Prefil) or Celevac (Methylcellulose) or giving the patient steatorrhoea with Xenical, Orlistat. (If you do use this, then supplement vitamins, stop if weight loss isn't continuing and warn against pill failure due to malabsorption.)

Newer agents which show some promise include:

Lorcaserin, Belviq (Serotonin RA),

Phentermine/Topiramate SR Qsymia (Sympathomimetic amine and long acting "neurostabiliser"),

Naltrexone/Bupropion SR Contrave Mysimba (Opioid antagonist and antidepressant),

Liraglutide (GLP-1 Agonist) Saxenda, Obese or overweight-with-a-co-morbidity patients and

Canagliflozin (SGLT-2 Inhibitor).

Weight reduction surgery:

(Usually available on the NHS if BMI>40 and weight loss on diet and exercise is not maintained for 6m). Alternatively if the BMI is 35+ and there are associated medical complications (Type 2 DM etc).

Gastric bypass (Gastro enterostomy/Roux en Y),
Vertical or horizontal shrinking gastroplasty,
Gastric balloon,
Gastric sleeve: Midway between a band and a bypass. Can be converted to a bypass if necessary.
Gastric band: with a fluid filled access port under the skin of the chest. (Introduced laparoscopically). **See the diabetes section**. These surgical options all work and "Cure" Type 2DM.- But many patients put the weight back on as soon as the reversible procedure is reversed, some put weight on after a period anyway, many become depressed with or without weight gain.

Calcium in food:
Cheddar 100g 800mg,
Camembert 100g 380mg,
Milk Semi skimmed 1pt 730mg,
Milk Full Cream 1pt 700mg,
Double Cream 100gr 50mg,
Yoghurt 125gr 225mg,
Butter 100gr 15mg,
Milk Chocolate 100gr 220mg,
Plain Chocolate 100gr 40mg,
Muesli 55gr 110mg,
Chapatis 110gr 66mg,
White bread 55gr slice 55mg,
Wholemeal Bread 55gr slice 15mg,
Cornflakes 55gr 2mg,
Canned sardines in oil 100gr 550mg,
Canned pilchards 100gr 300mg,
Cod, poached 100gr 30mg,
Prawns 100gr 55mg,
Pork sausages 100gr 55mg,
Stewed mince 100gr 18mg,
Chicken 100gr 10mg,
Broccoli 100gr raw 100mg,
Spring greens 100gr 90mg,
Baked Beans 100gr 45mg,
Tomatoes raw 100gr 15mg,
Dried figs 100g 300mg,
Orange 100gr 40mg,
White wine 1 glass 14mg,
Red wine 1 glass 7mg,
Coffee/Tea Insignificant.

Calcium

Minimum daily requirement	0-8 years	600mg,
	9-14 yrs	700mg,
	15-17yrs	600mg,
	>18yrs	500mg,
	Pregnancy	1200mg,
	Breast feeding	1200mg,

Smoking, taking oestrogen and alcohol all deplete calcium stores.

Excess dietary calcium alone is not beneficial. It reduces Magnesium and Vitamin D levels and thus can become self defeating if the idea of calcium supplementation had been to strengthen bones. Long term excess dietary calcium alone increases prostate cancer risk and is believed to thicken and harden blood vessel walls and increase renal calculi.

Vitamin C:

Is used intravenously in some cytotoxic regimes to increase the anti tumour effect. It is said to act as an immune booster. It does shorten the duration of colds and some viral infections when taken as a supplement with zinc acetate or gluconate and also improves the healing of wounds, reduces cataract risk and may reduce atheroma formation. Vitamin C supplementation increases iron absorption but large doses orally can cause GI symptoms and kidney stones.

Vitamin D: (See "Pathology")

Is a steroid hormone but not really a vitamin as it can be made in the skin. It seems possible that many of us in cloudy countries (the dark skinned, the fully covered in clothing, the very young, breast feeding, pregnant and over 65s) are virtually always deficient.

The tolerable upper intake level is said by some authors to be 4000 IU/day and it seems likely that most westerners would benefit from supplements of at least this kind of dose. The current standard recommended daily dose has been a tenth of this up until now. **(400 IUs= 10mcg.)** Many safe supplementary doses are over 10,000Us (often guided, especially in the USA by blood levels.) One article I read said you would have to take 40,000 – 100,000IU/day for "many months" before adverse overdose effects occurred (Janet Zand Blog*.) Other expert references say it is just about impossible to take too much vitamin D orally. Supplements should be Vitamin D3 cholecalciferol not D2 ergocalciferol.

Bright sunlight 15-30 minutes a day yields enough Vitamin D in the skin for most bodily purposes. – Unless we cover ourselves completely with clothes or sun block. Indeed, the 400 Us recommended as our RDI can be obtained by standing outside in a loincloth in bright sunshine without sunblock for 18 seconds!! (Barefoot and Reich. The cancer Factor) but who does that these days without sun block anyway? – and at least 2,000-10,000Us are made in the skin from 15-20 minutes of midday sun (Separate ref.*)

So how much Vitamin D should we be supplementing?

For the whole population, a study in summer 2014 showed the average dose to cause an increase in 25 OH Vit D was 4707 IU/day. (Values for ambulatory and nursing home patients were 4229 and 6103 IU/day). Factors that influence the change in Vitamin D levels are the starting level, BMI, age and serum albumin. The race of the patient does not make much difference and the somewhat complicated equation to work out the dose is:

Dose of Vit D in IUs/day to affect a given change in 25 OH Vit D:

Dose= [(8.52-desired change in 25 OH Vit D level) +(0.074xAge) – (0.20X BMI)

+(1.74X Albumin concn) − (0.62X Starting serum25 OH Vit D concn)]/(-0.002)

This equates to 5000Us needed daily to correct deficiency and maintenance is 2000Us/day at least.

Should everyone take extra Vitamin D?

Various references suggest 4,000 − 10,000Us/day to treat and prevent bowel cancer (Nutrient Insider Jan 2015, Vit D Council) and up to 10,000 Us a day protects against deterioration in biopsy positive prostate cancer for instance. A plethora of clinical conditions is now associated with low levels of the vitamin. This is not the same as being able to prevent the conditions by supplementing large populations or at risk groups however and many vitamin D "applications" are currently works in progress. We were almost certainly ill advised when we made generations of patients fearful of getting a suntan. New (2016) evidence shows that long term avoidance of sun exposure is on a par with obesity and smoking or drinking too much as an increased lifestyle risk.

The trouble is that we are all now paranoid about skin damage and melanoma and rarely allow the sun to make this pseudo vitamin in our skin for us. If we are black it is even worse. Several hundred thousand years ago we evolved in African fish eating coastal communities in a hot climate, then moved northwards and westwards and away from the coast. As a consequence we all seem to be suffering from chronic Vitamin D deficiency today. Ricketts is an up and coming disease within populations that have skin covered with melanin or clothing and have emigrated from hot to cold climates. But It isn't only bones that might benefit: supplementing vitamin D seems to reduce a vast and unrelated number of morbidities: Vitamin D has a finger in almost every bodily pie. It is epigenetic and affects at least 200 human genes. Over the last few years Vitamin D deficiency and supplementation have been found to influence dozens of apparently unrelated conditions and bodily functions from dementia to prostate cancer. For instance,

One authoritative study showed that at a level of Vitamin D between 12-20 ng/mL (30 to 50 nmol/L), (low) there was a 17% higher risk of dying from **any** cause compared with the "reasonable levels" of greater than 20 ng/mL (50 nmol/L). For those with low levels of less than 12 ng/mL (30 nmol/L), the risk of dying increased to 71 percent higher than that experienced by subjects with "reasonable levels".

Low to reasonable levels compared gave a 42% greater risk of dying of cancer, a 39% greater risk of dying of cardiovascular disease and a 250% greater risk of dying of respiratory disease.

For bone health 40nmol/li seems to be an adequate serum level of 25 hydroxy vitamin D though.

It seems that Vitamin D triggers and arms the immune system and helps reduce the incidence of various cancers − such as colon and breast. In prostate cancer − eCholecalciferol supplementation 2,000 Us daily stabilises PSA in Bx positive and treated prostate cancer, (Univ Toronto 2014) though high calcium diets increase prostate cancer. Vitamin D has been shown to improve histology in between prostate biopsy and prostatectomy. Vitamin D helps improve the control of infections, the management of diabetes, modify the progress of MS, metabolic syndrome, improves balance, reduces falls and dementia and with calcium supplementation reduces fractures. The latest research shows that low levels of Vitamin D affect cognition and memory and are linked to both depression and schizophrenia. Supplementing Vitamin D does not, it seems, improve depression. There are Vitamin D receptors in memory areas of the brain, the hippocampus and dentate gyrus.

Active vitamin D regulates nerve growth factor and reduces amyloid cortical neuronal damage. The optimal Vitamin D level to prevent dementia is 50nmol/li (possibly, some researchers think, 75nmol/li)

Other reputable studies have shown decreased incidences of Alzheimer's, Parkinson's and Hypertension with Vitamin D supplementation. Vitamin D deficiency makes melanomas more malignant (melanomas not related to sun exposure do have a worse prognosis) – all very confusing given the sun avoidance mantra of the last 30 years – but it does seem that our sun overavoidance may well have done our species, whether pale or dark skinned, more harm than good. Low levels are associated with faster rates of cognitive decline in older (normal) adults and with Macular Degeneration. It affects circulation, acute coronary death, Vitamin D deficiency in one study increased total CVD 27% with a 62% increase in fatal CVD: (Perna Schottker. Dec 2013 J Cl Endoc and Metab).

Overall death rates over a 13 year period (Am J Clin Nut Sept 014) are lower in people with higher levels of vitamin D and it protects brain function after cardiac arrest.

In August 2014 an Iranian study was published showing some improvements in childhood asthma with Vitamin D supplementation but doses were 100,000 U IM initially and 50,000 Us orally each week. They didn't say if the patients were Vitamin D deficient to start with. This effect has been noticed before in a British Study and it was postulated then that Vitamin D affects T Cells (TH17 cells) involved in the inflammatory response in asthma.

A major Danish study published in Dec 2014 related the genes associated with permanently low levels of vitamin D and higher mortality (30% higher generally, with a cancer mortality 40% higher) thus seemingly establishing a one way causal relationship.

Vitamin D appears to act as an anti inflammatory on prostatic cancer via the gene GDF-15.

At the risk of becoming boring, another study in 2014 showed that, in patients with OA knee, (with pain and X ray changes) those with low Vitamin D levels saw their disease progress over a 4 year follow up period and the lower the vitamin D levels the worse the deterioration in pain and arthritis. Supplementing Vitamin D reduces OA knee pain although I doubt that it reverses OA itself. Vegetarians tended in another 2014 study to have worse knee OA than dairy, fish and meat eaters. Yet another reason to be omnivorous.

Yet more: There is a vitamin D receptor on the cell nucleus and this activates part of the genome.

This may modulate up to 2000 genes, some related to inflammation and cellular mutation, both of which are, of course at the route of cancer development. For every 10ng/ml increase in serum Vitamin D the relative colorectal cancer risk drops by 15% (Gandini 2011, Jenab 2010). Other studies have found an association between low vitamin D levels and colorectal cancer incidence and mortality. Chronic recurrent headache may be a symptom of vitamin D deficiency and it may be worth checking levels in this situation. A paper published in the BMJ in Feb 2017 showed a reduction in URTIs with vitamin D supplementation although the NNT was 33. If the patients had a pre existing severe deficiency, the number needed to treat was only 4. (Martineau et Al)

Goodness knows why Vitamin D seems to improve almost every bodily function – unless, because of our evolution around and subsequent migration away from the sunny equator many of us at higher latitudes are now too pale and too deprived of sunshine to function properly. Many people take vitamin supplements but if you are not a vegetarian and you are still going to take extra vitamins, Vitamin D is the one to supplement.

Vitamin D Sources:

Whole milk: 1/3 pint	0.06ug
Semi skimmed milk: 1/3 pint	0.02ug
Cheddar Cheese: 3.5oz	0.26ug
Butter: 3.5oz	0.76ug
Eggs: 3.5oz	1.75ug
Margarine, supplemented: 3.5oz:	7.15ug
Liver, raw: 3.5oz	4.5ug
Tuna, canned: 3.5oz	5.8ug
Salmon, raw, Pacific: 3.5oz	12.5ug
Salmon, raw, Atlantic: 3.5oz	none.

Calcichew D3 Forte 1250mg CaCo3=500mg Ca and 400IU Vit D3 (=5mcg cholecalciferol) Dose is 2 daily.

A sustained intake of 1250ug Vit D/**day (50,000 IU) can cause toxicity**. But note that a piffling 400IU is the current recommended daily intake!

Supplements can come as Vitamin D2 and D3. D2 is the synthetic, less active form. D3 is three times more potent and far more bio available.

Vitamin D3 is in some foods and made in the skin when UVB reacts with 7-Dehydrocholesterol. Birds and furry animals make it in oily skin secretions and absorb it orally from grooming oil from their skin coverings! Indeed sheep lanolin is the source of much commercial Vitamin D.

It is then hydroxylated twice, once by the liver to Calcidiol (25 OH Cholecalciferol or 25 OH Vitamin D), – the level of which is the best guide to Vitamin D status, then in the kidneys to Calcitriol (1, 25 OH Vitamin D) if the kidneys are functioning properly. This twice hydroxylated vitamin D is the most active metabolite of the vitamin.

Amongst other things active Vitamin D then promotes intestinal calcium absorption, promotes bone resorption by stimulating osteoclasts and is, despite this seeming paradox, important for proper bone formation. It has many other roles. There are Vitamin D receptors in the heart, liver, stomach, skin, brain, pancreatic B islet cells, thyroid, parathyroids, adrenals and various immune cells.

Deficiency is generally considered to be 30-50nmol/li 25(OH) D and 50-100nmol/li is considered optimum in most studies.

There is some evidence that *most western adults* are Vitamin D deficient and that supplementing Vitamin D has multiple health benefits other than those related to bones (see above). It is now believed that significant Vitamin D deficiency is very common in the UK, especially in the overweight and dark skinned. In older patients Vitamin D deficiency is associated with falls and huge initial top up doses are safe. For instance 10,000 Us/day for 2 weeks followed by 2000 Us/day in winter and 1000 Us/day in summer (and this assumes 20 minutes a day of sunshine exposure).

To estimate the amount of Vitamin D lacking:

40x (75 – (patient's level) x patient's weight (kg)) eg a 70kg person with a Vit D level of 20 would need 154,000 Us or 10,000 us/day for 15 days, followed by the 1000Us or 2000us on whether it is summer or winter.

So: 2000U/day for 2months then 1000U/day is reasonable for most people!

Vitamin D toxicity is over 375nmol/li – impossible with sensible dosing.

Vitamin D3, Fultium-D3 colecalciferol, 800IU and 3200 IU capsules are intended for pregnant or breast feeding Vitamin D deficient women.

Vitamin E:

When I was training, Vitamin E was a poor cousin of the other vitamins, preventing sterility in rats. It seems to be coming of age now however, with a variety of recognised metabolic influences.

Most products purporting to be Vitamin E are Alpha Tocopherol. Tocotrienols are the other form of Vitamin E and appear to have many of the anti cancer, anti lipid and neuro-protective effects that Tocopherols lack. So just as with other vitamins, it is important to be clear about which form is being consumed/administered. Vitamin E seems to affect the growth of various cancers – breast, liver, pancreatic cancer. It is in various dietary oils as well as asparagus, avocado, kiwi, broccoli, sweet potato, tomatoes etc. It has anti oxidant, fat metabolism, tissue repair, neurological and visual functions, possibly slowing the rate of intellectual decline in Alzheimer's disease (as long as there is no bleeding history, CCF or coronary artery disease). It does not seem to prevent Alzheimer's. Various studies (Cancer Treat 2007 33 and Int J Vit Nut Res 83 (2)) have shown a protective effect against chemo-therapy peripheral neuropathy.

In the SELECT trial (of men taking Vitamin E and or Selenium or placebo) there were more cases of prostate cancer in the group of men taking Vitamin E alone. (2011)

In men, Vitamin E supplements in the presence of a low Selenium level may actually increase the risk of prostate cancer. (JNCI Feb21 2014 etc.) Vitamin E levels are reduced in patients who have Metabolic Syndrome and its absorption is increased by cow's milk.

Vitamin K:

Phytomenadione, Konakion MM (10mg to reverse the anticoagulation of coumarins, 2mg to all neonates to prevent haemorrhagic disease of the newborn). This is 0.2mls orally (one ampoule) or 0.1ml IM at birth with the oral dose repeated at 1 week. In exclusively breast fed babies this oral dose is repeated monthly until they are on formula or solids.

High vitamin K2 intake protects from cardiovascular disease, aortic and coronary artery calcification. One Dutch study showed that (2016) the third of the study population with the highest level of K2 intake were 57% less likely to die from cardiovascular disease, 52% less likely to get severe aortic calcification and 20% less likely to have coronary artery calci-fication than the third of the population with the lowest intake. Vitamin K2 is important for bone health and should probably be given simultaneously with coumarins (in a regular dose regime to enable warfarin stabilisation) which otherwise cause osteoporosis.

Vitamin K levels in various foods: (for Anticoagulated patients)

Low levels: Green beans, cauliflower, celery, mushrooms, onions, green peppers, potato, tomatoes, most fruits including apples, blueberries, lemons, oranges, peaches, most meats, including beef, chicken, ham, pork, turkey, fish, including mackerel, shrimp, tuna, most vegetable oils, butter, most cheeses, eggs, yogurt, coffee, tea, milk etc.

Moderate Levels: Asparagus, avocado, red cabbage, green peas, iceberg lettuce, margarine, olive oil, gherkins.

High Levels: Broccoli, Brussels sprouts, cabbage, raw endive, kale, lettuce, mustard and cress, parsley, spinach, watercress, mayonnaise, canola and soybean oil.

Vitamin K supplementation reduces markers of inflammation and insulin resistance.

Vitamin B12:

Cyanocobalamin tabs (Only prescribable if there is a dietary deficiency, then endorse FP10 "**SLS**").

Dose is 1-6 daily (Up to 6 in pernicious anaemia). Can be prescribed for vegans, in dietary B12 deficiency, post gastrectomy (no Intrinsic Factor), Megaloblastic Anaemia, Tropical Sprue,

B12 deficiency is very common in vegetarians as there is no plant food source other than fortified milks, cereals and other foods. Most vegans do not consume enough B12 from fortified sources to avoid heart disease or pregnancy complications. (VeganHealth.org)

The injection is

Hydroxocobalamin 1mg/ml.

Dose in macrocytic anaemia without neurological symptoms: Initially 1000ug IM alt days for 1-2 weeks, then 250 ug weekly until blood count normal, maintenance 1000ug every 2-3m.

With neurological symptoms (SACD) 1000ug IM alt. days "as long as improvement is occurring" then 1000ug IM every 2m. Since you cannot overdose on water soluble B12 it seems logical to give more than this regime if in doubt rather than less.

B12 shots were regularly used by 30's film stars and Hitler as an energy boost and they did gain some sort of subjective enhancement by this – although presumably they were not macrocytic or B12 deficient.

Cancer and Diet:

Boron, magnesium, zinc, Saw Palmetto, lycopene, red grape polyphenols, turmeric, (curcumin), resveratrol, rosemary, ursolic acid from apple peel (all four reduce risks of prostate cancer), selenium, omega 3 oils, citrus pectin and a large number of other food constituents have genuine and demonstrable effects in preventing various cancers. Many are active against established cancer and the effects of all these should be part of the knowledge base of a well informed GP.

There are more potential carcinogens in a cup of coffee, probably over a thousand, than the pesticide residues we get in a year. Some of these compounds might either be carcinogenic or on the other hand have anti cancer activity. Individual constituents might have these clinical effects alone or in concert and as it turns out, drinking coffee has beneficial effects on a variety of biological outcomes and survival. This is after years of being a bit of a health pariah. On the other hand, if you want to drink something really healthy, green tea and red wine are now actively under investigation as anti amyloid and anti Alzheimer's as well as having anti cancer properties. If only green tea tasted as good as coffee. Green tea also dissolves oxalate crystals and can reduce or dissolve this type of kidney stone if used frequently enough. Thankfully green tea is available as tablets.

Cancer cells are constantly forming in the body and being destroyed by the body's defences. In the average adult one ml. of peripheral venous blood contains 5 billion red cells, 10 million white cells and approximately 10 metastasised tumour cells.

We have known for decades that aspects of our modern diet cause or contribute towards our modern disease epidemics including cancer. What we have also been realising is that diet and what we eat can help not just in the management of diabetes, heart disease, gout, migraine, hyperlipidaemias and so on but in cancer treatment too.

Various studies have shown a healthy diet, various foods, supplements and exercise can have a profound effect on cancer behaviour at the cellular level, the body's ability to defend itself against "background cancer" and affect the incidence and prognosis of many tumours.

Cancer cells, once they have lost their programmed limit on division, need to be able to promote local inflammation and new blood vessel growth to implant and grow. They produce inflammatory mediators which block cell apoptosis (suicide) and paralyse the host's Natural Killer Cells. These inflammatory markers are a reflection of disease activity and tumour aggression in many cancers. Our own defences, including the "Natural Killer Cells" are sensitive to the effects of diet, exercise and stress.

Cortisol and catecholamines increase inflammatory factors and thus "fertilise" cancer. Various dietary substances antagonise them, for instance Catechins in green tea and Resveratrol in red wine.

Cancer cells have to generate new blood vessels, angiogenesis, to permit implantation and extension of primary and secondary tumours. A variety of foods antagonise this by being anti angiogenic – for instance: various mushrooms, green teas, some spices and herbs.

Cancers, most types of cancers, are increasing in frequency. Our refined, processed diet and the huge number of new chemical products we are exposed to may be part of the reason for this. – Who knows? It's not just the variety of separate questionable molecules in something as bland as a cup of coffee, think of the plastics, paints, volatile organic compounds (the new car smell), the dry cleaning vapours, non stick pans, cosmetics, cleaning products, flame retardants, hydrocarbon exhaust gases, PCBs, solvents, pesticide residues, think of the food we store, cook and microwave in plastics that didn't exist sixty years ago when cancer was rarer let alone 300,000 years ago when our genes were settling down into a modern pattern. Many of these chemicals are oestrogenic and many cancers are oestrogen sensitive including the obvious ovary and breast but also various lung cancers and brain tumours. 15% of fragrances are said to be oestrogenic. 13 Xeno oestrogens (compounds that mimic oestrogen – they are either synthetic or natural) are associated with prostate cancer and are present in sun tan lotions, nail varnish, etc. A woman will swallow up to 4kg of lip stick in a lifetime. A million new chemical entities have been released into the environment since the second world war and by definition, none have long term safety data. The most dangerous place for exposure to toxic chemicals and solvents? Your home. There is no environmental surveillance or health and safety department at home.

Think of the way we grow and feed livestock and ourselves. Over half of our calories come from sources that didn't exist when our hunter gatherer genes were forming – white flour, refined sugar, vegetable oils and trans fats. Little of our food contains the natural Omega 3 Fatty Acids, vitamins and minerals that have been shown to suppress tumour formation. Refined sugar and insulin like growth factor (the latter released when we eat high glycaemic index foods) stimulate cancer growth and inflammation. A low cancer diet would include a lot of Omega 3 Fatty Acids and very little "unnatural" Omega 6 which is ubiquitous in modern diets. (Outdoor fed cows and chickens are higher in Omega 3, indoor fed livestock are higher in Omega 6). It would have lower glycaemic index foods. It would include dark chocolate – the darker the better, and very little refined flour and sugar. It would include a lot of wholegrain cereals, pulses, natural fruits (particularly red fruit), red wine, garlic, onions, shallots, blueberries, raspberries, cherries and a variety of brightly coloured fruit and vegetables. Overall these are the best anticancer foods.

Specifically: Pomegranate and its juice reduce the risk of developing and the spread of established prostate cancer. Red wine contains polyphenols including resveratrol which blocks 3 stages of cancer development. Especially good are Burgundies and Pinot Noir. (Sorry, only one glass a day is enough for this effect). Dark chocolate; (>70% Cocoa) contains antioxidants, proanthocyanidines and polyphenols which slow cancer growth and limit angiogenesis. (One square has more effect than a glass of red wine). Dairy products eaten at the same time neutralise the effect, so milk chocolate doesn't work. Some cocoa products contain polyphenols, flavanols, which as well as improving general vascular function have been shown to improve cerebral blood flow and mental function possibly even affecting cognitive decline and dementia (Cocoa via, AAAS 2014, Int J Med Sc Dec 2014).

Cancer rates are proportional to the meat and milk consumption and inversely proportional to vegetable consumption of a country. Rates are also reduced by a population that eats Omega 3 rich fish. Fish fingers and calamari won't do.

As mentioned, green tea tastes horrible but you can get it in tablet form now and it is very anti cancer in its effect, containing polyphenols and catechins. Many studies have suggested that green tea consumption can lower the risk of multiple cancers, including cancers of the pancreas, colon, stomach, ovary, bladder and prostate. Soy reduces the progress of oestrogen dependent tumours (because of its isoflavones and phyto oestrogens) being a hundredth as active as natural oestrogen itself but blocking the body's oestrogen receptors. Turmeric is the strongest food anti-inflammatory agent (active ingredient curcumin) and black pepper increases its absorption 2000 times. Gastro intestinal and a variety of other cancers are much rarer in India where it is consumed in significant quantities.

Various mushrooms; Button, Shiitake, Maitake, Karawatake, Portobello and Oyster mushrooms stimulate the immune system and protect against breast and colon cancer.

Various brightly coloured berries have anticancer properties: These include raspberries and strawberries, which contain Ellagic acid, which antagonises tumour blood vessel growth. Ellagic acid is also present in hazelnuts, pecans, walnuts, cherries, blueberries and cranberries. Cinnamon and ginger contain anticancer agents. Blueberries have a reputation for being full of anti oxidants but blackberries probably pip them at the post in this regard.

Various herbs, spices and vegetables are also anti cancer: mint, thyme, marjoram, oregano, basil and rosemary, (contain the nice smelling terpenes which help prevent cancer spreading and carnosol in rosemary enhances some chemotherapies). Parsley and celery are angiostatic.

Ginger, cabbages, sprouts, broccoli, cauliflower (avoid boiling), garlic, onions, leeks, shallots, chives likewise have all been shown to have antitumour effects.

Highly coloured fruits and vegetables containing Vitamin A and lycopene inhibit cancer cell growth: – carrots, yams, sweet potatoes, tomatoes, apricots, beetroot.

Tomatoes are particularly good at antagonising prostate cancer (lycopene) but they must be cooked (a good excuse for ketchup). Cooking in olive oil helps the release of the active agent.

Soy blocks oestrogen sensitive cancers (there is a lower incidence of breast cancer in Asian women who have had soy in their diet since adolescence).

Omega 3s reduce cancer growth and metastases, diminishing the incidence of various cancers in oily fish eaters. That is the eaters of oily fish. The bigger the fish, the less likely it is to be polluted, apparently. Marine Omega 3 is better than vegetable Omega 3 and Omega 6 is not good at all. Omega 3s also improve memory believe it or not.

Selenium is said to boost our own Natural Killer Cells, Vitamin D reduces various cancers. B vitamin supplementation, ie Folic acid, reduces homocysteine levels relative to increased cysteine and reduces colorectal cancer (and strokes).

So diet is important in the causation, maintenance and outcome of various cancers. Other factors like personality, marriage, religious faith and exercise are also important and probably additive in their beneficial or negative effects. Exercise is one of the few things known to reduce lung cancer incidence in smokers who give up smoking but also in the incidence of various other cancers. We should, as G.P.s be suggesting, if not prescribing healthy varied diets of colourful fruits and vegetables, spices and herbs, red wine and dark chocolate, mushrooms and oily fish. But then we probably ought to be suggesting this and consuming it ourselves everyday anyway.

It is absolutely shameful that until a short time ago the nutrition departments of major cancer hospitals were advising patients to eat high carbohydrate, empty calorie diets to prevent catabolism and just to keep their weight up. Carbohydrate rich diets, especially refined "white" diets simply feed the cancer. Comfort foods offer only cold comfort in cancer.

It is also worth mentioning that although many legitimate studies have demonstrated the beneficial effect of say, Selenium or Green Tea, Boron or Lycopene in various cancers, few trials show that supplements of the agent are as effective as the food that contains it in its natural state.

Milk, Lactose, Lactase, Lactose Intolerance:

Cow's milk (and the cow's milk based formulae derived from it) was the baby food designed by nature for baby cows.

70% of Western Europeans have lactase in their guts as adults and can readily digest cow's milk. For the rest of the world only 25% of adults are able to digest lactose as adults and the figures are even less for the indigenous populations of Africa, E and S E Asia and Oceania.

In America 75% of Black, Jewish, Mexican and Native Americans are lactose Intolerant and 90% of Asian Americans are Lactose intolerant. I presume this means we have had dairy cows domesticated for more generations and have consumed their products for longer here in Europe. Cheese from cow's milk is lower in lactose and is easier to digest than "raw milk".

The figures for lactose intolerance for different nations are:

Swedish: 2%,
Europeans in Australia 4%,
Swiss 10%,
American Caucasians 12%,
Finns 18%,
African Tussi 20%,
African Fulani 23%,
American Blacks 75%,
Australian aborigines 85%,
African Bantu 89%,
Chinese 93%,
Thais 98%,
American Indians 100%.

http://www.foodreactions.org/intolerence.
Estimates of the age of the lactase mutation, encoded by the gene LCT, are that it is 5,000-10,000 years old.

Disaccharides:

Sucrose (cane, beet, table sugar) is Glucose/Fructose. Fructose is often called "fruit sugar".
Lactulose (a stool softener) is Galactose/Fructose,
Lactose (Milk sugar) is Galactose/Glucose,
Maltose is Glucose/Glucose,
Trehalose is Glucose/Glucose.

Soluble fibre:

Is good for everything from cardiovascular risk to IBS and bowel cancer: This is part of the high bulk, low irritant old fashioned "spastic colitis" diet and includes:
Peas, beans, fruits, oatmeal, high fibre cereals, porridge.

In terms of the amount of fibre, the recommended daily amount is 38grms for men and 25grms for women. The most constipated patients I have had have tended to be women and certainly IBS which comes in two types, one a slow transit type, tends to be commoner in women so I do not know why women require less fibre than men. An increase in 7gr a day in the diet reduces stroke risk 7% but the ideal amount of fibre equates to 8-10 helpings of vegetables a day.

Few foods diet:

There are very few patients who have **genuine** food allergies. Figures are hard to come by on serious allergies but as far as anaphylaxis goes approximately 20 UK citizens are said to die of anaphylaxis a year, 10 due to food allergy. In my career of about 6/7 years as a Paediatrician, 5 miscellaneous years as other sorts of doctors and over thirty years as a GP I have seen many cases of moderately severe allergy including to IV drugs but I have never lost a patient due to anaphylaxis. It is in fact very rare. Even those with proven (double blind challenge) milk allergy seem to lose the allergy after a year or so off cow's milk protein. Peanut allergy can obviously be severe in the very few and "intolerance" of various foods/urticaria etc are more common than true allergies.

If the patient insists that they have a genuine food allergy or allergies of some sort, RAST and skin testing are notoriously unreliable and you could recruit them into trying an exclusion diet regime once and for all to lay the ghost to rest. The whole process is so inconvenient and obsessional that the part time sufferer will either be put off pursuing what is an unlikely diagnosis, find a genuine food they can exclude from the diet at last or realise it isn't bothering them that much.

There are many exclusion diets including the Feingold diet for ADHD which excludes additives, colourings, aspartame, preservatives and natural salicylates etc. A simple few foods diet would include:
Rice, rice milk, lamb, turkey, broccoli, and peaches.
You then add one new food or drink each 2-3 days and keep a symptom diary. Then try and make sense of the results. I am assuming you have excluded PU or Inflammatory Bowel Disease by this point or tried appropriate treatments for these conditions without success.

A Typical Food Allergy hand out:

For 5 days eat only Lamb (including offal), fresh (not tinned) pears and liquidise them to make a juice with still spring water in bottles. This is the only fluid source initially. Use only sea salt. On the first day take an aperient to empty the bowel of potential residual allergens. Do not deviate from this diet in any way. Don't take even small amounts of tea or coffee etc. Use only sodium bicarbonate solution to brush the teeth. Don't smoke during this test. Don't take any tablets, even the pill, don't lick stamps or envelopes and expect to feel worse initially. Some symptoms: headache, tiredness, etc can be eased by bicarbonate of soda in warm water.

The initial foods tested will be broccoli, plaice, fresh pineapple and turkey. This is to find foods you are not allergic to and if you do not react to any food you can add it to the others that you are already able to eat.

Day 6 Broccoli.

Day 7 Plaice, fresh pineapple, turkey.

Day 8 Fresh tomatoes, fresh melon, beef grilled or roasted, no added fats.

Day 9 Tap water, rice, cod.

Day 10, Banana, soya beans.

Day 11 Cow's milk, cabbage, chicken.

Day 12 Indian tea, apple, yeast tablets (or baker's yeast powder, no other vitamins).

Day 13 Butter, leeks, pork.

If any of these are unavailable, try turnips, trout or avocado.

Symptoms normally occur within 4-5 hours of exposure, occasionally within 1 hour. They can last up to 3 days and during a reaction do not test for other foods. Symptoms of reaction vary a great deal and can be obvious or mild. Occasionally there may be a tachycardia as part of a food reaction. If the reaction is questionable it can be retested later. Never retest a food within 5 days of the original contact with it. Keep a food and symptom diary.

Next some more common allergens are tested:

Day 14 Eggs in the morning, potatoes in the evening.

Day 15 and 16 Wheat as wholemeal bread, assuming the yeast test was negative. Eat wheat at each meal for 2 days (It tends to cause a slower onset reaction).

Then on successive days:

Percolated or "real" coffee in the morning, mushrooms in the evening.

Cane sugar in various forms (Demerara).

Oranges   grapes

Beet sugar   lettuce.

Corn as corn on the cob and as corn sugar.

Onion   peanuts

Cheddar cheese   spinach.

White bread (if yeast was tolerated) coconut, garlic.

Plain chocolate (if not allergic to wheat, corn, sugars), grapefruit, dates,

Courgettes or marrow, French beans, cauliflower.

Rye bread (if not allergic to yeast, a 2 day test, slow reaction).

Black pepper, rhubarb, honey.

Instant coffee, (if not allergic to "real coffee"), asparagus, lemon.

Olive oil, parsnips, tinned carrots (if not allergic to fresh carrots and no added sugar).

Oats (porridge) – another 2 day test.
Monosodium glutamate, sprinkle on some meat, prawns or shrimps, Brussels sprouts.
Artificial sweetener tablets, herring, almond.
Malt extract – one whole day.
Avocados, red or green peppers, raisins.
Other foods are tested as above and any reaction noted.

The Feingold diet (for hyperactive children)

Suggests avoiding foods with naturally occurring salicylates as well as all artificial additives. if a good clinical response, individual foods can be added back to the diet after 4-6 weeks to see if the child reacts to specific items.

Natural salicylates are in almonds, apples, apricots, peaches, plums, prunes, oranges, tangerines, tomatoes, cucumber, blackberries, strawberries, raspberries, gooseberries, cherries, currants, grapes and raisins. All are excluded.

All food and drink containing artificial flavouring and colouring must be stopped. This includes monosodium glutamate, nitrates, vanillin, E numbers etc., most fizzy and bought drinks.

So avoid all artificial colours and flavours, instant and prepared breakfast cereals, cakes, biscuits, most packet puddings, soups, mixes, most processed meat products, frankfurters, salami, bacon, ham, commercial sausages, barbequed products, frozen fish/breadcrumbs with colouring, shop bought ice creams, yogurts (with colouring/flavouring). All shop bought sweets, all cider, wine, beer, cider and wine vinegar, all soft drinks, tea, margarine, salted butter, all mint flavouring, soy sauce, sauces, flavoured crisps, cloves, chilli sauce, coloured cheeses, aspirin, cough drops, pastilles, coffee, antacid tablets, all gravy mixes and stock cubes, caramel, saffron, annatto (orange colouring). Avoid BHT – an antioxidant in fats, egg-bread, dyed wholemeal bread, etc.

You can allow: Any cereal without artificial colouring and flavouring, all homemade bread, sweets, bakery, fresh meat and poultry, white fish, jellies with permitted fruit juice and plain gelatine, bananas, grapefruit, lemons, pears, pineapple, guava, melon (although some of these do contain salicylates), tapioca, rice, long spaghetti, plain yogurt, homemade puddings, *Seven Up*, milk, eggs, white cheese and unsalted butter, pure cooking oils and fats, homemade or bought jams without artificial C and F, honey, white vinegar, all fresh vegetables.

Quite a difficult diet to stick to as nearly everything has to be made from scratch and most bought treats are not allowed. It can make a dramatic difference in SOME children with ADHD/behavioural problems.

Salicylates in food:

These can not only affect behaviour in some children but many of these foods contribute towards allergies of various kinds, chronic and recurrent urticaria, oral allergy syndrome etc.etc.

High levels are in: Asparagus, celery (powder), dill powder, currants, dates, raisins, prunes, blueberries, raspberries, cherries, oranges, aniseed, cayenne, cinnamon, curry powder, chinese five spices, garum masala (a blend of ground spices), honey, liquorice, peppermint, mace, mixed dried herbs, mustard, oregano, paprika, rosemary, sage, tarragon, turmeric, thyme, Worcestershire sauce, allspice, bay leaf, chilli, cloves, ginger, mint, nutmeg, black pepper, pickles, almonds, pistachios, peanuts, chestnuts, macadamia nuts, pine nuts.

Fairly high levels are in: Tea, coffee, apples (especially Granny Smith), various berries, citrus fruits, nectarines, dried fruits, figs, guava, grapes, kiwi fruit, peaches, pineapple, plums, broccoli, chicory, endive, gherkins, mushroom, peppers, radishes, water cress, chewing gum, wine, rum, port, Tia Maria, Benedictine, Drambuie, cola etc.

The Mediterranean diet:

The Mediterranean diet is the reason for the French Paradox: Good cardiovascular health despite smoking and a high fat diet: It is high in fruit and vegetables, -lower in processed foods and is often based on local produce, wheat products, such as bread, pastry and pasta, fresh fruit, salads, pulses, grains and vegetables, white meat, poultry, fish and olive oil. Add red wine, drunk in regular moderate amounts with its anti oxidants and there is a significant (and proven) benefit on cardiovascular risk, cancer incidence, Parkinson's and Alzheimer's. Also add in all that sunshine, and Vitamin D of course and probably a less sedentary lifestyle (?). There is probably also a benefit to suffers of Rheumatoid arthritis. So tell your patients to stop buying processed and convenience foods (ie burgers and fried chicken) and to start sourcing their own food. To substitute olive oil for heavy fats and butter, to avoid hydrogenated vegetable oils (they will have to look at the cartons of everything) and saturated fats. Lots of fish and chicken, almost no processed red meat, (twice a month only) lots of exercise, primarily plant based foods, vegetables, whole grains, legumes and nuts, herbs and spices instead of salt for flavouring. Canola oil and olive oil (and flax seed oil and various others) are probably healthier oils than butter-at least they were considered so until January 2015 and the recent rehabilitation of dairy fats. Also drinking wine, especially red wine in "moderation" seems to be positively beneficial. Obviously the average British city dweller isn't going to find all of that advice practical but some of it may turn out to be cheaper and easier than they think. The Mediterranean diet has also been shown to be beneficial in terms of preventing both depression and cognitive decline. But if they really want to get into the lifestyle, learning a foreign language later in life is also supposed to stave off cognitive decline so why not suggest your older patients celebrate Brexit by learning French, Spanish or Italian too?

The Ketogenic Diet:

Fasting stops epilepsy in the majority of children suffering from Grand Mal epilepsy. A ketotic diet has the same effect especially during added fluid restriction. If the acidosis is reversed by giving alkaline salts, the anticonvulsant effect is lost. This was first used as a treatment for epilepsy in the early decades of the 20th C. The diet consists of very low carbohydrate and very high fat, the fat being converted to ketone bodies, much like after prolonged vomiting. The fat calories are increased to around 85-90% in an average ketotic or ketogenic diet. MCTs are more ketogenic than long chain triglycerides and are often supplemented as a calorie source in the diet. Children and adults with epilepsy benefit, even if they try the less stringent Atkins diet, even after fit frequency has reduced and the diet has been stopped. The diet can be used as an adjunct in the rare event of polypharmacy with conventional drugs being ineffective.

Renal Failure Diet:

This is usually a high carbohydrate and low protein diet (0.6g/kg) despite the bad reputation that carbohydrate (substituting for fat) calories now have.

Reduce total meat intake as this reduces acid load and reduces the rate of progress of the failure.

Monitor serum phosphate with a view to giving a phosphate lowering agent.
Monitor calcium with a view to giving calcium and Vitamin D.
Reduce total Na intake from between 2 to 6gr.
Monitor K and pH.

Red Meat:

The consumption of too much red meat has been linked to a number of negative health issues over the years but the science on this has been weak and the data indirect. Meat is receiving a bit of a rehabilitation these days. The problems previously associated with meat have included cardiovascular disease, diabetes and a number of cancers. On the other hand, exclusively vegetarian diets and diets whose protein is solely from fish and white animal meat are frequently deficient in some vitamins and minerals. We evolved as omnivores. Vegetarians do however develop less bowel cancer (17% less) though interestingly fish eating vegetarians, pescovegetarians, have a much lower incidence of bowel cancer, – 43% lower. The red meat of today is not the red meat we evolved to digest however and our guts and livers to metabolise. Today cattle can live indoors for much of the year, be fed grain or concentrated feed rather than the natural diet of grass and their meat is frequently processed after slaughter to preserve or flavour it. It is this manipulation, the unnatural diet fed to livestock, the curing, smoking, the addition of nitrites and other agents to the meat, which further alienate some forms of red meat from our metabolism.

In terms of cardiovascular mortality it is processed meat, ham, bacon, sausages, minced meat in readymade products not red meat per se that is linked to mortality. The risk of new onset heart failure and death from heart failure increases by 8% and 38% for every 50gr daily increase in processed meat intake.

BUT Note:
100 grm (3 1/2 oz) of beef which is 10% fat, 20grm protein, has
25% RDA Vit B3, Niacin
37% RDA Vit B12, Cobalamin (unavailable from plant sources)
18% RDA Vit B6, Pyridoxine
12% RDA Iron, (high quality haem iron, better absorbed than plant iron)
32% RDA Zinc and
24% RDA Selenium.

Red meat is also rich in Creatine and Carnosine which are often deficient in a vegetarian diet and are needed for muscle and brain function. If the cattle had been grass fed then the meat is likely to be richer in Omega 3 fatty acids as well as more Vitamin A and E.

Red meat per se has not been shown in some very large studies to increase the risk of diabetes or CVS disease.

Red meat may be linked weakly with a higher incidence of some cancers and this may be to do with the way it is cooked rather than the meat itself. At high temperatures meat breaks down and can form Heterocyclic Amines (HAs), advanced Glycation End Products (AGEs) or Polycyclic Aromatic Hydrocarbons (PAHs) all of which may be carcinogenic. One common problem when comparing different diets is that a low meat diet group is usually inevitably a high carbohydrate diet group and high carbohydrate fed populations generally do far worse in almost all health related parameters than meat eaters.

There are no proper controlled trials which link red meat with harm in humans, especially grass fed and non overcooked, un: burnt, scorched, bar b qued, roasted and un processed meat.

FATS: Fat: 1gm protein=4 calories, 1gm CHO= 4 calories, 1gm Fat= 9 calories

I was brought up by parents who had such poor teeth in childhood that they had complete dental clearances in their teens and wore dentures all their lives. They remembered Rickets in their neighbourhoods as they grew up in the 1920's and 30's and believed the Milk Marketing Board's later propaganda about calcium and strong teeth and bones. Who can blame them? So we had Gold Topped milk, cheese and cream with everything, my mother cooked with cream and butter. So fat was not an issue as I grew up ten years after the war. Indeed there was still rationing just before I was born and so our treats were lardy cake, beef dripping on toast, clotted cream when we could get it, crackling on pork, a fry up (in lard) for breakfast and anyway, olive oil didn't exist in the UK much before the 70's. Nor did the concept of safe and harmful fats. If you were successful you tended not to be thin.

No wonder my parents' generation were all overweight, hypertensive and all waiting to die from their clogged main arteries.

Unfortunately the dairy products that were and still are delivered to their doors and were fed to us at school daily are suspected of increasing the risk of cardiovascular disease and of ovarian, prostate, ovary, breast and colorectal cancers too. I concede that in the last few years and even in the course of writing this book, the fat mantra: Saturated, dairy, solid and animal fat – all BAD, unsaturated, vegetable and oils – all GOOD has been shown to be far too simplistic. That cooking with vegetable oil isn't necessarily healthy, that eating butter, meat and cheese isn't always unhealthy and, like life, fat is complicated.

Thus:

Saturated fats and Health:

Saturated fats (saturated fatty acids) in the diet increase LDL-C which is supposed to be a CAD risk marker. They also however affect particle size, increase HDL-C and decrease triglycerides. They have a neutral effect on Total: HDL cholesterol. They increase LDL-C but **reduce** the LDL particle number. These various risk indices contradict each other. Meta analyses have shown no direct link between saturated fat in the diet and subsequent CVS risk. **Saturated fat intake is (shockingly) NOT associated with all cause mortality, cardiovascular disease mortality, total CHD, ischaemic stroke or even T2DM. There is a "Trend of association with CHD mortality" But given how much time we have all been proselytising against cholesterol, animal fat, dairy products and saturated fat for decades, this news (2015) was like hearing that smoking was good for you.**

Total Trans fat was in the same meta analysis, associated with a one third increase in all cause mortality, 28% increase in CHD mortality, 21% increase in risk of CHD, but not ischaemic stroke or T2DM.

As we all know now, the medical profession is currently doing an about turn on the health dangers of milk, meat, cheese, butter, cholesterol and saturated fat and admitting that the cholesterol guidelines which we have all used as gospel in giving dietary advice for decades were plucked out of thin air. After all, if it tastes good or feels good, doctors generally advise against it, from unrestricted sex to excessive red meat and wine. So why wouldn't fried food, cheeses, cooking with saturated fats, putting cream onto puddings and having lots of meat be bad for you? It certainly sounds like it should.

But a systematic review and meta analysis (Harcombe, Baker, Cooper, Davies,

Sculthorpe, DiNicolantonio, Grace 2015) showed no basis for the dietary fat guidelines of 1977 and 1983.

Many authors regard the modern cardiovascular epidemic as a result of sloth, obesity and sugar/carbohydrate (especially refined carbohydrate) intake and not the result of butter, cheddar cheese or the occasional steak. In a more recent confirmation of the reversal of orthodoxy, the US Library of Medicine database (Pubmed) was searched for studies looking at the risk of dying from a raised LDL over 60 years of age. In a total of 19 studies involving 68,000 patients there was in fact an **inverse relationship** between LDL and mortality. The reverse of what we have all been led to believe. The lower the LDL the higher the chances of dying, the higher the LDL the lower the rate of heart disease death and any cause death. The conclusion was "Our study provides the rationale for re evaluation of the guidelines recommending reduction of LDL cholesterol in the elderly as a component of heart disease prevention strategies". In other words, statins in the over 60's may be causing heart disease.(Ravnskov U et Al BMJ Open 2016 Jun 12.6 (6):e010401).

Sugar and trans fats as well as processed meats are the new saturated fat and cholesterol. As with so many factors in medicine, if something is new in our evolution, if our bodies haven't had millennia to adapt, to a food, an activity, an infection, a treatment, a behaviour, a chemical, a custom, a diet and so on then it will probably cause harm to many of its consumers, users or adherants.

Saturated fats have no double bonds between carbon atoms in the fatty acid chain and come mainly from animal sources including dairy.

Poly unsaturated and mono unsaturated fatty acids (PUFAs and MUFAs):
Polyunsaturated fats have 2 or more double bonds and are called Omega 3 or Omega 6 FAs depending on where the first double bond is. They include plant sourced Omega 6 FAs (including linoleic acid) and plant and animal Omega 3 FAs (alpha linoleic acid and the fish oils, eicosapentaenoic acid and docosahexaenoic acid).

Monounsaturated Fats have one double bond. Those with a double bond in the "Trans" configuration are called "Trans fats".

MUFAs come from plant oils, olive and sunflower etc, nut sources, avocado and seeds. The saturated fatty acids from meat and dairy sources are qualitatively different – with dairy the less risky. Higher intakes of dairy saturated fat seem, counter intuitively, to reduce both cardiovascular and diabetes risk. (MESA, EPIC-InterAct Studies).

The EPIC trial clarified the meat cardiovascular culprit as processed, not red meat, processed meat being a negative factor for CVD and diabetes risks. If saturated fat is replaced in the diet by polyunsaturated fat, then CAD decreases, if it is replaced by carbohydrates then CAD risk increases and if it is substituted by monounsaturated fat then the benefits are uncertain.

The goal of 7% of total calories is a general guide for calories from saturated fat and the ideal diet is and always has been a Mediterranean one of colourful vegetables and fruit, fish, particularly oily fish, poultry, some meat, olive (etc) oils, whole grains and seeds, leaves and very little refined carbohydrate, white flour or indoor raised animal flesh.

Hydrogenated Oils (synthetic trans fats): Are entirely artificial, having been invented in the 1890s. By hydrogenating a vegetable oil you can extend the shelf life of the fat before it goes rancid and make a fat that is a liquid oil at room temperature into a solid. Trans fat consumption is a cardiovascular risk factor independent of saturated fat consumption.

It raises LDL and lowers HDL, the risk of stroke and T2Diabetes are increased. Trans fats may also increase various cancers including colon and pancreas. Hydrogenated fat is entirely synthetic and unnatural. There are just a few natural trans fats.

The FDA in America announced the start of a ban on trans fats in June 2015. This would take 3 years. Many European countries have done likewise and there are calls for a complete ban in the UK. We are down to 0.6% of dietary energy in the form of trans fats currently (2015) but these are said to be concentrated in the diet of the "poorest" in society as they tend to occur more in convenience foods and pre processed foods. In America the PHOs, partially hydrogenated oils, must be removed from manufactured foods by the end of that period. They are in all sorts of processed foods – vegetable shortening, margarine, crackers, cereals, biscuits, doughnuts, pizza, crisps, snack foods of various kinds, salad dressings, commercial fats, fried foods etc – and in no natural foods.

There is one *natural* trans fat that we consume by eating meat from cud chewing animals – conjugated linoleic acid. This is not harmful.

Saturated Fats:

For decades there always seemed to be a clear relationship between saturated fat intake (particularly of processed meats), blood cholesterol level and cardiovascular morbidity. High saturated fat intake resulted in: high total cholesterol, high Tgs, high LDL, low HDL, High Total/HDL ratio – and all these seemed to increase the risks of cardiovascular disease and stroke.

Saturated fat includes triglycerides in animal fats and nuts (palmitic and stearic acids), lauric and myristic acids in vegetable fats and dairy products. Saturated fats tend to be animal fats, dairy products, ghee, suet, lard, meat, but they do include many vegetable products too, including coconut oil, cottonseed oil, palm kernel oil, chocolate etc.

Unsaturated Fats:

Which are Polyunsaturated and Monounsaturated are fatty acids where there is at least one double bond in the fatty acid chain. A monounsaturated fatty acid has one double bond, a polyunsaturated one has more than one double bond but is more prone to going rancid than the saturated or mono unsaturated fat molecule.

Polyunsaturated fats are liquid at room temperature, for instance Soybean, Sunflower, Safflower oils. Surprisingly they may make atheroma worse in post menopausal women so monounsaturated fats are the only really safe fats from a cardiovascular point of view.

Monounsaturated fats are oils that include olive and walnut oils. High levels tend to lower insulin resistance.

The percentage of monounsaturated fats:
Olive oil 73%,
Rapeseed oil 60%,
Hazelnuts 50%,
Almonds 35%,
Cashews 28%,
Brazils 26%,
Sesame seeds 20%,
Pumpkin seeds 16%.

Olive oil, especially unmodified "virgin" olive oil, reduces the incidence of various cancers and reduces heart disease. This is part of the Mediterranean diet we all seem to aspire to, along with the variety of fresh fruit, vegetables, fish, red wine, relative lack of obesity and presence of exercise.

Other oils of interest are **Omega 3 oils**. Fish or marine Omega 3 oils are long chained, flaxseed, linseed and oil of evening primrose are short chained omega 3. There are also omega 6 and some omega 9 oils. These are all essential oils. If livestock, cows, poultry etc are bred inside or fed on stored feed the proportion of omega 3 fats in their flesh decreases compared with outside or "organically" reared animals. Omega 3 oils are anti inflammatory and have a number of positive health (cardiovascular and anti cancer) benefits. They also lower LDL. Insulin resistance and dietary fat intake may well be connected via the mechanism of inflammation: Omega 6 fats being pro inflammatory and Omega 3 and 9 anti inflammatory.

Omega 3 oils also reduce aggression in children.

Fat and Food:
Only 1/3 of serum cholesterol is from the diet so even stringent diets have less effect than statins.

Exercise increases HDL.
Oil of all kinds is 100% fat.
Lard 99%,
Butter 82%,
Margarine (all kinds) 80%,
Double cream 50%,
Cream cheeses 50%,
Fried streaky bacon 45%,
Stilton 40%,
Grilled streaky bacon 36%,
Cheddar 34%,
Parmesan 30%,
Grilled lamb chops 29%,
Ben and Jerry's Chunky Monkey ice cream 28%,
Pork pie/luncheon meat/liver sausage 27%,
Processed cheese 25%,
Camembert/Edam/cheese spread 23%,
Roast leg of pork 20%,
Fried beef burgers 17%,
Smoked mackerel 16%,
Fried fish fingers 13%,
Grilled rump steak, grilled kippers 12%,
Cod fried in batter 10%,
Dairy ice cream 7%,
Tinned ham, gold topped milk 5%,
Cottage cheese, silver topped milk 4%,
Steamed plaice 2%,
Steamed haddock, yogurt 1%,
Skimmed milk <1%.
The worst food from cereals: savoury cheese biscuits, croissants, puff pastry.
The worst fruit and vegetables: crisps, chips, avocados, olives.

The best nuts: walnuts, the worst coconut.

The worst fish: fish roe.

The worst meat: visible fat, crackling, sausages, pate, duck, goose, streaky bacon, meat pies and pasties.

The worst eggs and dairy: hard cheese, stilton, cream cheese, egg yolks, mayonnaise.

The worst fats: Butter, dripping, suet, lard, oils which are not high in polyunsaturates or any oil above its smoke point when cooking.

The worst spreads etc: Peanut butter, chocolate, toffee, fudge, butterscotch, lemon curd, mincemeat.

The worst drinks: cream soups.

Weight reducing diets and surgery:

In 1993 the American National Institutes of Health Expert panel reviewed decades of diet studies and found depressing outcomes. 90-95% people regained 1/3 – 2/3 of the lost weight within a year of losing it and all of it within 5 years of dietary loss. The outcomes for children, however, should they have weight reduction surgery, are far better. Apparently an adult's appetite is fixed and very difficult to alter permanently. The long term picture is slightly better if they have gastric bypass surgery: Then they lose 2/3 of their excess weight within a year with only 10-20 pounds regained over the following 10 years. 80% of diabetics operated on in this way are cured of their diabetes. With gastric banding however, after two to three years many women develop depression and self harming as if they do not become psychologically adjusted to being slimmer for some reason.

"Natural" POISONS

PLANTS: Usually Alkaloids (eg. Atropine, Vincristine) or Glycosides (Digitalis)

The following are poisonous (plants, seeds, berries, roots):

Ergot	)	Broom	Ragwort
Lorchel	)	Lucerne	Groundsel
Clavaria	)	Clover	Lily of the Valley
Inocybe	)	Vetch	Solomon's Seal
Agaric (Fly)	) Fungi	Laurel	Bluebell
Ink Cap	)	Cotoneaster	Meadow Saffron
Sulphur Tuft	)	Mezereon	Snowdrop
(False) Death Cap	)	Mistletoe	Daffodil
Panther Cap	)	Ivy	Cuckoopint
Bracken		Hemlock	
Yew		Cowbane	
Marsh Marigold		Dropwort	
Hellebore		Parsley	
Monkshood		Bryony	
Larkspur		Mercury	
Baneberry		Sponge	
Wood Anemone		Caster Oil Plant	
Columbine		Buckwheat	
Common Buttercup		Rhubarb	
Spearwort		Beech	
Celandine		Oaks	

Corn Poppy etc	Rhododendron
Rape	Azalea
Wild Radish/Mustard Seed	Horseradish
Sorrel	Privet
Holly	(Deadly) Nightshade
Flax	Henbane
Box Tree	Thorn Apple
Buckthorn	Potato, Tomato (parts of)
Lupin	Figwort
Laburnum	Foxglove

Probiotic supplements:

(Yoghurt, kefir, miso soup, various proprietary supplements, Yakult, Actimel and sauerkraut etc)

Seem to improve colic and toddler diarrhoea in children, to slightly drop blood pressure, to improve H Pylori eradication with antibiotics and may reduce the incidence and recurrence of some cancers.

They may speed recovery from antibiotic diarrhoea and are certainly more palatable (to think about) than the increasingly fashionable **Faecal Transplants** (Faecal Microbiota Transplants) used for:

Clostridium Difficile infection,

Crohns and UC,

Chronic constipation,

IBS,

ME,

CFS,

MS,

Trimethylaminuria and

Post antibiotic diarrhoea.

etc.

See sections on Microbiota, Infection, Antibiotics.

16: Driving:

The up to date rules (which change quite regularly) for various medical conditions and Group 1 and 2 driving are on the DVLA's website or via their very helpful drivers medical enquiry line 01792 761119 or for further information: The Medical Adviser, Drivers Medical Group, DVLA, Longview Rd. Swansea. SA991TU. Phone 01792 782337 or E Mail medadviser@dvla.gsi.gov.uk or access DVLA "At a glance".

The Risks of Driving:

One death every 6-7million passenger miles, 27x greater than by rail. Flying is 10 times safer than rail travel with a fatality rate of 1 fatality every 2,000,000,000 person miles flown or a fatal accident ratio (in the USA) of 1 per million flights.

Obviously it is possible to manipulate the figures a bit as most car journeys are not trans-continental and don't have 250 passengers to reduce the risk statistics, so here are comparable figures:

per billion hours:	per billion kilometres:
Bus 11	Air 0.05
Rail 30	Bus 0.4
Air 31	Rail 0.6
Water 50	Van 1.2
Van 60	Water 2.6
Car 130	Car 3.1
Foot 220	Space Shuttle 16.2
Bicycle 550	Bicycle 44.6
Motorcycle 4840	Foot 54.2
Space Shuttle 438,000	Motorcycle 109

Road Traffic Accidents:

In 2011, 1,901 people died in R.T.A.s in the UK, that is 1780 vehicles on the road per death. 40 years ago the figure for total deaths was 8000.

In the UK we may have a government and police force that seem obsessed by safety but to put our driving in perspective, we have half the number of accidents that the impulsive French have and a third of the over emotional Italians.

Driving (DVLA Guidelines): In brief:

For a standard licence (Group 1) you don't need to notify the DVLA about

Diabetes controlled by tablets or drugs without hypoglycaemia and without visual or limb complications.

Angina, infarct or myopathy with full recovery and without symptoms,

TIA/CVA where there is no one month residual deficit,

Reduced vision limited to one eye,

-as long as driving ability is not affected by any of these.

But if in doubt, notify.

Sight:

You used to have to be able to read in good light (with glasses/contacts) a car number plate at 20m, (65' 7") and have acuity >6/12. In 2011 the EU dictated that this requirement could be reduced to:

Reading a number plate at 57' or 17.5m. In 1937 when the driving test was introduced it was 75' or 23m. If the patient uses glasses they can wear them for the test.

When the EU loosened the vision standards for Group 1, they also allowed Group 2 drivers to work wearing glasses and a loosening of rules relating to diabetes and epilepsy.

Group 1: (Normal Driving Licence)
Vision must be better than 6/12, ie 6/9-6/12 in at least one eye with
Visual Field at least 120 degrees in one eye.
Must notify Glaucoma. Must be able to read a standard number plate at 17.5m.

Group 2: (Large goods vehicles, passenger carrying vehicles, horse boxes and often taxi drivers)
At least 6/60 in each eye and corrected must be 6/9 or better in one, 6/12 in the other. Any field defects, diplopia, or patients with single eye vision are banned.

These recommendations were reviewed to: An acuity if necessary with lenses of 6/7.5 in the better eye and at least 6/60 in the other. Glasses must not be stronger than +8 dioptres. Plus the group 1 requirements **in 2013.**

Epilepsy:

The EU defines epilepsy as two or more epileptic seizures less than five years apart. The government regards epilepsy relating to Group 2 drivers as two or more seizures less than 10 years apart.

Group 1:
6 months fit free after first, solitary unprovoked and any further fit. (Same for an unprovoked LOC with normal cardiac investigations) – *provided the driver has seen a specialist and undergone EEG and brain scan and it is thought to be of low recurrence risk.* The 6 months is at the recommendation of the specialist but **if the patient has had a first unprovoked fit the period off driving is usually 1 year.**

During treatment changes or cessation of treatment 6 months before driving again.

If no cause found after first ??fit DVLA must be informed and no driving 1 year.

Sleep attacks: Stop driving one year. If the patient only has sleep related seizures for one year they can then drive. This followed the above EU directive, it was 3 years until 2011.

Changing/stopping medication: If stopping medication, stop driving while that is happening and for 6 months after. If a further fit, medication must be restarted at the effective dose, driving stopped six months and the DVLA Informed. The same applies if a fit while changing medication.

Anyone who continues to drive in contravention of these rules is effectively without valid insurance or licence.

GPs have a duty to tell the DVLA if they believe that a patient is continuing to drive despite being informed of these rules. They should inform the patient of this.

Rarely (i.e. after a head injury or CVA) a seizure may occur which is highly situational and unlikely to recur and the DVLA may make an exception to its rules.

Group 2:
Must be seizure free off medication 5 years and had the appropriate assessment and considered to have a good prognosis.(<2% risk off treatment/yr).

Isolated seizures (First and only single seizure with no history or seizures limited to a 24hr period).

This stops the patient driving 6 months (Group 1) – but only if the EEG is normal, it was a solitary fit, no abnormality had been detected and the specialist assessment is completed. Otherwise it is one year. etc or 5 years (off medication) (Group 2). How you as the GP determine that a first seizure is an isolated seizure rather than the first seizure of many and therefore a 6 months rather than 12 months ban, – I don't know. I usually phone one of the helpful DVLA medical advisors and discuss what advice to give. I also do my best to speed up the specialist assessment. Or advise the patient to go privately. The loss of a the freedom to drive is extremely disruptive even if the patient's living does not depend on it and neurology waiting lists are amongst the longest in the NHS.

Seizures not affecting consciousness: (Simple, partial or focal, the patient is fully aware and reactive). If these are the only seizures then after a year the patient may reapply for a licence.

Provoked seizures: You can usually drive 3 months after encephalitis, meningitis, after a head injury you can drive soon too. All seizures must be notified to the DVLA apart from provoked vaso vagal faints.

Epileptic attacks while asleep or falling asleep: Stop driving at least a year. The patient can apply for a licence if the last attack was over 3 years ago and no awake attacks have happened since.

Presumed LOC or altered awareness with seizure markers:

Group 1

6 months off driving assuming the driver has been seen, assessed and given a good prognosis by a specialist.

Group 2

5 years off driving assuming an assessment and clean bill of health (and good prognosis) by a specialist.

On withdrawal of medication: Stop driving until the patient has been off medication and fit free 6 months.

T.I.As and Strokes:

Should not drive 1m and only drive then if recovery is satisfactory. No need to inform DVLA if no residual neurological deficit. If multiple TIAs may need to stop driving until 3m after last attack.

Seizures at the time of a cortical vein thrombosis require 6 months off driving.

Neurological disorders:

Driving in such conditions as Parkinson's will depend on whether "driving is impaired".

Psychiatric Disorders:

In Dementia with poor short term memory, disorientation, lack of insight and or judgement then you must say that they are permanently unfit to drive. You have an absolute responsibility to the other road users who could be hurt, injured or killed by your patient.

Mania/hypomania: Stop driving acutely and don't restart after an acute episode until stable for at least 3m. This increases to 6 months off driving if the patient has had 4 or more episodes of mood swings in the previous year.

Acute psychoses: No driving in the acute episode. Only drive if stable and well for over 3 months.

Chronic psychoses: Stop driving, must have been stable at least 3m, stuck to the treatment regime, without S/Es and subject to the consultant's favourable report.

Coronary Artery Disease:

Myocardial infarction: Avoid driving 4 weeks, notify the DVLA.

After CABG stop driving 4 weeks at least.

Angioplasty stop driving 1 week or 4 weeks if procedure unsuccessful.

Valve conditions: GP to discuss, driving will be based on symptoms and triggers.

Angina at the wheel: Stop driving until satisfactory control of symptoms.

Arrhythmia: Cease driving if the arrhythmia causes "incapacity". Restart driving when cause sorted for 4 weeks (2 days at least after a successful catheter ablation).

The DVLA must be informed of any condition that may cause a sudden attack of disabling giddiness or fainting (ie the conditions which necessitate an indwelling defibrillator or pacemaker).

Group 2:

Cannot drive within 3m of CABG, MI, angioplasty or any episode of unstable angina. Cannot drive if the angiogram shows extensive disease or impaired LV, angina or heart failure – even if symptom free on medication, or confirmed peripheral vascular disease, eg aneurysm, cardiac ischaemia, dissection of the aorta, if BP>200/110 or in treated hypertension if BP>180/100, or if medication might affect driving, if a pacemaker is present, if acquired valve disease, or any significant arrhythmia within 5 years (heart block, SVT, VT, AF, atrial flutter), cardiomyopathy, heart lung transplant, Marfan's, complex congenital heart disorders. Relicensing 3 or more months after MI, angioplasty, CABG provided the driver can safely complete the first 3 stages of the Bruce Protocol *off treatment for 24 hrs* without symptoms.

Note: **The Bruce Protocol** is a standardised regime of graded exercise on a treadmill. The grade of this is increased every three minutes thus:

Stage	minutes	%Incline	Km/hr	MPH
1	up to 3	10	2.7	1.7
2	6	12	4.0	2.5
3	9	14	5.4	3.4
4	12	16	6.7	4.2
5	15	18	8.0	5.0
6	18	20	8.8	5.5
7	21	22	9.6	6.0

Hypertension/Heart Failure: Can continue driving unless symptoms are "distracting".

Pacemaker implant: Stop driving 1 week at least.

PCI (Percutaneous Coronary Intervention): Stop driving at least a week.

Driving and diabetes:

Treated by diet: Neither type of licence holder needs to inform the DVLA.

Diabetes treated by Sulphonylureas and Glinides (Repaglinide, Nateglinide, etc): Group 1 drivers don't need to tell the DVLA, Group 2 drivers do.

These drugs may increase the risk of hypoglycaemia with some otherwise benign diabetic medications.

Diabetes treated by other tablets and non insulin injections: Group 1 drivers don't need to tell DVLA, Group 2 drivers do.

Diabetes treated with insulin: All drivers must tell the DVLA but Group 2 drivers can now use insulin.

The DVLA must be informed if the diabetic patient has more than one episode of severe hypoglycaemia (ie requiring the assistance of another person) within 12m, if they have a poor awareness of impending hypos, one episode of disabling hypoglycaemia while actually driving or another condition which affects their driving. If the patient has frequent hypos or reduced awareness they should inform the DVLA and stop driving. Can resume driving "when awareness/control achieved."

In 2013-4 some rules changed and to summarise:

Group 1 vehicles

Drivers must inform the DVLA if they are taking insulin. Drivers of group 1 vehicles (cars and motorbikes) using insulin must have an awareness of hypoglycaemia, have adequate blood glucose monitoring, not be a danger to the public and meet eyesight standards.

Patients must inform the DVLA if they have had two episodes of hypoglycaemia requiring assistance from another person in a year. You should advise patients **not to drive** if they have had an episode requiring admission to A&E, treatment by paramedics or assistance from a partner/friend who had to administer glucagon/glucose because the patient could not do this.

The patient does not have to report an episode of hypoglycaemia if they were conscious of it and able to take appropriate action independently.

Patients taking insulin temporarily (less than three months), for example due to gestational diabetes, need not inform the DVLA as long as they are under medical supervision and not at risk of disabling hypoglycaemia.

Group 2 (Professional) vehicles

Since 2013 drivers on insulin or oral medication that can induce hypoglycaemia can drive a group 2 vehicle (bus and lorry) provided they:

Have had no episodes of hypoglycaemia requiring the assistance of another person in the past 12 months – (if they have, they must stop driving.)

Have full hypoglycaemic awareness (that is, are able to avoid the onset of hypoglycaemia by taking action after warning symptoms.)

Can demonstrate regular blood glucose monitoring **at least twice daily** with a meter with memory function – and provide these records on demand.

Have no other debarring complications of diabetes, such as eye problems.

The DVLA will arrange an annual review by an independent diabetic consultant, who must examine three months of blood sugar readings, which the patient collects on a blood glucose meter.

If patients change from oral hypoglycaemics to insulin, they must tell the DVLA and stop driving group 2 vehicles until the requirements are met.

Again the GP's overriding responsibility is to the innocent road user or pedestrian who may be killed, injured or maimed by the unreasonable and unrealistic diabetic. I remember falling out with one patient who I counted as a reasonably good friend up until he presented with large gash on his forehead sustained during a sudden hypo one evening at home. It turned out that this was the second episode, one having happened at work six months earlier. This LOC was followed by a fit and confusion before his wife could get some sugar in to him. There had been no warning. He was very inconvenienced by the thought of informing the DVLA when I told him the rules and I saw him driving his wife and children a few days later. He had made no adjustment to his treatment and

I reasoned was still a danger to himself and others. The subsequent consultation by phone and shouting match at the surgery were basically reasoned threats from me on behalf of the community. His response was of course, he needed his car for work and to get the kids to school and he was no danger to anyone, he would sue me for lost earnings etc etc... you know the sort of stuff. The GP **must** consider the safety of someone's child on a bike, or a mother pushing a buggy on the pavement or driving her children home from cubs or school. If these innocents were made victims by you, the GP's inaction – how responsible would you then feel?

After all, neither a car nor a driving job are a basic human rights and we all know of tragic episodes from the national news where vehicles have mown down numbers of innocent people in the street when the driver had fallen unconscious at the wheel. In a few cases it appears, having failed to declare previous similar episodes to his employer. Unforgivable. In America they go to jail for life. Here it appears that they often escape prosecution.

Alcohol:

UK legal driving limit rules:
80mg % in Blood,
35ug in Breath,
106mg/ml in Urine.

Driving and alcohol/drugs:

Licence withheld until patient free of problems

>6m (persistent alcohol or cannabis misuse, amphetamines other than metamphet-amine, ecstasy, psychoactive drugs) or

>1year (alcohol dependency, heroin, morphine, methadone, cocaine, metamphetamine, benzodiazepines.)

17: ODD DRUGS:

"One of the first duties of the physician is to educate the masses not to take medicine"
Sir William Osler

Or possibly only the right medicine in the right dose, for the right duration at the right time.

At any time 8000 NHS beds are said to be occupied by patients suffering drug side effects and the NHS spends £1Bn/year treating them.

I believe in the importance, the crucial role in our interplay with the patient and his illness, of drug therapy. Think of the reasons that bring patients to doctors: Infections, pain, various deficiencies, hypertension, inflammation, autoimmune excess, glandular over or under activity, depression, mood disorders, neoplasia, nearly everything except decrepitude and wear and tear can be addressed with a pharmacological agent prescribed by a doctor. Specific, targeted and active therapies are what separate us from the medics of every century before the 20th. Agreed, many aspects of normal existence, shyness, acne, hair loss, lack of libido and so on are medicalised as soon as a drug therapy is found and promoted for them but think of life a hundred years ago when people frequently died of otitis media, strep skin and throat infections, myxoedema, TB, childhood gastroenteritis, or suffered with gout, heart failure, angina or migraine for miserable years on end.

The agent we prescribe may be effective, ineffective or have a negative effect. It was announced in 2015 that "hospitals" are the third biggest killers in the US after cancer and cardiovascular disease and much of that morbidity must be through direct drug side effects. For most of us however, drugs are wholeheartedly beneficial agents- in my forty years I remember very few deaths in my patients directly from drugs other than Warfarin.

There are the dual effects of the pharmacological effectiveness of the therapy we prescribe and "promote" but also the power of the tablet as the doctor's ambassador, a reminder of the influence and ongoing support of the doctor himself. Thus it is always important to explain what each drug is expected to do, what if any side effects there might be, certainly playing down their likelihood but how to cope with them and within limits, what is the drug's mode of action: "The blood pressure comes down because the drug relaxes the blood vessels, makes your kidneys pass more water, counteracts the effect of adrenaline" and so on. It is so important to make an investment of yourself in the treatment you prescribe and be rationally (slightly over) optimistic about the outcome.

So I regard drugs as beneficial tools, our emissaries doing good in the alien no man's land of the patient's body on our behalf. Many however, in medicine and medical journalism believe that "Big Pharma" has too much influence within the medical profession due to its financial and funding power. One source quotes 82% of doctors' medical information as coming from the pharmaceutical industry itself. If that is the case it says much about the apathy of my colleagues in not seeking more independent and reliable data. It is also a comment on the poverty of medical education from primary and secondary care non promotional sources. Especially since every doctor regards most published trial data with a dose of cultural disbelief. Indeed, as one who has a more than average interest in some effective alternative pharmaceutical treatments, especially in the field of cancer, I am saddened that so many (especially American) independent writers use the term "Big Pharma" as if it were synonymous with corrupt capitalism and any patient benefit was accidental.

Through functional MRI scanning we are only now learning how the placebo effect turns on the body's own endorphins, releases natural cortical opiates and so genuinely does relieve pain at pain receptors and not just at "a psychological" (imaginary) level. Even stranger: studies have shown that many patients respond to placebos that they have previously been told contain no active drug, but are also interviewed supportively and as part of that interview process are informed that many patients do naturally respond to placebos. Indeed GPs ought to be able legitimately (as we used to) unashamedly prescribe placebos. As you read this book you may argue that my multi vitamins in glandular fever or Betnesol nose drops in Glue Ear are no more than placebos. I would argue that if they improve the patient's symptoms, do no harm AND don't cost much....why are we arguing?

Clearly, prescribing, dispensing, administering, thinking about and consuming drug treatments is far more complicated than just doling out a drug that plugs into a receptor site and stimulates a bodily response.

The ability to make up my own mind about which drugs were best for my patients without being controlled by restrictive hospital drug policies and pharmacopoeias was one of the main reasons I swapped careers into General Practice over three decades ago. The penny pinching (in many cases it is only pennies) then crept from hospitals into General Practice. I now despair at the prescribing incentive schemes as part of QuoF, PIS schemes and at the proscriptive prescription controls at the behest of Local Prescribing Committees which invariably encourage drugs with the worst collection of adverse reactions (Simvastatin, first wave ACEIs, relatively ineffective antibiotics, CCBs with nasty flushing and tingling, poorly tolerated generic drugs and so on) just because they are cheap. I write elsewhere that by far the best mid range pain killer taken by the elderly for decades was Co-Proxamol. Then this combination analgesic became tainted by its risk when taken in overdose with alcohol. This was only ever done by the psychiatrically unwell young (and something the elderly virtually never did) and it was finally priced out of the running by the restricted number of manufacturers prepared to make and indemnify it and by the cheap constipating and brain-fogging alternatives. It was therefore effectively banned by default but finally by cost.

Likewise there is no addictive potential for a patient in taking an occasional temazepam or the more rational middle half life (but now too expensive to be prescribed) lormetazepam. Instead the standard wisdom of most local prescribing committees is that is that we should prefer the hang-over causing and metallic tasting Z drugs. They have a different effect on "sleep architecture" and were originally thought to have lower dependence and next day adverse effects. Both these beliefs are now being revised. As long as the frequency of the prescription and the mental state of the patient are supervised properly by the prescriber there will be no problem of addiction to hypnotics in the vast majority of patients on benzodiazepines. But one reason the Z drugs are in favour is because GPs were not thought capable of effectively counselling, supervising or disciplining their patients on benzodiazepines. Interestingly Zolpidem is now not considered quite the paragon it once seemed and I suspect the same will be true for all Z drugs: Zolpidem has had various caveats attached to its prescribing because of dangerous adverse effects occurring the morning after. These include bizarre behaviour, agitation, "sleep driving", as well as sedation and confusion etc. Patients are advised not to take top up doses in the night (far more common than we doctors are ever aware of) or to drive within 8 hours of a dose due to these dangerous driving side effects the next morning.

It is associated with increased visits to A and E and appears to be metabolised slower in women. Women are far more likely to ask for sleeping drugs than men in the first place. I have had elderly patients who had serious and recurrent morning or night time falls beg for bigger doses of Z drugs and even claim they had lost prescriptions- no doubt all due to early hours top up doses after early morning waking. Google Zopiclone or, I suspect any Z drug and you will find addiction is a real problem with them too and now an increased risk of dementia with long term use.

Drug authorities always assume the lowest common denominator exists amongst GP prescribers and that we had better be restricted to what are considered intrinsically safer drugs. This is rather than letting us make up our own minds about what is best for the patient, taking prescribing responsibility and with it the duty of proper supervision. A subtle form of disenfranchisement and professional restriction which, like our endless protocols and guidelines is resulting in the lowest common denominator mind set of GP and the blandest, standardised, most inflexible and unresponsive service to the patient. A self fulfilling prophesy of low professional expectation linked to restricted independence.

There are shared care guidelines for dozens of drugs which may be initiated by hospital specialists then the care taken over by GPs. Methotrexate, Lithium, and maintenance steroids are the better known.

The GP has to be familiar with the drug's adverse effects and monitoring and I have often heard my whingeing colleagues complain about the awesome and burdensome responsibilities of this. Nonsense. If it is in the patient's interests- and it always is, then surely the GP should be prepared to take on any responsibility to assist?

I personally have no problem, given the right patient, starting certain drugs with which I have become familiar but for which GP initiation is not generally recommended - and which happen to be of particular use in psychiatry. -Lithium, most of the atypical antipsychotics, Ritalin, other ADHD drugs and so on. The reason for this is that my local psychiatric and adolescent mental health services have been poor and unsupportive for decades so I and my GP colleagues have had to some extent become primary and secondary care mental health services. The truth is that either I had to become familiar with essential secondary care drug treatments or the patient just wouldn't get treated. There is also a very real factor of GP morale which has become obvious over the last ten to fifteen years. The less flexibility and independence, the fewer choices and decisions that each doctor allows himself or herself to make, the less professional pride he or she will get out of their job. These days there are undoubtedly larger numbers of my colleagues who do family medicine, simply as a job of convenience. They are less than fully committed to the life and ethos of General Practice than my generation was. It is an inevitable consequence of part time working and of non partnership GPs, of doing a fewer sessions and having no connection with the practice as body, a unified family. By ethos I mean an individualism and independent attitude to focus on the best interests of each person on your list of patients. Proscriptive prescribing, controlled by outside influences is just one factor in the progressive depersonalisation, enforced disengagement and deterioration of the quality of Family Medicine and the morale of the GP. This is thanks to a fundamental change in the identity of the GP, their professional control and independence.

More and more my prescribing is being controlled by a priority list of factors with cost at the top and what I consider to be best interests of the patient at the bottom. I was never asked to take the Hippocratic Oath but just as it includes a promise never to perform an abortion, it omits any mention of cost or generic "equivalents" in treatment deliberations. It does not say always consider the cost of treatment above effectiveness or acceptability of treatments.

Generic equivalent: That is an interesting phrase. Are generic drugs really identical, equivalent, to branded similar products? Reuters news agency reported what I have suspected for decades as a doctor and as a consumer in April 2014. That many US doctors were becoming concerned at the quality of generic drugs (in this case supplied by Indian manufacturers) -"Following a flurry of recalls, of import bans and recalls by the FDA" These included the wrong drugs and differing doses of drug in the same packets. My concern is a bit more subtle: I have as a prescriber and as a consumer seen drugs that previously worked at one specific dose stop working as soon as the "generic equivalent" was substituted. This has been the case using non sedating antihistamines, PPIs, H2 antagonists, antidepressants, anti inflammatories, antibiotics, analgesics, even anti depressants. I can't help wondering if cheap foreign imports have quite the same quality controls that they do in the hyper inspected, over scrutinised west. Do all generics actually work?

Back in 2011/12 the total UK healthcare budget was £112Bn. Around 11% was the drugs budget. Of this, 8% was primary and 3% secondary care. It is worth noting that 68% of the total bill is staffing salaries/wages. This only leaves 21% of the £112 Bn to actually spend on patient activity. How much have GP prescribing costs increased, say over the last 5 years? This has been a steady increase- in absolute terms of healthcare costs and prescribing costs. In relative terms expenditure on prescribing is rising in relation to the rest of healthcare.

What percentage of drugs is generic? About 65-75%.

What follows is a random set of useful facts about various drugs:

Drugs, where they come from; Different phase trials:
- Phase 0: Pharmacodynamics and Pharmacokinetics,
- Phase 1: Screening for safety,
- Phase 2: Establishing the testing protocol,
- Phase 3: Final testing,
- Phase 4: Post approval studies.

Of the drugs that make it into MIMS,
For every 10,
7 are not profitable for the manufacturer,
2 break even,
1 makes money (sometimes a lot).

Total adverse drug reactions:
NSAIDs 30%,
Diuretics 27%,
Warfarin 10%,
ACEIs 7%.

New drugs are far more likely to have their adverse reactions reported than older, well establish drugs. Familiar drugs with known adverse reactions tend to have those reactions ignored as if drug reporting were simply a way of discovering new and previously unknown adverse reactions. Do we ever report bleeding on warfarin, indigestion on indomethacin, ibuprofen or steroids? An international study of spontaneous adverse drug reporting found a median under reporting in 37 studies of 94%. So ADR reporting is not a very reliable way of tabulating the real side effect profile of harmful drugs.

Under-reporting of adverse drug reactions: a systematic review. Drug Saf 2006 29 (5) 385-96.

Interesting odd drugs you might have forgotten about:

Benzodiazepines, half lives:

	Anxiolytic	Hypnotic	Anticonvulsant	Amnesic	Sedative*	(0-5) Half Life
Alprazolam Xanax	x				2	12-15 hrs
Chlordiazepoxide Librium	x				2	7-14hrs
Clobazam Frisium	x		x		0	36-46hrs
Clonazepam Rivotril			x		5	22-44hrs
Diazepam Valium etc	x		x	x	4	14-90hrs
Flurazepam Dalmane		x		x	4	24-48hrs
Lorazepam Ativan	x	x	x	x	5	9-22hrs
Lormetazepam Noctamid		x			1	8-12hrs
Midazolam Hypnovel		x		x	0	1.5-2.5hrs
Nitrazepam Mogadon		x	x	x	4	18-33hrs
Oxazepam	x				3	6-24hrs
Temazepam Normison		x			1	4-10hrs
Triazolam (not in UK)	x	x	x	x	1	2-4hrs

Available abroad and taken for jet lag because of rapid onset and short action. Various cognitive day after side effects, potential teratogen, anterograde amnesia, has been abused as a date rape drug. For Flunitrazepam see page 558.

*The extent of sedation as a result of daytime therapy with anxiolytic or in the case of hypnotics, residual sedation in the morning following nocturnal treatment.

Lorazepam: Ativan. Short to medium duration benzodiazepine. Has all 5 benzodiazepine effects: anxiolytic, amnesic, sedative/hypnotic, anticonvulsant and muscle relaxant. It has a high addictive potential and a strong anti anxiety effect. I prescribe it but never for more than a couple of weeks. It also has a potent amnesic effect so it is used as a premed orally or IV. It is a reliable anti convulsant, needing to be repeated less often than diazepam given IV and can be used in alcohol withdrawal treatment regimes.

Side effects include sedation, addiction, disinhibition, suicide, amnesia and all the therapeutic effects which may occur to an unwanted degree.

Ativan was prescribed at twice the American dose here in the UK and this and its relatively short half life led to significant early problems with withdrawal symptoms.

Other competing BDZs had longer half lives and so their withdrawal symptoms were attenuated.

The Z Drugs: Half lives:

Zolpidem 2.5 hrs (residual next day sedation in some),

Zolpidem CR 2.8 hrs,

Eszopiclone 6 hrs (fewer next day hangover effects than Zolpidem),

Zaleplon 1 hr (few residual next day effects),

Zopiclone 5 hours.

Other hypnotics:

Ramelteon 1-2.6 hrs (a melatonin receptor agonist),

Suvorexant Belsomra An orexin receptor antagonist, which alters the signalling of orexins, neurotransmitters responsible for regulating the sleep wake cycle.

SSRIs

The half life issue is interesting and applies to SSRIs too: Fluoxetine has a long half life, with significant residual drug persisting in the patient for weeks and therefore "withdrawal" being less of an apparent issue. It is well known that Paroxetine can be difficult to discontinue and this is due to its relatively short half life. I am never sure whether recurrence of that sense of despair and anxiety, lack of self esteem, symptoms of depression and the very reasonable wish to continue or restart the medication is actually "true withdrawal" or a recurrence of the pre existing depression. A desire to stay well, a bereavement for the wellness, a proof of something akin to "serotonin deficiency" which the SSRI has treated in just the same way as insulin treats diabetes. Given the relative long term safety of SSRIs, the lack of tachyphylaxis and the way they transform patient's lives, I have no real ethical dilemma in prescribing very long term or even life-long treatment with a stable dose regime of an SSRI in a patient with regular supervision, after discussion. I do see patients on antidepressants every 2-3 months long term, and more frequently initially, obviously. Surely it is simply a question of the least harm?

	Half Life	Withdrawal reports (Yellow cards from a 2010 paper)
Fluvoxamine	17-22 hrs	1%
Fluoxetine	4-16 days	6%
Sertraline	22-36 hrs	6%
Paroxetine	21 hrs variable	84% (I have never been unable to get a patient off this)
Venlafaxine	5-11 hrs	2%
Citalopram	1.5 days	<1%
Dutonin	up to 24 hrs	>1%

Undoubtedly the yellow card system has highlighted an exceptional number of patients with physical symptoms of Paroxetine and other SSRI withdrawal ranging from nausea, dizziness, tremor to sweating, the symptoms beginning 1-4 days after discontinuation of therapy in the case of Paroxetine. Neonatal withdrawal symptoms of babies born to mothers on SSRIs have also been described and so physical dependence **is** real as well as emotional dependence.

Antidepressant classes and side effects:

	Sedation	Anticholinergic	Nausea	Hypotension	Cardiac S/Es	Fatal O/D
SSRIs						
Citalopram	0	0	++	0	0	+
Escitalopram	0	0	++	0	0	+
Fluoxetine	0	0	++	0	0	0
Fluvoxamine	+	+	+++	0	0	0
Paroxetine	0	0	++	0	0	0
Sertraline	0	0	++	0	0	0
TCADs						
Amitriptyline	+++	+++	++	++	+++	+++
Clomipramine	++	+++	++	+	++	+
Dosulepin	+++	++	0	++	++	+++
Doxepin	++	+	+	++	++	++
Imipramine	+	++	++	+++	++	+++
Lofepramine	+	++	+	+	+	0
Trimipramine	++	+++	+	++	++	++
Trazodone	++	+	+++	++	+	0
NaSSA						
Mirtazapine	++	0	0	+	0	0
SNRI						
Venlafaxine	+	0	++	0	++	–
NARI						
Reboxetine	0	+	+	0	+	0
MAOI						
Phenelzine	0	+	++	+++	+	++
RIMA						
Moclobemide	0	+	+	+	0	0

Nortriptyline is a useful and underused TCAD. It works in major depression, nocturnal enuresis, (<3m total course). Some prescribe it in panic disorder, IBS, migraine (where it works well in a low dose, with Topiramate), in chronic pain/neuralgia, including TMJ pain. It CAN help improve ADHD symptoms and improve smoking abstinence.

Other Useful random drugs:

Bumetanide: Loop diuretic 1-5mg daily a "stronger diuretic" in heart failure:

Omeprazole: Use this if other PPIs are causing diarrhoea (especially Lansoprazole). Protons are hydrogen ions of course. Proton pump inhibitors are widely prescribed, taken bought OTC and have been linked, when prescribed continuously for prolonged periods to a number of unexpected (and rare) complications. These include:

Serious gastro intestinal infections, including by C Difficile, Salmonella, Shigella and Campylobacter. Possibly upper respiratory infections. Malabsorption of Vitamins including B12, Vitamin C and minerals including magnesium, iron and probably calcium, increasing osteoporotic fracture risk. These complications are rare and seen more often in the elderly, malnourished, hospitalised, dialysed and frail.

An increased risk of dementia. The 2013 PLOS ONE study linked PPIs to an increased production of beta amyloid proteins characteristic of Alzheimer's disease. In 2016 a JAMA Neurology study of 74,000 German patients >75 years found PPI users were 44% more likely to suffer dementia than non users.

An increased risk of renal problems. A 2013 BMC Nephrology study found patients with the rather vague diagnosis of "kidney disease" were twice as likely to be on PPIs than those without "kidney disease". Long term treatment with a PPI was associated with a 20-50% increased risk of CKD. The theory is that blood vessel endothelial cells break down cellular protein detritus using stored acid. This is part of normal cellular housekeeping. PPIs hinder all hydrogen ion production not just that in gastric oxyntic cells and so some cells become stuffed with debris they normally remove dissolved in acid. Where there are many blood vessels (kidney and myocardium) this backlog becomes functionally significant.

Chloral Hydrate, Welldorm 707mg 1-2 nocte for adults, suspension if necessary in children.

Midazolam: 10mg inj in 2ml. Injection in endoscopy and premed.

Likewise:

Nozinan, Levomepromazine: 25mg in 1ml (Some analgesic properties too).

Promazine, Sparine: 50mg/ml in severe psychomotor agitation.

Trifluoperazine, Stelazine: 1mg, 5mg tabs, Syrup and soln. Anxiety, agitation.

Buccastem Prochlorperazine: Sublingual 3mg for nausea, sickness and dizziness. Not desperately effective but swallowed tablets are vomited or not absorbed and a lot of British patients aren't keen on Domperidone suppositories. – And even these are now generic, hard to come by and expensive. What other options are there?

Pericy(i)azine: A phenothiazine used in schizophrenia and in severe anxiety/agitation. 5mg for anxiety increasing to 75mg (adult, divided doses) for psychosis. Can be used from children to the elderly.

Olanzapine and Quetiapine: can be used in severe anxiety or agitation.

Motion sickness:

Cinnarizine 15mg, Stugeron (OTC) 1-2 TDS

Scopoderm Patches: 1.5mg, last 72 hrs.

Varicose Veins:

Some patients find Antistax Red Vine leaf extract Capsules (OTC) helpful. – Stranger things have happened.

Hirudoid Cream and Gel (THF Salicylate, Ethyl Nicotinate, Hexyl Nicotinate) certainly do help alleviate uncomfortable varicose veins, as does Transvasin cream/gel. (which has the same contents as Hirudoid).

Extrapyramidal drug side effects can be treated using:

Orphenadrine Disipal, Procyclidine Kemadrin: Benz(a)tropine, Cogentin and (dystonia, akathisia, Parkinsonism, tardive dyskinesia, etc) **can be caused** by:

Fluphenazine, Flupenthixol, Haloperidol, Trifluoperizine, Chlorpromazine, Sulpiride, Risperidone, Metoclopramide (especially if you are unwise enough to prescribe them in sub teenagers) Prochlorperazine, Amitriptyline, Paroxetine, Carbamazepine, Methyl Dopa, Lithium Tardive Dyskinesia: Rx Tetrabenazine with a small dose of Haloperidol.

"Real Alternative" Treatments:

Green Tea (as tablets) contains Catechins and Polyphenols which are anti cancer molecules.

Red Wine (etc) contains Polyphenols and Resveratrol which are said to be anti cancer.

Turmeric, a cooking spice contains Curcumin which is one of the most effective anti cancer molecules, especially active with black pepper which aids its absorption.

Blueberries, black currents, black berries and other brightly coloured berries contain anthocyanidins which, again, are anti cancer, promoting cancer cell apoptosis (suicide).

Raspberries, strawberries and cherries contain Ellagic Acid (Polyphenols and Glucaric Acid), as do cranberries, cinnamon and

Dark Chocolate (>70% cocoa) contains proanthocyanidins and polyphenols which have a demonstrable anti cancer effect.

Pomegranates have a specific anti prostate cancer effect as does the Lycopene in gently cooked tomatoes.

Many herbs and spices including ginger are anti inflammatory and anti cancer as are the cruciform vegetables and Omega 3 oils.

Most of these foods' effects are demonstrable, recorded in numerous blinded trials, but very poorly known and promoted amongst my medical colleagues, particularly my oncology colleagues. We should be telling all our cancer patients about them and trying to get **all** our patients to permanently change their diets to incorporate active, healthy foods.

Bromelain is a mixture of pineapple enzymes (Proteases) – So is Papain which can also be used, which may help soft tissue bruising and swelling (after surgery, episiotomy etc) settle quicker. Used on the continent for this, in arthritis and as an aid to digestion. I have found it to work for post episiotomy and post surgical swelling pain and bruising.

Antidotes:

N-Acetyl Cysteine for paracetamol (Methionine has been used with more S/Es). Activated charcoal.

High dose atropine for organophosphate insecticides.

Sodium Nitrite, Sodium Thiosulphate or Dicobalt Edetate, Hydroxycobalamin for Cyanides.

Digoxin specific FAB Abs.

Flumazenil for benzodiazepines.

Naloxone for opioids.

IV Benzodiazepines for cocaine toxicity, also can give nitrates, Labetalol.

Other Interesting Drugs:

Fenofibrate reduces triglycerides as does Nicotinic Acid.

Unusual Hypnotics:

Melatonin:

3-12mg for Children with ADHD and adults with shift work and jet lag. The safest antioxidant. It can be used in insomnia caused by B Blockers, BZD withdrawal and stopping smoking. It reduces growth in metastatic breast cancer (in some small trials).

Terminal Care:

Bone Pain: Etidronate 800mg/day, steroids (especially in myeloma). Old fashioned: Disprin (aspirin) and nepenthe (literally a "potion that induces forgetfulness"). Originally morphine elixir but any contemporary morphine suspension would do.

Anticoagulants in pregnancy:

Heparin in first 6-9 weeks then oral anticoagulants 16th-36th week then heparin again. Heparin throughout can cause osteoporosis. Anticoagulation in some studies caused 7% congenital abnormalities, S.B. or abortion 16% if oral throughout pregnancy.

Paracetamol Toxicity:

at a dose level of 150mg/kg. Antagonists are Methionine (it was once suggested that this should be combined with OTC Paracetamol tablets) and Acetylcysteine (given as an antagonist in overdose as well as activated charcoal etc).

While we are on the subject of paracetamol (acetaminophen in America) it may not be as benign as we have all thought since it was discovered in 1852. It is analgesic (probably by reducing prostaglandin production in the CNS) and anti pyretic (via the hypothalamic heat regulating centre) and it has a well known narrow therapeutic index in overdose. A 2015 systematic review found that it had some unexpected side effects and its long term use was linked to increased mortality, – the risk of MI and stroke being increased up to 68%, of gastric ulcers and bleeding by 49% and mortality by up to 63%. All pretty hard to believe given the numbers of patients who consume large amounts regularly. Good old Paracetamol has had a bad press over the last few years, being found ineffective in back pain combination analgesics four times daily, in and out of favour with NICE and in one study linked to asthma. It quadrupled the risk of liver function abnormalities in another study. The only trouble is that anti inflammatories are far worse when it comes to bleeding and drug interactions, potent analgesics have significant central side effects, the most patient friendly combination mid range analgesic, (and with a lower dose of paracetamol) – Co Proxamol, has unjustifiably been withdrawn from its most benefitted patients via cost and theoretical overdose restrictions. And later life can be a very painful time.

Opiate withdrawal:

Lofexidine, Britlofex. Alpha adrenergic agonist, takes 7-10 days, 0.2mg BD gradually increasing, maximum 12 daily, slightly sedative.

Adrenergic Receptors:

Cardiac β1,
Adipocyte β1,
Vascular smooth muscle β2,
Bronchial smooth muscle β2,
Uterine smooth muscle β2,
Leukocyte β2,
Vascular α1,
Kidney α2,
CNS (Lowers BP) α2,
Adipocyte α2,
Platelet α2.

Methotrimeprazine: Is one of my most useful and adaptable drugs, as a GP who supervises hands – on pain management at home-when patients with cancer choose to end their days there. Also known as levomepromazine or Nozinan, it is a sedative antiemetic often used in terminal care but it also has useful profound analgesic properties. It is a congener (related by origin, structure or function) of Chlorpromazine with poor anti psychotic but good hypnotic, analgesic and antiemetic properties. It is sedative and all these effects make it ideal for use in terminal care where it can be incorporated in a syringe driver regime. Interestingly it can act as a local anaesthetic, an analgesic in cancer, post herpetic neuralgia and MI pain. It is a very useful drug. Certainly worth having a couple of ampoules in the visiting bag along with the Diamorphine.

Date Rape Drugs:

I have had a number of patients ask me to investigate if they could have been the victims of "date rape". One was a female student at a UK university, another a male air crew member overnighting in a hotel in South America. I think it is likely that they had both been drugged and sexually abused and that "spiking of drinks" seems to be quite common at university, some crowded pubs and some teenage parties. You have to make an assessment about the circumstances and suggest involving the police and even if necessary the local AIDS prophylaxis team if the situation warrants it.

Various drugs are used to incapacitate the potential victim in these attacks and these include

Alcohol.

GHB Gamma hydroxy butyrate (also called "Liquid Ecstasy") is actually a CNS depressant, colourless and odourless but it is **salty** to the taste. Small doses are said to be a stimulant and aphrodisiac. It is (rarely) used medicinally – in narcolepsy. It produces a short coma like sleep. 1 in 5 rape victims is unable to remember the assault and 70% say they felt unable to physically resist if they *can* remember.

GHB can be tested in urine – but only within 8-12 hours. It is detectable in hair for some months however.

Overdose can cause death through respiratory depression and cardiac arrest. Alcohol and other sedatives multiply its effect.

Benzodiazepines:
Flunitrazepam – Rohypnol*,
Temazepam*,
Midazolam*,
*Soluble in alcohol.

Flunitrazepam causes anterograde amnesia (the victims cannot remember events while under the influence of the drug) and it prevents them from resisting. The effect can start in 10 minutes and peaks at 8 hours. It causes sedation and euphoria in 20-30 minutes. Peak plasma levels in 45 minutes. It is very fast acting. It is colourless odourless and tasteless. It has a half life of 18-26 hours. It has an active metabolite (like diazepam) which lasts 36-200 hrs.

It causes confusion, drowsiness, lowered inhibitions and amnesia.

Flunitrazepam can be detected in urine for 5days and in hair for a month.

Non Steroidal Anti-inflammatory Drugs: The classes:

Salicylates: Aspirin, Diflunisal.
Propionic Acid Derivatives: Ibuprofen, Naproxen, Ketoprofen.
Acetic Acid Derivatives: Indomethacin, Etodolac, Diclofenac. Nabumetone.
Enolic Acid Derivatives: Piroxicam, Meloxicam.
Fenamic Acid Derivatives: Mefenamic Acid.
Selective COX-2 inhibitors: Celecoxib, Etoricoxib.
Also:
Pyrazolones: Phenylbutazone.
Benzotriazine: Azapropazone.

NSAIDS and CVS risk (See Cardiovascular section):

COX-1 and COX-2.: Things you may have forgotten:

Cyclo-oxygenase is an enzyme involved in the inflammatory response and other metabolic pathways. There are two types, 1 and 2. COX-1 is in most tissues, it maintains stomach lining and is involved in renal and platelet function. COX-2 is mainly present at sites of inflammation.

Generally it is therapeutically useful to inhibit COX-2 but not COX-1.

Regular NSAID use is associated with a 10% increase in cardiovascular death, non fatal MI, non fatal stroke as opposed to not taking NSAIDs. This is OVERALL, for the group as a whole. Different types of NSAID however, constitute different risks: Thus:

for Coxibs (COX 2 selective) CV risk increases 13%,

for Non COX selective (Greater COX 2 than COX 1 selectivity) eg Naproxen, Diclofenac increased risk is 17% although most physicians still regard Naproxen as amongst the safest NSAID as far as CVS risk is concerned.

for Non COX Selective (Greater COX 1 than COX 2 selectivity) eg Ibuprofen, Ketoprofen, Indomethacin, there is no increased risk. (WHI analysis).

Indeed Aspirin consumption reduces the CVS risk associated with COX 2 inhibitors but not with non COX 2 inhibitors.

Regular long term NSAID use reduces Vitamin B6 levels and can lead to deficiency with a list of potential secondary complications. AmJ Clin Nut2013 Oct 23.

Regular long term aspirin consumption reduces thrombotic cardiovascular risk, it also reduces the risks of developing a number of cancers, of bowel, oesophagus, breast and stomach as well, surprisingly, as the progress of emphysema (MESA-lung study – this is the Multi Ethnic Study of Atherosclerosis). It may or may not make macular degeneration worse. It is the classic example where large studies of the same drug in the same clinical situation come to opposing conclusions.

SUMMARY: THE LATEST FDA (2015) RECOMMENDATION

With a history of MI there is an increased risk of cardiovascular events with COX-2 inhibitors and non-selective NSAIDs. Both are contraindicated in patients with an acute MI. Caution in patients with stable Ischaemic Heart Disease.

For patients with acute MI, Coronary A Disease, or risk factors for Cardiovascular Disease:

Aspirin (81mg) in all patients, add a PPI, if on NSAID, monitor BP, oedema, renal function and GI bleeding. I presume 81mg=75mg to you and me.

Acetaminophen (paracetamol), aspirin, tramadol, narcotic analgesics, (short term)
Non Acetylated salicylates
Non COX-2-selective NSAIDs (Naproxen)
NSAIDs with some COX-2 selectivity
COX-2 selective NSAIDs

Circulation 2007:115:1634-1642

Stroke: Ibuprofen and diclofenac have the highest risk of stroke

Cancer and conventional drugs:

Naltrexone:

Is a drug used in opiate withdrawal. But it is an extremely interesting drug which is used in low doses to reduce the risks of cancer recurrence. Some studies suggest that up to 60% of cancer patients with a variety of tumours may benefit. The mechanisms may be via adrenal endorphin production, by altering opiate receptors on tumour membranes or by stimulating NK (natural killer cell) numbers. Also known as LDN (low dose Naltrexone).

Other drugs that have a proven effect against cancer include:

Aspirin which reduces metastases and improves survival in a number of cancers,

Cimetidine which, alone among the H2 antagonists reduces metastatic spread of bowel and other cancers, including during surgery,

Metformin which improves the prognosis in many cancers,

Clomipramine, which aids the effect of Temozolomide (used in Glioma treatment) etc,

There is also a plethora of supplements from Omega three oils and Vitamin D to Curcumin, Resveratrol etc that help reduce cancer severity and recurrence.(See diet section etc).

Prescribing Dilemmas:

Independent prescribers may prescribe any licensed or unlicensed medicine for any medical condition within their area of competence. Prescribing and clinical responsibility are linked.

Patients referred privately are expected to pay the full cost of the treatment they receive and any drugs prescribed at a private consultation should be the responsibility of the patient. The private prescription costs cover a particular condition and one episode of care. However although you **are** within your rights to do this, I do think you have to be a particularly mean spirited doctor to force your patient to pay for their privately prescribed drugs under these circumstances. If the patient has seen a doctor privately, he is effectively paying for that service twice, through compulsory taxation to provide the service to others and through private premiums for him and his family. You cannot opt out of blanket NHS payments. Why should he have to pay the exorbitant cost of a private drug when the hopelessly unfair NHS system excludes the vast majority of people from paying anything on irrational and outdated rules? The whole prescription payment system is unfair – let's face it.

GPs may issue private prescriptions to NHS patients for drugs not available on the NHS and for drugs to treat indications not covered by the SLS (Selected List Scheme) conditions. These include certain travel vaccines, antibiotics for future traveller's diarrhoea, acetazolamide (altitude sickness) etc.

A private prescription for a named patient-preferred branded drug may not be issued if the NHS permits the generic prescription. I have never charged my patients for private prescriptions. I believe it is morally unjustifiable to charge someone for a prescription which you are telling them they must take as well as charging them for the consultation. They will have to pay the pharmacist for the drug when they collect it but charging them for the scrip and for the consultation is like charging them twice for the same therapeutic advice.

Unlicensed use of drugs must be justifiable, supervisable, recognised by conventional medical opinion and the patient apprised of any adverse effects.

For instance: HPV: If the GP decides that the patient's behaviour justifies vaccination outside the national immunisation programme then this is not a situation where a private scrip can be issued, this is a GMS service.

The NHS ceases responsibility for patients travelling abroad. In Europe patients should carry the EHIC card. Usually no more than three months of a regular medication should be given and in the case of CDs, a covering "Personal Licence" may be needed. GPs are not required to provide NHS scrips for prophylactic medication (sea sickness or anti diarrhoeal medication). A private prescription should be used for "just in case" medication such as Ciprofloxacin for backpackers.

Emergency Travel Kits can be purchased and contain sterile needles, sutures and dressings.

Travel Vaccines which are available on the NHS: Include Typhoid, Hep A, Polio, Cholera.

Private scrips can be issued for Hep B, Meningococci A, C, W135 and Y, Japanese Encephalitis, Rabies, Tick Borne Encephalitis, Yellow Fever. GP s may charge patients (one of the rare occasions) directly for these.

Travel advice is, of course, given free.

If the patient spends more than three months abroad then they should register with a doctor and obtain top up drugs there.

Anti malarial drugs, advice and the supply thereof are all private and chargeable. If the patient is doing a charity walk, cycle ride or marathon don't for goodness sake charge them for anything. In fact go out of your way to suggest cream for saddle sores, sun burn, get your travel nurse involved if appropriate.

Controlled Drugs: Generally prescriptions should be for no more than 30 days. Any longer prescription should be recorded on the patient's notes.

Three months worth of CDs necessitate a personal licence. Fewer than three months' worth will need a letter from the prescriber including the patient's name, address, DOB, the dates of exit and return, the country visited, a list of the relevant drugs with doses and totals. The drugs should be in the original packaging, in hand luggage, with the licence and or covering letters. The patient is also advised to contact the relevant country's Embassy, Consulate or High Commission to clarify the rules for that particular country.

Any patient staying abroad for three months should reregister with a doctor in the country they are visiting.

Borderline food and dietary supplements should be limited to patients with the specific conditions listed in the BNF (dysphagia, gastrectomy, IBD, malabsorption, liver disease, disease related malnutrition, metabolic disorders, renal failure, some specific skin disorders etc). I suppose the commonest situation would be in cancer where it would be entirely inappropriate to deny the patient a selection of what are after all pretty unpleasant tasting high calorie, high fat or high protein supplements. I prescribe whatever the patient wants and let them see if there is anything they can stomach. The same isn't true for thin patients in nursing home situations where a cheaper and probably more palatable alternative would be higher calorie extra drinks (with ice cream or sugar), extra snacks etc.

Complimentary Therapies: Few, other than osteopathy are supported by proper robust evidence based data so I would never prescribe homeopathic medication, aromatherapy treatments, herbal medications, etc even though I am aware that some herbal medicines contain active ingredients. Some of these are potentially very dangerous. Homeopathic medication is listed in neither MIMS nor the BNF so my response to Prince Charles would be that I was unwilling to be responsible even for the absence of effect as I knew nothing about the treatment. And homeopathic medication still costs money despite being water.

Infertility: I offer to prescribe half the total cost of the drugs of any couple going for private infertility treatment. As long as they are married.

These are the reasons:

They are saving the NHS money if they are referring themselves and at 20% a cycle the NHS often fails to provide potentially excellent parents with a wanted baby.

They are victims of an unfair and unpredictable and distressing situation which they have asked me, their GP to help with.

Private infertility treatment is extremely expensive, emotionally draining and not very reliable.

Generally I like my patients, I care about their wellbeing and I want them to value me as much as I try to do them.

This is one way in which the patient will value your empathy and support in a practical way for decades.

My only caveat is that I need to be sure that the couple is committed to staying together. Since unmarried couples with children are 4X more likely to separate than married couples, I take a lot of persuading to feel as committed to the unmarried who say they want children compared with the couple who have made that formal commitment in front of friends, family and the state. We are an evidence based profession. If any couple feels hard done by when I refuse, then the evidence of their statistical prognosis together is readily available and easy to access.

Erectile dysfunction. The NHS rules on this are clear and the qualifying conditions are listed under "Urology". The majority of prescriptions though are now from sympathetic GPs for men who are failing in confidence, or in prowess, starting a new relationship after some time away from "the fray" or after an emotional trauma – etc. Male doctors prescribe more than female, interestingly, or perhaps it is that male patients consult male doctors more often (if they get a chance) about that sort of problem. The drugs work and have relatively few side effects. Viagra is now OTC which takes some of the pressure off the poor beleaguered GP but it **is** always worth going over the side effects, C/Is and risks and checking the BP in any man who mentions E.D to you. Also: how long is a man supposed to carry on having sex for? Just because drugs exist to cause erections, shouldn't we be thinking about the moral and ethical dimensions of elderly men who can barely walk or think straight in their 80's or 90's still expecting to bother their poor wives in this *artificial* way? And shouldn't the partner be interviewed alone for her opinion? Is your approach the same with gay couples? Lesbian couples ? How many other drugs have no purpose but pleasure, self indulgence? We cannot pretend we are treating illness or suffering here, Viagra is not exactly what the NHS was conceived for.

A group of drugs is found to cause priapism as a side effect and an erection becomes a human right? I have to admit, just because a drug exists, it doesn't mean it should be readily and freely available or as some people think, a RIGHT for everyone who wants it.

Prescribing for yourself or your family: This is where I have a serious ethical disagreement with the GMC and its current official guidance. I think it is out of contact with reality, reason, practicality and implies a mistrust in the average member of the medical profession which is unjustified and unreasonable. I explain this elsewhere in the context of a GP who was suspended for a year, lost her practice (partly through the subsequent actions of a malicious partner) and her reputation and all because she prescribed a Fentanyl patch for her terminally ill sister at a weekend. The alternative was to force a much beloved sister with breast cancer and secondaries to travel twenty miles and sit in a virus infested waiting room for a doctor who was stranger to top up her prescription. I feel The GMC (which usually has few or **no GP members** and if you look at their credentials are totally urban and out of touch with non city General Practice) overreacted excessively.

I see absolutely no reason not to prescribe for your own daughter's earache or for you to refrain from delaying your wife's period while you are on holiday or not to treat a family member's back strain while they cannot easily see their own trusted GP. The GMC, however, seems to fall over itself to suspend GPs who do this while ignoring the huge numbers of GPs who care less about their patients than their family medical businesses or their own childcare timetable, who have given up listening to or caring for their patients in any meaningful sense and whose credentials, English skills and qualifications are unfit for purpose.

I know from the experience of my own family that trusted GPs who are available, competent and familiar with that patient's previous problems are a dwindling resource in inner cities, in practices with many part time GPs who work limited hours. I feel very strongly that provided the doctor is not prescribing psychoactive, addictive drugs, unmonitored controlled or strong analgesic drugs, the following advice is mostly just plain wrong. But here it is:

The GMC says that family members should be registered with a different practice, as should practice staff and that wherever possible all conditions should be treated by an objective (other) GP.

I see no reason not to prescribe for your own family. Or if a family member falls ill in the evening or at the weekend I see no reason why you shouldn't phone a local medical friend, tell them what to prescribe and let them fill in the T/R form next morning or on Monday. I guess that is what most of us do anyway. The end result is that you are prescribing isn't it?

Prescribing Errors:

Come in many forms.

Some studies have found that up to 80% of prescriptions contain some kind of error. These errors can include the wrong patient, drug, strength, dose, formulation, frequency or quantity.

Wrong drug: Being inaccurate or wrong about what a drug does or having poor handwriting so that the wrong drug is dispensed.

Bad hand writing still occurs very frequently and many drug names are easily mistaken for one another. Penicillin and Penicillamine, Hydroxyzine and Hydrallazine.

Wrong formulation/frequency (a confusing variety of extended release, or slow and extended release formulations of a drug and therefore giving the wrong formulation at the wrong frequency).

Assuming "slow release" or "extended/delayed release" mean the same absorption rate for all drugs (twice a day, once a day etc).

Ignoring electronic warnings through red flag fatigue. A common enough drug software problem which ignores the human frustrations of obstruction and delay when writing dozens of prescriptions a day.

Failure to make dose alterations based on changing or newly reported renal function.

Misplaced decimal points, mixing up of ug and mg, especially dangerous with Digoxin and drugs with a narrow therapeutic Index.

Confusing shorthand and abbreviations.

Continuation of drugs that are no longer necessary. A common problem when patients are discharged home without proper summaries from hospital. Inappropriate discontinuation of longstanding treatments on admission by junior staff who do not know why a particular regime was commenced by the GP ("SHO Syndrome").

Overseas visitors: NHS Treatment is available to patients registered with a practice who are going to stay at least 6 months. E.U. patients who hold an EHIC, patients who require immediate, essential treatment (which the doctor does not think can be delayed) patients holding an E112 for a specific condition only, patients holding an E128, patients allocated by the HB (or equivalent), certain refugees and asylum seekers.

All others may be charged for private treatment.

Occupational Health Vaccines: Hepatitis B needed by certain occupational and educational groups should be provided by the employer or education establishment via Occupational Health Departments or funded via the practice by the employer. There are some situations where individuals at risk (volunteers working with mentally disabled teenagers and adults, prison visitors etc) might not be funded but provide a socially useful service and where I would not have a problem writing an NHS scrip for a Hep B Vaccine.

Locums: Who wrote that scrip?

Because locums flit from practice to practice and there are 17,000 of them active in the NHS in 2016, they tend to prescribe using the absent partner's or even borrowed on-long-term-loan prescription pads. Thus the printed name on the pad is irrelevant and the signature is often undecipherable. The prescription has a Doctor's Index Number (DIN) (Prescription Number) which has been assigned to each British GP working in England and Wales by the Health and Social Care Information Centre. Each six digit DIN is tied to the GP's practice being assigned by their employing organisation. Therefore it is very difficult to identify locums who are responsible for any given prescription. Officially the prescription came from the absent partner.

The GPC has suggested a sensible solution which is to have personal prescriptions with an individual doctor's own GMC number on them. These could be paired with an organisation number to identify the practice that the GP was attached to at the time the prescription was issued. Problem solved.

The Visiting Bag:

When I qualified nearly 40+ years ago, the average G.P. was the boy scout of medicine. Prepared to deal with every medical situation that work and life could present. Even in commuter belt England in the second decade of the 21st century, all my experience tells me that neighbours still fall off step ladders, neighbour's children fracture collar bones playing in the garden, you come across men with broken necks, still alive, in wrecked cars on the way home from work, people in pubs have fits, friends and their guests have asthma attacks and that the out of hours service does not provide adequate immediate home care. Certainly the ambulance service, burdened as it is with ferrying patients to casualty out of hours that we GPs used to see and reassure does not arrive promptly at any time of day or night anymore.

So you have a choice as a G.P. – You can turn away and pretend, as many do, that General Practice is an all elective and desk bound job or you can do what the public expects of you: Treat pain and illness and give sensible referral advice based on how the patient responds to your immediate treatment. You can put a prescription pad and a stethoscope in your handbag but to do the job properly you do need a proper set of tools.

My visiting bag contains:

Tongue depressors, a bright pocket torch, a nasal speculum, Band Aids and Medi Swabs, an adult Guedel's Airway, a Resusciade, a selection of syringes (5mls the most useful) and needles (21g, green needles the most useful), latex examination gloves, KY jelly or similar, glycerin suppositories and Micralax Microenemas, (Micolette), Voltarol 100mg, Motilium 30mg and Paediatric Paracetamol suppositories (Alvedon 125mg), 75mg soluble Aspirin tabs, GTN Spray. (Coronitro is small, but keep an eye on the expiry date), Glucogel.

A MIMS – Although this is now available as an App in my i Phone, which is much lighter to carry, a variety of changing Aid Memoires in the form of an old PDA, my prescription pad folder with FP10s, a pad of Med Certs, a few private prescriptions (hardly ever used) and compliments slips (I always put through the letter box if I call in on a "house bound" patient who happens to be out).

Paper instructions on:

Parenteral doses of emergency drugs, Adult advanced life support algorithm, Mini Mental State examination, Treatment of anaphylactic shock algorithm, A list of symptoms and signs of specific diseases in children as well as the Traffic Light System for identifying the likelihood of serious illness in children (see paediatric section), Guidelines for the management of infection in primary care from our local H A.; My own protocol for missed pills and contraceptive advice as this seems to change frequently, Guidance on the use of anti flu treatment, A risk assessment tool for the evaluation of occupational exposure to HIV.(and local HIV contact phone no.); The ABCD2 scoring system and the CHADS scoring system of strokes and AF, Algorithm of treatment of patients with acute stroke and TIA, Algorithm of adult choking treatment, Summaries of the law on clarification and confirmation of unexplained deaths, The Eligibility of overseas visitors to receive free primary care, Phone numbers of OOH and unregistered dental services, Phone numbers of all my partners, local surgeries, D/Ns, CMHT, local hospitals, ambulance services etc etc, My cover rota.

Surgery headed note paper, envelopes, EDD calculator, Drug Interaction Alert, a Guide to Drugs in Breast Milk (The i Phone can usually access "Safefetus.com" which does much the same thing). A list of Tubigrip sizes, spare pens, a "Crocodile" which is a device for safely cutting off the tops of ampoules) and (because I once fished out a beer can ring pull from a croupy child's hypo pharynx), a pair of ENT elongated forceps, as well as sharp scissors, a pair of splinter forceps, a scalpel and blades (disposable scalpels are poor substitutes for the real thing), a Jobson Horne probe (lots of aural foreign bodies over the years) and suture material. You look really feeble if you can't stitch a neighbour's cut at the weekend and they have to spend 6 hours in casualty with the drunks. Stethoscopes, adult and neonatal, a sphygmomanometer, a patellar hammer, a mini auriscope/opthalmoscope set (although actually the latter has NEVER significantly contributed to a decision as to whether to admit a patient from home or not), a urine multitest Dipstix kit, (10 tests), a digital thermometer, transcutaneous oxygen monitor (very overrated as this depends as much on peripheral circulation and temperature/hydration as it does on oxygenation and several studies in sick children have shown how unreliable they can be), a tourniquet, a selection of Butterflies and Venflons, cotton wool balls, micropore tape.

Drugs:

I carry:

For the nebuliser: Salbutamol, 5mg in 2.5ml, Atrovent 500mcg in 2mls, Pulmicort 0.25mg/ml 2ml nebules (for croup etc).

Oral: Penicillin V, Erythromycin, Cefadroxil and Co Amoxiclav (my antibiotics of choice for OOH UTIs or LRTIs), Norfloxacin (Prostatitis), Timethoprim, Solpadol Tabs, Half Inderal LA, EC Prednisolone 5mg, Soluble 5mg Prednisolone, Propranolol Tabs 40mg, Furosemide tabs 40mg, Cyclizine tabs 50mg, Diazepam 5mg Tabs,

Co Dydramol, Co Codamol (500/30), Codeine Phosphate 30mg, Dihydrocodeine 30mg, Tramadol 50mg, Lormetazepam 1mg, Maxalt Melt (Rizatriptan), Ranitidine 150mg and Omeprazole 20mg, Chlorpromazine Tabs 50mg, Haloperidol Tabs 1.5mg, Diazepam 5mg.

Minims Tropicamide, Fluorescein, Amethocaine.

Controlled Oral Drugs: MST 10mg Tabs, Diconal Tabs, Pethidine 50mg tabs.

A one drop blood glucose testing kit, lancets and test strips. (e.g. One touch Ultra).

Rectal Diazepam 10mg (Stesolid).

Injectables:

Naloxone (Short shelf Life, but still works long after the expiry date), water for injections (2x10mls), Benzyl Penicillin 600mg dry powder, Cefuroxime (Zinacef) injection for the supposedly penicillin allergic, Adrenaline 1:1000 **at least** 2 in date ampoules, Glucagon 1mg (oral glucose gel just isn't enough sometimes), Chlorpheniramine 10mg in 1ml, Hydrocortisone 100mg in 1ml (at least 2 ampoules), Buscopan 20mg/ml 1ml amps, Atropine 600mcg in 1ml, Hypnovel/Midazolam (terminal care, aggression, panic and anxiety states), 10mg in 2mls, Nozinan 25mg in 1m, Haloperidol injection 5mg in 1ml, Chlorpromazine inj 50mg in 2mls, Depixol inj 20mg, (you might not necessarily expect these to be present in an emergency bag but the domiciliary psychiatry services I have had contact with over the last 30 years have been so inaccessible, so inconsistent and often so unhelpful that after they have finally come, deliberated and gone, a systemic injection of one of these drugs has been of huge benefit to the patient and their relatives and temporarily substituted for absent duty psychiatric services), Diazepam inj 10mg in 2mls, Stemetil 12.5mg in 1ml, Metoclopramide Injection 10mg in 2mls (avoid under 14-15 years old because of dystonia), Cyclizine 50mg inj. in 1ml, Furosemide 50mg in 5mls, Sodium Chloride inj 0.9% 2ml amps, Glycopyrrolate 200ug in 1ml (terminal care "secretions"), Kemadrine 5mg/ml and Aminophylline 250mg in 10mls (which is out of date and I haven't used in over 10 years because the nebuliser is usually so effective.) IV Glucose 10g in 20mls (50%),

Systemic pain killers: Diclofenac, Voltarol Inj 75mg in 3mls.

Controlled Drugs:

Pethidine Injection: 100mg in 2mls. Diamorphine 10mg dry powder amps,

You may think that all this is GP overkill but the VERY LEAST a real GP carries with them at all times in terms of systemic drugs are: Benzyl Penicillin and Water for Injections, Adrenaline, Hydrocortisone, Diamorphine, Diazepam, and Furosemide. I just don't see how you can pretend to be a doctor without having these basic systemic tools at your constant command.

GPs and Systemic analgesic Drugs:

(Non controlled alternatives: Tramadol injection 100mg in 2mls. Tramadol is an opioid agonist, not fully antagonised by Naloxone, more effective in surgical than dental pain, in terms of strength 50mg orally = Co codamol 30/500. Parenterally it is equivalent to Pethidine, approx 1/10 that of Morphine. Can increase seizures and per operative recall but causes less constipation than codeine.

Meptazinol injection is likewise not controlled but not very strong either.

Systemic analgesics (Controlled):

Morphine, Diamorphine, Methadone, Pethidine, Dihydrocodeine, Buprenorphine, Oxycodone, Pentazocine, Fentanyl.

Harold Shipman:

Was a British trained GP, who as a junior doctor killed approximately 15 patients including a 4 yr old and was known to have been cavalier with the doses of systemic drugs (including Diazepam) that he administered. As a GP is thought to have killed some 250 of his patients. His "unlawful killings" took place between 1970 and 1998 when he was finally arrested. Altogether 800 of his patients died during his medical career and were investigated, I presume this number is related as much to the practice age demography and the type of hospital jobs as to his cruel and murderous behaviour. His victims were mainly previously well elderly women who he killed by administering intravenous Diamorphine. He was known to have been a Pethidine addict himself in his early career when he had forged scrips which led to his being expelled from one GP partnership. He was treated for his addiction before the GMC permitted him to start practising again. He became a partner in Hythe, Manchester, killing 70 patients, then a single handed GP – by all accounts very popular, with a good practice prescribing profile and a huge list of 3,500. He was at one time Secretary of the local LMC and there was a 1 year wait to get on his list.

The high death rate amongst his patients and the suspicious circumstances (previously well patients, he had visited earlier in the day and had left the door on the latch so that he could return to "discover them" etc), led to suspicions being raised by a GP who was asked to sign Part 2 Cremation forms and by a local Undertaker. The police undertook a superficial investigation and found insufficient evidence to proceed. He then forged a will and this was instrumental in his final detection.

Harold Shipman denied the murders until the end. He hung himself in prison. The subsequent enquiry under Dame Janet Smith addressed the question why no one in authority had noticed what Shipman had been doing despite the existence of numerous concerns being expressed by various colleagues both medical and non medical during his career.

The net result of the enquiry was a series of burdensome and to be honest, irrelevant recommendations. Certainly they were irrelevant if the aim was to prevent psychopathic doctors using their position to murder patients. The bottom line for the practising GP is that Harold Shipman has resulted in:

1) Appraisal: This is an annual "Cornerstone of Revalidation". This was a political response to address the public revulsion at what had happened and to regulate a previously self regulated profession. It didn't construct a system for detecting dangerous doctors but resulted in a way of managing post graduate training and formalising professional reac-creditation of GPs. **Not the point in Shipman's case AT ALL**. It consists of the recording and "reflecting" on the appraisee's year of learning activity by discussing the varied forms of personal development undertaken. It is frequently a mentoring and support session and highly unlikely to uncover occult rogue doctors.-The most challenging thing that can be said for appraisal is that another doctor is suggesting alternative ways and means of keeping up to date.

It is, exactly what many of us hoped it would not become. – The Royal Colleges and their Deaneries setting agendas and standards for what makes a good doctor. In hospitals and in GP. In practical terms it is the completion of one of three electronic standardised Toolkits which prevent you from demonstrating your individualism in any way. It includes (included) the highly dubious or often totally pointless multisource feedback questionnaires and standardised audits amongst a series of data recording compulsory tasks. They are time consuming, structured and fiddly standardised software boxes but the process is ticking boxes nevertheless. Also it is incredibly expensive at around £500-550 per appraisal. **What is isn't is a way of finding unsafe doctors.**

Go to a course on appraisal or revalidation and the appraisers, of which I was one for ten years, will use terms (and I quote) like:

Appraisal is: "Part of a drive for quality in our healthcare systems,

About improving the governance of medical practice,

Intended to bring doctors into a structured process and encourage self reflective practice,

"A chance to celebrate good practice". (Celebrate? What have we come to as a profession that quiet satisfaction at a job well done has become a celebration?)

A positive affirmation of a doctor's professionalism"

-BUT *"It is NOT a new way to raise concerns about a doctor or a way of detecting another Harold Shipman"* (KSS Conference 2014)

Well, given the fact that the Francis enquiry about the Mid Staffordshire cruelty concluded that: "The more box ticking there was and management supervision of previously independent medical professionals the less committedly and caringly they did their job", you have to wonder why appraisal and revalidation are supposed to improve standards in this form and why they were constructed like this as a "Response to the Shipman scandal". But more importantly why all the academics who now control the process fall over themselves to emphasise how it isn't a way of weeding out bad doctors. Don't the patients have the right to expect exactly that after the publicity the government expended at the start of medical appraisal? Don't the patients have the right to expect improved safety as the goal of appraisal for their huge ongoing at least £550 per doctor a year cost?

Over a five year appraisal cycle, five separate annual files (each recording 50 or more one hour periods of documented "learning") will be considered sufficient for a 5 year Revalidation and Relicensing – Reaccreditation, before the granting of a Licence to Practise.

If it were designed as a response to or to detect a psychopath who was murdering his patients, it would have missed Shipman by a mile.

Cost:

There are, according to the GMC 235,170 doctors with full registration in the UK (2016).

Doctors on the GP register: 67,836.

Doctors on the specialist register: 87,869.

Total number of doctors on LRMP 281,138 (List of Registered Medical Practitioners). Cost of appraising just GPs annually at least £34 million (£500 X 67,800).

2) A longer and more intrusive Part 2 Cremation Form. The most intrusive part of the extra Shipman bureaucracy is the necessity to telephone grieving relatives to try subtly to find out if they had any suspicions about the death itself without upsetting them still further. If the death took place in a nursing home there is likewise a duty to talk to the nursing team involved to find information about the final days of the patient's life. This is often impractical given shift rotas, team responsibilities, holidays and so on and you may need to get some history related second hand by members of staff who weren't actually directly involved. So not only does this upset relatives and potentially introduce an element of suspicion, since they will not know who you are, phoning them up and asking about their doctor's handling of their loved one, but much of the information you glean is hearsay, subjective and inaccurate.

3) More intrusive controlled drug management. The more rigid stock control of CDs has been the most patient-harmful result of the Shipman aftermath. When I entered General Practice 30 years ago, every GP carried controlled drugs as a normal tool in their bag. I have asked colleagues from my own and other local practices and at recent post graduate meetings which of them had injectable controlled drugs in their bags? I was shocked at the result: Only 10% of my colleagues now carry Pethidine or Diamorphine with them. This is in my opinion a professional act of mass cowardice and betrayal which is beyond precedent. It is as a result of the "burdensome" new CD regulations and the fear of being labelled as a potential murderer and not a potential carer. The suffering, pain, fear and distress that this has already caused is immense. We seem to have forgotten that we are supposed to put the **patient's needs and potential needs** uppermost, not our own sensitivities, or the misplaced concerns and the potential suspicions of relatives or officious administrators.

The new Strengthened CD audit trail includes:

An **Accountable Officer** who now asks every the GP to fill in a form (Declaration and Self Assessment form) regarding his use of CDs.

Typical questions: (Do you prescribe, hold stock, dispose of CDs, do you have SOPs for CDs, do you have SOPs for significant events involving CDs, have there been any complaints about your prescribing of CDs, have there been any significant events involving CDs, are returned medicines ever reused, do you supply addicts, do you maintain records of administration, are all CDs kept under lock and key, do you keep CDs in your bag, how often do you date check your CDs, do you keep an up to date CD register, do you keep unused patients' stock etc.?)

All these questions, of course, rely on the honesty and probity of the individual and you would expect a dishonest doctor to lie to cover his tracks so I find the Declaration and Self Assessment a little pointless. How do you think Harold Shipman would have answered these questions?

Every practice has to write up a **SOP for the use of Controlled Drugs** at the surgery. I wrote my own practice's SOP and although it was all blindingly obvious to anyone who has given a few doses, the whole point of real life as a front line GP is *flexibility*. So by definition there is nothing standard about the use of a drug with a relatively low therapeutic index and for which you would have to write various caveats. These might include: use in severe pain but also in cardiac failure and its associated dyspnoea as well as severe and intractable cough (for which Diamorphine was first manufactured). So "Standard" isn't really appropriate when every operating procedure has to be considered on its separate merits.

The Safer Management of Controlled Drugs (Record Keeping) Act 2006 includes:

Strengthened record keeping ("the audit trail") throughout the NHS and private sector. There are now computerised systems for monitoring excess prescribing (eg the ePACT system) and whether maximum licensed doses are being exceeded, more than 30 day prescriptions are being issued and whether the CD is routinely prescribed in GP.

Records for schedule 2 drugs (Opiates, Amphetamines, Barbiturates) to be kept in a Controlled Drug Register, a CDR – All "Healthcare Professionals" who hold a personal stock of CDs must keep their own CDR and maintain it. These records must include the date the supply was obtained, name and address of the supplier, the amount obtained, name, form and strength of the CD.

For CDs supplied to patients or practitioners, the register must include the date, the name and address of the recipient, the quantity, the name form and strength of the CD supplied.

The following information is likely to be necessary later: Running balances, (this was recommended by the Shipman enquiry and is considered good practice), prescriber identification number, or the name and professional registration number of the dispenser.

Regular running balance checks should be made – I tend to do this every time I give an injection of a CD, the responsibility being that of the GP not a non clinical member of staff.

The paper records must be kept for 2 years, 11 years if on computer.

Other requirements for dispensers are to obtain proof of identity of the person collecting the drug, to record this in their drugs register etc.

There are denaturing kits available for the destruction of old CDs. (Usually from the Medicines Safety and Controlled Drugs Manager at the PCT/Commissioning Group).

The destruction of old CD stock must be witnessed by authorised staff (for most practical purposes this will be the Prescribing Advisor at the PCT/Commissioning Group) but the list includes:

A Chief Dental Officer,
Supervisors of Midwives,
Senior Officers in NHS Trusts,
Chief Executives of NHS Trusts, (!)
A Primary Care Trust Chief Pharmacist,
A Registered Medical Practitioner,
Medical Director of a Primary Care Trust.
etc.

This role used to be performed by a Police Controlled Drugs Liaison Officer.

The proposed Patient Drug Record Card is not yet a legal requirement.

All this is particularly applicable to Diamorphine, the most useful Terminal care drug and Harold Shipman's murder weapon of choice.

Up until these regulations, the fate of every ampoule of Pethidine and Diamorphine in the possession of a GP should have been recorded in their own Controlled Drug Register. Mine goes back to the early 80's when my trainer gave me two ampoules of Diamorphine which were duly recorded at the start of the book. So far I haven't ever been inspected by the Drugs Squad officer during my career (41 years, 32 in GP)) but perhaps Shipman will change the frequency and intensity of that like he has changed nearly every other aspect of the CD GP/trust/self regulation environment that existed before.

The practical Rules for Controlled Drug use in practice are (This is from the MPS):
1) Keep CDs in a lockable cupboard/safe.
2) Maintain a CD register (written (2 years) or electronic (11 years)) which includes:
3) A running balance of stock and
4) Entries on the correct page (separate sections for Pethidine, Diamorphine etc).

The CD register must be bound, contain class sections for each CD, have the name of the drug specified at the top of the page, entries in chronological order, no blank lines, in ink without cancellations/alterations, be kept for a minimum of 2 years after the last dated drug was given. This can be computerised.

New CD entries must record the supplier, the date, the amount, name, form and strength.

For CDs supplied to patients, the record must include the date, the name and address of the recipient, the amount, the person collecting the drug if not the patient, plus or minus proof of identity of the person collecting the drug if not the patient.

5) Try to have 2 members of staff (at least one clinical member) check the stock that comes and goes. This can be done monthly.

6) Keep individual registers for your bag CDs. Given that so few of us carry CDs now most practices leave the CD book to the individual doctor and let him obtain, store and dispose of stock.

7) Check expiry dates regularly as with all other injectable drugs (although there is evidence that virtually all drugs are effective months or years after their expiry dates*).

In any life threatening situation, the fact that a systemic drug is out of date should never prevent you from administering it if you do not have access to an in date alternative. I know of no drug that becomes toxic, only less effective as it ages and most, including opiates seem to work for decades past their shelf life expiry. The general advice though is try not to use if discoloured or precipitated.

Basic rule: Never leave needles, wrappers or ampoules of drugs you have administered to patients at their home. I know of a colleague who valiantly and successfully treated acute heart failure in an elderly patient in her 90's with IV Furosemide 2 months out of date. By doing so, he avoided an admission, 24 hours on a trolley, hospital acquired infections, sleeplessness, malnutrition and all the misery of hospital. He then received a letter of complaint from the patient's daughter. She had noticed the expiry date on the Furosemide ampoule was 2 months out of date.

8) Have expired stock disposed of by an authorised witness. (PCT, >Commissioning Group etc)

The net result of these bureaucratic regulations was not to make life safer for patients from rogue psychopathic GPs but to make pain relief in real emergencies and accidents cruelly, agonisingly and tragically delayed.

*Expiry dates are the time that the manufacturer is prepared to guarantee the full potency of a drug up to. It is not the date after which the drug loses potency. If you think about it, it is clearly in the manufacturer's interests to give a short expiry duration rather than a long one. The shorter, the more often the drug will be replaced and the more of the drug they will sell. Usually there are no reasons why drugs, most of which are perfectly stable if kept in reasonable storage conditions, shouldn't last many multiples of their given expiry dates. The American FDA conducted a study at the millennium on a large stock pile of their military's drugs. These represented a huge financial investment. They looked at 100 prescription and OTC drugs and found 90% were just as effective 15 years after the expiry date as they were new. Many were good 25 years later. This does not apply to Nitroglycerin, liquid oral medications including antibiotics, insulin and I would add drugs that are clearly visibly denatured, discoloured, or that you have kept in the "labile thermal environment" of your car boot (trunk in America). I would only advise that if you are administering "out of date drugs" do not leave the blister pack, box or ampoule with the expiry date for the patient to see.

(Second opinion: Pomerantz MD. Recycling Expensive medication. Why not? MedGenMed 2004 6 (2) 4 and etc Feb 2017)

18: Ear, Nose and Throat:

Some Anatomy:

The confusing jaw lymph glands are:

The submental glands, just medial to the anterior ramus of the mandible on each side, drain the lower lip, point of the tongue and floor of the mouth then drain backwards to the submandibular and submaxillary glands (which are the **same** names as the associated salivary glands).

The Middle Ear:

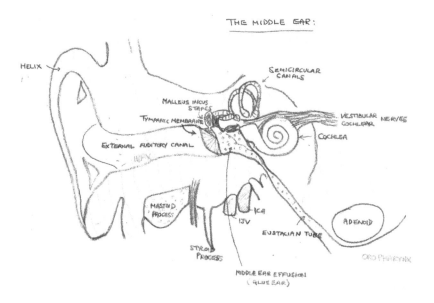

Sudden Deafness:

Wax is the commonest cause,
Otitis externa,
Acute otitis media, purulent or secretory,
Trauma to middle or outer ear,
Otosclerosis,
Presbycusis (old age deafness),
Vascular accidents to inner ear,
Infections including Mumps, Rubella, etc.
Drugs: Salicylates, streptomycin, neomycin, kanamycin, quinine, chloroquine, phenytoin.

Useful drugs ENT:

Otitis Externa:

Most drops are C/I in perforated ear drums.

Locorten Vioform: (Clioquinol/Flumetasone) (AF, S). Otomize: (Dexamethasone Acetic Acid, Neomycin), (S, AS, AB). Sofradex: (Dexamethasone, Framycetin, Gramicidin) (S, AB). Gentisone HC (Gentamicin and Hydrocortisone) (AB, S). Otosporin (Polymyxin B, Neomycin, Hydrocortisone) (AB, S). Clotrimazole (Canestan) 1% solution (AF).

Note: Antifungal AF Antiseptic AS AB Antibiotic Steroid S

In otitis externa, good aural toilet is needed to keep the canal as clean and dry as possible. Pseudomonas is the common organism, Staph if there is a boil. Aspergillus and Candida are the common fungi. Otitis Externa can be "malignant" and extremely painful, requiring admission especially in the immunocompromised and diabetics. Topical Acetic Acid is anti fungal and antibacterial. Topical aluminium acetate drops are antibacterial and anti inflammatory.

On otoscopy it is very important to view the 'attic' as this is where sinister problems begin. Wax is only made in the outer 1/3, do not falsely identify cholesteatoma as wax against the drum. The common bacteria are pseudomonas and staph. So a good idea is to do a swab on second presentation, gentle ear toilet and drops – Gentisone is good in staph and pseudomonas, Cipro and Ofloxacin good for pseudomonas. In perfora-ration aminoglycosides can cause ototoxicity if used for >7d. Fungal infections are due to immunodeficiency or overuse of antibiotics. Locorten has anti-fungal and anti-bacterial actions. Sometimes Canesten drops are needed for 6wks to clear candidal infections. Sudden hearing loss is an ENT emergency, give Prednisolone/Betahistine and Aciclovir and refer or review soon unless it is clearly just wax.

Otitis Media:

80% resolve within 4 days without antibiotics so treat the pain, especially in the first 24 hours. Apparently the stated NNT is 20 over 2 year old children and 7 between 6 and 24 months to relieve one episode of pain between 2 and 7 days. It took only a few years of Family Medicine to lead me to doubt the provenance of those sort of figures. You soon get to know the many children on your list who genuinely suffer with their ears and you do see so many bulging red drums (not the pink injected drums of mildly unhappy children with colds). This is in children in utter misery with earache who are better in 24 hours after a bacteriocidal antibiotic but aren't without it. Antibiotics undoubtedly reduce pain, reduce the risk of complications. How many mastoiditisis from middle ear infec-tions have you seen?, something which were two a penny 50 years ago. They reduce the very rare risk of intracranial spread of sepsis etc. They do, however undoubtedly contribute to resistance, the spurious perception of antibiotic allergy (earache, URTI and rashes are common bedfellows) and to sterile middle ear effusion – glue ear. They prevent nature's myringotomy, the perforated drum.

The writers on this subject say that bilateral symptoms and the presence of a discharge are indicators that antibiotics are more likely to be effective. Often the hard pressed GP and the vaguely ill child with pink drums and a past history of nasty OM collide in an evening surgery. This is a good time for a sympathetic consultation, a prescription and instructions to get the antibiotic but not to use it if the analgesics work and if there is no discharge etc etc. – It does seem a good situation for a time delayed prescription and a sympathetic hearing.

I often get the chemist to dispense a bottle of dry powder and instructions to patients I trust, given the decades long shelf life of dry antibiotics and the reassurance a bottle can give when previous episodes of earache have caused utter misery. It is worth mentioning in these days of antibiotic nihilism that the American commentators (Hoberman Medscape March 2017) comment that a 5 day course of Co Amoxiclav is associated with a higher risk of clinical failure than a 10 day course in young children with AOM but there "Was no difference in the rates of middle ear effusion, recurrence of AOM, or colonisation with resistant bacteria" in the 5 and 10 day treatment groups.

A few other points: In America the standard guidelines suggest the above ten day course of Co Amoxiclav in children with symptomatic acute OM. This is my antibiotic of choice.

A few other points: Haemophilus is an extracellular pathogen so macrolides don't work very well since they concentrate in cells.

The main bacteria in OM are Strep pneumoniae, Moraxella catarrhalis and Haemophilus influenzae.

Glue Ear, serous otitis media, is a very common and under diagnosed condition in damp climates particularly in the cold and cool months. It may even be the result of the rhinorrhea of Summer hay fever. So you may see it all year round. Up to 20% of under two year olds have it at any given time in the UK and up to 80% of all children will have had the condition by the time they are 5 years old.

Deafness and its complications, intermittent earache and even developmental and speech delay are symptoms. Poor speech, absent startle to loud noises or the converse, - a startle reaction to siblings or parents who the child hadn't noticed were in the same room and "gave them a start" are signs.

It is commoner where parents smoke and there is a family history.

If glue ear persists for more than 3 months or affects speech development, refer for grommet insertion which is dramatically curative. In the mean time Carbocysteine, topical nasal steroids and nasal inflation devices (Inflating a balloon through the affected side's nostril), eg Otovent do no harm.

Topical Nasal "Antiseptics": Bactroban, Naseptin, Fucidin. These are useful in a variety of situations including recurrent staphylococcal sepsis of other parts of the body – (recurrent Impetigo, Staph. spots, axillary or perineal boils etc) when you want to remove the reservoir of infection. Also useful in this situation is to advise a few capfuls of disinfectant in each bath for a month to help eradicate perineal carriage and the perianal application of an anti-staphylococcal cream. If the suggestion that the patient should bathe in disinfectant is a bit too much for them to swallow, prescribe Chlorhexidine Soln. (Hibiscrub) as it doesn't smell like or have the associations of household disinfectants.

Nasal polyps: Flixonase Nasules 400ug OD/BD, Application: The patient is on their back, head must be tilted right back, (hyperextended), usually lying down, head over the end of the bed, looking at the skirting board.

Chronic Rhinorrhoea: A common GP problem and something nearly all children suffer from ("post nasal drip and morning cough with occasional mucous vomiting") from a few weeks of age to school entry. Undoubtedly some of us exude more catarrh than others and many people find excluding dairy products reduces the quantity and thickness of this. Many adults also have the *watery* runny nose of Vasomotor Rhinitis* and this is very difficult to treat. Surgery is drastic and often not the cure. Exclude polyps and try topical Iptratropium, Atrovent, spray, topical steroids and cromoglicate. House dust mite, grass pollen, tree pollen, mould spores, pet fur, many occupations, nasal polyps etc –these are all causes of excess catarrh. I have seen it follow and persist after chemotherapy treatment. Presumably because of some damage to the patient's immune system.

Post nasal drip cough in children can be improved acutely by a **FOOT UP** posture. **Most "health professionals" get this wrong and advise the head up position. This is better for croup and upper airway obstruction not post nasal drip.** The head down, feet elevated position is so that catarrh is swallowed not inhaled. Prescribe topical nasal steroids as well. The head must be hyperextended when the drops are instilled so they bathe the adenoidal pads at the back of the nasal cavity and several drops or sprays need to be used or they will just be swallowed with the catarrh.

Other treatments: Topical decongestants eg Xylometazoline etc for up to a week, again, give generously with the head in extension in older children and adults topical Ipratropium, Rinatec.

Vasomotor Rhinitis*:

Non allergic runny nose that can be like a tap being turned on in response to environmental temperature and humidity changes, smells (perfumes etc), eating strong tasting food (curries, peppers etc). ALWAYS look with a good light and a nasal speculum (every GP should have several although I have done many locums in surgeries where they didn't exist) to exclude the unexpected polyp or rare tumour etc. Treatment: Topical Anti inflammatory: Sodium Cromoglicate, Rynacrom. Anticholinergic, Ipratropium Rinatec. Antihistamines: Azelastine, Rhinolast, or any of the five or six topical nasal steroids. Some claim success from a dairy free diet, non-sedating anti histamines and leukotriene receptor antagonists (e.g. Montelucast, Singulair)

Acute sinusitis:

Like Otitis Media, many are viral. 70% are said to resolve in 7-10 days without antibiotics, 84% with antibiotics. The Cochrane review on the subject shows that high dose Amoxycillin (and apparently Phenoxymethyl Penicillin) are as effective as other antibiotics. I am not sure which patients they were looking at or how they diagnosed sinusitis. This is often a vague and non specific condition which can present with symptoms of rhinorrhoea, disturbed balance, distorted hearing, halitosis, visual symptoms, cough, nausea, reflux, general malaise, facial pain, dental pain and so on. It doesn't always present acutely. We are not good at identifying and localising pain from our sinuses, especially the ethmoids and I have seen patients with significant unattributed quite severe and chronic malaise which in retrospect was due to occult sinus infection. Add to this GP quandary, the current pressure to avoid broad spectrum antibiotics and the often impractical **point of contact testing** – for instance lab based tests which may need to be done on home visits, Friday evenings, with *miserably ill* feeling patients needing a decision *now*, for part time doctors doing house calls, or the surgery pathology collection run being inflexible, mid morning and the hospital miles away, or on a last visit or late afternoon appointments. Or portable kits which disagree with clinical findings and the patient's clinical state-Will you take the risk? **Treat the patient not the test result.** Also: consider the current rapid rise in Scarlet Fever, Purulent Tonsillitis, and "Sepsis Deaths" in children and Community Acquired Pneumonia due to GPs refusing antibiotics to genuinely sick, septic patients. The American guidelines on sinus disease advise consideration of the patient's treatment preferences and experience. These will be for the broadest spectrum and highest dose bacteriocidal antibiotic. In other words the quickest acting and most reliable antibiotic if my own experience of maxillary sinusitis is anything to go by. Throw these into the decision mix and I just do not accept that non GP bacteriologists or epidemiologists can understand the real issues we face. Damned if we do, but real dangers for the patient if we don't.

Anyway, you do have to relieve pressure (nasal sprays – vasoconstrictors and steroids together for a few days before stopping the former) and treat what can be severe pain at the same time as giving effective broad spectrum antibiotics. I would assess the systemic "unwellness" of my patient and factor in any previous prolonged episodes, admissions or complications but high dose Penicillin or Amoxicillin are probably not the top of my list of antibiotics. Co Amoxiclav, Doxycycline, Haemophilocidal Cephalosporins or even combinations of antibiotics would be more appropriate.

I think, as in the patients with Otitis, you soon work out who has real symptoms and who gets genuine recurrent disease. Presumably these patients have small sinus openings, so that infected exudate cannot vent into the nasal cavity. It has always seemed silly to me that humans squeeze the front of the nose while blowing it into a tissue or handkerchief, thus increasing intra nasal pressure and forcing infected mucoid discharge from the nasal airway into the paranasal sinuses. No other animal blows its nose with a socially acceptable mop. Perhaps sinusitis sufferers have anatomical susceptibilities or thicker discharge, chronic colonisation with more virulent organisms, allergies, dustier work or home conditions, or other specific harmful factors.

There are always patients who are quicker off the mark in consulting and who exaggerate their suffering. Assessing this is part of being a GP.

Please don't assume all patients are the same just because some academic has looked at a lot of data and wants you to stop using your common sense.

In keeping with the seemingly endless clever medical acronyms:

The SNOT-22 (Sino-nasal outcome test) is a patient questionnaire which gives a rough subjective assessment of upper respiratory (mainly nasal) symptoms and includes scores for

Loss of smell/taste, Cough, Difficulty falling asleep, Fatigue, Waking up at night, Sneezing, Ear fullness, Waking up tired, Post nasal Drip, Reduced concentration, Reduced productivity, Nasal obstruction, Thick nasal discharge, Sad, Need to blow, Ear pain, Lack of a good night's sleep, Frustrated, Restless, Irritable, Dizziness, Runny nose, Facial pain/pressure, Embarrassed.

Each parameter is scored 0 – 5 (No problem<---->as bad as it can be) (Download from ENT UK).

Sinus infection – to treat or not to treat?

We GPs are constantly bombarded with demands from regulating authorities, prescribing groups and health departments to reduce our antibiotic prescribing – particularly in patients who "just have minor infections or coughs and colds". 2015 was the lowest rate of GP antibiotic prescribing for many years but we do not have the reciprocal figures for children admitted with bacterial meningitis following OM or URTI, septicaemic elderly patients admitted after missed or ignored UTIs, LRTIs or cellulitis, community acquired pneumonia, quinsies and so on. We know childhood "sepsis" deaths, the worst forms of bacterial tonsillitis and Scarlet Fever are increasing. We are supposed to be falling out of love with these life saving drugs now and to be seeing them as sinners as well as saints. We are told that drug resistance is increasing and that the number of available new effective antimicrobials is not. In fact in the community, in the vast majority of patients with normal immune systems, antibiotic resistance to the available GP antibiotics is actually very rarely, if ever a problem. GPs are not the cause of most MRSA or C Difficile hospital super infections. Drug resistance is more the fault of vetinary prophylactic antibiotic practice on farms and the ubiquity of antiseptic washes, wipes and gels than GPs who treat painful ears and throats with penicillins. As someone who has been hospitalised with agonising maxillary sinusitis on three occasions, I have some sympathy for the patient who does not want to reprise this experience if they have suffered it before. I have no sympathy at all for the dogmatic, protocol bound (usually young) GP who simply repeats an "it's a viral infection" mantra over and over again to his (her) miserable, suffering patients. Especially patients who haven't been properly examined.

The American Academy of Otolaryngology-Head and Neck Surgery Foundation in April 2015 produced new clinical guidelines which for the first time recognise that **Bacterial sinusitis is**

1) Impossible to exclude or confirm clinically in the surgery. 2) Can be extremely unpleasant, protracted, acute or chronic and complicated. 3) Often the patient recognises their own symptoms early and deserves early and effective treatment. 4) That the usual knee jerk antibiotics at weak GP doses can be a waste of time in sinusitis.

They say in their report that one in five courses of antibiotics in the US is for a sinus infection and the decision to prescribe or not should be a *SHARED* one between doctor and patient. They say an approach of "watchful waiting or antibiotics" is appropriate. But the important thing for me is that they say *Listen to the patient*. Shared decision making should be applied to giving antibiotics, analgesics, topical nasal steroid sprays and nasal saline irrigation. They also say (hurray) that Amoxicillin with Clavulanic Acid can now be recommended instead of the previous (what I regard as fairly unreliable) first line Amoxicillin. They recommend anterior rhinoscopy (-a nasal speculum and a bright light), nasal endoscopy or CT (not practical for General Practice) are also appropriate – but then the report IS American.

In the UK I suggest it is essential to share the decision making with the patient, accepting that they usually know from experience if antibiotics (and which antibiotic) have helped the same symptoms in the past. If you are convinced the patient is over reacting to what is clearly an uncomplicated viral infection you could employ a post dated prescription. And don't be dogmatic. Your responsibility is to the well being of the patient not the Prescribing Committee audit results.

Hay Fever:

Can be all year round with tree pollen, grass pollen, mould spores, especially with hydrocarbon pollutants coating the airborne allergens and acting as co irritants.

Early tree pollens: Jan Feb Mar: alder, hazel.

Mid/Late trees: Mar April, silver birch.

Grasses: May – July.

Nettles and other weeds: July-Sept.

Moulds are persistent or intermittent.

Steroid nasal sprays:

44% of Beconase is systemically absorbed but only <1% of Nasonex, Avamys etc are systemically absorbed. 8% of the population are said to have a tendency to epistaxis with topical steroids. (I would say it was considerably more than this). A preliminary saline douche helps nasal steroids work. Most take up to 48 hours to start to work.

Sore Throat: Symptomatic treatment:
Strefen Lozenges, Flurbiprofen: One sucked every 3-4 hours.
Difflam, Benzydamine: Spray and oral rinse (used as a gargle). Good old soluble aspirin in warm water gargled and swallowed (with an H2 blocker).

Glossitis:
Infections: H. Simplex, apthous ulceration, Strep Infection, Candida, Syphilis; Allergy, topical and systemic; Local irritants, including dentures, plates, teeth, tobacco, alcohol; Iron deficiency; B12 deficiency; Lichen Planus; Pemphigus; Sjogrens Syndrome, etc; Idiopathic.
Rx: Baking soda mouth wash and Listerine. Corsodyl, Difflam (retained in the mouth a couple of minutes every 3-4 hours).
Apthous ulceration: Folic acid or folinic acid orally or topically.

Petechial spots on palate:
Scarlet Fever, Rubella, Glandular Fever.

Vertigo:
Vestibular dizziness is always rotatory vertigo, nearly always on head extension, nearly always BPPV. If the vertigo lasts "hours" it is more likely to be vestibular migraine. Only 1:200 of patients with BPPV are not improved by a consultant run Epley clinic.

Vertigo, a wide variety of treatments:
Cinarrizine, Dimenhydrinate, benzodiazepines, Promethazine, Prochlorperazine (not long term), Cyclizine, sometimes steroids in acute vestibular neuronitis.
Serc, Betahistine 8mg 16mg init. 16mg tds – said to be safe in pregnancy.
Arlevert is Cinnarizine and Dimenhydrinate, 1 tds in labyrinthitis and vestibular vertigo.
BPPV:
Characteristically worse on lying rather than standing. Usually self limiting (approx 6m). Unilateral.
Causes:
Head Injury, migraine, age, idiopathic (50%), viral infections, CVA, Menieres.
The Epley manoeuvre is supposed to move debris from the semicircular canals to the insensitive "sump" of the utricle where it can cause no hair cell stimulation and vertigo. The procedure is limited by
Modern surgery design, which prevents getting at both sides of the couch,
Time, which allowing for explanation, reassurance, frailty, physical limitations, nystagmus and recovery can take 10-15 minutes,
Nausea. Some patients do feel sick during and shortly after the manipulation. Some of the problems can be avoided by a dose of Serc, Stugeron or Stemetil an hour or so beforehand.
Afterwards, do not let the patient drive home and make sure they sleep angled at 45 degrees for two nights. Also they should try to keep the head vertical for the same length of time. For one week after they should avoid extreme head extension or rotation (avoid swimming, sit ups, visits to the hair dresser, DIY, etc).

The Hallpike test:

(To show paroxysmal vertigo, the test causing nystagmus, **the fast phase towards the affected ear).**

With the patient sitting on the couch, turn the patient's head to 45 degrees. Quickly bring patient to lying position with head extended over end of couch. **This is the Hallpike position.** Keep there for 30 seconds*. Classically there is a rotatory nystagmus to the undermost ear (may only last 1 minute). On repetition the reaction is reduced. On sitting up there is a recurrence of vertigo and nystagmus to the opposite direction.

The Epley Manoeuvre is the cure but the various techniques do vary somewhat:

With the patient sitting upright rotate the head either 45 or 90 degrees to the **affected side.** Wait 30 seconds. Slowly (self administered) or quickly (done by a therapist) lie the patient flat, head off the end of the couch. The neck is now 30 degrees extended; the affected ear is facing the ground. Wait 30 seconds (to 2 minutes) again. This is the Dix Hallpike position.

Then rotate the head towards the good ear slowly and wait another 30 seconds (or 2 minutes) maintaining the 30 degree extension.

Keeping the head stable relative to the body, get the patient to roll over on to their shoulder while rotating the head another 90 degrees in the direction they are facing. They are now looking down at 45 degrees. Wait another 30 seconds (to 2 minutes).

(Sometimes an extra section is added: Now turn the head again, this time toward the good ear. They will now be looking at the floor with chin near their shoulder. Wait another 30 seconds. This is not used in many descriptions of the manoeuvre).

Now slowly sit patient up keeping the head rotated 45 degrees. Wait 30 seconds.

Some descriptions add: Finally centre and flex the head gently in one movement and wait another 30 seconds.

Epley suggested a collar and remaining erect for 2 days (or not lying flat).

Tell patient not to sleep on bad side 2 days.

The Semont manoeuvre simply involves rapid rotation of the patient from lying on one side to the other.

The Epley Manoeuvre can be taught at home with the patient doing it three times each night for a week.

Contraindications to Epley and other similar manoeuvres:

Severe carotid stenosis, unstable heart disease, severe cervical spondylosis, advanced Rh A.

Vestibular Rehabilitation Exercises:

Cawthorne – Cooksey Exercises:

These are designed to encourage vestibular compensation in situations of dizziness, vertigo and incoordination affecting the middle ears, neck, head and vision.

They are designed to relax neck and shoulder muscles, improve eye/head coordination, improve general balance, coordination and movement as well as down regulating the head movements that cause dizziness.

In Bed or Sitting:

1) Eye movements up and down then side to side then focussing on a finger moving from 3 foot to 1 foot away from the face. Doing these movements slow at first then quickly.

2) Now head movements: Bend the head forwards and backwards then turn from side

to side. First slowly then quicker and finally with eyes closed.
Sitting:
Eye and head movements as above:
Shoulder shrugging and circling.
Bending forwards and picking things up from the ground.
Standing:
Eye, head and shoulder movements as before.
Changing from sitting to standing with eyes open/shut.
Tossing a ball from hand to hand (above eye level).
Tossing a ball hand to hand below knee.
Changing from sitting to standing and turning around in between.
Moving about (in a class).
Circle about a central person who throws a large ball and to whom it is thrown back.
Walk across a room with the eyes open then with them closed.
Walk up and down a slope with the eyes open and then with them closed.
Walk up and down steps with the eyes open and then closed.
Any game which involves stooping, stretching and aiming-such as bowling or basketball etc.
My thanks to Mr James Fairly of The ENT Kent Partnership for his advice regarding the various ENT exercises and manoeuvres.

Acoustic Neuroma:
Is very rare and most are managed by watchful waiting. If 2cm or larger, can damage the Trigeminal nerve. It is a benign Schwannoma of the acoustic nerve and makes up less than 1 in 10 of primary brain tumours.
The symptoms are hearing loss, tinnitus, both unilateral, vertigo, unilateral facial numbness, parasthesiae or pain.
Treatment is by radiotherapy, steriotactic radiosurgery, or conventional microsurgery.

Menières syndrome:
Paroxysmal rotational vertigo, fluctuating but progressive deafness, unilateral or bilateral tinnitus and "fullness" in the ear or ears. Usually unilateral, this can alternate its side but the hearing loss can become permanent. Head injury and whiplash are associations. Nystagmus, vomiting, sweating and sometimes sudden drop attacks may occur.
Differential diagnoses include: MS, acoustic neuroma, dysautonomia, hyper and hypothyroidism, Cogan's syndrome.
Treatment traditionally includes salt restriction, diuretics, avoidance of alcohol, caffeine and tobacco, labyrinthine sedatives and ginger. Middle ear steroid injection, decompression of the semicircular canals, gentamicin or surgical labyrinthectomy or vestibular neuronectomy. Vestibular rehabilitation.
Most patients do eventually recover.

Temperomandibular joint pain/dysfunction:
This is said to bother 30% of adults at sometime. 10F:1M. The TMJs are two of the 4 joints in the body with cushioning semilunar cartilages (like the knee joints) and the only joint designed to dislocate in use.
The commonest cause of pain is an internal derangement, presumably a trapping of the synovium (?) or the mobile disc or part of it within or just outside the joint. The disc

is free in normal conditions to slide forwards and backwards but not, unless its attachments are damaged, sideways. Local disease (tumour) or referred pain (cervical OA) can also be an underlying cause. In practice teeth grinding due to stress is often a factor and trauma has occurred in up to 25% cases. This may be trauma due to dental or anaesthetic manipulation.

TMJ dysfunction is most common in younger women between 20 and 40 years. It may have been going on for months or years. The books say severe degenerative changes can occur in the TMJs even in children. If this is true it is very rare these days.

Pain on eating and talking, the jaw getting stuck on yawing, clicking, headache, tinnitus, vertigo, etc are the symptoms.

How the jaw works: When the jaw opens, the mandibular heads rotate about a common horizontal axis in combination with a forward and downward sliding movement in contact with the lower surface of the articular discs. Simultaneously the discs move forward and downward on the temporal bones. On closing the mouth the mandibular heads glide backwards then hinge on the discs which are held forwards by the lateral pterygoids. Then these relax and the discs glide backwards and upwards on the temporal bone. No wonder the system breaks down occasionally.

Investigation is preferably by MRI (for soft tissue), CT (for bone),

but a plain X Ray will show early arthritis too.

Some specialists units will do arthroscopy/arthrography.

The treatments:

Most patients respond to amitriptyline at night, a bite plane (– like a gum shield which stops gritting and grinding of teeth at night) fitted by the dentist and jaw exercises.

If necessary, surgery via discal plication, discectomy or implant is the last resort. The implants may be Teflon, Silicon, Silastic or various bodily tissues.

This in my experience is only appropriate in the very worst cases.

In very severe cases a condylectomy may be performed or reduction osteotomy of the articular eminence.

The differential diagnosis includes myofascial pain syndrome, OA, synovitis, Rh A, sepsis, gout, tumour, cervical spondylosis, mandibular head avascular necrosis, upper jaw dental pathology, malocclusion, etc.

Acute sensorineural hearing loss:

The ENT equivalent of Bell's Palsy. Preceded by hearing distortion plus or minus tinnitus. Cause unknown. Give 60mg prednisolone daily for 1 week or dexamethasone injection to the middle ear twice weekly. With Aciclovir. This is an ENT emergency (so presumably due to an occult Herpes virus infection).

19: GASTROENTEROLOGY:

One finger in the throat and one in the rectum makes a good diagnostician.
William Osler.

The Acute Abdomen:

In an average practice with an average list you will see:
2-3 acute appendices a year,
2 renal colics a year,
1 biliary colic a year (but getting commoner due to obesity),
1 intestinal obstruction a year,
1 case of peptic ulcer complications (but diminishing due to PPIs),
A strangulated hernia every 2 years,
An acute pancreatitis, an ectopic pregnancy and another gynae. emergency each every 4 years,
A congenital pyloric stenosis every 10 years.

Abdominal pain: Visceral or Muscular?

The Carnett Sign (1926): Find the abdominal point of maximal tenderness, place your hand(s) on that point and ask the patient to cross their arms and sit up or lift head and shoulders of the couch. If the pain is exacerbated then it is likely to be musculoskeletal rather than intrabdominal.

Acute Gastroenterology, who sees what:

Severe abdominal pain (even suspected pancreatitis) >the surgeons.
Upper G I bleeds and haematemesis are generally dealt with by endoscopy and the physicians are generally the endoscopists these days.
Lower G I tract problems other than bleeds >the surgeons.
All melaena >the physicians.
Diarrhoea and bleeding >the physicians.
Fresh bleeding P.R. is the province of the surgeons.

The Mouth:

Recurrent Apthous ulcers:
Sometimes 5mg Folic acid daily for a month helps, exclude iron and vitamin deficiency, exclude Coeliac disease and Crohn's disease.

Irritable Bowel Syndrome:

With "Non ulcer dyspepsia" it is probably the commonest significant abdominal condition seen in General Practice. It is very common, (supposed to be 1:20 GP consultations and affects 10% of the world population). It is hard to treat, has no diagnostic tests or clinching history and can breed a contemptuous familiarity than can lead even competent GPs to miss surreptitious serious background conditions. So beware assuming abdominal pain is just IBS. But note that low grade (Mast Cell) inflammation is present in colonic biopsies in two thirds of patients.

One morning surgery, one of my life long IBS sufferers mentioned that he had a slightly worse pain than normal in roughly the normal distribution. This was during a routine consultation for something else. I asked if I could examine his abdomen and he had a liver full of secondaries from a new bowel cancer. He was a fit man in his mid 50s and died soon after. His diagnosis was a shock to us both. Another 80 year old lady who had consulted monthly with abdominal pain for over 20 years and an IBS diagnosis had a rectal carcinoma missed by the GI surgeons and myself until it began bleeding. It was impalpable PR and it presented already locally spread and entangled in the sacral plexus.

IBS is said to be migraine of the gut. Indeed new research is finding a common situation where sufferers of one condition have the other as well. The figures were in a 2016 study where IBS, according to strict diagnostic criteria occurred in 54% of migraine sufferers and 28% of patients with episodic tension type headache. In addition, 36% of patients with IBS had migraine and 22% of patients with IBS had tension headache. (Am Acad Neurol Mtg April 15 2016. Abstr 3367).

Sufferers generally differentiate between the constipated and the rapid transit types and there are roughly 2 women for every 1 man affected. About a third suffer the constipated, a third the diarrhoea predominant and a third the mixed type. The older the patient group, the more equal the sex ratio. Since overall, the patients are more likely to be women, it is no surprise that IBS sufferers with abdominal pain are more likely to consult than patients with non IBS abdominal pain. Men are far less likely to consult with any symptom than women. Up to 10% of the population suffer at some time and it constitutes up to 70% of referrals to gastro-enterologists. Definitions include "Pain 3 days a month for 3 months" etc (I would have thought the symptoms are generally far more frequent than this though). It is commoner between 20 and 40 years of age but can occur in older patients. Classically there is pain relieved by defaecation, abdominal distension, the passage of mucus, tenesmus and incomplete evacuation. These are called "Manning's Criteria".

Never assume a new onset of abdominal pain in anyone over 40 is IBS until you have excluded other more serious causes (like ovarian or bowel cancer, Coeliac Disease, inflammatory bowel disease, diverticular disease etc).

There is a very high incidence of sexual abuse as children in IBS sufferers, more common in women than in men. 50% follow a stressful event and 20% follow a GI illness of some kind. The patients are more likely to have had a hysterectomy and a cholecystectomy, fibromyalgia, CFS, TMJ dysfunction, than the general public.

Red Flags are:

Age>50, nocturnal symptoms, male sex, weight loss, rectal bleeding, FH of ovarian or bowel cancer, changed bowel habit (looser/more frequent) >6 weeks, anaemia (all iron deficiency anaemia over 50 yrs is bowel cancer unless specifically excluded), abdominal or rectal masses, investigations:

FBC, ESR, CRP, stool M, C and S, Giardia, faecal calprotectin (Inflammatory bowel disease), reducing substances, U and Es, TFTs, LFTs, TTG (tissue Transglutaminase), Coeliac Abs,

Advise low fibre diet during flare ups. Despite the old advice, simply increasing bran in the diet probably makes it worse. You need soluble fibre, see below for detailed dietary advice.

Drugs: Antispasmodics: e.g. Mebeverine (Colofac 135mg) is probably the most consistent. Spasmonal, Alverine 60mg. Pro-Banthine, Probantheline 15mg. Merbentyl, Dicyclomine, Dicycloverine 10/20mg. Buscopan, Hyoscine for colic, gut spasm, 10mg ii qds. Not <6yrs. >6 yrs i qds.

Peppermint oil: Colpermin, Mintec (beware reflux via relaxation of the lower oesophageal sphincter).

Low dose Amitriptyline for the frequent stool version of IBS, Citalopram or other SSRI for the slow transit type. Can also try Cholestyramine – 1 sachet daily, slowly increasing.

Some specialists prescribe Rifaxamin, an antibiotic for traveller's diarrhoea for 4-12 weeks in refractory IBS.

In a recent American review (2015), Loperamide was suggested for diarrhoeal symptoms, (but not "global symptoms", the pro-secretory drugs Linaclotide (Constella) and Lubiprostone (Amitiza) in constipation predominant IBS and to increase stool frequency in chronic idiopathic constipation. For chronic constipation, they also suggest polyethylene glycol (Macrogol, Movicol, Laxido etc).

Most sufferers are convinced that diet has some influence on either the symptomatology or the treatment of this condition.

Our primate guts evolved to cope with a diet of foraged fruit, wild vegetables and nuts, some edible roots, small animals, shell fish, crustacea and fish once we had over the last few hundred thousand years developed spears and nets to catch them. We were controlling fire and so presumably cooking meat so the protein was more digestible over 120,000-250,000 years ago, indeed there is some evidence of our ancestors roasting food over a million years ago.

It is only the last few thousand years we settled to a more efficient agrarian immobile life and cultivated genetically selected grasses (flour, rice, wheat, barley, oats and bread and related products etc), ate the seeds and grains of these, consumed ruminants and their lactations (meat and milk), and other domesticated animals. Wheat protein, Gluten, Gliaden, (and carbohydrates, primarily indigestible short chained components, FODMAPS-fermentable oligo, di, mono saccharides and polyols) are thought to be responsible for the symptoms. It is only a for few hundred years that we have eaten the boiled sap of cane or root vegetables as refined sugars or eaten processed foods. Our guts can be forgiven therefore for not having evolved the enzymes and mechanisms to digest these new energy and protein sources. Thus some of us are intolerant of a "normal" modern diet and suffer fermentation, irritation, distension, pain, bloating, diarrhoea or constipation as a consequence. Despite the sensation and sometimes appearance of bloating, IBS sufferers do not actually generate more gastro intestinal gas than non sufferers.

The best way of improving the symptoms is by getting back to the diet our guts were designed for.

Dietary and other advice: There are various approaches:

Avoid canned drinks, caffeine, alcohol, dairy products, wheat, and other "grains", which our guts are not up to digesting. Reduce high fibre, yeast, potatoes and onions, citrus fruit, – but not all at once unless you are trying a formal exclusion "few foods" diet (of: – rice, rice milk, lamb, turkey, broccoli, bottled water and peaches).

Some try probiotics with or without the "FODMAP" diet – This, as mentioned, stands for Fermentable Oligo Di and Mono saccharides And Polyols. The idea is to eat foods with a low "FODMAP" value to reduce gas and fluid distension of the gut.

This particular diet avoids various grains, apples, mangos, pears, peaches, plums, prunes, fructose containing foods, rye and wheat, lactose, various vegetables (beans of various sorts, artichokes, cabbage, cauliflower, mushrooms, onions etc), sorbitol, xylitol and a host of other daily foods.

You can treat the symptoms:

Bloating: Bloated IBS sufferers do not produce more gastro intestinal gas. They do have weaker abdominal muscles though. Oats and golden linseeds are said to reduce bloating, as does *reducing* fruit, fruit juice and "**resistant starches**" (pulses, whole grains, sweet corn, bran, reheated potato and maize, oven chips, crisps, waffles, part baked and reheated breads, pizza bases, processed foods, bought biscuits and cake, ready meals containing pasta or potato, dried (but not fresh) pasta in the diet.

The advice for the **constipated type** of IBS used to be to give the patient bran. But this is "insoluble fibre" – now called "resistant starches" and can make what was called "Spastic colitis" or some IBS worse. What the patient needs (and what WAS actually advised before the high fibre 60s and 70s) is a soft "low irritant diet". In the old days that often meant low bulk but now the best of both worlds is a high bulk, low irritant, high soluble fibre diet. This is without pips, husks, peel and nuts but with lots of water and bulk in the form of soluble fibre.

Soluble fibre: Use	Insoluble fibre(-resistant starches) – avoid
Oats, golden linseed	Wholegrain bread
Barley	Bran
Rye	Cereals
Bananas	Nuts and seeds
Apples (etc)	
Root vegetables (carrots, potatoes etc)	

IBS-C has also been found to respond to Melatonin (up to 60mg/day).

Dietary management of the **diarrhoeal form** of IBS: Drink plenty of non caffeinated drinks, reduce fizzy drinks, no regular alcohol or no more than 2Us in one day, no more than 3 cups of caffeinated drinks per day, limited insoluble fibre – whole grains, bran, cereals nuts and seeds except golden linseed, avoid the skin, pith and pips of fruit and vegetables, no more than 3 portions of fresh and dried fruit a day, 1 small glass of fruit juice, make up the deficit with certain vegetables, reduce resistant starches (see above) avoid sugar free sweets and sorbitol, try probiotic yogurts, reduce high fat foods.

The opposite advice holds for constipation in IBS – increase whole grains, fruit and vegetables, (slowly) and again, oats and golden linseed are likely to be tolerated best, increase fluids, and try probiotics in post infection IBS.

Hiatus Hernia

HIATUS HERNIA

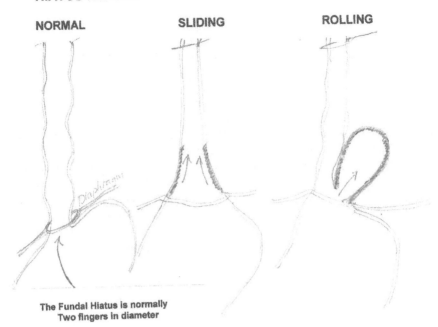

NORMAL **SLIDING** **ROLLING**

The Fundal Hiatus is normally
Two fingers in diameter

Inflammatory Bowel Disease:

Ulcerative Colitis:

Continuous mucosal inflammation
of the colon without granulomata on Bx.

Affects the rectum and a variable extent
of the colon,
In continuity,
Relapsing and remitting,
Occasionally only the rectum,
Crypt abscesses,
Pseudopolyps,
Diarrhoea, blood and mucus

Crohn's Disease:

Discontinuous transmural inflammation,
often granulomatous. Affects any part of
GIT.
Distribution: Terminal Ileum 30%,

    Colon 30%,
    Ileum and colon 30%,
    Anal lesions, can spare rectum.

No bloody diarrhoea,
Symptoms depend on distribution,
Pain, mass, malabsorption, fistulae,
perianal disease.

Montreal Classification:

E1 Proctitis (rectum only),
E2 Left Sided (colon distal to splenic flexure),
E3 Extensive (extends proximal to splenic flexure).
Both present with bloody diarrhoea.

Investigations:
Stool cultures, CDT (Carbohydrate Deficient Transferrin, – which is normally a test for excess alcohol consumption),
Faecal Calprotectin (distinguishes IBS from IBD),
CRP – a predictor of severity and response more helpful than ESR,
FBC,
Albumin (inversely proportional to inflammation).
Sigmoidoscopy.

Fine Ulceration, double contour on XR, strictures rare, fistulae very rare, mucosal polymorph infiltrate, glandular destruction.

Cobblestones, rosethorn ulcers, strictures common, fistulae can occur, transmural inflammation, granulomata, cholangitis.

Disease activity assessed by **Truelove and Witts** Criteria:

	Mild	Moderate	Severe
Bloody stools/day	<4	4 or >	6 or >
Pulse	<90	</= 90	>90
Temp	<37.5C	</=37.8C	>37.8C
Hb	>11.5	>/=10.5	<10.5g/dl
ESR	<20	</=30	>30mm/hr
or CRP	N	</=30	>30mg/li.

Treatment:
Severe IBD: IV steroids (100mg Hydrocortisone qds), Heparin (there is an acute DVT/PE risk despite the bleeding).
If steroid unresponsive, Cyclosporin, Infliximab, ?Vedolizumab, colectomy.
Mild to moderate disease: Oral and topical Mesalazine (eg suppositories) plus or minus topical steroids and oral steroids if unresponsive.
Mild to moderate IBD: Oral steroid treatment:
Simple regime: Prednisolone (I prefer prednisolone plus an H2 antagonist or PPI), 40mg/day for 1 week then reduce by 5mg/day every week.
Plus or minus eg: An aminosalicylate: eg ASA, – Mesalazine, Asacol 800mg TDS, Pentasa supps. 1 nocte.

Maintenance of remission:
Oral 5-ASA/topical 5-ASA in L sided disease. 80% patients prefer oral treatment. Considered safe in pregnancy.
Azathioprine if >2 relapses in 12m Don't forget TPMT level (or Mercaptopurine, Infliximab).
Monoclonal anti-TNFα is used in severe Crohn's and in Europe the monoclonal antibodies Infliximab and Adalimumab.
Conditions linked to inflammatory bowel disease: pericholangitis, sclerosing cholangitis, bile duct carcinoma, gallstones, CAH, cirrhosis, fatty change, amyloid, apthous ulcers, E.Nodosum, Pyoderma Gangrenosum, acute arthritis, conjunctivitis, episcleritis, uveitis, sacroileitis, ankylosing spondylitis, polyarthritis.

The Bristol Stool Form Scale:

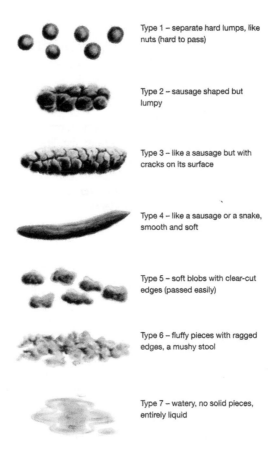

Type 1 – separate hard lumps, like nuts (hard to pass)

Type 2 – sausage shaped but lumpy

Type 3 – like a sausage but with cracks on its surface

Type 4 – like a sausage or a snake, smooth and soft

Type 5 – soft blobs with clear-cut edges (passed easily)

Type 6 – fluffy pieces with ragged edges, a mushy stool

Type 7 – watery, no solid pieces, entirely liquid

Heliobacter Eradication:

It is a singular fact that a bacterium is responsible for peptic ulcer disease and that you can treat it with antibiotics. Barry Marshall and Robin Warren got the Nobel prize for discovering this. Barry Marshall, an Australian gastroenterologist, by drinking a Petri dish of live bacterial culture. But no wonder it attracted a certain amount of disbelief when he promulgated the idea in the mid 80s. However, three quarters of the world's population are infected, 90% of patients with a PU are infected and also gastric cancer is strongly associated with Helicobacter Pylori. 85% of infected people suffer no symptoms however. Bizarrely, Helicobacter infection is **negatively** associated with Barrett's oesophagus. Up to 2/3 of HP infected patients have concomitant upper GI thrush infections, perhaps as a result of multiple triple and quadruple antibiotic anti HP regimes which have been ineffective. Imagine what that has done to their microbiome. Like all bacteria, HP develops resistance in time to the antibiotics that used to kill it. Peptic ulcer disease was actually something quite rare in Victorian post mortems unless they were "stress ulcers" but PU disease was virtually an epidemic in the west in the 60's 70's and 80's. A variety of antibiotic and PPI combinations has been suggested to eradicate the infection. These are less and less effective. For instance:

Amoxicillin 500mg qds, Metronidazole 400mg tds and Omeprazole 20mg daily all for 2 weeks,

or Omeprazole 40mg daily with Amoxicillin 750mg bd for 2 weeks,

or Omeprazole 40mg daily with Amoxicillin 500mg tds and Metronidazole 400mg tds all for 2 weeks.

or Clarithromycin 500mg tds and Omeprazole 40mg od for 2 weeks,

or Omeprazole, Amoxicillin and Clarithromycin high dose for 1 week,

or Omeprazole 40mg od, Clarithromycin 250mg bd, Metronidazole 400mg bd for 1 week.

or Lansoprazole 30mg bd, Clarithromycin 250mg bd and either Amoxicillin 1gr bd or Metronidazole 400mg bd – this gives 90% eradication.

If all this is ineffective then you could try a PPI, De-Noltabs (Tri potassium di citrato bismuthate) and Metronidazole.

The Breath Test:

Helicobacter Pylori infection can be diagnosed by antibody tests, by identifying the organism in biopsies taken during endoscopy, or by the non-invasive breath test that identifies bacterial production of urease enzyme. The test involves swallowing radiolabled urea which is split into ammonia and carbon dioxide over 20-30 minutes by H Pylori. The isotope labelled carbon dioxide is then measured in exhaled breath. Antibiotics must have been stopped a month before and all acid suppressing medication two weeks before the test.

Eosinophilic Gastroenteritis:

Although this is not a common illness, as a statistical quirk I seem to have had a disproportionate number of patients with this condition and I was never completely convinced that it wasn't just a histological description of allergic inflammation.

It is "rare"-, there have only been 300 cases described in the last 70 years apparently. Defining it (with any diagnostic precision) seems to be a problem. It is a condition in which gastoenterological symptoms are associated with eosinophiic infiltration (20 or more per HPF) in various layers of the GIT.

Male patients slightly outnumber females, patients usually present in their 20's. There is a history of atopy, raised IgE and peripheral eosinophilia.

It may be due to occult allergy, infection or immune reactions.

The symptoms include diarrhoea, upper abdominal pain, bloating, anorexia, dysphagia, weight loss etc. The precise symptoms and complications (iron deficiency, malabsorption, steatorrhoea etc), depend on which layer of the bowel and which part of the gut are affected.

The treatment may include oral steroids, cromoglicate, (Nalcrom), elimination diet, montelukast.

It may be worth a trial of antiparasitic medication (mebendazole) if infestation is thought to be a possible cause.

Infantile Colic:

There is some evidence that probiotic drops (Lactobacillus Reuteri) from day 1 reduce colic, the development of "long term visceral hypersensitivity" and "mucosal permeability" and reduce the development of subsequent childhood (you've guessed it) IBS.

Infacol is Simeticone, an antiflatulant, antifoaming, non absorbed treatment for colic which has not been shown in RCTs to have any positive anti colic effect. The best you can say for it is that it is safe and that many mothers think it helps. It helps more if you are sympathetic, understanding, give the baby a proper examination and send off the stool for a few tests (including reducing substances and possibly culture). I hesitate to suggest a trial of Lactase drops but these are now available OTC and marketed for colic.

Probiotics

As well as colic there is some evidence in favour of probiotic use in H Pylori eradication, IBS, functional GI symptoms and possibly in reducing diarrhoea after viral gastro enteritis and antibiotic diarrhoea. There are more alien bacterial cells in your biome than cells that make up **you** and the complex and intrinsic way in which they interact with multiple body systems is coming to light constantly these days. Their alteration or relative absence seems to have significant negative effects undreamt of in the recent past. (See section on Microbiome).

Reflux oesophagitis:

Heartburn, waterbrash, (sour or tasteless regurgitation), odynophagia, (painful swallowing), (which most of us erroneously call dysphagia), dysphagia (difficulty swallowing), halitosis, loss of dental enamel, occasional severe chest pain ("oesophageal spasm") are common gastric reflux symptoms in adults. Rarer are cough, throat clearing and hoarseness.

There used to be little evidence that long term PPI therapy prevented oesophageal cancer in patients with Barrett's oesphagus. Barrett's increases the risk of oesophageal cancer 30-125X but even so, only a small proportion of patients with Barrett's will get cancer. The difficulty is therefore who to screen because the first symptom of cancer is usually dysphagia and by the time the patient has difficulty with dysphagia it is often too late to save them.

However in a recent meta analysis (Gut 2014:63 1229-37), the authors did find that 2-3 years of PPI use reduced OAC (Oesophageal Adenocarcinoma) or high grade dysplasia by 71%. There was no decision on H2 antagonists but on acid suppression, inflammation suppression and efficacy I would assume frequent H2 antagonists would work but not quite as well as PPIs – and antacids less well again. I presume highly selective vagotomy would be the most effective at switching off acid but then again complete achlorhydria has its own risks.

Anti-Reflux Surgery:

The symptomatic success rate for anti reflux surgery such as laparoscopic fundoplication etc, (**You may have forgotten**: a plica is a plait or fold and in this procedure, the gastric fundus is gathered around the lower oesophagus as a wrap before being sutured in place) can be up to 90%. Other techniques are the injection of a synthetic polymer submucosally, the laparoscopic insertion of a wrap around mesh, a necklace of magnetic beads, endoscopic radiofrequency ablation of the oesophageal mucosa, endoluminal gastroplication, etc but the relapse rate can be up to 50% at 5 years for these.

Oesophageal cancer can be a complication of reflux oesophagitis and hiatus hernia – the difficulty for GP s being that many people with endoscopy proven reflux and 45% Barrett's patients are totally asymptomatic, 40% of oesophageal cancer patients have no GORD Symptoms but at least 20% of the population have GORD symptoms (look at your PPI costs). Conversely, many, perhaps most patients who complain bitterly about heartburn have little to show for it on endoscopy.

Barrett's is when the normal squamous epithelium of the lower oesophagus becomes columnar due to intestinal metaplasia. About 1:20 (5%) of adults with reflux symptoms have Barrett's. So the theory is that GORD >Barrett's >adenocarcinoma of the oesophagus. It used to be said that approximately 0.5% of Barrett's oesophagus patients developed cancer per year. Actually the newer data suggest it is more like 0.12-0.14% and a *total* of only 5% of Barrett's patients die of oesophageal cancer. This certainly puts the risk in perspective. The risk depends on whether it is short (<3cms) or long segment and other factors like obesity and sex (premenopausal women are protected, overweight men and women aren't). Wine apparently has a slight protective effect despite being a potent cause of heartburn. The incidence of Barrett's in populations varies a great deal in the various published studies, from 0.5-15%! It is twice as common in men and oesophageal cancer is 3.5X commoner in men, – with white men and Hispanics being more affected than other races.

The **ABSENCE** of H Pylori increases Barrett's oesophagus and reduces gastric cancer (H Pylori is the cause of a third of UK gastric cancer) puzzlingly.

Obesity is a definite risk factor (visceral obesity, related to abdominal circumference). There is an increased rate of the more dangerous long segment (>3cms) Barrett's in Metabolic Syndrome. Interestingly the visceral adipose itself has been shown to have a direct effect on cell proliferation and reduced cell apoptosis (cell suicide) in Barrett's derived cancer. Fat really does kill you.

Some gastro-enterologists believe reflux patients should be endoscoped 2 yearly. This simple approach is actually a bit more complicated now: If there is no dysplasia, a 3-5 year endoscopy depending on the length of the Barrett's segment, the sex of the patient, their weight, and other risk factors is probably OK. With low grade dysplasia a one yearly endoscopy is fine. In some departments Barrett's can be treated with Radio Frequency Ablation, like reflux is itself in some centres. The trouble is that screening so far hasn't been shown improve survival, certainly not in a cost effective way.

Eating an apple late at night is, ironically, supposed to reduce gastric reflux symptoms, I am not sure how. It doesn't work for me. Obviously, extra pillows and phone books under the legs at the top of the bed have their own problems if the patient has cervical spondylosis or obstructive sleep apnoea or ankle oedema. Strawberry extract reduces the microscopic lower oesophageal histological changes of acid reflux, Deglycyrrhinised Liquorice helps eradicate H Pylori which reduces reflux symptoms (even if that presumably increases the risk of Barrett's!) and even Melatonin, the hormone used in jet lag and ADHD has been shown to reduce the effects of both acid and bile reflux.

Domperidone, a prokinetic, which I have always found a useful adjunct in patients with bloating, reflux, heartburn and dysphagia is now no longer recommended for use outside of actual vomiting, because of cardiac side effects. I have never seen a whiff of a cardiac side effect with this drug at any dose at any age.

PPIs and interactions:

PPIs cause a possible increase in osteoporosis related fractures, a 16% increase in MI (not seen in H2 antagonist users), a twofold increase in cardiovascular mortality, a reduction in the effectiveness of bisphosphonates, they may cause hypomagnesaemia, possibly calcium and Vitamin C malabsorption, reduction in absorption of branch chain amino acids, Vitamin K2, silicon, boron, strontium, calcium, and zinc. They cause a decrease in the effectiveness of Clopidogrel, a possible increase in some infections including Clostridium Difficile and Pneumonia but the advantages given the weak associations of risk far outweigh the disadvantages. Also some increase in arrythmias, B12 and iron deficiency, (PPIS can be used as an adjunct in haemochromatosis and do reduce ferritin levels). They can also cause restless legs syndrome. They increase the incidence of asthma in babies when taken in pregnancy. A Danish observational study presented at the American Heart Assn 2016 Scientific Sessions reported a dose related increased risk of ischaemic stroke with all 4 PPIs investigated. The comments made at the presentation were that PPIs reduce Nitric Oxide production and this causes endothelial dysfunction-the underlying process in many PPI side effects.

Of the PPIS, the most likely to have a drug/drug interaction (usually via competing liver metabolism, – Cytochrome P450) is Omeprazole followed by Lansoprazole. Pantoprazole is the least likely. Possible interactions involve Digoxin, Warfarin, Ciclosporin and iron. It is probably better to use Pantoprazole with Warfarin despite the cost. Likewise with Clopidogrel. So as usual, the cheap and cheerful first line generic drugs, the drugs first off patent, encouraged by national guidelines and local prescribing committees, are the least safe overall. This applies to almost every class and group of drugs.

If the patient suffers diarrhoea with a PPI, change them to Omeprazole or Pantoprazole.

Interestingly PPIs are supposed to increase the absorption of Creon (pancreatic enzymes) when prescribed for malabsorption due to **Pancreatic Insufficiency/Pancreatectomy.**

While we are on the subject of **pH:**
Gastric Juice:

If you are interested is pH	1-2.5
Lemon juice	2.1
Coca Cola (no wonder it dissolves the enamel from your teeth)	2.6
Bananas	5.1
Milk, **surprisingly, is still slightly acid** at	6.1
Blood is alkaline at	7.4
Sea water	7.9-8.3
Egg white	8.3
Milk of Magnesia	10.5

Constipation:

Laxatives:

There seems to be an overlap between osmotic, bulk forming and stimulant laxatives, some agents doing several things in the lumen and to the musculature of the bowel and being classified in various ways. But to generalise:

Bulk forming:

Sterculia, Normacol, with Frangulia (Normacol plus) taste quite nice, take with water. Ispaghula, Fybogel.
Methylcellulose, Celevac.

Osmotic:

Lactulose,

Macrogol (Polyethylene glycol):

1-8 sachets a day to clear impaction or to prevent chronic constipation. Klean – Prep, Laxido, Movicol, Movicol Paediatric. Dose can be spread over the day and not known to be harmful in pregnancy and breast feeding.

(Studies in animals have shown "reproductive toxicity" in that sensitive species for gut acting drugs, the rabbit. There have been no human suspicions of teratogenicity. – It is not actually absorbed).

Magnesium Sulphate.

Softeners:

Liquid Paraffin,

Docusate.

Stimulant laxatives:

Bisacodyl tabs and suppositories,

Senna,

Castor Oil,

Sodium Picosulphate,

Liquid Paraffin.

The prokinetic SSRA (5HT4 receptor agonist) Prucalopride, Resolor can be used in chronic female constipation when other treatments have failed. I am not sure why **women only** – except that the NICE guideline says that chronic constipation is 2-3X more common in women than men and they must be thinking about cost.

Does this strike you as sexist nonsense or have I missed something here? Can you imagine the howls of protest if it were restricted to men ?

Stimulant combination laxatives:

Co – Danthramer: Dantron/Polaxamer "188" 1-2 caps nocte (or liquid). Now restricted to terminally ill patients because animal testing showed liver and GI tumours in mice and rats. This wasn't the case when I first prescribed it in the 70's and 80's.

Co-Danthrusate: Dantron/Docusate, Normax. 1-3 caps at night and liquid.

Manevac: Senna and Ispaghula.

Enemas: (Enemata):

Sodium Phosphate, Bisacodyl, Glycerol.

The Fleet enema is sodium acid phosphate enema 133ml.

Micolette, Micralax, Relaxit are sodium citrate containing micro enemata. The Relaxit can be used in children but you don't push the nozzle in so far as with adults!

Children and constipation:

Provided there are no grounds for suspicion, (myxoedema, late meconium, possible Hirschsprung's, signs of actual obstruction etc.) Try starting with Lactulose, increase the dose until there is at least one soft stool a day without straining. Then if this is not working add Senna liquid at night, or Movicol paediatric (gradually increasing the number of sachets from 2-6 if necessary and reducing again, using the higher dose for 3 days, spread throughout the day to relieve impaction). If this is not working, try Picolax sachets, eg at 1-2 years 1/4 sachet bd etc.

Paediatric Docusate solution is said to be more effective than Senna: eg Docusol Paed. Soln. TDS as an adjunct to Lactulose.

Safe in pregnancy: (Merec Bulletin)

Lactulose, Methyl Cellulose, Celevac, Sterculia, Normacol, with Frangulia (Normacol plus), Ispaghula, Fybogel, Senna, Magnesium Sulphate, Liquid paraffin, Docusate.

So in adults for constipation for short term use, try Movicol sachets, 2-8 PRN or Picolax sachets, 2 nocte plus ongoing lactulose to prevent recurrence.

Causes of Constipation:

Inadequate roughage or fluid, any cause of Ileus, aluminium containing antacids, anticholinergic drugs (Parkinson's drugs), antidiarrhoeals, analgesics (Codeine, opioids and related dugs), antitussives, antihistamines with intrinsic anticholinergic activity, CCBs, calcium, Clonidine, diuretics, iron, MAOIs, phenothiazines (anticholinergic), TCAS (anticholinergic).

Bowel Prep:

Picolax half to one sachet 10-12 hours before, half to one 2-4 hrs before procedure.

Appendicitis:

An acute appendix can still kill in the UK and can still be missed by even a competent doctor. I remember being on call, covering three practices one weekend and visiting a total of 24 patients at their homes. This was during a gastroenteritis epidemic and when a normal weekend for GPs was 80 hours continuous duty. I was fairly bored with being phoned by and going out to see people who complained of severe abdominal pain but had relatively mild tummy upsets. Then I was called by a family who I had already seen on the Saturday, once again on the Sunday evening. I was fairly reluctant to go until they quoted my own words back at me "But doctor, the pains **are** now constant, **not just** before bowel actions or vomiting and they **have** moved downwards from the tummy button". I reluctantly went and found the (teenage) patient with a rigid abdomen and a burst appendix. Appendices do get inflamed and rupture during episodes of viral gastroenteritis and other unrelated abdominal conditions and this is one of the many diagnostic traps that are set for GPs to fall into. Don't ever resent going and looking at the patient twice. There are no golden rules about appendices.

I have heard colleagues reassure patients with abdominal pain over the phone, saying "No, it isn't an appendix because you aren't vomiting. **This is wrong**. You can have an advanced, even perforated appendix without vomiting. My daughter of 34 years did.

Appendicitis in children:

The patient may not be febrile but IS usually tachycardic. As mentioned elsewhere, nausea and vomiting may not necessarily be present and just because you saw them yesterday and they seemed to have gastro enteritis it doesn't mean the diagnosis hasn't changed overnight to an inflamed or burst appendix.

Things you may have forgotten:

Don't forget that a retrocaecal appendix doesn't necessarily demonstrate rebound and guarding in the R.I.F. (Always do a rectal examination if you are not sure but suspect the diagnosis.) Also an appendix which is entirely pelvic will not trigger abdominal rigidity.

Appendicitis tends to happen in people who have a sluggish colon and fewer bowel actions per week as they are said to be susceptible to appendicular faecoliths.

Mesenteric adenitis is the great mimic of appendicitis, the swollen glands being adjacent to the appendix and becoming swollen during a variety of unrelated viral infections.

The combination of raised WBC, RIF pain and tenderness, guarding, rebound, fever, nausea, anorexia and so on lead to a presumptive diagnosis (assuming a negative MSU and if appropriate, pregnancy test etc). Often an ESR or CRP can help clinch the diagnosis although these would be raised with the white count in salpingitis too.

Unless perforation has taken place, these days, IV rehydration, IV antibiotics and strong analgesia are given first until the patient is settled. The elective appendicectomy being done during the hours of daylight or the appendicitis may be treated by IV antibiotics alone with a 30% recurrence rate in the following year. When I did my surgical house job we made the presumptive diagnosis and we went straight in. It always seemed to be in the small hours. I still have a slight problem with today's delayed surgery for what is a potentially lethal condition. I can't believe waiting while the pus bathes the peritoneum and all those peritoneal adhesions are formed a risk worth taking. IV antibiotics do not prevent all septicaemia and what is all that broad spectrum antibiotic doing to the microbiome?

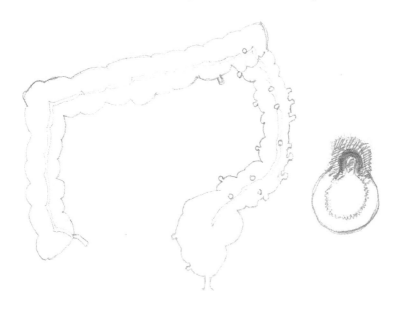

Diverticular Disease diagram (DD 1)

Diverticulitis:

40% people over 60 year have colonic diverticulae. These are usually asymptomatic but if one becomes infected then the usual symptoms are lower abdominal pain, (L>R), fever, sometimes rectal bleeding and diarrhoea or constipation. Complications can include diverticular abscess, peritonitis, fistulae or haemorrhage. Treatment depends on the severity and the presence of complications which are, thankfully, rare. Most cases are treated at home with oral fluids antispasmodics, non constipating analgesics and:

Antibiotic Treatment:

Co Amoxiclav, Cefalosporin plus Metronidazole or Ciprofloxacin PLUS Metronidazole
If Clostridium Difficile is present:
Metronidazole and Vancomycin (-the latter can be given orally and systemically and is

also used in pseudomembranous colitis and staphylococcal enteritis).

Bowel Cancer Recent staging and Prognosis: (and up to 2002): 5 year survival

Duke's A, or stage 1 The innermost lining of the bowel/rectum, no further than the muscle layer 93% (83%)

Duke's B, or Stage 2 Through the muscle layer 77% (64%)

Duke's C, or Stage 3 Spread to lymph nodes 48% (38%)

Duke's D, or Stage 4 Distant spread 6% (3%)

The figures in brackets are from over a decade ago showing how prognosis and treatment are improving.

American Joint Committee on Cancer:

Stage 1 93% More malignant than a polyp but still the innermost layer.

Stage IIA 85% Through the muscle layer not outside the colon.

Stage IIB 72% Through the colon wall but not outside the colon.

Stage IIIA 83% Inner and middle layers of colon wall and 1-3 nodes plus local tissue OR 4-6 nodes.

Stage IIIB 64% Through all the wall layers plus 1-3 nodes OR through the muscle and/or outer layer plus 4-6 nodes OR in the inner and middle layers (could be the muscle layer) plus 7 or more nodes.

Stage IIIC 44% Through all wall layers plus 4-6 nodes OR through the muscle layer and/or outer layer of colon and 7 or more nodes or the cancer is in all layers of the colon and has spread to adjacent organs plus or minus nodes and tissue around them.

Stage IV 8.1% Distant metastases: IVA May have gone through the bowel wall, possibly affecting local nodes and organs and one organ not adjacent to the colon or abdominal wall. IVB as IVA but spread to more than one organ not adjacent to the colon or abdominal wall.

Alternatively:

T1 2 3 or 4 (tumour extent, 3 being up to the bowel wall, 4 being through it).

N 0 1 2 etc (N 1 is 3 or fewer nodes).

M 0 1 2 etc. (number of metastases).

Roughly speaking 2/3 of large bowel cancers are colonic and 1/3 are rectal.

to reduce the incidence of bowel cancer by half, (37 to 20/100,000) the treatment may increase pancreatic cancer 60% (6>12/100,000) as a side effect.

Bowel Cancer Screening:

Is via faecal occult blood testing (even though, ironically, our Biochemistry department withdrew the test from GPs a few years ago as it was "no better than tossing a coin" according to our Consultant when used in patients with anaemia as a test to exclude significant gut bleeding!)

The screening test which seems to regularly pick up asymptomatic bowel cancer in my patients starts >60 years and up to 75 years and is every 2 years.

FIT for purpose?

Faecal immunochemical testing has an overall accuracy for detection of CRC (Colorectal Cancer) of 95% and 79% sensitivity, 94% specificity (Lee et Al 2016). FIT has been shown to have a greater sensitivity in detecting advanced adenomata and CRC than standard guaiac-based faecal occult blood testing (gFOBT).

Anal Fissure:

Common causes are 2-10% cancer (gastric/colorectal,)
20-30% adenomata,
Diverticulae,
Haemorrhoids,
Inflamm. bowel disease,
Angiodysplasia of colon,
SCA, (Sickle Cell).
Marathon runners.

Fissures are supposed not to heal because they cause auto ischaemia via spasm due to the pain and the lack of blood prevents their own healing. Hence there is a vicious circle of constipation>split mucosa>pain>spasm>ischaemia>failure to heal>pain>spasm etc. This circle can be broken by relieving the spasm with ointments that relax the internal anal sphincter (the ointments contain GTN, (Rectogesic) Diltiazem, and topical analgesics, Scheriproct, Proctosedyl, etc)

A long time ago a procedure known as Lord's procedure or the anal stretch was performed for chronic anal fissure and haemorrhoids. This damaged the internal anal sphincter, sometimes permanently, but relieved the spasm that caused the perpetuation of the fissure.

Coeliac Disease: Gluten Enteropathy.

An allergy to the gliaden fraction of gluten in wheat, barley, oats (some patients) and rye. Rice, soy and corn (maize) are tolerated. Wheat, like milk, has only been a part of the human diet for a few thousand years and so allergy to it hasn't died out yet. (-i.e. killed its genetic carriers) – Indeed, the incidence may be as high as 3% in people who complain to the GP of gastrointestinal symptoms.

1: 200 of the general UK population and up to 6% of patients with type 2 diabetes may have Coeliac. Coeliac Disease can begin in the first year of life with muscle wasting, abdominal distension and foul, loose stools. It is said to be commoner in children who have frequent early "infections". Oddly, these do not have to be GI infections. Children with 10 or more respiratory tract **or** GI infections between 0-6m and between 6 and 18m have a 30% increased risk of Coeliac disease. There is often a secondary lactase (disaccharidase) deficiency and hence milk intolerance. It can present in teenage and young adulthood with abdominal symptoms, oral ulcers, tiredness, appetite loss, bloating, nausea, steatorrhoea etc, and needs to be excluded in CFS and IBS patients.

Dermatitis Herpetiformis, delayed puberty, osteoporosis and thyroid dysfunction are associated.

There is in the untreated an increase in adenocarcinoma and lymphoma (NHL) of the small bowel. There is a characteristic absence of villi on jejunal biopsy and this with the immunology is diagnostic.

There is an association with hyposplenism so consider pneumococcal and influenza vaccines.

Pathology: Bloods: Anti endomysial antibodies (which are IgA) are more reliable than anti gliaden antibodies (IgG and IgA) but the patient needs to have been eating gluten for at least 2-6 weeks before the antibodies reappear after a gluten free treatment period. You can also test anti Reticulin Abs and also useful are anti-tTG antibodies. Do a total IgA to make sure the patient makes sufficient IgA to give a positive endomysial test. If not the IgG – tTG can substitute.

HLA DQ2 or DQ8 are strongly associated. There are weak associations with Type 1 Diabetes, Down's Syndrome and Turner's Syndrome.

There are multiple deficiencies, of Iron, fat soluble vitamins, B12 etc all due to chronic steatorrhoea.

Dietary supplements are advised, of iron, folic acid, vitamins A, D and K, B vitamins, B12, bisphosphonates, Ca, (presumably Mg supplements too) and HRT are needed as well as a strict gluten free diet.

Some gluten free products are prescribable. I limit my gluten free prescibing to a few staples and no desserts. I can see that prescribing bread and pasta may be reasonable given their cost but I have a slight problem with the whole range of gluten free food (desserts, sweets, etc) available. After all, it is perfectly possible to eat a full nutritious diet without cereals and this is the only group of people apart from those in receipt of foreign aid for whom the tax payer buys food. Keep an eye on bone mineral density.

Dyspepsia:

A tumour must be excluded in the presence of weight loss, dysphagia, food getting stuck, post prandial nausea, vomiting or melaena, jaundice and in anyone over 50 with iron deficiency or a change in the pattern of any chronic abdominal symptoms. It is very easy to dismiss the dyspeptic patient as it is such a common symptom and **nearly always** benign. In this regard I differ with the view of some biochemists and find occult blood tests very useful and very reassuring. Along with the USS, stool culture, Coeliac tests, HP serology, Faecal Calprotectin, LFTs and FBC, there are not many other screening tests that GPs can resort to in the patient with abdominal pain. All other patients would probably be treated symptomatically with either an anti acid approach (PPI/H2 antagonists in biggish doses and PRN antacids) and/or an anti Irritable bowel regime. All patients with gastro-enterological symptoms need a symptomatic review with regard to response to treatment and bitter experience has led me to do a few simple screening tests relatively early even in the most classic dyspeptic or irritable bowel patient. Certainly I like to see them soon after the first prescription and then fairly frequently especially if they are on a repeat prescription of any GI drug.

General Rules:

Dyspepsia:

Below 55 years Reflux Symptoms	No reflux or alarm symptoms	Alarm symptoms	Over 55 years Endoscope (2WR if Alarm sympts)
4 Wks PPI	HP Serology (or etc)	Haematemesis, weight loss, dysphagia, anaemia. **Refer 2 WR.**	
No response or relapse ENDOSCOPY	Neg Pos Symptomatic Treat............>Asymptomatic>No action treatment, >Symptomatic Exclude HPagain. consider other causes.		

Helicobacter serology remains positive after Helicobacter eradication and the breath test is said to be more reliable. Triple therapy is up to 90% effective at eradication but don't forget all infections can recur.

Alternatively:

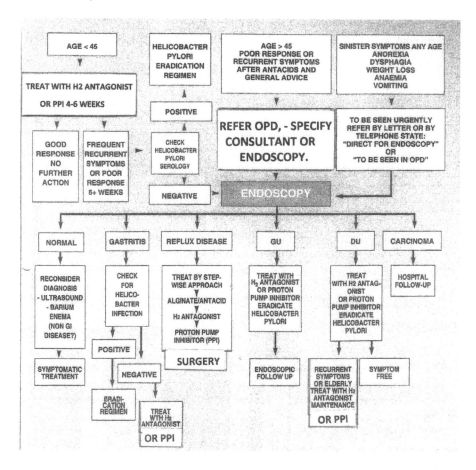

Diagram: Guidelines for dyspepsia: (GFD 1). (Adapted from The Surrey and Sussex Trust, -Thanks to all the Gastroenterologists who helped draw it up)

(2014, Nov) Guidelines for H. Pylori Eradication:

Initially, if a patient is positive for HP give a 7 day BD course of a PPI, Amoxicillin 1Gr. and either Clarithromycin 500mg or Metronidazole 400mg.

If allergic to penicillin, give 7 days of BD PPI, Clarithromycin 250mg and Metronidazole 400mg.

If allergic to penicillin and has had previous exposure to Clarithromycin give 7 days of BD PPI Bismuth, Metronidazole 400mg and Tetracycline 500mg.

Second Line treatment:

If patients still have symptoms after initial eradication treatment, give:

7 days of BD PPI, Amoxicillin 1Gr plus whichever of Clarithromycin 500mg or Metronidazole 400mg that wasn't used first line.

If the patient has had previous exposure to Clarithromycin and Metronidazole, give a 7 day BD course of a PPI, Amoxicillin 1Gr, a quinolone or tetracycline 500mg.

If allergic to penicillin (and not previously exposed to a quinolone) give 7 days of BD PPI, Metronidazole 400mg and Levofloxacin 250mg.

If allergic to penicillin and previously exposed to a quinolone give a PPI, Bismuth and Metronidazole 400mg and Tetracycline 500mg.

Refer to a Gastroenterologist if second line treatment is ineffective.

Bovine lactoferrin and probiotics (the original paper says Lactobacillus Acidophilus, L Salivarius and L Casei via lactic acid or an autolysin production) improve eradication rates as does quadruple therapy. The probiotic discovery can only be good given the broad spectrum and high doses of antibiotics being used here and our current paranoia about antibiotic resistance, GI super infections and harm done to our microbiome. Lactoferrin, found in many exocrine fluids but especially colostrum is antibacterial, antiviral and antiparasitic. It is structurally similar to Transferrin and also has anti cancer as well as anti allergic properties. It is fascinating stuff.

PPI Therapy:

PPI standard doses are: Esomeprazole 20mg, Lansoprazole 30mg, Omeprazole 20-40mg, Pantoprazole 20-40mg, Rabeprazole 20mg.

There may be some long term risks but there are many old wives' tales about PPI treatment: eg:

Community acquired pneumonia – a small relative risk, secondary to the **reflux** of acid and aspiration and not due directly to the PPI.

Effect on calcium metabolism: (hip fractures) but PPIs actually reduce osteoCLASTIC activity (osteoclasts are driven by a proton pump) not BLASTIC activity. So Urinary Calcium in PPI patients is actually **lowered.** But many PPI patients have their calcium metabolism interfered with by thiazides and other drugs that they are taking concomitantly – anticonvulsants, benzodiazepines etc. So this is not a significant risk due to the PPI.

Lowered absorbed Magnesium **may be**. It may be rational to supplement magnesium in long term PPI users. If you are interested, the Magnesium content of bottled water varies tremendously. The highest level I have seen is in the slightly alkaline tasting San Pellegrino from Italy (Mg 50mg/li) perhaps you should suggest PPI users who drink bottled water look for one with a high Mg++ such as that.

C.Difficile: Recent evidence does NOT show a relationship between PPIs and C Diff. It is an acid resistant spore anyway! so it would be independent of anything we do to the stomach pH.

Clopidogrel Interaction. Clopidogrel is a pro drug and both it and PPIs use liver Cytochrome P450.

In fact Clopidogrel and Statins compete for the same enzyme too. There isn't usually a clinically significant issue here but give the PPI in the morning and the Clopidogrel in the evening and there should be no theoretical interaction either. This is because of Clopidogrel's half life – the active metabolite having a half life of about half an hour.

Many other potential side effects, including an increased risk of asthma in the baby of a mother who takes a PPI during pregnancy have been suggested in recent years.

Bariatric Surgery:

Is indicated >BMI 40kg/SqM or 35kg/SqM with co morbidities.

Obesity causes type 2 diabetes, hypertension, dyslipidaemias, sleep apnoea, CVS disease, various cancers, steatohepatitis, reflux, gallstones, pseudotumour cerebri, OA, infertility and incontinence to name but a few.

The obesity cancers are *oesophageal adenocarcinoma, M.M., cancers of the gastric cardia and colon in men, the rectum in men, biliary tract, pancreas, post menopausal breast, premenopausal endometrium, ovary and kidney. Feb 28 Online BMJ 2017.

The long term picture of permanent weight loss is better with gastric bypass (etc) surgery than with any diet, exercise or appetite suppressant treatment. Patients generally lose 2/3 of their excess weight within a year with only 10-20 pounds regained over the following 10 years. 80% of diabetics operated on in this way are cured of their diabetes, 83% patients with sleep apnoea get better, CV risk drops 72% by 5 years. Overall there is 30-40% drop in all cause mortality. Can you think of any drug treatment or any treatment at all that comes close to having this kind of overall benefit?

The Operations:

Intra gastric balloon (for BMI 27-35)
Laparoscopically Adjustable Gastric Banding:
A restrictive procedure. A silicone inflatable band is placed around the cardia just below the gastro oesophageal junction. There is a subcutaneous port which adjusts the band and produces a sensation of satiety.

Patients lose about 50% of their excess weight after this. Suggested in 2014 by NICE in all Type 2 diabetics with BMIs>30.

Roux-en-Y Gastric By-pass:
The stomach is effectively transected and most of the lower part is isolated laparoscopically while connected to a blind tube of duodenum and jejunum and therefore bypassed, the upper part forming a 20-30ml pouch which connects to the small bowel.

After this procedure patients lose 60-70% of the excess weight in 2 years and most of it stays off.

Sleeve Gastrectomy:
60-80% of the stomach is resected leaving a small sleeve of the lesser curve.

Biliopancreatic Diversion:
(With or without duodenal switch) bypasses most of the small intestine and causes malabsorption.

A number of female patients develop self harming and depression within two to three years of gastric banding, having lost the weight initially. There are several dietary deficiencies that can occur after bariatric surgery. Thiamine, (presenting as Wernicke's Encephalopathy if vomiting is not treated with Thiamine as well as fluid rehydration) B12, folate, Vitamin D, Vitamin E and copper. There is a variety of potential neurological complications that can follow also. These range from encephalopathy, optic neuropathy, to polyneuropathy and so on. J of Obesity, 2012.608534, 8pp

20: Geriatrics/Old age medicine: (See other sections)

Old age is the most unexpected of all things that happen to a man.
Leon Trotsky

If you are over sixty and you wake up in the morning with nothing aching, you're dead.

Demography:

Life expectancy in the UK was 77.4 years (m) and 81.7 (f) in 2010. It had increased to 79.1 (m) and 82.8 (f) by 2014.

This is slightly worse than Japan (79.3 and 82.7 years in 2010) but a lot better than the world's worst place, the Central African Republic, (45.9 and 44.5 years).

16.5% of the population is >65 years old in the UK compared with 27% of those in Monaco and 0.9% in the United Arab Emirates. All the really low figures for the elderly are in the "developing world". China is 8.9%, Canada 16%, USA 13%. Old age, putting aside the absence of destructive behaviour traits, is inherited and associated with various alleles. These include FOXO3A, SIRT1, CETP, TP53, with a variant of FOXO3A having borderline significance. Longevity is how long you live but healthspan is how long you live in optimum health.

Multimorbidity is the rule: 40% Canadians over 80 years old have 4 or more chronic conditions and the complexities of managing multiple conditions in older patients is said to be one of the main challenges facing British General Practice in the mid teens of the 21stC. There are at least 20 chronic conditions to which the elderly are prone and so clinical guidelines tailored to specific clinical situations where there are so many variables would be impractical. This is where the Geriatrician and GP have to use their common sense in management and prescribing decisions. It is also where national guidelines for GPs to have management plans for their elderly patients are out of touch with reality. There are just too many variables, too many things that can go wrong in the same patient and all the altering morbidities are interdependent.

When is it right to ignore guidelines for the benefit of the majority?

Over recent years many sources I have read have suggested ineffective, or even NO treatment be given to the elderly disturbed, disruptive patient in hospital wards or nursing homes. Many suggest that no physical restraint, no isolation from other patients or residents and no pharmacological sedatives are ever appropriate when one irrational individual continuously shatters the safety and peace of a ward. I can only say that the authors of such guidelines can never have worked in, spoken to the staff of or tried to sleep in nursing homes, residential units or wards where disturbed, confused, ranting or threatening residents or patients are present. They can make life absolutely miserable, upsetting, frightening and intimidating for residents, other patients and staff. It is utterly wrong that only the rights of the victims in these, very common situations be ignored. GPs are on the horns of the same treatment dilemma here as in terminal care – with too little or too much pain relief. To treat or not to treat the disruptive disturbed irrational patient – to sedate or not to sedate, that is the question. – And how much drug to give? The desperate relatives often asking for a sedative "cosh" to give them respite. The alternative is a possible risk of violence at home or mistreatment by end of tether staff in a residential setting. I have even seen other patients take the law into their own hands on a unit when an irrational, often aggressive, unpredictable and frightening patient who was affecting the health of many and who was utterly inaccessible to reasoning was ignored by staff. The demented screaming old man was locked in a side ward and the exhausted patients had their first night of relative peace for days.**

Senile confusion, psychosis and paranoia.
Very important to exclude a cause – of which UTI and LRTI are the commonest but clearly there are many bacteriological, biochemical and other causes:
Including atypical presentations of:
Stroke, acute abdomen, C.C.F., M.I., respiratory failure (or hypoxia of any cause), anaemia, diabetes, thyroid disease, renal failure/damage/UTI, septicaemia, hepatic failure/damage, malignant disease, drug side effects, electrolyte disturbance.
One possible treatment: (Assuming the cause (all the above) has been addressed): Quetiapine, starting at 25mg nocte.

Dementia:

Aggression in Dementia:
Many alternatives, some controversial. Can try Valproate, (although Depakote was the subject of some FDA concern in America) Quetiapine, Trazadone, Sertraline, even Risperidone.

Depression and agitation in the elderly:
Sertraline and Quetiapine is a reasonable combination.

**Dementia and disturbing all the other residents, in an otherwise well elderly patient and no physical cause can be found and all reasonable screening tests (FBC, ESR, TFTs, U and Es, LFTs, MSU, full examination for causes of pain, Temporal A.s, OA, reflux, cardiac pain, biliary, renal or digestive pain, constipation, anal fissure, etc) – especially if the nursing home or hospital staff (or family) say something has to be done and you have no choice but to prescribe something.
Try Mirtazepine 15mg and Quetiapine 50mg daily.

Senile Vaginitis, Atrophic Vaginitis:
Ovestin, Orthogynest, Estriol vaginal Cream.

Falls:

Falling at home is a symptom of illness and frailty in the older population, a marker of vulnerability and one of the commonest reasons for prompting permanent residential or nursing home care. It can, as we know, be the cause of an injury, admission and rapid decline in hospital for some older patients.

Up to 30% of over 65 year olds fall significantly each year. An analysis of 79,000 patients in 159 studies back to 1946 (Cochr. database Syst Rev 2012 Sep 12:9:CD007146.) showed that intervening to offer group exercise therapies reduced the risk of falling by 29%, exercise schedules given at home improved falls 32%, Tai Chi and balancing exercises 29%. Taking away trip and fall risks in the home environment (carpets, slippery floors, trailing extension leads etc) reduced risk of falls 19%. Poor vision is a major fall risk. Unsurprisingly, cataracts are at the top of this list but multifocal glasses are too. I found it almost impossible to walk down stairs when I was first prescribed these as the distance lens is at the top of the frame, close-up lens at the bottom, the stairs are a blur and you need to tip your head right down to see the floor ahead. They cause untold neck pain and related complications! Removing cataracts reduced falls 44% and substituting multifocals with single lenses also reduces rates of falling. The most effective intervention though was stopping all psychotropic medication which reduced falls 66%. This is however a bit of an unachievable gold standard given the frequency of depression, insomnia, severe anxiety, dementia and chronic pain in the elderly population.

A 2016 paper (Circulation: Cardiovascular Quality and Outcomes DOI:10. 1161CIRCOUTCOMES .115. 002524.) showed that falls were much commoner up to two weeks after starting, changing or intensifying antihypertensive treatment. I would imagine with some treatments even longer. (ie alpha blockers). No surprise there but salutary to remember that blood pressures often peak in the surgery. So when we try to comply with contemporary NICE or other cardiovascular blood pressure guidelines to reduce blood pressure to the minimum compatible with consciousness we should remember this: that falls cause nursing home admissions, that few residents ever go home once they are a resident in a nursing home and life in residential care is shorter, more medicated, more frustrating, less varied and less stimulating than independent life at home.

21: HAEMATOLOGY: (SEE PATHOLOGY SECTION, HAEMOGLOBIN, ELECTROPHORESIS, HAEMATINICS ETC)

Highly selected topics:

Blood Groups

The ABO gene is on chromosome 9.

The proportions of the ABO groups (see below) are roughly the same in all races except Native Americans who are virtually all group O.

Why does the rest of the world's population have this diversity of blood groups? It turns out that different ABO groups confer protection against various different forms of gastro enteritis, a number of other infectious diseases and systemic disorders. AB confers a powerful resistance to Cholera which O does not. Group O however confers (like Sickle Cell Haemoglobin and Thalassaemia) a slight resistance to Malaria. There must have been strong evolutionary selection pressures caused by various prevalent diseases in the past to have resulted in today's mixture of worldwide ABO groups.

Also there are secretors and non secretors of the ABO protein (who either secrete a soluble form of the ABO protein into their saliva and gut secretions or not) and they are susceptible to different diseases:

For instance: The Non secretors: are more likely to develop meningitis and UTIs, less likely to get Flu and RSV.

There is also a difference in the respective clotting risks of different blood groups. Venous thrombo- embolism having an incidence rate of 1.8 in the non-O groups compared with group O blood. Similar risks rates apply for PE and DVT but are slightly higher for pregnancy and abortion related VTE. (X2.22)

Arterial events are higher in non-O blood groups although the relative risk at around X1.1 is less than that of venous clotting.

Group O has the lowest risk of dementia, AB being significantly higher. O has a lower overall risk of heart disease, AB is the highest.

In the UK	O+	A+	B+	AB+	O –	A –	B –	AB-
	37%	35%	8%	3%	7%	7%	2%	1%

A +, of course, is the universal recipient, O- the universal donor.

Iron Deficiency: (see Iron in "Pathology")

Replacement:

Iron: Ferrous Sulphate (cheap and cheerful) 200mg BD/QDS,
Ferrous Gluconate 300mg 1-2 TDS,
Liquid Iron eg Sytron can be given at any age. 10mls is equivalent to 55mg Fe
<1yr 2.5ml BD, adult 10mls TDS.

Never dismiss iron deficiency as purely dietary. It is one of the commonest presenting features of bowel malignancy and bleeding and **usually requires investigation**.

Current BSG (British Society of Gastroenterology) guidelines suggest upper and lower GI endoscopy in non anaemic iron deficiency over the age of 50. I would add anaemic iron deficiency to this recommendation since anaemia can just be the end result of a chronic GI blood loss.

Thalassaemia: (Aut Rec) Alpha, Beta, Major, Minor (Trait – partially expressed or carrier), Intermedia:

A condition which is characterised by dysfunctional globin chains in the Hb molecules of erythrocytes. Like Sickle Cell Hb, it may offer some protection against Malaria.

What you may have forgotten:

You may remember that the haem is attached to 4 chains of globin which is in 2 pairs. In normal adult Hb there are two alpha and two beta chains.

Foetal Hb has two alpha and two gamma chains (Hb F). Other haemoglobins have two alpha and two other (which are the same as each other) globin chains.

Alpha Thalassaemia causes dysfunctional Alpha chains and Beta Thalassaemia affects the Beta chains of the haemoglobin. The abnormal haem leads to premature haemolysis of the erythrocyte, a **microcytic hypochromic anaemia despite a raised iron**, poikilocytosis, polychromasia, low MCHC, target cells visible and nucleated red cells on the peripheral film.

Classic Thalassaemia is Beta chain Thalassaemia and the different severities are due to homo or heterozygosity.

Thalassaemia major then, is usually homozygous beta chain Thalassaemia. Both parents will have the heterozygous Thalassaemia minor form. The reduced erythrocyte Hb A is made up for by Hb F and HbA2. If the patient has another abnormal Hb as well and is heterozygous for (eg) Hb S and Hb F then their symptoms are as severe as a straight forward homozygous Thalassaemia major. The FBC is as above, the Hb electrophoresis shows the abnormal, predominantly foetal Hb and there is a raised bilirubin.

So in the major (homozygous) form, infants fail to thrive from about the age of one and have abnormal facies too.

Homozygous Alpha Thalassaemia can cause hydrops and death in utero.

Thalassaemia minor, the heterozygous Beta chain type form is much milder with a hypochromic anaemia, normal or high serum iron. There is raised Hb A2.

Alpha and Beta Thalassaemia traits cause mild anaemia or no signs or symptoms.

There is also a Thalassaemia "Intermedia" based on clinical severity.

Most sufferers of Thalassaemia are from the Mediterranean area but sufferers can come from any location. Carriers:

1:1000 White British,
1:7 Cypriots,
1:12 Greeks,
1:10 Gujeratis,
1:25 Pakistanis etc.

Beta Thalassaemia is the commonest type around the Mediterranean, the Middle East and India. Alpha Thalassaemia occurs in Southeast Asia, India, the Middle East and Africa.

The treatment of the more severe forms includes transfusion and chelation therapy (now orally in the form of deferiprone). Splenectomy if hypersplenism occurs. There is the possibility of a matched donor marrow transplant for some.

The symptoms and signs include failure to thrive, hepatosplenomegaly, frontal bossing, malocclusion, pallor, jaundice, iron overload (Haemochromatosis, Diabetes etc), various endocrinopathies.

The classic laboratory findings are of a microcytic hypochromic anaemia with replete iron. Hb electrophoresis shows the abnormal Hb. Serum iron is raised, saturation raised (up to 80%) and ferritin is raised too.

Skull X Ray shows the "Hair on end" appearance. Complications apart from Haemochromatosis include unusual and serious infections (due to raised iron levels), gout, osteoporosis, liver cancer, CCF.

In untreated Cooley's anaemia (B Thalassaemia major) the mortality rate is 80% before the age of 5.

22: Hormones:

"I don't know what's happening to me. – They're called hormones"

T. Mafi

Thyroid Disease:

Hyperthyroidism: Rx: Carbimazole 20-60mg OD Initially until euthyroid. Then 5-15mg a day for 6-18m and tail off, watching TFTs (as well as LFTS and WBC).

Children: 5-15mg daily, initially.

Can be given in a bigger dose with concomitant Thyroxine.

Examine the thyroid regularly and do at least one USS at start of the course.

Alternatively: Propylthiouracil 200-400mg daily initially until euthyroid then maintain on 50-150mg daily watching TFTs. Can be given in pregnancy. Both Carbimazole and Propylthiouracil can be used in breast feeding mums.

Propranolol and Nadolol are the best beta blockers for quick symptomatic control.

Growth Hormone:

Adult GH deficiency is rare but it does exist, leads to lethargy and tiredness and is part of the work up for "CFS". (Also it is just worth a thought in depression!)

Normal Random Growth Hormone levels: Men: <5 ng/mL (<226pmol/L), Women: <10ng/mL (<452pmol/L) and Children 0-20 ng/mL (0-904pmol/L).

Treatment: Sub cut inj. 150-300mcg (0.45-0.9IU)/day. Adjustments are based upon IGF-1, median dose is 0.4mg (1.2IU). S/Es: H/A, fluid retention, arthralgia, myalgia, carpal tunnel syndrome, parasthesiae, etc.

Sex Hormone Treatment:

"Oestrogen deficient women are nothing but the walking dead"

Marie Hoag

"The women's health initiative standards for HRT are nothing but an embarrassment to all physicians, and I'm not sure why they have not retracted all the statements that came out of that joke of a study."

Marie Hoag

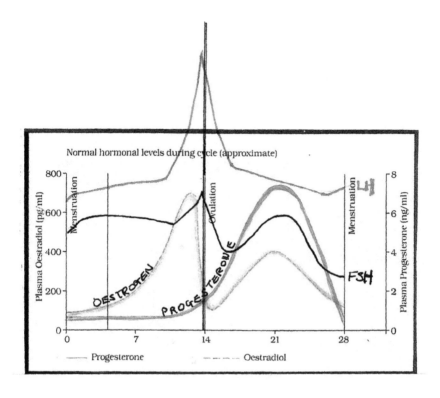

Diagram: (HNMC1) Hormones of the menstrual cycle.

Hormones of the normal menstrual cycle:

The environment seems to be awash with hormones and I don't just mean teenage television and pop DVDs. It isn't just the medical and dental professions that are excluding males. Male fresh water fish and reptiles are becoming feminised or hermaphrodite just swimming in open rivers and ponds. In the area of human health, sperm counts have dropped 20% in 25 years and hormone sensitive cancers are rapidly increasing in incidence. Oestrogen is a potent carcinogen for various cancer lines, not just breast, uterus and ovary for which there are testable receptors. There are Xeno oestrogens in plastics and many industrial compounds that we are exposed to each day. Testicular cancer has increased 80% on the last few decades; breast and prostate cancers are rising in incidence likewise.

There are Alpha and Beta oestrogen receptor subtypes. Alpha stimulation tends to encourage cancer cell growth; beta cell stimulation generally has the reverse effect. Synthetic oestrogens stimulate both while plant oestrogens (phyto-oestrogens) preferentially tend to stimulate beta oestrogen receptors.

Phyto-oestrogens include soy, red clover, (isoflavones) and black cohosh. There is some controlled trial data that suggests a rhubarb extract, Rheum Rhaponticum reduces hormonal anxiety and hot flushes via an interesting focussed SERM like action.

By the time river water reaches the sea it has been drunk by someone three or four times and it contains significant synthetic HRT, contraceptive hormone conjugation and excretion products. These did not exist 50 years ago. They are not effectively removed by the filtration and detoxification processes used by water companies and along with a host of industrial and other contaminants are present in drinking water as it emerges from the tap. This is unless you can afford a reverse osmosis filter or ozone treatment filter to oxidise all the non H2O content of the tap water. Indeed many anti cancer and exclusion diets suggest glass bottled spring water as the sole source of hydration.

Testosterone Deficiency:

Supplements in women (!) for lack of libido in a very selected group (oophorectomised, hysterectomised and receiving oestrogen therapy). Intrinsa 300ug Testosterone patches, are no longer available but Testogel and Sustanol are sometimes used instead. In the US those prescribed testosterone constitute a much larger clinical group.

Menopausal testosterone deficiency can cause dry and itchy eyes in a significant number of women.

In Men, Testosterone Undecanoate Injection (Nebido), every 10-14 weeks, capsules (Restandol), buccal Testosterone (Striant), Sustanon injection 3 weekly as well as gel (Testim, Testogel – 50mg/5gr, Tostran) and an implant etc. can be used to treat androgen deficiency. There is quite a debate about whether Testosterone supplements are a good thing or not. They seem to slightly increase the number of monthly orgasms but not do much for erectile dysfunction. In terms of general health, the evidence is a little contradictory:

The American FDA issued a warning in February 2014 that Testosterone treatment carried a significant cardiovascular risk. Indeed a published analysis of 27 studies showed all of the 14 not funded by the pharmaceutical industry indicated an increased risk with strangely, none of the industry sponsored studies showing the same risk! One study showed a doubling of heart attack risk within 90 days of the first testosterone prescription for men over 65. This increased risk was even worse for younger men with a history of heart disease. (Reuters Feb 25 2014).

In the other corner of this debate is a series of longitudinal population studies which have shown that in men with the co morbidities of cardiovascular, respiratory, renal disease and cancer, a low testosterone is a biomarker of increased mortality risk! This is certainly true of Klinefelter's syndrome in which their hypogonadism is associated with increased death rates from diabetes, cardiovascular disease, respiratory disease and cancer. It is more complicated than just a low serum level however, as individual androgen receptor sensitivity does vary. Circulating and inflammatory cytokines suppress testosterone levels via the hypothalamic pituitary testicular axis and so the low testosterone levels may be secondary to (ie a marker of) disease severity in all these associated conditions. Other situations which produce inflammatory cytokines include obesity, atherosclerosis, diabetes, COPD, inflammatory arthritides. Some acute illnesses also suppress the HPA and reduce the level of testosterone and these include infection, infarction, inflammation, surgery and other types of trauma.

Testosterone replacement has been shown to greatly improve survival in hypogonadal men (Barnsley, up to a twofold improvement in survival).

Low testosterone promotes intimal media thickness – and it may be via this mechanism that it encourages cardiovascular disease through atherosclerosis. So if you are supplementing testosterone for significant deficiency symptoms, (weakness, reduced muscle bulk, fatigue, mood changes, lack of motivation, depression, reduced concentration) do it gradually and assess the CVS risk first.

The latest study of normalising testosterone levels in older men is wholeheartedly in favour of replacement therapy: Aug 2015 Eur Heart J. A large study looked at 83,000 "veterans" with low testosterone levels. Those patients who achieved normalisation of testosterone levels on treatment had a 47% reduced mortality, an 18% lower MI benefit and a 30% stroke benefit compared with patients who did not achieve normalisation. You have to prescribe enough testosterone and check the level though.

But a 2017 systematic review of 150 controlled trials, commenting that $4Bn were to be spent on testosterone supplementation in the US this year, found no conclusive evidence it improved mood or cognitive function and mixed results for sex and cardiovascular outcomes. In four "recent" papers in JAMA and JAMA Int Med, testosterone was found not to affect memory but to increase Bone density, Hb and non calcified coronary plaque volume.

A few other points about Testosterone: Symptomatic male hypogonadism is said to occur in anything from 2-40% of US >65 year olds in different studies. Testosterone prescriptions tripled from 2001-2010 in America so that 4% of American males over 65 are on now the hormone. Both high and low levels of testosterone have been associated with increased risk and aggression of prostate cancer (Morgentaler et Al 96).

OR

Venlafaxine can be used to treat hot flushes in men experiencing androgen deprivation as can medroxyprogesterone with the anti androgen Cyproterone.

Progestogens:

Progesterone: Cyclogest suppositories. 200mg. 400mg. An effective non "happy pill" treatment for post natal and premenstrual depression for women squeamish about taking SSRIs. For PMT, use vaginally or rectally days 12-26. For post natal depression 200-400mg od/bd from 12th day until periods begin.

Norethisterone: 5mg.

Postponement of periods: 1 tds from 3 days before expected date of menstruation.

For dysmenorrhoea: 1 tds from day 5 to 25 then 8 tablet free days.

For menorrhagia and PMT: 1 TDS From day 19-26 inclusive.

Progesterone only HRT is 5mg Norethisterone daily.

Norethisterone as part of combined HRT is usually as Micronor 1mg on day 15-26 of the cycle.

Oestrogens:

Oestrogen patches. Estraderm, Evorel, 25, 50, 75, 100ug/24hrs. Used in PMT and HRT. Twice weekly with an oral progesterone in HRT eg Norethisterone 1mg day 16-28 OR with Medroxyprogesterone 10mg day 14-28 – if the patient has a uterus.

Premenstrual Syndrome:

Mood and memory changes, weight gain and fluid retention, migraine headache, breast tenderness, bloating, abdominal and bowel symptoms with sudden relief at the onset of menstruation.

Many other conditions, such as IBS, migraine, vaginal thrush, eczema, etc can be cyclically worse premenstrually and some women will be eternally grateful if you can help alleviate their symptoms.

PMT **is** an odd condition. It may be due to a relative excess of oestrogen or rapid fluctuation in oestrogen levels in the two weeks before menstruation. It can respond to either progesterone or oestrogen supplementation, to an SSRI or even to Vitamin B6 (Pyridoxine) supplements.

Menopause:
Mean age is 51.3 years, (some sources say 53 years) mean duration 4 years.

Hot flushes: and the suffering female population:

11% at 38 years,

60% at 52-54 years,

30% at 60 years,

15% at 66 years,

9% at 72 years!

The patient can stop contraception 1 year after the last period. (Most people say carry on with contraception for 2 years if the menopause starts before age 50 and for 1 year if it starts after age 50).

Hormone Replacement Therapy H.R.T.
Not for healthy women without symptoms. It increases the risk of breast, endometrial and ovarian cancers as well as arterial and venous thrombo-embolism. Give the lowest dose for the shortest time and review at least annually. (I do 3-6 monthly) Don't use HRT first line for long term prevention of osteoporosis over the age of 50. Can be used if intolerant of other treatments.

Can be used in younger women with a premature menopause, to treat menopausal symptoms or for osteoporosis prevention to the age of 50.

Total mortality is no better and no worse for a woman on HRT or off it. Probably in the UK 20-50% of 45-70 year olds take HRT (-I suspect this wide range depends a lot on where you live and when these results came out. We are currently in a low uptake period.)

I have always found contraception and the menopause a bit of a problem, having had at least two patients with gonadotrophin proven menopausal symptoms then on HRT become pregnant.

One summary might be: (See above)

If a woman >50 years in the menopause needs contraception, give for 1 year.

If a woman <50 years in the menopause needs contraception, give for 2 years.

Or you might advise an IUCD and it stays in for "The foreseeable future".

Cancer and hormones
The discussion about HRT might include an assessment of how bad the climacteric symptoms are, how significant the osteoporotic risk is and: the extra breast cancer risk with HRT – which is the main worry of women who think about benefits and risks.

Oestrogen stimulates the oncogene Bd-2 (oestrogen sensitive). Progesterone down regulates the same gene. Progesterone also up regulates P53 – a tumour suppressor gene.

Unopposed oestrogen increases the risk of endometrial, breast and ovarian cancers.

Oestrogen also stimulates prostate cancer.

Natural progesterone reduces breast cancer risk. Synthetic progesterones increase breast cancer risk.

Testosterone activates the P53 apoptosis (cell suicide) gene (but methyl testosterone does not).

The risk in different studies varies a bit so some of these are slightly different having come from different sources:

One study for instance showed:

Extra breast cancer risk with HRT: (Epinet)

2/1000 over 5 years
6/1000 over 10 years
12/1000 over 15 years

Put another way:	Breast Cancer Risks:		Endometrial cancer
Baseline (No HRT)	10/1000/5yrs	20/1000/10yrs	
Increased risk of			
combined HRT X2	6/1000/5yrs	19/1000/10yrs	?10yrs <2
Oestrogen alone			
HRT X1.3	1.5/1000/5yrs	5/1000/10yrs	4/1000/5yrs 10/1000/10yrs
Tibolone HRT X1.45			

Generally speaking you can say that:

HRT Increases breast cancer risk, endometrial cancer risk and very slightly (X1.8 for sequential HRT for 10 years but none for CC HRT) ovarian cancer risk.

In a more recent meta-analysis from the Collaborative Group on epidemiological studies of Ovarian Cancer published in 2015, they found one additional ovarian cancer case for every 1000 users of HRT over 5 years, starting near age 50 and one extra ovarian cancer death for every 1700 users. The UK guidelines state that ovarian cancer risk may rise with long term use at the moment.

In another report on the same group's research, the findings seem to be much more alarming: "Women who use HRT even for a short time are approximately 20% more likely to have had ovarian cancer than those who have never used HRT". The more recent the therapy, the greater the risk, even with less than 5 years use. If they had stopped HRT but were still within 5 years of using it then they had a 23% increased risk. The cancers were associated with oestrogen only and oestrogen/progesterone combinations. So the later report from this umbrella group is far more alarming than the previous one above.

ERT* and Tibolone have lower breast cancer risk than combined HRT.

HRT increases VTE, CHD and CVA but reduces colorectal cancer.

or put another way:

WHI showed oestrogen/progesterone combinations increase breast cancer, VTE, CVA, heart disease.

Oestrogen alone shows no increase in breast cancer or heart disease, but increased CVA, increased VTE.

Raloxifene (Evista) reduces breast cancer, reduces breast density, reduces endometrial cancer, increases VTE, CVA, reduces vertebral #.

Tamoxifen increases uterine cancer, increases cataracts, increases VTE.

(J. Clin Onc.Sept 1 2008, Vol 26.4151-4159.)

* American for (O)estrogen Replacement Therapy

99% women have gone through the change by 55 years and although the average age is getting later – it is usually said to be 53.

Continuous combined therapy or Tibolone (Livial) are often recommended after 55 years.

Various alternatives to HRT are taken by women who wish to avoid conventional hormones and their possible side effects.

These alternatives include Black Cohosh (black snakeroot) an American plant with pretty white flowers (and some serious liver reactions in the unlucky),

Vitamin E,

Vitamin C,

Dong Quai (Angelica Sinesis),

Sage,

Flavonoids,

Isoflavones from Soya/Tofu (-phytoestrogens).

Several of these alternatives to HRT contain known carcinogens, compounds that affect cell growth factors and new blood vessel formation, some chelate minerals, increase the risk of cancer metastasising, have a variety of significant side effects and may contain other plant material harvested simultaneously. "Organic" isn't synonymous with "safe".

In the extensive alternative literature on treating cancer, all forms of synthetic oestrogen (horse oestrogens and non bio identical oestrogens) as well as non bio identical progesterone ("progestins") are associated with increased cancer risk. Basically that is all the hormones we prescribe women for contraception and HRT. The cancers are particularly but **not only** breast, endometrium, ovary and prostate.

Plant oestrogens on the other hand, phytoestrogens, have weak oestrogenic activity in human beings and bind to and block oestrogen receptors. The phytooestrogen subgroups are

Isoflavones – (genistein, biochanin, daidzein, formononetin), coumestans, flavanones flavones, flavanols, lignans, chalcones.

These are found in legumes, citrus fruits, seeds, grains, cereals and various vegetables. Beans, chickpeas, lentils and fermented soy products seem to be particularly good sources.

Oestrogen comes from other sources than by prescription:

Xenooestrogens are now in the food we eat – in pesticides, (breast cancer deaths dropped in Israel between 1976 and 1986 after a ban on various organochlorine pesticides and this was after a 25 year period of gradual increase) insect sprays at home and in the garden, traffic fumes, contaminated ground water near land-fills, eating artificially fattened dairy food, solvents, plastics and some soaps.

Central obesity. Fat is an endocrine organ and increases breast cancer risk.

So does alcohol consumption.

Supplementing "natural" progesterone which can be done trans-dermally in a cream form counteracts the carcinogenic effects of these various oestrogenic influences. An increasing number of your peri-menopausal patients may ask you to prescribe (-for instance "Endau") a progestogenic transdermal HRT. Natural progestogens have many benefits compared with synthetic progestin molecules and certainly do not have the cancer potential of oestrogenic HRT.

Cancer and the Pill: In 2017 a 44 year long study was published which involved 46,000 women who had at some time taken the COCP. "Ever" use of the pill was associated with reduced colorectal endometrial, ovarian, lymphatic and haematopoietic cancer. An observed increase in breast and cervical cancer during current and recent users "appeared to be lost within 5 years of stopping oral contraception". There was no increased risk of new later life cancers once off the pill. The cancer benefits, lasting at least 30 years, balanced the cancer risks.

Breast Cancer:

In terms of breast cancer, the risk probably begins 1-2 years after starting HRT irrespective of the type, drops off as soon as HRT is stopped and is back to normal 5 years after treatment.

More recent evidence suggests that HRT has little increase relative risk of breast cancer death and the breast cancer risk is similar to that of statins!? Either way, being obese or drinking alcohol are said to be bigger risk factors and we should make sure we get things in proportion. It is a great irony to be discussing the risks of HRT with a 20 stone woman who drinks the best part of a bottle of wine a day.

The various studies relating to HRT and breast cancer are complicated and can be confusing. Obesity for instance has caused >50,000 breast cancers in the last 10 years on its own – and HRT saves 3 lives/1000/5years from hip fractures averted and 3 from colorectal cancer prevented/1000/5years.

The two main HRT studies are a bit flawed for general interpretation, the WHI (Women's Health Initiative, 1993-1998) study involved 162,000 obese and older, 50-79 yrs, mid west Americans. The results may not be relevant to peri-menopausal British ladies. They tended to take equine rather than synthetic oestrogens. Then there was the Million Women Study which ignored the changes in HRT treatment of 40% of the women studied. They contradict each other in terms of breast cancer risks for oestrogen only HRT.

The first of these, the WHI study found a 2% increase risk in breast cancer risk per year of use, the oestrogen only arm being quite favourable for breast cancer and CVS disease, but the arm being stopped because of increased stroke risk. The continuous combined HRT arm patients were 1.24X more likely to suffer breast cancer in the study's 5.6 yrs.

The CC (continuous combined) HRT arm of WHI was stopped because of poor risk benefit (stroke, CVS, breast cancer.)

Overall breast cancer increased from 30 to 38 cases per 10,000 women after 5 years HRT use, coronary heart disease increased from 30 to 37 and stroke from 21 to 29.

Another way of putting breast cancer risk in perspective to the patient would be:
Menarche before 11yrs Risk 3,
Menopause after 54yrs Risk 2,
Perimenopausal BMI >35 Risk 2,
First Child after 40 yrs Risk 3,
High intake of saturated fat Risk 1.5,
Oestrogen Progesterone HRT Risk 2,
Oestrogen HRT 1.3,
Tibolone HRT 1.45.

Risk factors for breast cancer were early menarche, late first pregnancy, late menopause (defined as >50), obesity and 2Us alcohol/day. Apart from the alcohol, all these are oestrogen exposure related.

So: For Breast Cancer, Increased risks from HRT use:
WHI E+P X1.09
     E X0.99 (a reduction !!)
Million E+P X2
     E X1.3.

The Million women study was UK based, women 50-64 yrs and showed an increased breast cancer risk,

(Background 50/1000, ERT 55/1000, combined 60/1000 with the risk returning back down to normal 5 years after HRT treatment.)

OK I agree this is a confusing and frequently contradictory area. But the battle lines of ignorance and bias were exemplified in my opinion by a female (honorary) Scottish Gynaecologist speaking for NICE on the Today Programme 12th November 2015. This NICE's representative said that a generation of doctors had grown up frightened by studies linking HRT to breast cancer. This is definitely not true if my experience of colleagues, registrars and new GPs is anything to go by. She went on to say that GPs do not give "Correct evidence based advice, – Like NICE does" – the implication being that thousands of poor women were suffering intolerable climacteric symptoms because GPs were putting the fear of God into them about cancer risks" and the poor patients were missing out on a valuable treatment due to the GP's ignorance.

What clap trap. There was more: That GPs should tell the patient the risks, mention that being overweight and their half a bottle of wine each night is a bigger risk than the HRT (does the esteemed Honorary Professor have any experience of General Practice or life outside academia?-probably not – I'm pretty sure most of us would have done that already): and she continued: That 20% of women had "Quite significant symptoms" but only 10% of menopausal women were on HRT in Scotland. Well, what does that discrepancy imply? What are quite significant symptoms? They don't sound too awful do they? Does the doctor ever have to see patients dying with pulmonary emboli or breast cancer and have these patients with significant symptoms tried any alternative treatments first? Does she, like most consultant Gynaecologists have a slightly narrow clinical perspective? Does she know that no one dies of hot flushes, however bad they are?

No, I doubt as an honorary Gynaecologist that she has ever supervised the terminal care of friendly and familiar patients whom she has looked after for years, now dying of breast, ovarian or endometrial cancer at home. Perhaps it is a case of once she has done the diagnostic laparotomy and biopsied the cancer, her job, being a Gynaecologist, is over.

As GPs, our purview is wider; it is the life, wellbeing and survival of the whole person – and sometimes their terminal care too. And in the back of our minds that "Oestrogen plus progestogen risk = breast cancer times two" statistic. Yes, the menopause can cause miserable symptoms but so could the treatment of it and it may not be such an easy decision for a doctor with the holistic and long term responsibilities of the GP. Finally she said that HRT given to a million women might only cause 6,000 extra cancer cases. But what about strokes and coronaries, DVTs and PEs? The only thing she missed out given the tone of her hectoring was how the poor female patients were being neglected by a male dominated profession – BUT as it happens, General Practice is now dominated by female doctors, all of them obsessed by evidence based medicine and in my experience quite able to decide with patients what is or isn't the right treatment.

This just illustrates that NICE spokespeople, like nearly all TV consultants, GMC committee members, and virtually all public academic "experts", – everyone who publically wrings their hands about the knowledge or skills of GPs should do some General Practice themselves, leave their metropolitan ivory towers and go a walk in the real patient world occasionally.

And while we are on the subject, Testosterone frequently gets a good press particularly in the US medical literature in terms of male wellbeing, cardiovascular health and so on, – when do we hear academics on the today programme encouraging GPs to prescribe testosterone to menopausal men?

In the latest published study on "ERT" (Oestrogen replacement therapy), ERT after 50 years of age was associated with an increase in ovarian cancer risk of 1.3X. This is for Serous and Endometroid tumours and it increased with duration of use (Lee Ness Roman et al Obs Gynecol 2016;127. 828-8*.)

Blood vessels and HRT:

The HERS study (The Heart and Estrogen/Progestin Replacement Study) showed that in the first year women on HRT suffer more coronary events than placebo but this dropped to less than placebo by years 3 and 4.

Up to 60 years of age oestrogen reduces CVS disease by 50%. (Oestrogen ("E") and progesterone ("P") together make no difference). VTE is increased by 2-3X but mainly in the first year of use.

Early on, HRT appears to increase CVS risk but paradoxically by year 4 it is reduced by 40%. – I said some of the data were confusing.

Trans dermal HRT reduces the CVA risk and obviously, as in all treatments, start with the lowest effective dose.

Note: IF there is a personal past history or FH of thrombosis, do a clotting screen. Apparently there is a 25% risk of thrombophilia. (Factor 4 Leiden deficiency is present in 4% of the white population).

Oestrogen only HRT:

is fine in hysterectomised and oophorectomised women who cannot develop endometrial cancer and therefore do not need to worry about unopposed oestrogen. Don't forget the Mirena coil gives endometrial protection in the owners of a uterus. The latest study shows the risk of unopposed oestrogen on ovarian cancer to be 1.3X*.

Estradiol: Oral: Climaval, Elleste Solo, Progynova.
Patches: Elleste Solo MX, Estraderm MX, Estradot, Femseven etc.
Pessary: Estring.
Gel: Sandrena, Oestrogel.
Vaginal Tab: Vagifem.

Other oestrogens: Estradiol+estriol+estrone = Hormonin
Estriol: Gynest Cream, Orthogynest Pessaries.
Conjugated oestrogens: Premarin

Make sure the patient is on a progestogen as well if she has an intact uterus.

Cyclical or Sequential HRT:

comes in a monthly or 3 monthly form and is for the younger patient with regular periods.

Tablets:

Estradiol with Dydrogesterone: Femoston
Medroxyprogesterone: Tridestra.
Norethisterone. Climagest, Clinorette, Elleste Duet, Novofem, Trisequens.
Norgestrel. Cycloprogynova.

Oestrogen with Norgestrel. Prempak-C

Patches: Evorel Sequi Fem Seven Sequi.

Continuous Combined HRT:

designed for post menopausal women (amenorrhoeic >1 year or >54 yrs) causes less endometrial hyperplasia (<1%).

Estradiol with   Drospirenone. Angeliq.
                        Dydrogesterone. Femoston Conti.
                        Medroxyprogesterone. Indivina.
                        Norethisterone. Climesse. Elleste Duet Conti. Kliofem.
                        Kliovance. Nuvelle Continuous.

Oestrogen with medroxyprogesterone. Premique.

Patches: Evorel Conti. Femseven Conti.

Evista: Raloxifene. A selective oestrogen receptor modulator (A SERM, which of course should really be a SORM). Oestrogenic effects on bone but anti oestrogenic at the uterus and breast. Increased risk of VTE and hot flushes. Reduced risk of breast Ca. Lowers LDL.

Tibolone, Livial. Improves bone density and libido.

Tibolone:

LIFT Study: Mean age 68, 4,300 women. Endometrial cancer risks similar to HRT. Breast cancer risks similar to ERT, X1.45 (Ger Med 2005), reduced vertebral fractures, increased CVA risk, avoid in history of breast cancer.

Improves libido and vasomotor symptoms (weak androgenic action).

Progestogen only HRT:

Progesterone: Utrogestan.

Norethisterone 5mg daily helps combat vasomotor symptoms.

Transdermal Progesterone: Pro-gest cream. Protects against breast cysts, is diuretic, mildly antidepressant, increases libido and reduces hot flushes, ? increases bone density?

A lot of patients and therapists are keen on progesterone only HRT (particularly transdermal and "natural" progesterone which they differentiate from synthetic progestins in terms of chemistry, potential adverse effects and benefits). eg Endau cream, progesterone from yams, soybeans etc.

These are said to be the relative advantages:

Oestrogen Effects:	Progesterone effects:
Breast cysts stimulated	Protective
Increases fat stores	Helps metabolise fat
Water and salt retention	Diuretic
Thyroid hormone antagonistic	Facilitates Thyroid function
Increased thrombotic tendency and CVA	Normalises clotting
Decreased libido	Increased libido
Impaired glucose metabolism	Normalises blood sugar levels
Zinc loss, copper retention	Normalises both
Slight reduction in bone loss.	Increased bone density.

The Endometrium:

Is less stimulated by CCHRT (<1% Hyperplasia),
ERT and Tibolone increase the risk of endometrial cancer.

The Risks and Benefits of H.R.T.

Reproduced with the permission of Drug Safety Update (September 2007)

Marginal notes:

* Background incidence from: Hospital Admissions in England (HES) for stroke and VTE; WHI trial for CHD; the International Agency for Research on Cancer (IARC) for ovarian cancer and endometrial cancer; and from never-users in the Million Women Study for breast cancer.

† Best estimate and range based on relative risk and 95% CI.

‡ Risk ratios and 95% CI from: meta-analyses of randomised controlled trials (RCTs) for stroke; meta-analyses of RCTs and observational studies for VTE, endometrial cancer, and ovarian cancer; meta-analysis of RCTs and observational studies in Europe only for breast cancer; and from Women's Health Initiative (WHI) trial for CHD.

§ European studies have generally identified higher breast-cancer risk than North American studies and may be due to differences in prevalence of obesity.

|| Progestogen added for 10 days or more per 28-day cycle.

¶ Estimates from placebo groups from the conjugated equine oestrogens (CEE) and CEE plus medroxyprogesterone placebo arms of WHI trial.

** Menopausal symptom relief is not included in this table, but is a key benefit of HRT and will play a major part in the decision to prescribe HRT.

NS non-significant difference.

O+P oestrogen-progestogen. `

Age range (years)	Time (years)	Background incidence per 1000 women in Europe*	Oestrogen-only HRT — Additional cases per 1000 HRT users†	Oestrogen-only HRT — Risk ratio (95% CI)‡	Oestrogen-progestogen HRT — Additional cases per 1000 HRT users†	Oestrogen-progestogen HRT — Risk ratio (95% CI)‡
Cancer risk						
Breast§						
50–59	5	10	2 (1–4)	1·2 (1·1–1·4)	6 (5–7)	1·6 (1·5–1·7)
60–69	5	15	3 (2–6)		9 (8–11)	
50–59	10	20	6 (4–10)	1·3 (1·2–1·5)	24 (20–28)	2·2 (2·0–2·4)
60–69	10	30	9 (6–15)		36 (30–42)	
Endometrial						
50–59	5	2	4 (3–5)	3·0 (2·5–3·6)	NS	1·0 (0·8–1·2)||
60–69	5	3	6 (5–8)		NS	
50–59	10	4	32 (21–48)	9·0 (6·3–12·9)	NS	1·1 (0·9–1·2)||
60–69	10	6	48 (32–71)		NS	
Ovarian						
50–59	5	2	<1	1·1 (1·0–1·3)	<1	1·1 (1·0–1·3)
60–69	5	3	<1		<1	
50–59	10	4	1 (1–2)	1·3 (1·1–1·5)	1 (1–2)	1·3 (1·1–1·5)
60–69	10	6	2 (1–3)		2 (1–3)	
Cardiovascular risk						
Venous thromboembolism (VTE)						
50–59	5	5	2 (0–4)	1·3 (1·0–1·7)	7 (5–10)	2·3 (1·8–3·0)
60–69	5	8	2 (0–6)		10 (7–16)	
Stroke						
50–59	5	4	1 (1–2)	1·3 (1·1–1·4)	1 (1–2)	1·3 (1·1–1·4)
60–69	5	9	3 (1–4)		3 (1–4)	
Coronary heart disease (CHD) (Background: Oestrogen¶ / O+P¶)						
50–59	5	14 / 9	NS	0·6 (0·4–1·1)	NS	1·3 (0·8–2·1)
60–69	5	31 / 18	NS	0·9 (0·7–1·2)	NS	1·0 (0·7–1·4)
70–79	5	44 / 29	NS	1·1 (0·8–1·5)	15 (1–32)	1·5 (1·0–2·1)
Benefits						
Colorectal cancer (Background: Oestrogen¶ / O+P¶)						
50–59	5	6 / 3	NS	0·9 (0·7–1·1)	NS	0·9 (0·7–1·1)
60–69	5	10 / 8	NS		NS	
Fracture of femur (Background: Oestrogen¶ / O+P¶)						
50–59	5	0·5 / 1·5	0	0·6 (0·4–0·9)	NS	0·7 (0·5–1·0)
60–69	5	5·5 / 5·5	−2 (−3 to −1)		NS	

Table: **Risks and benefits of HRT**

Risks of HRT (Taken from Drug Safety Update 2007)

Atrophic vaginitis: When treating topically, (Estriol cream, Ortho-Gynest pessaries, Vagifem vaginal tablets (now 10ug), Ovestin, Orthogynest etc) – it is wise to stop treatment for 2 weeks every 3 months.

Vagifem 10mcg daily for 2w then 2x per week long term is very safe and is the lowest dose available.

Hot Flushes:

Clonidine, Testosterone, Various antidepressants, Gabapentin, HRT, Norethisterone, Tibolone: Not recommended >60 years but does improve libido., "Alternative" Medicines:

Black Cohosh (but potential severe liver adverse reactions), Menopace: «21 nutrients» vitamins B6, B12, B1, Soya Isoflavone, Vit C, Mg, Zn, Vit D, etc, Red Clover, Promensil (from Red Clover Isoflavones),

Isoflavones are converted to phyto-oestrogens in the body which are structurally similar to oestradiol. They may protect against prostate and breast (etc) cancers by blocking oestrogen receptor sites. Some oestrogens are potent cancer stimulators. Red clover decreases fertility in sheep and some bird species but interestingly has never been shown to have any objective effect on menopausal symptoms despite its weak oestrogenic receptor affinity.

Vitamin E 400 IU BD, Vitamin C 2-3Gr/day, Dong Quai (Angelica) which is also used by some for PMS and dysmenorhoea. Interacts with anticoagulants.

Sage (Isoflavonoids).

Isoflavones from Soya/Tofu.

-On the other hand, soya (phyto-oestrogens) reduce breast density, reduce oestradiol, oestrone, reduce the incidence of prostate cancer, endometrial and breast cancer.

Surgery and Venous thrombosis

Should stop oestrogens 4 weeks before surgery.

Gynaecomastia in Men:

Causes:

Hermaproditism/Pseudo hermaphroditism, Endocrine: Normal puberty (75% resolve in 2 years). Neonatal hypothyroidism, (neonatal due to breast feeding and consumption of maternal oestrogen). Thyrotoxicosis, Acromegaly, testicular atrophy, testicular, pituitary and adrenal tumours, Klinefelters Syndrome, Hyperprolactinaemia, Cirrhosis, Ca. bronchus, malnutrition, Renal failure, paraplegia;

Various drugs – Sex Hormones, Spironolactone, Amphetamine, Reserpine, Digoxin, Methyl Dopa, Cimetidine, Ketoconazole, Growth Hormone, Gonadotrophin Releasing Hormone Analogues, HCG, Flutamide, Finasteride, Risperidone, CCBs, opioids, Omeprazole and related drugs.

Libido in Women:

Various drugs have been suggested if the patient (rather than the partner) really has a problem and wants it solved.

These include:

Testosterone in various forms including patches, gel and depot injections, Tibolone and Bupropion (Zyban). If vaginal dryness is an issue Replens and Sylk are prescribable moisturisers.

Endocrine Disruptors in the Environment: (Medscape, ENDO 2015)

Never in the evolutionary history of human beings have we been exposed to so many compounds that interfere with so many metabolic pathways. Given mankind's endless ingenuity for discovering effective and powerful new chemicals, drugs, plastics, industrial compounds, solvents, active agents of all kinds it is not surprising that some have long term damaging effects on us as well. Humans have discovered 50 million separate chemical compounds. Most since the second world war.

Endocrine systems in the body are known to be disrupted by a number of chemical agents: Indeed, if the definition is an exogenous substance that causes adverse health effects in an intact organism or its progeny, secondary to changes in endocrine function, these substances would include: pharmaceuticals, industrial solvents, some personal care products, aluminium can plastic linings, flame retardants, plasticisers, pesticides, various environmental pollutants, a multitude of environmental chemicals including diethylstilboestrol, polychlorinated biphenyls, (PCBs), dioxins, perfluoroalkyl compounds, solvents, phthalates, (food wraps, cosmetics, shampoos, flooring), Bisphenol A (BPA) (which is deemed safe at all ages by the European Food Safety Authority and has been banned from baby bottles by the FDA), dichlorodiphenyldichloroethylene, organophosphate/organochlorine pesticides and polybrominated diphenyl. I have heavily edited the potential full list of compounds. The full list is much, much longer. The hormone systems that are disrupted include those for oestrogens, androgens, thyroid, PPAR, retinol and aryl hydrocarbon pathways etc.

So to minimise your personal harm, always remove food from plastic containers before microwaving it, don't microwave in cling film, do not drink or eat from aluminium cans, or from plastic bottles that have become warm, allow plenty of fresh air in the house – by reducing its thermal efficiency. (This will improve the children's asthma too), scrub new pots and pans before cooking in them, especially non stick pans, drive new cars and paint your house with the windows open. Try not to spend long periods breathing in varnish, hair spray, polish, petrol, car exhaust, dry cleaning fluid, new carpet or other solvent fumes, however nice they smell.

The population effect of these chemicals may be an increase such conditions as ADHD, lowered IQ and to cause other neurological harm, autism, obesity, diabetes, infertility and some forms of cancer.

23: Immunisations/vaccinations:

There are 25 vaccinations available worldwide (2015). The word vaccination is derived from vacca, the latin for cow. This is of course because cowpox pus from Blossom the cow was used by Edward Jenner to protect his patients from Smallpox.

There are various historical infectious diseases resurgent in the UK in the teens of the 21st Century. Scarlet Fever, probably because doctors have been lazy and unselective in their response to pressure to reduce antibiotic prescribing. If you don't examine pharyngitis patients properly and you are determined to refuse antibiotics to EVERYONE with a painful throat how could you not miss Scarlet Fever, Diphtheria, Quinsy or possibly even worse? (see other sections). TB is resurgent because of our pattern of mass migration and patients' reluctance to finish courses of drugs. Pertussis and Measles because every parent thinks them self an armchair epidemiologist and misunderstands risk. Diseases I thought science had just about eradicated. I hadn't predicted the short memories and gullibility of both doctors and patients.

There has been an epidemic of Measles going on in the 21st century in our advanced western society. Children, adolescents and some adults will suffer this particularly unpleasant illness. Some will be damaged permanently and a few will, no doubt, die from a highly infectious virus which we should have eradicated decades ago. Indeed whole civilisations have been worse than decimated by measles in the not too distant past, something it is all too easy to forget.

This epidemic is the result of what seems to have been one biased researcher who was subsequently discredited but who seemed to have been cooperating with vested interests and whose data and research was subsequently discredited. Andrew Wakefield was eventually struck off. World class epidemiologists made it publically clear that the MMR vaccine did not cause autism, just as 25 years earlier the statistics and the same sort of epidemiologists showed no relationship between Whooping Cough Vaccine and brain damage. However a media bandwagon of disreputable and unbalanced scare mongering led to parents ("Daily Mail Epidemiologists") deciding to exercise their right not to vaccinate their children. I watched the Whooping cough public debates and cleared up some of the paediatric fall out over long nights and weekends on call as a registrar in the 70's. Unvaccinated toddlers coughed their hearts out, popped lungs and cerebral blood vessels simply because their parents knew nothing about risk/benefit and so their children suffered the consequences. Then I saw the same depressing and predictable pattern of uninformed, entitled, opinion broadcast and listened to and the "no smoke without fire" culture spread, do its harm and cause its measles deaths thirty years later.

The low point for me was a BBC radio consumer programme which pitched an internationally renowned epidemiologist against a landscape gardener who's only argument was "We wouldn't be having this programme if there wasn't some suspicion against the vaccine so why should I take the risk?" There was no discussion of the concept of the risk/benefit ratio which is overwhelmingly in favour of every single vaccine or cross examination of the parents about what he or she knew of the effects of Measles, Mumps or Rubella infection. They didn't ask if the parents knew what dangerous diseases these were or what the side effects of untreated infection were and how likely their unprotected child was to suffer death or permanent harm through their decision not to vaccinate.

Some mildly challenging questions followed from the same reporters in the same programme five years later when the predictable epidemic happened and the same parents were queuing round the block to get their children vaccinated. Unfortunately no one asked the questions "What gave you the right to think you were an expert in Epidemiology, Infectious Diseases, Community Medicine, Paediatric Intensive Care, Risk Benefit Ratio, Herd Immunity" and "Do you think parents like you should have the legal right to risk the lives and brains of their children and the children of others on nothing more than a whim?"

In other words irresponsible reporting, dangerous and ignorant parents, a liberal society which although it has laws to prosecute parents who assault and brain damage their children, allows a parent's wilful ignorance of the true facts to result in the same outcome through their dangerous misguided inaction. Even worse, unvaccinated, their child will almost certainly get measles at some time and as the various components of MMR are less than 100% effective, their child may give other, immunised children the infections and possibly cause **them** serious harm too. Random non accidental injury to the children of other parents too.

Why cannot society compel parents to protect their children and others by immunising them, especially since every single vaccine controversy in the last 30 years has caused death and damage by scaring over anxious parents but has subsequently been shown to be a false alarm? Why can't we let the people who understand the statistics and who know how to judge the research make the recommendations on vaccination and then make them **compulsory**? We did this with seat belts, with every controlled drug, with speed limits and so on.

Immunisation scares are irrational and local. The MMR vaccine scare was only seen in the UK until Andrew Wakefield went to the USA and now some ethnic groups over there are blaming their local incidence of autism on vaccination as well. They quote the absence of autism in the Amish community (who do not vaccinate) as evidence. Here the MMR story generated 1200 articles in one year and peaked between 1998 and 2003. You rarely hear about it now. In France in the 1990's there was a public fear that Hepatitis B vaccination was linked to M.S. The same vaccine was used internationally without similar anxieties being expressed elsewhere. In the USA another concern has been voiced regarding Thiomersal*, a mercury containing preservative, which is rarely mentioned in Europe where there is more interest in mercury amalgam in dental fillings. In the developing world, the WHO's attempt to eradicate polio has been violently and cruelly opposed by Muslim extremists in Nigeria and Pakistan who, it is said, believe the vaccine will make them sterile. In Kenya Christian fundamentalists are also opposing some vaccinations apparently also because of fertility fears.

Polio:

Wild **Polio** remains infectious in Afghanistan and Pakistan.

In 1988 there were 350,000 cases in 125 countries and the global effort to rid the world of polio began then. In August 2015 Africa had, for the first time in history been polio free for one year.

Unfortunately new cases arose in Ukraine in 2015, the first European polio in five years. It arose from the mutated attenuated virus used in vaccination.

There had been reports in the literature in the weeks before this news that highly mutated polio strains originating from vaccines had been isolated from sewage samples from Slovakia, Finland, Estonia, and Israel. All bore the molecular fingerprint of "iVDPVs" vaccine derived polio viruses excreted by immunodeficient patients. Researchers suggested that such patients be given anti viral treatment to stop viral replication.

Herd immunity:

This probably has to be around 90% to keep diseases suppressed but varies depending on the infectivity of the organism. If immunisation rates drop lower than this level then not only are the unimmunised population at risk of infection but, since most immunisations are less than 100% effective (one MMR is 95% and two are about 99% protective for measles) then even some of the immunised population are put at risk.

Thiomersal*: Just like Whooping Cough, MMR and so on, Thiomersal, the ethyl mercury containing anti bacterial preservative that is in some vaccines became the subject of a newspaper panic in 2001. It is used to inactivate killed vaccines and as an anti microbial and antifungal agent. Prior to its use some vaccines had historically become contaminated, with patients dying of staphylococcal sepsis.

Fears were expressed that the mercury might cause harm to the vaccine recipient – specifically autism. (The later DTP and TT.)

In the United States and the European Union, Thiomersal is no longer used as a preservative in routine childhood vaccinations. Several vaccines that are not routinely recommended for young children do contain Thiomersal, including DT (diphtheria and tetanus), Td (tetanus and diphtheria), and TT.

The routine immunisation schedule from Autumn 2017

Age due	Diseases protected against	Vaccine given and trade name		Usual site
Eight weeks old	Diphtheria, tetanus, pertussis (whooping cough), polio, Haemophilus influenzae type b (Hib) and hepatitis B	DTaP/IPV/Hib/HepB	Infanrix hexa	Thigh
	Pneumococcal (13 serotypes)	Pneumococcal conjugate vaccine (PCV)	Prevenar 13	Thigh
	Meningococcal group B (MenB)	MenB	Bexsero	Left thigh
	Rotavirus gastroenteritis	Rotavirus	Rotarix	By mouth
Twelve weeks old	Diphtheria, tetanus, pertussis, polio, Hib and hepatitis B	DTaP/IPV/Hib/HepB	Infanrix hexa	Thigh
	Rotavirus	Rotavirus	Rotarix	By mouth
Sixteen weeks old	Diphtheria, tetanus, pertussis, polio, Hib and hepatitis B	DTaP/IPV/Hib/HepB	Infanrix hexa	Thigh
	Pneumococcal (13 serotypes)	PCV	Prevenar 13	Thigh
	MenB	MenB	Bexsero	Left thigh
One year old (on or after the child's first birthday)	Hib and MenC	Hib/MenC	Menitorix	Upper arm/thigh
	Pneumococcal	PCV	Prevenar 13	Upper arm/thigh
	Measles, mumps and rubella (German measles)	MMR	MMR VaxPRO[2] or Priorix	Upper arm/thigh
	MenB	MenB booster	Bexsero	Left thigh
Two to eight years old[1] (including children in reception class and school years 1-4)	Influenza (each year from September)	Live attenuated influenza vaccine LAIV[3]	Fluenz Tetra[2]	Both nostrils
Three years four months old or soon after	Diphtheria, tetanus, pertussis and polio	DTaP/IPV	Infanrix IPV or Repevax	Upper arm
	Measles, mumps and rubella	MMR (check first dose given)	MMR VaxPRO[2] or Priorix	Upper arm
Girls aged 12 to 13 years	Cervical cancer caused by human papillomavirus (HPV) types 16 and 18 (and genital warts caused by types 6 and 11)	HPV (two doses 6-24 months apart)	Gardasil	Upper arm
Fourteen years old (school year 9)	Tetanus, diphtheria and polio	Td/IPV (check MMR status)	Revaxis	Upper arm
	Meningococcal groups A, C, W and Y disease	MenACWY	Nimenrix or Menveo	Upper arm
65 years old	Pneumococcal (23 serotypes)	Pneumococcal Polysaccharide Vaccine (PPV)	Pneumococcal Polysaccharide Vaccine	Upper arm
65 years of age and older	Influenza (each year from September)	Inactivated influenza vaccine	Multiple	Upper arm
70 years old	Shingles	Shingles	Zostavax[2]	Upper arm

1. Age on 31 August 2017.
2. Contains porcine gelatine.

3. If LAIV (live attenuated influenza vaccine) is contraindicated and child is in a clinical risk group, use inactivated flu vaccine.

All vaccines can be ordered from www.immform.dh.gov.uk free of charge except influenza for adults and pneumococcal polysaccharide vaccine.

Immunisation
The safest way to protect children and adults

NHS

Diagram Routine Immunisations 2017 (See CRI 1 and 1a)

Selective immunisation programmes

Target group	Age and schedule	Disease	Vaccines required
Babies born to hepatitis B infected mothers	At birth, four weeks and 12 months old[1,2]	Hepatitis B	Hepatitis B (Engerix B/HBvaxPRO)
Infants in areas of the country with TB incidence >= 40/100,000	At birth	Tuberculosis	BCG
Infants with a parent or grandparent born in a high incidence country[3]	At birth	Tuberculosis	BCG
Pregnant women	During flu season At any stage of pregnancy	Influenza	Inactivated flu vaccine
Pregnant women	From 16 weeks gestation	Pertussis	dTaP/IPV (Boostrix-IPV or Repevax)

1. Take blood for HBsAg at 12 months to exclude infection.
2. In addition hexavalent vaccine (Infanrix hexa) is given at 8, 12 and 16 weeks.
3. Where the annual incidence of TB is >= 40/100,000 – see www.gov.uk/government/publications/tuberculosis-tb-by-country-rates-per-100000-people

Additional vaccines for individuals with underlying medical conditions

Medical condition	Diseases protected against	Vaccines required[1]
Asplenia or splenic dysfunction (including due to sickle cell and coeliac disease)	Meningococcal groups A, B, C, W and Y Pneumococcal Haemophilus influenzae type b (Hib) Influenza	Hib/MenC MenACWY MenB PCV13 (up to two years of age) PPV (from two years of age) Annual flu vaccine
Cochlear implants	Pneumococcal	PCV13 (up to two years of age) PPV (from two years of age)
Chronic respiratory and heart conditions (such as severe asthma, chronic pulmonary disease, and heart failure)	Pneumococcal Influenza	PCV13 (up to two years of age) PPV (from two years of age) Annual flu vaccine
Chronic neurological conditions (such as Parkinson's or motor neurone disease, or learning disability)	Pneumococcal Influenza	PCV13 (up to two years of age) PPV (from two years of age) Annual flu vaccine
Diabetes	Pneumococcal Influenza	PCV13 (up to two years of age) PPV (from two years of age) Annual flu vaccine
Chronic kidney disease (CKD) (including haemodialysis)	Pneumococcal (stage 4 and 5 CKD) Influenza (stage 3, 4 and 5 CKD) Hepatitis B (stage 4 and 5 CKD)	PCV13 (up to two years of age) PPV (from two years of age) Annual flu vaccine Hepatitis B
Chronic liver conditions	Pneumococcal Influenza Hepatitis A Hepatitis B	PCV13 (up to two years of age) PPV (from two years of age) Annual flu vaccine Hepatitis A Hepatitis B
Haemophilia	Hepatitis A Hepatitis B	Hepatitis A Hepatitis B
Immunosuppression due to disease or treatment[3]	Pneumococcal Influenza	PCV13 (up to two years of age)[2] PPV (from two years of age) Annual flu vaccine
Complement disorders (including those receiving complement inhibitor therapy)	Meningococcal groups A, B, C, W and Y Pneumococcal Haemophilus influenzae type b (Hib) Influenza	Hib/MenC MenACWY MenB PCV13 (to any age) PPV (from two years of age) Annual flu vaccine

1. Check relevant chapter of green book for specific schedule.
2. To any age in severe immunosuppression.
3. Consider annual influenza vaccination for household members and those who care for people with these conditions.

Immunisation
The safest way to protect children and adults

NHS

It doesn't feel that long ago since the 70's when I started medicine, when children had only 6 childhood routine vaccines, none against croup, infectious diarrhoea or flu, when we could only dream of a meningitis vaccine let alone seven. When HPV just wasn't yet a problem and nights on call were punctuated by stiff necked and seriously ill children and those gasping with croup. Now an average child will receive over 49 vaccine doses before school entry and be protected against many of the killing and maiming diseases of a few decades ago, as well as those of past centuries.

2 months: Includes the new 6 in 1 vaccine, Dip, Tet, Pert, Pol, Hib and Hep B. Pneumococcal (PCV) vaccine (13 serotypes), Meningitis B vaccine (73% protection with some protection against invasive Men C as well) and oral Rotaviral vaccine.

3 months: 6 valent vaccine, Rotavirus Oral vaccine.

4 months: 6 valent vaccine, Pneumococcal, Meningitis B vaccines.

1 year: Hib, Meningitis C, Pneumococcal, MMR, Meningitis B.

Age 2,3,4,5,6,7,8 years: Flu vaccine in the Autumn, despite its poor efficacy of late. Started 2014, the aim being to roll out the vaccine to all children up to sixteen as well as at risk groups to eighteen.

3yrs 4m: Dip, Tet, Pert, Pol, MMR. Theoretically this is "a preschool booster".

12-13yrs: GIRLS only: (unless the logic of universal vaccination and herd immunity wins the day as in other countries) HPV vaccine. Two or three jabs over 6m to 2 yrs. Overwhelming numbers of patient groups and over 95% of doctors and dentists support a gender neutral immunisation regime given the common aetiology of throat and mouth cancers. 1 in 9 American men already have oral HPV (Web M.D. Oct 17)and when America sneezes......Also, of course, if you eradicate the infection from all boys the vaccination of girls would be unnecessary! Chicken and egg, herd immunity.

14yrs: Dip Tet Pol Meningitis A,C,W,Y.

65yrs: Pneumococcal.

65yrs: Flu

70yrs: Shingles.

Pregnant Women: (originally 28-38wks >16 wks in 2016)

Vaccinations in pregnancy:
Currently Flu and Pertussis vaccinations are recommended in the UK. The latter is to protect the baby prior to its first Pertussis vaccine at 2 months and this now only comes as a combined vaccine (with Dip Tet and Polio) (28-38 weeks changed to 16 weeks in 2016)
The former is to avoid pneumonia in the mother and perinatally in the baby and to reduce the miscarriage risk.

HPV Vaccine
In 2015 the Joint Committee on Vaccine and Immunisation announced that GPs should be vaccinating men under the age of 45 who have sex with men. That of course raises some awkward questions for GPs: Do we know all the homosexual and bisexual men on our lists? Are they all "out". Do "MSM" (Men who have sex with men) all

want their doctors to know who they are and have the fact written on their records? If we don't know who they all are, should we be asking all men who consult us if they have sex with other men in the spirit of liberalism, openness and public health? Are we prepared for the occasionally antagonistic, even aggressive response from some of the straight men we have upset who exclusively have sex with women? I have often mentioned how out of touch and undemocratic such " representative bodies" as the RCP and GMC are and how their agendas have little to do with most doctors' or patients' best interests. But this very question of intrusive, politically motivated, often medically irrelevant questioning sums up the problem: The Telegraph front page 16/10/17 described the conflict; "GPs to defy NHS diktat on patient's sexuality". -The Chairman of the College of Medicine saying that GPs would refuse to follow guidance from NHS England instructing us all to record everyone's' sexual orientation, since it was irrelevant and potentially offensive. The Rcgps chairwoman, of course, replied that it could be important when making a diagnosis and when we were recommending treatment. Well, yes I agree in the tiny number of recurrent Pneumocystis or Kaposi's Sarcoma patients or patients with multiple infections who have come from abroad. But isn't that part of the very problem? If we ask everyone we cause offence to many but we are acting in a politically acceptable way, if we are selective about who we ask, targeting the most likely, then we are by definition likely to question more black people, recent migrants, and the minority people who seem overtly to be gay. I need hardly say how that would go down with the RCGP, The GMC, the DoH, The BBC, etc.etc

Free NHS Travel Vaccines include:

Hepatitis A,

Typhoid,

Cholera.

Note: aP is Acellular Pertussis. (There is also a whole-cell, wP vaccine-of killed purified B Pertussis. These vaccines tend to have more side effects both local and systemic, than acellular vaccines but perhaps slightly greater efficacy).

As far as pertussis vaccination is concerned WHO recommends a 3 dose primary course at 6, 10 and 14 weeks then a booster at around 2 years (1-6 years at any rate).

Hepatitis and TB

Non routine immunisations for at risk babies:

At birth, 1 month, 2 months, 12 months Hepatitis B Hep B Vaccine. In thigh.

At birth, Tuberculosis BCG I.D. upper arm.

Meningitis Vaccinations:

Are capsular polysaccharide vaccines and all recommended in Asplenia.

Quadrivalent meningococcal vaccine ACWY (W135) recommended for Muslims going to the Hajj (major pilgrimage) and Umrah (minor pilgrimage) adults and children >5yrs.

Haemophilus Influenzae Type B:

There are 6 H.I. types but 99% human disease is B. Of total infections, 60% are meningitis, 15% epiglotitis. The vaccine is effective >2m. 99% effective after 3 doses.

Meningococcal (Neisseria Meningitidis):

Vaccines exist against capsular types ACWY and B. Corynebacteria, Neisseria

Meningitidis.

Under 2 years Group B predominates, between 14 and 18 years group C is more prevalent with more clusters.

Group B is 2/3 disease. Bexsero* is: A Sero group B vaccine (the most severe meningitis in the UK is epidemic septicaemic group B meningococcal disease), is a 4 antigen "4CmenB vaccine" which protects against various sero group B strains and has been given since June 2014 at 2, 4, 6, and 12 months. Those of us who lived and practiced in the decades before this new vaccine know what a profoundly vindictive disease it is for those that succumb and many who survive. These patients can lose infarcted limbs, digits, noses, ears, slough skin and suffer permanent neurological sequelae. The vaccine's broad antigenicity may cover meningitis C too. Local pain and pyrexia (effectively prevented by paracetamol) are common side effects. Note: Another vaccine designed for adolescents (rLP2086) will be available soon. This is bivalent.

"Trumenba" is the B serotype vaccine in the USA (after 3 doses 82% of patients have antibodies to 4 different N Meningitidis strains).

Group C is 1/3 disease. Vaccine>18months. Disease can affect school age children and young adults.

Group A is <2% UK disease. Vaccine >3 months. Routine vaccination was not until recently recommended to prevent UK meningitis due to the strains, low incidence and age groups at risk. Single dose lasts 3-5 years.

A group ACWY vaccine was introduced for the 3.3m adolescents (14-18 year olds) from 2015 after an increase in an aggressive form of Men W since 2009 with 117 cases in 2014. The upper age limit changed to "Up to the 25th birthday" in 2017.

Pneumococcal. Strep Pneumoniae:

The vaccine covers 80% of UK strains. Prevents 60-70% pneumococcal pneumonia but its value in preventing meningitis is limited. 5 yearly vaccination in at risk populations, single dose. This is probably a life-long immunisation unless the patient has an immune problem in which case 5 yearly boosters are needed. Age ranges: Pneumovax from >2years, Prevenar from 6 weeks-6m and adult.

Given in Asplenia, Coeliac Disease, Sickle Cell, CRF, Nephrotic Syndrome, immunodeficiency, HIV, CCF, chronic lung and chronic liver disease including cirrhosis, both types of diabetes.

Rotavirus:

Just about every child in the world has been infected by their 5th birthday and there are 5 subtypes, prosaically called A, B, C, D and E. A is the commonest and causes immunity after infection. Death is rare in advanced countries but hospitalisation is common and cross infection between children (not adults who are usually immune) is frequent. The oral vaccination is safe but seems to carry a small risk of intussusception.

Hepatitis A Vaccine:

Havrix monodose. Virus antigen (inactivated) stat, then booster 6-12m later, then booster within 5 years. Immunity lasts 10 years

Hepatitis B Vaccine:

All Hep B surface antigen preparations for active immunisation. If the titre is >10 U after primary immunisation then you almost certainly have permanent protection. (PHLS

BBV1 2000). Then a single booster at 5 years is recommended in health care workers and regular testing is unnecessary. If no response at all to vaccine, try another manufacturer's vaccine.

Many recommend if protected, a single booster at 5 years ? – with a booster at the time of significant exposure. Chronic carrier: Test for HBcAg (HSE Circular 1996) Non responder: HBIG and consider booster vacc. at time of significant exposure.

Note:

Stuff you will have forgotten:

Hepatitis Core Ag shows natural Infection.

Surface Ag and E Ag = Infectious.

Surface Ab (after immunisation, infection) = Protective Ab, not infectious.

So if the individual is immunised Anti – HBs Ab assesses level of immunity.

If non immunised, HBsAg taken to indicate the presence of infection.

If non immunised and exposure occurred >20 weeks ago HBsAg and Anti HBc Ab because 90% of infected individuals clear HBsAg within this period.

Efficacy of vaccines:

An American epidemiological study of the history of and the period 2011-2013 showed:

Vaccine	Prevaccine cases	Cases in 2011-2013	Reduction %
Measles	502,282	288	99.6
Mumps	186,000	404	99.6
Polio	16,316	0	100
Rubella	47,740	4	>99.6
Diphtheria	206,000	0	100
Pertussis	147,271	48,277	68
HiB	20,000	9	99.2

Immunoglobulins:

IgG is the only immunoglobulin to cross the placenta. Various subclasses perform different functions from neutralising toxins to fixing complement. Most gamma globulin given therapeutically is IgG.

IgM (macroglobulin) is the first response immunoglobulin and most gram negative antibodies are IgM.

IgA is secreted in saliva and various bodily secretions and contains the antibodies for such infections as Brucella, Polio and Diphtheria.

IgD – a cell bound antigen receptor on B Lymphocytes.

IgE – Secreted by the respiratory and gut epithelium. It is raised in atopic disease and may protect against infestations/parasites.

Other Vaccines

Stuff you may have forgotten:

You may remember that vaccines are **Active**: i.e. live attenuated, killed (inactivated), an isolated antigen, the toxoid or **Passive**: i.e. The specific or pooled immunoglobulin.

Thus:

Killed: Rabies, Pertussis, Plague (killed Yersinia Pestis), Salk polio (injection), Typhoid (injection), Influenza.

Live attenuated: MMR (all three), oral polio 3 types of live attenuated virus, (Sabin vaccine) gives intestinal and humoral immunity-this was not given in the USA where the risk of catching wild type polio is low and the tiny risk of live vaccine reaction not thought worth the risk of live vaccination. Rotavirus live oral vaccine, Typhoid (oral vaccine), Varicella virus vaccine, Yellow Fever, Hepatitis A, BCG – (Living avirulent Mycobacterium Bovis – which can also be used as intravesical advanced Bladder cancer treatment – as non specific immunotherapy).

New guidance (2015) has been issued for **Live Vaccines:**

Vaccine combination:	Advice:
Yellow Fever and MMR	Minimum 4 week interval, not the same day.
Varicella and Zoster vaccine, MMR	Same day or minimum 4 weeks.
Tuberculin (Mantoux) and MMR	Delay MMR until the Mantoux has been read - once it has been given, unless measles protection needed urgently. Likewise if a recent MMR has been given, delay tuberculin 4 weeks.

All current live vaccines-BCG, rotavirus, live attenuated influenza, oral typhoid, yellow fever, varicella zoster, MMR, and Mantoux testing (tuberculin) – all can be given at any time before or after each other than the above combinations.*

Specific antigens: Meningococcal vaccine is the capsular antigen of N Meningitidis, Haemophilus Infl. B is the capsular polysaccharide, the Pertussis acellular vaccine is purified antigenic components of the organism.

The Pneumococcal conjugate vaccine contains up to 23 capsular serotypes of Strep Pneumoniae. Typhoid is from the Vi capsular polysaccharide. Anthrax is a killed avirulent organism. Hep B (surface antigen). Lyme vaccination is a preparation of an outer surface protein. The polio injection contains the inactivated poliovirus 80 D antigen units.

Toxoids: Diphtheria and Tetanus.

*Note: Thus if you are giving a live vaccine like polio, give it one month before or two months after gamma globulin or some another live vaccines which stimulate an antibody response. You can give live vaccines together or three to four weeks apart because a live vaccine stimulates a non specific Interferon surge which lasts a few weeks and stops some live vaccines entering cells and triggering an immune response for a few weeks. That is the theory anyway – but if that were completely true wouldn't we die of viraemia if we got two viral infections a few weeks apart?

Diphtheria:
There were 5000 deaths in the former Soviet Union in the last decade of the 20th C from a resurgence of Diphtheria. Children and adults require a low dose i.e. 0.1ml single antigen vaccine if over 10 years of age. Td vaccine is Tetanus plus 0.1ml paediatric Diphtheria and should be given unless the 5th dose Tetanus has already been given. Avoid the bigger dose of Diphtheria Ag over 10 yrs. A monovalent vaccine is not available.

Tetanus:
Only introduced in 1962. Td vaccine replaced Tet. for school leavers in 1994. Td should now be used for primary immunisation of adults and adolescents who were previously unimmunised against Tetanus. Where booster doses of Tetanus are indicated following a tetanus prone wound or for the purposes of travel, 5 doses of Dip or Tet give lifelong immunity.

Boosters are only indicated following a tetanus prone wound if the patient has not had 5 doses in all, and for travellers to areas where no assistance will be available following a Tetanus prone wound and the last dose was >10 years.

Polio:

I remember seeing huge "Iron Lungs" in a ward in the hospital that my older brother was incarcerated for six weeks of intravenous antibiotics when he developed osteomyelitis in the early 60's. My parents described the horrors of the disease poliomyelitis and how they had known of children who had been infected. But they told me how all their children had been given drops on the tongue to protect them from that infection and his was only a bone infection, not one of the spinal column that would paralyse him.

I have never seen an active case of polio because world-wide vaccination is well on the way to eradicating it – except for areas where religious bigotry prevents immunisation campaigns. The claim is that the drops on the tongue are a way of sterilising the indigenous population of certain areas by "the West". There are three areas where polio is currently endemic, Afghanistan (80 Cases 2011, 37 in 2012, 14 in 2013, more cases reported in 2014), Pakistan and Northern Nigeria, all in areas controlled by Taliban, Boko Haram or similar religious extremists who think that the vaccine has some form of toxin in it which causes sterility. Dip, Tet and polio are all given systemically now as part of the 6 in 1 vaccine.

Passive:

Zoster Immune Globulin. VZV IgG or Measles (normal) immunoglobulin.

(Usually via the Consultant microbiologist). Should be given <10 days after first exposure in order to attenuate the disease. Significant exposure is face to face at least 15 minutes.

Active:

Chicken Pox: Chicken Pox vaccine is part of the routine schedule in some countries but not the UK.

Interestingly, an adult over the age of 15 is 10X, an Adult over 50 is 100X more likely to die from Chicken Pox than a child so you could argue that some are vaccinating the wrong age group anyway. Also it IS possible for contacts to catch Chicken Pox from a vaccinated individual so there is a definite downside to the mass vaccination of populations against Varicella.

Even without vaccination 90% of British adults grow up immune from the natural infection and it is actually very rare indeed for a healthy child to die of Chicken Pox. Here it is offered to patients for whom Varicella infection constitutes a particular risk:

Those who have had chemotherapy or HIV or people in close contact with them,

Pregnant women,

Non immune healthcare workers,

In adults two doses give 75% immunity, it is 90% in children.

Varilrix, Varivax. Over 1 year of age, 2 separate doses. Active immunisation of adults and adolescents against Varicella Zoster.

Other Specific Vaccines:

Shingles:

1 in 3 adults gets shingles if unvaccinated. However, it is a bit strange, if the V Zoster/H Simplex viruses are antigenically the same, that the lifelong immunity of Chicken Pox infection doesn't do the same job as a Shingles (H Zoster) immunisation in suppressing the Shingles that it (the Chicken Pox) causes.

Zostavax: Single dose of V. Zoster virus to the over 50 yr. olds to prevent Shingles and PHN. Or reduce its severity.

Typhoid:

Typherix Typhim Vi one dose IM/Deep SC repeat 3yrly.

Vivotif Live oral strain Ty21a S. Typhi.

Rx 1 cap, days 1, 3 and 5. Protection in 7-10 days. **Annual** Booster of 3 doses. Avoid in the immunosuppressed and in acute gastro enteritis. Organism not excreted in faeces.

Measles:

Modification of symptoms: Gamma globulin (Normal immunoglobulin) 0.02ml/kg into opposite deltoid at time of immunisation. This can be given to immunocompromised patients, babies, pregnant women in contact with Measles. Different preparations are different strengths-doses? Kabiglobulin is 16%, the DHSS is 8%. Kabiglobulin is pooled immunoglobulin with antibodies to whatever the donors of blood had antibodies to. Hep A, Measles, Rubella, Mumps etc. The effect of normal immunoglobulin lasts only 3-4 weeks.

Mumps/MMR:

History: Pluserix and Immravax contained the Urabe strain and caused a transient mild meningitis. Now withdrawn. MMR II has the Jeryl Lynn strain. Jeryl Lynn Hilleman was the daughter of a Merck research doctor from whom he got the culture for the original vaccine. Contains 3 live attenuated vaccines. Avoid pregnancy within 1m. (Priorix and M M R Vax Pro). Give other live vaccines elsewhere in the body or wait 4 weeks.

Avoid MMR in the immuno-suppressed, in allergy to egg, allergy to Kanamycin, Neomycin. Patient can get a mini Measles 5-14 days after the vaccination. Two MMR doses give 99% efficacy against Measles and if given within 72 hours of exposure it can prevent infection. See previous note on Mumps regarding effectiveness and duration of Jeryl Lynn vaccination.

MMR reactions:

MMR is a live attenuated vaccine and reactions are more likely after dose 1 than 2 (at 12-15m and 3-5 yrs respectively). The vaccines CAN in an emergency be given 4 weeks apart. Reactions can include fever, malaise and rash at 1 week, febrile convulsions in 1:1,000, parotid swelling, ITP is possible though less so than after Mumps itself. There were rare episodes of meningo-encephalitis after the original Urabe vaccine (fully recovered) but none after the new Jeryl Lynn strain. Contraindications include: Immunosuppression, malignant disease, high dose steroid treatment, another live vaccine within 3 weeks, high temperature and allergies to any of the vaccine constituents including Neomycin. Avoid pregnancy for a month (though there have been no reported foetal side effects). Protection to Dose 1) is 60-90%. To dose 2) is 95%. Under 1 year of age the vaccine may not work as the mother's antibodies counteract the vaccine antibody response.

Measles Immunisation:

From time to time outbreaks or spontaneous cases of Rubeola, Morbilli, Measles, occur. Measles IS Misery. There were cases in unvaccinated "travellers" in Surrey in 2006 with epidemics at that time in such countries as the Ukraine, Greece and some Pacific Islands. Then there was the Wakefield Scare, with the fallacious accusation of an association between MMR and autism and subsequently inflammatory bowel disease. Although the accuser and the false message have been completely debunked since, there are still ethnic communities in the USA who with Wakefield's support continue to cling to MMR as one cause for mental ill health in their children. We still have the fall-out from the unimmunised cohort and at least one Measles death has now come to light. Unsurprisingly the non vaccinating parents were subsequently desperate to get their offspring protected, queuing sometimes out into the streets for scarce MMR vaccine doses.

The death rate in Measles is about 0.3%. It is higher in the weak, malnourished, sick from other reasons, immune deficient, those with AIDS, and so on. Life threatening adverse reactions occur in less than one per million vaccinations (<0.0001%) and there is no association with autism. We can expect more deaths and long term harm to surface from this shameful episode. I am sure this period will become an object lesson in biased reporting both in the medical and general press, with irresponsible national radio and TV coverage. In combination with gross public ignorance of the facts and an abject political failure to confront this apparent basic human right of parents, the results were disastrous for children. Thousands of parents put their children at risk causing direct and serious damage through their own stupidity and government inaction. It is an almost exact repeat of the Whooping Cough hysteria of the 70's and 80's. There are still adults, patients I am seeing in my surgery now with paroxysmal coughs for 3 months and developing permanent bronchiectasis because their parents read somewhere in the late 1970's that there might be a 1 in 300,000 risk from vaccination against Pertussis.

There is a complete public lack of understanding regarding the concept of risk/benefit ratio. Putting butter on your toast, taking the train, chewing gum, drinking coke or a glass of wine, playing squash, getting out of bed, going to exotic countries, taking any medication, crossing a road – all these things have a quantifiable statistical risk. But then there is a harm in staying in bed, not exercising, not riding a bike, not taking your medication, failing to be immunised, failing to gain knowledge, experience, never going out or crossing a road.

My analogy of the risk of immunisation is that it is similar to the risk of teaching your child how to cross a busy road. You wouldn't dream of letting your child discover the hard way how dangerous a busy road can be without first standing with them many times, holding their hand and showing them how to look both ways and wait for a gap or using a Zebra crossing. Only when they were confident, protected and safe would you let them take the risk alone. However there must be a handful of children (and adults) killed or injured every year while learning to cross the road with their parents. We just don't know how many hundreds are saved by the national learning process that all responsible parents submit their children to. Risk/benefit, just like vaccination.

1 in 300,000 risk of vaccination of a severe neurological reaction – does that sound much? The High Court decided in the end it was this or less. The risk of death though, from not vaccinating your child is (from various sources) several times more than if you do have the child vaccinated. This is calculated from populations and the number of notified

cases of whooping cough who actually die from it. I calculated the risk in my part of the country at the time of the Whooping Cough scare of not vaccinating your child so I could give a proper risk benefit ratio to any parent who actually wanted to know the truth:

72% of the deaths are under 1 year, (including younger siblings of the unimmunised), 27 dead between 1977 and 1979, up to 40% mortality under 5 months, mortality up to 1:1000 overall, 2% under 1 year dead.

So I calculated the risks of getting Whooping Cough in semi rural Sussex in the early 80's if the child were unimmunised and over an observation period of 5 years and it came down to about 1:4, on my list, higher if you had an unimmunised sibling. So there you had it: If my patients didn't immunise their child against Whooping Cough they were swapping a theoretical 1:300,000 risk for an actual 1:4,000 risk of death. Risk benefit in a nutshell.*-a 75x greater risk of dying by denying your child the vaccine. It must be similar for Measles.

I return to the intrinsic need for society to confront this injustice and to look after the general good of all. That the safety and health of the community trumps the human right of the individual to do harm through ignorance or whim. Particularly if it is harm to those that cannot yet speak for themselves. So all children, even Daily Mail Epidemiologists and Southern Irish and European travellers should carry immunisation cards by law which show they will not be a danger to the innocent children of others or to the immuno-suppressed or vulnerable innocent bystander and show that they have been immunised.

*Just to illustrate how useful lawyers and politicians are when they get involved in emotional medical issues, time has shown that 1:300,000 is probably an overestimate of any harm that pertussis vaccination causes. BUT approximately 300 years worth of compensation was paid out (£6m) within the roughly first 10 years after the "Vaccine damage compensation campaign". I wonder if any has subsequently been paid back?

See Measles (Infections)

Mumps:

The aseptic meningitis symptoms that follow Urabe strain Mumps vaccination were around 1:11,000 at 3 weeks. Natural Mumps meningitis incidence after Mumps is around 1:400. Many more children than this with mumps develop meningism. The Urabe strain was then withdrawn because of the aseptic meningitis and febrile convulsion side effects and substituted by the Jeryl Lynn vaccine (Priorix).

Pertussis:

Has been covered extensively elsewhere in this section and in "Infections and anti-biotics". Suffice to say the vaccine damaged children scandal caused many deaths and injuries due to the safe Pertussis vaccine being unfairly pilloried in the 70's. Now another epidemic of deaths is happening because the weaker acellular vaccine is being actively resisted by pregnant women and by Bordetella Pertussis itself. New born infants of vacci-nated mothers have a 91% reduction in risk of catching whooping cough. Yet another wave of Whooping cough deaths is underway (2014-5) affecting the unprotected newborn and very young.

In 2012 there were 10,000 confirmed cases – the last "peak" being only 900 in 2008. A subsequent surge killed 14 babies under three months and up to the end of march 2015 there had been 11 deaths of young babies since a new vaccination drive was started by the DoH – the majority babies of unvaccinated mothers – hence the move to vaccinate all pregnant women at 28-32 weeks.

The new acellular 2004 vaccine may be part of the problem. It contains specific bacterial surface proteins acting as antigens and does not promote as long an immune response as the whole cell vaccine used to. Also these specific surface proteins on the Pertussis organism are mutating at a faster rate than some of its other surface proteins and so the bacteria are evolving quickly to evade any vaccine stimulated immune response. Evolution and Natural Selection.

In this infection arms race our options are to improve the range and variety of surface proteins in the vaccine, to add novel adjuvants to the vaccine or even to go back to a killed whole cell vaccine. But with only 60% of eligible pregnant women taking up the vaccine, the epidemic and the deaths seem likely to continue.

Tuberculosis:

In 2005 school age BCG vaccination was stopped and "targeted" vaccination was commenced (this varied between PCTs). The Mantoux likewise replaced the Heaf test. The target of the immunisation were the high risk immigrant communities mainly in our cities. After a century of decline in numbers in the UK, TB has been increasing since the late 1980s. It is commoner in immigrants, the homeless, immunodeficient and prisoners. However because the UK is now Europe's TB hot spot, anyone with a persistent cough, weight loss and malaise, particularly if they live or work in a city must be considered and investigated for TB. It is infectious and in places like Birmingham and London people work, play, learn and travel in packed crowds so it isn't only ethnic communities who get TB.

The BCG will be for all babies in areas where TB incidence exceeds 40/100,000.

In low risk areas (<40/100,000 person years) a selective immunisation policy takes place: i.e. immunising if parents or grandparents come from a high risk area, (>40/100,000), and previously unvaccinated new immigrants from high prevalence areas. Some PCTs immunise if the patient is in contact with a case of TB or if travelling to a high risk area for 3m. Different PCTs therefore offer selective or universal immunisation and some vaccinate all children on post natal wards, some in the community in the first month. In other words the system is not consistent and it remains to be seen whether the abandonment of universal BCG after Heaf testing will have an impact on the further rise of British TB in the 21st century. Given the UK's current TB incidence and risks, ending general immunisation seems as rational as demobilising the only armed forces you have on the eve of an invasion.

The vaccination is given in the L upper arm – you cannot give any other vaccination in this arm for 3m. You cannot give polio inj. at same time.

Note: BCG is Bacille Calmette-Guerin – a strain of attenuated bovine TB. It is at best 80% effective for 15years. Probably 60-80% in UK. Effectiveness varies enormously depending on where in the world the vaccine is given.

In a 2016 study, TB rates were 3.3/100,000 person years in the unvaccinated and 1.3/100,000 years in the vaccinated with 40% protection persisting 40 years. (Median F/U 41 years!) BCG appears to be more effective at preventing some forms of TB (TB meningitis in children) than others (adult pulmonary TB).

Except in neonates a Tuberculin test is done before the BCG. This is because of the risk of a severe local reaction and if the test is positive the patient needs to be screened for active TB.

Note BCG is 25% protective against Leprosy. Interestingly it is also used in a variety of other conditions from bladder cancer (and other cancers) to Type 1 Diabetes and M.S. Presumably it works as a non specific immune stimulator. In 2017 a way of testing the

Tubercle bacillus' DNA at speed became practical and opened the door to rapid typing and accurate assessment of drug sensitivity.

Hepatitis A:

Avaxim, Epaxal, Havrix etc. One dose stat then booster 6m to up to 3-4 years later depending on vaccine.

Hepatitis A and B:

Twinrix Ambirix Typically: Stat, 1m and 6m.

Hepatitis A and Typhoid Vaccinations:

Hepatyrix, ViATIM. Hepatitis booster 6-36m later, Typhoid booster 3yrs later.

Hepatitis B:

Now part of the childhood immunisation schedule and the six in one jab. Separate vaccines: Engerix, HBVax PRO etc : Stat, 1m and 6m. If recent Hepatitis B exposure, use rapid schedule (Stat, 1m, 2m, 12m or "the very rapid schedule" is stat, 1 week, 3 weeks, 12m) – with hepatitis immunoglobulin given at a different site at the same time as the first immunisation.

Responders have titres >100 US. Repeat titre in 3-5 years. Poor responders: (<100US) give booster and retest. Non responders (<10US) give full primary course again and retest. "Never responders" (<10US despite further primary courses) are assumed to be vulnerable to Hepatitis B infection.

Human Papilloma Virus: HPV

Known to be one of the causes of cervical and throat cancer. There are three vaccines currently available and they cover different strains of the HPV virus. There are up to 40 strains of HPV. They cause verrucae and cancers of various parts of the perineal region and genital tract in men and women as well as of the oropharynx and anus. The high risk HPV viruses are not those that cause warts elsewhere in the body.

Gardasil HPV 6 11 16 and 18 can be given at intervals of 0, 2 and 6m (or even stat, 1m, 3m if necessary).

Cervarix 16 and 18 covers 70% cervical cancers. A new (2015) vaccine "Gardasil-9" covers, as you would expect, 9 strains of HPV. This new version of Gardasil 9 covers HPV 6, 11, 16 and 18 (the same as Gardasil) as well as types 31, 33, 45, 52, and 58. These latter five are responsible for approximately 1 in 5 cases of cervical cancer. Collectively, all these types are responsible for 90% of cervical cancers.

Nearly 100% of cervical cancers, 90% of anal cancers, 70% of vaginal cancers, and 15% of vulval cancers are caused by HPV and persistent infection with certain types of HPV has also been linked to malignancies of the mouth and throat. The quadrivalent vaccine covers the infections that cause throat cancer.

If you are interested:

Common warts:	HPV 2 and 7
Verrucae:	HPV 1, 2, 4 and 63
Flat warts:	HPV 3, 8 and 10.
Anogenital warts:	HPV 6, 11, 42, 44 etc
Genital cancer:	HPV 16, 18, 31, 45 (there are many others)
Oropharyngeal cancer:	HPV 16.

You can make up your own mind whether the initial decision to fund the narrow spectrum vaccine was the right one. In Australia they vaccinate boys and girls which makes sense if you think about where the girls get the perineal infection in the first place (chicken and egg). Michael Douglas' announcement that his throat cancer may have been contributed to by HPV, oral sex and his number of partners just illustrates the carcinogenic potential of this virus at sites above the waist too. HPV Vaccine: In 2015 the Joint Committee on Vaccine and Immunisation announced that GPs should be vaccinating men under the age of 45 who have sex with men. But not as yet young boys who will grow up to be men who have sex with women.

Duration of Immunity:

Tetanus: At least 10 years. For most injuries and after the primary course and a couple of adult boosters it is lifelong. However, for travellers to areas with no access to doctors and who haven't had a tetanus booster for >10 years, give an extra booster anyway.

Human Tetanus Immunoglobulin 250-500 IU IM can be given if a dirty wound, a puncture or devitalised wound occurs for "immediate" protection.

Typhoid: 3 years
Cholera: 6 months
Polio: 10 years
Yellow Fever: 10 years
Hepatitis A: 10 years.

Malaria (see travel section)

General notes:

Antimalarials to be taken from one week before to **at least** one week after the trip.
Chloroquine and Proguanil are OTC
Adult doses: Chloroquine 300mg weekly
Proguanil 200mg daily
Mefloquine (Lariam) 250mg weekly. One week before to 4 weeks after return. Contra indicated in epilepsy, F.H. of epilepsy, significant history of psychiatric disorder. Face to face counselling recently (2016) advised by the MoD. Interactions with various drugs, BBs, Digoxin, CCBs, Quinidine etc. Avoid in pregnancy, lactation etc etc. Maximum 3 months Rx (as usual, 1 week before til 4 weeks after the trip is over).
<15kg Not Recommended,
<20kg 1/4 tab
<30kg 1/2 tab
<45kg 3/4 tab
>45kg 1 tab
Children's doses for most antimalarials:
<1year 1/4 the adult dose
1-5 years 1/2 the adult dose
6-11 years 3/4 the adult dose
>12 years give the adult dose.

Don't prescribe Mefloquine to <2 year old children, babies and potentially child bearing women (avoid pregnancy for 3m after course). However they can take Chloroquine (Avoclor, Nivaquine) and Proguanil (Paludrine), but not Mefloquine (Lariam) or Doxycycline (avoid pregnancy for 1 week and don't give <8 years).

In Epilepsy: Avoid Chloroquine, Mefloquine. – Doxycycline 100mg/day is best if visiting areas where these are recommended.

Long term travellers: Could give Quinine 600mg TDS for 3 days followed by Fansidar tabs (Pyrimethamine and Sulphadoxine) X3 stat if they develop a fever.

Influenza Vaccine:

>65 years, pregnant (reduces maternal pneumonia, miscarriage, perinatal pneumonia in the baby), long stay care home residents, main carers, healthcare workers/social care workers, patients with chronic respiratory disease (especially treated with inhaled steroids), chronic heart disease, CKD, chronic neurological disease, DM (drug or insulin treated), splenectomy, Sickle Cell Anaemia, HIV, steroid Rx, chemotherapy.

Nasal Influenza vaccine: eg Autumn/winter 2015/6 etc Nasal spray children aged 2-8 offered flu vaccine.

Some studies show that Flu vaccine is relatively ineffective. That its formulation is, of necessity based on old data, (the 2014/5 flu had mutated to AH3 by January 2015, not covered by the vaccine) and so, due to the rapidly changing antigenicity of flu, it is out of date by the time it becomes available. Worse still, some research from America has shown that vaccinated patients actually get worse flu for longer than unvaccinated patients. Certainly for what it is worth, whenever I was given the flu vaccine – which I was annually for several years, I felt achy, shivery and ill for a week every year and eventually ignored official advice, eschewing the jab. I never really experienced 'flu in the years before during or after having the vaccine. I can't really say it prevented much "Flu-like illness" in my patients. The only exception to this general observation is pregnant women whose babies need all the protection they can get – even if it is partial.

At one point, reports regarding the 2014/5 flu vaccine said it was preventing only 3% of flu infections anyway. Subsequent data from Public Health England announced that the vaccination regime had been 34% effective in preventing flu in vaccinated patients. This must make it the least effective vaccine that has ever been given nationally. The latest American audit of the 2016/7 flu vaccine showed it was 61% effective against A and B strains at ages 6m - 8yrs, 19% 18-49 yrs and 25% >65yrs. The UK winter death rate figures announced in April 2016 were the worst ever and approximately equally attributable to dementia and pneumonia/flu.

A 2017 report isn't even that positive (34%) about the benefits of flu vaccine: (Skowronski, Chambers et Al: A Perfect Storm: Impact of Genomic Variation and Serial Vaccination on Low Influenza Vaccine Effectiveness During the 2014-2015 Season. Clin Infect Dis. 2016. Jul 1:63 (1) reported in "Second Opinion Feb 2017): The report showed that if you had regular annual flu vaccination, the effect was to reduce your immunity and increase the likelihood of you catching flu, not to protect you. Absolutely counter intuitive and the only vaccine I have ever heard of that makes you susceptible to a disease- but the figures were: If you had the vaccine once it increased your risk by 16%, if had it in 2013 and 2014 you were 32% more likely than unvaccinated patients to catch flu, and if you had it each year from 2012- 2015 you were 54% more likely to catch flu than if you declined the vaccine. Utterly shocking I know but even more shocking, since this is a reputable journal and a reputable study is why don't we all know this, why aren't we all discussing it and why will we go ahead with vaccinating and extending the programme (2017) to the morbidly obese (£6.2m)?. And it seems that this will not only be without benefit but positively harmful.

24: INFECTIONS:

Medicinal discovery, it moves in mighty leaps,
It leapt straight past the common cold and gave it us for keeps.

Pam Ayres

The UK statutory notification system for infectious diseases (also called Notifications of Infectious Diseases or NOIDS) is a system whereby doctors are required to notify a "Proper Officer" of the local authority (such as a Consultant in Communicable Disease Control) if they are presented with a case of a serious infectious disease. The Proper Officer then sends a report to the Centre for Infections of the Health Protection Agency (HPA) in Colindale, north London (used to be The Communicable Disease Surveillance Centre).

This is our equivalent of the American CDC which we see so often in Hollywood pandemic disaster movies.

By the way:

www.healthmap.org shows world maps with the areas of outbreaks of:

Vectorborn, Gastrointestinal, Respiratory, Animal, Skin and Rash, Other Alerts, Neuro, Fever/Febrile, STD, Environmental, Haemorrhagic and MRSA/Hospital Based infections worldwide.

80% of the planet's biomass is microbes. In fact your own gut microbiome consists of 90 trillion bacterial cells. You only consist of 7 trillion cells. There has been life on earth 3.8Bn years. These were at first unicellular organisms. It took over a billion years for these single celled organisms to evolve into successful multicellular organisms. Then 570m years ago arthropods appeared, fish 530m years ago, land plants were 475m years ago and mammals not until a mere 200 million years ago.

There have been 5 major extinction episodes during the period of life on earth so far:

Ordovician

Devonian

Permian

Triassic and

Cretaceous – and the demise of the dinosaurs happened at just the right time for we mammals to move into their vacant niche. These events have been both extraterrestrial and environmental.

Many think that the population of the planet is currently unsustainable and that the high human density of cities and mass transit systems is asking for a large scale epidemic. Add to this the migration and mixing of large numbers across continents at work and play in densely packed cities and another mass extinction seems a likely result. Think of our crowding together in education, on transport, as spectators, in high density housing, think of our intensive farming and the close proximity and density of farm animals to each other and to people. Consider the ease and frequency of international travel and large scale population shifts, all of these being the right ingredients for another infectious mass extinction event. Think of the lax health supervision of international migration and immigration and the public health fall out that has already happened. This may take the form of a mutated virus or resistant bacterium which spreads too quickly for mass vaccination to be effective. However, the three most serious public health crises in Britain today are due not to mutations of infectious organisms but wholly or mainly due to political decisions. The decision to open our borders to mass migration and resulting in the current tuberculosis and hepatitis B epidemics and the much of the perpetuation of HIV.

If you have reason to suspect an exotic or inexplicable infection, discuss with your Local Health Protection Team or phone 01980 612 100 (Porton Down).

Hand washing: You may have sat through various "teaching sessions" on infection control in the last year or two which included the standard dogma that bare forearms, dispensing with ties, using antiseptic hand washes and gels are necessary to cut down cross infections in hospitals and in General Practice. Perhaps you found the whole process a bit patronising and unconvincing. Perhaps you suspected that simple cleanliness and regular hand washing without the dermatitis-promoting and skin-drying effects of gels and soaps might be just as good? Along with the seemingly harmless and usually highly motivated advice comes the logical corollary that all surgery decorations, fomites, pictures, toys and books be removed. Goodbye toybox, family photos, flowers and reference books. Hello plastic keyboard cover, no hand shaking and a reduction of actual *touching* the patient to a bare minimum. The sterile consulting room indeed.

This is actually nonsense and has no clinical evidence to support it. In fact much research information specifically contradicts this new infection control dogma. The private sector where most doctors wear ties and many wear jackets while consulting has the lowest infection rate in UK healthcare. A 2015 paper from Korea showed that antibacterial soap is unnecessary too. The most common antibacterial agent in soap was Triclosan and the study compared the effects of washing with Triclosan containing soap and plain soap on 20 bacterial strains. After 20 seconds washing at 22 deg C, there was no significant difference in antibacterial activity between the two. Then volunteers' hands were contaminated with bacteria culture and washed with plain and medicated soaps again. Again the antibacterial agent added nothing extra to the soap's antibacterial activity. (Kim, Moon, Lee etc J Antimicrob Chemoth Sep 2015). This is fairly academic now as Triclosan has been banned in the EU (and in initially in Minnesota) as it was an "endocrine disrupter" and believed to be a carcinogen. From Sept 2016 the FDA banned it nationally, and 18 other antiseptics which were leading to the creation of antibiotic resistant organisms, in the US in antiseptic washes as it had also been found to be ineffective as an antiseptic.

Add to this the growing threat from treatment resistant bacteria – many strains becoming resistant not only to antibiotics but to antiseptic agents as well and you see the problem. The bacteriocidal gels on every corridor and ward, on cruise ships, in surgeries and hospitals are presumably hastening the development of a truly "Khan type" genetically modified untreatable superbug. Of course no anti bacterial will kill viruses. Soap and water is more effective at preventing Norovirus cross infection than spirit gels too. You can't help wondering whether we should just go back to self discipline and soap and water in General Practice at least.

General Infections in the Community and standard treatments:

Pharyngitis: Penicillin V/Erythromycin/Clarithromycin.

Otitis media: Amoxycillin/Erythromycin/Clarithromycin.   Alternatively   Co Amoxiclav or a Cefalosporin.

Sinusitis: Amoxycillin (big doses) or Oxytetracycline, Erythro/Clarithromycin, Doxycycline or Co Amoxiclav or Ciprofloxacin plus Metronidazole. (Or, again, Co Amoxiclav, big doses).

Lower Respiratory Infections: Amoxycillin or Oxytetracycline or Doxycycline or Co Amoxiclav.

Community acquired pneumonia: Same as for LRTI but treat for 10 days not 5 days. Thus: Acute bronchitis: Amoxicillin or Doxycycline.

Acute exacerbation of COPD (30% viral 50% bacterial, the rest unknown).

Amoxicillin, Doxycycline, Clarithromycin, or if no better>Co Amoxiclav or Levofloxacin.

A study from Cardiff University published in 2014 showed that antibiotic courses failed in the community 15% of the time. They looked at 11m prescriptions issued between 1991 and 2012 and saw a slight rise in the failure rate from 13.9% to 15.4% over the period of the study. They used this to emphasise the need for tighter control and more focussed antibiotic prescribing. But only a 15% failure rate? That's not bad in the community where we don't usually have quick access to bacteriology and use a best guess approach. I wonder what the failure rate in secondary care would be? Somewhat higher I would imagine.

New evidence ("Straight to the point") suggested in July 2015 that GPs might measure CRP using "point of care testing" in the newly acronymed **CRP-POCT**. This is to try to differentiate viral from significant bacterial upper respiratory infections. How reliable, available and effective is this likely to become across the surgeries of Britain? A Cochrane review of CRP-POCT in six randomised trials led to a reduction of 41% in the quantity of antibiotics prescribed. How much longer and how much more pain and suffering did these patients experience though ? This technique can result in a defendable 5 minute decision as to whether antibiotics are appropriate (in case of complaint or litigation). However, I suspect the newly qualified dogmatic doctor in declining an antibiotic, as many seem to, while ignoring thick sputum, pus on the tonsils, cervical lymphadenopathy, the patient's past experience and an ill, septic patient is still pretty unreasonable, uncaring, silly and risk taking.

Procalcitonin (confusingly called PCT) is another indicator of "invasive bacterial infection". It is a prohormone with 116 amino acids and its level rises rapidly, in 4-6 hours, in response to bacteria, fungi and malaria but not viral infections. Levels correlate with subsequent mortality rates (see Pathology). This could be a PCT-POCT. (which will no doubt colloquially become known as picked pocket).

The front pages of many news papers in late August 2015 declared "**Threat to GPs over antibiotics**"

"-GPs are prescribing 10m courses of antibiotics for coughs colds and minor infections said the director of NICE," (but nationally 41.6m prescriptions for antibiotics in total were issued in 2013-2014) advising GPs to delay prescribing for URTIs, LRTIs and UTIs. He suggested those who did not stick to new delayed prescribing guidance should be brought before the GMC and even eventually struck off. Since the GMC has few or no GPs in it, it will be ignorant of why antibiotics are prescribed in this medical arena and why GPs feel obliged to do so. He suggested that prescriptions carry diagnoses so that pharmacists could challenge doctors' instructions and monitor needless prescriptions. – Really?

This whole area is, of course, hugely problematic. Pharmacists want nothing less than being set at loggerheads with their GP colleagues. They do not have the time, experience or expertise to comment on the appropriateness of every course of antibiotic that passes their counter. GPs (and I have been one for more than three decades) are often subject to a protracted, morale sapping official complaints procedure if they refuse an antibiotic to which a patient feels entitled. One such complaint about my refusing a patient her "normal penicillin" (to a Spanish T/R) went as far as a dozen letters, an interview with the Ombudsman's representative and a year of uncertainty before it petered out and the complaint was dismissed. Was it worth the aggro? There were of course no official congratulations for me at the end of it for my prescribing Puritanism or official open criticism of the patient. I stuck to my guns and continue to do so about giving or declining antibiotics but if the patient disagrees, what you may regard as self evident good practice may take a long time to be accepted by the complaints authorities. Many patients have experienced miserable illnesses in the past due to infection, want to avoid a repeat at all costs and will never forgive the GP for refusing what seems to them such a little indulgence. They will hold this against the GP every time they meet for years to come. After all it isn't like casualty or outpatients where you tell the patient No and never see them again. Also NICE says: refuse antibiotics for minor infections like UTIs and LRTIs? UTIs cause confusion and distress, incontinence, failure to cope and septicaemia at both ends of life and LRTIs are still probably the most common terminal event on death certificates. Minor infections? Aren't they what all major infections begin as?

"I quit school in the sixth grade because of pneumonia. Not because I had it but because I couldn't spell it"

Rocky Graziano (Boxer)

Pneumonia is a disease that often flies under the radar of not just the public but even the global health community. It kills more children under 5 years old every year than AIDs, Malaria and Measles combined.

Mandy Moore

"Sepsis"

This term has been used by journalists over the last few years when what they actually mean is progressive infection or septicaemia. It was a lead item after NICE updated its guidelines in July 2016 on the "Today" programme on Radio 4. It was said in the report that 10,000-40,000 people die each year with this diagnosis. To most doctors listening, the inaccuracy, vagueness and inappropriateness of the term which is used like a precise diagnosis rather than a common terminal event for multiple conditions or a vague general description of infection just serves to indicate how little that reporters understand the problem they pretend to be explaining. Have any of them the slightest medical experience ? However, listening to the frequent sad stories of small children whose chest infections were missed by out of hours call handlers and GPs – none of whom presumably knew the family (ie that they weren't frequent callers or panickers), or the history (ie that the parents had called a number of times over the preceding days, spoken to various doctors who hadn't communicated or that at each call the condition of the child had become worse) was a sad reaffirmation of the inadequacy of emergency out of hours GP cover today. Minor chest infections, like those of UTIs, soft tissue infections, URTIs, even meningitis, can start as a minor treatable conditions, easily nipped in the bud but unpredictably decompensating in some patients, adults or children and becoming an overwhelming septicaemia, – a "SEPSIS". I presume that in the days when GPs were more willing to treat coughs with wet chest signs and painful red throats or ears with antibiotics, fewer of these infections reached a critical mass that overwhelmed the patient's immune system. I also assume that our profession's current antibiotic aversion is one of the reasons for the apparent increase in septicaemia. As it is for Scarlet Fever. Like I say throughout this book, good Family Medicine works best with named patient lists, full time GPs, a lack of locums and part time or sessional doctors (or at the very least excellent communication and handover within the practice) and doctors with at least one Paediatric training job. It really worked best when GPs did their own out of hours cover. But it mainly depends on familiarity, knowledge, accessibility and a willingness to re examine sick patients from top to bottom again and again. Also when I was a trainee my Trainer told me that if a sick child's parents asked for help twice you **had** to see them and make sure you had a good reason not to refer them in. Most of the time that second examination confirms you don't need to send them in. But it doesn't always.

Community acquired pneumonia:

The common organisms are: only established in 1/3 cases but of those isolated: Strep Pneumoniae, Haemophilus Influenzae, Moraxella Catarrhalis, make up 50%. Mycoplasma Pneumoniae, Chlamydophila Pneumoniae, Chlamydophila Psittaci, Coxiella Burnetti and Legionella Pneumophilia make up 15%. Influenza A and Rhinoviruses constitute up to 30%. Staph Aureus is a rare cause.

Assessing severity can be done by **"CURB-65 Score"**:

CURB-65 Score	Severity	Management
Confusion of new onset Abbreviated mental test score </= 8	Score 0-1 Low 30 day mortality <3%	Manage in the community
Urea >/= 7mmol Respiratory rate >/= 30/min	Score 2 Moderate 30 day mortality 9%	Consider hospital admission
BP <90 syst or 60 diast Age >/= 65	Score 3-5 High 30 day mortality 15-40%	Hospital ITU/High dependency

Amoxicillin, Co Amoxiclav, Clarithromycin or Doxycycline – or combinations thereof.

A 2015 study showed adjuvant steroid treatment reduced mortality 3%, the need for ventilation 5%, and reduced hospital stay by 1 day in CAP. (Annals of Int Med, Meta Analysis Aug 2015). The article says that inflammation may initially clear bacteria but "Ultimately contributes to sepsis and end organ failure". So systemic steroids can be effective even though not currently part of conventional clinical guidelines.

What is Mycoplasma Pneumoniae? The smallest free living organism, unusual amongst our host of bacterial adversaries in lacking a cell wall.

It is the organism that causes Atypical Pneumonia. (Other causes are Psittacosis, Q Fever and Legionella). A different Mycoplasma can cause Pelvic Inflammatory Disease. Interestingly it may cause carcinogenic chromosomal transformation of cells, – certainly, this has been shown in vivo. It used to be called the Pleuro-Pneumonia like organism. Mycoplasma causes 7-10% of community acquired pneumonia and occurs in epidemics every 3-4 years.

It commonly affects children, young adults, in Autumn and Spring. The infection is slow in onset, a hacking cough developing, with flu like symptoms, contagious for 10 days or more, IP 14-21 days, up to 28 days and it lasts from a few days to 3-4 weeks. On examination: focal crepitations are common. Patients can also have a red throat and cervical lymphadenopathy. As you can see, there is a lot of variability. It can mimic bronchiolitis in small children which is why wheezy toddlers should usually be given macrolides not Amoxicillin or other cell wall antibiotics. There is a dry cough, often a wheeze and 10% develop frank secondary pneumonia. Complications include otitis media, haemolytic anaemia, pneumonia, rashes.

Erthromycin, Clarithromycin, Azithromycin all work if you need to treat it, penicillins etc don't as the organism has no cell wall.

CXR is usually worse than the clinical symptoms suggest, showing such things as bronchopneumonia, plate-like atelectasis, effusions and lower lobe infiltrates. Patchy changes.

Cold agglutinins are positive in 50-70%, as a bedside test: Put a few drops of blood in the citrate of a prothrombin tube then put the tube in a fridge for 10 minutes: Cold agglutinins show as a coarse granular appearance that clears on warming in the grip of your palm – but there are more specific CFT and immuno assays etc. WBC is usually N.

Ureaplasma organisms

The family *Mycoplasmataceae* contains two genera that infect humans: *Mycoplasma* and *Ureaplasma*, which are usually referred to collectively as mycoplasmas.

Ureaplasma and Mycoplasma organisms may cause Nongonococcal/non Chlamydial urethritis in men. Mycoplasma organisms may contribute to 10% of pelvic infection, can cause severe perinatal infections of babies, both may cause endometritis, arthritis, neonatal pneumonia, meningitis, PID, urethritis, pyelonephritis, infections of patients with immune deficiency and so on.

Azithromycin or Doxycycline are generally the treatment if Ureaplasma organisms are considered to be the cause of infection. Clindamycin can be used in Mycoplasma if it is Tetracycline resistant but it is not as good against Ureaplasma. Macrolides, fluoroquinolones, or tetracyclines are the DOCs (drug of choice) for *Ureaplasma* infections. A single 1-g dose of Azithromycin is approved for treatment of urethritis due to *Chlamydia Trachomatis* and works as well clinically as 7 days of doxycycline in persons with urethritis due to *Ureaplasma* species. Fluoroquinolones are effective against both organisms usually in the UGT.

Urinary Tract Infections:

In uncomplicated UTI (no fever or flank pain), if the dipstick is negative (– nitrite and leuks) the test is said to be 95% reliable. **This has not been my experience** and cannot be relied upon in children.

Rx Trimethoprim or Nitrofurantoin (both bacteriostatic) both for 3 days in women 7 days in men (often ineffective despite your prescribing committee's preferences).

Do MSU if no better soon,

UTI in pregnancy, children and in men, do MSU. Nitrofurantoin, Trimethoprim, or second line Cefalexin/Amoxicillin each for 7 days.

Recurrent UTI in women (>3/year) Nitrofurantoin 50mg or Trimethoprim 100mg, post coitally or once nocte (equally effective).

Acute pyelonephritis: MSU. Co Amoxiclav 14 days, Ciprofloxacin 7 days, Trimethoprim (if sens.) 14 days.

Catheterised: UTI only treat if fever and abdominal pain are present as well as positive MSU.

Gastro Intestinal Infections: (See Gastroenterology section)

H Pylori: Lansoprazole 30mg BD, or Omeprazole 20mg BD, or Pantoprazole 40mg Bd, Ranitidine Bismuth Citrate 400mg BD, (Unavailable now in US and I couldn't find it in any of my local UK suppliers) Plus 2 antibiotics: Amoxicillin 1gr BD, Clarithromycin 500mg BD, Metronidazole 400mg BD, Oxytetracycline 500mg QDS for 7days or 14 days in relapse.

See Gastroenterology section for a fuller list and beware, H Pylori often recurs. Eradication not supposed to be helpful in reflux per se. However 8% "NUD" patients benefit so why not give it a try? See Gastroenterology section.

Clostridium Difficile gastroenteritis: C Difficile lives harmlessly in the GI tract of 10-15% of all adults. Spread by air born spores. Stop oral antibiotics and PPIs, D/W Microbiologist, Rx Metronidazole 3-5 days then? Vancomycin.

Travellers' Diarrhoea: Ciprofloxacin 500-750mg a single dose for travellers to remote areas given clear instructions.

Rifaximin-a (Xifaxanta) 200mg TDS for 3days. It can be used in non bloody, <8 stools in 24 hours, no systemic symptoms, Travellers' Diarrhoea.

Worms: Threadworms: Mebendazole >2 yrs, Piperazine/Senna (Pripsen) 3-12m. Giardiasis. Metronidazole.

Genital tract infections:

Vaginal Candidiasis: Clotrimazole 10% 5gr vaginal cream, or 500mg pessary or Fluconazole 150mg orally.

Bacterial Vaginosis: Metronidazole 400mg BD 7 days (or 2gr stat if not pregnant) or Metronidazole vaginal gel 5g daily 5 days (topical is just as effective).

Chlamydia Trachomatis: Treat partners and refer to GUM clinic. Doxycycline 100mg BD 7 days, or Oxytetracycline 500mg QDS 7 days, or Erythromycin 500mg BD 14 days/ QDS 7 days or Azithromycin 1gr stat.

Trichomonas: Treat both partners, refer to GUM clinic: Metronidazole 400mg BD 7 days or 2gr single dose. Clotrimazole 100mg pessary daily 6 days.

Pelvic Inflammatory Disease: Metronidazole 400mg BD and Ofloxacin 400mg BD or Metronidazole TDS and Doxycycline 100mg BD – all for 2 weeks. Must exclude Gonorrhoea and Chlamydia.

Acute Prostatitis: Ofloxacin 200mg BD or Norfloxacin 400mg BD, or Ciprofloxacin 500mg BD or Trimethoprim 200mg BD, **28 days for all.**

Threadworms; Mebendazole 100mg stat or Piperazine under 1 year. Repeat 2 weeks.

Soft tissue/Skin infections:

Severe Impetigo: Flucloxacillin or Erythro/Clarithromycin 7 days. Add topical Fucidin/Bactroban.

Cellulitis: Amoxicillin and Flucloxaciilin or Erythromycin or Co Amoxiclav (especially if severe or facial or secondary to an infected bite of any kind – asses tetanus/rabies risk and treat appropriately etc). If penicillin allergic try Metronidazole plus Oxytetracycline, or Metronidazole plus Erythro/Clarithromycin.

Scabies: Permethrin 5% cream X2 applications, a week apart.

Dermatophyte infection of finger nails: Amolrofine paint twice weekly for 6m (toes 1 year).

Terbinafine tabs 250mg daily for fingers 6-12 weeks, for toes 3-6months. Send clippings for mycology first – exclude psoriasis, trauma etc. I find the daily application of Terbinafine cream to soft nails (Before the gym or after a bath), especially the nail folds, works almost as well.

Zoster: Shingles and Chicken Pox: Aciclovir 800mg 5X daily or Valaciclovir 1gr TDS 7 days. Herpes Simplex has different dosage regimes.

Conjunctivitis:

Chloramphenicol or Fucithalmic are the usual stand bys. How genuinely useful they are in most conjunctivitises, how accurate our diagnoses are and how much gets in the eye for how long are different questions. Alternatives include: Ciprofloxacin drops, (ulcers, bacterial infections). If Trachoma, bacterial infections, etc Azithromycin, Azyter drops, Gentamycin, Genticin drops, Tobramycin (bacterial) Tobravisc or Tobradex with steroid. Also Levo/Mo/and O-floxacin drops (bacterial) and Aciclovir, Ganciclovir in H. Simplex infections.

Assess allergy, viral, abrasion, dendritic ulcer and of course, internal eye disease. Possible need for short term steroid, NSAID drops (like Ketorolac, Acular), antihistamine drops or Cromoglicate.

Other useful eye drops include Otrivine-anthistine (antihistamine and vasoconstrictor) and a multitude of antihistamines, Azelastine, Emedastine, Epinastine, Ketotifen, Lodoxamide, Nedocromil, Olopatadine, Cromoglicate etc.

Petechial spots on palate:

Scarlet Fever
Rubella
Glandular Fever.

Gingeval/Dental abscess:

Amoxicillin 500mg TDS or Metronidazole 400mg TDS both of which are available from the dentist. Co Amoxiclav is now too.

Other common Infections:

Herpes Simplex causes cold sores
Herpes Zoster causes Shingles
and
Varicella Zoster Chicken Pox:

IP 10-21 days   No prodrome Cropping   Rash Fades
<---------------------> <-------------------------> <------------------------------->
        <--Infectious1-5 days before spots til lesions dry--->

10-21 day IP. Waves of spots, Trunk mainly, Contagious 1-5 days before spots until all blisters scab over, dew drops on a rose petal. Foetal Varicella affects brain, eye, spinal cord, hypoplasia of limbs, motor/sensory deficits, skin damage,

Vaccine lasts 5 years, there is anti varicella Immune Globulin, avoid aspirin in infected children (Reyes syndrome). Complications in adults include pneumonia, purpura, encephalitis, fasciitis, secondary bacterial infections. Remember Reye's and Guillain Barre.

Rx: Idoxuridine, Herpid Solution Apply QDS for 4 days.

Aciclovir: Safe in children and pregnancy:

Varicella or H. Zoster: 800mg 5x daily 7 days,

H.Simplex 200mg 5x daily 5 days,

Long term suppression 400mg BD,

H.Simplex in immunocompromised 400mg 5x daily,

Genital Herpes in the immunocompetent: 200mg 5x daily 5 days,

Children: (Varicella) <2 yrs 200mg QDS 5days,

2-5 yrs 400mg QDS 5days,

>6yrs 800mg QDS 5days.

Also Penciclovir, Valaciclovir, (H. Zoster, H.Simplex type 1 and 2, V. Zoster. EBV, Human Herpes Virus 6) Famciclovir etc.

Post Herpetic Neuralgia:

Carbamazepine, Venlafaxine, Valproate, Clonazepam, Axsain Cream, Oxycodone, Periciazine, Clonazepam, Clobazam (SLS), Phenytoin, Dosulepin, Steroid and local anaesthetic injection to dorsal root ganglion.

Also the Shingles vaccination: Offered to the over 65s (a single dose being 50% effective).

Actinomyces:

On HVS or smear may be secondary to IUCD. A branching Nocardia Bacterium/ Fungus. If symptomatic Rx Penicillin. Can usually ignore. Can cause Actinomycosis.

Listeria:

Listeria Monocytogenes. Gram Pos Bacillus. This is so widely distributed in the environment that exposure is inevitable to us all and 1:20 of us carry the bacillus in our guts at any given moment. Can cause Flu, septicaemia, meningitis, midterm abortion. IP 2 days to 6 weeks. Diagnosis on blood culture. Serology unhelpful. Do a blood culture if a pregnant patient is pyrexial >38 Deg C for >48Hrs. Organism killed at 70deg C for 2mins but is relatively unaffected by refrigeration at or above 6 deg C. Don't refrigerate blood culture. Sensitive to Amoxicillin and Erythromycin.

If pregnant or immuno-compromised, patients should avoid soft ripened cheeses, Brie, Camembert, blue veined cheeses, all pates, cook-chilled meats, ready to eat poultry unless piping hot. Up to 18% of some pre-cooked chilled packaged foods are positive for Listeria. In 2015 a report was published in the USA proving an outbreak with deaths was due to caramel coated apples. Hard cheese, processed cheese, cottage cheese and cheese spreads are fine.

PREGNANT patients – avoid lambing time with sheep – (Listeria, Toxoplasma, Chlamydia), – Note: Amoxycillin is usually effective against Chlamydia. Also avoid silage – This is a Listeria risk.

There were only 24 cases of materno/foeto transmission in 700,000 births in 1990.

Glandular Fever, Infectious Mononucleosis:

An Epstein-Barr Virus infection (which is a herpes virus) which may be the cause of Burkitts Lymphoma as well.

50/100,000/year. 1/1,000 at 15-25yrs. Infects >90% of the world's population. Lifelong latent infection and immunity after primary illness. 4-7 week incubation period. EBV is shed >6m after acute infection then intermittently for life.

5% develop CFS,

50% have splenomegaly,

Palatal petechiae (between hard and soft palate),

Maculopapular rash,

Mild thrombocytopoenia,

Mildly raised ALT/AST in half of uncomplicated cases.

Monospot heterophile antibody test is not immediate but positive at 1-2 weeks.

This is called the kissing disease but that is the only funny thing about it. It often presents as an exhausted miserable teenager, usually about to take exams, with no idea whom he or she has caught it from. They have a sore throat (sometimes agonisingly sore) so that they cannot even swallow saliva, – the nasal gaping mouthed talking with wincing as they try to swallow is characteristic. It is hard not to feel sorry for these, normally ebullient extrovert patients. Look for posterior cervical lymphadenopathy and try to feel the liver edge and splenic tip (I always examine the abdomen in a teenager with pusy tonsils). You might even do the Monospot/Paul Bunnell and LFTs before you see them again. Many will prescribe antibiotics but if you do, avoid Amoxicillin/Co Amoxiclav/Ampicillin which can give a generalised rash "The poor man's Paul Bunnell". This, by the way, occasionally results in the persistence of a delayed reaction to penicillin long after recovery from the Glandular Fever.

If the patient cannot swallow fluids due to pain or has signs of respiratory obstruction you can consider admission but I have managed to avoid this three times in the last 30 years by giving IV Hydrocortisone (on two successive days in the worst case) with a dramatic improvement.

The tiredness that follows glandular fever is genuine, prolonged and deserves sympathy. To reduce the risk of habituation and reinforcement, I use strong positive reinforcement, right from the start, regular reviews, graded exercise despite the tiredness, strong multi-vitamins which I believe do help despite the hippiness of that sort of approach and even, rarely, SSRIs. The worry is of course that susceptible patients may develop CFS.

Giardiasis:

Giardia Lamblia, a protozoan, causes nausea, anorexia, watery, foul diarrhoea, abdominal pain and distension. Can lead to chronic diarrhoea and malabsorption but can also be asymptomatic. Treatment with Metronidazole and Paromomycin (not absorbed) – both can be used in pregnancy. Mepacrine.

Clostridium Difficile:

Metronidazole and Vancomycin (– the latter can be given orally and systemically and is also used in Pseudomembranous colitis and Staphylococcal enteritis).

Food Borne Botulism:

(Anti toxin from Health Protection Agency 020 8200 6868).

Signs and symptoms occur from 6 hrs to 36 hrs after ingestion of contaminated food. Initially there are nausea, vomiting, abdominal pain, – subsequently neurological signs and symptoms. Double (6th N palsy) and blurred vision are common, dysphasia, dysarthria, autonomic dysfunction leading to dry mouth, hypotension, retention, constipation.

Then descending weakness/paralysis, hypoventilation (as in Guillain Barre). The patient needs to be admitted urgently for blood gases and if necessary, assisted ventilation.

So look for dysphagia, dry mouth, diplopia, dysarthria, weakness, but not usually fever, loss of reflexes or altered conscious state.

Aeromonas Hydrophila. A pathogen of fish which can cause gastro-enteritis or cellu-litis and can be a cause of chronic diarrhoea. Can respond to Trimethoprim, some cepha-losporins and Ciprofloxacin.

Meningitis:

Prophylaxis:

Haemophilus Influenzae B: Antibiotic prophylaxis: The standard UK vaccination regime includes HIB at 2, 3 and 4 months. BUT if an unvaccinated child under 4yrs lives in the same house as the patient, give prophylaxis to everyone in the house including the patient.-Unless already treated with the highly penetrative Ceftriaxone which eradicates carriage.

Normal Haemophilus prophylaxis for adults and children >12 yrs is:

a stat dose of Ciprofloxacin 500mg.

An alternative is Rifampicin prophylaxis thus:

Adults and children >12 yrs 600mg once daily 4 days,

Children 3m-12 yrs: 20mg/kg once daily 4 days, max 600mg.

Children 1m-3m: 10mg/kg once daily 4 days.

Note that dosing of prophylactic Rifampicin for this indication is once daily, it is BD in meningococcal infection.

Pregnant contacts are, however, treated the same if using:

Ceftriaxone 250mg stat dose IM (-Not licensed so will need "counselling").

Antibiotic prophylaxis can be given to all household members and room contacts where there are children <3yrs. Also playgroup contacts where there are >2 cases.

Note: That Haemophilus Influenzae vaccination began in '92 and Note also that Erythromycin has fairly useless anti – Haemophilus activity.

Meningococcal meningitis, ie Neisseria Meningitidis:

Meningococcal prophylactic Antibiotics:

To eradicate nasal carriage (this stops spread but not infection) of the N Meningitidis, give Rifampicin to all household contacts, family and non family, all people who sleep near the index case (dormitories etc), girl/boy friend (kissing), school children in contact >4 hrs in an enclosed space, healthcare staff who may have had exposure to respiratory droplets, (arbitrarily often given as within 3 feet but would you risk 4 feet or 6, or 10? Also the index case will need prophylaxis unless already treated with Ceftriaxone (to eradicate nasal carriage). Ceftriaxone has particularly high nasal and saliva penetration and so eradicates the significant infection as well as the carriage.

In all groups including the pregnant:

Ciprofloxacin orally: Adults 500mg one dose stat, Children 5-12 yrs 250mg stat, 1month – 4 years 125mg stat.

Alternatively:

Rifampicin orally:

Adults 600mg BD 2days,

Children 1-12 yrs 10mg/kg (max 600mg) BD 2days,

Neonates and infants <1 yr 5mg/kg BD 2days.

Prophylaxis of meningococcal meningitis in pregnant contact: Ceftriaxone 250mg IM stat (one dose) – not licensed so needs to be "counselled".

Meningitis is likely to occur, if it is going to, within the first 5 days of acquiring a new strain of N Meningitidis and is unlikely after 7 days. Nasopharyngeal carrier rates are 10% of the overall population going up to 25% in the late teens and early 20's. The idea of antibiotics is to eradicate the strain from the carrier and reduce the risk of infecting friends and family.

There are harmless strains of Neisseria (Lactamica and some Meningitidis) in the nasopharynx and the eradication of these may lead to a worse strain taking up residence. Better the devil you know.

If group A or C meningococcal meningitis, vaccinate close contacts within 2 weeks until chemoprophylaxis complete BUT Group C meningococcal vaccine is ineffective <2yrs and Group B organisms cause 2/3 infections. There is now at long last: the following effective meningitis vaccination against the scourge of meningococcus B:

Meningitis B Vaccine, Bexsero (Novartis) IM: 73% protection, 3 injections, 2-5 months, later booster 12-24m. Two injections for older children (>6m) with later boosters up to the age of two. No boosters after this age. This routine schedule inclusion was proposed and under what seemed interminable negotiation between DoH and Novartis when writing this paragraph in March 2014. Finally introduced June 2015.

I don't yet know what the recommendations for family and other contacts of the wild infection will be will be but I suspect they will be similar to those of meningococcus A and C.

Acute Meningitis:

Meningococcal Meningitis:

Immediate Rx: 50mg/kg Penicillin G (Benzyl Penicillin),
>10yrs 1.2Gr Penicillin,
1-10yrs 600mg,
Infant 300mg Stat.

If genuinely allergic to Penicillin, IV Chloramphenicol can be given. I carry Cefuroxime as the wait to get a purpuric child to hospital for IV second line antibiotics is worth the miniscule risk of allergy to cephalosporins. Of people who think they are allergic to penicillin 10% **are** and of these, 5-10% have a cross-reaction to cephalosporins. Meningococcal meningitis kills within minutes and whenever I have seen a drowsy or febrile child with a purpuric rash I have taken blood into a syringe, swapped syringes, put the Penicillin back through the same needle/Venflon/Butterfly followed by a bolus of Hydrocortisone. They die of septicaemia and adrenal shock if they do die. The paediatric SHO will put the blood sample in a blood culture bottle if he knows what he is doing or a sharps bin if he doesn't (I **have** seen this happen despite my telephone and written explanations). Dial 999 first, don't bother waiting for the interminable switchboard and Registrar to answer the phone before you have transport organised.

Meningococcal prophylactic antibiotics: See above

To eradicated nasal carriage of the N. Meningitidis, give to all household contacts, family and non family, all people who sleep near the index case (dormitories etc), girl/boy friend (kissing), school children in contact >4 hrs in an enclosed space, healthcare staff who may have had exposure to respiratory droplets, (arbitrarily often given as within 3 feet but how far would you risk?) Also the index case will need prophylaxis unless already treated with Ceftriaxone (to eradicate nasal carriage). Ceftriaxone has particularly high nasal and saliva penetration and so eradicates the significant infection as well as carriage.

In all groups including the pregnant:

Ciprofloxacin orally: Adults 500mg one dose stat, children 5-12 yrs 250mg stat, 1month – 4 years 125mg stat.

Alternatively:

Rifampicin orally: Adults 600mg BD 2days, children 1-12 yrs 10mg/kg (max 600mg) BD 2days, Neonates and infants <1 yr 5mg/kg BD 2days.

Prophylaxis of meningococcal meningitis in pregnant contact: Ceftriaxone 250mg IM stat (one dose) – not licensed so needs to be "counselled"

Things you may have forgotten: regarding Meningitis, Prophylaxis and Vaccination:

Hib and the Pneumococcus are vaccinated against now, Group C meningococcal vaccine is part of UK routine childhood vaccination shedule X3 from 3 months and there is at last an effective vaccine against Group B. This is Bexsero which is 73% effective and has been in the UK routine vaccination schedule from June 2015. This is a 4Ag 4CMenBVacc. immunisation, usually at 2, 4, 6 and 12 months (depending on age at first). Under 2 years Group B infections predominate but between 14 and 18 years Group C is more prevalent, occurring in more clusters. I spent much of my 80 hour weekends and duty nights on call as a Paediatric SHO and Registrar in the 70's and 80's doing lumbar punctures on babies, toddlers and children. Often four or five a weekend. It looks like my successors might have other things to do on their brief 12 or 18 hour weekend shifts soon.

Epidemiology:

W. Europe: Epidemic disease, small numbers, mainly septicaemia and children.

Sub Saharan Africa: Epidemics, mainly young adults and meningitis.

Case fatality in UK stuck at 10-20%.

In UK mainly Group B over the last 20 years much smaller numbers of Group C and Group W135.

So: Group B 2/3 of total disease, Group C 1/3 of the total disease, (school age children, young adults). Group A <2% UK disease, the vaccine can be given >3months, a single dose protects 3-5 yrs.(Routine group A vaccination not generally recommended in the UK because of the strains and low incidence in the at risk age groups).

In Africa most Meningococcal meningitis is Group A.

Meningitis vaccinations are all capsular polysaccharide vaccines and all are recommended in Asplenia.

H. Influenzae: There are 6 types but 99% human disease is B. Of the total infections, 60% are meningitis, 15% epiglottitis (pre vaccination). The vaccine is effective over the age of 2m and after 3 doses. Recommendations: <13 months 3 doses. In Asplenia and 13-48 months 1 dose.

Pneumococcal: Strep pneumoniae vaccine: Covers 80% UK strains, ineffective less than 2 yrs of age prevents 60-70% pneumococcal pneumonia but less effective against meningitis. 5 yearly vaccination of at risk population.

Haemophilus Influenzae B Meningitis:

Prophylaxis is Ciprofloxacin, Ceftriaxone or Rifampicin (See above).

Pneumococcal meningitis:

Strep. Pneumoniae is carried nasally in up to 10% healthy adults and up to 40% healthy children. Various Co Factors make an aggressive infection more likely; asplenia, HIV, Flu, smoking, COPD etc. It is second commonest in the UK to Meningococcal meningitis. It is vaccinated against as part of the routine childhood vaccination program.

Treatment: The strep. used always to be Penicillin sensitive though this is not now always the case. If you don't have time for sensitivities (which presumably, treating suspected meningitis or pneumonia, you won't) try:

Vancomycin and Cephalosporins, Levofloxacin. Possible high dose penicillin and an Erythromycin group antibiotic (a macrolide).

B Haemolytic Strep in pregnancy:

Can be up to 30% carriage, 1:1000 babies/year get neonatal disease. Mothers need prophylactic I.V. antibiotics pre delivery. DO treat strep UTIs in pregnancy. There is an increased risk if PROM>18 hrs. If a carrier, risk to baby is 1:300 and oral antibiotics don't eradicate the infection or carrier state.

Chronic/recurrent Staphylococcal skin sepsis:

Painful recurrent boils or obvious Impetigo (golden, scaly, weeping crusts) often need oral Flucloxacillin or Erythromycin for 10 days but if there seems to be nasal farunculosis or the condition is recurrent, do nasal swabs and prescribe topical nasal "antiseptics" as well: Bactroban, Naseptin, Fucidin. These are useful in a variety of situations including recurrent staphylococcal sepsis in of other parts of the body – (recurrent Impetigo, Staph. spots, axillary or perineal boils etc) when you want to remove the reservoir of infection. Also useful in this situation is to advise a capful of disinfectant in each bath for a month to help eradicate perineal carriage and the perianal application of an anti-staphylococcal cream. (Even something like Savlon will do). If the suggestion that the patient should bathe in disinfectant is a bit too much for them to swallow, prescribe Chlorhexidine Solution. (Hibiscrub) – as it doesn't smell like or have the associations of household disinfectants.

Impetigo:

Commoner in the Summer, erythematous macules, >thin walled vesicles and pustules >honey coloured crusts. Can be circinate with lesions anywhere. The usual cause is Group A b Haemolytic Strep with superinfection with Staph. Treatment is a Penicillin type antibiotic effective against Staph, Erythromycin etc

Topical treatments:

Retapamulin Cream, Altargo. Sodium Fucidate, Fucidin. Mupirocin, Bactroban. Bacitracin and Polymyxin, Polyfax.

Hibiscrub topically or in the bath for a month in recurrent Impetigo.

Cellulitis:

Amoxicillin and Flucloxacillin,

Co Amoxiclav,

Levofloxacin 500mg/day for 5 days is said to have 98% overall success.

Salmonella:

Check stools in an infected patient until one is negative or in the case of a food handler, three negative. Antibiotics are not given unless the patient has an artificial joint or heart valve or other foreign body in which case Ciprofloxacin or Azithromycin can be given for a week.

Salmonella can infect all sorts of food. "Salmonella" is actually 2000 different bacteria. Clinical infection is usually from faecal contamination (animals or human). Acquired from contaminated meat, poultry, eggs, milk, vegetables.

A 2015 outbreak in the US killed four, hospitalised 160 and made thousands ill. It was from imported cucumbers.

Campylobacter Jejuni:

Bloody diarrhoea 5-7 days. The commonest gastro enteritis prompting admission in the UK. 2/3 shop bought chicken grows Campylobacter. 280,000 Britons affected each year (but only 28% of a 2014 FSA survey had heard of it).

Reservoir in poultry, untreated milk and water. Sensitive to Erythromycin, (these days usually Azithromycin) and some quinolines.

Blastocystis Hominis:

An interesting organism of unknown pathogenicity.

An anaerobic protozoan, in 20% stool samples – used to be thought of as "probably harmless" but nowadays suspected of causing a diarrhoeal illness in some with abdominal pain etc. There are 9 or 10 species of Blastocystis found in humans but considerable doubt as to how much they are the actual cause of disease. Pigs, dogs, other humans and possibly other animals may be the infecting reservoir in any individual case. Infection is faeco-oral. There is some suspicion that it may cause chronic IBS Symptoms. If you are concerned and do get a positive stool culture in a patient who persists in not getting better, Metronidazole or Trimethoprim/Sulfamethoxazole may help.

Toxoplasma gondii:

See pregnancy and pathology section. A protozoan parasite who's main host is the cat but can infect a variety of other hosts including man. Toxoplasmosis is one of the myriad of classic flu like illnesses and one of at least three Glandular Fever like illnesses but is usually mild and undiagnosed. It can of course cause serious harm to the foetus or the immunocompromised.

Contact with soil, eating undercooked and cured meat and (probably) contact with cat faeces are infection risk factors. All to be avoided in pregnancy.

The life cycle is a sexual phase within cats then an asexual phase in any warm blooded host. Here the parasite becomes intracellular and damages muscle, brain and other tissue, being resistant to immune attack. The infected cells burst, release tachyzoites and the infection continues.

In human infection the acute flu like infection can be from days to weeks long and then leads to a latent stage. The infection can be asymptomatic but in the immunocompromised, acquired Toxoplasmosis can involve a glandular-fever like illness, a fulminant infection with encephalitis or a chronic form with retinochoroiditis, uveitis etc. The congenital infection causes extensive system wide damage to the foetus: – CNS damage, choroidoretinitis, hepatosplenomegaly, jaundice, a maculopapular rash, thrombocytopenia, cerebral calcification, hydrocephalus, microcephaly, spontaneous abortion, etc

In an amazingly clever evolutionary self enhancing quirk, toxoplasma infected rodents lose their fear of cats, are more likely to get caught, eaten and the parasitic life cycle perpetuated. You have to hand it to evolution sometimes.

Toxocariasis: (Dog and Cat Roundworm):

Is included not because it is common in UK practice but because I used to confuse Toxocariasis Catis with Toxoplasmosis. Both are cat parasites, human infection is caused by contamination with cat faeces, both cause uveitis, choroidoretinitis and they sound similar.

Toxocariasis Canis and Catis are however totally different organisms from the unicellular Toxoplasmosis – they are a nematode worm, the infection of human organs being with the larva, with a different outcome and implications.

The contamination of soil and sand boxes with cat faeces is common to the two infections however. Up to a quarter of children's sandpits are infected. The larvae pass through the gut and into the body of the unsuspecting child, lodging in almost any tissue. The larvae damage tissue via a granulomatous reaction but remain mobile and alive for some months.

There may be systemic symptoms – fever, cough, (recurrent pneumonia is possible), wheezing and you may find hepatosplenomegaly and eosinophilia, urticaria. Visceral Larva Migrans. Other clues are choroidoretinitis, ocular larva migrans (decreased visual acuity, floaters, uveitis, optic neuritis and other ophthalmic symptoms), hyperglobulinaemia. The infection is self limiting and settles in the healthy host after 6-18m. Albendazole, Thiabendazole and steroids can help.

Regular worming of pets, washing of vegetables, proper disposal of cat and dog faeces, wearing of gardening gloves all help to reduce the risk. Or, of course, get a dog.

Worms:

Threadworms (Pinworms) cause abdominal pain, vaginitis and discharge in toddlers, perianal itching and frequency. Tell the parents they can sometimes see the slowly writhing threads of white cotton by looking perianally at their dozy child at about 11.00 pm with a torch or do the Sellotape test. This is just applying a few inches of sellotape to the perianal skin, folding it up and asking microbiology to look for eggs.

Personal hygiene and frequent cleaning/washing of fomites and the hands of playmates eventually stops recurrence.

Pripsen (Piperazine and Senna) is licensed from 3m, repeat the dose after 2 weeks, safe in pregnancy and if feeding is avoided for 8 hours after dose, while breast feeding.

Vermox, (Mebendazole) licensed over 2 years. Repeat after 2 weeks. A virtually tasteless tablet. Both are OTC.

Cryptosporidium:

Another protozoan, with infections common after heavy rainfall. Found in the guts of humans and farm animals. Infections arise from visits to farms, person to person, feeding lambs, from contamination with farm yard manure, eating undercooked meats, drinking unpasteurised milk, river/pond water contamination, occasionally through swimming pools. It is a common cause of waterborne diarrhoea. The normal concentration of chlorine and the filters in public pools are not effective at eliminating cryptosporidium. Some water authorities have resorted to advising prolonged boiling or the UV treatment of water.

The infection is commonest in the 1-5 year old group and is one of the commonest causes of paediatric diarrhoea and traveller's diarrhoea. IP 2 – 14 days. The diarrhoea lasts 1-4 weeks. It is less common under 6m or over 45 years. There is abdominal pain, low grade fever and profuse watery diarrhoea. The standard wisdom is that there is no need to treat or check repeat samples as long as the diarrhoea clears up, which it will in an immunocompetent patient. The cysts however may be shed by some infected individuals for weeks after symptoms resolve. The mitochondria are DNA free (unusual in cells with a nucleus). Children and the immunocompromised are particularly susceptible. Oocysts are resistant to chlorine, most disinfectants and bleach but not to boiling for 1 minute, freezing, drying or Hydrogen Peroxide. Interestingly, even some bottled water (from lakes and rivers) may not be free from infection. Generally, spring, well or underground sources are a bit safer. The oocysts are 4-6um in diameter-so presumably they have been through the equivalent of a 0.1 – 1 micron microfilter – which should see to most other G.I. infectious organisms, Giardia included.

Outbreaks can occur occasionally from the contamination of public water supplies – after periods of heavy rainfall or agricultural contamination. It can be difficult to prevent, to detect and to treat. The otherwise reliable Chlorine seems impotent against it.

Paromomycin may be effective in some clinical cases.

Probiotics:

These days this is taken to mean a food substance or culture containing non pathogenic organisms with some sort of theoretical health benefit when taken orally.

Obviously a great deal of marketing nonsense is claimed for these products which give your gut flora an injection of "good bacteria". They MAY help improve some clinical situations like post antibiotic diarrhoea (including C. Difficile associated diarrhoea) and candidiasis. There have been postulated beneficial effects in the areas of colonic cancer risk, blood pressure (milk fermentation may produce ACEI like molecules apparently!), general immune stimulus, IBS and so on but they may also increase some forms of allergy. Two sub types of microorganisms are usually used: Lactic acid producing bacteria and bifidobacteria. In special circumstances, extract of human faeces have been used. In terms of foods, sauerkraut, Miso soup, yogurts, soft cheeses, Kefir, sourdough breads, probiotic drinks and sour pickles are all probiotic.

In the UK Actimel and Yakult are the commonest OTC products. Many probiotic tablets and capsules are available from the Internet, with a variety of doses and strains of organisms.

Diverticulitis:

Treatment is Co Amoxiclav, or a Cephalosporin plus Metronidazole, see Gastroenterology section.

SARS:

Severe Acute Respiratory Syndrome. First case was recognised in 2003, occurs in pandemics. Death Rate 4-10%. I.P. 2-10 days. Coronavirus, zoonotic, from bats. Sudden high fever, dry cough, dyspnoea, headaches, diarrhoea, respiratory distress. Beijing, Guangdong, Shanxi, Hong Kong, Toronto, Hanoi, Singapore, Taiwan. Spread by droplets, stools, surfaces. Usually fairly close contact (mainly family members, healthcare staff). 800 deaths, 8,000 infected in 2003.

CXR shows pneumonia with infiltrates. The treatment is steroids and antibiotics. But no *specific* treatment.

Yosemite: Hantavirus infection:

Yosemite National Park is a beautiful Californian National park. It has crystal clear, freezing cold rivers, wild bears, famous sheer rock faces, (Star Trek's El Capitan), sky high waterfalls and a newish viral infection called Hantavirus.

The Hantavirus causes Hantavirus Pulmonary Syndrome (HPS) with an up to 30% mortality. The recent outbreak was linked to a specific set of cabins in 2012. The virus is spread by deer mice urine and faeces and the infection occurs in poorly ventilated spaces. It is thought the outbreak was linked to a population surge in the park's mice.

The infection is similar in symptomatology to The South American Andes Virus (which is also a Hantavirus).

Novel Coronavirus:

A novel severe respiratory infection originating in Qatar, Saudi Arabia. Fever, cough, dyspnoea, IP 7 days, Contact the HPA fever service 0844 7788990 if you suspect this or any of the unusual infections mentioned.

Chikungunya:

An alphavirus common in the Caribbean and tropical Americas, India, the Far East and Africa. A mosquito borne infection causing high fever, rash, headache, muscle and joint pains. It is now being spread by local mosquitoes in Italy, the USA (Florida) and the UK (295 cases in the UK in 2014). 2-12 days after the bite the symptoms develop and there is no specific treatment. It is not usually fatal in the healthy.

Chikungunya, Dengue fever and West Nile Virus are said to be amongst the infections which will increase in future years in the UK due to "climate change".

Chikungunya, Yellow Fever and Dengue (390m/year) are spread by the Aedes Aegypti mosquito's insanitary feeding practices. As is:

Zika virus infection:

This flavivirus first described in 1947, is also spread by mosquito bites (Aedes aegypti and Aedes Albopictus) and consists usually of a typical viral infection – fever, rash, arthralgia and conjunctivitis. The acute infection usually lasts from "several days to a week or so". Viral shedding up to 15 days in urine and (AUG 2016) *at least 180 days* in semen. Possibly a lot longer. The duration of viraemia is uncertain. In may 2015 the infection in Brazil occurred for the first time but was found to be linked to Guillain Barre syndrome and to teratogenic effects in pregnancy. The main negative pregnancy associations were microcephaly, eye abnormalities (chorioretinal and optic nerve abnormalities) and miscarriage.

It is rare for a mother to infect her child after delivery, even breastfeeding. It can be spread, as you would expect if mosquito saliva and blood are vectors, through sex and transfusions. There is currently no treatment or immunisation. GPs should advise patients not to conceive for 4 weeks after returning from a Zika infected area (14 day IP plus 14 day viraemia.)

There are 25 South American countries from Barbados to Venezuela and other areas including American Samoa, Samoa, and Cape Verde where Zika has occurred. In Feb 2016 WHO announced a global Zika emergency for Brazil, partly stung perhaps by the criticism of its tardy Ebola handling the year before. In July 2016 the first infections spread by native United States mosquitoes took place in Florida. It was widely predicted that various other Gulf states would soon be home to indigenous Zika infected mosqitoes. The UK and other European countries have now (2016) seen citizens infected during travel abroad.

Flu, Influenza:

The First World War killed 21m people. The world Flu pandemic (Spanish Flu, A Zoonotic virus from wild birds) that followed, killed between 20 and 50m. 220,000 in the UK alone. 3-5% of the world's population. At least 10-20% mortality of those infected partly, it is believed due to an excessive immune reaction in the young. That was before international air travel.

If you are interested in modern art, the brilliant Austrian modernist Egon Schiele, lost his wife and unborn first child to the "Spanish Flu" in October 1918. He died of pulmonary complications himself aged 28 on the day his spouse and child were buried.

Treatment: Amantadine, oseltamivir, zanamivir.

Zanamivir, Relenza. (Influenza A and B) 2 inhalations BD for 5 days. For adults who present within 48 hours of the onset of the illness or 36 hours of exposure. This is the one to use in pregnancy.

Oseltamivir, Tamiflu Adult 75mg BD for 5 days. Start within 2 days of the first symptoms. Prevention 75mg a day. Not used in pregnancy but can be given to breast feeding mums. <1 year: 3mg/kg bd 5days. Caps, susp. soln. There is surprisingly little independent data of its effectiveness and what there is may have been for the wrong infection, drug company sponsored and somewhat biased. Apparently 60% of the research data on Tamiflu was never published (Today programme 2013).

Viral infections labelled "Flu" are actually proven flu in only 1 in 8 out of season and 1 in 3 in season. The other "Flu" infections are other respiratory viruses. I don't know how many are proper flu in "man flu" or in woman "flu".

Under 6m give olseltamivir soln 15mg/ml 2mg/kg bd or od as prophylaxis.

6m-1yr 3mg/kg bd 5days or OD as prophylaxis,

Rx:	Proph:
<15kg 30mg BD	30mg OD
<23kg 45mg BD	45mg OD
<40mg 60mg BD	60mg OD
>40Kg 75mg BD	75mg OD

Some recent reports (April 2014, a Cochrane Review reported on Radio 4) suggest that Tamiflu, stockpiled by the British Government at enormous expense (£424m), reduces the duration of 'Flu by no more than half a day and is no more effective at alleviating symptoms than paracetamol. They also mentioned the difficulty in getting clinic data from Roche and problems with trial designs and conduct.

PHE countered this (late 2014) by saying that the data for neuraminidase inhibitors was from RCTs on healthy adults not those at high risk. More recent evidence was more positive, suggesting that NAI (Neuraminidase Inhibitors not Non Accidental Injury) treatment in severe cases can reduce the likelihood of dying by 25% compared with no treatment.

Amantadine, Symmetrel, (Lysovir) is an anti Parkinson's drug which is used in the prophylaxis and treatment of Influenza A. Actually it was, historically, the other way round, an anti viral that was found to help Parkinson's patients. Treatment: 100mg daily for 4-5 days. Prophylaxis 100mg, also once daily. NICE does not now recommend Amantadine for the prophylaxis or treatment of Influenza because all seasonal flu is resistant.

Flu, vaccination and genetic mutation:

Two thirds of the circulating flu viruses in 2014-2015 (Influenza A), H3N2, differed from the H3N2 component of that year's vaccine. Therefore the vaccine was only 23% effective in protecting against laboratory proven H3N2 infection. The vaccine was even less effective (12%) in younger recipients aged 18-49. Indeed some research seemed to suggest immunised patients developed symptoms worse and longer than the unimmunised. (CDC Morbidity and Mortality Jan 16 2015). This situation is likely to recur annually with conventionally developed vaccines. There are however newer vaccine development techniques which will target more stable core flu antigens and these should lead to vaccines which are valid against multiple flu viruses, year after year. For even more surprising flu vaccine information see the final section of the immunisation chapter.

H1N1: Swine Flu

Named after the two surface proteins **Haemagglutinin** and **Neuraminidase** that are on the surface of the virus. Hence the H and the N abbreviation. These are two very useful surface proteins that help the Flu virus propagate: the haemaggluttinin (H) helps it penetrate a victim cell and enter and the Neuraminidase (N) enables a newly made virus particles to get out of the cell again. Influenza originated primarily from birds. The H5N1 appeared in humans in Hong Kong in 1997. It was endemic in Chinese open air chicken markets before this. For the most part most H5N4 flu remains a bird infection. Humans do not generate new viruses. Every so often a strain will however make the evolutionary leap to be a human disease (like the 1918 H1N1 disease). This can happen when two flu strains infect the same cell and trade genes with one another. The H5 and H7 sub groups tend to be more aggressive in people and birds. These are part of the Influenza A sub group of viruses and the H5 N1 designation refers to the RNA genetic structure expressed. Swine influenza virus is any strain of the influenza family of viruses that is endemic in pigs.

H5N1 might mutate into a form that transmits easily from person to person. If such a mutation occurs, it might remain an H5N1 subtype or could shift subtypes as did H2N2 when it evolved into the Hong Kong Flu strain of H3N2.

H5N1

Avian influenza A (H5N1) was found in poultry in Egypt in 2006 and a variety of potential travel destinations since; human cases and deaths were also reported. It usually cannot transfer from human to human, living in the lower respiratory tract, not the upper airway. It was also noted in Viet Nam in 2004, 2005. Travellers should avoid all direct contact with birds, including domestic poultry (such as chickens and ducks) and wild birds and avoid places such as poultry farms and bird markets where live birds are raised or kept. For a current list of countries reporting outbreaks of H5N1 among poultry and/or wild birds, view updates from the World Organization for Animal Health.

Up to 50% human mortality in infected human patients. Apparently it would take only 5 mutations of the virus to allow it to become airborne.

H9 viruses can become airborne as can:

H7N9

The latest (2013) avian flu. China, 2013 etc. The big worry again being if the virus mutates to spread from human to human instead of from bird to bird and bird to human.

'Flu vaccine types: are based on predicting which "mutants of H1N1, H3N2, H1N2 and Influenza B will proliferate in the following season.

2004/5 A H1N1, A H3N2 and B
2005/6 A H1N1, A H3N2, B
2006/7 A H1N1, A H3N2, B
2007/8 A H1N1, A H3N2, B
2008/9 A H1N1, A H3N2, B
2009/10A H1N1, A H3N2, B
2010-2015 ,, ,, ,,
2015 – 2016 WHO recommended: Northern Hemisphere: H1N1 H3N3, Bx2

(Southern Hemisphere: H1N1, H3N2, Bx2).
H3N2 kills a lot of elderly patients.

The 1889-90 Pandemic H3N8 or H2N2 (1 million dead).
1918 pandemic H1N1 (20-50m dead).
1957-8 H2N2.
1968-69 H3N2.
1977-78 H1N1.
2009 pandemic H1N1 pdm09.
The antivirals currently advised in acute flu infection in the vulnerable are Oseltamivir (Tamiflu), Zanamivir (Relenza) and Peramivir (Rapivab).

MERS
Middle Eastern Respiratory Syndrome Coronavirus (MERS-Co V):
First identified in 2012 in Saudi Arabia and the majority of cases originate in the Arabian peninsula – although a Korean outbreak has also taken place. Same family as SARS, a greater than 40% mortality (2013). Similar symptoms to SARS. Can spread person to person with close contact, to health care workers and in between patients. It seems that contact with camels is an infection risk but the virus is genetically similar to a bat Coronavirus. The symptoms range from none, to fever, cough, dyspnoea, pneumonia, sometimes diarrhoea, respiratory failure. The complications being worse in the elderly, those with concomitant illness and the sick. There is no vaccination and treatment is currently supportive.

Norovirus: (Norwalk like virus):
Winter vomiting virus, the commonest form of UK gastro enteritis. Faeco-oral or person to person, aerosol contamination. Infectious from as soon as the patient begins to feel ill, some can remain infectious for up to two weeks after apparent recovery. As few as 5 virus particles can cause an infection. Virus killed by heating. **Very** infectious. IP 1-2 days, diarrhoea, vomiting and flu like illness. Hand washing and alcohol rubs partly effective at reducing cross infection. Soap and water better. A million cases a year in the UK. It is rarely a life threatening illness in the otherwise fit unless the patient is at the extreme ends of life in terms of age. Headache is common and the Kaplan criteria help in making a clinical diagnosis during an outbreak: Thus:
Vomiting in more than a half of symptomatic cases
Mean IP of 24-48 hours
Mean duration of illness 12-60 hours and
No bacterial pathogen in the stool culture.

West Nile Fever:
Can now be contracted in America, North and South, the Caribbean, Canada, parts of Europe as well as Africa and so on but originally described in Uganda. A mosquito borne Arbovirus. Mortality 3%, most infections being subclinical but it did kill nearly 300 Americans in 2012. IP 3-15 days, complications include aseptic meningitis, encephalitis, flaccid paralysis, rash, lymphadenopathy, nausea, abdominal pain, diarrhoea, pharyngitis, etc. There is no specific treatment.

Dengue fever:
A Flavivirus, spread by female mosquitoes which bite by day. Common in Central

and South America, India, SE Asia and parts of Africa. 2-5 days after the bite there is a biphasic fever, then severe headache, arthralgia and myalgia. There may be a maculopapular rash, lymphadenopathy and lethargy. Bloods show eosinophilia, raised LFTs and a positive RT-PCR and IgM. Other flaviviruses are Yellow Fever, Japanese Encephalitis and West Nile Fever. Complications include Haemorrhagic Fever and Dengue shock syndrome. There is no specific treatment and DEET is the best Mosquito repellent.

Ebola: ("EVD")

First described in 1975/6, there are four viruses which cause this viral haemorrhagic fever (similar to Marburg Disease from which Ebola diverged genetically a few thousand years ago). The different varieties of Ebola can infect humans, other primates, dogs, pigs and have a case fatality of between 35% and 90%. The mean is about 70%. The reported figures vary but at least 5,000-11,000 people seemed to have died in 24 outbreaks since it was first described in 1976 up until "The worst acute medical crisis in modern times" in 2014. In fact the latest estimates were 11,000 deaths in that outbreak alone. This was mainly in Sierra Leone, Guinea and Liberia in West Africa. Other countries were affected to a lesser extent, by travel associated transmission and localised transmission (Nigeria, Spain, USA, Mali and Senegal). Most outbreaks are in Africa but monkeys from the Philippines have been affected too. The symptoms are of a high fever, a flu like illness, a sore throat, D and V, headache, sometimes seizures, coma and other serious CNS and psychiatric symptoms. There are signs of cutaneous bleeding – petechiae, purpura, haematomata etc, then a collapse and eventually death is due to DIVC and multiple organ failure.

The IP is 12-25 days (some say 2-21 days). Most patients feel ill within 8-9 days. The wild reservoir appears to be in fruit bats but once infected, there is person to person spread and contact with infected animals such as sick or dead infected primates can cause the disease too. Spread is via body fluids and prevented by proper barrier nursing/isolation. The main risk to medical staff seems to be on removing their protective clothing. There is no specific treatment. Those who survive 2 weeks have a better prognosis. A gene based immunotherapy using protein covered extracts of RNA was showing some promise in Aug 2014. Zmapp ("Zeemapp") is a collection of three monoclonal Ebola antibodies providing passive immunity.

A vaccination was hastily manufactured (Oct 2014), given to volunteers and brought in to service in 2015. In December 2016 a vaccine, rVSV-ZEBOV had been found to be highly effective in final stage trials. The West African outbreak killed 11,000 people by the time it seemed to have died down. Some survivors appear to remain infectious via Ebola staying active in various bodily fluids. Male survivors need to have semen tested at least three times before unprotected sex is safe or advised abstinence for 6m. Ebola virus is also said to persist in tears, CSF, testes, aqueous humour. There are 17,000 Ebola survivors and 20 cases suspected as being sexually transmitted. It may persist in semen and possibly tears for much more than 6 months. After the epidemic had settled, 61% of Ebola cases were found to have been caused by 3% of patients.

Typhus: (Various Rickettsia):

I add this as much out of historic and literary interest as medical relevance.

Typhus is a collection of killer Rickettsial diseases which has affected battles, sieges, prisons and social history around the world throughout the centuries. Spread by insects, lice, mites, rat fleas and ticks, various forms of Typhus are recognised – Epidemic, Scrub,

Murine, Australian etc. They result in high temperature, myalgia and headache up to 3 weeks after the inoculation by insect bite. About a week later a central rash appears, spreading centrifugally to the limbs. Meningo encephalitis, confusion, delerium and coma follow with a 60% death rate without antibiotics. The treatment is Doxycycline, Chloramphenicol etc. It is mentioned in many Victorian novels, ravaging the work-house in which Jane Eyre grew up. It is endemic in Russian literature of the 19th C. Anne Frank died of Typhus in Bergen-Belsen concentration camp. There is a vaccine.

Typhoid (Salmonella Typhi)

Called Typhoid because it resembled the infection of Typhus but is an infection due to Salmonella Typhi 1-4 weeks after the oral ingestion of the organism. It is a faeco-oral infection. Abdominal pain, headache, but NOT usually diarrhoea and vomiting is NOT severe initially. Occasionally patients may remain asymptomatic while being infectious while many develop a rash which may include rose spots. The various stages of the infection are: Fever, with epistaxis, exhaustion, bradycardia, delirium with Rose Spot rash, diarrhoea, wet chest bases, (positive Widal Test), possible GI haemorrhage or perforation, encephalitis, pneumonia and various "metastatic infections".

Typhoid vaccine, both oral and injectable exist, a number of antibiotics are effective (Ciprofloxacin, Cefotaxime, Azithromycin etc etc) and oral rehydration is critical.

Prince Albert was one victim.

Malaria:

300m cases a year world-wide 600,000 – 1m deaths (different sources) these are mainly babies in Sub Saharan Africa.

In July 2014 GSK applied for approval for the first antimalaria vaccine. RTS, S. The final stage trials showed that for 6-12 week old babies, the vaccine offered only 30% reduction in infectious episodes after 4 immunisations. It is the first anti parasitic vaccination.

1300 children die a day in Africa from Malaria.

For current malaria prophylaxis, other travel vaccination and advice, good maps of endemic areas etc, http://www.traveldoctor.co.uk takes a lot of beating.

Some recent research suggests certain bacteria in the gut microbiome protect against severe infections. (Villarino et Al. Composition of the gut microbiota modulates the severity of Malaria. PNAS. Feb 2016 DOI: 10 .1073/pnas 1504887113). The different blood groups offer degrees of protection – which may be one reason why they exist.

Tuberculosis:

Current testing regime for household contacts of TB: (NICE)

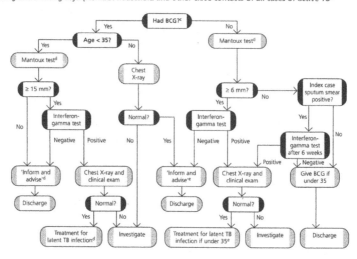

Testing and treating asymptomatic household and other close contacts of all cases of active TB[b]

NICE Clinical Guideline 33

Nice Clinical Guideline 33

Legionaires' Disease: (Notifiable:Contact Environmental Health)

Pneumonia caused by the Gr. Neg Legionella bacterium (various species within the genus). The bacterium has a symbiotic relationship with water borne amoebae and thrives at temperatures between 25 and 45 degrees C. The infection tends to occur wherever water is used to cool air conditioning systems and in the atmospheric aerosols produced. This includes air conditioning and cooling towers, humidification systems, nebulisers, even fountains and freshwater ponds etc. Occasionally, soil can become infected. The infection was first described after an American Legion meeting in Philadelphia in 1976. A sixth of the 180 who were infected died in that outbreak. The infection is usually recognised and dealt with better these days. In 2010 in the UK there were fewer than 40 deaths from 360 known cases despite there probably being dozens or hundreds of mild infections nationwide. IP 2-19 days. There is a milder Legionella infection, Pontiac Fever, which does not involve pneumonia.

The classic symptoms are those of Flu, cough, dyspnoea, fever, myalgia, rigors, confusion. Serious complications include pulmonary or renal failure and septic shock.

Patients are at higher risk if they have pre existing lung disease, immunodeficiency, over 50 age, smoke, have diabetes, drink heavily, have cancer, have a heart or liver condition.

Legionella antigens are present in urine.

The infection responds to quinolines (Levofloxacin) and macrolides (Azithromycin, Clarithromycin).

If the infection is recognised and treated soon the mortality rate can be as low as 5%.

Lyme Disease: Borrelia Burgdorferi/Afzilii/Garinii

A spiroch(a)ete. Tick borne, -the most common tick borne northern hemisphere disease, named after a town in Connecticut. Ticks are second only to mosquitoes as the commonest insect vector of disease in man. Several hundred cases in the UK every year-813 in 2008. As Lyme is not notifiable the total is probably much higher. A stunning 300,000 cases in the USA diagnosed in 2013! Returning travellers are 15-20% of the total. An initial fluey illness with Erythema Migrans, a bull's-eye rash at the site of the bite. The annular erythema gradually spreading outwards is then followed by the secondary stage. An early systemic phase including neurological and cardiac symptoms is followed months later by central and peripheral nerve symptoms, muscle and joint as well as dermatological disorders.

The diagnosis is by serology. The treatment: Doxycycline (200mg/day for 1m, some say 100mg BD 14-21 days) or Amoxycillin, a big dose, for a long time. So a lot of antibiotics however you look at it.

The symptoms depend on the time post bite and whether the infection has been aborted with antibiotics. **Beware:** There is a phase before the immunology becomes positive during which the patient may feel wretched with headache and myalgia and have a good idea that they have Lyme. The rash then confirms it, the immunology may even be last. If there is a strong suspicion, a compatible travel history and the patient is ill, just start the antibiotics.

Erythema (chronicum) migrans 5-28 days after tick bite, flu like symptoms, tiredness, myalgia, headache, fever, neck stiffness,

Some weeks later:

myalgia, tiredness, inflammatory arthritis, facial palsy, numb peripheries, poor memory, poor concentration, even changes in personality, sometimes meningitis.

Late – months or years later:

tiredness, poor memory, poor concentration, lowered mood, cardiac complications, parasthesiae, joint pain, rashes.

Coxsackie Virus: (One type of Enterovirus):

Hand foot and mouth (Coxsackie A16 and Enterovirus 71):

Virus in blister fluid, saliva and stools. 3-7 day IP. Low grade fever and headache. Vesicular lesions on hands and feet, occasionally buttocks. The mouth lesions are yellow ulcers with red borders, on tongue, lips, gums, buccal mucosa and palate. Lasts 3-10 days, aseptic meningitis a rare complication:

(Enterovirus 71 can cause paralysis, meningo-encephalitis, pulmonary oedema, myocarditis).

Other Coxsackie infections:

Cardiomyopathy, M.E., Herpangina group A, Summer grippe, Pleurodynia (Bornholme disease) Coxsackie B, Aseptic meningitis, Severe neonatal infection.

Coxsackie is a town in Greene County New York, named after the native American for "Owl's hoot". This was where the virus was first isolated. Pieter Bronck was one of the first Coxsackie settlers (In the "New Netherlands" area). The Bronx in New York is named after him.

Human Parvovirus:

B19 **Slapped cheek or 5th Disease**, Erythema Infectiosum. Erythematous raised rash on cheeks, lace like symmetrical pruritic maculopapular rash on external surfaces, palms, soles, buttocks. Resolves in 10-12 days. Can cause foetal hydrops or adult Glandular Fever type illness. 50-60% of adults have had the disease at sometime and are immune. By the time the rash appears the infectious period is over. The symptoms of the infection are usually fairly mild with headache, fever and arthralgia.

If infected in the first 20 weeks of pregnancy, 9% risk of miscarriage. If infected 9-20 weeks, there is a 15% risk of miscarriage and also a 3% risk of hydrops (treated by intrauterine transfusion).

Koplik's spots may be noted in Parvovirus infection just as in Measles.

Roseola Infantum, Exanthem Subitum-Sixth Disease

Herpes Virus Types 6 and 7.

I.P. 9 days. Common cause of febrile convulsions in children. High fever, sub occipital lymphadenopathy, morbilliform rash.

Mumps:

IP 15-25 days from contact until the start of Parotitis

```
<--------------------------------------------><---------syptoms 7-10 days------->
             <--Infectious 2-7 days before and several days after parotitis-->
```

The mumps can mean a fit of melancholy or sulking, depression in spirits. Mumping is also cheating, taking bribes, bad behaviour or overreaching. I presume parotitis is called "Mumps" because of the lowered mood rather than the bad behaviour. Mind you there was the MMR scandal – that was pretty bad behaviour.

I.P. 15-25 days, exclude from school for 5 days after swollen glands. Parotid swelling in 95%, usually bilateral, occasionally unilateral, 30% cases subclinical.

Complications: Orchitis 20%, oophoritis 5%, aseptic meningitis 15%, encephalitis (clinically significant) 1:6000, permanent deafness 1:15,000, pancreatitis 5%. ITP and increased risk of first trimester miscarriage, no harm to foetus otherwise.

Confirmation of infection is via an HPA saliva testing kit, specific IgM or viral culture from saliva. There is no increased teratogenicity but there is an increase in miscarriage in the first trimester of pregnancy.

Pertussis: (Whooping Cough)

IP 6-20 Days   Catarrhal, paroxysmal, convalescent, 6-8 weeks, often longer

```
<------------------><--------------------------------------------------------->
```

"The one hundred day cough"

Bordetella Pertussis, Gram negative rod, (but also a parapertussis and adenovirus possible interaction). IP 6-20 days, highly infectious, most deaths <1 year, various stages: Catarrhal, paroxysmal, 2-4 weeks, – Paroxysmal cough and whoop, convalescent stage. Marked peripheral leukocytosis.

Complications: Pneumonia, bronchiectasis, O.M., S.A.H., I.V.H., hernias, etc. Erythromycin can shorten infectivity and can abort the disease if given early enough.

Prophylaxis for Close Contacts:

There were >8,000 UK cases of Whooping Cough notified in 2012 (Heath Protection report), 38,000 in Australia in 2011, >8,800 in New Zealand since 2011, >40,000 in the USA in 2012 etc.

Treat with Erythromycin/Clarithromycin. Erythromycin 50mg/kg/day in 3 doses for a child, or 500mg tds for 10 days in adults – and finish incomplete courses of vaccination. Macrolides are only of any use in preventing transmission if given within 21 days of exposure so they should only be given within that window unless you are treating a secondary infection.

See Paediatrics and Immunisation – The highest mortality and complication rate of infection is <6m of age, especially those not fully vaccinated and most deaths are <3m.

People born before 1996 did not routinely receive a pertussis preschool booster and so most adults and older children are only partially immunised. This means they can catch it but also they present a risk of transmitting whooping cough so should receive chemoprophylaxis if in contact with an index case.

Confirmation of infection can be done by sputum culture. The per-nasal swab is however, pretty unpleasant to perform technically. Sputum is viscid and hard to come by – or by serology for polymerase chain reaction (PCR) testing. The oral fluid test (from your Health Protection Unit) is done brushing along the gum line as in DNA sample collecting etc. This is the anti PT IgG test and is for anyone coughing for more than 2 weeks.

Immunity is waning in the adult population and Pertussis is now a common cause of persistent cough in adults. They can have mild symptoms but they are still infectious. Do the tests on any adult with a persistent cough, not just on children.

More advice on management of the various contacts, how long to keep them isolated and off school etc. from your local Health Protection Unit.

Pregnant women are now recommended to have their immunity boosted between 28 and 38 weeks so that their newborn child is not at risk before their 2, 3 and 4 month routine immunisations kick in.

In 2012 there were 10,000 confirmed cases – the last "peak" being only 900 in 2008. This latest surge killed 14 babies under three months, hence the move to vaccinate pregnant women. By June 2015 the figures showed 1,744 cases for the year. The newborn of immunised mothers have been shown to have a 91% reduced risk of contracting pertussis. The uptake in White British, Chinese and Indian ethnic groups being good, the lowest in "Black and other ethnic groups" according to the DOH.

The new acellular 2004 vaccine may be part of the problem. It contains specific bacterial surface proteins acting as antigens and does not promote as long an immune response as the whole cell vaccine. Also these specific surface proteins on the Pertussis organism are mutating at a faster rate than some of its other surface proteins and so the bacteria are evolving quickly to evade any vaccine stimulated immune response.

In this infection arms race our options are to improve the range and variety of surface proteins in the vaccine or to add novel adjuvants to the vaccine. But obviously the patient has to get on and have the vaccine first.

Scarlet Fever:

(Also known as Scarlatina although many people use this to describe any sore throat and pink rash)

<- IP 12 hours to 7 days-><-Illness 2days-><- Rash lasts 3-4 days--><desquamation up to 1m->

In 2013 there were 4,600 scarlet fever cases. These then started rapidly increasing, apparently surprising everyone with 15,600 cases in 2014, reaching 17,586 by 2015. These were the highest weekly totals in 33 years. Just for once this infectious disease resurgence was not due to poor immunisation uptake levels. Between 1900 and 1930 Scarlet fever was a common serious infectious illness with levels topping 100,000 a year. There is no new 21st century strain of organism involved, – it is the same strep now as a hundred years ago. These numbers are continuing to rise in all four countries of the UK (2016). Expert bacteriologists were said to be "flummoxed" in one medical journal. Well, they must be easily flummoxed. In April 2017 it was announced that community disease surveillance had detected that tonsillitis admissions had increased by more than any other common illness over the previous few years, a staggering 68%. For at least the last five years primary care physicians have been systematically brow beaten and blamed by everyone from national news paper journalists to politicians, local prescribing groups to hospital bacteriologists because of their prescribing antibiotics for "routine" infections. Although clearly not the main cause of resistant hospital and community infections, GPs were seen as an easy targets compared with factory farms, vetinary practices, OTC antibiotics abroad and multiple and prolonged hospital antibiotic regimes. For decades GPs had been prescribing Penicillin V if they had any sense – and broader spectrum antibiotics if not for the thousands of community patients they saw each year with painful red throats and cervical lymphadenopathy. The more compliant and unquestioning almost instantly and unselectively stopped when told to do so. Unfortunately, the message that many GPs garnered from this constant criticism is that most, if not all patients, no matter how ill, no matter how bad their pharyngitis, no matter how gross their cervical lymphadenopathy, or their chest signs, ONLY HAVE A VIRUS INFECTION. The question is not why is Scarlet Fever now becoming so common but why was it so rare for the last several decades? The answer is the same one as to why was quinsy, intracranial abscess, pulmonary abscess, empyema, erysipelas, Rheumatic Fever and all the post streptococcal illnesses relatively rare for the last few dacades? Because GPs had been relatively generous with penicillin. No need for flummox any more. Indeed I wrote to one medical journal at the start of the epidemic explaining it and predicting other "puzzling" increases in community bacterial infections (ie deaths from paediatric "sepsis") which will come to light over the next few years.

Scarlet fever is a pharyngitis and fever caused by Group A B Haemolytic Strep infection. The organism produces a toxin which causes the erythema – hence the scarlatiniform rash. It is spread by droplet transmission and infections are usually in Winter and Spring. Roughly 10% of the infected population develop scarlet fever.

The symptoms include sore throat, headache, fever, vomiting, abdominal pain and then the rash appears a couple of days after the first symptoms. Apart from the exudative tonsillitis there are soft palate petechiae and tender cervical nodes, a pink face with perioral pallor and the scarlatiniform rash. The Pastia sign is lines of confluent petechiae along skin folds. The rash then fades after 3-4 days and peeling of the palms begins.

The tongue goes from "white strawberry" (a white coat with red papillae) to the "red strawberry tongue" which is the raw appearance after desquamation.

Complications include quinsy/abscess, generalised or upper respiratory sepsis, OM, Rheumatic Fever, post streptococcal Glomerulonephritis, pneumonia etc and the treatment is Penicillin for 10 days.

Differential diagnoses include:

Fifth disease, Rubella, Rubeola, Tonsillitis, GF, Erythema Toxicum, toxic shock, Kawasaki, drug side effects, rat bite, acute LE. etc

By 2016 Scarlet Fever levels were increasing and set to break annual records for the third successive year. This was, according to various Department of Heath announcements and academic articles, as I said, inexplicable. Scarlet fever is an unpleasant illness with a number of unpleasant post streptococcal sequelae and had been a relatively rare condition in the three or four decades up until 2010. The medical news paper headlines in early 2016 expressed bafflement and confusion at this resurgence of an old fashioned illness. Why was it happening? The reappearance of this all but forgotten historic scourge followed hard on the heels of the national daily news papers criticising GPs and casualty doctors for failing to recognise "SEPSIS". They portrayed this vague term as if it were a single condition, which badly trained doctors were failing to recognise and treat, showing photographs of numerous toddlers who had been seen with early symptoms of "infection", sent off "without lifesaving antibiotics" only to die at home".

Their message was clear. Doctors, far from over treating nearly all patients with antibiotics as they once did – and causing "resistant superbug infections" were in fact now withholding appropriate antibiotics when they could be saving lives. From one extreme to the other.

Indeed, there was a very definite propaganda war whose purpose was to restrict GP antibiotic prescribing, which had won over virtually all newly qualified and inexperienced junior doctors by the mid teens. Especially those who had little experience of paediatric intensive care or significant hospital experience of sepsis. By 2015/2016 our GP journals were full of praise for practices which off loaded the management of minor infections to nurse practitioners who had rigid diagnostic protocols and a mission to refuse antibiotics to as many patients as possible. The patients all hated this of course and gave uniformly negative feedback to these practices – but these partnerships did reduce their antibiotic prescribing. I wrote to one medical magazine which had a front page headline on The Scarlet Fever Epidemic and a smaller article about just such a parsimonious practice next to it. I asked for the practice's Scarlet Fever, quinsy, COPD complications and post Streptococcal glomerulonephritis rates.

The reason Scarlet fever is coming back is the same reason more children are dying of septicaemia and intracranial abscess, AND I would imagine older patients dying with bronchopneumonia, septicaemia, getting post streptococcal complications, possibly even Rheumatic fever. It is simple and obvious. We are now not prescribing sufficient antibiotics. GPs are not thinking for themselves enough, they don't treat each patient individually enough, they don't strip off and examine every patient with a temperature to exclude serious infections and instead too many of us assume every patient with a febrile illness these days has a benign infection. Because we have been told we must reduce our antibiotic prescribing we simply refuse antibiotics to virtually every patient. Because of this nihilistic mind set, I am sorry to say, many of us don't even examine patients thoroughly enough to exclude a serious infection. At least, so say my patients and the front pages of many papers.

It seems that a large number of GPs are good at implementing policies – prescribe less, prescribe more, without understanding and applying the right rules to the right patient. It is hard to properly assess 40 febrile patients each day and decide which of them needs an antibiotic. It takes time, experience, patience and skill. But that is what good GPs do. Clearly too many of us are over diagnosing viral infections, taking unforgivable and lazy short cuts and missing Scarlet Fever and septic children at the moment and that is at least as bad as giving every viral pharyngitis patient a course of penicillin.

Well, this may be overstating the case a little but isn't that far from the truth. The failure of today's GP and hospital doctors to examine patients thoroughly is dealt with at length elsewhere. Also the over dependence on point of care testing investigations which have many "inapplicabilities" and impracticalities and can over reassure if done too early in an illness or not repeated often enough.

In my opinion my profession's most difficult job is and has always been to see endless numbers of relatively well patients and to assess them properly, giving antibiotics to all those who have signs of bacterial infections and an open door or a prescription with instructions to those who have poor histories, susceptibilities, or inadequate supervision. In these days of poor out of hours cover the consultation has to include a full examination, a management plan and instructions for the next few days. A simple "It isn't a bacterial infection, it doesn't need an antibiotic" has caused the "Sepsis" deaths and the Scarlet fever epidemic. It will also be causing a spike in the incidence of purulent OM, quinsy, meningitis, purulent LRTI and so on, very soon.

Erythema Multiforme:

A "hypersensitivity" reaction to drugs and infections etc. Common in childhood. Causes include Herpes virus, Mycoplasma, Coxsackie, Echo and Influenza viruses etc. Mumps, Salmonella, Diphtheria, Haemolytic Strep, TB. Also penicillins, tetracyclines, sulphonamides, barbiturates, aspirin, some vaccines, as well as collagen diseases etc !! Obviously no one in their right mind would be giving aspirin or tetracyclines to children.

Stevens Johnson Syndrome is where the skin and two mucous membranes are affected. The rash is symmetrical, it crops, mainly on the limb extensor surfaces, but this can involve anywhere except the scalp. The rash can be macular, papular, nodular or urticarial. There can be bullous lesions or bizarre urticarial plaques. Intradermal haemorrhage and petechiae are common, Iris or Target Lesions are pathognomonic. Oral lesions in 25% rapidly become ulcers. Skin lesions crop for up to 3 weeks and any treatment is directed at the cause (eg steroids etc).

Toxic Epidermal Necrolysis (Lyell Disease):

Is a hypersensitivity reaction with the same causes as E Multiforme. There can be a 25% mortality though. Fever malaise and local erythema as well as skin tenderness are seen, there can be bullae and peeling of large sheets of skin (with the Nikolsky sign). The conjunctivitis and oral lesions are similar to Stevens Johnson Syndrome.

Staphylococcal scalded skin syndrome (Also called toxic epidermal necrolysis but this is Ritter Disease):

A prodrome, then erythema of the face, neck, axillae and groins, wrinkling bullae and Nikolsky sign again. Facial oedema and perioral crusting. The treatment is the staphylocidal penicillins, not steroids.

Thrush/Fungal Infections:

Nail infections include Trichophyton Microsporum and Epidermophyton.

Oral Treatments:

Fluconazole, Diflucan caps: (Also for cryptococcal and coccidioidomycosis infections). Chronic/recurrent vaginal thrush, Fluconazole 50mg od for 1 week each cycle.

For oral and oesophageal thrush, 100-200mg daily until better. Various dosage regimes for other susceptible infections.

Has been used in breast feeding mothers (150mg stat plus or minus 50mg bd for 10 days).

Itraconazole, Sporanox caps: Indications also include Aspergillosis. Exacerbates the oedema of Calcium Channel Blockers, interacts with Warfarin, Statins, etc.

Dose for simple vaginal thrush 100-200mg daily or more commonly 100mg ii BD for 1 day.

Pityriasis Versicolor 100mg caps 2 daily for 7 days.

Tinea Corporis 100mg 1 cap OD for 15 days or 200mg OD for 7 days.

Tinea Pedis/Manuum 100mg 1 cap OD 30 days.

Oropharyngeal Candidiasis 100mg – 200mg Caps OD 15 days.

SPORANOX PULSE:

2x100mg Caps BD for 1 week then no treatment for 3 weeks.

Rx 2 cycles of the above for Tinea of Finger nails,

3 cycles for Toe nails.

Ketoconazole, Nizoral: Use if intolerant to the two above, 200-400mg daily.

Griseofulvin 500mg, 1000mg Interactions with OCP, anticoagulants, avoid in pregnancy. The only licensed option in children, however Terbinafine is considered first line in children because of efficacy and shorter treament.

Lamisil, Terbinafine 250mg daily (and a cream is available). Effective against the cell walls of Dermatophyte fungi. Can be used down to 4 years of age by mouth. Finger nail infections: 90% clear in 6 weeks, Tinea Pedis skin infections take 6 weeks, toe nails 82% have responded in 3 months. 1:250,000 have significant liver problems.

Nails grow at an average rate of about a one cm in 3 months, though there are many factors that influence the rate. Index fingernails grow faster than little fingernails and toe nails are a quarter the speed of fingernails (ie 1mm a month). You should be able to review progress and see new normal looking healthy nail at the Lunula at 3 months and decide whether the fourth month of treatment is necessary.

Lamisil cream is good for thrush, Pityriasis Versicolor, Ringworm, Athlete's Foot. It can also eradicate chronic fungal nail infection if rubbed into the nail bed daily, diligently after baths or the gym (soft nails, so more porous) for a few months.

Tioconazole, Trosyl, solution is applied twice daily to infected nails. Amorolfine, Loceryl, lacquer is applied twice weekly (I suggest Monday and Thursdays usually so patients don't over treat or forget).

Nystatin Susp 100,000 Us/ml. 1ml QDS.

Daktarin oral gel, Miconazole. Always worth trying in the common clinical situation of the steroid inhaler using asthmatic with heartburn. Particularly if broad spectrum antibiotics have been given too. Swallowed steroid frequently causes oesophageal thrush and the symptoms can be dramatically relieved with this orangey mash-potatoey tasting gel.

Vaginal thrush:

Pessaries:

Clotrimazole, Canestan, 200mg X3 or 100mg X6. 500mg x1. Canestan Combi (500mg Pessary and cream). Make sure the male partner uses the cream twice a day for a week, under the foreskin, or mention that the symptoms will come back.

Econazole, Ecostatin, Gyno-Pevaryl: Pessaries (150mg) and cream.

Fenticonazole. Gynoxin vaginal capsule. 200mg, 600mg, cream.

Splenectomy:

Risk of infection from Strep Pneumonia(e), Neisseria Meningitidis, Haemophilus Influenzae, etc, which is lifelong. Give daily Penicillin prophylaxis to age 16, some say for life but at least for the first two years after – particularly if young – all a bit confusing and different authoritative sources are contradictory.(Penicillin 125mg OD or BD up to

6 yrs then BD from 6-16 yrs, Erythromycin 250-500mg BD if Penicillin allergic). There is no consensus as to whether a BD dose is actually better than once daily in childhood. In adulthood the risks of infection 2 years after splenectomy have reduced to a point where regular antibiotics may not be advisable so there is no black and white position on this either. Over 2 years, immunise with 23 valent Pneumococcal polysaccharide vaccine, revaccinate in 5-10 years. (Pneumovax 2). Also recommended is vaccination against HiB and Meningococci Groups A and C-Meningivac – Boost 3-5 years. Also at higher risk of Malaria. Vaccinate against flu annually too because of the risk of piggy back infections. Some sources say you should make sure the splenectomised patient has a supply of antibiotics (Amoxicillin is suggested as it is absorbed quicker than Pen V and has a longer shelf life) with instructions to take at the first sign of a raised temperature, if the patient is no longer on regular prophylaxis.

Our local DGH handout on splenectomised patients recommends for all surgically splenectomised patients and patients with **"functional hyposplenism"** (this can happen in situs inversus, glomerulonephritis, SLE, RhA, graft vs host disease, sarcoid, alcoholic liver disease, hepatic amyloid, some patients with coeliac and inflammatory bowel disease etc) that all patients should have the pneumococcal vaccine 5-10 yearly, they should be kept up to date with HiB vaccine, Meningococcal and flu vaccines, their notes documented and they should have lifelong antibiotics.

Also that if the patient presents febrile and unwell, **hospital admission** should be considered after a blood sample taken (send the syringe in with the patient) and before the IV bolus of Penicillin G is given – (as in meningococcal septicaemia). Bear in mind that if you are treating the patient at home, Amoxicillin **is** actually absorbed better than Pen V. Also don't forget that malaria is a much more serious infection so emphasise the importance of proper prophylaxis and preventative measures abroad, that dog bites should be treated promptly with Co Amoxiclav and that even tick bites need to be taken seriously.

Given the possible effects of life-long antibiotic prophylaxis on the patient's gut flora (biome) and what we now know are the previously unexpected health consequences of even short courses of antibiotics, I wonder if anyone has looked into the adverse effects of lifelong antibiotics in this clinical situation?

Zoster Immune Globulin: Z.I.G.in potential Varicella Infection:

Named patient basis for those at risk of severe infections, (chemotherapy, Leukaemia, cell mediated immunity problems, pregnant mothers, steroid treatment, neonates, HIV etc). Given as a single IM dose, 125Us/10kg body weight. Within 4 days of contact, protection lasts 4 weeks.

Generally held and managed by the BTS.

A.I.D.S/H.I.V.

Is a single stranded Zoonotic RNA Virus originating in central African chimpanzees which makes RNA using reverse transcriptase. HIV has a surface glycoprotein which binds to the CD4 antigen on the cell surface of the host and this antigen is an essential part of the mechanism of the infection.

Characteristics of the infection include opportunistic infections and neoplasms. Persistent generalised lymphadenopathy is epidemiologically associated with AIDS.

Pneumocystis Carinii pneumonia   Cervical cancer
Cerebral (etc) Toxoplasmosis   Kaposi's Sarcoma

Cryptosporidial diarrhoea   Lymphomas
Chronic thrush infections
Coccidioidomycosis
CMV
Herpes Simplex and Zoster
TB
Recurrent pneumonia
Recurrent Salmonella septicaemia
Other conditions related are:
HIV dementia and wasting syndrome, progressive multifocal leukoencephalopathy.

35 million people "live with HIV" although global AIDS related death and new infections have fallen by a third in the last decade "Raising hopes of beating the killer disease by 2030" Said the UN in August 2014.

H.I.V. Prophylaxis: Initiate from 1 hour to 72 hours after presumed infection risk, (**Can** be begun up to 2 weeks after) continue for 28 days.

The actual risks after a needle stick injury are extremely low: 3/1,000 percutaneous, <1/1,000 mucocutaneous (Eye, nasal and oral mucosa etc). There were 150,000 needle stick injuries reported in the U.K. in 2000. The latest official figure is 600,000-800,000 annually of which half "go unreported" HHS.gov

There is a slightly greater risk if actual blood or deep injury from the source were involved, a hollow needle transmitted the body fluid, or a vein or artery were known to have been punctured. Obviously the source can be assessed for likely risk of having been a carrier of HIV or any of the Hepatitis viruses. The at least 5 or 6 needle stick scratches I have received over my 40 years were from patients I considered to be of extremely low risk. It is amazing how easy it is to scratch yourself with a suture needle or while blood taking or injecting if you aren't focussing 100% on what you are doing.

Current PEP (post exposure prophylaxis 2015) is

One Truvada tablet (245mg Tenofovir and 200mg Emtricitabine) one tablet OD (this is the tablet currently used also as **pre exposure prophylaxis**: PrEP, a daily pre exposure prophylaxis regime for high risk individuals)

plus

Two Kaletra tablets BD (these are 200mg Lopinavir and 50 Ritonavir). Possible drug interactions.

This regime is for occupational and non occupational exposure and should last for 4 weeks if possible – there are many side effects.

Check HIV status (antibody with EIA) 12 weeks after the end of the prophylaxis.

Alternatively:

4 weeks of Zidovudine (600mg/day in 2-3 divided doses) (ZDV or AZT, as in Dallas Buyers' Club) and Lamivudine (150mg BD)

Expanded   regime: As   above   plus Indinavir 800mg tds. Nelfinavir 750mg TDS,

Interferon Ribavirin prophylaxis decreases risk by 40%.

Start as soon as possible but may be effective up to 2 weeks.

Risk assessment Tool after a sharps injury: (a guide)

Injury

Superficial, No inoculation   0

Inoculation	2
Condition of sharps	
Clean	0
Contaminated	1
Type of sharps	
Solid	0
Hollow	1
Used for	
Sutures/IM/SC	0
Venous/Arterial access	1
Route of entry	
Skin intact	0
Skin broken	1
Mucous membrane	1
Deep penetration	2
Volume of blood	
<0.1ml	0
>0.1ml	1
Source patient	
Unknown	0
High risk behaviour	2
HIV pos	3

Score:	Risk rating:	Recommendation:
8-10	Highest risk	Yes
4-7	Increased risk	Consider prophylaxis
1-3	No increased risk	No

Non occupational exposure risks in descending order of actual risk:
Blood transfusion
Receptive anal intercourse
Receptive vaginal intercourse
Insertive vaginal intercourse
Insertive anal intercourse
Receptive oral sex.

Needlestick Injury: (Various sources of information)
Risks: Following percutaneous exposure to single positive source:
Hepatitis B 1:3
(HBeAg pos and needle-stick injury risk 19-30%
HBeAg neg and needle stick injury risk is 2-5%)
Hepatitis C 1:30
(Some sources say 2% risk after percutaneous injury)
HIV 1:319.

Infections from needlestick injuries:
Hepatitis B and C, D and G,
HIV,

HTLV I and II,
CMV,
EBV,
Parvovirus B19,
TTV (Transfusion-Transmitted Virus),
West Nile Virus,
Malaria,
Prions (incl. TSE, Transmissible Spongiform Encephalopathy).

Four healthcare workers are known to have died after occupationally acquired HIV infection, 17 healthcare workers were infected with Hepatitis C between 1996 and 2009.

Tuberculosis: T.B.

Rx: Initial phase: Rifampicin, Pyrazinamide, Isoniazid, (-Rifater) and Ethambutol for 2 months (Unless at low risk of Isoniazid resistance, when can omit Ethambutol).

Continuation phase: Rifampicin and Isoniazid (Rifinah, Rimactazid) for 4months.

Delamanid (Deltyba) is for multi drug resistant TB.

Migration and public health:

Arguably three of our most serious public health hazards, one of which we thought we were controlling fifty years ago are due to mass international migration. HIV, TB and Hepatitis B.

Unlike the quarantine procedures of New York's Ellis Island in the past, the UK has failed to screen the majority of immigrants, let alone quarantine migrants from endemic areas for infectious diseases and only slowly and piecemeal come to terms with the consequences. For instance: 95% of new Hep B cases in the UK over 2009-13 have come from abroad. It is an eminently preventable disease but our prevalence rate of 0.5% is low and this does not make it cost effective to introduce mass vaccination as the US did with such success from 1991.

US immigrants are first examined by a panel doctor of whom there are 600, based abroad. They are screened for a variety of infectious illnesses including TB. There is a list of "Communicable diseases of public health significance" – including TB, syphilis, leprosy, etc which, if present, require a waiver before the sufferer can be admitted. There is also, on the CDC website a long list of 15 immunisations which are preferred.

At present in the UK the DoH only vaccinates high risk groups (health workers, police officers, ambulance crew, families of chronically infected carriers, IV drug abusers, prisoners and prison staff, travellers to endemic areas and babies at risk from A/N screening). HBV carriage in London antenatally is 1%. The rate amongst the three largest migrant groups is 4% though migrants are interestingly not even mentioned as an at risk group on the NHS Choices website. This is not for the first time that the politics of sensitivity trumps accuracy, patient welfare and well, *the truth* in official health information. Eastern European migrant communities have similar rates of 4% of Hepatitis B and in the absence of a new compulsory triple test for all immigrants the only way of preventing ever increasing rates of Hepatitis B and the various associated liver diseases and cancers seems to be universal vaccination.

Isn't it time all migrants were screened for the "big three" infections before being granted any right of entrance? When will the right to life and health of the community as a whole trump the political sensitivities of the minority groups linked to a particular public health problem?

Hepatitis HbsAG prevalence in 161 countries was examined by WHO in 2015: Seroprevalence was 3.61% worldwide with the highest endemicity in Africa (8.83%) and the Western Pacific region (5.26%). The prevalence ranged from 0.2% (Mexico) to 13.6% (Haiti) in the Americas and 0.48% (Seychelles) to 22.4% (South Sudan) in Africa. Globally 248m individuals are HBsAG pos.

Likewise, London is now the European centre for TB and drug resistant TB. Every day 7 Londoners develop TB. I need hardly tell you that this disease was disappearing from the UK until it opened its borders to unscreened immigrants from every part of the world.

Literature of the last three hundred years is full of the death and suffering this disease caused before effective drugs became available. Art and Literature of the last few centuries is full of the acid fast bacillus, for both protagonists and subjects: La Boheme, The Lady of the Camelias, La Traviata, (Nicole Kidman in Moulin Rouge), The Constant Gardener, Crime and Punishment, Les Miserables, Angela's Ashes, Doc Holliday, Emily Bronte, Elizabeth Barrett Browning, Robert Burns, Chekhov, Robert Heinlein, Keats, DH Lawrence, Orwell, Ruskin, Walter Scott, Robert Louis Stevenson, Dylan Thomas, Gauguin, Elizabeth Siddal (Millais' Ophelia), Chopin, Purcell and so on.

A new report in 2014 disclosed the fact that the UK will have more TB than the USA (Population 62m. versus 317m. ie five times bigger than us) by 2015. TB is second only to HIV as a world "Single agent killer" with 8.6m people ill and 1.3m deaths each year. A report in 2015 gave it equal billing.

2 Bn people in the world have latent TB.

The drug resistant regime consists of 19 pills daily, 14,000 in all, if the patient is compliant, with a variety of permanent possible side effects – neuropathy, renal and hepatic damage, visual and hearing impairment.

In 2012 there were 8729 cases in the UK, with approximately one person dying each day. Although many indigenous Londoners and residents of other cities are contracting TB from their fellow city dwellers due to mass transit, social and work contact, 7 out of 10 sufferers were born outside the UK. The areas where the infection is commonest is, of course, where immigrants from certain parts of the developing world settle en masse. Haringay, Brent, Newham, Birmingham, Coventry, Manchester, Leicester (Public Health England). If you happen to live in those high risk areas but are from the host population, under current rules you and your children probably won't be given a BCG. I repeat, it is a medical imperative now, surely, that all prospective settlers from these areas should be screened for all the three killers above **before leaving their homeland.**

The Health Protection Agency reported in 2014 that 31,800 black African men and women have HIV infection in the UK. This is a prevalence of 26/1000 African born men and 51/1000 African born women. Of the 1,522 black Africans newly diagnosed with HIV in 2012, 66% men and 61% women were diagnosed at a late stage of infection. – Begging the question How many others had they infected?

Antibiotics:

In 1990 there were 18 drug companies actively working on new antibiotics. By 2013 there were 5. No new antibiotic families have been discovered between 1987 and 2017. (See page 678 for new developments.) Given the brevity of the exclusive licence, the ease with which drug licences are suspended due to post marketing side effects and the cost of drug development you can hardly be surprised that drug companies are focussing on more lucrative areas like chemotherapeutic, anti inflammatory, anti hypertensive, novel oral anti coagulant, lipid lowering, anti diabetic, inhaler drugs and other chronic disease modifying agents. None of these are usually given for a week and then stopped.

Research is now taking place into active immunisation against resistant strains of Salmonella and Staph Aureus rather than further strides in the antibiotic arms race.

We are constantly reminded to be more selective with how and when we prescribe antibiotics as "Bacterial Armageddon" is around the corner. The explosion of resistance from small populations of genetically evolved organisms is, of course, Natural Selection in action. Half of all the antibiotics prescribed however are dished out to increase the yield of animals in the farming industry worldwide and not the fault of doctors at all.

The last new class of antibiotic was discovered in the 1980s and if you think about it there is little incentive for drug companies to find new molecules that are more effective. Antibiotics are used for short periods and in small quantities. We doctors are all encouraged to prescribe generic alternatives, preferably traditional, familiar and cheap ones. Why would a drug company try to make a new type of antibiotic when the non generic life span of new drugs, even those which are given in long courses is only a few years? Very few people take antibiotics for long periods and therefore they are not an obvious money spinner.

More recently it turns out that the increase in antibiotic prescribing to children may be one reason responsible for the increased incidence of eczema and possibly asthma. It appears that a course of antibiotics in the first year of life increases the risk of eczema 40% with each subsequent course increasing the incidence still further by 7%. This may not however be a result of a disordered microbiome and due to the antibiotic as originally thought. Recent data suggest that it is the infections not the antibiotics that are used to treat them that are most likely the trigger for the later development of asthma (see Respiratory and Paediatrics).

Despite an increase in the hospital level of antibiotic prescribing, GPs reduced their level of antibiotic prescribing by 3.5% in 2013 (though it was still 4% higher than in 2010) according to PHE in 2014.

Antibiotics fail in 1 in 7 cases, a 12% rise in 20 years with antibiotic resistant infections killing 25,000 in Europe each year.

The backlash from patients was inevitable (December 2015) and was that they resent having to put up with agonising throats, UTIs and ear aches, which sound trivial but can be extremely unpleasant, let's face it. Patients often suffer unpredictable complications of bacterial infections before their GP will take them seriously. We know Scarlet Fever and paediatric septicaemia are increasing and I wonder what the rates of serious systemic sepsis, quinsy, intracranial extension and so on there are now compared with ten years ago? Or maybe patients don't like the way some GPs just fob them off dismissively and offer nothing in the way of symptomatic treatment or a timed prescription. The quick "you're wasting my time consultation". Public Health England may be patting us on the head but lower antibiotic prescribing is directly associated with worse patient satisfaction scores in GP patient surveys for practices and doctors. This came from a 2015 study involving 7,800 practices. Patients were less satisfied with frugal antibiotic prescribers – practices prescribing 25% fewer antibiotics getting lower satisfaction scores.

So much for the value of patient objectivity of their doctor's skills and of feedback questionnaires. Or maybe there **is** more to it than that: wouldn't it be interesting to see if the frugal prescribers had more patients attending A and E or the OOH services and being prescribed antibiotics by other doctors or who were admitted with complications?

And Bacterial Resistance:

In 2015 PHE analysed 24,000 samples from 2012-2015 to assess bacterial resistance trends.

Colistin resistance was found in 15 samples including Salmonella and E Coli.

Serious drug resistant threats were said to be C Difficile, Carbapenem resistant Enterobacteriaceae and Gonorrhoea. Drug resistant Campylobacter, fluconazole resistent Candida, multidrug resistant Pseudomonas, drug resistant Shigella and Salmonella, MRSA, Vancomycin resistant S Aureus, Erythromycin resistant Gp A Strep and Clindamycin resistant Gp B strep.

Stop press: News of a new antibiotic came in 2015: Teixobactin which was extracted from a soil organism and appears to have activity against MRSA, C.Diff and possibly even TB. For some reason researchers believe bacterial resistance will take decades to develop against this agent. Let's hope its use is restricted to human treatment and not the treatment or growth enhancement of farm animals. It is envisaged it will be administered systemically.

A brief look at the Antibiotics/Anti Infection Drugs currently available:

Penicillins,

Penicillinase resistant penicillins Flucloxacilin etc.

Broad spectrum penicillins Amoxicillin, Co Amoxiclav etc.

Antipseudomonal penicillins Piperacillin with Tazobactam etc.

Mecillinams Pivmecillinam.

Cephalosporins.

Cefradine 500mg BD QDS.

Cefpodoxime Orelox 100mg 1-2 bd.

Cefaclor Distaclor 250mg 375mg 500mg.

Cefuroxime Zinnat Orally and the very useful Zinacef systemically, a broad spectrum cefalosporin for most infections, UTIs, URTIs, soft tissue etc. Gonorrhoea 1Gr Single dose.

Cefadroxil Baxan, Adults 500mg-1g BD. The best guess first line in complex UTIs especially when you can't wait for sensitivities.

Carbapenems

Other Beta Lactams (The beta lactams being the penicillins, cephalosporins, carbapenems, and monobactams).

Tetracyclines Tetracycline, Doxycycline etc.

Aminoglycosides Gentamicin, Amikacin, Tobramycin, Neomycin.

Macrolides: Erythromycin, Clarithromycin, Azithromycin (arrhythmias in patients with co morbidities a side effect with the latter).

Clindamycin.

Chloramphenicol.

Sodium Fusidate.

Vancomycin.

Teicoplanin.

Daptomycin.

Linezolid.

Polymyxins.

Sulphonamides.

Trimethoprim.
Antituberculous anti leprous drugs.
Metronidazole Tinidazole.
Quinolones: (Nalidixic Acid was the first). Tendon pain and occasional rupture are side effects. Ciprofloxacin, Ciproxin. Ofloxacin, Tarivid (LRTI, UTI, Gonorrhoea.) Norfloxacin Utinor – Pretty good if you suspect prostatitis, give for at least 10 days. In cystitis, 3 days. Ciprofloxacin is the treatment of choice these days for Gap Year traveller's diarrhoea (given some fairly strict written caveats) and is also effective against Anthrax, Haem Infl, M. Catarrh. Strep. Pn. Mycoplasm, Legionella, Chlamydia, Gonorrhoea, (single dose). Levofloxacin, Tavanic. Skin, soft tissue infections, UTIs, sinus infections, LRTIs, incl Haemoph. Inf, Mycoplasma, Chlamydia.

Trimethoprim: Not advised in pregnancy because it is an inhibitor of folic acid and there are concerns about even the short term inhibition of this in the growing foetus. However as far as I can see, it has only been the combination in Co Trimoxazole that seems to have caused clear demonstrable harm in pregnancy. It can be given from age 6 weeks onwards (25mg bd).

Bacterial Vaginosis:

Something fishy going on:

Gardnerella: Present in 20% swabs of the vagina. Fishy odour, itching, grey, green or brown discharge. Encouraged by an alkaline vaginal pH just like thrush, so give the usual advice about letting the introitus get some fresh air, avoiding local deodorants, douching, tights and as semen is alkaline, using a condom. Treatment is not necessary just because the swab is positive but may be impossible to refuse if there is a smelly discharge. It is commoner in pregnancy but does not adversely affect the baby.

Topical treatments include: Clindamycin cream, an applicatorful nightly X3-7, "Caution in first trimester" – though not actually licensed for pregnancy.

Metronidazole vaginal Gel, Zidoval, used once at night X5.

Oral: Metronidazole (although, again, avoid in first trimester if possible. (Medscape)). Amoxicillin is safe in all trimesters if the patient is not penicillin allergic.

Trichomonas: A protozoan infection with 70% unaware of their infection. I.P usually 1-4 weeks, but can be longer. Urethritis in both sexes, vaginitis, – with a long term increased risk of cancer – both of the cervix and prostate, (-cancers are often due to chronic inflammation), white, yellow or green discharge, which, like GV, is fishy. It may be fishy to the sufferer but the cause is straight forward, – sex. TV is an STD. TV can increase premature labour, increase the risk of other STDs like HIV and although half of men expel the infection spontaneously. Women do not.

Metronidazole, oral 2000mg once ! or topical or Tinidazole. Must treat both partners.

Antibiotics in Pregnancy

Antibiotics taken during pregnancy account for only 1% of congenital malformations. Virtually every data sheet for them has the unhelpful caveat that benefits and risks must be balanced. How do you do that when two reports of malformations in pregnant rats followed the intraperitoneal instillation of huge doses of Metronidazole in the first trimester of the rat pregnancy but your patient is 32 weeks, human and has a horrible Trichomonal or Gardnerella discharge?

Categories:

In America, and since most of the information is indirect, from animal studies and probably overcautious, they use 5 categories of risk:

- Category A: Studies in pregnant women do not demonstrate any risks to the mother or foetus.

- Category B: While animal studies show no risk, human studies are inadequate or animal toxicity has been noted, but the studies on humans show no risk.

- Category C: Animal studies indicate toxicity but studies in humans are inadequate.

- Category D: There is evidence of human risk.

- Category X: There have been reported foetal abnormalities in humans.

Obviously, in all classes of drugs, the benefits of antibiotic use must always outweigh the risks.

Commonly used antibiotics

Penicillins (Category B): All the penicillins including Co Amoxiclav are said to be safe throughout pregnancy though you may need to use higher doses due to the larger extra cellular fluid volume.

- Cephalosporins (Category B): This group has not been well studied in the first trimester and should therefore not be considered the first line of treatment in this stage of pregnancy. Generally, these drugs are considered safe. I regard cephalosporins as safe in pregnancy.

- Sulfonamides (Category C): Can cause hyperbilirubinaemia in the newborn perinatally if given in the 3rd trimester. Can cause Haemolysis in G6PD deficiency. Co Trimoxazole should be avoided in the first trimester as it has been associated with foetal cardiovascular defects.

- Tetracyclines (Category D): Tetracyclines can harm the mother and foetus: The pregnant mother can develop liver fatty necrosis, pancreatitis, kidney damage. Tetracyclines can adversely affect foetal growth, discolour and damage dental enamel (and colour bones). Deciduous teeth are affected unless the antibiotic is given near term when the crowns of the permanent teeth are affected.

- Aminoglycosides (Category D): Aminoglycosides if used in the presence of low Mg, Ca or with CCB treatment may result in neuromuscular blockade. Streptomycin and Kanamycin can cause foetal deafness. Gentamicin appears not to do this.(Category C)

- Nitrofurantoin (Category B): Safe except in G6PD deficiency.

- Quinolones (Category C): Possible first trimester administration problems, ?? – Spina bifida, limb defects, hypospadias, inguinal hernias, eye, ear, skeletal and cardiac defects. Higher incidence of LSCS for foetal distress. Cartilage damage of weight bearing joints in animals.

- No human studies and no human teratogenicity. High affinity for bone and cartilage.

- Metronidazole (Category B): Although it is recommended to avoid this during the first trimester, (possible mutagen – this is controversial) there is no *known* association with foetal damage.

- Macrolides (Category B): These agents, including Azithromycin, have not been associated with birth defects and are considered safe for use in pregnancy.
- Clindamycin (Category B): This drug has not been associated with birth defects.
- Vancomycin (Category C): No congenital abnormalities have been attributed to use of vancomycin based on limited data.

Dental (etc) Prophylaxis: (to prevent S.B.E., Sub-acute Bacterial Endocarditis):

Who really knows if this is actually necessary?

In any given patient, the presence of a vulnerable heart valve may be uncertain, the risk of an adverse reaction to the medication unpredictable and even the protective value of antibiotics unknown. Even whether antibiotics actually do prevent SBE seems in question these days. This area is one of many where the prevailing wisdoms of my medical youth have been turned upside down. – In my opinion inappropriately. Antibiotics **are** amongst the safest drugs we prescribe, SBE is an awful, deceitful disease and often almost impossible to diagnose, particularly early. So why take the risk of withholding what may be a life-saving medication from a vulnerable patient? This by the way, includes the patient who is just having their teeth scaled. The American Dental Association currently recommends prophylactic antibiotics for patients with a variety of specified heart conditions but has reduced the target group, as we did, in 2007/8. Patients with prosthetic joints need not take antibiotics but the heart diseases and target patients are:

Patients with prosthetic valves or prosthetic valve repairs,

Those with a PH of SBE,

Cardiac transplant patients with a valvulopathy,

Those with congenital unrepaired cyanotic heart disease including those with palliative shunts,

Those with a prosthetically repaired congenital HD.

Note that if a patient is already on an antibiotic for any reason, you should use a different class of prophylactic antibiotic.

However:

You don't have to look far to find authoritative sources, less narrow minded and saying that:

Also at moderate risk are those with:

Isolated ASDs and previous surgical repairs of ASDs or PDAs,

Bicuspid aortic valves (which are very common and often undetected),

Acquired valve disease including Rh. heart disease, MS, Calcific AS,

Hypertrophic cardiomyopathy,

Mitral regurgitation and prolapse

and **high risk** procedures are said to include:

Tonsillectomy, bronchoscopy, GI surgery, biliary and urological surgery, prostatic and cystoscopic surgery, even urethral dilatation.

(Patient Trusted Medical Information and Support web site).

Apparently, tooth brushing, flossing and even chewing exposes patients to the risk to SBE. Despite this, NICE and the American dental and medical authorities have decided that the risk of taking antibiotic prophylaxis outweighs the potential benefits for many patients. They also give the unhelpful statement "The data are mixed as to whether prophylactic antibiotics prevent IE". (Infective endocarditis)

The NICE Guidelines remind us that bacteraemia follows not only dental procedures but Obs and Gynae procedures, including giving birth, Any bladder or UGT procedure, Any upper or lower GI procedure, Any respiratory or ENT procedure. They advise all patients with infection prone hearts to pay strict attention to dental hygiene and all articles on the subject stress that non prophylaxis is a world minority view.

But they still say antibiotic prophylaxis is unnecessary with these procedures. This, even though they concede that the rate of SBE has been increasing over time and to quote NICE again "**with a higher rate of increase after the publication of the (***revised***) NICE guideline**".

So there we have it. A rare killer disease. Almost impossible to diagnose and prove, (how often have you actually seen the retinal haemorrhages, Roth's spots, transient petechiae, Osler's nodes and other signs in SBE? and would you recognised them?), no quick diagnostic test, just interminably slow blood cultures, vague early clinical signs and a rapid, untreatable late clinical deterioration. So do you still want to refuse an at risk patient even a slim chance of avoiding that fate and would you actually be safe medicolegally if they were subsequently found to have died of SBE?

Anyway the prophylaxis is:

3gr orally 1 hour before, and 1.5g orally 6 hrs later.

If allergic to penicillin or the patient has had amoxicillin in the last month, Clindamycin 600mg 1 hour before plus 600mg 6 hrs later, or

If enterococcal organisms are potential pathogens then alternative appropriate antibiotics +/- Gentamicin (etc) may be substituted

Erythromycin 1.5Gr orally before and 500mg 6 hrs later.

For children 5-10 years half adult dose

<5 yrs, a quarter adult dose.

aged 1, 1/4 adult dose even though endocarditis is very rare below the age of 2.

To this can be added a mouth wash of Chlorhexidine retained for 1 minute.

By the way, all this applies to the urethral and gynaecological in-patient procedures too. Except the mouthwash, obviously. (– For instance: Ampicillin and Streptomycin 30 mins before and 6 hrs after **some say**).

Always avoid bacteriostatic antibiotics as prophylaxis.

Individual useful Antibiotic Regimes

In Diverticulitis: Co Amoxiclav or
    Metronidazole and Ciprofloxacin.

In Chlamydial Infection: Azithromycin 1 Gr Stat dose,
    Doxycycline 100mg BD 7 days,
    or Ofloxacin 200mg BD 7days.

In Bacterial Vaginosis: Metronidazole, 400mg tds orally or topically as vaginal gel (Zidoval) 1 applicatorful nocte X5. Tinidazole 500mg (Fasigyn, 4 stat then 2 daily for 5 days).

    Clindamycin orally 300mg qds or cream (Dalacin Cr 1 applicatorful nocte X7).

Infectious Diseases:	Incubation Period (Days)	Isolation
Campylobacter		Exclude from food handling but no need to exclude from school/nursery. Can return to school when well.
Chicken Pox Varicella:	Day 10-21	Infective 5 days before the onset of the rash until 7 days after appearance of rash or 6 days after the last crop of spots.
Cholera	Hours-5 days	Variable.
Cytomegalovirus*:	20-60	During acute Infection, probably infectious for life.
Diarrhoea and vomiting (including "food poisoning").		Do specimens if food handlers, who can return to work when one stool neg, children can return to school when symptoms resolved.
Diphtheria	1-6	Until bacteriologically negative (2-3 weeks). Family and case investigated by CCDC exclude from food handling and school until throat swabs neg.
Dysentery (Shigella)	1-7	24 hrs after the end of diarrhoea.
Erysipelas	1-2	Until Clinical recovery. B Haemolytic Gp A Strep upper dermis skin infection "St. Anthony's fire".
Fifth Disease*1 (Slapped cheek)	7-28	While unwell, though infectious period not known rash may be prolonged.
Giardia/Cryptosporidium		No need to investigate contacts. Exclude food handlers while unwell. Return to school when well.
Glandular Fever	14-50	While the patient is unwell, especially when febrile.
Gonorrhoea	2-14	During the infection.
Hand foot and mouth*3	3-7	During the acute phase. Hygiene important. Stool excretion several weeks.
Hepatitis A	14-42	Before and roughly 10 days after infection. Generally stool specimens not needed, can handle food 7 days after the onset of jaundice and can return to school when fit, at least 7 days after onset of jaundice.
Hepatitis B	42-175	Isolation of no value.
Herpes Simplex, cold sores.		Infectious through direct contact with moist lesions Very infectious until treated.
Impetigo		Exclusion until 48 hours of treatment completed.
Lice (head or body)		Infectious while patient still infested.
Measles	7-21	Until clinical recovery. Infectious a few days

		before until 4 days after onset of rash.
Meningococcal meningitis	2-10	Until meningococci absent or 24 hrs after start of antibiotics.
Mumps	14-25	3 days before swelling until swelling subsides (some say 7 days after).
Pertussis, Whooping Cough*4	7-21	Until completion of antibiotics or 7 days after exposure until 3 weeks after the onset of symptoms. Erythromycin reduces infectivity.
Mycoplasma*5	7-21	Uncertain.
Pneumococcal Pneumonia	1-3	Uncertain.
Poliomyelitis*6	7-35	Several weeks after initial infection. CCDC will investigate outbreak. All contacts to avoid work/school for 21 days or until clinically recovery. Close the class, contacts should be vaccinated or boosted. Nearly eradicated except in areas of the world where religious fundamentalists prevent immunisation.
Rabies*7	10-730	IP depends.
Ringworm (usually a fungal skin infection)		Incubation period varies.
Tinea corporis Incubation period 4-7 days		Usually Trichophyton or Microsporum fungal genera. Isolate until at least 2 days after treatment well under way (some authors say completed) but with oral and topical treatment, infectivity is likely to be less? Contagious until "the tiny blisters heal".
Rubella. German Measles*8	14-21	Until clinical recovery or: 7 days before rash until 4 days after.
Salmonella Infections		Contacts investigated if symptomatic. Food handler contacts investigated even if asymptomatic. Food handlers must have 3 neg stools, can consider return to school of asymptomatic excretors, discuss with CCDC.
Scabies (Mites)		Varies, may be infectious several weeks if not treated until mites and eggs destroyed. Exclude children until 24 hrs post treatment.
Scarlet Fever (Strep throat, Scarlatina)	2-5	Until clinical recovery or 10-21 days after the onset of the rash.

(New evidence suggests strep throats actually clear bacteriologically within 24 hours of oral penicillin and the American recommendation is that is with a **simple strep throat** they can go back to school on treatment after 24 hours. Ped Inf DisJAug 20 2015).

Shigella Dysentery		Investigate contacts if they have symptoms, food handlers need 3 neg stools. Generally contacts must be excluded from school or nursery until situation clear or 2/3 neg stools. (d/w CCDC).
Syphilis	10-90	Stages 1 and 2 and during relapses.
Tetanus	2-50	Not communicated between humans.

Threadworms enterobiasis		Exclusion is not warranted although they are infectious while worms are still alive in intestine.
Tuberculosis		Infectious up to 14 days after initiation of treatment. Exclusion for same period. Notifiable.
Typhoid (S.Typhi) and Paratyphoid (S.Paratyphi)		Investigate family and contacts. Exclude food handlers. Discuss with CCDC (3 Neg specimens). Exclude cases from school/nursery.
Typhoid Fever	7-21	Some become long term carriers.
Varicella See "Chickenpox" above.		

*CMV is a human herpes virus which is drawn to the salivary glands, may cause fatal disease in the immunocompromised, hydrops in utero. It has the ability to remain latent in the body like others in its class. It is a member of the TORCH complex (Toxoplasmosis, "Others", [ie Coxsackie, Syphilis, VZV, HIV, Parvovirus B19], Rubella, CMV, Herpes Simplex 2.

*1 Fifth Disease is Erythema Infectiosum (Parvovirus B19, also called the Erythrovirus), causing Slapped Cheek Syndrome. This may also include a fine body rash, covering also the upper arms and legs. Once the rash appears the infectivity ends. As with CMV there is a risk of hydrops particularly in the first trimester, older children and adults may get joint pains.

It is called 5th Disease because it was described historically 5th in line:

1) Measles, 2) Scarlet Fever 3) Rubella 4) Duke's Disease (Staphylococcal scalded skin syndrome, Ritter's Disease) 5) Fifth Disease 6) Roseola.

*3 Can be excreted in stools several weeks. The commonest HFM viruses are the Coxackie A and Enterovirus 71 intestinal viruses. This is different to the Foot and Mouth that decimated British cattle in 2007. HFM occasionally kills patients, usually in the far east in epidemics.

*4 Antibiotics do not directly improve Pertussis but do reduce the period of infectivity and also the frequent secondary chest infections, middle ear infections etc. The four stages are the IP, the catarrhal stage, paroxysmal stage, then the convalescent stage. Infectivity is maximum from the catarrhal stage and up to 3-4 weeks after the onset of the paroxysmal cough.

*5 Mycoplasma Pneumoniae lacks a cell wall and is one of the causes of Atypical Pneumonia (ie not Strep type pneumonia). Generally the patient has fairly few physical signs despite patchy consolidation on the CXR and often looks better than the symptoms would make you think. This is the main reason to treat a wheezy cough in spring and autumn with Erythromycin or other macrolide and not the ubiquitous Amoxicillin.

*6 Polio is most infectious 7-10 days before and after the onset of symptoms but the virus is excreted in the faeces for several weeks after the initial infection.

*7 The IP of Rabies depends upon how long it takes the virus to reach the CNS after a bite. The usual IP between bite and flu like symptoms is 2 – 12 weeks. Some have recorded IPs as long as 6 years!

8* Third Disease if you like! Although considered to be a benign disease as long as you don't give it to your unimmunised foetus, Rubella was the cause of the saddest loss of a child during my long paediatric career. This was when I had to turn off the ventilator on a beautiful little two year old curly headed girl who was in a vegetative state following

Rubella encephalopathy. The whole family, their vicar and I myself were in tears. Thank God for the MMR.

CCDC Consultant for Communicable Disease Control (or equivalent).

Notifiable Diseases: (GPs tell the local consultant in communicable diseases and he or she informs the Health Protection Agency) "Urgently" means by phone rather than by form.

Phone Number of Consultant in Communicable Disease Control..................

Currently over 30-35 notifiable diseases in total: (May need occasional updating, – feel free):

Acute encephalitis (not Scotland)

Acute viral meningitis (not Scotland)

Acute bacterial meningitis (urgent)

Acute poliomyelitis (urgent)

Acute infectious hepatitis (not Scotland, urgent)

Anthrax

Botulism

Brucellosis (urgent if UK-acquired) Gram Neg Cocco-bacilli, Brucella abortus

Cholera (urgent) Vibrio Cholerae bacteria

Diphtheria (urgent) Corynebacterium Diphtheriae

Enteric fever (Typhoid or Paratyphoid) (urgent)

Food poisoning (not Scotland, urgent – if clusters or outbreaks) actual or suspected

Haemolytic-uraemic syndrome (urgent). E Coli 157, occasionally Strep Pneumoniae

Infectious bloody diarrhoea (not Scotland unless E.coli 0157, (urgent)

Invasive group A Streptococcal disease (Scotland any Necrotising Fasciitis, urgent)

Scarlet Fever (not Scotland) Group A Strep Pyogenes

Legionnaires' Disease (not Scotland, urgent) Gram neg aerobic bacterium, Legionella Pneumophila usually

Leprosy (not Scotland or N Ireland) Mycobacterium Leprae

Malaria (not Scotland, urgent if UK-acquired)

Measles (urgent) Rubeola, a Paramyxovirus Morbillivirus

(Meningitis)

Meningococal septicaemia

Mumps A Paramyxovirus

Plague (urgent) – Yersinia, Pasteurella Pestis infection

Rabies (only urgent if seen at time of bite rather than with symptoms)

Rubella, Rubella virus

Severe Acute Respiratory Syndrome (SARS) (urgent) Coronavirus

Smallpox (urgent) Variola viruses, the last case was 1977

(Scarlet Fever)

Tetanus (urgent if iv drug user) Clostridium Tetani

Tuberculosis (urgent if health worker, case cluster or multiple drug resistance) Mycobacterium TB

Typhus (Various Rickettsia bacteria, arthropod vectors)

Viral Haemorrhagic Fever VHF (urgent), Various RNA Viruses

Viral Hepatitis

Whooping Cough (urgent in acute phase), Bordetella Pertussis bacterium.

Yellow Fever (urgent if UK-acquired) – a Flaviviridae mosquito borne virus.
AND SEE BELOW
Sometimes it may be necessary to notify such diseases as chickenpox in a nurse or doctor or Parvovirus B19 in someone in contact with pregnant women, suspected Carbon Monoxide poisoning etc. Just ask yourself if the infection will need chasing up or puts others at risk. Needlestick, HIV, CJD are all notified separately.

Older and some other lists include:
Dysentery (amoebic and bacterial)
"Infective Jaundice"
Lassa Fever
Leptospirosis
Marburg Disease
Ophthalmia Neonatorun (The concern is Gonorrhoea or Chlamydia in other words) but can also be due to HSV, (Herpes Simplex), Staph Aureus and various Streps
Paratyphoid Fever
Polio
Relapsing Fever
Scabies
Typhoid Fever
I daresay you might want to notify (and discuss some of these as well) anyway.

Target Chlamydia

Is the Government's screening campaign for young people, providing swabs for girls and urine specimen pots for boys. These are included with free post and packing and the patient is phoned or texted with their result within a few days. Generally it has worked very well. It has found a staggering 8% of the young people who did the test proved to be positive.

Chlamydia can be transmitted by oral as well as conventional sex. It can infect the rectum as well. The trouble is that 70% of infected women and 50% of infected men have no symptoms.

The symptoms when present are dysuria, urethral or vaginal discharge, pelvic inflammatory disease, epididymo-orchitis, rectal discharge or bleeding, irregular vaginal bleeding, 2% develop arthritis.

Investigations are first catch urine in men and a vulvo vaginal or endocervical swab in women. Symptomatic women should be tested for Gonorrhoea as well. Treatment:

Azithromycin 1gr stat (OK In pregnancy or use Erythromycin 500mg BD 14 days) or Doxycycline 100mg BD 7days are the alternative treatments. Obviously avoid Doxycycline in pregnancy.

There is a 10% risk of infertility in women after the first infection, 20% after the second, 40% after the third. Don't forget Opthalmia Neonatorum and pneumonia in the babies of infected mothers – so a test for cure after treatment is essential in pregnancy.

There are, by the way a number of Chlamydial Infections and subtypes:

The "Serovars" A-C cause Trachoma, D-K are genital infections but can also cause conjunctivitis, L1-3 cause Lymphogranuloma Venereum. L2 can cause proctitis in homosexuals especially in association with HIV.

Infections in Pregnancy, Neonatally and in Childhood:

Note: IgM goes up acutely, IgG later. So a current or recent infection is usually

indicated by a specific IgM. IgG crosses the placenta.

Chickenpox (Higher risk of pneumonia and encephalitis/hepatitis to the mother. The baby may be born with Foetal Varicella Syndrome, if acquired before 28 weeks and may show:

Hypoplasia or loss of a limb,

Cicatricial (scarred) lesions in a dermatome distribution,

Hydrocephalus,

Microcephaly,

Horner's syndrome,

Cataracts,

Choroidoretinitis,

Micropthalmia,

Growth retardation,

GI structural defects,

GU structural defects.

Develop shingles (28-36 weeks) or may be born with chicken pox (>36 weeks)

Genital Herpes.

```
                    10-14 days          3-4days
Measles: <----------IP----------><----Prodrome------><-------Rash--------------->
              9<--------------infectious-------------------->5
```

From time to time outbreaks or spontaneous cases occur. There were cases in unvaccinated "travellers" in Surrey in 2006 with epidemics at that time in such countries as the Ukraine, Greece and Pacific Islands. Then there was the Wakefield Scare, the fallacious accusation of an association between MMR and autism and subsequently inflammatory bowel disease. Although the accuser and the false message have been completely debunked since, there are still ethnic communities in the USA who with Wakefield's support continue to cling to MMR as the cause for mental ill health in their children. We still have the fall-out from the unimmunised cohort and at least one Measles death has now come to light. Unsurprisingly the "Daily Mail epidemiologist" parents subsequently queued around the block to get their offspring protected.

Measles, Rubeola is a paramyxovirus. The IP is 10-14 days, it is highly infectious and the symptoms are high fever, catarrh, conjunctivitis, cough and the characteristic generalised maculopapular rash which is retro auricular initially. You may see the salt grain Koplik's spots opposite the back teeth on the inside cheeks 3 days before the rash but these are often not there or are missed. The patient is probably infectious for a further 5 days once the rash has appeared.

The complications are bronchitis, otitis media (very common), encephalitis, the lethal pan encephalitis and sub acute sclerosing pan encephalitis. The death rate in developed countries is about 0.3%. It is higher in the weak, malnourished, sick for other reasons, immune deficient, those with AIDS and so on. Life threatening adverse reactions occur in less than one per million vaccinations (<0.0001%) and there is no association with autism. We can expect more deaths and long term harm from this shameful vaccine confusion. I am sure this period will become an object lesson in how biased publishing both in the medical and general press, irresponsible national radio and TV coverage and gross public ignorance of the facts can coincide to harm innocent children. Add to this the abject

political failure to confront the apparent basic human right of parents to put their own children and those of others at risk through stupidity and inaction once the ignorant but opinionated mob gets going. It is an almost exact repeat of the Whooping Cough hysteria of 30 years before. There are still adults, patients I am seeing in my surgery now with paroxysmal coughs that last for 3 months, who develop bronchiectasis because their parents read somewhere in the late 1970's that there might be a 1 in 300,000 risk of some sort of side effect through vaccinating against Pertussis.

I return to the intrinsic need for society to confront this injustice and to look after the general good of all. That the safety and health of the community trumps the human right of the individual to do indirect harm through ignorance or whim. Particularly if it is harm to those that cannot yet speak for themselves.

Rubella,

| | 14-21 days | 2 days | 3 days |

German Measles <---------IP------------><---Prodrome---><-------Rash---->
<-Infectious 1 week before to -->
1 week after the start of the rash

German Measles: RNA virus. Contracted in the first three months of pregnancy or one month before conception may result in miscarriage or the baby suffering: (The risk drops between 12 and 20 weeks.)

Congenital Rubella Syndrome which includes:

Cataracts, glaucoma, deafness, PDA, Pulmonary A stenosis and other cong. heart defects, interstitial pneumonia, microcephaly,

Intellectual delay, schizophrenia and autistic spectrum disorders, motor disability, hepatosplenomegaly, blood and bone disorders, Diabetes.

There is little or no prodrome in Rubella but there is obvious lymphadenopathy, cervical, posterior auricular and sub occipital. Joint pains may be present and the fine rash which starts on the face and neck spreads to the trunk and limbs. Several paediatric infections show petechial spots on the hard palate and these are present in Rubella (Forsheimer's spots). Neuritis, encephalitis and thrombocytopoenia are rare complications. The last child whose ventilator I switched off died of Rubella encephalopathy.

Group B Strep which can cause septicaemia, pneumonia and meningitis in the neonate. 30% carriage, 1:1000 babies a year get neonatal disease, mums need prophylactic IV antibiotics pre-delivery. Do treat Strep UTIs in pregnancy. Increased risk if premature ROMs >18 hrs. If a carrier, the risk to the baby is 1:300. Oral antibiotics don't eradicate infection/carrier state.

Hepatitis B: Vertical transmission occurs in 90% where the mother is Hep B e Ag pos and 10% where mothers are surface Ag pos e Ag neg. 90% infected infants become chronic carriers. Infants are vaccinated and given Hep B immunoglobulin at birth, reducing the transmission by 90%. Possibly this can be further improved by giving the mother Lamivudine in the last month of pregnancy.

Breast feeding has no negative effect on the risk.

Hepatitis C transmission to the baby is less if the mother is HIV negative and has not abused IV drugs or had blood transfused (<18%). Transmission is higher if the Hep C RNA titre is >1million/ml, transmission doesn't happen if the levels are undetectable.

There is no current prevention treatment given.

HIV/Aids: Only 2% mother to child transmission of HIV occurs in pregnancy. The rest happens during blood transfer at delivery or during breast feeding.

1 in 450 pregnant UK mothers is HIV pos.

Mother to child transmission more likely in:

Higher levels of maternal viraemia,

HIV Core Ags,

Lower maternal CD4,

If the primary infection took place in the pregnancy,

Chorioamnionitis,

Other STDs or Malaria co existing,

Instrumental procedures around delivery,

ROM >4 hrs,

Vaginal delivery,

Preterm birth,

Female babies,

Older mother,

First twin,

Less likely if:

High levels of HIV neutralising Ab,

Elective LSCS,

Zidovudine (etc) treatment,

No instrumental delivery,

Drugs:

Three antiviral combination treatment from 20-28 weeks unless needed earlier for maternal reasons. ZDV is given to the baby for 4-6 weeks.

A planned vaginal delivery may be offered to women on high dose combination anti retroviral treatment with low viral loads.

Breast feeding increases mother to child transmission 15% and should be avoided. With a combination of all these treatments the risk can be as low as 1%.

Genital Herpes: If there are no symptoms of an impending outbreak then a vaginal delivery may still be possible. Most gynaecologist would offer antiviral therapy from 36 weeks. However if a genital infection has been acquired late in the pregnancy or there are warning symptoms of a new eruption (with viral shedding) an elective LSCS will be offered. If there are no maternal antibodies to be acquired by the foetus (i.e. a new infection), the risk if transmission is up to 50% via vaginal delivery.

Listeria: Usually a D and V type illness, it can cause meningitis and a more severe generalised infection. Pregnant women are 20X more likely than the general population to get Listerial infections. Killed by proper cooking, the organism can be present in soft cheeses, (unpasteurised), blue veined cheese, luncheon meat, patés and meat spreads, smoked salmon, pre packed sandwiches etc. If acquired in pregnancy the maternal illness is usually mild with flu like symptoms, rarely it can cause serious CNS complications. It is more dangerous to the baby however – causing miscarriage, neonatal pneumonia, meningitis, septicaemia, micro-abscesses, with a mortality of 25%. Ampicillin and Erythromycin are effective.

Fifth Disease, Erythema Infectiosum: (Slapped Cheek): Parvovirus B19 can cause foetal death, hydrops (5% of infected pregnancies) due to anaemia, necessitating an intrauterine transfusion. There is only a 1% chance of a non immune exposed mother passing the infection onto her baby. Neither the cheek nor lacey general rashes in adults are always typical so any fluey illness with joint pains should raise your suspicion and prompt a blood test during pregnancy.

Swine Flu: (H1N1) Causes a 5X increase in miscarriage, spontaneous abortion or perinatal death due to congenital defects. Premature labour is more common. It can be vaccinated against and this is recommended for all pregnant women. If infected, the antivirals, Zanamivir, Relenza or Olseltamivir, Tamiflu can be given for what they are worth (See "Bad Pharma by Ben Goldacre").

Toxoplasmosis: The protozoan, Toxoplasma Gondii. Once infected, the parasite remains in the host, usually dormant. Women and their pregnancies are safe if they have antibodies at the onset of pregnancy – however this is not routinely tested for. In France it IS requested 3-4 times in pregnancy. About 1,200 pregnant women a year are infected in the UK. They give this to 480 babies (40%), 10% seriously. This is 20X more common than Rubella. Spread via cat faeces, cat litter and food contaminated by cats, undercooked meat and poultry and from unwashed fruit and vegetables. There is also a risk from contact with sheep at lambing time. 30% of 30 year olds and 50% of 70 year olds show signs of past infection. Most infected patients are asymptomatic and it is not usually dangerous to a healthy adult. 1:10 feel fluey with pyrexia, lymphadenopathy, headache, myalgia and sore throat. Some develop encephalitis or even retinochoroiditis. There is even a suspected link to some cases of schizophrenia. Immunity is life-long.

Treatment: Azithromycin, Clindamycin, Spiramycin, (60% effective at preventing placental transfer of Toxoplasmosis. In France cord blood in then tested before proceeding to second line therapy). Prednisolone, Sulfadiazine, Pyrimethamine, Folinic Acid. If a pregnant patient becomes fluey, do this and the various other titres.

Infection confers lifelong immunity.

If a woman contracts the infection in pregnancy there is a 40% chance the foetus will be infected. It is less likely to cross the placenta early in the pregnancy but more likely to cause serious harm. However the infection can cause damage at any stage in the pregnancy.

The risks are: Abortion, hydrocephalus, chorioretinitis, brain damage, the biggest risk being between 12 and 26 weeks.

Pregnancy and lambing. Various infective risks:
Ovine chlamydiosis,
Toxoplasmosis,
Listeriosis.

Post infectious syndromes you will have heard of:
Rheumatic Fever,
Post streptococcal Glomerulonephritis,
Erythema Nodosum,
The various viral exanthem rashes.
PAN,
SBE (Splinter haemorrhages, haematuria etc),

HSP,
Goodpastures Syndrome (Haemoptysis and haematuria, caused by drugs and some viruses),
Reactive arthritis,
Stevens Johnson Syndrome,
Erythema Multiforme,
DIVC.
-to name but a few.

The Gut Microbiota: (Microbiome)/Faecal transplants etc.

We are, each of us, a network of coexisting cells, most of them, numerically, bacterial and in our gut, all usually working together and totalling 100 trillion in all. The bacteria, viruses and fungal cells in and on our body outnumber our own 10 to 1. 70% of our faecal bacteria are stable over any given year and only minor changes will take place over a five year time scale, even perhaps during a lifetime. Assuming we leave them in peace. Our bacterial populations are roughly similar to those of the people we live with and crucial to all sorts of what at first sight seem totally unrelated conditions and diseases.

There is increasing evidence that the billions of bacteria (from 1000 species), viruses, archaea (no nucleus) and eukaryotic (containing a nucleus and other membrane bound organelles) microbes living in commensal harmony with us inside our guts are responsible for a great deal more than fluid and vitamin absorption. The living microbiome (which weighs 1kg) is reflected by our oral cavity bacterial population and influenced by breast feeding, the mode of our birth delivery, our education, gender, diet, antibiotic history and many other factors. Babies born by Caesarean section have completely different gut flora to those "contaminated" by the commensals of their mothers' genital tracts. They grow up to have increased incidence of obesity, asthma and auto immune diseases. Indeed, the process of **vaginal seeding** – using wet swabs removed from the mother's vagina to wipe around the new born baby's mouth, eyes and facial skin is now popular in some countries in order to kick start a more normal microbiome. Hopefully the secretions don't contain Herpes simples viruses, Gonorrhoea, Chlamydia or Group B Strep of course.

If you don't want your child to get allergic spectrum disorders or asthma, bring them up on a farm or with a dog. Certainly don't try to keep them dirt or contamination free. Children lacking four types of bacteria, Faecalibacterium, Lachnospira, Veillonella and Rothia (Flvr) in their microbiome at three months are at high risk of developing asthma, the same is true at one year.

Gut bacteria are responsible absorbing vitamins, for digesting otherwise indigestible dietary components, (eg Xyloglucans) and liberating short chained fatty acids from dietary fibre (important in cancer and immune regulation in the gut).

The microbiota has been shown to affect immune development and programming, influencing a variety of inflammatory conditions both gastro intestinal and systemic, producing various enzymes and proteins from bacterial DNA and RNA which are involved in several bodily metabolic pathways. It affects gut absorption and stimulates some gut receptors, making vitamins and short chain fatty acids, influencing many conditions including anxiety and depression. It is greatly influenced by antibiotics, caesarean section, breast feeding (which provides staph, strep, lactic acid bacteria, enterobacteria and bifidobacteria etc) prebiotic foods and probiotics.

The microbiota can produce a proatherosclerotic compound, TMAO (Trimethylamine

– N-oxide) thus increasing the risk of adverse cardiovascular events (this is avoided by consuming a vegan diet).

C Difficile infections, inflammatory bowel disease and IBS can often be improved or even prevented by altering the microbiome. This counter intuitive approach has even been used to treat various mental illnesses. The microbiota has been shown to influence rheumatoid arthritis, blood pressure, colonic cancer proneness, obesity (thin people have a more diverse but possibly a specific microbiome which thrives on a healthy diet than the overweight), diabetes and the immune response to amyloid plaques in Alzheimer's. The prevailing wisdom was that antibiotics in infancy even led to obesity in later life but it appears this is not so, according to a paper in January 2017, Lancet Diab and Endocr. It turns out that it isn't the antibiotic but in a parallel to the asthma association, it is the infection for which the antibiotic is prescribed that causes the obesity. The sort of oral bacterial colonisation a patient has can influence coronary artery disease, the presence of methanobreibacter species increases the risk of diabetes. H Pylori can cause ulcers and gastric carcinoma but it may affect the incidence of Alzheimer's disease also.

Gut bacteria influence brain development and function. They may play a role in the development of MS by activating T and B lymphocytes which damage cerebral white matter. Parkinson's Disease is commoner after H pylori infections. Autistic children have been shown to have different gut bacteria to normal children. The link between gut bacteria and disease may be through various different mechanisms. These may include an effect on absorption, through triggering an immune response, stimulating afferent visceral nerves and so on. Clearly however, the gut and its living contents can no longer be considered solely a passive portal for the transfer of nutrients.

The puzzling relationship between previous courses of antibiotics and a number of subsequent illnesses including Diabetes and Juvenile Rheumatoid Arthritis can be in part explained by an effect on the gut micro flora (20/7/2015 Pediatrics). A relationship has also been found between antibiotics used in the first year of life and asthma development by the third year but in this case it may be that wheezing below twelve months may have been misdiagnosed as infection and treated with antibiotics instead of anti asthma medication.

My relative intellectual resistance to the whole microbiome/biota story is the number of papers warning of dire long term consequences from what have been for decades, a common and essential part of the doctor's armamentarium: standard courses of antibiotics. As GPs, we just **don't see** patients with COPD, splenectomies, recurrent UTIs, Cystic Fibrosis, recurrent diverticular disease, Lyme Disease, immune defects, or repeated SBE prophylaxis etc who frequently have large doses, prolonged prophylactic or repeated antibiotic treatment going on to suffer serious unrelated ill health as a side effect of their antibiotics. So it does seem that a temporary alteration of the Microbiome either recovers very quickly or cannot *really* be that bad for you. – And should further research on such new areas as treating chronic unremitting back pain with three months of Co Amoxiclav prove positive, are we going to prioritise the patient's microbiome and the bacterial herd sensitivity or the patient who may have no other cure for his suffering?

In any event this is a new and exciting medical subject with connections to almost every systemic disease, undreamt of even ten years ago and may turn out to be a 1 kg alien but symbiotic, even essential organism living within us.

25: Legal issues:

The Abortion Act 1967

This was David Steele's private member's act, becoming law from 1968, making abortion up to 28 weeks legal. It may not seem comprehensible today but I remember the parliamentary debate and the public controversy about morality, promiscuity, democracy, at what gestation independent life and pain sensation began, religious faith, what would happen to the next generation of teenagers. Indeed, the difference in social and "moral" attitudes in so short a time is partly due to the changes imposed on society by the abortion act itself. Even as a 16 year old I realised there were profound questions being asked, not being taken seriously and not really being answered in the debate. Parliament proved that it didn't understand statistics, risk, human behaviour, adolescent sexual activity, peer pressure, foetal development way back then, much as it is largely ignorant of how most medical issues are felt and practiced by society today. It was out of touch with the British people and much else related to health and the young and it was absolutely ignorant about the number of healthy pregnancies that would soon be aborted, routinely, without challenge on the NHS. The gestation was changed subsequently to 24 weeks from 1990. The arguments, which I remember hearing as a sixteen year old at the time, were mainly about ending the number of deaths from back street abortions. In 2017 the BMA without reference to its members or the profession voted to lobby for abortions to be simply a matter of maternal choice, like cutting hair or your toe nails and completely outside the criminal law. Thus permitting gender specific abortions, removing any concept of the sanctity of human life and making an even greater farce of the weighty arguments put forward to justify the original bill. The BMA after the strike and this pronouncement must be the least democratic, the least representative, the most rigidly political and the most inward looking of all professional bodies in the UK now.

But originally any mention of a woman's domain over her own body or her right to choose were not the issues. It was about saving adult lives.

Between 1967 and 1970 the rate of maternal deaths due to botched abortions dropped from approximately 30/million to 15/million. So I assume the Act, at best, saved far fewer than 15 or so lives per year for a few years. Far fewer. Some estimates are a handful or less per year at the start. With the ready availability of walk in casualty units and since at least the 70's, effective powerful antibiotics and laparoscopic surgery, probably even fewer than this. Currently this is at the cost of 200,000 aborted foetuses each year – the vast majority of them potentially normal human beings. There is also the parallel cost of a profound moral change in attitudes regarding the importance of the unborn child and personal sexual behaviour in our society. Every GP sees depressing numbers of teenagers who frequently get drunk and have unprotected sex with semi-strangers at parties knowing that abortion is free and no questions asked if the inevitable happens. They duly turn up for an emergency appointment the next day because the "Morning after pill" is free from the GP. Every GP knows of women who also use abortion as lazy contraception and have had several terminations. This is despite free, effective, safe and universally availably birth control and the "morning after pill" over the counter. These were not around in 1969. These days very few of those women who would have been aborted in back streets would actually die as a consequence. Most of the mortality was from haemorrhage or sepsis. These would be avoided now thanks to effective broad spectrum antibiotics and walk in casualty units. And hopefully avoided altogether by readily available contraception and if necessary, the post coital contraceptive. Thus we are using abortion as a form of secondary birth control for the lazy and the feckless and the original humanitarian life saving argument doesn't apply.

If the abortion debate were happening today as it has been in the Republic of Ireland, it would have shifted from saving maternal life (It is legal even in the ROI to abort to save the mother's life) to the woman's right to choose what happens to her body. The proto human of course, always dies. But doesn't the woman choose whether to have sex, choose whether to access free and universally available birth control, especially a barrier method and choose whether to ask for the post coital contraceptive afterwards? Does she really want the right to choose to be completely irresponsible too? The right to make a life through not taking a simple precaution then the right to take that life? That is her "Right to choose". A foetus isn't the only thing she has been risking after all. Apparently the Irish have exported their problem to us over the years with 162,000 women travelling to the UK for an abortion between 1980 and 2014.

What we have now in the UK then is De Facto abortion on demand, for every woman who wants it – whatever her reason (or objectively, no reason at all). The justification, using the mealy-mouthed words of the act is that a normal pregnancy puts a healthy woman's life at slightly more risk than a termination of that pregnancy. So any pregnancy is safer terminated.

You could argue that we all ought to debate this situation again since what the pro abortion supporters denied would happen, has happened: abortion on demand and mass abortion for the convenience of healthy women who are having healthy babies but don't want them at the moment. Very few maternal lives having actually been saved at all. The free availability of abortion without restriction has led over the years to its increasing popularity as a form of lazy default birth control.

And what the anti abortion lobby warned would happen **has** happened: abortion on request of huge numbers of healthy foetuses (**8,400,000** since the act became law (8m DoH Stats in 2013)) – **this is the exact population of London** and next to no benefit for the genuinely desperate woman of the 1950s who today would have used the morning after pill or IUCD. Back street abortionists would have been put out of business by now by the morning after pill. Worst of all is the change in sexual morality that sex without conse-quences has contributed to. Couples of all ages have sex far earlier in their relationships and now a quick recourse to bed is expected and normal. We see a change in attitude to sex around us that therefore permeates our culture from the ubiquity of Internet pornography, including child pornography on line, to grooming of vulnerable children and teenagers, from teenage sexting to revenge porn and adult dating websites for the unfaithful married. If the state takes away the risk, why not?

The current libertarian abortion free for all is a women's right to choose:

a) Not to use hormonal contraception in its multiplicity of types.

b) Not to use barrier methods of contraception in its many assorted variations.

c) Not to wait until her partner could or would be willing to choose b) (for mutual health reasons).

d) Not to wait until the relationship had developed a bit further than the first or second meeting so that she might be able to access a) or b).

e) Not to access the over the counter Post Coital Contraceptive.

f) Not to get to know a potential sexual partner well enough before agreeing to sex in order to discuss the implications, risks or meaning of sex or to discuss the desirability of infection and pregnancy risk free sex.

g) But her right, having chosen a) to f) instead to choose termination of pregnancy. This of course is the right to be irresponsible with your body and dismissive of your ability to create another human body and generally speaking I would not regard that as something a state funded health care system should indulge. (Think of obesity and smoking, immunisation and drug abuse).

Of the 200,000 women seeking termination annually in the UK, up to one third have had a previous abortion and at least half haven't bothered taking any contraception. (Today programme 28/4/14).

Interestingly however this free, libertarian consensus on abortion was severely challenged in September 2013 when it transpired that Daily Telegraph reporters had managed to procure abortions on request from a couple of (as it happens, Asian) Manchester gynaecologists. The reporters clearly stated to the doctors that their reasons for wanting to terminate the pregnancy was the female gender of the foetus. The Sunday Times ran an eloquent half page article on this situation which quoted angry MPs denouncing the failure of both the GMC to take action against the doctors and the DPP to prosecute them. Female MPs and other commentators said they were "Pro choice" but against aborting babies on the grounds of their (female) sex. This was the thin end of some sort of wedge.

Now think about the hypocrisy of this situation. It is the classic liberal mental intellectual contradiction. I mentioned the background of the doctors advisedly.

It is OK to abort 200,000 normal babies every year, 100,000 of them healthy girls presumably. But if you go to the gynaecologist wanting to abort one healthy girl because she is a girl then it suddenly becomes immoral and illegal. If you are the gynaecologist and you abort, say 1,000 health baby boys and girls every year, 500 of them presumably girls then it is just "abortion on demand" as usual and OK under the abortion act. But if, just before you give the premed to one of the patients she mentions that the only reason she is there is because she wanted a boy not a girl then it suddenly becomes a crime.

Surely the problem here is that abortion of healthy proto people on demand is wrong, aborting all healthy infants just because the mother hasn't been organised enough to prevent conceiving is wrong. That is true whether the mother knows she is ending the life of a boy or a girl. And the more we do it, the more the demand will be. The situation was clarified somewhat by an amendment to the Serious Crime Bill in 2015 making Gender Abortion illegal. So sexism does trump a woman's right to choose. A woman can kill her own proto boys and girls indiscriminately but not selectively.

Confidentiality:

All doctors are bound by an unwritten (and actually unsigned) code of confidentiality regarding medical information divulged during a consultation.

Hold on though......Having said all that, and since the previous section is about the number of abortions done each year, and since the Hippocratic Oath includes "I will never cause an abortion", it is obvious that doctors don't always take a lot of notice of lawyers and the law or even stick to their own undertakings and codes. I wonder how BOUND by confidentiality we actually are. I never took an oath of confidentiality. 99% of my work does not require it, indeed it requires excellent and accurate communication of patient information *with others*, especially people who are strangers to the patient. Like consultants and therapists. And after consulting I detail the patient's problems by dictating their history in a letter to my secretary. This is then read by at least three or four other administrators before it is seen by the person to whom the letter was directed. So this confidentiality is NOT ABSOLUTE, IS relative, and often IS ignored by us doctors. If this information relates to criminal or potentially antisocial or socially dangerous activity ("my boyfriend has several illegal weapons, I hurt my hand mugging an old lady last night", "I keep fainting at the wheel of the lorry I drive" "My memory is going and they say I've got Alzheimer's but I'm damned if I'm stopping driving") then the bounds of confidentiality are loosened.

The World Medical Association's International Code of Medical Ethics states that a physician shall respect a patient's right to confidentiality but **it is ethical to disclose confidential information** when the patient consents to it or when there is a **real or imminent threat of harm to the patient or others** and this threat can only be removed by a breach of confidentiality. My experience is that, over a career, absolute confidentiality needs to be stretched or broken many times to protect the lives and safety of your patients and of the public.

The law assumes that doctors will share confidential information with medical students and other doctors involved in that patient's care and even that some "civilian" administrative staff will have limited access to that information as part of their role. It is assumed that the patient knows all this. Laws controlling confidentiality information are now under the umbrella of the Convention of Human Rights, Article 8, which says that everyone has a right to respect and family life (see later). This covers correspondence and personal data. There is however a caveat that the duty of confidentiality is suspended in the interests of national security, **public safety**, the well-being of the country or the **prevention of disorder of crime**, protection of health or morals, or **the protection** of rights and freedoms **of others.** So if you think about it there are many circumstances under which medical confidence may be suspended. Confidentiality is in fact a *relative term*. Doctors must also disclose information to the courts if ordered to do so; they must disclose information related to any terrorist activity, any notifiable disease, facts about births and deaths. This is on top of the ethical duty to disclose information spontaneously if others or "society" are in danger. Practically this usually means if your patient has an unrecognised drug or mental health problem, a transmissible disease or carries on driving when he or she has a physical, mental or substance problem which makes them a risk to others. Confidentiality, Data Protection and the law say that a breach of confidence is not actionable if the public interest in the disclosure outweighs the public interest in the non-disclosure. As so often, the advice is unhelpful and the decision is delegated to the doctor making his mind up on the hoof. You often find that is the case with lawyers and an issue of medical law. (See Gilligan Competency).

This whole area was brought into stark, horrible contrast in Scotland just before Christmas 2014. I have personally had at least three patients have sudden episodes of loss of consciousness at the wheels of vehicles. As soon as I knew, when they came to seek a diagnosis, as I dictated the letters to the neurologists and EEG departments, I immediately wrote to the DVLA, informing the patient in the surgery that I had no alternative but to do so and telling them it was illegal for them to drive.

Just before Christmas 2014, Harry Clarke, a Glasgow bin lorry driver suddenly became unconscious at the wheel of his vehicle and ploughed into a pavement full of shoppers killing six and seriously injuring many others. It subsequently transpired that he had lied about previous episodes to keep his licence and get the job. I do not know whether any of his medical attendants might have prevented the deaths by informing the DVLA when he first had an episode and not trusting him to self report his condition. It seems extremely unlikely that **no** GP, specialist or A and E doctor knew about Mr Clarke's previous episodes. This should now be a statutory requirement for all doctors, – to report a sudden loss of control of a vehicle to the DVLA. On pain of striking off. In the USA a driver who did the same and killed even more innocent pedestrians at a bus stop was sentenced to life in prison. Our judiciary is far too liberal ever to reflect public anger at this sort of avoidable death in the same way. Inexplicably, no action has so far been taken against this driver by the Scottish courts. Having performed numerous pre employment medical examinations I know that a great deal of the "assessment of suitability" is based on the patient's own history and "Trust". This doctor patient interaction has become even more manipulatable now patients have access to and a partial right of veto over their GP's medical reports.

In the case of children and the dead, disclosure of confidential information has to be in the patient's best interest. The doctor has to decide what that is of course.

Should you tell the wife of a philanderer who has acquired HIV not to sleep with him? The law is now beginning to say yes, even if the patient tells you not to. In the last thirty plus years I have written to our Chief Police Constable informing him of illegally held weapons, patients regularly driving drunk the following morning, to the DVLA regarding patients driving following hypoglycaemic or epileptic convulsions. In these circumstances, as well as numerous instances of patients having sex with under-age children in which I involved the social services, I felt my duty to 'society' outweighed that of 'confidentiality'.

When others' lives or welfare are at stake, trusting the patient to do the right thing just isn't enough.

Sex and children:

A child under 13 years cannot consent to sexual intercourse and if sex has taken place it has been by definition, rape. You **must** involve Social Services and or the Police.

Access to Medical Reports Act:

The patient can ask to see any report for employment or insurance purposes prepared in the previous 6 months and can:

1) Decline consent to a report being submitted,

2) Give consent but request to see it before it is released. The patient has 21 days to approve the report. After this the doctor can send off the report anyway (assuming approval). After viewing it the patient can request in writing that the report be amended. The doctor may not agree. The patient may then withdraw consent, ask the doctor to attach the patient's own views, agree to the report being issued unchanged.

The doctor may refuse to show the report or part of it if he considers there are special circumstances (if he considers it would seriously harm the physical or mental health of the patient or others, if it indicates the medical practitioner's intentions in respect of the patient or if it reveals information about or the identity of someone who has given the doctor information – unless that person consents, or is a health professional involved the case and the information relates to or has been provided in that capacity.)

3) If the patient does not want to see the report (This hardly EVER happens these days) they may request a copy up to 6 months after.

Any charge from the provision of access is the patient's own responsibility.

Data protection: (1984, 1994, 1998) See below

The data protection Act 1984 allows access to any personal record held on computer or on paper and the right to correct or amend that information. There is a 40 day release period.

Under the Data Protection Act Certain principles have to be obeyed in handling sensitive information:

These are the Caldicott Principles:

Caldicott Principles

The Caldicott Report set out a number of general principles that health and social care organisations should use when reviewing their use of patient information and these are set out below:

Principle 1: Justify the purpose(s): Every proposed use or transfer of personally identifiable information within or from an organisation should be clearly defined and scrutinised and with continuing use regularly reviewed by the appropriate guardian.

Principle 2: Do not use personally identifiable information unless it is absolutely necessary.

Personally identifiable information items should not be used unless there is no alternative.

Principle 3: Use the minimum personally identifiable information.

Where the use of personally identifiable information is considered to be essential, each individual item of information should be justified with the aim of reducing identifiability.

Principle 4: Access to personally identifiable information should be on a strict need to know basis. Only those individuals who need access to personally identifiable information should have access to it.

Principle 5: Everyone should be aware of their responsibilities. Action should be taken to ensure that those handling personally identifiable information are aware of their responsibilities and obligations to respect patient/client confidentiality.

Principle 6: Understand and comply with the law.

Every use of personally identifiable information must be lawful. Someone in each organisation should be responsible for ensuring that the organisation complies with legal requirements.

A Caldicott Guardian is an individual, a senior member of each NHS organisation whose responsibility it is to make sure that patients' data is kept secure.

Who can have access to information about a patient?

Parental access to children's notes can depend not only on marital state but if born before 1/12/2003, only the mother's husband or the male named on the birth certificate can have access to the child's history and notes.

Unmarried fathers only count after Dec '03. Some of us wonder why attitudes changed in 2003. The commitment of unmarried couples to staying together doesn't seem to have.

By the way, when registering a father on the birth certificate, he must actually be present or be the legal husband if not physically present at registration to be named on the certificate.

You may think that the law used to be unreasonably harsh on the male parent who hadn't formalised his relationship with the commitment of marriage. If you do, consider the statistics: unmarried parents are 4X more likely to split up than married couples and thus leave the children with a single parent who becomes dependent on the tax payer.

So far it seems that gay male couples who get married go on to divorce at the same rate as heterosexual married couples but at half the rate of lesbian couples who get married.

Principles of the Data Protection Act 1998

The act contains eight "Data Protection Principles":

These specify that personal data must be:

1. Processed fairly and lawfully.
2. Obtained for specified and lawful purposes.
3. Adequate, relevant and not excessive.
4. Accurate and up to date.
5. Not kept any longer than necessary.
6. Processed in accordance with the "data subject's" (the individual's) rights.
7. Securely kept.
8. Not transferred to any other country without adequate protection in situ.

Data Protection Act 1998 supersedes

Access to Health Records Acts 1990, (>2002:)

Patients or their representative have a right of access to their records within 21 days of their request, unless the information released may cause serious harm to the physical or mental health of the patient or someone else.

or

Unless the information would disclose information given by or relating to a third party. People with parental responsibility can apply for the records of children for whom they are responsible.

The GP is the "Data Controller" and you can charge a limited fee (currently a maximum of £50 for copies and £10 for simply viewing the notes). If the patient feels that the notes are inaccurate or wrong they can **complain** through the complaints procedure and you can add a note giving your view and theirs and whether you agree.

The BMA says you should keep clear, accurate, legible and contemporaneous records (not, of course, add to them after things have gone wrong) which report the clinical findings, decisions, information given to patients and drugs or treatment prescribed. Personal views about the patient should only be included if they have a bearing on the treatment. If the patient expresses views about future disclosure to a third party, these should be recorded.

If there are problems relating to the withholding of information (and you must take a reasonable time to read all the notes to protect your previous self and others who wrote notes – THIS OFTEN JUST DOESN'T HAPPEN) then refer the patient to The NHS Complaints Procedure or The Information Commissioner's Office:-

Wycliffe House, Water Lane, Wilmslow, Cheshire, SK95AF. 01625 5457000.

The problem with data protection in General Practice is that good family medicine sometimes depends upon the doctor having informal often "secret" conversations about the worries, illness, behaviour, prognosis of one member of the family with another member. "How can I help my mum if I don't know what's wrong with her?" "I can't sleep with worry about my teenage daughter, is she really going off the rails/sleeping around?" "Doctor is it drugs or just teenage moodiness"? I know of some particularly narrow minded colleagues who would not even reassure one parent that their child wasn't suicidal or on hard drugs (-they weren't) because of "Data Protection". I went to a lecture on the subject where I was told not to call patients over the waiting room PA by name, because of "Data Protection". Local pharmacists have told me that they have been advised not to call patients names out to the shop interior to collect their prescriptions because of "Data Protection". Data Protection Law (or its application) has become the medical profession's "Human Rights" Act – misused, misapplied, misunderstood, abused, hated by all but lawyers and used as justification by everyone as an excuse for professional laziness and inactivity.

This is the most misused and misunderstood bogeyman of soft medical politics of the last decade and does patients far more genuine harm than good. Indeed, in 40 years I cannot remember a single occasion when a patient of mine actually suffered by having medical or personal information divulged to a third party against their "interests" or against their will. It is a huge holy cow to politicians, the Legal Profession and to many in our profession now, especially those in research and administration. Even anonymised data is protected as if each bit were the life of a child. But was "Data Protection" legislation really of benefit to significant numbers of patients, what harm does data access do and is complete data protection really necessary?

I once phoned another GP who had just registered my daughter (who was in her late twenties) as a patient in London so that I could give him a brief past history prior to her notes arriving. She had been registered with various doctors at home and abroad. Her history was quite complicated and I knew it well. I had my daughter's full consent. He refused to take the call as (to quote the receptionist) "He never talks to any third party, even other doctors, it's "Data protection". – What total nonsense.

It turned out he was not a particularly meticulous, effective or attentive doctor – just as these first impressions had suggested he might not be. He never took more than the vaguest, most unconcerned interest in my daughter's (and I believe his other patients') care. She said he always did the minimum he could when he did see her.

Sometimes data needs to be a little vulnerable and unprotected in the best interests of us all – as in the case where social services were not allowed to tell a gas supplier that a vulnerable old couple were not coping at home but refusing their help and were at risk. The couple died of hypothermia in their freezing flat with the heating cut off and the unpaid bill contributed to their deaths. Data protected – couple dead, lawyers happy, job done.

For my daughter's new GP, "Data Protection" was just a good excuse. The truth was he was too lazy to spare ten minutes to pick up the phone; probably his daily working life was too chaotic and he couldn't be bothered to spare the time talking to a colleague. "Data Protection" was used to cover his laziness and disorganisation, shirking of responsibility, his avoidance of a meaningful Duty of Care. It was his way of avoiding work and so in the end the patient suffers, the doctor's time is saved, Data Protection, job done.

Always remember our prime duty is to the well being of the patient and that may some-times mean telling a teenager's parents that they don't need to worry and the depression/self harming/volatile behaviour **is** going to improve. – "No the teenager isn't doing drugs or there is treatment in hand that will help them to improve, or they will get off drugs, fight their depression, their self harming and they won't be like this forever so don't kick them out of the home yet. Give them a little longer to get better".

Data protection Act stretched a bit: – Patient protected. Family cared for. REAL Family Physician's job done.

Access to Health Records act 1990:

Gives the right to see the health records written after Nov 1991. (Data protection applies to all records back to the patient's birth).

Information that may be withheld: Personal information about other people, requests for information that are manifestly unreasonable, far too general or would require unreasonable resources to answer.

You don't HAVE to tell a patient if information has been withheld from them in their own or someone else's interests.

An estranged parent may demand access to a child's records (this is often the case in custody battles and in legal conflicts over care). You can ask to see the shared custody document if your understanding is that the other parent has custody. I would pass this before your defence organisation to ensure you are not infringing the father's rights.

Male health records must be kept for 10 years after death, a woman's records for 25 years after the last live birth.

What do you do if a patient denies his/her history? You can annotate the records with the patient's amended version, sign and date it without opinion but you must not delete or remove the pre existing notes, physical or electronic. You can add "Patient does not believe this to be true" – after all, doctors **are** fallible. Future readers of the notes must make up their own minds.

This whole area of patients' access to their history has a chequered past. On the surface it is a human rights issue and we should all know what is being said about us behind our backs.-Correct? Well, of course not, not if we know what is in our best long term interest and that of our families. Medicine doesn't work if there isn't two way trust. Particularly Family Medicine.

One of my patients was a very senior and very stressed nurse in a managerial position in our local Trust. Very soon after joining my list she made a formal complaint about me when I refused to nod through a prescription of some third line cephalosporins she requested for what she described as "upper UTIs with negative MSUs". She said that this and various other (dubious) diagnoses had been made for her after extensive investigations, several negative laparoscopies and cystoscopies at various London hospitals. She and her house husband berated me, a humble GP, for *presuming* to take over her management after all the "suffering" she had been through. I did not find any abnormal physical signs and never managed to obtain a positive MSU or confirmatory test of a physical disease of any kind in her or her notes. To cut a long story short, her son then developed non specific abdominal pain in his early teens and in my referral letter to the Paediatric Gastroenterologist I said:

"This is ironic as his mother suffers from a similar non specific abdominal pain, probably similar to IBS and related to her stressful job, but which has been labelled without much evidence as "renal pain". Johnny finds life with a stressed mother who works long hours very difficult and all his tests are negative, just as were his mum's".

I felt very strongly that I should not be intimidated by the parents and that the Paediatrician who actually worked with and knew the mother should know the whole family background and be able to make up his mind with all the evidence. Unfortunately the mother saw the referral letter on a computer in outpatients at the hospital and you can imagine what this did to my hard built up relationship with her, her husband and the anxious son. She felt her history was irrelevant. I thought it was crucial.

Interestingly she and her husband subsequently split up. It turns out she had been having an affair and their relationship had been rocky for some time. The husband and son were devastated. They have now all moved out of the practice area and presumably gone their separate ways. But it is a typical General Practice story and in retrospect, the pieces, including her anger at me, all add up – The abdominal pains in mother and son, the complaints, the resentment at not being taken at face value, the husband's protectiveness, her self – justification, the child's unhappiness, her unhappiness, both expressed with physical symptoms, the brittle relationships and the willingness to attribute blame elsewhere – towards me. All GPs will recognise this situation and their role as sometime innocent victim.

Never forget that the Human Rights Act (which see below) gives even the humble GP the right to speak his mind (Freedom of Expression) if he feels strongly about an issue like this and if you feel you can defend your point of view ethically do not be pushed around by someone misdirecting their anxiety or guilt. (The Right to Freedom of Thought and Expression and not to be treated in an Inhuman or Degrading way). As long as the views you hold are based on a well reasoned case and you can justify them to a third party.

Freedom of Information Act 2000

Does not cover personal information.

The Freedom of Information (FOI) Act entitles anybody to ask a public authority in England, Wales and Northern Ireland, including Government Departments, for any recorded information that they keep.

A list of organisations covered by the Act is available at the Information Commissioner's website: http://www.ico.gov.uk/

This Act gives greater access to information about how decisions are taken in Government and how public services are developed and delivered.

The FOI Act operates alongside the Data Protection Act, which allows people to access information about themselves (e.g. personnel records, or information held by credit reference agencies) and the Environmental Information Regulations, which give people access to information about the environment.

You can ask to have any recorded information. This could be in the form of e-mails, notebooks, videos or tapes.

In most cases a response must be made in 20 working days of receiving the request and if it cannot, an explanation should be given (at least by local, national and statutory bodies).

The information should usually be given unless there is a good reason for not doing so (e.g. your request relates to someone else's personal details). The exemptions are listed in the FOI Act.

A reason must be given for declining your request. If you do not find the reason persuasive, you can ask the body to reconsider its decision and if the request is still declined you can ask **the Information Commissioner's Office** to review that decision.

The Information Commissioner's Office is an independent body that enforces the FOI Act and the Data Protection Act. For more information, visit the Information Commissioner's website.

I got much of the information regarding the sexist and racist (-anti white male) selection processes of most medical schools by sending FOI requests to their FOI officers. It took an average of several weeks for them to reply and some of the replies were disappointing if you believe the profession should reflect the population of the nation it serves. One University of London medical school showed a 33% white intake in 2013/14 saying this reflected its local area. Most Medical Schools were admitting 70% female medical students: I wonder whether every medical school reflects only the racial demography of its local area and whether that is what universities are supposed to do? Only a half of the Medical Schools in the UK, all of whom I wrote to twice, quoting FOI, responded to my officially couched request for demographic information on their student intake. If you look at the wholly unrepresentative racial and sexual make up of medical students from those who did reply you may draw your own conclusions about those who chose to keep their intake populations secret.

The point being: The FOI act isn't always as effective as you might assume at freeing up what should be accessible information to those who request it.

A Receiver:

Is an individual or organisation responsible for dealing with the management, termination or administration of a patient's financial affairs. This is clearly defined in the order appointing them, eg – by the Court of Protection when the patient is no longer capable of managing their own affairs and in subsequent further orders. A receiver may be required to provide a report once yearly recording income/expenditure. The receiver can be responsible for the patient's tax affairs.

General Power of Attorney:

Is granted to a trusted person for a limited time scale and while an individual still has "mental capacity" so that decisions can be taken and documents signed on a patient's behalf – for instance during a protracted stay in hospital or abroad.

Enduring Power of Attorney:

Was replaced by Lasting Power of Attorney in October 2007. There are two types of Lasting Power of Attorney –related to Property and Financial Affairs and Health and Welfare. Currently it costs approx £110 to register a LPA.

Lasting Power of Attorney "LPA":

Lasting Power of Attorney is arranged while the individual has mental capacity to decide, so that an individual chosen by the patient can:

Manage their financial affairs in the event of an accident or incapacity,

Ensure the decisions made on their behalf are what they would have wanted,

Make decisions according to their wishes with regard to any medical treatment,

Ensure any care they receive is in line with what they would have expected.

Ensure the people making decisions on their behalf are chosen by them in advance, not the **Court of Protection:**

This is usually arranged through the "Office of the Public Guardian". The form can be obtained from them and is valid once stamped by them – Helpline 0300 456 0300. Note: The "Donor" is the patient; The "Attorneys" are usually the relatives.

If an adult is incapable of giving consent then they may have conveniently:

1) Made a previous LPA, they may have:

2) Previously appointed a proxy decision maker ("while capacitous") or you or their relatives may:

3) Ask the court to make the decision.

In practice most medical decisions are actually made by the medical team on the patient's behalf and if they are in the patient's best interests they will be upheld by the courts.

Section ten:
The power of attorney begins as soon as the form is filled in, provided under Schedule 1 of the act. When filling in the form it is necessary to specify the starting and ending dates. Section 10 of the Power of Attorney Act provides details on when and how this power is applied. A general power of attorney is a very short document whose form is prescribed by section 10 of the Powers of Attorney Act 1971; it is for this reason that they are often referred to as "Section 10 Powers of Attorney".

An LPA can be cancelled when no longer needed

Read more: http://www.ehow.com/info_10063957_section-10-power-attorney-act.html

Help can be obtained from customerservices@publicguardian.gsi.gov.uk 0300456 0300

Consent: (Your defence association help line can be useful!)
Who can give consent? Different references say the usual different things: BUT legally everyone under 18 is considered a child for the purposes of most medical decision making.

BUT confusingly the age level drops by 2 years and possibly by even more when **"Gillick competency is taken into account – i.e. A child has the capacity to consent to medical treatment when *he or she* achieves sufficient understanding to enable him or *her* to fully understand what is proposed...."**

Everyone over 16 is usually presumed to be competent to give consent unless shown otherwise. If a child under the age of 16 has sufficient understanding and intelligence to enable them to fully understand what is proposed then they can give consent. You should ask yourself: Can they comprehend and retain information material to the decision and use and weigh up the information in the decision making process particularly as it relates to whether to have the intervention in question? This all sounds much easier in theory than it is in practice.

Young people aged 16 and 17 can sign consent forms as can "Legally Competent" younger children but you or they may like a parent to countersign the form. A competent 16 or 17 year old on the other hand can be overridden by a person with parental responsibility or a court. This principle of overrule is based on the best interests of the child being paramount. If a child is not able to give consent themselves then someone with parental responsibility may do so and you should always try to involve the parent unless the child expressly declines this. If a patient is mentally competent but physically unable to sign a consent form, complete the form and ask an independent witness to confirm that the patient has given their consent.

If a patient has no capacity for informed consent then the doctor always acts in THE BEST INTERESTS OF THE PATIENT. If the patient is unable to give valid consent then the doctor acts anyway – if the treatment is lifesaving.

A parent can always consent for a child (<18yrs) but not for another adult (even with learning disabilities).

So you might need a court order (via Social Services) and in the case of contraceptive provision (other than depot) you would do well involving a gynaecologist too.

However, if an adult with learning disabilities is felt unable to appreciate the implications of sex or contraception then they cannot give consent to sex either – and Social

Services should be involved.

The DOH does a "Seeking consent, working with children" publication which summarises giving and obtaining consent with children.

In the case of an adult with dementia, the same principles of law apply. If the patient is incapable of consent and/or seriously ill, act in their best interests-otherwise a court order (via S.S.) may be necessary. This can all be very unwieldy if the patient has multiple serious medical problems and it is reasonable to take the management decisions in what you perceive to be the patient's best interests. You can't always practice medicine strictly to legal principles. Act with common sense and reason.

The court can overrule parental decisions just as it can overrule decisions made by someone previously given Power of Attorney.

A child under 13 cannot consent to sex. Anyone younger than this has been raped and any sexual activity must be reported to Social Services or the Police. Clearly there are situations where a child under 16 may be having a sexual relationship with an older person, especially someone in a position of trust where it would be reasonable to breach medical confidentiality on behalf of the child's long term emotional and (dare I say it?) moral well being. I had a family on my list a few years ago where the daughter of 14 was sleeping with the same man as the mother. He seemed to be a temporary lodger of no fixed abode and they seemed to be taking turns. I got Social Services to investigate via a case conference. The result was that the daughter was taken into care and both mother and daughter gave me a tirade of abuse at the case conference for interfering with their cosy *"Menage a trois"*.

A "competent" 13 year old can consent to an examination and treatment. Discuss with colleagues what is in the child's interests if in doubt.

There are increasing numbers of sexual abuse cases involving adults suffering dementia. Some of them involving staff at care homes. Do not be afraid to voice concerns of what you may consider inappropriately sexualised or affectionate behaviour between staff whether male or female and residents. Warning signs may be a change in previously contented behaviour by the resident or unexplained aggression, fearfulness, unwillingness to be undressed, bathed or alone in their room.

A competent ADULT Jehovah's Witness can refuse a life saving transfusion for them self and a mentally competent adult can insist that the doctors turn off their ventilator under certain future conditions. As long as they understand the consequences. "Autonomy is respected unto death" except that the law is currently a little vague about assisting and accompanying someone during their suicide (Debbie Purdy's case was that she, as a severe MS sufferer wanted to know if her husband would be prosecuted for assisting her suicide. It was considered a breach of her human rights for this not to be clarified.) What DID lawyers do before Human Rights? What will they do if and when the UK ceases to be bound by The European Convention on Human Rights after Brexit?

The doctor has to be acting with the express or *implied* consent of the patient – for instance while performing physical and especially during intimate examinations. I take this for granted thirty times a day especially in the patient's home. Indeed it only becomes an issue when we make it one. This works provided the patient is given the freedom to decline, the examination is done gently, sympathetically and consensually, – in other words *professionally* and stopped immediately there is any sense of reproof or discomfort.

Most new registrars have been made to feel paranoid regarding intimate examinations by their trainers, as if every patient whose breasts they check for lumps is going to accuse them of sexual assault. So they ask every patient they wish to examine if they would like a **chaperone**. My generation of doctors never even considered this. Doing so has the following consequences:

The patient assumes the doctor could be immoral, incompetent, inexperienced or a potential sexual predator, or why else would they need supervision?

The presence of a third party, usually a receptionist or a busy nurse, destroys the continuity, flow and relationship normally built up in the consultation. The whole dynamic of the interaction is ended. Like a cameraman at a marriage proposal, a stranger in the confessional.

Introducing an outsider reduces the patient's trust and confidence in the previously assumed experience and reliability of the doctor – he must be new at the job, lacking in confidence, needing back up and support.

So the doctor often learns not to undergo all the bother of examining the patient and either makes a diagnosis without enough information or admits the patient to hospital unnecessarily where the SHO or registrar will do the examination with an embarrassing entourage of strangers attending, ensuring an intimidating clinical experience for the poor recipient but almost no risk of litigation for the doctor.

Physical contact is part of the ritual of the consultation, usually purposeful but even if it is just a pat on the arm or the small of the back. It reminds the patient that a doctor is more than an administrator. He or she has a potential but benign dominion over body and mind.

So I firmly believe that examination should form part of most consultations, even if it is brief and superficial and that it should be assumed that no chaperone is needed unless the patient asks for one. The chaperone quandary could be avoided with a notice in the waiting room saying no chaperone is normally offered but if desired can be provided (or some such).

I have used a chaperone twice in 40+ years and each time it was when I knew the patient had accused a previous doctor of sexual assault. So far no one has accused me of lewdness or creepiness or inappropriate behaviour. But then I have never been guilty of such things and I tend to consult with a mixture of light friendliness and serious distance which has taken four decades to develop.

What is **INFORMED consent**? You should, in explaining a procedure or treatment to a patient mention all the common and reasonable risks and disadvantages so that they can make a sensible decision. We all know though that almost every minor operation or course of drugs has a small risk of serious harm or death and that explaining all those possibilities would make the preamble to most procedures impractically long and frightening and probably put everyone off even the safest procedure. Patients usually have no concept of risk/benefit ratio (see immunisations). In the UK up until now "The Bolam test" has applied (the doctor will have discharged his obligation if he counsels the patient in a way that would be endorsed by a responsible body of medical opinion) but this defence is now beginning to change towards a demanding, less medically indulgent and more American system.

The Bolam Test has been used to help the courts decide in a variety of medical spheres of litigation – not just the adequacy of counselling. Surgical mistakes, unwanted side effects of treatment, obstetric disasters, GPs not telling parents about children on the pill or husbands with STDs. What do reasonable GPs normally do? – That was the basis as to how it was assessed.

Recently things have changed a little against doctors in that the gold standard is no longer what an average bunch of doctors in your speciality would do but what a reasonable patient would consider important and what evidence based medicine suggests is best. These are not necessarily the same as what doctors might tend to do en masse, as the judge now decides what constitutes an average patient and what evidence base to select. So the outcome is less familiar and is constantly changing compared with what a group of average doctors might actually do.

The modification of the Bolam defence was based on a decision made in the Bolitho v Hackney Health Authority case – that you couldn't just refer to commonly held opinion within the profession, it had to be *responsible* opinion.

The Bolam case though **was** a real one if you want to know, (1957, Bolam v Friern Hospital Management Committee) and the "Endorsement by a responsible body of opinion in the relevant speciality" concept has been used in courts as the parameter to judge all sorts of decisions in a variety of professional activities. After all, what do judges know about Cardiology, Paediatrics, Ophthalmology, Orthopaedics, Neurology etc? Who are they to decide between two arguing medical experts?

"Informed consent" is a moot point though. Do you mention the negligible risk of fat necrosis when you are injecting a shoulder? (I have done hundreds and never had this complication though if I were injecting Victoria Beckham or Claudia Schiffer I suppose I might feel obliged to mention it) or the 1:1000 risk of dying of a Pulmonary Embolus after a herniorrhaphy? Do you mention the 1:300,000 chance of a neurological reaction after Pertussis vaccination and at the same time the 10-100 times greater risk of death from actual whooping cough if you don't have the vaccination? I would imagine the parents of the many children who were killed or brain damaged by whooping cough **infection** and who will be similarly damaged by Measles **infection** might have a reasonable case to sue their GPs because they *were not informed loudly enough of the risks of* **not having** *the routine vaccination*. Watch out Andrew Wakefield!

Mental Capacity Act Code:

The Mental Capacity Act 2005 introduced:

A New Court of Protection from 2007 (contactable 24 hours a day by the clinician).

A New Office of the Public Guardian.

A New Independent Mental Advocacy Service (2007) whom local NHS authorities must appoint on behalf of some patients to make serious medical decisions and a Code of Practice.

The Act also sets out rules on Advanced Decisions to refuse treatment and Lasting Power of Attorney (LPA) covering new areas or a Court Appointed Deputy (CAD) to make decisions for situations when the patient will be unable to make their own decision.

The five key principles in the Act are:

Every adult has the right to make his or her own decisions and must be assumed to have capacity to make them unless it is proved otherwise.

A person must be given all practicable help before anyone treats them as not being able to make their own decisions.

Just because an individual makes what might be seen as an unwise decision, they should not be treated as lacking capacity to make that decision.

Anything done or any decision made on behalf of a person who lacks capacity must be done in their best interests. There is a "Best Interests checklist".

Anything done for or on behalf of a person who lacks capacity should be the least restrictive of their basic rights and freedoms. (You could read "The Children Act" by Ian McEwan if you want to get an idea of how complicated assessing a minor's rights can be).

A Lasting Power of Attorney is a legal document which states who will make decisions in lieu of the patient if and when they lack mental capacity. (An Enduring Power of Attorney already existed relating to property and money, The Lasting Power of Attorney now covers health, welfare, property and money.)

The Court of Protection can appoint a Deputy to act in your best interests if you have No Lasting Power of Attorney.

The Public Guardian supervises the Deputy.

Two stage assessment of Mental Capacity:

1) Does the patient have a temporary or permanent disturbance of brain function?

If that is the case, does it stop them making the relevant decision when they need to make it?

2) The person cannot make the decision if they cannot:

Understand the nature of the decision, the information and consequences involved.

Remember that information.

Weigh up the pros and cons in order to make the decision in a normal balanced way.

Communicate their decision.

The patient's best interests are the core of the act, try to get the patient involved as much as possible, refer to the patient's past wishes and decisions on the matter, talk to everyone involved and keep good notes on the process.

Try to involve potential future changes in circumstances in any decision. If an **ADVANCE DECISION** is recorded in the medical notes **it is confidential**. This will cause some difficulty and may need to be negotiated to be clear about the patient's actual wishes, who is allowed to know etc.

You should, in any record of advance written decisions include full details of the patient, the GP and if they have a copy, a statement saying the document should be used if the person ever lacks the capacity to make decisions, a clear statement of the decision, the treatment to be refused, the situation in which the decision will apply, the date, the patient or representative's signature, the witness' signature.

A standard mental capacity act assessment form is included.

Mental Capacity Assessment and Best Interests

What procedure or treatment does the person have to make a decision about?

What information have they been given by you or others about the procedure or treatment and risks involved in consenting to it or refusing it?

You should assume that the person has capacity to make the decision unless they are giving you cause to doubt it. What is causing you concern that they lack capacity?

Does the person have an impairment of, or disturbance in, the functioning of their mind or brain?		If yes, briefly describe
YES	**NO**	
		If no, the MCA does not apply

Whose opinion have you asked for to help you decide about capacity?

Does the person have a general understanding of: what decision they need to make, why they need to make it and the likely consequences of making, or not making, this decision?

Explain your decision
Yes –
No – Explain why you think they cannot understand this

Is the person able to retain the information long enough to make the decision?

Explain your decision
Yes –
No – Explain why you think they cannot retain the information

Is the person able to use and weigh up the information relevant to this decision?

Explain your decision
Yes -
No – Explain why you think they cannot weigh up the information

Can the person communicate their decision by talking, using sign language or any other means?
Explain your decision Yes – No – Explain why they cannot communicate
IMPORTANT - If you have answered 'NO' to any of the above 4 questions then the person you are assessing is deemed to be lacking in capacity.
Before making a decision in someone's best interests, because you have assessed them as lacking capacity to make this particular decision, consider:
Even if the person lacks capacity, can the decision be delayed until they regain capacity? *Explain your decision (if yes don't proceed)*
Do they have an advance decision which covers this issue? If they do then you should follow the guidance in this document.
Before deciding on best interests ensure that you have done whatever is possible to permit and encourage the person to take part, or to improve their ability to take part, in making the decision.
Consider the person's past and present wishes and feelings (in particular if they have been written down).
Explain what you took into account (eg family or friends' assertions re the patients wishes)
Consider any beliefs and values (e.g. religious, cultural or moral) that would be likely to influence the decision in question and any other relevant factors.
Explain what you took into account
Who else have you asked about what is in the person's best interest and what did they say? Does anyone disagree with the decision?
Explain (eg GP or other professionals who knows the patient)
What have you decided is in their best interests? Include details of any restrictions or restraint that may be necessary.

Advance Care Planning:

Advance directives, Advance Health Care Directive, Living Wills, may include instructions to withhold treatment from oneself given a future hopeless situation but they cannot include instructions to end life ("No antibiotics" but not "A lethal injection" please).

Advance care planning needs to be done when the patient has mental capacity. Advance care planning is a key process of discussion between an individual and their carer provided it enables planning and provision of needs and preference based care for those people approaching the end of life. This involves the identification of patients who may require additional supportive care at this stage in their lives, the holistic advanced planning of that care and recording of the patient's preferences and the planning of any agreed care.

An Independent Mental Capacity Advocate IMCA service.

This was set up under the Mental Capacity Act in 2007.

Assesses a patient's ability to decide such matters as an advanced directive. A local IMCA can usually be found on the Internet and they are intended to help people without family or support.

Advanced Directive:

A lawful decision generally is one that the patient has made while having mental capacity or one that is in the patient's best interests if they do not have the capacity to decide for them self.

An Advanced Directive is made while the patient is "capacitous", to cover treatment alternatives which they may not physically or mentally be in a position to express a choice about later but they know in advance what the decision would be. It is usually a statement that requests the medical team not to be heroic, not to attempt resuscitation or life prolonging treatment in the event of an incurable terminal illness. This of course should be the natural and normal state of affairs for most elderly patients and certainly those with chronic life diminishing illness, especially those with cancer, serious neurological illness and so on. The life expectancy of successfully resuscitated patients is very poor whatever their background. We, the medical profession should make these decisions without legal documents telling us what is in the patient's best interests. For instance it should also be normal not to attempt resuscitation in the seriously disabled, very dependent young adult – shouldn't it? – or should it? But how do we assess quality of life when we are constantly balancing what we perceive to be the relatives' pressure to prolong life endlessly these days against what we see often as an uncomfortable, joyless, totally hopeless and dependent existence. Cared for usually by a succession of disinterested, poorly paid strangers. But then again, talk to the parents of some seriously disabled young adults and they will tell you of the simple pleasure, fulfilment and feedback both sides of the partnership can sometimes get.

Note:

A **POLST** is a Physician Order for Life Sustaining Treatment (in the USA) which provides greater insight and ability to care or to plan for the care of those patients unlikely to live a year.

DNAR and Tracey Vs Cambridge University Hospital NHS Trust:

Clin Med Vol 14 .571

The Appeal Court decision in this case was that the patient's human rights under article 8 (The right to a private or family life – although what they really mean is a right to perpetual existence I suppose?) had been breached, as a decision not to resuscitate her had been made without consulting her first. This decision places a responsibility upon clinicians to consult before filling in a DNAR form except in very limited circumstances. The patient, Janet Tracey had metastatic lung cancer, chronic lung disease and was admitted to hospital with a serious cervical fracture. She had previously been given a prognosis of no more than 9 months and subsequently failed two extubations. After a "successful" third extubation Mrs Tracey subsequently deteriorated and died. The family brought the case against the Trust and the Secretary of State. No doubt you feel as confused, angry and frustrated by this complaint and this situation as I do. It is hard to imagine someone suffering more, with a worse prognosis or quality of life or for whom any decision to resuscitate would be more wrong.

This decision means that you should normally discuss whether or not to attempt resuscitation with the patient personally. If you consider that resuscitation will fail, the patient cannot demand it, but you should still tell the patient the clinical decision has been taken. Only if the discussion will cause physical or psychological harm to the patient may it be omitted. However: Let's get real: If you consider resuscitation would be wrong and the patient demands you do it then the discussion where you say you won't resuscitate them will inevitably cause psychological harm. What planet do lawyers live on?

In practical terms the question will usually be (and this is a classic example of the gulf between the idealism, lack of grounding and unreal expectations of lawyers (judges) and the realism and practicality of (doctors)) – Will resuscitation stand any chance of being successful or of giving a meaningful life (with spontaneous respiration, a lack of pain, but with awareness and some pleasure and fulfilment – "a quality of life") or will it fail and perpetuate a dependent, bleak, blank, unpleasant, painful or miserable existence? So do you want to spend time you usually cannot spare, having a surreal conversation in which there is only one sensible humane outcome but you are duty bound to offer two alternatives to a patient who is usually sick, bewildered, confused and in no real mental or emotional state to make the decision? The truth is you and I know very well that the way you pose the question often begs the answer.

This is classic lawyer's stuff, classic human rights getting involved in medicine nonsense. Is there a basic human right to misery and pain?

A Typical Advanced Directive, Living Will or Health Care Directive:

This advanced decision or directive allows the patient to provide instructions for medical care and treatment should they become incapable at a future date while they are still able to make decisions for them self. It provides an opportunity to discuss the treatment with family and medical staff.

Governing Law (eg England, Scotland)
Your Information:
Name, Address, DoB
Date
Advance Statement of Values and Beliefs

An Advance Statement is a description of your views and beliefs that you wish to be taken into account if health care decisions are being made for you. While such a statement is not binding on medical professionals, it could provide them with the kind of information they need to make decisions for you when you are no longer able to do so for yourself. This feature is optional.

I wish to include a statement of my basic values and beliefs:

Living Will

Below, you can select what kinds of treatment you would or would not want to receive if you should be diagnosed with a terminal condition. If you would prefer to specify something different about a particular kind of treatment, select "or" and type your instruction in the space provided.

Terminal Condition

If my condition is determined to be terminal and with no hope of recovery, I would like the following done:

Life Support:

I DO NOT w ant to be kept alive by artificial life support. ▼

or I do want to be kept alive by artificial support

Tube Feeding:

I w ant tube feeding. ▼

Or I do not wish to be fed by a tube

CPR:

I w ant to be given CPR if my heart s tops beating. ▼

or I do not wish to be resuscitated

Intervening Illness:

If I develop another illness, I w ant that illness to be treated. ▼

or I do not wish any interval illness treated

Persistent Unconsciousness

If I am persistently unconscious with no hope of recovery, I would like the following done:

Life Support:

I w ant all possible life prolonging procedures. ▼

I do not wish to be kept alive artificially

Tube Feeding:

I w ant tube feeding. ▼

I do not want to be tube fed

CPR:

I w ant to be given CPR if my heart s tops beating. ▼

I do not want to be resuscitated

Intervening Illness:

If I develop another illness, I w ant that illness to be treated. ▼

I do not wish to have any illness treated

Severe and Permanent Mental Impairment

If I am severely and permanently mentally impaired, I would like the following done:

Life Support:

| I w ant all possible life prolonging procedures. | ▼ |

I do not wish to be kept alive artificially
Tube Feeding:

| I w ant tube feeding. | ▼ |

I do not want to be tube fed
CPR:

| I w ant to be given CPR if my heart stops beating. | ▼ |

I do not want to be tube fed in this situation
Intervening Illness:

| If I develop another illness, I w ant that illness to be treated. | ▼ |

I do not want any interval illness treated
If my behaviour becomes violent, disruptive or disturbed I wish it to be controlled by drugs even if that might shorten my life.
Likewise if I am suffering pain, I wish it to be adequately treated whatever the effect on my physical condition or lifespan.
Other Treatments
□

I wish to express the following feelings about certain treatments:

Organ Donation
□

I want to give directions about organ donation.
Additional Instructions

You may want to provide instructions about other issues that concern you. Some examples are:
– Who you want to be with you during your final moments.
– Who you would prefer not to be present during your illness.
– Who will care for your pets during your illness.
□

I want to include additional instructions.
Signing Details
Date
Name and number of witnesses:
A witness should be at least 18 years of age, should not be a spouse or partner, should not be entitled to any portion of your estate and should not be your health care provider, an employee of your health care provider or an employee of a nursing home or care facility in which you are a resident.
Where will the document be signed?

The Court of Protection:

Was also set up under the Mental Capacity Act and is designed to advise and adjudicate for patients who are unable to make treatment or financial decisions for themselves. Applications can be made by letter but it is theoretically accessible 24 hours a day.

The Public Guardian

Again is a new office under the Mental Capacity act and is tasked with supervising LPAs, deputies and coordinates with police and SS in cases of abuse of people with limited mental capacity.

Life prolonging care:

A competent adult can refuse life sustaining treatment and if his medical attendants believe his quality of life is so poor that his best interests are served by withdrawing life prolonging care then the court usually supports that decision. (See the legally protracted, false hope filled, expensive and extremely sad life of poor Charlie Gard.) It is slightly different when treatment is commenced with the express purpose of killing the hopeless patient and this of course is where the post Shipman suspicions, the Liverpool Pathway cruelties and the apparent new found lack of trust in the inherent well meaning of nurses and doctors in our patients' hours of need may have created a frightening mix of anxiety and foreboding in dying patients.

The courts are supposed to apply a "Best Interests" test and thankfully this doesn't always include continuing to live and suffer. In law there is no difference between withholding and withdrawing treatment. If there were, it could easily discourage doctors from starting a life saving but not guaranteed treatment which might leave the patient alive but severely damaged.

Compensation:

After a medical error or accident, most angry patients and relatives seek their retribution to be paid in the form of a fine, financial compensation theoretically levied against the "guilty party" as a punishment. Retribution against the people responsible for the harm they or their loved ones have suffered. The fallacies in this legal merry go round are that most of the time the doctor did not intend to cause the damage, not in the way a thief or a felon sets out to commit a crime, the hospital and doctor are not going to pay the compensation themselves and the money often comes out of funding for further patient services thus making those services worse for the next patient. The prime focus of their legal team is to seek compensation for their client in the form of cash. If a wage earner has died or been injured and so is unable to earn a living or someone requires private care this might be justified. Usually however the ongoing medical care is to be provided by the state, free. Thus the financing is irrelevant.

The way the process proceeds is by accusation, blame, cover up and denial. The legal and medical professions have no concept of the other's motives or self justification. In short they are suspicious of, resent and misunderstand one another.

I have never understood why there seems this and only this form of settlement through the courts. Most claimants say in interviews that all they want is for other patients not to suffer as they have done. Simply an acknowledgement of error and a public apology from the closed ranks of self justifying professionals. But then they never, never decline their compensation cheques and by draining the NHS of resources they are ensuring worse care for other patients.

I read these stories with despair. The legal profession always wins, (always gets paid), the NHS, the patients and the tax payer always lose. It is now a staggering seventh of the NHS budget that is paid in compensation. £15.7Bn in 2012. Think how much extra care that could provide. Parliament is ruled by lawyers and so things are unlikely to change anytime soon. Punitive litigation and compensation have been shown throughout the world to have no beneficial effect on clinical standards or doctors' behaviour. Lawyers have no real interest in improved health care. If they did they would encourage lower compensation payments. It is retribution and recompense pure and simple. What does improve standards is when clinicians analyse their accidents and mistakes and make organisational changes, particularly staffing, cover and SOP changes to their routine work as a result. This is done best through routine clinical meetings to openly discuss what went wrong or could have been done better in a mea culpa atmosphere of constructive "no blame".

Compensation to the parents of brain damaged babies is paid assuming a future life of privately funded care, adaptations made to houses, often full time carers and so on.

I can see how having privately funded nurses all day is nicer than having the NHS District Nurse or Social Services but why do you deserve Rolls Royce care when the person next door who didn't sue has to put up with the same care as all the other NHS brain damaged babies? You get the better service for life because of "negligence"; they get the common or garden service because of bad luck. In all likelihood it was bad luck in both cases.

Doesn't that imply the NHS is providing a pretty poor service? And think of the harm that siphoning those millions into your baby's private care does by depleting the funds available so that planned treatments for other sick patients can no longer be afforded? £6m-£10m pay outs to the parents of brain damaged children are common now and the NHS bill for compensation is £18bn and rising ("Negligence payouts bankrupting NHS – Independent 31/8/2013"). An unbelievable £56Bn set aside for compensation claims in Dec 2016 (Express Online front page). A senior staff nurse on ITU earns £32,000 so that one £6m pay out could fund 187 senior ITU nurses. Isn't something very wrong here?

Given the fact that we have a state health care system and a Welfare State you could wonder why we have a system that pays any medical litigant large sums of money under any circumstances. The "victim" shouldn't need to pay for reasonable care and they should get sickness and or unemployment benefit if medical negligence leaves them unfit to earn a crust.

Compensation was never, I believe, designed to make up for dented pride, inconvenience or hurt feelings. Compensation is supposed to put patients back in the position they would have been but for the medical negligence that took place. It is supposed to cover things like pain, suffering, loss of earnings, (If that is EVER possible to predict), the cost of appliances, cost of care and the loss of amenity – for instance the amenity of your leg below the knee is worth £150,000. All these sums though should be to a basic agreed level assuming the state will cover most of the family's needs anyway. The current type of multimillion pound pay outs are unsustainable, unjustifiable, promote defensive (bad, inappropriate and expensive) medicine and are harming the care of thousands in the intensely cash limited organisation we work in, the NHS.

Human Rights Put simply: (and simplistically)

The right to life.

The right not to be tortured or treated in an inhuman or degrading way.

The right to be free from slavery or forced labour.

The right to liberty.

The right to a fair trial.

The right to no punishment without law.

The right to respect for private and family life, home and correspondence.

The right to freedom of thought, conscience and religion.

The right to freedom of expression.

The right to freedom of assembly and association.

The right not to be discriminated against.

The right to peaceful enjoyment of possessions.

The right to an education.

The right to free elections.

The problem, of course, is how you interpret these 14 slices of motherhood and apple pie.

26: THE LIVER:

Hepatitis B: The complex serology:

The Hepatitis B Surface Antigen HBsAg is part of the infecting virus. The Hepatitis B Surface Antibody HBsAb or anti-HBs is the patient's protective antibody, does not indicate infection or infectivity but does indicate immunity or vaccination.

Hepatitis B Core Antibody HBcAb or anti-HBc. This antibody does not provide protection against Hep B but shows previous exposure.

Surface Ag	Core Ab	Surface Ab	Clinical Interpretation
Neg	Neg	Neg	No exposure.
Pos	Neg	Neg	Early acute Hepatitis B.
Pos	Pos	Neg	Acute infection or carrier.
Neg	Pos	Neg	Persisting infection or early seroconversion/convalescence.
Neg	Pos	Pos	Recovered, immunity developing.
Neg	Neg	Pos	Immune to Hep B.

	HBe AG	HBsAG	HBeAb	HBSAb
Acute	+	+	−	−
Vaccinated	−	−	−	+
Non Hep Carrier	−	+	+	−
Chronic Hepatitis (Infectious)	+	+	−	−

Put another way:

HBsAg pos	Anti HBe Ab pos	Core IgM Neg	Low risk Hep B carrier.
HBsAg pos	HBe Ag pos	Core IgM Neg	High risk Hep B carrier.
HBsAg pos	HBe Ag pos	Core IgM pos	Acute Hep B infection.

or another:

HBsAg	neg Susceptible
anti-HBc	neg
anti-HBs	neg

HBsAg	neg Immune due to natural infection
anti-HBc	pos
anti-HBs	pos

HBsAg	neg Immune due to vaccination
anti-HBc	neg
anti-HBs	pos

HBsAg	pos Acutely infected
anti-HBc	pos
IgM	anti-HBc pos
anti-HBs	neg

HBsAg	pos	Chronically infected
anti-HBc	pos	
IgM	anti-HBc neg	
anti-HBs	neg	

HBsAg	neg	Interpretation could be resolved infection (most common)
anti-HBc	pos	pos anti – HBc, thus susceptible
anti-HBs	neg	Low level chronic infection
		Resolving acute infection.

To check immunisation, check Hep B Surface Ab. Immunisation does not protect recipient against pre-existing disease complications or potential recipients of his blood from infection.

Vaccination: (**Engerix B, Fendrix, HB Vax PRO**) Stat, one month, one year. Check Ab response – if low give further dose, if still low, only 50% respond to a further primary course. If good initial response (>100MIU/ml) probably never need another booster.

HBeAg positivity indicates infectiousness in HBsAg pos individuals.

Core Ab indicates natural infection.

Hep B virus has 3 antigenic components:

Surface Ag (persistence>6m means carrier status) – No protective Anti HBs (Hepatitis B surface Ab)

Core Ag

eAg

We should exclude HBeAg+ carriers from exposure prone procedures – indicates active viral replication. Also infectivity of Hep B carriers is related to the concentration of HBVDNA.

HBeAg pos and needle-stick injury risk 19-30%

HBeAg neg and needle stick injury risk is 2-5%

Note: **Twinrix** Vaccine is Hep A and Hep B vaccine. Gives 10 years protection against A and up to 5 yrs against B. Give Stat 1month and 6 months.

Anti viral therapy:

Hepatitis C: Beta or alpha interferon and Ribavarin for 24 weeks.

Hepatitis B: Interferon alpha and Lamivudine. These days most hepatitis B patients are migrants from Eastern Europe or Africa.

Hepatitis C:

They started screening donated blood for Hep C in 1991. This was after 7,500 patients had become infected by foreign blood products, leading eventually to 2,400 deaths mainly from Hepatitis C and HIV and an inquiry announcement in July 2017. This has been described as the NHS' greatest disaster and cover up.

In 2003 there were either 60,000 or 200,000 known infected individuals in the UK – I have read articles which quoted both figures – but up to 5X as many were suspected of having the infection (That is 1 in 100-200 of the population!) In 2002 there were 1000 Hep C positive blood donors

These patients should receive Hep A and B vaccination.

Of 100 exposed, 80 develop chronic Hepatitis C, 60 get long term liver inflammation and 16 will develop cirrhosis over the subsequent 20-30 years. 1-2 may get liver cancer.

Sexual transmission is less than 5% in stable partners. Vertical transmission to children is 6% unless they are HIV co infected. Hepatitis C is not transmitted in breast milk.

Hepatitis C currently affects 0.4% of the British population (7 per average GP list). The majority of patients are infected by blood contamination. Needle-stick injury carries a 2% risk. 10-30% have a "sporadic" infection with no known cause. Household contacts should not share toothbrushes or razors and should cover open wounds. The infected must notify their insurance companies.

The confirmed clearance of Hepatitis viral RNA suggests a cure. Antivirals are used if fibrosis and or significant inflammation are present on biopsy. e.g. Peginterferon alpha and Ribavirin for 24-48 weeks or B Interferon and Ribavirin.

HCV is in 6 serotypes, 2 and 3 being more sensitive to treatment.

Specialist HCV units exist in various parts of the UK Including The Royal Free, St Marys, Kings College, Addenbrookes, etc.

Hepatitis C affects 3% of the world's population, but less than 0.1% of the UK donor population. Worldwide, 100m are carriers. In Europe the prevalence is 0.5-2%. Infection is parenteral, sexual or perinatal. Average transmission rate after percutaneous injury is 1.8%. The transmission risk is higher during viraemia (when there is a pos polymerase chain reaction for HCV RNA). If the PCR is neg but the patient is Ab pos then they have cleared the infection and there is no long term risk of liver disease unless they are reinfected.

Hepatitis E:

80% British pigs carry Hepatitis E, 10% British sausages are positive and French sausages carry 700,000 viruses per gram. Sausages must be cooked at 70C for at least 20minutes to kill the virus – a temperature and duration not reached by many Bar B Ques. This is of significance to the under immune (those on steroids, chemotherapy or with HIV etc) as Hep E is normally a relatively minor infection with a mortality around 1-3% but much more serious in the vulnerable. There were 660 confirmed cases in the UK In 2012 but it is increasing in frequency and many cases go unrecognised. In the Far East it is considered so much a growing problem that China has produced a vaccination.

Haemochromatosis:

The commonest recessive condition, 1:200. Commoner in Northern Europeans and descendants. The human haemochromatosis protein is also known as the HFE protein. The HFE gene (High Fe, iron) on the short arm of chromosome 6 is at location 6p22.2. There are 37 allelic variants.

Transferrin >55% (M) >50% (Premenopausal F)

(N adult 2 – 4.0 g/L (200-400mg/dl), maternal 3.0g/L).

Transferrin Saturation is also raised in haemochromotosis Normal Fem 12-45% Male 15-50%

Serum Ferritin only rises after liver stores are full. TIBC may be low but can be normal. It causes cirrhosis, hypopituitrism, cardiomyopathy, diabetes, arthritis and pigmentation.

May occasionally be secondary to too much iron administration (transfusions, haemolysis, supplements).

Treatment: Venesection.

Abnormal Liver Function Tests:

Bilirubin, albumin, transferases, (which are non specific and are present in skeletal and cardiac muscle and RBCs), GGT (elevated with ALP in cholestasis or if elevated alone suggest induction of liver enzymes), ALP (from bone as well as the bile ducts where damage or pressure causes raised GGT as well) – Isoenzyes differentiate the source. ALP is raised physiologically in growth as well as in bone damage and also comes from the placenta in pregnancy.

Causes:

Drugs including paracetamol, isoniazid, troglitazone, ketoconazole, phenytoin (hepatitis), co amoxiclav, erythromycin, TCAs. ACEIs are cholestatic.

Fatty Liver Disease which is probably the commonest contemporary cause of raised LFTs.

Alcohol (AST: ALT 2:1), viral hepatitis, auto immune hepatitis, biliary disease which may be secondary to stones, cholecystitis, obstruction, etc., tumours, primary and secondaries, lymphoma etc., Haemochromatosis, Sarcoid, CCF, Primary Biliary Cirrhosis, Primary Sclerosing Cholangitis, Progressive Familial Intrahepatic Cholestasis, anorexia (AST, ALT),

Ischaemia of liver but including MI (AST, ALT), α1 Antitrypsin Deficiency, Wilson's Disease, Glycogen Storage Diseases, non hepatic causes: Coeliac, haemolysis, hyperthyroidism.

The bloods for a liver work up include not just enzymes but:

Immunoglobulins (IgA, alcohol, IgM antimitochondrial antibodies in PBC, IgG autoimmune liver disease), serology, virology (CMV, EBV, Rubella, HIV etc), FBC, electrolytes, TFTs, iron studies, copper studies, alpha fetoprotein, alpha 1 anti trypsin, clotting studies, auto immune profile, imaging.

Non alcoholic fatty liver disease, NAFLD, NASH Is the commonest cause of liver dysfunction in the western world. It is part of the Insulin Resistance, obesity, Metabolic Syndrome spectrum and can respond to the same treatments as Type 2 DM i.e. diet, Metformin and thiazolidinediones. It is associated with hypertension and hyperlipidaemia.

The worst type of NAFLD is:

Non alcoholic steatohepatitis, NASH – is a common cause of cirrhosis. The associated hepatocellular injury of NASH can lead to cirrhosis, liver fibrosis or hepatocellular carcinoma as well as an increased cardiovascular risk. In this, alcohol consumption is by definition low (<2g or 25ml/day) and the condition is usually asymptomatic. There is no currenty approved treatment for NASH but weight loss, pioglitazone, angiotensin receptor antagonists, Vitamin E and Obeticholic Acid are being assessed.

Various drugs can cause NAFLD and these include:

Amiodarone, Tetracyclines, Aspirin (Reye's syndrome in the young), steroids, Methotrexate, Tamoxifen, Some antivirals.

Overall, the treatment of NAFLD is similar to that of Type 2 DM and Metabolic Syndrome. A calorie and fat restricted diet, Metformin (which will help reduce the incidence of various cancers too!) thiazolidinediones, high dose vitamin E, statins and even ONE glass of wine a day all have their place. Coffee consumption reduces the severity of steatohepatitis in NAFLD. Daily coffee consumption should be encouraged in these conditions. (You may remember that coffee enemas are part of the Gerson treatment in cancer and are said to "detoxify" the liver, regular coffee consumption is also considered one way of counteracting various fatty liver disorders).

Some authorities blame wholesale consumption of fructose for NAFLD. Fructose is the most soluble sugar, found in fruit, some vegetables, honey, table sugar, Agave syrup etc. It is a monosaccharide often bonded to another monosaccharide, glucose, forming the disaccharide sucrose, table sugar.

Co Enzyme CQ10 supplementation reduces LFTs and inflammatory markers in NAFLD.

I said NAFLD was the commonest cause of abnormal LFTs but I was excluding patients on statins in that statement and that only applied to liver enzymes. Bilirubin alone is frequently abnormal – as in Gilbert's Syndrome-unconjugated hyperbilirubinaemia*.

NAFLD and NASH (Non Alcoholic Steatohepatitis) have no definitive aetiology or therapy, or even evidence based clinical guidelines. However the WGO, (World Gastroenterology Association) Guidelines (2014) say:

NAFLD is excessive Tg accumulation in the liver (steatosis), – some of these patients develop liver cell damage (steatohepatitis), excessive local fat and this is NASH. Histologically it is similar to alcohol damage. There is no short term morbidity but if progression to NASH takes place then there is the increased risk of cirrhosis, liver failure and cancer.

Gilbert's Syndrome:*

This is benign Aut. Rec. unconjugated hyperbilirubinaemia. (Indirect bilirubin is unconjugated/Direct bilirubin is conjugated). The gene is on the long arm of chromosome 2 (2q37). The enzyme which is reduced is uridine disphosphate glucuronosyl transferase 1A1. It conjugates bilirubin.

Bilirubin:

Unconjugated:

Due to haemolysis, (check the Coomb's test), drugs, Gilbert's and the very rare Crigler Najjar syndrome.

Gilbert's syndrome is very common. Back in the days when house jobs and long weekends meant up to 80 hours unbroken on call over each weekend, inside under fluorescent lights surrounded by sick patients and yellow curtains I became aware that my normal sallow pallor was complimented by an icteric tinge to my sclerae. I immediately assumed that I had acquired infectious hepatitis or was haemolysing. I was immunised against Hep B and HIV didn't exist. I sat down in the ward coffee room with 4 other junior staff bemoaning my fate. The medical registrar told me not to be an idiot. I needed some sunshine and all I had was Gilbert's syndrome, as indeed had he and it turned out, one other of the 4 doctors present. Three out of five doctors with Gilberts syndrome.

This was a bit of a statistical quirk as it is actually affects somewhere between 5 and 10% of the population. The condition is benign and due to underactive glucuronyl transferase. This enzyme renders bilirubin water soluble so it can be excreted in bile.

Irinotecan (a cytotoxic drug used in lower GI cancers) is not metabolised properly by patients with Gilbert's and they also have a higher rate of gallstones. On the plus side though, having a slightly raised bilirubin seems to significantly protect you from cardiovascular disease and you share at least one thing with Napoleon.

Conjugated:

Raised in the equally rare Dubin-Johnson and Rotor syndromes. As well as with various chronic liver diseases

Gallstones:

15% of us will develop gallstones at some time in our lives. Gallstones are precipitated out from a variety of bile constituents: Cholesterol in the UK, bile pigment or calcium are other constituents that can precipitate and build up the stone. Only 10% show up on XR. Oestrogen increases cholesterol excretion in bile (-hence female, fat, fertile), but inherited factors, pregnancy, damage to the terminal ileum, weight loss, metabolic syndrome and cystic fibrosis also increase the risk of biliary stones.

Stones present with pain or infection-cholecystitis or cholangitis, common bile duct stones can obstruct and cause jaundice and further down pancreatitis, they can obstruct the ileum causing ileus and long term they are one risk factor for gall bladder carcinoma.

Investigations: LFTs – Alk P'ase, bilirubin, GGT, also WBC, amylase and lipase. CRP, ESR and clotting. USS.

Interestingly, small stones may be worse (a bigger long term risk of pancreatitis) than bigger stones in the asymptomatic.

The treatments depend on the clinical situation: Antibiotics (Co amoxiclav), analgesics and anti emetics in the acute situation, cholecystectomy (usually laparoscopically and electively). ERCP or open surgery for CBD stones. Despite the Lower fat and high fibre diets of vegetarians and their lower BMIs, data from the EPIC study (2017) surprisingly showed they have an increased risk gall stones (HR 1.22 P=.006).

Weil's Disease:

This is a form of Leptospirosis, a bacterial infection usually causing 'flu like symptoms but occasionally causing a more severe infection. IP 7-12 days. It is via contact with animal urine contaminated soil or water. The portal of entry is any mucous membrane, swallowed water or damaged skin.

Various forms of Leptospirosis are spread by cattle, dogs, pigs, rodents, amphibians, reptiles. The usual symptoms are biphasic, with myalgia, pyrexia, H/A, nausea, vomiting, cough and flu symptoms initially. One tenth of patients deteriorate and develop a more severe illness with meningitis, oedema, hepatitis, tachycardia, dyspnoea, anuria, bleeding, confusion, seizures, encephalitis, haemoptysis, jaundice and this is called Weil's disease. Once established, Leptospira organisms may be found in blood, urine and CSF. There are serological tests including immune assays to confirm the infection and it responds to Penicillin, Doxycycline, Ceftriaxone.

27: Miscellaneous:

Alternative treatments:

Acupuncture:
Needling through the skin has been used in Traditional Chinese Medicine (TCM) according to maps (meridians) and an idea of physiology (the life force energy, qi) which clearly don't exist. At least in terms of having physical structures that are anatomical and demonstrable by dissection or scanning.

Cochrane reviews show some effect in the limited areas of post operative and chemo-therapy sickness and idiopathic headache. NICE have recently excluded acupuncture from treatment for back pain. The process of puncturing the skin and moving needle tips in subcutaneous tissue may well release endorphins which relax muscle spasm locally for a while and may have some psychological benefits. You can imagine how difficult it is to do a controlled double blind study to genuinely assess the effect of acupuncture (-you would have to give general anaesthesia and then do the acupuncture, comparing outcomes). Random siting of needles can be as effective as putting them in traditional meridians. There is some beneficial effect on pain and nausea which are, of course highly subjective states, but not in most objective and quantifiable diseases. False acupuncture needles (that the patient thinks they can see being pushed into their skin but in fact retract within themselves, the needle sliding back into the shaft) have been used with local anaesthetic skin cream in controlled trials of IBS. The "acupuncture" was effective in a significant proportion of affected people. This tells you more about IBS than acupuncture really.

Reflexology:
Another unbelievable and placebo based treatment based on qi. (Qi but Not I.Q.). Here areas of the hands, ears or feet are stimulated and said to be able to influence distant parts of the body – having specific areas related to the different organs and working through reflex or possibly circulatory effects. Obviously, a basic grasp of anatomy known since the 17th C should correct any misunderstanding about why a nice person rubbing your hands feet or ears would make you feel better. Especially if they take the time to ask you personal questions, sympathetically, while appearing understanding and caring.

We are only beginning to fathom the power of the placebo effect. I describe elsewhere how research has shown that even when patients are told both that they are being given an inactive treatment but also "Some people with your condition respond to this inactive treatment and improve", significant numbers of patients do get better. What is more they relapse when the inactive treatment is stopped. Horizon BBC2 Feb 17 2014. Obviously however, the placebo effect has limits. It doesn't make solid tumours, infections, broken bones, genetic or traumatic injuries better.

Iridology:
Again this is a tribute to the imagination and hopefulness of people rather than their commonsense or rational mind. Here it is believed that medical conditions cause observable changes in the iris and aid diagnosis and treatment. There are different areas of the iris that relate to specific parts of the body-for instance, looking at the L eye, the heart is at 3 O'clock, the sciatic N about 5 O'clock, the rectum about 7 O' Clock and the oesophagus about 9 O'clock. All rigorous investigation as to whether irises change in response to

illness or whether Iridologists can in fact differentiate ill people from healthy have shown they don't. It is hard to imagine any evolutionary benefit having such a complex complete set of pointless feedback wiring would have. – AND if internal sickness were visible to the outside world, wouldn't evolution have made each one of us evolve the ability to read each other's eyes so we didn't make the mistake of having offspring with someone with a hidden genetic disorder?

Marry her? You must be joking, she is going to get Huntington's, you can see it in her irises, just take a look.

Homeopathy:

Most people (apart from Prince Charles) are well aware of the utter madness of Homeopathic theory. – That is: By giving an extremely diluted solution of something you can effect a cure for the condition that the agent normally causes in the patient – or that further dilutions of that agent make the final product even more effective through the ability of the solvent to remember the solute when no solute remains. There is a bit more to homeopathy than that, some involving herbal or vitamin treatments but most just as irrational and unproven.

My own personal experience of homeopathy was of a series of night visits to the child of our well known local homeopath about 30 years ago whom he had refused to vaccinate against whooping cough. I advised him that this was a dangerous course but he insisted that the best treatment would be a homeopathic medication. The child developed a severe 3 month paroxysmal cough, secondary pneumonia, subconjunctival haemorrhages, hypoxic fits and perforated ear drums and had to be admitted at least once for oxygen, antibiotics and (standard treatment at the time), steroids and sedatives. I remember my frustration at picking up the pieces of what I considered an irresponsible and dangerous parent and a child who was eventually left with bronchiectasis permanently and lucky not to be more severely damaged. All for an unscientific, irrational and dangerous myth.

Can someone explain why a parent that starves or neglects their child or refuses a life saving transfusion on religious grounds has that child removed after a case conference and a court order but a parent who injures the child, sometimes permanently, by refusing a life saving vaccination and treats them with nothing more than a fairy tale is allowed to keep him? In what way are they any different?

Tired all the time: TATT:

Elsewhere I make it clear that iron deficiency in all patients over 50 is bowel cancer until you have excluded it. Just putting the patient on iron without a preliminary examination, including an RE, and blood tests, a few OBs, iron studies, probably other things too – TFTs, LFTs, U and Es, FBC, coeliac antibodies etc (see Pathology) is reprehensible. Let's assume you have excluded another physical cause to your satisfaction. Even in the presence of a "normal iron" the chronically and puzzlingly tired patient can respond to iron treatment. We know that there is a great range of *normal* iron within the population.

Treatment with Ferrous Sulphate once daily in women with low normal iron status improves symptoms 50% apparently. I would tend to try multivitamins (Forceval usually) tds for ten days (which does contain iron and trace elements) then od for a month after doing the usual investigations – what have you got to lose?

Sarcoid:

Granulomatous nodules in virtually any organ (mainly lungs and lymph nodes).

Most cases clear spontaneously but a few develop chronic lung disease and various other complications. Tiredness and other systemic symptoms with breathlessness are common symptoms. E. Nodosum, dry eyes, bilateral hilar lymphadenopathy, progressing sometimes to interstitial lung disease are all possible.

Most people have pulmonary involvement. Also hepatomegaly, skin plaques, lupus pernio, (florid pink lumpy lesions of the nose, cheeks and rest of face and nothing to do with systemic lupus), heart involvement (arrhythmias), parotitis, cervical lymphadenopathy, facial palsy etc.

It is not known whether sarcoid is mainly genetic or post infectious, or a bit of both. It is probably an excess and inappropriate immune response to some ?infecting stimulus. That was the theory when I first read about it in my first medical text book in 1970 and that is still the theory today. Sarcoid granulomata produce Vitamin D in the form of 1 alpha 25 (OH) 2 Vit D which results in hypercalcaemia. I remember theories that the granulomata were a reaction to pollen grains or air borne foreign bodies or even mycobacteria of some sort when I was training. Vitamin D and prolactin levels are raised as a secondary effect and sarcoid is associated with, well, nearly everything-Thyroid disease, autoimmune disease, Coeliac Disease, various infections and cancers. ACE levels are monitored in the supervision and diagnosis of Sarcoid. The levels are raised in active Sarcoid.

The C1 esterase inhibitor level is also raised (it is low in hereditary angiooedema).

Mastalgia:

Treatment: Oil of evening primrose. Topical Ibuprofen Gel.
Pyridoxine 100mg OD,
Ascorbic Acid (neither have any side effects),
Tamoxifen which usually works very well.
Bromocryptine,
Goserelin,
Danazol (many unpleasant side effects).

Compression Hosiery:

Pressure:
Class 1: 14-17mm Hg
Class 2: 18-24mm Hg
Class 3: 25-35mm Hg
In prescriptions you should specify "The Manufacturer" and "Made to Measure stockings open toe below knee". – And remember if the support is tight enough to prevent the (usually frail and elderly) patient putting them on then they are going to need help.

Chilblains

This is cold damage to the extremities, particularly associated with damp cold injury. It affects toes but also involves ears, even the nose sometimes. The toes become red, itchy and painful, the symptoms lasting sometimes several weeks. Some people are more susceptible than others and it can rarely be a marker of connective tissue disease. Topical fluorinated steroids help itch, vasodilators such as Nifedipine or Diltiazem hasten healing and of course reduce the risk of recurrence. These lesions are cold ischaemic injury and can cause long lasting pain and visible painful induration. They can hurt and drag on for much more than the trivial name and reputation suggests.

Like so many common and "trivial" conditions we see every day, cold sores, haemorrhoids, in growing toenails, quinsy, shingles, post herpetic neuralgia, etc, they can be highly debilitating and very unpleasant indeed.

Raynaud's: (Syndrome, Phenomenon and Disease)

This is extremely common, extremely annoying and usually unrelated to general vascular health. Exclude connective tissue disorders, SLE, Systemic Sclerosis, AF, stop smoking and in men suggest avoiding vibrating tools. 9/10 of Raynauds phenomenon is "primary" rather than secondary to other conditions. The condition often leads to ischaemic damage (chilblains etc) to the peripheries even in the presence of good peripheral pulses. The vasoconstricted white finger, toe, ear or tip of nose is accompanied by numbness, then on warming, a tingling, throbbing, blueness and the redness of vasodilatation follow. The environmental temperature does not have to be particularly cold. Indeed, sometimes the patient will find that they can escape symptoms in very cold weather only to get them later in a slightly warmer but still cool environment.

Treatments vary from regional sympathectomy at one extreme to alternative medicine, which includes acupuncture, Niacin (nicotinic acid), fish oils, (containing GLA), ginger, oil of evening primrose, gingko biloba, Vitamins E and C etc at the other. (Omacor, Maxepa or Epogam are good sources of the appropriate oils). In between there are conventional drugs:

Calcium channel blockers, Nifedipine (Adalat retard), Amlodipine, Diltiazem, ACEIs, Captopril, Enalopril, Lisinopril, etc, AIIRAs Losartan, Valsartan, SSRIs, Fluoxetine, Sertraline, Paroxetine, GTN patches.

IN an emergency IV prostacyclin (Iloprost) can be administered.

Raynaud's Syndrome can be secondary to:
Autoimmune/Rheumatological disorders:
Vasospastic conditions:

Dermatomyositis,	Arteriosclerosis,
Sjogren's,	Migraine,
Takayasu's	Prinzmetal's angina,
Temporal Arteritis,	Thrombangitis Obliterans.
PBC,	
SLE, RhA, Scleroderma.	

Odd Treatments:

Soft Tissue Infections:

i.e. Cellulitis: Amoxicillin in big doses has better tissue penetration than Flucloxacillin, Erythromycin, Clarithromycin, or Clindamycin but often needs to be given for at least 14 days with elevation and rest. However I find Co Amoxiclav better than any of these in terms of response, recovery, freedom from side effects AND complications.

After Vasectomy, infection is common and a good combination is Cefradine and Metronidazole for 5 days.

Hypersalivation/Drooling:

Responds to Atropine 600mcg 1-2 nocte. Or Hyoscine (OTC as Kwells 300mcg, can be used in children from 4 years, also as a treatment for motion sickness).

on the other hand:

Dry mouth, Lack of saliva:

Pilocarpine 5mg TDS.

Nausea/Vertigo:
Buccastem, Prochlorperazine 3mg, 1-2 bd/tds (max qds) sub lingual absorption, used in Menieres, not very effective in my experience, but can be used in the nausea/vomiting of migraine.

Diarrhoea after Cholecystectomy:
Cholestyramine, Questran which is usually prescribed to lower cholesterol, often helps. This is an ion exchange resin, a bile acid sequestrant which can stop itching in liver failure and can also help reduce the diarrhoea in the rapid transit form of IBS.

Flying

Air Travel: Contraindications:

(Cabin pressure is 6,000 – 8,000 feet (1828-2440m) above sea level) Note: Ben Nevis, the UK's tallest peak is 1344m so a pressurised cabin is equivalent to almost twice this altitude.

Respiratory Disease:
Patients who can walk 50m on the flat without oxygen at a steady pace and without dyspnoea or needing to stop should not find cabin pressure difficult.

Airlines will provide extra oxygen if forewarned, at an extra charge. Nebulisers are not permitted on take-off or landing.

For children with Cystic Fibrosis and other chronic lung diseases and an FEV1<50% predicted, a hypoxic challenge test is recommended. If the SpO2 falls below 90% during the challenge, supplementary in flight oxygen is recommended. Passengers may carry small oxygen cylinders with them provided they seek permission first (they may be charged). All flights to and from the USA carry bronchodilator inhalers in their medical kit.

Pregnancy >35 weeks international,

36 weeks internal.

Clearance after 28 weeks. Some airlines ban twin pregnancies after 30 weeks.

Neonates not under 48 hours,

Infectious diseases,

Offensive passengers,

Terminal illness if likely to die in flight,

Uncompensated heart failure,

Recent MI (within 21 days of an acute episode of ischaemia). Patients should be "Able to walk 80m and climb 10-12 stairs without symptoms."

With heart failure, as a rough guide the patient should be also be able to walk 80m and climb 10-12 stairs without symptoms before flying.

Severe respiratory disease – If a patient can walk 100yds without severe dyspnoea then OK to fly.

All infectious diseases,

OM,

Recent middle ear surgery is a C/I until the middle ear is dry and aerated normally.

Sinusitis.

Pneumothorax: The "Arbitrary" 6 week rule has been discarded. A minimum delay of 1 week after full radiographic resolution on CXR is advised before flying or 2 weeks after traumatic pneumothorax or thoracic surgery.

Not less than 10 days after abdominal surgery or GI Bleed.

Colostomies may need extra dressings.

Not less than 14 days after chest surgery.

Dyspnoea at rest is a complete contraindication to flying. Breathlessness after 50m walk on the flat – the patient should be seen and issued with a "Fitness to fly Certificate".

Not less than 7 days after eye surgery or penetrating injury.

No long haul flight within 3 months of hip or knee replacement.

Epilepsy may be more likely-notify airline.

Non ambulant cases with cerebrovascular disease,

Patients prone to confusion must be accompanied,

Stroke if less than 10 days, some say 21 days,

Epilepsy if less than 24 hrs,

Brain surgery under 10 days.

Diabetic patients only if they can manage their own medication.

Severe anaemia (Hb<8gm/dl).

Various psychiatric disorders.

After the introduction of air to body to body cavities for at least 7 days. At altitude sea level gases can increase their volume by 30%.

Others: Wired jaws, middle ear surgery? Sickle Cell ? Within 7 Days of Tonsillectomy.

There is a higher risk of DVT in lung cancer.

Careful assessment of the cardiac risk of children with Down's syndrome before flying is suggested.

Traveller's Thrombosis. Economy Class Syndrome, Flight related DVT.

Staying still in one position with the knees flexed, possibly sleeping, possibly becoming dehydrated is not exclusive to flying. It happens on long coach journeys, even in theatres. Getting up and walking about is not always practical even on long flights especially if you have a seat near the window. You can try to exercise your calf muscles while seated, avoid too much caffeine and alcohol and drink plenty of other fluids. Any increased risk factor: previous thrombosis, hormone therapy, BMI, age over 60, pregnancy, malignancy, cardio-respiratory disease, other chronic illness, thrombophilia, varicose veins, should have led to the flight socks and Aspirin/PPI/Ranitidine discussion if the flight is over 4 hours.

There are some exercises that reduce the risk of DVT significantly and are easy to do sitting:

Gently lean the head to one side: Rest for 3 seconds and breath out. Repeat on the other side. Repeat the cycle 3 times.

Lift the hands. Breathe in deeply and hold for 3 seconds. Place the arms behind your head. Breathe out. Repeat three times.

Bend the foot upwards, spread your toes and hold for 3 seconds. Point the foot downward, clenching the toes and hold this for 3 seconds. Repeat 3 times.

Do these if you can every half an hour.

Wearing graduated Class 1 below the knee graduated elastic compression stockings definitely reduced the signs and symptoms of DVT in one study of flyers over 50 yrs.

Fear of Flying: (See Jet lag, light and sleep in SLEEP section).

In Britain 9 million people suffer.

I find a private prescription for Xanax, Alprazolam, 250ug 500ug, 1 about half an hour before flying gives 4-6 hours relief. May need dose another mid Atlantic or half way to

Australia. It is supposed to relax without too much disinhibition.

Knowing:

Death rates per billion miles travelled:

Motor cycle 208

Car 9

Non Scheduled Airline 1.2

Bus 1

Rail 1

Scheduled airline 0.2

Doesn't help much! – patients usually reply that it's 4000 miles across the Atlantic in a plane but only half a mile on my motorbike to get the news paper.

Advice from Fear of Flying: Heathrow 025 125 3250 Manchester 061 832 7972.

Professional flyers and medication:

A pilot with a BP of 160/95 should be grounded until his BP is controlled, likewise for a further 2 weeks with every change of treatment.

Aviators and air traffic controllers may take:

ACEIs, A2RAs, CCBs, Some BBs (Atenolol and Bisoprolol, not Propranolol), Thiazides, Potassium sparing diuretics, But not: Centrally acting agents, Adrenergic blockers, Alpha blockers, Loop diuretics.

Diving (SCUBA) contra indications:

Inability to clear middle ear for whatever reason, perforated drum, previous stapedectomy?/inner ear surgery, tympanoplasty, radical mastoidectomy, Meniere's, labyrinthitis, impacted wax, tracheostomy, incompetent larynx or any other ENT condition which would render middle ear equalisation via the Valsalva difficult.

Past history of convulsion, relatively soon after a concussive head injury, I.C. tumour, history of TIA, or CVA, past history of spinal surgery with sequelae, past unexplained syncope, peripheral neuropathy, coronary artery disease, septal hypertrophy, valve stenosis, (but generally functionally insignificant incompetence is not a C/I), CCF, intra cardiac shunting, significant hypertension, angina (even well controlled) any type of myocardial ischaemia, significant arrhythmias, WPW, within 6m of SVT, significant heart block etc. a bowel-containing hernia, severe reflux, achalasia, (?hiatus hernia repair?), a history of spontaneous pneumothorax, COPD, pulmonary cysts, active asthma, Sickle Cell, various dental and jaw issues, diabetic issues (of monitoring and control), panic attacks, mental state and personality, pregnancy and otherwise use your common sense in advising the patient. If something goes wrong 20-30 metres underwater in the pitch black or poor visibility and cold and the patient has a sudden recurrence of a panic attack/hemiplegic migraine/SVT/sudden LOC etc, are they going to be at serious risk-and does half an hour of weightless "fun" in a wetsuit justify that risk?

You can always contact the British Sub Aqua Club etc for detailed advice.

Hiccups: (Hiccoughing)

All GPs who have been in practice a long time will have had patients who after 24 hours or more of intractable hiccupping no longer found it funny.

I have been required to give IM chlorpromazine for intractable hiccup but Haloperidol IM or IV can be used also. Other drugs include Metoclopramide, Epilim and Nifedipine. Always consider the cause of diaphragmatic or phrenic nerve irritation. Renal failure,

Diabetes, electrolyte abnormality, CVA, MS, brain tumour, reflux and so on. Other treatments include traction of the tongue, lifting the uvula with a spoon, stimulation of the pharynx with a cotton bud, gargling, sipping iced water, the Valsava manoeuvre, supra-orbital pressure, irritating the tympanic membrane or rectal examination!

Haemochromatosis:

Aut recessive, 1:300 northern Europeans. Only 5,000 out of the 250,000 in the UK with the condition have been formally diagnosed. The genes are H282Y and C63D, and 1:200 people in the UK have the genotype. 9M:1F. The basic problem is rapid gut iron absorption and accumulation in various tissues. Iron starts to accumulate from the 20's onwards. This causes cirrhosis, liver cancer, cardiomyopathy, diabetes mellitus, joint problems and pigmentation. Hence bronze diabetes. It also leads to reduced libido, arrythmias, heart failure, Addison's, hypoparathyroidism, excess tiredness.

Bloods: The HFE C282Y gene

IRON studies: Ferritin raised, (but this is raised in many conditions) Transferrin Index (Saturation is >50%), (>55% M, >50% premenopausal F). Serum Ferritin only rises after liver stores full. If the Ferritin is raised due to tissue damage or an acute phase response (ie not iron overload Haemochromatosis) then the fasting Transferrin saturation will be <50%.

Liver biopsy? Rx Venesection.

1:4 sibs are affected.

There is a Haemochromatosis Society and website. Detailed guidelines from the British Society for Haematology @ www.bcshguidelines.org (where inexplicably they spell it HEMOchromatosis!)

Antidotes:

(Other than gastric washouts and induced emesis):
N acetyl cysteine for paracetamol.
High dose atropine for organophosphate insecticides.
Sodium nitrite, sodium thiosulphate, dicobalt edetate for cyanides.
Digoxin specific FABs.
Flumazenil for Benzodiazepines.
Naloxone for opioids.
IV benzodiazepines for cocaine toxicity (can also give nitrates, labetalol).

CT versus MRI scans:

A CT scan is a computer enhanced X Ray but an MRI works on a completely different physical basis – using a magnet and external field RF (radio) pulse. Water in the body is induced to emit a radio signal which is then received and interpreted by the scanner. An MRI tends to resolve soft tissue lesions better than CT – for instance:cartilage, ligaments, brain etc while a CT scan is better suited for bone lesions, lung and chest imaging and detecting cancers. CTs take a few minutes while an MRI is up to half an hour to perform.

There is good soft tissue differentiation with CT if IV contrast is used. MRI intrinsically differentiates soft tissues. Metal implants are C/I in MRI scanning.

There is a small radiation risk with CT but no known biological hazard with MRI. There has been much debate about the number and dose of radiation of CTs used in recent years in the USA. A single CT scan subjects the human body to between 150 and 1,100 times the radiation of a conventional x-ray, or around a year's worth of exposure to radiation from both natural and artificial sources in the environment. Therefore, a single CT scan increases the average patient's risk of developing a fatal tumour from 20 to 20.05 percent. This will depend on the dose of radiation as well as numerous patient related factors.

CTA – CT Angiograms visualise blood vessels and are taking over from old style invasive angiograms with catheters and dye. Contrast injections and in the case of coronary angiograms, Beta Blockers are given during the scan. A CTPA (Pulmonary Artery) is used to exclude PE. Renal, aortic and cerebral AV aneurysms as well as lower limb arterial malformations and obstructions can be investigated by CTA.

Magnetic Resonance Imaging: MRI, NMR

During this, the body is exposed to a static magnetic field, intensity up to 2.0 TESLA (T) .I.E.>25,000X the earth's magnetic field. Variable lower strength magnetic field gradients are then applied. Radiofrequency energy i.e. 60MHz range applied to the body in short pulses. The tissues then absorb and reradiate electromagnetic radiation.

The radio signals emitted carry information about the physical, chemical and spatial properties of tissue. MRIs are very noisy for the patient even wearing headphones. Having one really is like being inside a dustbin while someone randomly attacks it with a club hammer.

PET Positron Emission Tomography scanning:

Is a functional not a structural scan and depends on the administration of a radioactive tracer (radionuclide) given IV, by inhalation or swallowed. The tracer is tagged to glucose, water, ammonia or some other natural and metabolically active molecule. The scan gives a colour 3D image of the positrons>gamma rays released as the tracer is broken down in metabolically active tissue. This is usually used to show areas of active cancer (etc) and is combined with a CT or MRI to give the locally relevant anatomy.

SPECT scan: Single photon emission computed tomography. A vascular investigation similar to PET but the tracer remains in the blood stream. The scan takes place after an IV injection of radioactive tracer.

Poisons:

Information on management of poisoning available to doctors via the TOXBASE website (National Poisons Information Service).

Dangerous Plants (etc): (useful information at the Poison Garden website).

Some parts of the following plants, trees and fungi are poisonous:

Ergot, lorchel, clavaria, inocybe, agaric (fly), ink cap, sulphur tuft, (false) death cap, panther cap, bracken, yew, marsh marigold, helibore, monks hood, larkspur, baneberry, wood anemone, columbine, common buttercup, spearwort, celandine, corn poppy, rape, wild radish, mustard, sorrel, holly, flax, box tree, buckthorn, lupin, laburnum, broom, lucerne, clover, vetch, laurel, cotoneaster, mistletoe, mezereum, ivy, hemlock, cowbane, dropwort, parsley, bryony, mercury, castor oil plant, buckwort, rhubarb, beech, oaks, rhododendron, azalea, horseradish, privet, (deadly) nightshade, henbane, thorn apple, potato, tomato, figwort, foxglove, ragwort, groundsel, lily of the valley, solomon's seal, bluebell, meadow saffron, snowdrop, daffodil, cuckoo pint, sponge plant.

Plants contain a huge variety of interesting toxins and potential therapeutic agents. We all know about willow and aspirin (willow's Latin name is Salix Alba – hence salicylates), quinine (from cinchona tree bark) both of which were said to illustrate the Doctrine of

Signatures (one aspect of which was that the cure can be found where the illness was acquired – in swamps and marshland). Then there are Foxglove and Digitalis, Feverfew and migraine etc. Plants and their extracts were the mainstay of apothecaries and herbalists long before any attempt to isolate the active ingredients or a scientific approach to illness developed. Yew produces the cytotoxic drugs Docetaxel and Paclitaxel as well as being very poisonous. This is via various alkaloids, ephedrine and a cyanogenic glycoside but it also contains a calcium channel blocker – the first in therapeutic use.

Poisoning and antidotes/treatments:

"Poison":	Treatment:
Paracetamol	Acetylcysteine/Methionine (restore glutathione levels)

The Rumack-Matthew nomogram is a graph of time after ingestion against paracetamol (acetaminophen) plasma concentration. It is a precisely 45 degree line, above which "treatment should be administered".
This and other therapeutic/toxic levels are available online from many sources including the very useful:
http://www.globalrph.com/labs_drugs_levels.htm

Organophosphorous and carbamate insecticides	Atropine. Competitive inhibitor at muscarinic receptors. Obidoxime, Pralidoxime.
Dystonic disorders and S/Es of various psychotropic medications; Phenothiazines, butyrophenones, metoclopramide, thioxanthines etc.	Benztropine
Hyperkalaemia and Hypermagnesaemia	Calcium Gluconate ,, ,,
Iron	Desferrioxamine
Cyanide	Dicobalt Edetate/Sodium Nitrite/Sodium Thiosulphate
Heavy metals: arsenic, copper, gold, lead, mercury	Dimercaprol
Copper, gold, lead, mercury, zinc.	Penicillamine Also DMSA, DMPS, etc.
Methanol	Ethanol: Inhibits metabolism of methanol to formaldehyde and formic acid.
Methotrexate, Trimethoprim,	Folinic acid
Paraquat	Fuller's earth/Magnesium Sulphate (to speed up transit of delayed release preparations)
B Blockers	Glucagon:Bypasses B1 and B2 receptors, stimulates cyclic AMP with positive inotropic effect.
Aminocaproic Acid/Tranexamic Acid	Heparin
Heparin	Protamine
Hypercalcaemia due to excess vitamin D	Hydrocortisone

Methaemoglobinaemia (from nitrates, phenols, primaquine etc.)	Methylene Blue (or Vit C in G6PD deficiency)
Narcotics	Naloxone
Anticholinergics	Neostigmine
Hypertension due to clonidine, methysergide, MAOIs, Phenylephrine etc.	Phenoxybenzamine a long acting alpha blocker or Phentolamine a short acting alpha blocker
B2 stimulants-ephedrine, theophylline, thyroxine	Propranolol.
Sulphonamides etc.	Sodium Bicarbonate (Forced alkaline diuresis)
Lead	Sodium Calcium Edetate
Hypertension due to ergotamine/methysergide	Sodium Nitroprusside
Coumarin and Indanedione anti-coagulants	Vitamin K
Digoxin	Digoxin specific antibody fragments.
Benzodiazepines	Flumazenil reverses central sedative effects.

Specific prescribing problems:

Doctors (Independent Prescribers) can prescribe any licensed medicine (a product with UK marketing authorisation) or unlicensed medicine for any medical condition within their clinical competence.

Patients referred privately are expected to pay for drugs prescribed privately by the specialist during that "episode of care". The GP is expected to prescribe for conditions which they continue to have clinical responsibility for – unless it is a drug not normally prescribed by GPs such as anti-TNF, fertility treatment (I normally work out half in terms of cost and prescribe that much on an FP10), Interferon etc.

All prescriptions for travel vaccines, antibiotics to be taken in the event of traveler's diarrhoea, or acetazolamide for altitude sickness are private scrips. So is Malaria prophylaxis. The GP is not **required** to prescribe for conditions that **might** happen abroad (such as tropical sprue, altitude sickness, etc).

Some travel vaccines are private prescriptions (which can be charged for) – Hepatitis B, Meningococcal A, C, W135 and Y, Japanese Encephalitis, Rabies, Tick Borne Encephalitis, Yellow Fever.

If you agree to give a branded rather than generic drug on the request of the patient (and in my opinion there are probably many situations in which this is better for the patient), you have to give it on an FP10, not privately.

Should you decide to prescribe a drug for a use outside that for which it is licensed, you will be judged (should things go wrong) on not only whether it is the sort of thing your peers would do but on whether it was a reasonable thing to have done and may be called upon to justify the prescription (see legal section) (antidepressants in IBS, Aspirin, Cimetidine, low dose Naltrexone, Metformin in cancer etc.) You must explain the unlicensed use, pros and cons as well as side effects to the patient.

Three months worth of maintenance drugs may be issued for patients travelling abroad. They are expected to obtain drugs to cover longer periods abroad themselves after the "normal scrip" has run out. – I will give 6 months worth of most long term drugs including the pill to take on "gap years" and voluntary work abroad. It can be hard to access good medical care and equivalent drugs abroad for this sort of absence and I wouldn't want a pregnancy or a diabetic ketoacidosis on my conscience.

Emergency travel kits (including needles and syringes) must be purchased by the patient.

If your NHS patient on long term medication spends long periods living abroad in their second home you are only required to provide "sufficient medication to cover the journey and to allow the patient to obtain medical attention abroad".

Controlled drug prescriptions are limited to 30 days (Including such things as Temazepam).

If the patient takes controlled drugs abroad for their own use they will need a covering letter from the GP. It should include the patient's name, address and DOB, the dates of travel (including the expected date of return), the country to be visited and a list of the drugs including doses and total amounts taken. CDs should be in original packaging and usually in the hand luggage. More than three months worth of CDs need a personal export and import licence.

Borderline substances – in the form of foods and dietary products may be prescribed for specific clinical indications – malnutrition, metabolic conditions, malabsorption and so on.

I don't prescribe complimentary, homeopathic or other non evidence based products. But it is the responsibility of local NHS organisations (presumably now commissioning groups) if they are willing to fund alternative/homeopathic "remedies" etc.

This is increasingly unlikely in the light of the Government's, NICE's and all independent evidence reviews finding no effect but that of placebo. This is a CCG summary which puts the position fairly clearly:

What evidence is there about homeopathy as a treatment?

"A 2010 House of Commons Science and Technology Committee report on homeopathy said that homeopathic remedies perform no better than placebos, and that the principles on which homeopathy is based are «scientifically implausible». This is also the view of the Chief Medical Officer, Professor Dame Sally Davies."

The report by the Government Science and Technology Committee reviewed evidence for and against homoeopathy and concluded that the NHS should cease funding homeopathy. It also concluded that the Medicines and Healthcare Products Regulatory Agency (MHRA) should not allow homeopathic product labels to make medical claims without evidence of efficacy. As they are not medicines, homeopathic products should no longer be licensed by the MHRA. The indications being that any beneficial outcomes of homoeopathy treatment are due to a placebo effect. The full report can be found at:

http://www.parliament.uk/business/committees/committees-a-z/commons-select/science-and-technology-committee/inquiries/homeopathy-/ (External link)

The Government responded as follows:

"We agree with many of the Committee's conclusions and recommendations. However, our continued position on the use of homeopathy within the NHS is that the local NHS and clinicians, rather than Whitehall, are best placed to make decisions on what treatment is appropriate for their patients – including complementary or alternative treatments such as homeopathy – and provide accordingly for those treatments.

"There naturally will be an assumption that if the NHS is offering homeopathic treatments then they will be efficacious, whereas the overriding reason for NHS provision is that homeopathy is available to provide patient choice. The Government Chief Scientific Advisor's position remains that the evidence of efficacy and the scientific basis of homeopathy is highly questionable."

The full Government response to the paper can be found at: https://www.gov.uk/government/uploads/system/uploads/attachment_data/file/216053/dh_117811.pdf

NHS Choices Website further comments on several individual pages that homeopathy is not recommended. Further evidence is available in the document downloads on this page.

NICE Guidance

NICE Guidance does not state anywhere that homeopathy is a recommended treatment.

Drugs available as OTC medication (for minor ailments): The GMC says that prescribers should only prescribe drugs to "meet the identified needs of the patient and never simply for patient convenience or simply on patient demand". This is a bit of a grey area. Although I have almost never prescribed Calpol for the parents of hot children, claiming it is a "practice policy" not to, I **have** prescribed for instance Ibuprofen in acute musculoskeletal pain and I do prescribe Gaviscon to pregnant patients. All are OTC. I suppose I don't want to encourage patients to expect the NHS to prescribe medications they should have at home as responsible people but acute unpredictable conditions prompting a genuine new consultation are a bit different.

So: Can I have some Nurofen for the next time I have a headache? – "No, buy it yourself."

Doctor, I have an acute severe lumbar strain and it really hurts "Here, have some Ibuprofen to take three times a day". On the other hand, go into a retail pharmacist, see how much they charge for a bottle of 500mls of Calpol and try not to be shocked.

Fertility treatment: Many couples going privately will find themselves stuck with private prescriptions for hundreds or thousands of pounds worth of drugs. I know many of my colleagues will be unsympathetic to the expense of this but I usually write NHS prescriptions for half the total cost.

The couple have shown their determination and commitment because the whole process, especially self funded, is draining, depressing, very costly and fraught with difficulty and disappointment.

I have a long term, sometimes life long relationship with many of the patients on my list and I want to be part of their personal supportive medical establishment, not another hurdle that they have to negotiate on their treatment journey.

They never forget your help and it is one of the few ways GPs have the freedom to be practical and caring in an ethical way.

Infertility treatment, although not really within the original remit of the NHS, can positively transform the lives of a couple who have been hoping and trying to conceive for years and suffering all sorts of associated stress, depression, misery.

Infertility and the absence of a baby often become an almost irrational focus for some couples and dominates all their daily activities, planning, self esteem etc. Since it is SO important, the GP is obliged as everyone's advocate and expert friend to be positively involved.

Prescribing implies responsibility and professional involvement. You may be called upon to deal with side effects and complications, so knowing the drug regime and prescribing it is the most effective way of being closely involved.

However I do want to see some sort of commitment to demonstrate that couples will be staying together. It is too easy just to let the tax payer enable two unmarried people to have a baby and then find that the State pays for that child and picks up the pieces when the couple decides to "separate" soon after. Bringing up children, as any parent knows, is far harder than begetting them. Marriage is a commitment and I talk to and make up my own mind about how committed to staying together the couple is. A judgment of Solomon, I know, but GPs make judgments about characters, risks, morality, trust worthiness and intentions from their unparalleled experience of people and behaviour everyday. Can I trust this parent to supervise their sick child at home? Is this patient really a suitable person to have a shotgun?, Is this 90 year old safe behind the wheel of a car?, Is this mother finally drinking too much to be a proper mother to her children? Would I trust this teenager/young adult as a carer of small children? Is this feckless couple likely to stay together long enough to conceive, care for, nurture, love and bring up a child through childhood, adolescence and all the way up to adulthood?

Other odds and ends:

GPs are advised by the GMC to register themselves and their family with other doctors for fear that drugs may be abused, prescribed without proper objectivity, addiction encouraged etc. I sincerely believe this to be an exaggerated fear and a highly unreasonable edict. Controlled drugs aside.

I have been indirectly involved in the case of a GP who prescribed controlled drugs (two repeat Fentanyl patches) completely ethically to her sister who was terminally ill and was suspended for a year for her pains. In the end this destroyed her professional life and reputation. I believe that a caring relative or loved one may be the best person to decide what to prescribe for a family member sometimes. After all, they may have thought, researched and investigated all the various alternative treatments for a specific condition at length in a loved one because of their personal and lifelong involvement.

Overseas visitors have a right to free care if they plan to live here at least 6 months, (they must register with a practice), patients from the EU with an EHIC, patients who need immediate necessary treatment who can't wait for their return home (EHIC not needed), patients holding an E112 for a specific condition and prescribed solely for this condition, approved refugees and asylum seekers. Some of this this may change after Brexit.

28: MUSCULOSKELETAL:

Bones:

There are 206 in an adult body but up to 300 in the new born. This is of no practical daily use to the GP but often comes up in pub quizzes. Since most of the GPs I know do go to pubs quite frequently it is worth trying to remember.

Schmorl's nodes:

These are often seen and commented on in plain X Rays of the spine and are visible on MRIs even if sometimes not on XRs (only about a third of the total are visible by conventional radiography). They are vertical disc herniations through the vertebral body end plates. They seem to be commoner in teenagers indulging in rough sports and complaining of back pain – the theory being that the end plate above the disc is weaker than the tough circumferential annulus at that age. As you get older horizontal (transverse or posterolateral) herniations are more likely. Pain indicates a freshly damaged vertebral end plate but rest usually settles the symptoms within a few months.

Rarer causes are: More significant trauma, osteoporosis, hyperparathyroidism, Schuermann's Disease, osteomalacia, infections, tumours.

CT versus MRI scans:

(MRI soft tissues, brain, cartilage, muscle, ligaments, CT bone, lung, chest, cancer):

A CT scan is a computer enhanced X Ray but an MRI uses a powerful electro-magnet and an external radio pulse. Water in the body is induced to emit a radio signal which is picked up and interpreted by the scanner. An MRI tends to resolve soft tissue lesions better than CT – for instance: cartilage, ligaments, brain etc while a CT scan is better suited for bone lesions, lung and chest imaging, and detecting cancers. CTs take a few minutes while an MRI is up to half an hour to perform – or even longer.

There is good soft tissue differentiation with CT if IV contrast is used. MRI intrinsically differentiates soft tissues. Metal implants are C/I in MRI scanning. but most non ferrous metals are safe, in fact brachytherapy needles are often inserted under MRI control.

There is a small radiation risk with CT but no known biological hazard with MRI. There has been much debate about the dose of radiation of CTs used in recent years in the USA. A single CT scan is between 150 and 1, 100 times the radiation of a conventional X-ray, or around a year's worth of exposure to radiation from both natural and artificial sources in the environment. Therefore, a single CT scan increases the average patient's risk of developing a fatal tumour 20%. This will depend on the dose of radiation as well as numerous patient related factors.

CTA – CT Angiograms visualise blood vessels and are taking over from old style invasive angiograms with catheters and dye. Contrast is used and for coronary arteries. Beta blockers may be co-administered.

Magnetic Resonance Imaging: MRI, NMR

During this, the body is exposed to a static magnetic field, intensity up to 2.0 TESLA (T) .I.E.>25,000X the earth's magnetic field. Variable lower strength magnetic field gradients are then applied. Radiofrequency energy i.e. 60MHz range is applied to the body in short pulses. The tissues then absorb and re-radiate electromagnetic radiation.

The radio signals emitted carry information about the physical, chemical and spatial properties of the tissues.

Other therapies:

The Alexander Technique:

Invented by a Tasmanian actor at the end of the 19th C. Hard to explain, it is about relearning movement and posture to make our bodily movements less cramped, controlled, forced, more relaxed. A course in the technique involves some gentle hands on correction of dysfunctional spine and limb positioning as well as education regarding movement and its anticipation, posture and relaxation. It can certainly improve longstanding neck and low back pain as well as root pain due to spinal postural dysfunction. You can sometimes tell people who have been taught the technique by the way they get up from chairs or from the floor and by how they "carry themselves".

Osteopathy:

This is a mechanical approach to physical therapy by which the osteopath massages, stretches, manipulates and realigns (with various degrees of force) misaligned facets, displaced SIJs, muscles in spasm and damaged joints often with a click, a "give" and a sense of instant relief. Dry needling (which is supposed to reduce local muscle spasm ? via endorphin release) and education are often included. It certainly usually works well for me and I have no reservation about recommending osteopathy to my patients with neck, back, limb and joint dysfunction. I do not accept the theoretical basis for cranial osteopathy, especially in babies. My only reservation is that with repeated stretching and correction of one recalcitrant spinal facet joint over a period of years (in any patient's spine over time, some levels become stiff but others hypermobile and "unstable"), – wouldn't the treatment itself increase the long term local instability?

Chiropractic:

Founded at about the same time as the Alexander technique, by D Palmer in America. (In Iowa – which can now claim two famous fanciful Americans if you include James Kirk the Star Trek Captain).

Chiropractors tend to use a gentler (and sometimes less believable) approach to mechanical back neck and other bodily pain. They use manipulation, exercise, ultrasound and sometimes acupuncture but also make "adjustments" using a small mechanical device that percusses the skin overlying a facet for instance. Some also believe that spinal treatment has beneficial effects on a multiplicity of bodily conditions from gynaecological to dermatological. This is where Chiropractic enters the realm of faith, magic and psychology rather than rational physical therapy like osteopathy and physiotherapy. It is where I part company with it. I warn patients who see chiropractors about the limited benefits of spinal physical therapy on other bodily systems and the impossibility of gentle tapping over the spine actually having a significant effect on the facet joints under several centimetres of fat, muscle and sinew below.

Cramp:

A painful muscle contraction with multiple causes and none.

Causes: Pregnancy, muscle overuse, hypocalcaemia, hypokalaemia and hypomagnesaemia, dehydration, PAD, (Peripheral Arterial Disease), exposure to or submersing the periphery in cold water, MS, renal, thyroid disorders, posture, various drugs including the

COCP, diuretics, statins, antipsychotics and steroids.

Responds to Quinine (or real tonic water/bitter lemon) 200mg/300mg tabs, heat, (or ice sometimes), stretching the affected muscle, massage, fluids.

Gout:

Things you may have forgotten: – The Metabolic Pathway:

Purine nucleotides

Which are found in the diet, with higher levels in anchovies, sardines, liver, kidneys, beer, gravy, shellfish, sweetbreads, asparagus, cauliflower, mushrooms lentils, bran etc. and form a number of crucial body molecules – Adenine, Guanine (-hence DNA/RNA), ATP, AMP, etc.

V

are broken down to **Hypoxanthine**

(Interestingly this and other "organic molecules" have been found in outer space and on meteorites)

V

Then via Xanthine oxidase (inhibitors include Allopurinol/Febuxostat)

To Xanthine

V

Then via Xanthine oxidase

V

To Uric Acid

(Uricosurics include Sulfinpyrazone, Probenecid etc I.V. Pegloticase is licenced for severe tophaceous gout and offers an alternative metabolic pathway via Uricase).

To be excreted in the urine or metabolised via Uricase (via Pegloticase) to Allantoin. **Incidence is 2/1000 but 15/1000 in 35-44 yr males.**

Very uncommon in premenopausal women because of the oestrogenic influence on uric acid kidney secretion.

2/3 of uric acid is excreted in urine, 1/3 in gut secretions.

Primary Gout (30%),

Secondary is said to be 70% eg:

G6PD deficiency, smoke inhalation, M.I., respiratory failure, inherited muscle disorders, increased purine intake, Psoriasis, malignancies, exercise, Infectious Monocytosis, haematogenous malignancies, haemolysis, Polycythaemia,

Decreased tubular excretion/secretion includes:

Decreased renal mass, dehydration, Diabetes Insipidus, diuretics, starvation, Diabetic Ketoacidosis, Ethanol, Toxaemia, various poisons including Lead, Ciclosporin, Pyrazinamide, Salicylates, Ethambutol, etc.

Lesch-Nyhan syndrome (X Linked recessive, self mutilation, writhing, grimacing, gout, megaloblastic anaemia) etc.

Offer prophylaxis if 2 or more flares a year (or if the patient has been seriously distressed by a previous attack). Aim to get the level of uric acid as near as possible to 300umol/li (300-360umol/li). Advise the patient that diet **is** an issue, avoid too much meat, avoid shellfish and beer if possible. Oddly, there is a potential advantage for gout sufferers: There is a 24% lower risk of Alzheimer's disease. This finding was published in the Annals of Rheumatic Diseases on 4/3/15 in which the Rotterdam study of 300,000 people showed an inverse relationship between risk of any type of dementia and previous uric acid levels.

In a recent study, **gout was found to be associated with sleep apnoea.**

You, like me, may say that the same patients who are overweight, lazy, probably smoke, eat bad diets and have metabolic syndrome are likely to have both and a whole lot of other unpleasant metabolic indices too. Their obesity obviously puts them at risk of OSA, but BMI was excluded in this study. Adjustment was made for BMI, hypertension, age, gender, alcohol etc and so we are left with a direct link between cardiopulmonary function and uric acid levels. Fascinating.

Zhang Y. et Al, Arthritis Rheumatol 2015. 67:3298-3302.

The Diet and Gout:

Red meat, Salmon, sardines, trout, Shellfish, Asparagus, Cauliflower, Mushrooms, Spinach, Lentils, Oats, Rhubarb, Fructose containing fizzy drinks.

BUT daily Vitamin C *lowers* Uric Acid.

Colchicine: 500mcg Used to be given 3 hrly until diarrhoea and vomiting or relief of pain in acute gout. Now the dose is less frequent at TDS and no more than 6-10mg per course. Some use 500ug bd with or without half dose NSAIDs for up to 6 weeks to reduce flare ups (with the initiation of Allopurinol).

Etoricoxib, Arcoxia, 120mg daily (with a PPI) usually settles the pain within a few days. – Or even an

Intramuscular steroid injection if the oral treatments are contraindicated.

Prophylaxis:

Allopurinol: (Inhibits Xanthine Oxidase) Start with 50-100mg/day titrating up. Average 300mg 1-2 daily (with uricosuric agent (eg Probenecid initially, or with NSAID until after hyperuricaemia is corrected) Maximum Allopurinol dose is 900mg/day.

Can also use Sulphinpyrazone 100-200mg OD or

Febuxostat, Adenuric 80mg OD, (120mg if Uric Acid >357umol/ml after 2-4 weeks).

Long term treatment of gout: Try to get urate below 300-360umol/li.

Pseudogout

Commoner in the elderly and after metabolic stress. (including recent operations or severe infection.) Appears as chondrocalcinosis on XR. Common sites are the wrist, knee and pubic symphysis. Usually you need to aspirate the joint fluid for the diagnosis.

Non steroidal anti inflammatory drugs, NSAIDS:

Various classes:

Salicylates: Aspirin, Diflunisal, etc.

Propionic Acid derivatives: Ibuprofen, Naproxen, Ketoprofen, Flurbiprofen etc.

Acetic Acid derivatives: Indomet(h) acin, Tolmetin, Sulindac, Etodolac, Ketoralac, Diclofenac,

Nabumetone.

Enolic Acid derivatives (Oxicams): Piroxicam, Meloxicam, Tenoxicam.

Fenamic Acid derivatives: (Fenemates) Mefenamic Acid, Tolfenamic Acid.

Selective COX-2 inhibitors: (Coxibs) Celecoxib, Etoricoxib.

Sulphonanilides: Nimesulide.

Fashions in NSAIDs come and go. At equipotent anti inflammatory doses all non selective NSAIDs risk roughly the same level of upper GI bleeding – Perhaps Ibuprofen less and Indomethacin and Piroxicam somewhat more. There is a high incidence of new

NSAID products being taken off the market due to unforeseen circumstances and new side effects appearing and warnings to consider. Now it is cardiovascular risk. Twenty years ago it was upper GI bleeding.

Naproxen and Ibuprofen are said to have a safer cardiovascular profile than Diclofenac. Specifically:

Currently I prescribe either Naproxen with a PPI or a COX-2 with a PPI if the patient needs an anti-inflammatory. It has to be said that many people's lives can be made absolutely miserable by joint pain without treatment. Mild to moderate analgesics and topical treatments just don't work for most patients with significant OA who want to try to keep active. They then enter the pain/weight gain/worse wear and tear/pain vicious cycle.

Diclofenac (Voltarol) comes as a suppository, useful for the self medication of renal colic and migraine (etc) and is combined with Misoprostol (a prostaglandin analogue) in Arthrotec (50 and 75mg + 200mcg) which induces labour (avoid in pregnancy) and is cytoprotective. Misoprostol is also in combination with Naproxen in Napratec.

Diclofenac increases the risk of arterial thrombosis and all non topical forms should be avoided in patients with IHD, PVD, cerebrovascular disease and CCF.

Ibuprofen interferes with the beneficial cardiovascular effects of aspirin if taken simultaneously.

A retrospective analysis was published recently of **2,700,000 individuals** included in 51 studies. The data set allowed analysis of **184,946 cardiovascular events**. The relative risks of cardiovascular events for several NSAIDs were calculated as follows:

Rofecoxib 1.45 (95% CI 1.33 – 1.59)

Diclofenac 1.40 (1.27 – 1.55)

Ibuprofen 1.18 (1.11 – 1.25)

Naproxen 1.09 (1.02 – 1.16)

Celecoxib 1.26 (1.09 – 1.47) – from a data subset

Etoricoxib 2.05 (1.45 – 2.88) – from a data subset

Etodolac 1.55 (1.28 – 1.87) – from a data subset

Indomethacin 1.30 (1.19 – 1.41) – from a data subset

The authors conclude that, "*among widely used NSAIDs, naproxen and low-dose ibuprofen are least likely to increase cardiovascular risk*".

Things you may have forgotten: COXIBS

Cyclo-oxygenase, COX, is an enzyme that forms various biological mediators, including prostaglandins, prostacyclin, thromboxane etc, from arachidonic acid as the precursor. There are COX 1, 2 and 3 enzymes. Most anti-inflammatories are unselective in their effects in inhibiting all these enzymes. They reduce inflammation, pain, clotting and temperature and as prostaglandins have a mucosal protective effect on the stomach, unselective NSAIDS can cause gastric erosions or bleeding too.

COX-1 is present in most tissues. It is protective in the GI tract.

COX-2 is usually localised in inflamed tissue (joints and muscle) and COX-2 inhibitors cause less gastric upset. A few have been withdrawn (Rofecoxib, Vioxx Valdecoxib, Bextra) because of an increased risk of thrombosis which is associated with COX-2s.

COX-3 is found in brain and heart tissue and is thought to be involved in centrally mediated pain.

Etoricoxib, Arcoxia, increases INR by 13%. Celecoxib, Celebrex, interacts with warfarin

– just as Refecoxib (Vioxx) did – prolonging the INR.

Ironically though, Coxibs (-as do long term high dose conventional NSAIDs and Diclofenac in normal usage) slightly increase the risk of thrombosis (3 additional events per 1000 patient years) and so are contraindicated in patients with ischaemic heart disease. At the moment, Ibuprofen and Naproxen are said to be safer.

The older Meloxicam, (so often used by vetinary surgeons) Nabumetone and Etodolac are preferential COX-2 inhibitors but not "selective".

All NSAIDS slightly increase the risk of heart failure and slightly increase BP and the risk of oedema.

Osteoarthritis of the Knee:

In an American study of various treatments published in 2015, **for pain**, all treatments helped a little after 3 months compared with oral placebo. Paracetamol alone had an almost insignificant effect. Celecoxib is not much better (though some other studies disagree with this).

Injections of almost anything into the joint were found to help relieve pain. Placebo injections were actually more effective than oral NSAIDs. Presumably though, they were putting injections of saline or sterile water which, due to their joint spreading, local vascular/inflammatory reaction, cushioning space occupying properties cannot truly be said to be a placebo. The very process of injecting, – putting new volume into a joint changes its mechanical and pain dynamics.

Orally, **for stiffness**, naproxen, ibuprofen, diclofenac, and celecoxib were better than placebo or paracetamol. Injected hyaluronic acid was better than injected placebo.

For function, all interventions were better than oral placebo except injected steroids. All the NSAIDs were better than paracetamol. Injected Hyaluronic Acid was better than injected placebo or steroids.

I find:

Intra articular preparations of Hyaluronic Acid can reduce pain in a proportion of recipients but the effect seems to be temporary. 5 injections is the course (eg Hyalgan).

Chondroitin and or Glucosamine: Faith in these two come and go. The very latest randomised controlled trial (2015) offered some support to the 2008 Glucosamine/Chondroitin intervention trial ("GAIT"), suggesting that the two together might offer significant pain relief to patients with moderate to severe OA knee, despite being ineffective against milder OA pain.

BUT if you are asked, there is a belief abroad amongst respectable alternative practitioners that Glucosamine SULPHATE (NOT necessarily Chondroitin alone which may just relieve some pain symptoms only) may help various symptoms of OA knee – at a dose of 1500mg a day. This is a bigger dose than most patients seem to take. There are few significant side effects although a small increase in diabetes with Glucosamine was observed once.

Osteoporosis Prevention/Treatment:

DEXA SCAN: Why the way these are graded and reported cannot be more rational (for instance PLUS scores are normal, NEGATIVE scores are osteoporotic, the more negative the thinner the bone, heaven knows) But:

Normal T Score: 0 to – 1 SD

Osteopoenia T Score – 1.0 to – 2.5 SD STANDARD TREATMENT: Weight

bearing exercise and 1000mg elemental Ca++ 400 IU Vit D Daily. (See below) This is *standard treatment.*

Osteoporosis T Score lower than – 2.5 SD. *standard treatment* as above plus HRT or bisphosphonates, etc.

I.E. a T score of – 2.5 or below.

General advice should be to get adequate exercise (weight bearing), increase dairy products especially now dairy fat has been re-evaluated, sunlight, HRT if appropriate, Vitamin D and many therapists advise Boron, Mg, Vitamins K and C, Zinc and Strontium supplements too.

So do a Dexa scan if:

>1350mg lifetime steroid use, previous fragility fracture (but if vertebral, give bisphosphonate anyway), Inflammatory Bowel Disease, Coeliac disease, Rh A, menopause <45 yrs, significant amenorrhoea in early life, underweight, immobile, smoking, Thyroid disease, Family History, Hypogonadism in men (i.e. on Zoladex etc).

Primary and secondary prevention of fracture:

Rx Alendronate >Risedronate/Etidronate >Strontium Ranelate.

Bisphosphonates all have oesophageal side effects and they vary in what part of the skeleton they protect.

For instance: Alendronate, Fosamax 70mg once weekly (full glass of water, stay upright for half an hour): Fosamax is associated with an increased risk of atrial fibrillation and ironically, oral anticoagulants can make osteoporosis worse.

As at writing (2012-17) it is thought that Etidronate reduces vertebral fractures but that both Risedronate and Alendronate reduce vertebral and non vertebral fractures.

Bisphosphonates are said by some independent medical writers to work by killing osteoclasts. These are of course the cells that break down old bone and permit the manufacture of new bone by osteoblasts. If the remodelling cells are no longer there the resultant bone is denser and more brittle. Therein lies part of the bisphosphonate bone problem. They also increase the risk of osteonecrosis by 3X.

They do however seem to cause (especially alendronate, risedronate possibly, but not etidronate) a reduction of all cause mortality 40% (30% in men!) in both sexes which is independent of fractures. Perhaps this is related to the beneficial effect they have on *malignant disease secondary spread* (Bliuc et al ASBMR Ann. mtg. 2016) perhaps in some other as yet unknown mechanism. (Should aspirin, metformin and alendronate be in every 60 year old's pill box?)

Strontium also has serious side effects (thromboembolism, skin reactions, increased risks of MI and other cardiac disorders) so it is contraindicated in patients with IHD, PAD, cerebrovascular disease and hypertension which is uncontrolled. It should only be used in men and women at high risk of fracture. – Although this conventional advice is contradicted by some specialists who prefer it to calcium supplementation which may have no effect on bone density at all but causes calcium kidney stones in the 5% of women who have hypercalciuria. Elemental calcium supplementation is also said by some to contribute to atheroma, that increasing naturally calcium rich foods such as dairy produce and fish is safer and more effective (see diet section), that osteoporosis rarely occurs in naturally calcium deficient societies and that magnesium supplementation may be more useful. So limit calcium intake to 500mg a day and supplement Vitamin D in patients with osteoporosis! Overall the recommendation is currently that strontium is only used in patients without a past history of cardiovascular disease as long as they are regularly assessed for symptoms of CVS disease and if there is no alternative. It is all a bit more complicated than the Milk Marketing Board used to tell us.

Ibandronate, Bondronat, Bonviva, is a once monthly tablet or quarterly injection for osteoporosis but is also used to "prevent skeletal events in patients with breast cancer and bone metastases"

Bisphosphonates can cause the awful osteonecrosis of the jaw, something all my dentist friends dread, especially if they are being used intravenously for cancer.

Calcium and Vitamin D: Where are we?

Although these supplements were long recommended to prevent osteoporosis, by 2010 several randomised trials had shown **no benefit for independent older patients and some harm**: (Renal stones, falls, significant raised risk of MI, GI symptoms, CVA, even increased hip fracture! etc). There is no association between calcium intake and reduced hip fracture. There is with calcified arteries and kidney stones though.

In the BMJ of Sep 2015 a meta analysis put the final nail in the calcium coffin of calcium supplements, confirming lack of benefit and significant harm. Neither calcium supplementation nor dietary calcium reduced fractures or increased bone mineral density. 30% of older women in many western countries still take calcium supplements though.

If these are prescribed for some reason other than osteoporosis, it is wise to co prescribe them with bisphosphonates to avoid the risk of precipitating osteomalacia.

Taking extra calcium is therefore not harmless -it often tends to cause more side effects than benefits. The Institute of Medicine still recommends 1200mg calcium a day for women over 51yrs for some reason (2016). The calcium limits I have seen recommended vary from 500mg to "no more than 2000mg- 2500mg/day" but it is sensible to co prescribe WITH Vitamin K2. This is certainly useful if you want to avoid bone disease related to oral coumarins when Vitamin K2 should be co prescribed at a steady dose so that warfarin can be stabilised. Oral anticoagulants otherwise can demineralise bone and increase soft tissue calcification. Vitamin K antagonises both side effects. This soft tissue calcification includes arterial calcification and the complications of hypertension, myocardial ischaemia and heart failure. Attitudes regarding calcium supplementation are still based erroneously on a NEJM study of 1992 showing reduced hip fractures in elderly women on calcium and Vitamin D. These were institutionalised, malnourished women with low vitamin D and not average healthy, mobile women in the community. The meta analysis of 2015 mentions the severe side effects, cardiovascular, renal calculi, hospital admissions for GI symptoms, chronic constipation and so on of giving calcium to large numbers of normal women in the real world.

Simple yogurt improves bone density independent of calcium intake.

But if you do chose to treat osteoporosis with calcium:

Calfovit, Calcichew D3 (500mg and 200ius)/Forte (500mg Ca++ and 400ius of D3, ie Cholecalciferol) can also be used in the treatment of bone secondaries. Calcidrink, effervescent Calcit Tabs, Sandocal, Adcal D3, Calfovit D3 sachets.

Bisphonphonates are likely to have a beneficial effect in post menopausal women with breast cancer, (July 2015) making the bones a more alien environment for metastases. I wonder whether aspirin, cimetidine and bisphosphonates, each of which can reduce metastases in various cancers might be additive?

Alternative Treatments:

Nandrolone decanoate inj 50mg every 3 weeks IM.

Strontium Ranelate 2gr sachet a day, – Contraindicated with a history of DVT and cardiovascular disease (you also need to watch renal function in CRF) – Make sure you top up calcium and Vit D.

Parathormone as Teriparatide, (Forsteo) – a daily recombinant injection, 34 of the 84 parathormone amino acids. This is given for no more than 2 years otherwise the net effect is decreased bone mineral density. Stimulates osteoblasts and is therefore the only treatment for osteoporosis that preferentially stimulates new bone formation so far (2013). All the others preferentially affect osteoclasts.(Bisphosphonates encourage osteoclast apoptosis for instance).

Colecalciferol, Calcitriol, Calcitonin.

Tibolone Livial a slightly androgenic HRT.

Raloxifene, Evista: An oral Selective oestrogen receptor modulator (SERM). Oestrogenic actions on the bone (reducing vertebral fractures) but anti-oestrogenic activity at the breast and uterus.(Reduces breast cancer risk). Causes hot flushes, increased risk of clots, VTE.

Higher risk of Osteoporosis:

Caucasian/asian, slender, smoking, alcohol, caffeine, FH osteoporosis, especially mother, premature menopause, lazy, endocrine disorders: hyperparathyroidism, hypogonadism, hyperthyroidism, DM, Cushings, prolactinoma, acromegaly, Addisons. G.I. conditions: IBD, Coeliac, malnutrition, gastric bypass, liver disease, anorexia, Vit D or Ca++ deficiency. Renal disease, CKD, hypercalciuria. Rheumatological diseases, Rh. A, A.S. SLE. Haematological disorders: M.M., Thalassaemia, Leukaemia, Lymphoma, Haemophilia, SCA, Mastocytosis. Gene disorders: C.F. Osteogenesis, Homocystinuria, Ehlers Danlos, Marfan's, Haemochromatosis, Hypophosphatasia. Porphyria, Sarcoid, immobilisation, pregnancy, COPD, HIV etc. Low calcium diet, parenteral nutrition. Oral anticoagulants.

Corticosteroid induced Osteoporosis: (T Score <1.5):

>7.5mg daily of steroids for 6 months EVER, >1350mg lifetime steroid ingestion.

Rx:

Alendronate, Alfacalcidol, Calcitonin, Calcitriol, Clodronate, Cyclical Etidronate, HRT, Pamidronate, Risedronate.

Indicators of Low BMD:

Low BMI (<22Kg/M2),

RhA,

Untreated menopause,

A.S.

Crohn's,

Prolonged immobility.

There is now a **Fracture Risk Assessment Tool. (FRAX)**

It looks like this and is readily available online: NOTE THE 3 UNITS of ALCOHOL PER DAY.

Calculation Tool

Please answer the questions below to calculate the ten year probability of fracture with BMD.
Country: UK

Name/ID:

Questionnaire:

1.
Age (between 40 and 90 years) or Date of Birth
Age:

Date of Birth:

Y:

M:

D:

2.
Sex

☐ Male

☐ Female

3.
Weight (kg)

4.
Height (cm)

5.
Previous Fracture

◉ No

☐ Yes

6.
Parent Fractured Hip

◉ No

☐ Yes

7.
Current Smoking

◉ No

☐ Yes

8.
Glucocorticoids

◉ No

☐ Yes

9.
Rheumatoid arthritis

◉ No

☐ Yes
10.
Secondary osteoporosis

◉ No

☐ Yes
11.
Alcohol 3 or more units/day

◉ No

☐ Yes
12.
Femoral neck BMD (g/cm²)

[▼] [   ]

Calculate
Clear

Print tool and information

Risk factors

For the clinical risk factors a yes or no response is asked for. If the field is left blank, then a "no" response is assumed. See also notes on risk factors.

The risk factors used are the following:

Age	The model accepts ages between 40 and 90 years. If ages below or above are entered, the programme will compute probabilities at 40 and 90 year, respectively.
Sex	Male or female. Enter as appropriate.
Weight	This should be entered in kg.
Height	This should be entered in cm.
Previous fracture	A previous fracture denotes more accurately a previous fracture in adult life occurring spontaneously, or a fracture arising from trauma which, in a healthy individual, would not have resulted in a fracture. Enter yes or no (see also notes on risk factors).
Parent fractured hip	This enquires for a history of hip fracture in the patient's mother or father. Enter yes or no.
Current smoking	Enter yes or no depending on whether the patient currently smokes tobacco (see also notes on risk factors).
Glucocorticoids	Enter yes if the patient is currently exposed to oral glucocorticoids or has been exposed to oral glucocorticoids for more than 3 months at a dose of prednisolone of 5mg daily or more (or equivalent doses of other glucocorticoids) (see also notes on risk factors).
Rheumatoid arthritis	Enter yes where the patient has a confirmed diagnosis of rheumatoid arthritis. Otherwise enter no (see also notes on risk factors).

Secondary osteoporosis	Enter yes if the patient has a disorder strongly associated with osteoporosis. These include type I (insulin dependent) diabetes, osteogenesis imperfecta in adults, untreated long-standing hyperthyroidism, hypogonadism or premature menopause (<45 years), chronic malnutrition, or malabsorption and chronic liver disease
Alcohol 3 or more units/day	Enter yes if the patient takes 3 or more units of alcohol daily. A unit of alcohol varies slightly in different countries from 8-10g of alcohol. This is equivalent to a standard glass of beer (285ml), a single measure of spirits (30ml), a medium-sized glass of wine (120ml), or 1 measure of an aperitif (60ml) (see also notes on risk factors).
Bone mineral density (BMD)	(BMD) Please select the make of DXA scanning equipment used and then enter the actual femoral neck BMD (in g/cm2). Alternatively, enter the T-score based on the NHANES III female reference data. In patients without a BMD test, the field should be left blank (see also notes on risk factors) (provided by Oregon Osteoporosis Center).

Notes on risk factors

Previous fracture

A special situation pertains to a prior history of vertebral fracture. A fracture detected as a radiographic observation alone (a morphometric vertebral fracture) counts as a previous fracture. A prior clinical vertebral fracture or a hip fracture is an especially strong risk factor. The probability of fracture computed may therefore be underestimated. Fracture probability is also underestimated with multiple fractures.

Smoking, alcohol, glucocorticoids

These risk factors appear to have a dose-dependent effect, i.e. the higher the exposure, the greater the risk. This is not taken into account and the computations assume average exposure. Clinical judgment should be used for low or high exposures.

Rheumatoid arthritis (RA)

RA is a risk factor for fracture. However, osteoarthritis is, if anything, protective. For this reason reliance should not be placed on a patient's report of 'arthritis' unless there is clinical or laboratory evidence to support the diagnosis.

Bone mineral density (BMD)

The site and reference technology is DXA at the femoral neck. T-scores are based on the NHANES reference values for women aged 20-29 years. The same absolute values are used in men.

© World Health Organization Collaborating Centre for Metabolic Bone Diseases, University of Sheffield, UK

My thanks to Ageeth Van Leersum Science Administrator and The International Oteoporosis Foundation at Nyon, Switzerland for their support and permission to reproduce this calculator.

With it you can calculate the 10 year risk of a fracture with a system online using

Country, Age, Sex, Weight, Height, previous fracture, parent fractured hip, current smoking, steroid treatment (currently, or more than 3months of >5mg prednisolone equ. in the past), Rheumatoid arthritis, secondary osteoporosis, IDDM, Osteogenesis Imperfecta, untreated hyperthyroidism, hypogonadism, prem. menopause, malnutrition, malabsorption, chronic liver disease, **3 or more units** of alcohol a day, femoral neck BMD, **(Ref: Univ Sheffield, WHO, Nat Osteoporosis Society).**

An Alternative approach to avoiding Osteoporosis:

Increase non burning sun exposure (Vit D); Take at least 2000 IUs Vit D daily as a supplement (plus or minus Vit K2); Probably increase dairy products, don't take calcium supplements; Increase Magnesium (reduce alcohol, increase seeds, nuts, grains, cereals, preferably "organic"); Impact/weight bearing exercise; Increase green leafy vegetables.

The Diet and Osteoporosis: It is not just calcium and vitamin D in the diet that are important for bone metabolism. Magnesium and potassium rich foods such as sweet potato protect bones as well.

Green leafy vegetables are calcium rich (as well as containing bone protective Vitamin K), any food rich in Vitamin C reduces bone loss, figs are calcium rich, salmon, tuna and fatty fish contain vitamin D and Omega 3 fatty acids both of which contribute to bone metabolism. Nuts, including almonds are calcium and protein rich, alternative "Plant milks" are fortified with vitamin D and calcium, tofu, calcium fortified juices, prunes and molasses are all bone protective foods. See diet section.

Rheumatoid Arthritis:

Affects up to 1.5% of the world's adult population, 600,000 in England and Wales. The highest incidence is in Native American populations (5%), Australia (2.45%) and the lowest rural Africa (0.1%). RhA affects the synovial joints, progressing to permanent joint damage and disability. There is a female preponderance, 3F: 1M, the commonest age at presentation being 40-60. Children suffer a form of RhA, – Stills Disease. Other body systems are affected. – Dry eyes, Keratoconjunctivitis Sicca, scleritis, episcleritis, atherosclerosis and increased heart disease, rheumatoid vasculitis, subcutaneous nodules, lung complications, fibrosis, effusion, nodular disease, bronchiolitis, osteopoenia and osteoporosis.

The cause of the underlying autoimmune reaction against the synovium is unknown. But once initiated, B lymphocytes activate helper T lymphocytes which release inflammatory cytokines (Including TNF-a) and interleukins into the synovial fluid. An inflammatory reaction is set up attracting macrophages and PMNLs and the whole joint becomes swollen. The swollen synovium (the Pannus) then erodes and damages the surrounding joint.

Risk factors:

Being female (2-3: 1); Age: (>40); Positive family history (various gene markers including an HLA marker in 60% and Tyrosine phosphatase N22 and PAD 14); Smoking doubles the risk of developing Rh A.; Post Infection?; Hormones (some have a protective effect – eg pregnancy); Geographical factors: RhA is commoner in developed/industrialised countries; Diet? Possibly a Mediterranean diet may be partially protective.

Symptoms/Investigations:

Pain, warmth, swelling and stiffness of one or more joints. Although it can affect any synovial joint, it typically involves the small joints of the hands, wrists and feet. The larger joints can be affected, shoulders, knees, elbows, ankles but of the spine, only the neck is affected. It is usually symmetrical (after a period of time). Fatigue, malaise and fever may be associated, morning stiffness, anorexia, weight loss. As the condition progresses, hand deformities become obvious (up to 60%). Much of the increased morbidity and mortality is in fact related to immunosuppressant treatment side effects and complications.

Investigations: Rheumatoid Factor is an auto antibody against IgG. It is positive in 60-70% of Rh A patients though it is not specific and is positive in other inflammatory conditions. ESR and CRP are raised. Osteoporosis is a common association, due to age, steroids, Cytokine induced osteoclast activation and so on, so bone scans are wise in patients with RhA. Anti CCP (Anticyclic Citrullinated Peptide) antibodies are positive auto antibodies in 60% of RhA patients. There is a tendency to anaemia.

The progress of RhA varies: 10% progress to severe disability, 10% remit permanently in the first 6 months. Some follow a chronic progressive course, some a relatively self limited disease. A worse prognosis is associated with seropositivity (Rh Factor and anti-CCP antibodies), several joints affected at diagnosis, rheumatic nodules, a persistently raised ESR etc. As many as half of all patients are unable to keep a full time job 10 years after diagnosis, depression is much more common than in the general population and life expectancy is at present 5-10 years reduced.

Treatment. Generally speaking, the early use of Methotrexate (a conventional DMARD – Disease Modifying Antirheumatic Drug) within 3 months of the onset. Some advise 2 DMARDS from the start instead of Mtx if response is inadequate. Early steroids can tide the patient over while the DMARD starts to work.

If the conventional DMARD is ineffective then move to a biological DMARD.

So the drugs include analgesics, NSAIDs, steroids, locally and systemically and **Conventional DMARDS**, Methotrexate, Sulphasalazine, Hydroxychloroquine, Leflunomide,

With worse side effect profiles are: Cyclosporine, Gold, Azathioprine and Penicillamine.

Biological DMARDS: See below for why they have such weird names):

TNF-α inhibitors: Etanercept, Infliximab, Adalimumab, Golimumab, Certolizumab.

Other biological DMARDs: Ritixumab, Abatacept, Tocilizumab, Anakinra.

Other therapies: Occupational, Physio, Podiatry and dietary are also important as is joint surgery when necessary.

Juvenile Idiopathic Arthritis (JIA), Juvenile Rheumatoid Arthritis (JRA):

Pre age 16 and lasting >6 weeks. Presentation is similar to RhA in adults.

Large joints are commonly affected with swelling and morning stiffness, sometimes polyarthritis, with systemic symptoms, or oligoarthritis (fewer than 4 joints) without systemic symptoms.

Girls 3:1 Boys – just like the adult version.

The two common extra articular complications in children are uveitis and growth disturbance. Up to 50% of children continue to suffer the condition into adulthood.

Treatment:

Azathioprine, Ciclosporin, Hydroxychloroquine, Methotrexate, Penicillamine, Gold, Sulfasalazine, Leflunomide, Arava.

Azathioprine: Initially 50-100mg OD, maintenance 2 – 2.5mg/kg/day. A pro drug for Mercaptopurine.

Pre-treatment: Do FBC, U and Es, creat. LFTs, consider TPMT (Thiopurine S methyltransferase) genetic testing or actual enzyme levels, avoid Rx if TPMT homozygous recessive or low enzyme activity. 86-97% patients have normal enzyme levels. Immunise against Influenza and give Pneumovax while on Rx.

Monitoring: FBC and LFTs weekly for 4 weeks and after dose increase, once all is stable, do 3 monthly U and Es and creat. at 1m 3m 6m and 12 monthly thereafter. Consultant advice: If WBC>3 then treatment is OK, do FBC, LFTs monthly for 3m then 3 monthly.

For instance:(eg in Ulcerative Colitis etc), maintenance dose 200mg/day,
If WBC 2.5 – 3.0 then 150mg/day,

If WBC 2.0-2.5 have a few drug free days, then 100mg/day,

If WBC <2.0 stop treatment.

S/Es Nausea, bone marrow suppression, hepatotoxicity.

Hydroxychloroquine: Plaquenil 200mg od initially 200-400mg/day maintenance. Also Chloroquine sulph. Nivaquine. 250mg OD initially, 250mg maintenance. *D/C in UK July 2014*

Tests: Baseline and 6 monthly eye checks (retinal damage and corneal opacities). Renal function and regular FBCs during treatment.

Sulfasalazine: Salazopyrin: 500mg OD, increase by 500mg/week. Maintenance 2-4 Gr/day.

Tests: FBC and LFTs at 3 weeks, 6 weeks, then 3 monthly. Nausea, GI upset, urine discolouration, rashes, leukopoenia, thrombocytopoenia, hepatitis.

Methotrexate: 2.5mg-5mg once weekly initially. Maintenance 5-15mg/week. FBC and LFTs every 2-4 weeks for 3m, then every 6-12 weeks. U and Es, creat. every 3-6m especially if on NSAIDs. Can co prescribe 5mg Folic Acid daily without compromising effectiveness. All sorts of interactions and S/Es. Avoid in alcohol abuse, avoid with Trimethoprim, Co Trimoxazole (But who prescribes Septrin these days?) S/Es include dyspepsia. Complications: G.I. disturbance, hepatic fibrosis, abn. LFTS, cough, dyspnoea, pneumonitis, macrocytosis. Give low dose folic acid daily and for 1-2 days after dose. In most co prescribing situations Folic acid is given at a dose of 5mg every week or so with Mtx.

80-90% patients are also taking NSAIDs. May interact with high dose aspirin.

If MCV >97 Refer.

If WBC <3.5, Neuts <2.0, plats <150, stop Rx and refer.

If serial decrease in WBC or plats stop Rx.

Rising MCV can indicate folate depletion.

Note: High WBC and plats may indicate active inflammation and a fall along with a lowered ESR may indicate a response to treatment.

Gold I.M. (Sodium Aurothiomalate, Myocrisin) 5-10mg test dose then 10-50mg weekly, until signs of remission, then 50mg every 2 weeks, maintenance 10-50mg/m. By two years, 6 weekly injections. Keep patient under observation for half an hour after injection. FBC and urine analysis weekly initially then monthly once stabilised. S/Es: Rashes, mouth ulcers, arthralgia, , thrombocytopoenia, proteinuria, nephropathy.

D-Penicillamine. 125-250mg daily initially slowly increasing to max 1.5gr/day. FBC and urine testing monthly. Consider Pyridoxine supplementation as Penicillamine increases its excretion and reduces B6 activity. S/Es: Rashes, mouth ulcers, loss of taste, thrombocytopoenia, proteinuria, autoimmunity.

Steroids:

In acute exacerbations, Methylprednisolone or Triamcinolone 80-120mg IM.

Biologics:(DMARDS, Disease Modifying Anti Rheumatic Drugs) (See above):

Abatacept,

Adalimumab (Humira),

Etanercept (Enbrel) A disease modifying drug for Rheumatoid Arthritis, Psoriatic Arthritis, and

Psoriasis. Twice weekly injection. This is one of the anti TNF drugs, 25mg twice weekly. Don't give live vaccines. Do FBC if patient is unwell.

Infliximab, (Remicade).
Anakinra, (Kineret).
Golimumab.
Certolizumab, Pegol.
Tocilizumab, etc.
Rituximab.
-So: these include tumour necrosis factor inhibitors, IL-6 inhibitors, B cell and T cell targeted therapies.
The nomenclature is as follows: of **Clonal proteins and antibodies**:
Ximab: Chimeric monoclonal antibody,
Zumab: Humanised monoclonal antibody,
Umab: Human monoclonal antibody.
Cept: Receptor-antibody fusion protein.
The anti TNF treatments can reactivate TB and opportunistic systemic fungal infections and as featured elsewhere for various beneficial effects, many naturally occurring compounds in Turmeric, Green Tea, Cannabis, Echinacea etc may also have anti TNF activity. Most patients see an improvement in their symptoms after a few doses. They reduce Rheumatoid activity but do not cure the disease.

Psoriatic Arthritis:

Affects up to 30% of psoriasis sufferers. It is seronegative (for Rh Factor) and male and female incidence is equal. The most common age of presentation is 30-55, usually but not always, after the onset of the skin disease. Children can be affected, girls median age around 5 and boys around 10.

There is a spondylo-arthropathy affecting the spine and peripheral joints, tendons and ligaments. T lymphocytes, TNF-a, Interleukins and vascular growth factors are involved in the inflammatory process. There is local bony proliferation not seen in Rh A. There are definite genetic and familial factors in PsA with a cluster of genes on chromosome 6 and HLA associations (B27, B7, Cw6, DR7). In a fifth of patients the joint changes precede those in the skin. Always look for nail and umbilical psoriatic signs but the common pattern of joint involvement is: Distal interphalangeal arthritis (unlike RhA). Asymmetrical oligoarthritis in the hands and feet and affecting fewer than 4 joints, often all the joints of one digit. Sometimes one large joint can be affected. Symetrical polyarthritis (mimicking RhA). Spondylitis (M>F) and sacroileitis. Arthritis mutilans affecting the finger joints.

Psoriatic Arthritis	Rheumatoid Arthritis
Preceded by psoriasis in 80-85%	Co exists with psoriasis in only 3/10,000
M=F	4F:1M
Asymmetrical usually	Often symmetrical
Dactylitis in up to half	Dactylitis unusual
(Dactylitis is inflammation of an entire digit, – finger or toe)	
DIP joints usually involved	DIP joints usually spared
Spondylitis in 50%	Spine not usually involved
Enthesitis (Insertion of tendons inflamed) in 40%, including Achilles tendon	Enthesitis rare
No Rheumatoid nodules	Rheumatoid Nodules in up to 30%

Seronegative in 85%	Seropositive in 85%
Nails commonly affected	Not
Bone erosion and formation at joints	Bone erosion and osteoporosis at affected joints
	Rare to see abnormal bone formation.

Joints less tender but redder
Up to 30% of psoriasis sufferers develop Ps A.

The extra articular manifestations include conjunctivitis, uveitis, aortic incompetence, nail lesions and cardiovascular disease.

Investigations: RhF, anti-CCP are negative (positive in only 15% with polyarticular PsA). ESR and CRP are elevated.

A worse prognosis is indicated by polyarticular disease, high initial ESR, being female, starting young, bad skin disease, being positive for HLA markers, steroid use.

Treatment: NSAIDs, steroids, local and systemic.

DMARDS, conventional, including Methotrexate, Sulphasalazine, Leflunomide, Cyclosporin, Azathioprine, Gold and

Biological, Etanercept, Adalimumab, Infliximab, Golimumab.

Alternative Treatments:

The excellent Arthritis Research UK puts out a wealth of independent information on musculoskeletal conditions and recently performed a review of the published information on "alternative and complimentary treatments" which only used published RCTs. Therefore you can put your faith in it. They looked at 33 alternative preparations in regular use for joint pain and musculo-skeletal pain. 40% of chronic pain sufferers in this class use alternative treatments, physical or medicinal.

The objective results were:

No alternative treatments helped PMR.

The treatments that objectively work in other inflammatory and musculoskeletal conditions:

In Rh A: Borage seed oil, Evening Primrose Oil, Fish body oil,

In O.A: Capsaicin, Devil's Claw, Ginger, Glucosamine, Indian Frankincense, Pine Bark Extracts, SAMe (S-Adenosylmethionone). But not Chondroitin.

Assessment of the acute Bad Back:

NICE guidance on bad backs, one of the commonest, worst handled and potentially deceitful situations that we GPs see, is pretty unhelpful and changes frequently. Don't forget an acute or chronic "bad back" is a symptom, not a condition, not a diagnosis. The latest NICE guidance (2016) suggests exercise as the first line of treatment. Confronted with the obese, out of condition, acute, severely uncomfortable patient with a "muscle or ligamentous type tear" (whatever that means) trying to get them to exercise will be a waste of time. I agree that aerobic exercise can help alleviate many minor back pains – a swim or a knock about in the squash court can help relieve the pain of a misplaced facet or impacted osteophyte. But most back pain sufferers are not going to be easy to persuade to move and some will even want house calls and the analgesics delivered. Pain, stiffness, inertia and lack of fitness as well as a culturally misplaced faith in "rest" will have to be overcome first. NICE classifies Yoga as exercise (!) and no longer considers acupuncture effective. I know there is no logical rationale to acupuncture, no anatomical or physiological basis, it is impossible to do randomised double blind controlled trials of acupuncture (you would have to anaesthetise the skin of both groups of patients and blind fold them before inserting the needles in the active group) but thousands of rational, normal, intelligent people do derive benefit from it for some reason and it has few side effects. NSAIDs have taken the first drug spot from paracetamol – as far as NICE is concerned but I would imagine by the time the patient is seeing you, he or she will have taken both OTC. NICE also says use codeine but not anti depressants, anticonvulsants etc. It is also critical of orthotics, massage and manipulation when used alone and basically advises just exercise, NSAIDs or codeine and psychological therapies.

The true incidence of back pain is much higher than has been reported, probably 10-20% with up to 70% still suffering at 1 year. It is the root of 37% of chronic pain in men and 44% in women, costing £12Bn a year. Hence the previous NICE guidelines on manipulation and CBT for all were just not affordable in the real world. Serious spinal pathology is present in 1% (#, infection, cancer, inflammation).

I think NICE is a little out of contact with Primary Care reality. **NICE – Not In Contact Exactly.**

I would suggest that back pain can be **severe and debilitating,** can very definitely respond to strong analgesics, which should be **supervised,** (up to and including such drugs as Pethidine, Oxycodone and MST and add Diazepam if there is significant spasm in the worst cases). This will enable the patient to exercise and undo some but not all of the mechanical causes of back pain. I do not share NICE's trust in NSAIDs for acute back pain other than as an adjunct therapy. Also I would usually suggest manipulation, particularly by a good osteopath or osteopathic physician if the signs and symptoms are of a mechanical back pain. Massage and manipulation nearly always help. Make sure you limit the number and duration of any controlled drugs you give but just because back pain is common it doesn't mean it is trivial. Don't be afraid to treat it effectively. Psychological therapies: not available in my neck of the woods. If NICE means CBT then this is obviously for chronic low back pain and I would definitely want to exclude a physical, anatomical, primary cause with various investigations. Once I had done that I would use a Tricyclic or SSRI. **NICE Not Impressively Clinically Engaged.**

"Red Flags": A PMH of cancer, raised ESR, weight loss, reduced haematocrit, failure to improve after 1m, age>50 and your clinical judgement.

So do an XR, a FBC and an ESR as initial investigations if worried, always do a general examination of the patient and ask about other symptoms. I can't over emphasise the need to examine all patients with back pain and to **regularly re-examine patients who return with back pain.** I despair at my lazy and burnt out chair bound older colleagues and my no touch, screen obsessed younger colleagues who can't be bothered or are frightened to get off their backsides and lay their hands on naked flesh. I hope that new research linking sitting for a living to increased cardiovascular, venous, and cerebrovascular disease will prompt my GP colleagues to get up and examine more patients out of survival self interest if not out of professional self respect.

Sciatica: Every patient thinks their leg pain, which we all get occasionally, is "sciatica" – though the true lifetime incidence of sciatic irritation pain is about 5%.

Dermatome coverage varies tremendously as do myotomes. These are not the same in everyone.

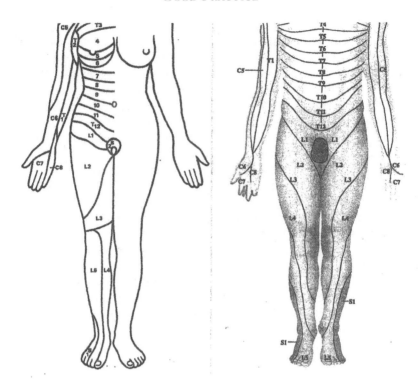

Diagram: How Dermatomes can vary.HDCV1

MRIs: Not as useful as we all think: Most of the population have disc protrusions at any given time, and 1:20 have root compression but carry on with day to day life regardless.

Surgery gives good immediate results but interestingly at one year the operated and unoperated-on groups are very similar in symptoms and function. For the risks of surgery read the excellent "Do no harm" by Henry Marsh.

Level of Herniation	Pain	Numbness	Weakness	Atrophy	Reflexes
L3/4 4th lumbar N	Low back, hip post/lat thigh ant leg	Antero-med thigh and knee.	Quads	Quads	Knee weak
L4/5 5th lumbar N	Over SIJ, hip, lat thigh and leg	Lat leg, Gt. toe web	Dorsiflexion Gt. toe, can't walk on heels, occ. foot drop	Little	Not usual
L5/S1 1st sacral N	Over SIJ hip, post lat thigh and leg down to heel	Back of calf, lat heel foot and toe	Plantar flexion of foot and Gt toe. Can't walk on toes	Calf wasting	Ankle jerk
Massive Midline protrusion	Low back thighs legs and or perineum. depending on level of Lesion Occ. Bilat.	Thighs legs feet and or perineum/ Variable may be bilateral.	Variable paralysis/ paresis of legs and or bowel and bladder ? incontinence.	?Extensive	Ankle jerk

The Keele STarT back screening tool is a prognosis assessment tool for acute back pain in GP. It includes physical and psychological aspects of the effects of the pain on the life of the patient to predict the prognosis.

| Pt name: | DOB: | Trial No: | Physio: | Date: |

STarT Back: For these questions, please think about your back pain over the **last few days.**

1st Time Score / 2nd Time Score / Change score

1. How **bothersome has pain spreading down your legs from your back** been in the **last few days**?

Not at all [0]   Slightly [1]   Moderately [2]   Very much [3]   Extremely [4]

2. How **bothersome has pain in your shoulder or neck** been in the **last few days**?

Not at all [0]   Slightly [1]   Moderately [2]   Very much [3]   Extremely [4]

For each of the following, please cross one box to show how much you agree or disagree with the statement, thinking about the **last few days.**

3. In the last **few days**, I have **dressed more slowly** than usual because of my back pain.

Completely disagree ... Strongly agree

| 0 | 1 | 2 | 3 | 4 | 5 | 6 | 7 | 8 | 9 | 10 |

4. In the last **few days**, I have only **walked short distances** because of my back pain.

Completely disagree ... Strongly agree

| 0 | 1 | 2 | 3 | 4 | 5 | 6 | 7 | 8 | 9 | 10 |

5. It's **really not safe** for a person with a condition like mine to be **physically active.**

Completely disagree ... Strongly agree

| 0 | 1 | 2 | 3 | 4 | 5 | 6 | 7 | 8 | 9 | 10 |

6. **Worrying thoughts** have been going through my mind a lot of the time in the last **few days.**

Completely disagree ... Strongly agree

| 0 | 1 | 2 | 3 | 4 | 5 | 6 | 7 | 8 | 9 | 10 |

7. I feel that **my back pain is terrible** and that **it is never going to get any better.**

Completely disagree ... Strongly agree

| 0 | 1 | 2 | 3 | 4 | 5 | 6 | 7 | 8 | 9 | 10 |

8. In general, in the last **few days**, I have **not enjoyed** all the things I used to enjoy.

Completely disagree ... Strongly agree

| 0 | 1 | 2 | 3 | 4 | 5 | 6 | 7 | 8 | 9 | 10 |

9. Overall, how **bothersome** has your **back pain** been in the **last few days**?

Not at all [0]   Slightly [1]   Moderately [2]   Very much [3]   Extremely [4]

STarT Back Screening Tool Website >
Using & Scoring the SBST

Using and Scoring The Keele STarT Back Screening Tool
The Keele SBST 9-item version

The Keele SBST 9-item tool is available in a number of languages, including English, Dutch, French, Spanish, Danish and Welsh. The questions it includes were selected because they are established predictors for persistent disabling back pain. They include radiating leg pain, pain elsewhere, disability (2 items about difficulties with dressing & walking taken from the Roland and Morris Disability Questionnaire), fear (1 item from the Tampa Scale of Kinesiophobia), anxiety (1 item from the Hospital Anxiety and Depression Scale), pessimistic patient expectations (1 item from the Pain Catastrophising Scale), and low mood,(1 item from the Hospital Anxiety and Depression Scale) and how much the patient is bothered by their pain (from Dunn & Croft 2005). All 9-items use a response format of 'agree' or 'disagree', with exception to the bothersomeness item, which uses a Likert scale. The Keele SBST produces two scores: overall scores and distress subscale scores (Hill et al 2008)

The distress subscale score is used to identify the high-risk subgroup. To score this subscale add the last 5 items; fear, anxiety, catastrophising, depression & bothersomeness (bothersomeness responses are positive for 'very much' or 'extremely' bothersome back pain). Subscale scores range from 0 to 5 with patients scoring 4 or 5 being classified into the high-risk subgroup

The overall score is used to separate the low risk patients from the medium-risk subgroup. Scores range from 0-9 and are produced by adding all positive items; Patients who achieve a score of 0-3 are classified into the low-risk subgroup and those with scores of 4-9 into the medium-risk subgroup.

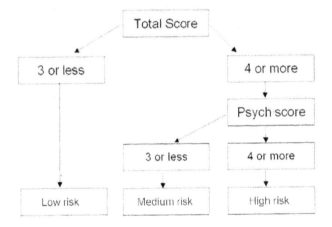

The Keele SBST 6-item version

The 6-item tool includes 6 of the same items as the 9-item tool, with 3 items excluded (fear, anxiety and pain elsewhere), making it quicker to use. However, our (unpublished) research indicates that it is only able to allocate patients to one of two subgroups (low-risk or high-risk). Patients who score 3 or more items positively have a high-risk of persistent disabling low back pain.

Instructions on embedding the 6-item Keele STarT Back Tool onto an EMIS system are provided here - 6-item EMIS tool

Using and scoring the Keele SBST clinical measurement tool

The 9-item clinical measurement tool is designed to help clinicians objectively measure the severity of the domains screened by the 9-item tool. When repeated measures are used this enables an objective marker of change over time to be made for individual items.
Cut-offs have been established for each item - to enable those using this tool to subgroup patients in the same way as the 9-item screening tool. The cut-off points that equate to an agree/positive score on the clinical measurement tool for subgrouping are:

Leg pain - 'moderately' or more
Shoulder/neck - slightly or more
Dressing - 5 or more
Walking - 5 or more
Fear - 7 or more
Worry - 3 or more
Catastrophising - 6 or more
Mood - 7 or more
Bothersomeness - 'very' or more

Its very easy to produce an acetate using these cut-offs that you place over the questionnaire to quickly enable you to score the clinical measurement tool for subgrouping purposes.

Using and scoring the generic condition tool

The 5-item generic condition tool is the 9-item psychosocial subscale modified to screen/identify distress in other conditions. S cores range from 0 to 5 with patients scoring 4 or 5 being classified as high psychosocial risk.

When using the tool please ensure the copyright and funding statement is maintained at all times.

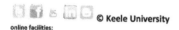 **© Keele University**
online facilities:

© Keele University 01/08/07 Funded by Arthritis Research UK

In chronic (1 year) back pain, MRIs disclose serious spinal pathology in 10%. So don't dismiss them all as heart-sinks.

Also it is worth noting that Danish researchers (Albert H et al. Europ Spine J. 22 (4) 697-707 2013) have now linked chronic back pain, disc herniation, Modic type 1 X-ray changes and chronic bacterial infection. More importantly they showed that antibiotics can relieve the back pain. Unfortunately it takes 100 days of Co Amoxiclav to clear the infection with Prop. Acnes and or Staph. so you can imagine what that does to your bowel habit, your microbiome, your oral, oesophageal and vaginal candida and presumably it increases the ever present chances of resistant organisms. It does however significantly improve the pain in up to 40% of sufferers.

Examination. All patients with back pain should be examined, even if briefly on just about every single occasion they consult. They don't **always** need to be laid on the couch but you do need to do a proper examination at the start and every so often after, as chronic occult conditions vary in their severity and clarity over time. Bony secondaries, osteomyelitis and osteoporotic crush fractures do progress and become more obvious if you stay alert for a developing condition.

Watch the gait, examine SLR, reflexes, (over 60's don't have reliable ankle jerks), test below knee motor and sensory neurology, – tiptoe walking tests S1, heel walking tests L5, irrespective of variation in dermatomes, the 1/2 web space is always L5. Dorsiflexion of the great toe is L5.

Rare complications of treatment:

Tendonitis and tendon rupture are rare complications of statins, quinolones (not so rare) and steroid treatment.

Orthopaedics/Sports conditions:

Shoulder

The Shoulder Muscles:

The Rotator Cuff consists of 4 muscles and these are the main stabilisers of the shoulder:

Supraspinatus, Infraspinatus, Teres Minor and Subscapularis.

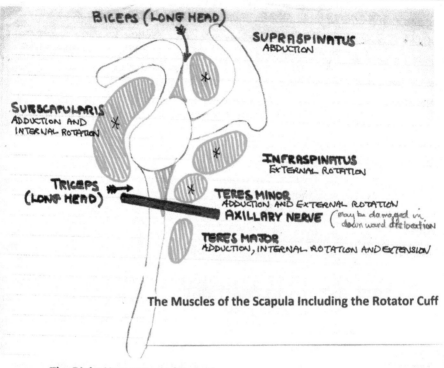

The Muscles of the Scapula Including the Rotator Cuff

The Right Humerus and Scapula

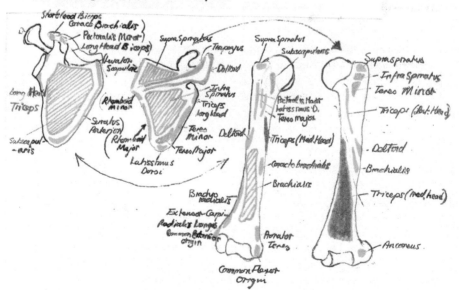

Muscles of the scapula (MOS1)

Shoulder movements are quite complicated. It is the joint that made me wish I knew what I was doing in my first year of dissection or maybe wish I had the chance of going back and doing some dissection mid GP career. It is a shallow ball and socket, with a huge range of movement but consequently the joint is prone to instability and dislocation. Perhaps it is the fact that we are supposed to be quadrupeds resting half our body weight on the shoulder that, like the opposable thumb, has resulted in mechanical difficulties due to adapting to an excessive range of movement. It is the easiest joint to inject (all GPs should be able to do this) and prone to two or three common acute and a similar number of chronic conditions.

SO: The shoulder movements are:

Subscapularis	Internal rotation
Infraspinatus	External rotation
Supraspinatus	Abduction
Teres Major	Adduction
Teres Minor	External rotation.

Elevation: The first 90 deg is all at the glenohumoral joint (Supraspinatus (first 15 deg) and deltoid muscles).

The next 60 deg is from rotation of the scapula (Serratus Anterior and upper Trapezius) In the final 30 deg the scapula is stationary, the movement is all glenohumeral and due to adduction of the humerus (Pectoralis Major).

Resisted movements:

Resisted abduction (arm at side of trunk) tests injuries of Deltoid (rare) and Supraspinatus (4 common sites of injury).

Resisted adduction tests the Pectoralis Major, Latissimus Dorsi, both Teres (lesions to all are rare).

Resisted Lateral Rotation implies an Infraspinatus lesion but if lateral rotation and abduction hurt then the Supraspinatus may be damaged.

If resisted lateral rotation and adduction hurt then we are looking at the Teres Minor. Resisted medial rotation is Subscapularis.

Capsular lesions: A dozen or more causes, traumatic arthritis, acute injury, OA, etc. The capsular pattern is a hard end feel and equal limitation of all 3 passive ROMs. Internal rotation is slightly limited, abduction more so but lateral rotation markedly.

Frozen Shoulder:

Adhesive capsulitis. Can be associated with M.I., CVA, diabetes, thyroid disease, as well as trauma, joint and capsular lesions. The commonest cause would be an acute, often minor injury, but a year of subsequent immobility and discomfort can be avoided by fairly vigorous initial capsule stretching and early attention by the GP +/– the physio. The patient can be shown how to stretch the joint within the limits of pain, (– prescribe appropriate analgesia). Don't forget that on examination 60 degrees of abduction are still possible due to scapular movement despite a locked glenohumeral joint and this can be seen by looking from behind as the patient abducts the shoulder.

If left for a month the joint is too painful to be passively stretched and it needs an injection of steroid. This can be repeated after a week and is actually one of the technically easiest for a GP to give. (The usual approach is posterior, less painful and less threatening). A frozen shoulder can be a potential risk after the fitting of a cardiac pacemaker since patients are told to avoid lifting their L arm initially. When they do stretch it they find there is a painful scar all around the pacemaker box and they therefore restrict their own shoulder movement. Tell your patients post pacemaker to rotate the shoulder and abduct it to the horizontal as much as discomfort permits from the start.

It is important to be sure that more serious trauma, infection in the joint, SLAP tears (Superior Labrum Anterior Posterior-in which muscle strength around the joint is not normal in *all* planes) have been excluded and if you feel insecure, a WBC, ESR, Alk P'ase and X Ray can be done within a few days first, or even, if you have access, a specialised shoulder USS. With a simple history, no systemic symptoms and normal resisted muscle strength in the various planes (document this to exclude the SLAP tear) the investigations are unnecessary 99% of the time.

SLAP tears:

What you may have forgotten:

The long head of Biceps originates at the supraglenoid tubercle of the scapula (where it fuses with the circular labrum around the joint) in the shoulder joint and inserts with the short head:

The short head of biceps originates at the apex of the coracoid process of the anterior scapula and swells with the long head into the fleshy belly of the biceps inserting into the tuberosity of the radius and ante brachial fascia (bicipital aponeurosis).

SLAP stands for superior labrum, anterior to posterior. When a tear of the labrum, the ring of cartilage around the edge of the glenoid cavity (which may actually be fibrous extensions of the biceps and triceps tendons) at the biceps tendon insertion occurs, this is a SLAP tear. It can be caused for instance by a sudden pull on the shoulder, an overhead strain (overhead throwing), or trying to lift something too heavy etc. Thus it can follow a weight lifting, a throwing or tackle injury.

The symptoms are: pain in the top of the shoulder, with significant sleep pain, weakness and a "catch" in the shoulder on overhead activities (somewhat like an acromnioclavicular joint problem).

The tear is diagnosed clinically or by USS or MRI (arthrogram). Treatment is surgical repair by arthroscopy as the labrum is poorly supplied with blood vessels and does not repair well if left alone.

Supraspinatus Tendonitis: (For tendonitis read tendinitis)

Whether or not this is the true pathological diagnosis, it is by far the commonest clinical chapter heading that over use shoulder pain gets given in General Practice. As mentioned, the shoulder is a dreadful design. It evolved from the forelimbs of our quad-ruped ancestors who only needed to walk, run, grab and occasionally protect their faces to be the most mobile, shallow joint in the body, capable of allowing us to reach above our heads, to do up bras, to reach, manipulate, throw stones and spears, climb, clamber, use tools, weapons, scratch virtually everywhere, remove parasites from our all over bodies and therefore some design compromises were inevitable. One is that range of movement and stability are mutually contradictory design parameters. This means the compact joint space leaves little room for long sliding tendons within it and one tendon, the supraspinatus, often rubs the inside surface of the acromnion and becomes inflamed when unfamiliar overhead repetitive activity takes place (painting ceilings, serving a tennis ball, using a screwdriver above the head etc).

It is the most prevalent shoulder tendinitis. The signs are painful resisted abduction, sometimes with painful resisted lateral rotation. Although a painful arc is common, this depends on which part of the tendon the inflammation is worst. If there is no painful arc, injection doesn't work, only local massage.

Bicipital Tendonitis:

Painful resisted elbow flexion and painful resisted supination. Local injection of steroid is to the tenderest spot and a small volume of steroid used.

Dislocated shoulder:

All GPs should be able to reduce this, like putting back a dislocated finger or patella, it is rewarding, often almost miraculous and if done properly convinces the onlookers that some doctors are still possessed of that mystique of skill and knowledge the public expect of them.

95% of dislocations are anterior. The patient, if relaxed and determined can reduce their own thus:

Bend the elbow to 90 degrees, internally rotate the arm so the forearm is across the abdomen, then slowly externally rotate the shoulder by pushing the fist of the affected arm outwards gently and progressively with the good hand. At 90 degrees (the forearm straight forward) the shoulder should pop in to the joint. If not, the patient can gently and slowly repeat the process until it does.

The doctor reducing the shoulder:

The arm should be resting alongside the trunk, hanging at the patient's side. Bend the elbow to 90 degrees. Internally rotate the shoulder so the forearm is across the lower abdomen.

Then slowly externally rotate the shoulder keeping the upper arm as static as you can. Just past 90 degrees the joint should reduce at which point you gently internally rotate the joint back towards the chest.

Alternatively you can have the patient prone lying on a bed, the arm dangling downwards toward the floor and gently and persistently pull the arm downward. The shoulder reduces after a while when they tire and if they relax. Hippocrates put his foot in the armpit and pulled

and the

Kocher 's techniques is: (two sources)

Elbow flexed and at the side of the body, arm in neutral position, externally rotate the upper arm, move upper arm anteriorly then internally rotate arm. Or

Traction, then abduction, externally rotation, adduction and internally rotation.

After the process advise NSAIDs and a sling and assess for damage.

Or simply: Tell the patient to relax, you won't make any sudden moves and will stop if he says stop, slowly abduct the arm to 90 deg and slowly externally rotate the shoulder. It should reduce.

Carpal Tunnel Syndrome:

Pain and parasthesiae over palmar aspect, radial half of hand, associated with pregnancy, myxoedema, Rheumatoid Arthritis, vascular shunts, trauma, Amyloid, Diabetes, Acromegaly, lipomata, ganglia, etc.

Signs: **Tinel's sign:** Tap the palmar aspect of wrist quite firmly with a patellar hammer. If positive, the patient will feel tingling or electric shocks over middle three fingers.

Phalen's sign: Maximum passive wrist flexion for 1 minute (or place the back of the two hands together in a "reversed praying" posture) and the middle three fingers go tingly or numb.

Treatment:INJECT depot steroid just lateral to Palmaris Longus tendon, distal to the palmar crease.

See end of section.

Finkelstein Test:

Hold the patient's thumb and push it firmly in an ulnar deviated direction with the wrist. A distal radial pain indicates **De Quervains tenosynovitis** – Abductor Pollicis Longus and Extensor Pollicis Brevis tendonitis.(You can also flex the thumb in the palm and then ulnar flex the wrist which will likewise cause pain).

De Quervains Syndrome:

Extensor thumb tendonitis usually due to overuse.

Tenosynovitis of the Extensor Pollicis Brevis and Abductor Pollicis Longus tendons. The pain is on radial abduction and thumb extension and is thought to be due to overuse. It is common in young mothers, possibly due to unfamiliar repeated lifting or hormonal changes or both. Splints help, so do Topical or oral NSAIDs. Usually a local steroid injection avoids the need for surgery.

Stenosing Tenosynovitis: (Trigger Finger):

This is when the tendon (always the flexor tendon) of for instance a finger or thumb exceeds the limiting diameter of the "retinacular pulley system" (the flexor tendon sheath). This is usually at the so called "first annular pulley ".

The affected finger is stiff to flex and extend and catches, suddenly releasing or in the later stages, needing to be straightened with a "give". Usually the sliding lump in the tendon can be felt as the target for the steroid injecting needle (infiltrated around the tendon). Local steroid injection, which is relatively easy to do, cures up to 2/3, for a while at least. Percutaneous needle release or open release cures 100%.

Dupuytren's Contracture:

Fibrosis and contraction of palmar fascia leading to finger contractures. 30% prevalence >65 Yrs. Can be related to diabetes, alcoholism.

Spine problems:

Neck Pain:

Neck and spine exercises: (See end of section)

McKenzie Retraction: Pull the chin in and push the head backwards. This stretches the back of the neck and is part of the Alexander Technique posture. 5-10 stretches every 2-3 hours. This can be done lying on a pillow.

Rotate the head slowly from one side to the other, then lateral flexion of the neck, moving the ear almost down to the shoulder on each side. If you have been a GP for any length of time and sat over a computer for six hours or more a day, this latter is virtually impossible. You can do this standing, gently dropping the shoulder you are pulling away from. Shrug shoulders up to ears for 2 seconds then down again. Rotate the neck against resistance (cheek against fixed palm) hold for a few seconds and relax. You can progressively move the hand away a few cms. at a time and push and hold again. This is not forceful but gentle pushing each time.

Using a walking stick or something of similar length, hold this in front of you, horizontally at arm's length. Then rotate the torso from one side to the other and back again. Repeat this without force, letting the rotation stretch your lumbar and thoracic spine about 20 times.

Posture:

Get the patient to walk looking straight ahead not down and in a relaxed occiput back and up position (double chin posture).

Sit with shoulders relaxed downwards and not rounded forward.

Adjust the work station so that the patient is not hunched over the desk but has feet flat on the ground, head up and eyes level (i.e. with a VDU screen) if possible. Hands should not be too low, usually the elbow should be at 90 degrees. Advise frequent shifts in posture.

When sitting watching TV try to have the occiput resting against something and have the TV directly ahead.

Pause Gymnastics:

A useful way of preventing postural pain and stiffness in people with repetitive jobs or operators of key boards or machinery.

Lateral flexion of the head a few times (ear to shoulder).

Retracting the chin (making a double chin).

Stand, place the palms of the hands in the small of the back and bend backwards at the waist.

Interlock the fingers, turn the palms to face away, stretch the hands up, palms facing the ceiling. Now stretch the arms back behind the head.

Straighten the arm at the elbow, flex the wrist up and stretch the arms back as far behind the body as possible.

Flex the wrist down so the palm is close to the forearm.

Do one or two stretches every 20 minutes.

Lumbar disc prolapse: Acute low back pain, refer if:

Severe sciatica (unilateral leg pain) and unilateral foot drop (weakness dorsiflexing foot).

Bilateral sciatic discomfort – sometimes, (VERY RARELY) a central disc with the propensity to cause permanent loss of sphincter control and impotence.

Refer to spinal/orthopaedic surgeon (or the neurosurgeon if you are lucky enough to have direct access) if

Cauda Equina Lesion:

Causes include:

Central Lumbar Disc L4/5 L5/S1, tumours, primary and secondary, trauma, infection including pressure from an epidural abscess, spinal stenosis worsened by lumbar OA, kyphoscoliosis and or spina bifida etc, Spondylolysthesis, haematoma, manipulation (incredibly rare according to my osteopath), IVC thrombosis, Sarcoid.

Presentation of Cauda Equina lesions: Some of:

Difficulty micturating, urinary retention (50-70%), decreased bladder and urethral sensation.

Severe LBP with pain in the legs, unilateral or (usually) bilateral sciatica and motor abnormalities, loss of reflexes depend on the root/s involved. Increased reflexes/up going plantars would indicate a cord lesion and effectively exclude a cauda equina lesion.

Loss of anal tone, faecal incontinence, bowel dysfunction, saddle and perineal anaesthesia, widespread weakness. Sexual dysfunction.

This is another area where our newly precious and diffident junior doctors with their personal rights and invasion of privacy agendas as well as their chaperone dependency may well find it impractical to examine the patient conscientiously and adequately. (see the sections on clinical errors due to doctors not examining patients' adequately and failing to notice bruises due to injury, or meningococcal infection). Will junior hospital doctors and GP s always find a chaperone out of hours, in late surgeries, when the nurse has gone home, when doing house calls, etc. so that they can slip off the underwear and test for perineal/buttock anaesthesia?

So: Red Flags:
Severe LBP with bilateral or unilateral sciatica,
bladder or bowel dysfunction,
anaesthesia/parasthesiae in perineal region/buttocks,
significant lower limb weakness,
gait disturbance,
sexual dysfunction.

Other back pain red flags:

Age <20 or >50.

Pain "not mechanical" (ie not movement and posture related, not relieved by position and rest etc).

Thoracic spinal pain.

Past history of steroid treatment, cancer, osteoporosis, HIV.

Systemic symptoms, generally unwell, weight loss, night sweats.

Progressive neurological deficits.

Structural deformity.

Constant/progressive pain.

Inflammatory character (worse after rest, in mornings, hot, red, tender etc).

Severe night pain.

Recent trauma.

Recent research has shown a small percentage of chronic severe low back pain following a disc prolapse is due to bacterial discitis and follows haematogenous implantation of usually "benign" and ubiquitous bacteraemia in an inflamed disc. These patients respond to antibiotics. (3 months of Co Amoxiclav).

Back pain exercises: (see end of section):

Tell the patient to lie on the carpeted floor with knees bent and a small book under the back of the head. Stay relaxed like this for 10 minutes a day.

Ask the patient to do 5-10 of the following exercises a few times (or more) per day:

Knee hugging: Lie on your back, pulling one knee up and then the other. Pull the knees into the chest so you are a ball, hold for 5-10 seconds and relax.

Leg stretches: Lie on your back and lift up one knee pulling with both hands cupped behind the knee. Then straighten the leg and hold for 5-10 seconds. Repeat with the other leg.

Lying on your back, slowly extend the hips, knees at 90 degrees, pushing down on the floor with the heels and with the elbows so that pressure is on the sacrum, then the lumbar spine, then thoracic spine and finally the body's weight is taken by only the heels and occiput. Then slowly lower the weight along the length of the spine again. Try to feel the weight at each separate spinal level.

Roll into a ball on your back with the knees flexed and the arms extended in a jacknife position. Then push down with the arms slowly rolling the body and putting pressure on the lumbar, thoracic, cervical spine and then the occiput. Then slowly down the spine again.

Half push ups: Lie face down on the floor, put your hands palm down on the floor in front of the shoulders and gently push the upper body up keeping the pelvis flat against the floor. Hold for 5-10 seconds and then slowly down again.

Knee rolls (lumbar rotation): Lie on your back with the knees bent. Soles flat on the floor. Gently rotate the knees to one side, push a little further, hold for a few seconds, then to the other side and hold again.

Arching and hollowing: Get on all fours, hands under shoulders, knees under hips. Then arch the back upwards with the head dropped, hold for 5 seconds then arch the lumbar spine down (tummy pushed towards the floor) lifting the head up and sticking the bottom out.

Bent knee sit ups, etc.

Ankylosing Spondylitis:

Schober's Test:

Mark L5, place one finger 5cms below, second finger 10cms above. Patient touches their toes-the gap should increase 5cms. It is less in, for instance, A.S.

The examination:

Stuff you may have forgotten:

Other Dermatomes:

C3 Upper shoulder
C4 Upper deltoid

C5 **Dermatome** lateral upper arm.	**Myotome** shoulder abduction.	**Reflex** biceps
C6 Lateral forearm and thumb.	Elbow flexion, wrist extension	Brachioradialis
C7 Middle and ring finger	Elbow extension, wrist flexion	Triceps
C8 Little finger	Finger flexion	
T1 Medial upper forearm and elbow	Finger abduction	Fingers
T2 Medial upper arm		
L1 Upper ant quads, upper buttock		
L2 Mid section of ant quads, postero-lat quads		
L3 Ant knee, postero-med knee		
L4 Medial calf, anterior shin, medial foot.	**Myotome:** Ankle dorsiflexion.	**Reflex:** Knee
L5 Lat Calf, middle dorsum of foot, great toe	Great toe extension	
S1 Lateral foot, heel, calf.	Knee flexion, eversion of foot.	Ankle jerk,
Little toe	Plantar flexion of foot	

Heel walking tests L5
Walking forwards on tiptoes tests S1,
Supine resisted knee flexion L2/3,
Supine resisted hallux flexion L4,
Supine resisted small toe flexion L5,
Supine resisted foot eversion L5 S1.

Useful Exercises: Diagrams: (My thanks to Arthritis Research UK and Nuffield Hospitals Physiotherapy Departments): (BPE, BPE2, NPE, KPE 1 2 3) (numbered 1>11)

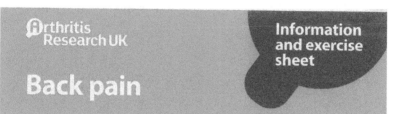

Back pain

Information and exercise sheet

The following exercises should be started gently and increased gradually, and you should not try to push hard to get rid of pain. A little discomfort is common when starting a new activity or exercise, especially if you have not been active for some time, as your joints and muscles get used to working again. Try each exercise in turn and find out how many times you can repeat it without feeling extra discomfort the following day. If you are not sure, try each one 5–10 times to start with. As your back gets used to the new exercise, you should gradually increase the number of times you do the exercise. If you are lucky, you may find a particular exercise eases your pain. If so, you should do more of this exercise and can use it as 'first aid'.

Sometimes you may experience a 'flare-up' or marked increase in pain. This can happen whether you exercise or not. For a couple of days you may be happier reducing the amount you exercise, but try not to stop completely. As the pain eases, try and build back up to the previous level quite quickly.

Exercises

1. Hugging knees to chest

Lying on your back with bent knees, lift one leg and hold on to it with one hand and then lift and hold the other leg. Pull both knees gently closer to your chest, hold for a count of 5, then relax your arms but don't let go completely. Repeat the hug and relax. Some people prefer to hug one knee at a time.

2. Leg stretches

Lying on your back with your knees bent, lift one knee and hold your thigh with both hands behind the knee. Gently straighten the knee that you are holding and hold for a count of 5. Repeat with the opposite leg.

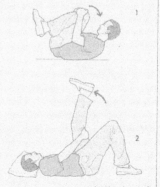

(continued overleaf)

This 'Information and exercise sheet' can be downloaded from the Arthritis Research UK website: **www.arthritisresearchuk.org/infoandexercisesheets**.

First published in Hands On, October 2007. Arthritis Research UK, Copeman House, St Mary's Court, St Mary's Gate, Chesterfield, Derbyshire S41 7TD. www.arthritisresearchuk.org. Registered Charity England and Wales no. 207711, Scotland no. SC041156.

3. Half push-ups

Lie on your front on a firm surface, with your hands under your shoulders, palms down. Look up and push up, lifting your head and shoulders up with your arms. Keep your hips on the floor. Hold for a count of 5 and then gently lower yourself back down. To start with, you may not be able to lift your shoulders far. As you become more flexible, work towards trying to straighten your arms, still keeping your hips on the floor.

4. Knee rolls

Lying on your back with bent knees, let your knees roll to one side, keeping your knees and feet together. Stay to one side for a count of 5 and then roll to the other side.

5. Arching and hollowing

Start on all fours, hands under shoulders, knees under hips. Arch your back upwards, letting your head drop, and hold for a count of 5. Then reverse this posture: lifting your head and looking up, relax your tummy and stick your behind out, holding for a count of 5.

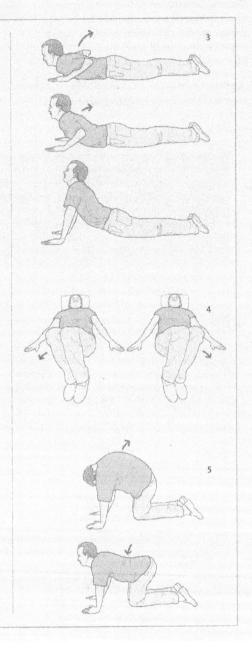

Back Exercises:(BPE BPE2)

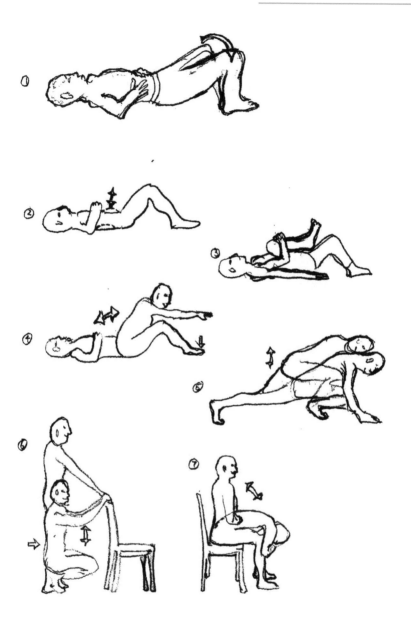

Back Pain Exercises:

1. Lie on back, hands on hips, knees bent, feet on floor. Rotate knees from one side to the other as far as they will go giving them an extra "Tweek" at the extreme end of range.

2. Lie on back, hands folded across chest, knees bent. Press the small of the back into the ground then arch the abdomen upwards holding each position for several seconds.

3. Lie on back, legs outstretched then pull the knees up to the chest holding them in position for several seconds. Then repeat using one leg at a time.

4. Lie on back, knees bent, feet tucked under the end of a bed or edge of a sofa. Perform bent knee sit ups 10-20 X.

5. Begin in a runners position, one leg extended backwards, one leg bent underneath, hands extended down onto the floor. Press down and forward several times, flexing the knee and pushing down onto the thigh. Reverse position with legs.

6. Stand holding the back of a chair, then squat on bent knees ensure the lumbar spine is arched forward. Stand and repeat.

7. Sitting on a firm chair, bend forward with chin between knees. Then slowly extend back to sitting position. Tense the abdomen all the time.

Quadriceps and knee exercises: (KPE)

Exercises
To be performed 2 to 3 times a day

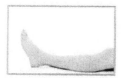

1. Ankle exercises (circling and pumping)

- Every hour pull your toes up as far as you can and point them down fully.
- Repeat for 1 minute

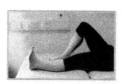

2. Static 'quads'

- Pull your toes up towards you
- Push you knee out as straight as it will go by tightening your thigh muscles (your 'quads')
- Hold for 3-5 seconds
- Repeat 5-10 times

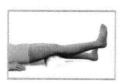

3. 'Inner range Quads'

- Place a rolled towel or blanket under the knee
- Pull your toes up towards you
  Push your knee straight levering against the towel/blanket to lift your foot off the bed.
- Hold for 3-5 seconds
- Repeat 5- 10 times

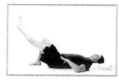

4. Straight leg raise

- Lying on your back
- Pull your toes up and lock the knee out straight.
- Keeping it straight lift the foot off the bed.
- Lift to about 20 cm (8 inches) and hold
- Hold for 3-5 seconds, and then slowly lower
- Repeat 5- 10 times

Strengthen the inner quads muscles

Repeat the exercise above with the foot turned out to make the muscles on the inner side of the thigh work harder. This may help with knee cap pain.

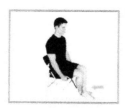

5. Knee flexion in sitting

- Sitting on a chair or bed
- Bend your knee as much as possible and place the heel of the good leg in front of the ankle of the operated leg. Gently ease back to bend the knee a little more and hold for 5 seconds
- Repeat 5 - 10 times

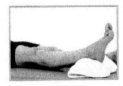

6. Passive knee extension

- Place a rolled towel under your heel.
- Allow your knee to hang out as straight as possible
- Sustain this position for up to 30 minutes if possible, occasionally taking your heel off the towel and bending it gently to stop it getting too stiff.

NB

A knee which will fully straighten is a more stable knee and will not hurt so much when you stand and walk. Over time you may have developed a habit of standing and walking with your knee bent, it is a good idea to break this habit and regain a knee which will fully straighten. If you are waiting for surgery to your knee your post operative recovery will be much quicker and less painful and you will also be more likely to achieve a better end result if you can achieve full extension before your operation.

Straight leg raising exercises:

'Oven glove' with cans of food or
Hand bag with bricks

Neck exercises (NE)

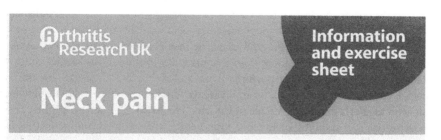

Ⓐrthritis Research UK

Information and exercise sheet

Neck pain

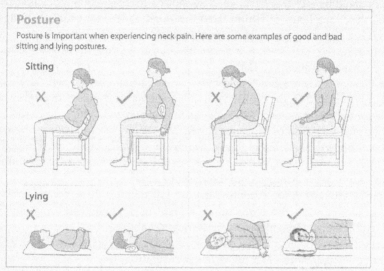

Posture

Posture is important when experiencing neck pain. Here are some examples of good and bad sitting and lying postures.

Sitting

Lying

Exercises

The exercises overleaf should be started gently and increased gradually, and you should not try to push hard to get rid of pain. A little discomfort is common when starting a new activity or exercise, especially if you have not been active for some time, as your joints and muscles get used to working again. Try each exercise in turn and find out how many times you can repeat it without feeling extra discomfort for the following day. If you are not sure, try each one 5–10 times to start with. As your neck gets used to the new exercise, you should gradually increase the number of times you do the exercise. You may find a particular exercise eases your pain. If so, you should do more of this exercise and use it as a 'first aid'.

Some aches or discomfort with exercise are normal and should be expected. However if an exercise makes your symptoms significantly worse, or you experience other symptoms such as dizziness, seek advice before continuing.

Sometimes you may experience a 'flare up' or marked increase in pain. This can happen whether you exercise or not. For a couple of days you may be happier reducing the amount you exercise, but try not to stop completely. As the pain eases, try and build back up to the previous level as soon as you can.

(continued overleaf)

Sitting:

While we are on the subject of posture, nature did not originally design us to be bipeds, to stand still for long periods, to ride a bike or to sit on a chair. We were hunter gatherers, always moving for most of our evolution, highly mobile apes before that and quadruped mammals before that. We were used to being constantly on the move and certainly not resting our weight on our Ischial tuberosities or standing still for hours on end. Prolonged sitting is associated with a 24% higher mortality from virtually all causes – and you don't just have to be in economy class on a plane or in a coach to suffer the consequences. Sitting "too long" is said to be more than 8 hours a day in the various studies concerning morbidity and complications of posture. These include various cancers – breast, colon, colorectal, endometrial and ovarian, cardiovascular disease and Type 2 DM, even among people who regularly exercise. (Annals of Int Med Jan 20 2015). Exercise **slightly** reduces the relative risk and standing or moving, even gently while at work mitigates the risk of sitting or standing still too. Meta analysis showed that those who exercised the least in between their long bouts of sitting fared the worst. Indeed all you have to do is get up from the sitting position and stand every half an hour to improve post prandial glucose metabolism just as effectively as a 5 minute bout of walking (in overweight postmeno-pausal prediabetic women). (2016)

But changing posture and "being busy" at work is not exercise and the British Heart Foundation in a 2017 report declared that 20m Britons were underactive. Women are 36% more likely to be underactive than men- 11.8m women and 8.3m men in the UK failing the Government guidelines which are currently 150 minutes of moderate physical activity a week and strength activities on at least two days a week. The laziest areas were the NW of England, Northern Ireland, Wales and the North East. The most active regions the South East, the South West, Scotland and the East of England.

Exercise Guidelines are currently at least 150 minutes of moderate aerobic activity (walking fast, mowing the lawn, riding a bike) or 75 minutes of vigorous activity a week,(aerobic activity, jogging, football, cycling fast etc).

Strength exercises on at least 2 days a week, (digging, gardening, yoga (?), weights etc).

Break up long periods of sitting with light activity.

Polymyalgia: P.M.R./(Giant Cell Arteritis):

Pain and stiffness worse in the morning. Affecting the neck, shoulders and hips. Inflammatory markers are up and there is often: Anaemia of inflammation, PMR with a normal ESR is possible but CRP is usually up. Weight loss, fever, synovitis are some-times present in PMR but they can also indicate a secondary reaction to malignancy, deep seated infection, (endocarditis/osteomyelitis) or inflammatory arthritides (RhA, spondy-loarthropathy, crystal arthropathy).

As long as there are no:

Severe headaches, scalp tenderness, jaw claudication, visual symptoms,

which might suggest **Giant Cell Arteritis** (ie Cranial or Temporal Arteritis). The HLA DRB1*04 allele is often positive in GCA but not PMR. But these are two condi-tions that "overlap" in a small number of cases.

PMR: Start steroids: Prednisolone 15mg daily and reassess in 2 weeks. Reduce to 10mg quickly then by 1mg every 4-6 weeks to 5mg then off steroids in 6-9m. Failure to respond in a few days should make you think about the other diagnoses. **If GCA intervenes, the treatment is much higher dose steroids**, to avoid blindness, started immediately, typically 60mg for 2-4 weeks, depending on the response. Then 40mg/day for 4-6 weeks, then a slow reduction to 5-10mg/day for up to 2 years monitoring the ESR and clinical response.

Start osteoporosis prophylaxis soon.

Fibromyalgia:

Affects 1-2% of the population according to some sources. That's 23 to 46 on my list which I find pretty hard to believe. I would have thought I only had a handful unless they were all keeping it to themselves or the definition was unhelpfully broad.

The definition actually is widespread pain of over 3 months duration affecting the axial skeleton and at least two contralateral quadrants of the body. This in itself would cover all sorts of unpleasant diseases which aren't Fibromyalgia – multiple secondary cancer, dermatomyositis, purulent skin infections, psychological conditions, rheumatoid and other forms of generalised joint and connective tissue diseases and so on. But in addition there have to be painful "trigger points" (11 of 18 of them) when they are pushed hard enough (or gently enough) to blanch a finger nail (-which **IS** quite gently).

Clearly the perception and the assessment of trigger point pain is highly subjective and as you treat more and more patients with fibromyalgia you do begin to wonder whether it is a separate condition at all or a convenient way of describing a chronically depressed and anxious group of mainly female patients who somatise their unhappiness in a particular way. It does have some common factors with I.B.S. and C.F.S. – particularly the patient type.

Not surprisingly, antidepressants help (improving fatigue, sleep, well being **and** pain – but not trigger point tenderness). I suspect the parallels with CFS, IBS, even with the scalp and neck tenderness of chronic migraine sufferers and other conditions is obvious. – Antidepressants relieving pain syndromes which may be the various specific physical ways that depression expresses itself. The trigger point sensitivity is of course subjective as is the tiredness in CFS and the abdominal pain in IBS. There is no objective way of measuring them. Fibromyalgia is defined by the number of trigger points but made better overall by drugs that do not reduce the trigger point sensitivity but instead treat depression.

From the practical GP's point of view the main issue is what makes the patient better – not the unwinnable discussion about what is the cause of the condition.

Hip conditions:

Usual ages at presentation:
CDH: 0-5 years
Perthē's: 5-10 yrs
SUFE: 10-15 yrs.

The "C Sign" – cupping of the hand over the hip joint from the side, is a classic indication of deep hip pathology. Hip joint pain itself though is usually referred to the groin, anteriorly, not laterally. Lateral hip pain (over the trochanter) is coming from the trochanter itself (bursitis), SIJ or the L/S etc.

Groin pain can come from the hip joint, the muscles around the joint, L5 S1 root, hernia, vascular or gynaecological causes.

Orthopaedic surgeons will tell you the commonest three causes of hip pain in GP are:

1) Trochanteric burstitis (can follow a contralateral back or knee problem-presumably putting excess strain on the opposite hip). The main treatment is directed at the cause and is physiotherapy.

I find deep injections of steroid the only practical and effective treatment but most orthopaedic surgeons say that these often fail and management must be physio.

Some orthopaedic surgeons say Trochanteric Bursitis as GPs understand it does not exist. This just seems to be another example of how we GPs see and treat a different type and spectrum of patient and disease to consultants and that not all secondary care wisdom is relevant to us. Don't you often sit in lectures, particularly by registrars and newly qualified consultants about bread and butter GP stuff and wonder what do they think they are talking about -And why isn't a year in GP a compulsory part of all specialist training?

2) Gluteus medius tear. This affects the elderly who are unable to abduct the hip lying on their side. The onset is with a sudden lateral hip pain and limp after a trip. The pain but not the limp then settles down. The Gluteus medius is a pelvic stabiliser and its damage causes a Trendellenberg gait, needing early repair. (So refer soon, at least within 6 weeks.)

(Note: **Trendellenberg sign**: Is positive when the hip abductors (Gluteus medius and minimus) are weak or paralysed or when the leg the patient is standing on causes pain (hip joint). This results in the unsupported side of the pelvis dropping. The hip supporting the weight is the affected hip.)

3) External Snapping Hip. Usually the Ileo-tibial band from the tibia to the iliac crest, young women 12-30 years. There is a loud snapping over the hip on rotating the leg with a hand on the trochanter. The treatment is physio. Tensor Fascia Lata stretches. Surgery leaves a big scar.

Hip Replacement:

Metal on metal:

The first (1938) hip replacement was metal on metal. The Common Ring and McKee replacements in the 1960's were metal on metal. Then Charnley invented the metal/poly-thene hip but the acetabulum tended to wear for younger patients who put a great deal of stress on their joints and metal on metal hip resurfacing was developed. With some resur-faced hips ARMS (adverse reaction to metal syndrome) started to occur so now the ASR, the anatomic surface replacement has been abandoned. The basic problem is that with some chromium alloys in metal on metal hip replacements and resurfaced joints there is excess release of local metallic ions. These cause soft tissue and bone necrosis. There is now tougher polypropylene as well as ceramic material for the socket and these are supposed to solve the problem.

Chromium

Normal   <134nmol/li
(Metal on metal joint replacements)

Cobalt

Normal   <119nmol/li
(measure both if concerned about metal on metal joint replacements).

Gilmore's Groin:

A tear of the external oblique aponeurosis where it inserts in the pubis. Common in footballers. The pain is on movement, in the groin and positional. There is a palpable widening of the external inguinal ring on the affected side, no hernia, but pain in the area on coughing, sneezing and squeezing the legs together. Core stability exercises, physio-therapy and surgical repair of the torn aponeurosis are the treatments.

Sports and Sports Injuries

New research (2017) suggests that exercise rates spontaneously diminish from the age of 7 years onwards, not from the mid teens, which is where government and educational "An hour a day" fitness schemes had been targeted. So human beings try to conserve energy as soon as they acquire any independence. Regular exercise has a multitude of health benefits: Amongst its benefits are:

Prolonging average life span, reducing cardiovascular disease, blood pressure, normalising abnormal lipid and glucose levels, reducing stroke risk, T2DM, Metabolic Syndrome, as well as the incidence and recurrence rate of a number of cancers, notably colon, breast and lung. Exercise is about the **only thing** that reduces recurrence in smoking related lung cancer.

Obviously it improves cardiovascular and respiratory function and "fitness", it controls weight, reduces stress, depression, anxiety, and improves or helps maintain cognitive function. It is supposed to delay cognitive decline and dementia. It stimulates normal bowel function, increases bone density and improves sleep quality.

Certain forms of exercise are better at some of these "gains" than others and some exercise is more traumatic than others too. High impact sports, Rugby, Tennis, Track and Field, Skiing all lead to joint injuries both acute and chronic. Indeed one British insurance company estimates that the average holiday skier has a 20% risk of a significant injury and a 5% risk of hospitalisation during a two week annual stay.

Stretching:

Despite the standard advice to stretch before and after exercise and the time spent religiously doing stretches after Body-Pump, "Circuits" and Legs Bums and Tums, there is no actual proof that muscle stretching has any effect at all on injury, performance (except a negative effect on muscle strength in power sports like weight lifting), recovery time, the PEMS (post exercise muscle soreness) or the DOMS (delayed onset muscle soreness) that we all suffer the day after.

The most effective anti injury regimes include strength training which reduces sports injuries to a third and overuse injuries to a half.

Tennis elbow, lateral epicondylitis

This is one of the commonest and most frustrating musculoskeletal conditions that GPs see. It is persistent lateral elbow pain made worse by clenching the fist or forcibly extending the elbow. It is a repetitive strain syndrome caused by repeated grasping with the elbow extended and forearm pronated or medial and lateral flexion of the wrist, or pronation and supination of the forearm as in back-hand at tennis, using a hammer, paint brush, gripping the neck of a guitar and so on. A particularly troublesome and persistent condition for which almost nothing often seems to help except rest and time. This is, it has to be said, poorly understood and very frustrating to treat with any of the 40 different treatment modalities available. Up to 10% of patients eventually require surgery. The pain comes from the common extensor origin on the lateral epicondyle of the elbow.

The extensor carpi radialis brevis (O: Lateral epicondlye I: to the base of the 3rd metacarpal – extends and abducts the hand at the wrist joint) is particularly vulnerable to shearing stresses during all wrist movements. It is this muscle that is the main site for pathological changes in L.E although a number of other wrist muscles' attachment sites have been implicated. A cortisone injection into the painful area can reduce the pain though sometimes only temporarily and surgically transecting the muscle may be necessary. There is no association with the dominant hand (it is often the guitar fretting hand for instance in which the wrist is cocked in an awkward position and the elbow of which suffers rather than the plectrum hand).

Signs and symptoms:

Lateral epicondylar tenderness and pain, pain on resisted wrist extension, painful resisted extension of the index finger, painful resisted forearm supination. Mill's test, – this is resisted wrist extension with the palm pronated while moving the hand sideways in the direction of the thumb-the pain is exacerbated. Or Maudsley's test – resisted 3rd digit extension (this is one of the most reliable tests) or Cozen's Test, resisted wrist extension with radial deviation and full pronation.

Of the many forms of physiotherapy which have been used, progressive muscle stretching (repeated medial flexion of the wrist with the forearm in the anatomical position) strengthening exercises and deep transverse friction over the muscle MAY help. So may repeated forced extension exercises of the fingers (splaying open the fingers with the hands stretched forwards, counter intuitively) and acupuncture. The lateral glide pressure technique over the painful area while the patient is holding a painful posture is another physiotherapy mainstay.(Get the patient to extend their forearm and wrist and massage the painful area laterally repeatedly with their own finger tips). Ultrasound, heat and massage almost certainly do not help a great deal.

In the differential diagnoses are radial tunnel syndrome and posterior interosseous syndrome. Several procedures may be unwittingly decompressing the PIN and thus relieving pain. Interestingly some studies associate tennis elbow with lower cervical spine hypomobility and improvement of symptoms with treatment to the neck (C56) so if they can afford it advise the patient to see an osteopath too.

Pulled elbow in a child:

Reduce by pushing the gripped forearm back toward the elbow and pronating. You should hear and feel the click. This is another trick, like shoulder and finger reduction and reducing dislocated patellae that **ALL GPs** should learn and be competent at.

Quadriceps exercises: Chondromalacia etc.

The theory is this: In some people the patella tracks to the outside (laterally) when the knee is extended due to an over activity of the lateral quads and a relative weakness of the vastus medialis. Thus there is "maltracking", possibly due to a shallow intercon-dylar groove and asymmetrical wear of the patellar articular cartilage, (worse on the lateral facet between the upper lateral surface of the patella and the lateral intercondlar articular cartilage). There are lateral knee pain, grating on standing and stiffness if the knee is held semi flexed for any length of time (i.e. driving). There is pain on taking weight on a flexed knee joint (going downstairs or walking down hill) and the joint grates, clicks, and can give way. It can sometimes feel mildly locked and therefore can be confused with a torn semi-lunar cartilage. It can be common in both the sporty (wear and damage to the cartilage) as well as the lazy (tall and thin with weedy thigh muscles). When acute, there can be an effusion and don't forget chondromalacia and retropatellar wear can coexist with other knee pathologies.

Testing for patellar pathology includes the patellar grind test (Clarke's sign). The patient is on his back, knee straight, you push down on the upper patella (upper pole in the thumb/first finger gap) while the patient contracts the quads. Grating and or pain is a positive sign and indicates retropatellar pathology.

The remedy (It slowly improves with age in teenagers) is to rebalance the knee (If you believe this theory) by building up the medial quads.

The Vastus medialis tends to come into its own towards the end of knee extension, (the Vastus lateralis is supposed to initiate extension) so in "Quads exercises" you need to preferentially build up the medial thigh muscles. This is done by using the muscles in extension (exercises extending the knee through the last 20 degrees – with weights on the ankle), straight leg raising with weights, tensing the quads with the leg straight, pushing the straightened leg down against a rolled up towel while sitting with the legs out straight on the floor, stepping up and down using the affected leg, on a book about 2-3" tall and: my osteopath tells me, straight leg raises with weights and the hip rotated slightly externally.

You could also tell the patient any movement or exercise that incompletely extends the knee without full extension will make it worse. When **cycling** the knee must be fully or nearly fully straightened on the down stroke-in other words the saddle must be as high as the rider can manage.

While we are on the subject of cycling, not only does the knee have to be almost fully extended on the downstroke but remember to adjust the saddle fore/aft position using a plumb line from the knee to the peddle spindle. This will get you the most efficient power transfer.

Other knee strengthening exercises include: Sitting on a firm chair, bend one knee, tucking the shin behind the calf of the other leg. Then push the posterior shin forwards, resisting the movement by pulling the anterior calf backwards. Push hard but keep both legs still and do this for 5 seconds several times. Sit in a firm chair and slowly stand up and then slowly down. Repeat several times and over a period of time, use smaller chairs. Step up and slowly down using one leg on the bottom stair, gradually increasing the height of the stair over a few weeks. Hold the back of a chair and slowly bend the knees and then straighten them while looking forwards over the chair. Gradually go lower but never squat right down. Wrap a bike inner tube or other elastic loop around your ankle and also around the corresponding chair leg you are sitting on. Then extend the knee and slowly relax it back to the starting position.

Hamstrings: lie on your back arching your lumbar spine and pelvis upwards but tilting the lower pubis downwards towards the floor, pulling your feet in towards your buttocks and holding this posture for 5-10 seconds. This can be improved by resting the feet on a Physiotherapy roll or rolling pin and sliding the feet forwards and backwards. This is hard work.

Torn knee cartilage:

Classically this takes place when a flexed knee is twisted as in a running turn, football tackle, a forced rotation at the knee playing high impact sports or a rotation of the joint while squatting etc. The usual history is of a painful click or catch felt in the lateral knee or popliteal fossa which causes the knee to give way, swell up and is sometimes associated with other damage, for instance a torn cruciate or lateral collateral ligament. Later the classic locking, clicking, giving way and swelling after some exercise can all start.

The signs are of joint line tenderness, a positive MacMurrays test, (Flexing the knee to 90 degrees and rotating the tibia a few degrees while grasping the foot.) There is a click very commonly when you do this test but in a torn cartilage, you can feel the posterior condyle "clonk" over the trailing edge of the meniscus and it can hurt. The menisci are often ragged at arthroscopy even in people without symptoms but a good tear (either bucket handle or parrot beak) can be trimmed and this usually resolves the symptoms. In the 1950's and 1960's the standard procedure was to take out the whole meniscus and this led moderately quickly to articular cartilage wear and osteo-arthritis in some famous footballers.

Ileotibial Band Syndrome:

A running injury, the ileotibial band is the extension of the tensor fascia lata that runs down the lateral side of the thigh inserting below the knee. It flexes, abducts and internally rotates the hip and stabilises the lateral border of the knee – sliding forwards and backwards on extension and flexion. It is an overuse syndrome, commoner in the bow legged.

Pain is over the lateral knee and lower lateral thigh.

Initial treatment is **RICER (Rest Ice Compression Elevation and Referral**), massage (including the gluteals.)

Pre exercise muscle stretches (Lateral bending, stretching the outer hip or crossing the legs and leaning towards the posterior foot and holding the posture for 30 seconds) as well as static quads exercises help. It is one of the few, if any situations where stretching before exercising achieves anything beneficial. Also, avoiding sudden sharp increases in running or cycling distances helps avoid this and most sports related injuries.

Anterior cruciate ligament:

A tear can be detected using the Lachman test. The knee is extended, just short of full extension then the examiner stabilises the thigh while pulling the tibia forward (upward). The movement should be relatively slight and a torn ACL allows a more extensive movement.

The anterior draw test is basically similar but the patient is lying supine and the knee bent to 90 degrees. Then the tibia is pulled anteriorly and the degree of movement again reflects the laxity (degree of damage) of the ACL.

Pronation problems and running:

Under pronation on running:

The outsides of each foot are the first point of contact. The ankle doesn't roll inward the normal 15% on taking the weight. This is commoner in runners with high arches you can see this from the lateral wear pattern on the shoes. **Pushing off is disproportionately done with the lateral toes.** Extra cushioning in "neutral" running shoes with more padding reduces possible lower leg injury.

Over/hyper pronation: Again, the lateral part of the heel makes the first contact on landing and taking the runner's weight and then the ankle rolls inward **more than 15%.** The arch tends to collapse on taking the impact. Finally on pushing off the **body's weight is on the inside of the foot** and the great and second toes do all the work. This causes less efficient shock absorbing and more likelihood of leg, knee and ankle injury. Pronation insoles distribute both the impact and pushing off pressures more equally. Typical secondary injuries include shin splints, Achilles Tendonitis, plantar fasciitis, metatarsalgia and knee pain. etc. The heel and front medial sole of running shoes are worn.

Knock kneed and flat footed patients tend to over pronate.

In the normal cycle the anterior foot is **flat** to the ground on pushing off.

Barefoot running:

Is becoming more popular here and in the USA.

There are significant differences in the way shoes make us walk and run compared with bare feet. After all, we evolved to do both bare foot. Shod runners strike the ground heel first but as you will soon find out if you start running bare foot you feel more comfortable if you make first contact with the forefoot to cushion the impact of landing. Shoes encourage heel first landing when legs are stiff. 6-8% of the body mass comes to an instant dead stop in that initial heel strike for a brief moment. In contrast, when the forefoot strikes, the ankle and mid foot cushion the impact and only 1.5% of the body's mass comes to a dead stop. Heel strikers will therefore suffer more traumatic hip, knee, back and tibial pain.

Shin splints: (Medial Tibial Stress Syndrome):

Made worse by excess subtalar pronation, high impact running, tight calf muscles. Pain is in the posterio-medial 2/3 of the tibia. It can lead to stress fractures of the tibia. Overpronation, external rotation of the foot on running and flat feet are risk factors. It needs to be differentiated from stress fracture and Anterior Compartment Syndrome. Rest, orthotics, physio, stretching and strengthening exercises (Tibialis Anterior) and anti inflammatories are the treatments. The last ditch surgical treatment is posterior fasciotomy.

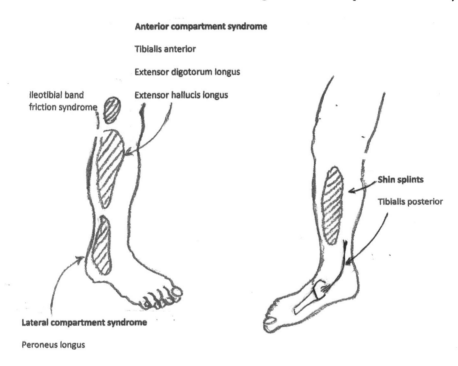

Diagram of Anterior Compartment Syndrome

Achilles Tendonitis:

The lesion is usually at mid tendon, all sides except the posterior surface can be affected. Massage and injection help, the latter is often temporary.

Haglund Deformity:

"Pump Bump", posterior heel bursitis common in women with a swollen lump over the posterior heel prominence. An underlying calcaneal exostosis forms with a bursitis on top. The usual treatments are applied followed by excision of the extra bone if necessary.

SHOULDER INJECTIONS

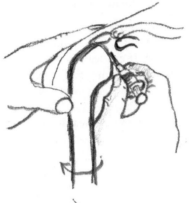

ANTERIOR

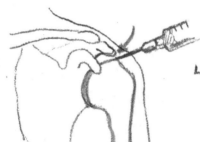

LATERAL

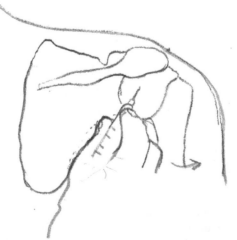

POSTERIOR

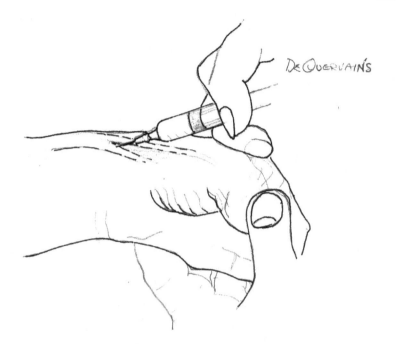

De Quervain's

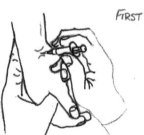

First Carpometacarpal Joint

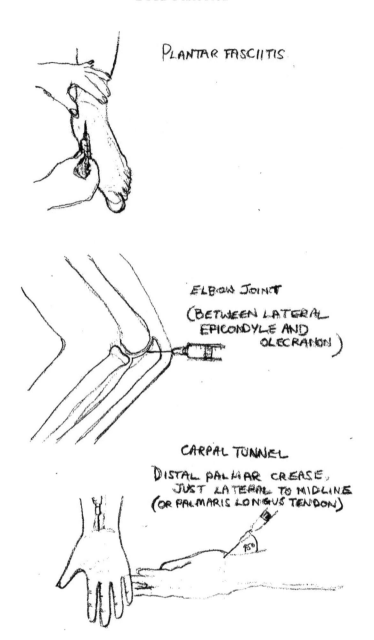

PLANTAR FASCIITIS

ELBOW JOINT

(BETWEEN LATERAL
EPICONDYLE AND
OLECRANON)

CARPAL TUNNEL

DISTAL PALMAR CREASE,
JUST LATERAL TO MIDLINE
(OR PALMARIS LONGUS TENDON)

95°

Diagram of shoulder, elbow, steroid, heel, wrist, knee, hip steroid injection techniques
(JI 1.2.3.4.). Flex wrist and oppose little finger against thumb to show the Palmaris
Longus Tendon (present in 85% of patients). Inject at distal wrist crease on ulnar side of
Palmaris Tendon.

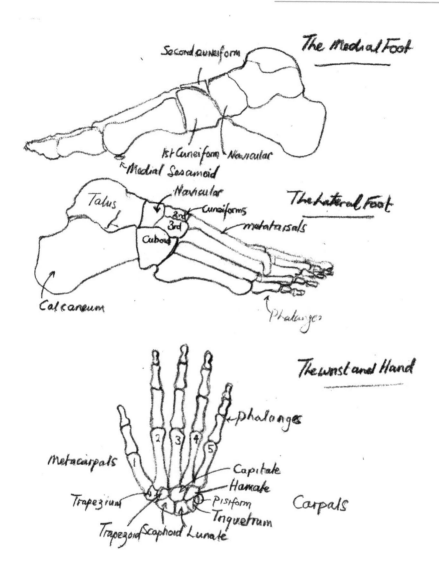

The Medial Foot

Second cuneiform

1st Cuneiform Navicular
Medial Sesamoid

Talus

Navicular
Cuneiforms

The Lateral Foot

metatarsals

2nd
3rd
Cuboid

Calcaneum

Phalanges

The wrist and Hand

phalanges

2 3 4 5

Metacarpals

Capitate
Hamate
Pisiform
Triquetrum

Carpals

Trapezium

Trapezoid Scaphoid Lunate

Diagram of bones of foot and hand (BFH1)

Feet:

Ingrowing toenail:

This is said to be caused by cutting rounded toenail corners which encourage concavity of the nail for some reason, a digging in at the edges and subsequent infections. Certainly in the long run you should encourage the counterintuitive sharp 90 degree corner nail paring and letting the nail grow a good couple of mms. proud of the skin. Also I read recently that careful scoring to thin the nail lengthwise down the centre of the convex surface reduces the flex and the tendency to dig in at the edges, allowing them to recover.

Toe Nails for patients:

A well cut toenail protrudes and is counter intuitively cut at right angles. If it is sculpted with a curve it becomes concave and ingrowing.

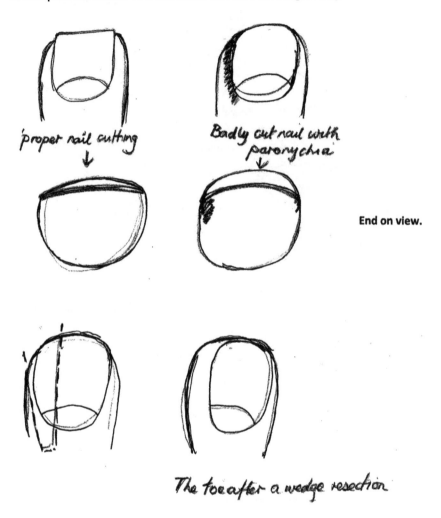

proper nail cutting ↓

Badly cut nail with paronychia ↓

End on view.

The toe after a wedge resection.

Zadek's procedure removes a wedge of nail and subcutaneous tissue down to the periosteum which is then phenolised. The removed nail does not grow back.

Diagram (TN1)

Hallux Valgus:

(Bunion) The toe is laterally deviated at the 1st toe MTP joint with the medial deformity causing pain, rubbing and increasing problems with getting shoes that will fit. Once it starts, it gets progressively worse. Pads and plasters as well as loose footwear help initially but when finding shoes to fit becomes impossible and foot symptoms affect mobility, some form of osteotomy, – straightening the first toe, is performed.

Typically these days this is a Scarf osteotomy where the metatarsal is cut, an Akin osteotomy where the proximal phalanx is cut and straightened, or a Lapidus procedure where there is a fusion of the first TMT joint with a distal soft tissue correction. This latter is done when there is a severe flat foot or a hyper mobile first ray.

Assessment is by standing X Ray (this shows the proper extent of the deviation).

Hallux Rigidus:

Is OA of the first MTP joint. Dorsiflexion, particularly, is painful and the joint is stiff, sometimes cracking. Temporary benefit arises from injecting the joint, removing the osteophytes but eventually the joint will probably have to be fused as it may be "rigid" but it hurts because it isn't rigid enough.

Forefoot pain:

Consider: Inflammatory arthropathy, **Metatarsal stress fracture** (often the second metatarsal shaft or neck but the X Ray may not be abnormal for 2 weeks).

Osteoarthritis of the second MTPJ is common in men and responds to injections, or debriding the joint. It presents with walking forefoot pain and tenderness on the dorsum of the joint on examination.

Metatarsalgia:

This is a generic term for plantar forefoot pain and it can be due to a number of causes. High heeled shoes, a high arched foot or long metatarsals, sesamoid pain, hammer toes, a tight Achilles, Hallux Valgus, excessive forefoot strike due to short calf muscles, pes cavus, weak flexors and so on. More often it is due to high impact exercise or injury.

Insoles and orthotics do help and sometimes steroid injections relieve specific areas of pain.

One of the common fore foot pains is from a benign fibrous swelling of the digital nerve where it is nipped between the heads of the 4th and 5th metatarsals (-or sometimes nerve 3/4 is affected) – a **Morton's Neuroma**. F10:M1, 30-60yrs usually, causing sudden sharp pains and tingling between the toes. In this the "Squeeze test" is painful but in my experience it nearly always is if you squeeze the forefoot hard enough in anyone.

When a patient presents with chronic pain and tenderness over the metatarsal pads in metatarsalgia or any foot pain, examine the running shoes (if they are a sports person) to make sure that the soles are still viable as a useful first step. Look at their normal shoes to see the tread wear. Then look at the naked foot with the patient standing and walking, then examine the feet, ankles and calves. Treatment options include prescribing arch and forefoot orthoses and exercises also help. Forefoot pads, or stiffeners, calf strengthening and injection to the painful metatarsal or between the metatarsals around the neuroma if present help too. Sometimes excision of the "neuroma" or ablation with various local injections is necessary.

Time and time again I have had friends, ex patients, family members, just people at parties and sometimes private patients come to me and relate totally *believable* stories about foot, heel or ankle consultations they have had with their GPs. They give a brief history to the doctor, the GP gives an erroneous standard diagnosis, refers them to an NHS information or exercise web site and sends them away. The GP, as is so often the case is glued to their seat and seems to know only two feet diagnoses. I ask if the GP got them to remove their socks or shoes and I get a puzzled look and a negative reply.

I mentioned this depressing fact to a foot and ankle orthopaedic surgeon and he confirmed that less than half of the referrals from GPs today include any examination information anymore.

When you look at the naked foot of the patient, get them to walk and stand on tip toe, squeeze the fore foot and Achilles tendon with them lying down and half the time, look at the huge verruca. Then the correct diagnosis may be obvious and has only taken 2 minutes more. Why are so many of my colleagues so lazy? Boredom? Lack of self respect, depression, their mind on their family or something else?

Advice and Exercises for patients with metatarsalgia:

Use square toed running shoes, (which do not squeeze the forefoot) not tapered shoes, elevate the feet after exercise, (+/– ice). Make sure mid soles have not exceeded 300 miles and increase the mileage or intensity of exercise slowly. Avoid higher heels in all shoes which increase forefoot pressure. Try forefoot/arch orthoses.

Achilles tendon stretches, (toes on a step, let the heels drop down) until uncomfortable then contract the calf muscles. Repeat several times.

Passive ankle stretches while sitting cross legged, flexion, extension and inversion planes, using the opposite hand and holding the affected ankle in the uncomfortable position for 10-15 seconds, then repeating the stretch several times.

Toe curls: stand feet apart – a hip's width and walk slowly, gripping the floor with the toes curled at each step. The patient should "pull themselves across the floor 6-10 feet distance grasping the floor with their feet at each step. Gradually increase the distance.

Hop downhill on a gentle slope (3%) 20 yards, looking straight ahead, do this carefully as it has the potential to put quite a strain on the forefoot rather than building it up. Then swap the foot and repeat.

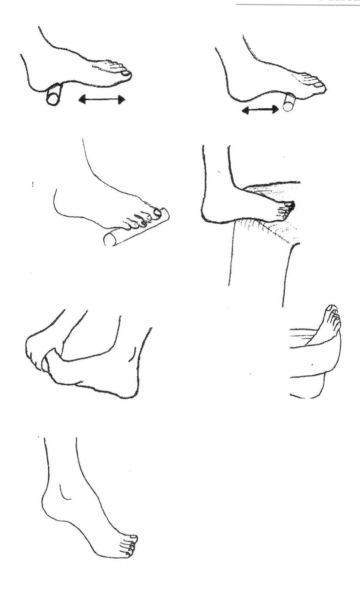

Foot Exercises: For Plantar Fasciitis, metatarsalgia etc.
Roll hard cylinder (broomstick etc) under heel and metatarsal area
Grip same tube /cylinder and hold for 10 seconds with toes
Stand with front of foot on edge of stair, lifting weight 10 X
Do heel toe exercises with both feet/ single foot
Stretch calf and deep sole muscles by pulling foot/toes upward and holding for
10 seconds

Foot exercises Diagram FE1

Sesamoiditis of the small bone under the metatarsal of the great toe can cause metatarsalgia of the first toe and is a traumatic or running injury. There is local pressure sensitivity and aching. Again, insoles (orthoses) and injections of steroids can help, sometimes excision of the Sesamoid bone itself. I went through 35 years of medicine without knowing Sesamoid bones in the feet existed.

Sesamoiditis presents with pain under the ball of the foot in patients who run or have high impact activities and high arched feet or thin padding on their forefeet. They have local marked tenderness under the metatarsals especially No 1. Pads, rest and steroid injections are the common treatments.

Plantar fasciitis:

Also called Policeman's or Shop Assistant's heel: The pain is under the Calcaneus and thought to be due to inflammation at the insertion of the longitudinal plantar ligament (which gives the foot shock absorbing and impact resilience). Some patients are flat footed.

The pain can be severe the first time the patient puts his foot on the floor in the morning and can be brought on by standing on a hard floor for long periods, by landing heavily after jumping – or even stamping when a curb etc is missed or by hard non cushioning footwear (eg safety shoes).

The heel hurts when squeezed from the sides or pushed hard with the thumb just anterior to the heel pad. 50% patients have a spur on X Ray but only 5% patients with a heel spur experience heel pain. Wearing trainers, using arch supports and padded insoles all help. Exercises can sometimes help:

Achilles tendon stretch (sitting on the floor, legs out straight, putting a towel under the toes and pulling up for 30-60 seconds, 3X on each side.

Wall push ups ie stretching the Achilles Tendon (extending the affected leg backwards while leaning forwards against a wall and "feeling the Achilles really pull") with the front knee bent. Do this 10X for about 20 seconds.

Stair stretches, with the front of the feet supported on the edge of a low stair, let the heels drop, pulling on the calf muscles. (Hold the hand rail to stop falling).

Dynamic plantar fascia stretches: Roll the arch of the foot over a cylindrical object, a rolling pin or a tin of beans. Allow the foot and ankle to move in all directions while rolling the cylinder forwards and backwards.

95% patients settle in 2 years conservatively. The surgery involves release of some plantar fascia and some nerve.

Most patients will opt for an injection (the lateral approach is the most humane) of steroid by their GP. It hurts but it nearly always helps. All GPs should be good at this.

Adult onset flat foot:

This is, I have to admit, a condition I had never heard of until I was reading up foot conditions for this book. It affects middle aged women and is all due to the degeneration and rupture of the Tibialis Posterior tendon. The Tibialis Posterior muscle originates in the calf, being attached to the posterior tibia, the tendon crossing under the medial malleolus and splitting, at the underside of the sole of the foot and inserting into the Navicular and the Cuneiform bones. It inverts the foot, maintains the arch and assists in toe standing.

It starts with inflammation of the tendon, medial malleolar pain, then the arch falls and the heel moves laterally. At this point the pain is in the lateral ankle. The patient cannot invert or tip toe. Then the tendon ruptures and subtalar arthritis develops.

The treatment depends on the stage and ranges from injection of the tendon sheath to rerouting a tendon, dividing the calcaneum or fusing the subtalar joint.

Is this cancer?

There are various things that patients come to the doctor about in distress, thinking the worst but having just discovered their own variant of a normal anatomy. The lumpy epididymis is one and the Xiphisternum is another.

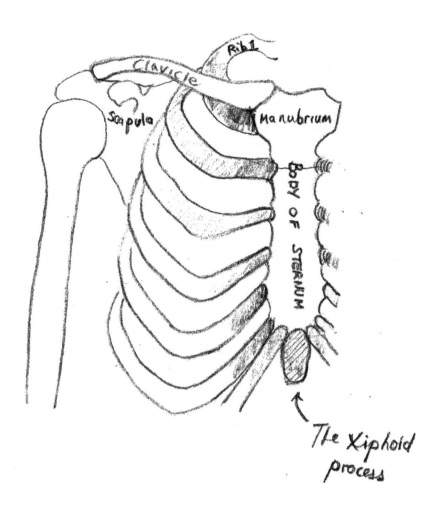

Diagram of the Xiphoid process (XPD 1)

The advantages of aerobic exercise:

In a large July 2014 study (J.of the Am College of Cardiology), 55,000 patients were followed up for 15 years with regard to their running habits. Even when other variables were excluded, the simple attribute of being a regular runner carried some significant health benefits. The summary I read unfortunately said "Running was associated with a significant lower risk of morality" but I think you know what they meant.

Conversely "not running" was almost as bad as having high blood pressure and accounted for 16% of all mortality and 25% of cardiovascular mortality. The study did not show any benefit from running a lot however. The lowest "quintile" was less than 51 minutes of running a week – not very much running at all – but even these patients did much better than non runners. Running further didn't improve the outcomes they looked at. The maximum all mortality benefit accrued from running as little as 6 miles (10km) a week. **The maximum cardiovascular mortality benefit was from running 5-10 miles, (8-16km) per week.**

Aerobic exercise in ex smokers significantly reduces lung cancer rates compared with non exercisers – by 25% in fact. Interestingly it doesn't reduce the risk of lung cancer in never smokers though.

A 2015 study compared yoga with aerobic exercise regarding systolic and diastolic blood pressure: Exercise was far more effective at reducing both and unlike yoga, improved bone and muscle mass, cardiac and sexual function. The researchers also commented that "more adverse effects took place during the yoga than during usual care". It is worth mentioning that lean body mass (specifically the limb muscle mass of over 60 year old men) as well as the dominant hand grip strength are related to bone density in this group.

Regular exercise of 2 hours of walking or cycling a week reduces admission and respiratory mortality in COPD by 30-40%.

Also, actual muscle mass is a predictor of longevity in adults. Some believe it to be a more important positive factor than the presence of absence of body fat mass. Indeed, a paper in the Am J Med. 2014 Jun: 127(6) 547-53 showed that in a group of older patients, those with the lowest muscle mass had a 20% higher mortality than those with the highest (pre existing) muscle mass. All were well at the start of the study – so the muscle mass wasn't lost due to illness. The deaths were from a whole variety of different causes. So resistance training for 1 hour, 3X a week could improve your older patients' survival by 20% over 6 years.

In a 2105 study it was demonstrated that when aerobic exercise improves cardiovascular fitness, cognitive abilities improve in parallel in patients with mild dementia. So "cardiovascular fitness should be a target for achieving cognitive benefit".

BUT, like too little exercise, over exercising appears to be harmful too. We have all heard of Olympic gold medal cyclists or rowers with osteoporosis due to a lack of weight bearing impacting on their bone architecture. Concentrating on one sport can cause damage to over stressed or ignored parts of the body.

We all see frequent training injuries in our healthier patients and the short and long term sequelae of both too much sport and too much treatment. We have all had young patients tragically die while out jogging or while doing a half marathon or a long cycle ride, without preliminary warning symptoms. In my patients I have been aware of marathon runners, triathletes and endurance cyclists with physiological bradycardias as low as thirty per minute, big baggy left ventricles with huge stroke volumes and a tendency to electrically twitchy hearts. They were slim and wiry but their hearts did not seem comfortable – like a racing car on the school run.

A number of recent papers show that relatively extreme exercise causes markers of inflammation to rise and leads to a disease state which it takes a while for the body to recover from. Endurance athletes are five times more likely to develop Atrial Fibrillation, thought to be due to cardiac scarring. Marathon runners can develop coronary calcification. – A huge and cruel irony if ever there was one. The American College of Cardiology published a study in Jan 2015 following 1000 healthy joggers and non joggers over 12 years. The best survivors were not those who exercised the most but those who jogged fairly slowly and **for less than two and a half hours a week.** Those who did more than four hours a week or no exercise were the least likely to survive. The "Ideal pace" was a **relatively slow 5mph** (8kph), 3x/week for their no more than two and a half hours a week.

The authors suggest heavy exercise remodels the heart and arteries which I suppose *leads to an arrhythmia prone heart at rest rates of relative bradycardia or even perhaps poor perfusion to a hypertrophied left ventricle at slow rates and low cardiac outputs?*

National guidelines currently suggest 150 minutes of "moderate intensity activity" a week. That is half an hour a day of sweaty activity with the weekend off. That is still the advice that I give – for as I look around at my fellow citizen in the high street and on the beach, very few of them seem to be underweight, walking up the stairs or riding the bike to work. Even in the gym car park most of the clients park as close as they can to the entrance so they don't have to walk too far to get to the gym once they exit their car.

29: Neurology:

Some functional anatomy you may have forgotten:

The Hypothalamus is part of the Limbic System, making releasing hormones for the pituitary but it is also involved in the developmentally ancient functions of controlling circadian rhythms, sleep and tiredness, thirst and hunger. It is involved in thermoregulation, heart rate and BP management, feeding, learning and memory, the management of some parenting and attachment roles. It sits above the pituitary.

Pituitary Hormones:

Anterior: ACTH, LH, FSH, Prolactin, GH, TSH.
Posterior: ADH (Vasopressin), Oxytocin.

The human brain has 100 billion cells and 100 trillion (10^{14}) neural connections. It became asymmetrical 2-3 million years ago. The brain, in proportion to the body has trebled in size in those 3 million years. Intelligence, 88% of which is with us when we are born, got our primate ancestors out of a lot of trouble, allowed them to plan for next year, to move away from dangerous territory and to more fertile or safer areas, to plan for warmth, shelter, protection and food. Thus clever genes survived and were passed down and less clever genes perished. But today society is actively trying to reverse that trend. We resuscitate babies born 4 months premature, sometimes with congenital abnormalities and subject them to intensive and supportive care despite almost inevitable neurological and developmental damage. We are actively protecting babies and children with known birth and genetic damage that will probably make them a societal burden and allow them to pass on their genes – the human right for all to have a family life. Meanwhile the least creative, contributive and intelligent in society generally tend to have the most children, the brightest and most talented the fewest. Better education and antenatal diagnosis may blunt this downward influence on cultural and intellectual development but the evolutionary progress that we have been used to over the rest of human history is not inevitable. "The secrets of evolution are time and death" (Carl Sagan). The medical profession is working to ameliorate half of that equation. Surely beneficial evolution will soon stall unless, you could argue, mankind starts actively using genetic engineering, some as yet undiscovered prenatal detailed screening, and/or some form of (dare it be mentioned?) eugenics.

But for the moment, society is at a stage of actively **reversing** evolutionary intellectual and genetic progress. So this is a bad time genetically for mankind. Perhaps refined antenatal diagnosis and gene editing put together with some means of reliably predicting and safely delaying premature labour will be the saviour of mankind long term.

Each side of the brain has a specialist as well as some common functions. It has evolved from the inside out. Deep down at its base the brainstem is managing our basic biological controls. Heartbeat, respiration and so on.

The higher functions evolved in three successive stages: On top of the brain stem is the R-complex, the seat of ritual, aggression, territoriality and social hierarchy. This evolved in our reptile ancestors hundreds of millions of years ago, hence "R". Deep inside us is the essence of dinosaur. Not so deep in some. Surrounding the R-complex is the Limbic system, the mammalian brain, – and this evolved tens of millions of years ago before mammals became primates. It is the source of emotions, moods, our concern and care for our offspring. Presumably this means that reptiles and amphibians don't have the same loving emotions and attachment for eggs that we evolved for our cute, clingy and dependent young.

Wrapped around all this history like a soft, corrugated grey crash helmet is the cerebral cortex. This evolved millions of years ago in our primate ancestors and just about coexists with the backward parts of the brain which predate it. It is 2/3 of the human brain mass and is where consciousness, intuition, critical analysis, ideas, creativity, mathematics, art, reasoning and science come into existence.

To quote Carl Sagan again: "The cortex regulates our conscious lives. It is the distinction of our species, the seat of our humanity". Civilisation is a product of the cerebral cortex. In terms of pure data stored, the brain data base contains 10,000X more raw information than our gene data base.

Cerebral Hemispheres

R	L
Generating Ideas, Random	Testing their Validity, Logical
Creative instincts, Intuitions, Pattern recognition	Rational/Analytic/Critical thinking
Analogies, 3 dimensions, Fiction, Art, Humour	Facts, Concepts, Language (in 95%),
Feelings, Imagination, Memories, Attention,	(Broca's and Wernicke's areas)
Intellect, Symbols, Abstract, Subjective,	Vocabulary, Grammar, Speech (mostly)
Holistic, Synthesising,	Visio-spatial, Image based.
Looks at wholes. Facial recognition.	Impulsive, Concrete, Objective
Sequential. Looking at parts	
Spatial awareness	Logical analysis and reasoning
Left side of body	Right side of body
Music rhythm	Maths, reality orientated
Damage:	
Visual perception, neglect of L side of body	Trouble speaking or understanding
L hemianopia, poor decision making. Impulsiveness	speech or written words. Slow careful
short attention span.	movements, R hemianopia.

The L and R hemispheres began to specialise 2-3m years ago. The L brain works faster! Everyone uses both sides of their brain – however artistic, creative, logical or rational they are.

The Hypothalamus gives us emotional reactivity, the Hippocampus shrinks on MRI in early Alzheimer's and is important in encoding new memories, envisaging how situations might pan out and in processing complex spatial and visual discrimination-amongst other functions.

There is a protein that affects hippocampal function called cAMP response element-binding protein – CREB, which affects our memory making ability and is lower in patients at risk of Alzheimer's. If you eat significant amounts of food at night, when your diurnal clock says you should be asleep, you have lower levels of CREB. Apparently this is one possible cause of poor memory storage.

Most R handed people have their speech centre in the L Hemisphere, so do most L handers.

Laterality: 10% of the population are L handed, 20% are L footed.

L handedness is commoner in homosexuals and commoner in men than women. (11.6% vs 8.6%)

It is commoner in the "gender confused". Hand dominance only becomes clear at the age of 18m to 2 yrs.

If both the parents are R handed, 8-9.5% children are L handed, if one parent is L and one R handed, 19.5% of the children are L handed. If both parents are L handed then 26.1% of their children are L handed.

According to official statistics L handedness is becoming more common. In 1900 it was approximately 3% of each sex but the teachers did use to force children to write with their right hands come what may in those days and perhaps reporting was a little biased.

Handedness varies internationally: Thus

UK and Canada 11.5%

Emirates 7.5%

India 5.8%

Japan 4.0%

	Cerebral L Sided Language	R sided Language
R Handers:	95%	5%
L Handers:	70%	30%

R eye dominant in 70%.

Normal neurology:

Vision:

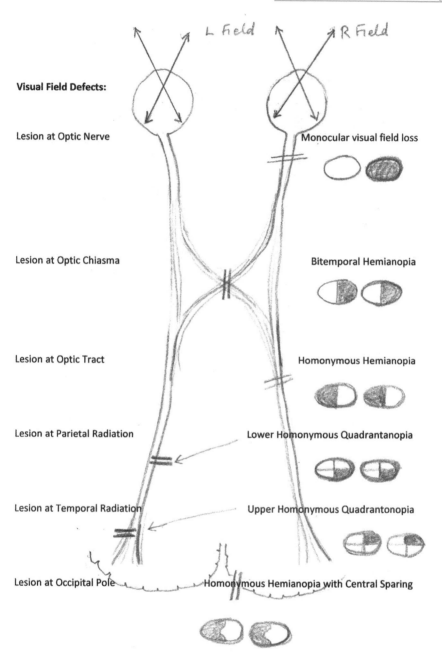

Visual Field Defects:

L Field   R Field

Lesion at Optic Nerve   Monocular visual field loss

Lesion at Optic Chiasma   Bitemporal Hemianopia

Lesion at Optic Tract   Homonymous Hemianopia

Lesion at Parietal Radiation   Lower Homonymous Quadrantanopia

Lesion at Temporal Radiation   Upper Homonymous Quadrantonopia

Lesion at Occipital Pole   Homonymous Hemianopia with Central Sparing

X3 Visual fields, Ocular palsy and External ocular movements

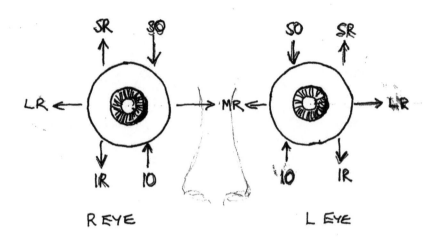

R EYE   L EYE

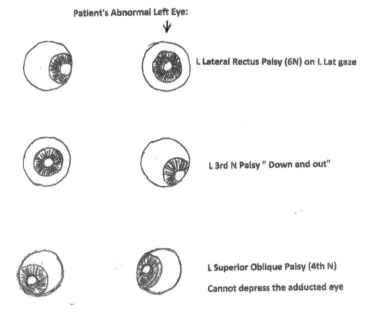

Patient's Abnormal Left Eye:

L Lateral Rectus Palsy (6N) on L Lat gaze

L 3rd N Palsy " Down and out"

L Superior Oblique Palsy (4th N)
Cannot depress the adducted eye

The superior and inferior recti are best assessed with the eye abducted. Likewise in adduction the obliques do the elevation and depression: The Inferior oblique elevates and the superior oblique depresses the adducted eye.

General Neurological Examination:

Cranial Nerves:

1 Olfactory: Smell.

2 Optic: Vision, visual acuity, fields, disc, fundus.

3* Oculomotor: All ocular muscles except Superior Oblique and Lateral Rectus (leaving the eye in the "Down and out" position when there is a complete 3rd N palsy).

      Ciliary muscle,

      Pupil,

      Levator Palpebrae.

4* Trochlear: Superior Oblique muscle (gives down and medial gaze).

5 Trigeminal: Sensation to face, teeth, corneal reflex, sinuses and ant. 2/3 tongue.

      Motor to chewing muscles, jaw jerk.

6* Abducens: Lateral rectus muscle (gives lateral gaze).

*Palpebral fissures, squint, diplopia, eye movement, nystagmus, pupils, PERLA?

7 Facial: Motor to face (expression and scalp) raise eye brows, frown, close eyes, smile, show teeth,

      whistle, platysma (pull down angles of mouth),

      Taste anterior 2/3 tongue (this is via the Chorda Tympani-which passes through the middle ear between the malleus and incus),

      Nerve to Stapedius. Ask about lacrimation and salivation, glabellar tap.

8 Auditory: Hearing of a whisper and balance. Romberg's etc

Romberg's test: (Romberg's sign) This tests for proprioception, middle ear disease or lower limb sensory ataxia.

      Get the patient to stand with feet together, hands at their sides and eyes closed, then watch for swaying. Be prepared to catch them if they fall. The test is positive if the patient falls when their eyes are closed.

9 Glossopharyngeal: Sensory to posterior 1/3 of tongue, pharynx, middle ear.

      Taste posterior 1/3 tongue.

      Also motor to some pharyngeal muscles.

10 Vagal: Motor to soft palate, larynx, pharynx. Ask about swallowing problems, dysarthria, examine

      soft palate, gag reflex (pharyngeal), sensation to back of tongue.

Sensory and motor to lungs, heart and viscera.

11 Accessory: Motor to Sterno-mastoid and Trapezius muscles.

      Accessory connection to Vagus.

12 Hypoglossal: Motor to tongue and hyoid bone depressors. Atrophy/fasciculation of tongue?

      Movements of tongue in all directions.

THE NERVE SUPPLY TO THE TONGUE

Glossopharyngeal IX Sensation to post third   SENSATION Lingual N V Sensation. ant two thirds
                                                          Mandibular branch

Glossopharyngeal IX Taste to posterior third   TASTE   Facial N VII Taste to ant 2/3 (Chorda Tympani)

Vagus X supplies the Palatoglossus muscle and   MOTOR   XII via Hypoglossal N

SENSATION via the Internal Larnyngeal N to the epiglottis/larynx
above the vocal chords as well as TASTE to the valleculae.

Diagram: Nerve Supply of the tongue

General Neurological Examination:

Cervical Column: Active and passive ROM,

Carotid Artery: Bruits and palpation,

Upper Limbs: Movements, tremor, fasciculation, muscle wasting, involuntary movements, tone, spasticity, rigidity (clasp knife, cog wheel, lead pipe),

Mobility: Active and passive movements, ROMs.

Power: Strength of different muscle groups.

Reflexes: Biceps C5, Radial C6, Triceps C7, Finger C8.

Cerebellum: Finger nose test, alternating upper limb movements. Heel, knee, shin test.

Abdomen: Reflexes: Epigastric: T 7-8, Mesogastric: T9 – 10, Hypogastric: T 11-12, Cremasteric: L 1-2.

Lower limbs: Appearance (muscle bulk, tone, fasciculation, posture etc). Active and passive movements, range and strength.

Toe extension is L5,

Reflexes: Knee jerk: L2-4. L4 Knee extension.

Ankle jerk: L5-S2. S1 plantar flexes foot.

L5 Lifts, dorsiflexes toes.

Medioplantar reflex L5-S2.

Adductor reflex: L2-4.

Also posture: Standing, walking (gait) etc. Sensation.

Note:

Two point discrimination: <6mm is normal. 6-10mm is fair, 10-15mm is poor.

Dermatomes, L4 Great toe,

        L5 Lat calf, mid dorsum of foot,

        S1 Little toe.

I used to think that dermatomes were fairly consistent but look at these two dermatome charts from different promotional material (when we used to be given it) from the last few years. There is a huge difference between the two so the upper lateral thigh for instance could be L2, L3 or L4! So presumably dermatome edges vary between patients considerably-as well as between reference charts.

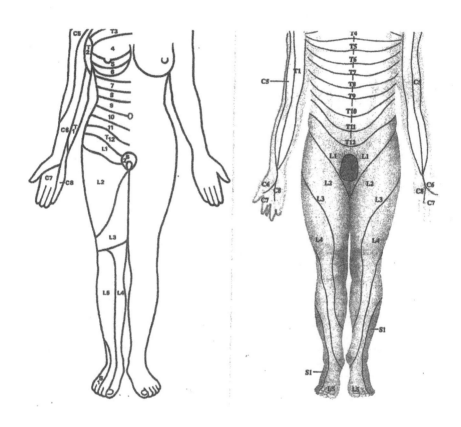

Diagram of Dermatomes

The Ear

Acoustic Neuroma

A benign schwannoma of the 8th cranial nerve. Can cause lesions in cranial nerves 5, 7 and 8 (cerebello-pontine angle.) Causes deafness, tinnitus and unsteadiness. Treated by (monitoring) radiotherapy or excision.

Rinne's Test:

Place the vibrating tuning fork on each mastoid and just as the patient says they can no longer hear it, put it in front of the ear. Normally air conduction exceeds bone conduction and they can still hear it in front of the ear. A "positive" test is normal (strangely). A negative test indicates conductive hearing loss, usually middle or outer ear disease (glue ear, wax etc). You can get false negative or positive tests in sensorineural hearing loss.

Weber's Test:

The vibrating tuning fork is placed in the mid line at the apex of the skull (some use the forehead or even the midline of the face!) In a normal patient the sound is heard symmetrically. If it is heard louder on one side then that side could have a conductive blockage or the other side could have a sensineural loss. Obviously this can be a little confusing unless the patient tells you which ear is deaf beforehand. You usually do a Rinne test at the same time to determine which scenario is more likely.

The Face

Facial Pain

Neuralgia of Trigeminal, Glossopharyngeal Ns, post herpetic etc.

Migrainous neuralgia (including cluster).

Trigeminal involvement in M.S.,

Acoustic neuroma.

Tumours (nasopharyngeal, pharynx, mouth, sinuses, Neurofibromatosis etc).

O.A., cervical or TMJ.

Fracture (mandible).

Dental pain (Inf. Dental N.).

Sinus pressure or infection,

Middle ear conditions including infection,

Aneurysm of post. communicating artery,

Temporal arteritis,

Superior orbital fissure syndrome.

Raeder(s) Syndrome: Paratrigeminal syndrome/neuralgia: Severe unilateral facial pain in Opth. Divn. of V, headache, with ipsilateral Horner Syndrome (oculosympathetic palsy), Atypical Facial Pain,

The commonest facial pains in General Practice are probably due to sinus and teeth infection, cervical OA and migraine. If the pain is tingly beware shingles and look for vesicles in the hair.

Bell's Palsy:

A paralysis of Cranial N 7, the Facial. Less than 1% are actually bilateral.

Some believe this to be a Varicella Zoster (Simplex) reactivation in the Facial Nerve and advise treatment with Aciclovir. Reactivation of Zoster in the nerve with or without vesicles is Ramsay Hunt Syndrome. The nerve becomes swollen and compressed in the facial canal but oddly the patient may complain of many anatomically inexplicable symptoms including unilateral limb weakness or sensory symptoms, facial sensory symptoms, headache etc.

You may have forgotten that the facial canal is the longest osseous canal that a nerve runs through in the whole body and presumably the Facial Nerve IS fairly vulnerable to compression because of this. Z shaped it runs from the internal acoustic meatus to the stylomastoid foramen.

You may also have forgotten: That there is a complete hemiparesis of the face in Bell's palsy. Remember that there is bilateral innervation of the forehead so if the facial paralysis is due to a stroke, the forehead is spared, if it is lower motor neurone, (ie Bell's) then it isn't. The other associated neurology with Bell's includes hyperacusis and loss of taste over the anterior 2/3 of the tongue on that side.

I give high dose prednisolone (plus a PPI) and Aciclovir just in case. The steroids have to be started within 3 days to make much difference but the prognosis is good.

Acute Convulsions:

Treatment:

Diazepam rectal (Stesolid) Adults 10mg, Elderly 5mg, Children, <1yr not recommended, 1-3 years 5mg, >3yrs up to 10mg.

Midazolam buccal solution – Buccolam Doses: 5mg/ml.
Child 300ug/Kg max 2.5mg up to 6m.
6m-1yr 2.5mg
1-5 yrs 5mg
5-10yrs 7.5mg
10-18yrs 10mg
Adult 10mg
Repeat if necessary after 10minutes. These come as prefilled syringes. It is a CD.

Multiple Sclerosis:

Second only to trauma as a cause of neurological disability in the young and middle aged. 80,000 in the UK are affected. A T-Cell auto immune condition affecting genetically susceptible people after an environmental trigger. (E-B Virus infection, low Vitamin D levels?, etc)

Demyelination is followed by actual loss of axons from the CNS. The clinical classification of MS is into:

Relapsing remitting MS (the commonest presenting form) which may progress to
Secondary progressive. There are also:
Progressive relapsing and
Primary progressive.

There is a dramatically increased incidence amongst ethnic populations moving from low to high incidence, usually first world areas. In a study published in 2016 about an ethnically diverse area of East London:

In a population of 907,000: 776 had MS. ie 111 per 100,000 (152 F: 70 M)
In the white population the incidence was 180/100,000.
In the black population it was 74/100,000. 29/100,000 in South Asians.

In Ghana the incidence is the highest of sub Saharan countries at 0.24/100,000 a tiny fraction of the incidence of Ghanaians in East London. The MS incidence in India (7/100,000) and Pakistan (5/100,000) are minute compared with their diaspora in London (29/100,000) so one has to assume a dietary or environmental cause or co factor is at work which is geographically dependent.

There have to be "lesions disseminated in both space and time" ie different parts of the CNS affected at different times of the illness. The less coffee consumed the higher the risk of MS. More than 6 cups a day for 5 years reduces your risk by 30% compared with non coffee drinkers (J of Neurology Neurosurg and psych. 20016:jnnp-2015-312431 DOI:10.1136/jnnp-2015-312431)

There are characteristic MRI changes but LP and evoked responses can contribute to the diagnosis too.

Relapse treatment:

Dexamethasone:

8mg daily for 1 week then reduce over a week.

Better prognosis: Women, early remissions, those presenting with mainly sensory symptoms.

Methyl Prednisolone 1 gr. IV for 3 days or 500mg orally for 5 days in disabling relapses.

There are no disease modifying drugs at present for progressive forms of MS.

Beta Interferon reduces exacerbations by a 1/3, reduces lesions on MRI, helps in secondary progressive relapsing disease, helps to reduce wheelchair boundness by 2 1/2 years. Extremely expensive.

Beta Interferon Rx in Multiple Sclerosis:

Our current local rules are:

Patients must have:

Neurologist diagnosis,

2 or more disabling relapses in last 2 years,

One relapse in the last year,

Functional recovery with minimal progression between relapses,

Can walk alone for 100yds.

Aware of diagnosis,

Accepts SC injections long term.

Don't refer:

Only one episode,

No relapses in 2 years,

Needs walking aid,

Contemplating or actually breast feeding or

pregnant.

<18yrs,

>50yrs,

Poor complier,

Hypersensitive to drug or components,

Depression or suicide attempt in past,

Decompensated liver disease,

Epilepsy,

Patients on immunosuppressives other than steroids.

As well as B interferon, Glatiramer Acetate (– a "random polymer" with an unknown action but is thought to shift T cells from a pro inflammatory state to a state that suppresses inflammation. It also resembles myelin and may act as a decoy for myelin antobodies) reduces relapses 30% but evidence for benefit in the long term is sparse. Generally Disease modifying Drugs are started after a few (2-3) acute episodes and before progressive MS Sets in. Fingolimod, Laquinimod, Teriflunonomod and Natalizumab etc are second line treatments.

Alemtuzumab is given as an infusion in relapsing/remitting MS.

In 2016 the newspapers were full of a new stem cell treatment which was said to "reboot" the patient's immune system and resulted in long term remissions in those who survived the treatment. Foetal stem cells have been used by clinics in MS treatment for some years (HSCT, autologous haematopoietic stem cell transplant) but this treatment was disclosed in a Canadian study published in the Lancet (June 2016) and consisted of aggressive chemotherapy, actually destroying the immune system rather than suppressing it first. This was then followed by stem cell transplant. Of 24 patients, one died from the chemotherapy but the others were effectively disease free after treatment.

Newer Treatments:

At least once a year over the last five years, new treatments for various types of MS have been announced and the prognosis and outcome for most patients have improved a great deal in my 45 year medical lifetime.

The MS Society lists 44 potential treatments for the various forms of MS. Some are for symptomatic treatment and are well known drugs, some are immune modulators.

For instance:

In Relapsing Remitting MS:

Daclizumab, Ocrelizumab, Cladribine, RPC 1063, Laquinimod, Ponesimod, Ofatumumab, (all immune modulators), Anti-LINGO-1 (repairs myelin). ATX-MS-1467 (stops immune damage of myelin), Minocycline (reduces the inflammation of infection of course), Raltegravir (anti viral), Amiselimod, Lipoic Acid (affects immune cells), Clemastine (repairs myelin), ALT 1102 (affects immune cells), Vatelizumab (immune modulator), Rituximab (discontinued).

Primary Progressive MS: Ocrelizumab (immune modulator), MD1003 (promotes repair of myelin), Masitinib, Fingolimod, (immune modulators). Fluoxetine (antidepressant), Ibudilast (reduces cell inflammation amongst other things), Laquinimod, Natalizumab, Rituximab (the latter discontinued, all immune modulators)

SecondaryProgressive MS: Siponimod, Masitinib, (immune modulator), MD 1003(myelin repair), MS-SMART (Amiloride, Fluoxetine and Riluzole -neuroprotective) - as is Simvastatin, MIS416, Tcelna, Lipoic Acid, (immune modulators), Ibudilast, (prevents apoptosis), Anti-LINGO-1 repairs myelin, Natalizumab, Rituximab (immune control again).

Optic Neuritis:

Phenytoin (neuroprotective), Anti-LINGO-1, (myelin repair), Amiloride, MD1003 (myelin repair).

Myasthenia Gravis:

There is a number of "myasthenias", all showing painless weakness. These include the Lambert Eaton Myasthenic Syndrome, congenital myasthenias and the main disease, Myasthenia Gravis.

This is an auto immune disease with antibodies to Ac Ch receptors at the neuromuscular junction. Fatigue of muscles with use is characteristic, often starting with the periorbital muscles. The first signs and symptoms are often therefore diplopia and ptosis. "Ocular myasthenia" may be the only extent of the condition in 15% of patients. Limb, axial, bulbar, respiratory muscles etc may be involved. Gait, speech, swallowing and breathing may be affected. The thymus is often abnormal (thymoma in 10%) and thymectomy can lead to a halt in progression. Other auto immune diseases are commoner (thyroid disease, diabetes, Rh A, SLE, MS etc). Chronic tiredness without actual weakness is not the picture of myasthenia.

There can be a transient perinatal myasthenia in babies of affected mothers so presumable an antibody or some immune agent crosses the placenta.

Muscular fatigability is evident on examination and on EMG testing and the antibody to the Ac Ch receptor may be positive on blood testing.

The Tensilon (Edrophonium) test or a similar challenge using Neostigmine (anticholinesterase) gives a transient improvement in muscle function. CXR to exclude a thymoma.

Treatments include cholinesterase inhibitors – eg pyridostigmine, also azathioprine, steroids, intravenous immunoglobulin (short term) and thymectomy.

The Lambert Eaton Myasthenic Syndrome: A tenth as common as MG, this begins >30 yrs of age, and affects the lower limbs more than the head and neck unlike MG. It can involve the arms and some autonomic functions. About 50% LEMS patients have small cell lung cancer due to smoking. It is associated with other auto immune diseases.

Spasticity:

Alternative treatments:

Tizanidine: Said to cause less weakness than Baclofen. 2mg initially slowly increasing to a maximum of 36mg daily.

Baclofen, Lioresal: 5mg TDS initially.

Essential Tremor:

Alternative treatments:

Propranolol, Primidone, Phenytoin, Gabapentin, Topiramate, Buspirone, Baclofen, Clonazepam.

Restless legs syndrome:

Causes:

Limb movement syndromes in peripheral neuropathy, pregnancy, dialysis, Parkinson's, renal disease, cramps, peripheral vascular disease, iron deficiency, secondary to caffeine, various drugs, gluten enteropathy etc.

Alternative treatments: are varied, complex, fraught with side effects and can be expensive:

Most authorities advise avoiding TCAs.

Top up iron if necessary and then go through

Gabapentin,

Ropinirole (Dopamine Agonist) 250ug initial dose at night,

Pergolide,

Pramipexole,

Cabergoline,

Benzodiazepines, (Temazepam, Clonazepam),

Opiates, (Codeine, Tramadol),

Clonidine,

Madopar, (Levodopa/Benserazide),

L Dopa, (Levodopa),

Sinemet, (Levodopa/Carbidopa).

Its significance:

An American study, reported in 2015 followed two matched groups of patients for eight years. One with and one without restless leg symptoms. There was a fourfold increase in stroke and heart disease in the restless leg group. There was also a threefold increase in renal disease. Over the study period, the RLS group members were 88% more likely to die. So, far from being a harmless, slightly strange disorder with a benign outcome and no objective serious signs, RLS seems to be a marker of arterial pathology and worth us taking seriously. Perhaps by paying close attention to BP and circulation, even considering aspirin and other prophylaxis?

Myopathy:

Proximal Myopathy:

PMR, Polymyositis, Dysthyroidism (usually hyper), Hypo/Hyper K+, Hypo?Hyper Ca++, Cushings, Drugs: Steroids, diuretics (low K+), Penicillamine, underlying disease: Bronchial Ca, myasthenia, Guillain Barrē.

Parkinson's Disease:

Slowness of movement, rigidity, postural instability, tremor (better with movement) in 70%, 4-6/second frequency, poverty of blinking, lead pipe or cog-wheel passive muscle movement, pill rolling, mask like face, monotonous voice, micrographia, drooling, constipation, urinary frequency and incontinence, sweating, dysphagia, dementia, flexed posture, festinant (short rapid steps, trying to catch up with the centre of gravity) gait, impaired arm swing, poor balance.

Neuropsychiatric: Poor problem solving, variable attention, bradyphrenia (slow thought), memory problems, poor recall of learnt information. Progressive deterioration of mentation to dementia.

Associated mood changes are depression, apathy and anxiety, OCD, bingeing, hyper sexuality, psychoses which may be associated with dopamine therapy. Visual or auditory hallucinations, sometimes paranoid delusions.

Sleep is disturbed and irregular, acting out dreams in some, insomnia etc.

Various autonomic symptoms, parasthesiae, loss of taste, loss of position sense, postural hypotension, urinary incontinence, ED, sweating etc.

Causes: Associated with rural areas, herbicides, pesticides, heavy metals, (and heavy metal rock musicians), head injury, atherosclerotic, post encephalitic, drug induced (Phenothiazines, Haloperidol, various hallucinogens, including LSD, Cannabis, Peyote, Psilocybe mushrooms etc, – So many of the rock stars of the 60's and 70's often seem to have quite severe Parkinson's if they are still alive), toxins, Manganese, (hence a link with welding and living near golf courses – Manganese is used in the sprays used to treat grass and is present in welding fumes), kernicterus, mid brain compression, post traumatic, syphilis, Wilson's Disease (Hepato-lenticular degeneration), hypoparathyroidism, idiopathic, etc. BUT Caffeine, Nicotine, and possibly NSAIDs may be protective? Loss of sense of smell is an early feature. 1-2% have a genetic LRRK2 mutation. Some suspect a prion aetiology. Lewy bodies are a non specific association. The associated dementia is the second commonest after Alzheimer's. PD is also associated with Acne Rosacea and both are associated with small intestinal bacterial overgrowth and H Pylori infection.

Treatment is basically Levodopa but patients develop fluctuations after 5 years so Dopamine agonists are used first. Bromocriptine, Pergolide, Ropinirole, Cabergoline, Pramipexole can all be used instead of or with Levodopa. Dopamine agonists can cause nausea, so Rx Domperidone.

For instance:

Treatment groups:

Anticholinergics: Benzatropine, Orphenadrine (Disipal), Procyclidine (Kemadrine) – these help reduce tremor.
COMT Inhibitors: Entacapone.
Dopaminergics: Amantadine.
Apomorphine: By injection to counteract "Off periods". Need to co prescribe Domperidone.
Bromocriptine: (Parlodel):(Dopamine agonist).
Cabergoline:
Co-Beneldopa: Levodopa/Benserazide (A Dopamine precursor and a Dopa-decarboxylase inhibitor) (Madopar) As: 50mg/12.5mg, 100mg/25mg and 200mg/50mg Caps. Also 50mg/12.5mg and 100mg/25mg dispersible tabs and also a controlled release 100mg/25mg capsule (Madopar CR).
Co-Careldopa: (Levodopa and Carbidopa) (a Dopamine precursor and a Dopa-decarboxylase inhibitor) (100mg/10mg, 100mg/25mg, 250mg/25mg and as Sinemet: 50mg/12.5mg (yellow tab), "Sinemet Plus" 100mg/25mg (yellow tab), 100mg/10mg (blue), 250mg/25mg (blue).
Also Sinemet CR 200mg/50mg (peach) and Half Sinemet CR 100mg/25mg (pink).
Levodopa, Carbidopa and Entacapone: Stalevo. Seven strengths of Levodopa from 50mg to 200mg.
Pergolide: 50 and 250ug tabs D1 and D2 Dopamine receptor agonist improves control when added to Levodopa 50mcg increasing to 3000mcg/day.
Pramipexole: Mirapexin: 88ug, 180ug, 350ug, 700ug.
Ropinirole: Requip. Starter pack then 1mg, 2mg and 5mg tabs. Delays the onset of motor complications. Lower incidence of dyskinesias than L Dopa and benefit more than 5 years. Can be used with or without L Dopa. Maximum benefit >10mg/day. Expensive.
Rotigotine: Neupro Patches: Starter pack then 2mg, 4mg, 6mg, 8mg.
MAO-B Inhibitors:
Rasagiline: Azilect 1mg.
Selegiline: Eldepryl 5mg, 10mg. This is an MAOI and delays the need for other treatments.

Alternative Therapy:
Some alternative practitioners suggest that supplementing the amino acid Cysteine improves Parkinsonian symptoms.

Suggested Regime:
First line: Dopamine agonist or Selegiline then Levodopa and Decarboxylase inhibitor, if on/off phenomenon then long acting Levodopa.
Can use Clozapine in Parkinson's paranoia as it improves the movement disorder as well as the paranoia. Entacapone can be used with other treatments to stabilise end of dose fluctuations.
or for an alternative view:
Younger, healthier patient: use a Dopamine agonist, Ropinirole (monotherapy or as an adjunct to levodopa), Cabergoline (not alone), Pergolide (second line as mono therapy or as an adjunct to levodopa), Pramipexole (alone or with levodopa).

Another Practical Regime of Treatment: (RCP)
Levodopa is still recommended as first line for most patients' motor symptoms in

combination with a dopa decarboxylase inhibitor. Thus: Co Beneldopa (Madopar) or Co Careldopa (Sinemet)

Dopamine agonists can also be a first line choice. The side effects include impulse control disorder in nearly a fifth of patients. Drugs include Pramipexole (Mirapexin), Ropinirole (Requip), Rotigotine (Neupro – a transdermal patch).

Monoamine oxidase type B inhibitors. Well tolerated, first line but not very strong. Some benefit may be conferred by starting early. Selegiline, (Eldepryl), Rasagiline (Azilect).

Anticholinergics eg Benzhexol, (Trihexylphenidyl) are no longer advised first line unless the patient's main problem is tremor and Amantadine a glutamate antagonist can be used when the patient has Levodopa induced dyskinesias.

Later in the illness when control is slipping and symptoms get worse again:

Wearing off and Levodopa Induced Dyskinesias (LIDs) can be dealt with by increasing the dosing frequency of Levodopa or by adding a second agent such as:

a Dopamine agonist.

a COMT inhibitor eg Entacapone (Comtess) and Tolcapone (watch LFTs), (Tasmar) there are combination tablets: (Stalevo),

an MAO B Inhibitor,

Complications of P.D. such as;

Depression are best treated with Pramipexole or Nortriptyline, Desipramine.

Psychosis with Clozapine,

Dementia, Rivastigmine.

Siallorrhoea with Botulinum toxin in the Parotid, Glycopyrrolate, or with Atropine eye drops under the tongue,

and constipation with Macrogol.

Clonazepam for REM sleep disorders, Melatonin for sleep.

Domperidone for nausea.

Headache:

Danger signals:

Sudden onset, severe, constant, lowered conscious level, H/O trauma, neurological deficit, visual loss, nausea, confusion, drowsiness, memory loss, fever >38°C, seizures, photophobia, age >50 yrs, increasing severity, frequency, duration, woken by headache, worse on coughing, sneezing, straining, exercise, (unless clearly migrainous), meningism, papilloedema, retinal haemorrhage.

Diagnostic features:

If the above are not present but there are nausea, vomiting, photophobia, visual, sensory symptoms then the diagnosis could be **Migraine with aura.**

If all the above but no visual or sensory symptoms then diagnosis: **migraine w/o aura.**

If daily symptoms, more than 2 hours, generalised, no vomiting or photophobia, analgesics not taken daily for most of the last 30 days, then diagnosis: **Tension Headache.**

If daily symptoms, unilateral with nasal symptoms, ptosis, lacrymation, conjunctival injection then diagnosis: **Cluster Headache.**

If daily, unilateral, no nasal congestion, ptosis, lacrimation, conjunctival injection, but raised ESR then possible **Temporal Arteritis.**

If daily, less than 2 hour episodes and analgesics or Ergotamine preparations taken more than once daily for more than 30 days, then consider **Rebound Headache (Analgesic withdrawal).**

So usual features:

Migraine: 15% population, (50% have "Muscle Tension" headache) Unilateral, throbbing, pounding, pulsing, aching, moderate, neurovascular, gradual onset, any time of day, prodrome or aura, lasts 4-72 hrs (*though in my experience, due to dehydration etc, total symptoms and malaise can take a week or 10 days to resolve*), associated photophobia, phonophobia, dysarthria, nausea, vomiting, mostly female, FH, common triggers: Light, fatigue, hunger, stress, alcohol, food etc.

Any migraine sufferer taking 12 or more triptan doses a month may have rebound headache as well and these patients are growing in number. Many of them are doctors. Some are friends of mine.

Episodic Tension Headache: (TTH): Bilateral, band like, pressure, squeezing, mild to moderate, onset and duration 30mins – days, any time of day, no prodrome or aura, no nausea, headache free between episodes, mild photo/phonophobia, any age, mainly female, often a FH, stress a common factor. Usually able to carry on as normal with the symptoms.

Cluster Headache: Always unilateral, sharp, boring, very severe, vascular, rapid onset (30-90mins), often same time of day eg at night, no prodrome, autonomic features on same side as HA, usually adult males, no FH. Trigger factors: stress, alcohol, tobacco. Last 15 mins-4hrs, see page 817.

Chronic Daily Headache (and Analgesic Withdrawal Headache): Location varies, but type of pain is similar to the originally treated HA, severity varies, cause unknown, gradual onset, anytime of day, often on waking, no prodrome, more than 15 days a month, patient can be anxious, nauseated, irritable, depressed, any age or sex, no FH, triggers are stress and regular analgesic, triptan or ergotamine use.

Note: Chronic daily headache and "analgesic overuse/withdrawal headache" have exactly the same characteristics. The only difference is that the patient takes regular analgesics in one and not the other. The sad logic is that treating AWH by getting the patient off OTC codeine and Ibuprofen will either leave them on long term alternative medication or with chronic daily headache!!

Temporal Arteritis: Unilateral but can be occipital as well as temporal in distribution, burning, aching, severe, continuous or intermittent, no prodrome, tender arteries, raised ESR, visual field loss, masseter claudication, PMR symptoms, age group over 50, FH not common, no triggers.

Sub Arachnoid Haemorrhage: Generalised or unilateral headache, constant, severe, **sudden onset,** severe any time, occasional prodrome or aura, patient can be drowsy, show neurological signs (25%), **stiff neck,** meningism, e.g. Kernigs, Babinski etc. Patient usually 25-50 but can be any age, FH rare, associated AV malformation, trauma to head.

Treatment:

Cluster Headache: Rx Valproate, Verapamil up to 160mg TDS Lithium, Methysergide, Steroids, breakthrough O2, Triptans, Ergot derivatives etc.

Chronic Daily Headache: (analgesic withdrawal headache) (>4hrs a day) – Reduce analgesia, Rx Dosulepin,/Amitriptyline, SSRI, Gabapentin, or Valproate or a combination of the preceding.

Migraine: Rx Propranolol, Pizotifen, Valproate, TCAs, Verapamil, etc (I find

Topiramate and Nortriptyline an effective combination in difficult migraine).

Prophylaxis:

Some advise if there are >4 attacks/month. I would say, as a sufferer, that if you get a patient with regular proper migraine lasting a day or more a month then you should seriously consider prophylaxis.

Other reasons to start prophylaxis:

Orgasmic migraine, Sexual Intercourse related migraine, Premenstrual migraine, Exercise migraine.

Patients suffering migraine with aura have a more than double risk of ischaemic (cardioembolic rather than thrombotic) stroke compared with those having migraine without aura.

Verapamil in a slow release form often in a large dose (120mg-240mg a day). Nimodipine, Nimotop, is an alternative 30mg TDS.

Clonidine: 25ug tabs 2-3 bd. I have never found this particularly effective but it can help in menopausal hot flushing. It comes as Dixarit-25ug and Catapres-100ug (the latter for Hypertension).

Pizotifen: Sanomigran. Still probably the most effective prophylaxis in childhood migraine but can cause daytime tiredness at first. Titrate the dose and give at night.

Others: TCADs, NSAIDs: (Voltarol 12.5mg, 25mg, 50mg, 100mg, or Indomet(h) acin 100mg supps before sex or exercise migraine). – also useful to prescribe to regular sufferers their own supply of suppositories to avoid house calls and permit self management of acute attacks at home. Phentoin, Feverfew – 3 small leaves of Tenacetum Parthenium daily. Some try Vitamin B2 (Riboflavin), Co Enzyme Q10 or Magnesium Oxide 200mg BD. Although I can see no harm in these, I cannot vouch for them either.

Non Selective Beta Blockers: Propranolol, Metoprolol, Nadolol, Timolol.

Methysergide. Deseril. Everyone knows about retroperitoneal fibrosis but it can be the only effective prophylaxis in severe migraine used for a few months. Treat for 6m and tail off.

Migraine Acute treatment:

Paracetamol 1gr plus Domperidone 10mg at onset.

Migramax (Aspirin and Metoclopramide) sachets.

Migraleve, Pink: Buclizine and Paracetamol, Codeine: 2 at onset then Yellow: Paracetamol and Codeine: 2 every 4 hours. (Buclizine is an anthistaminic, anticholinergic antiemetic).

Paramax, Paracetamol and Metoclopramide, tabs and sachets.

Tolfenamic Acid (Clotam Rapid) 200mg at onset, repeat PRN after 1-2 hours. This is an NSAID of course.

900mg soluble aspirin and metoclopramide combined are as effective as triptans.

5HT1 Agonists: Selective Serotonin Agonists:

Possible side effects: Chest pain.

Almogran, Almotriptan. Tabs.

Eletriptan, Relpax Tabs, 26 Hr half life.

Frovatriptan, Migard Tabs.

Naratriptan, Naramig Tabs, Long Half Life, No MAOI interactions, slow onset, low rate of recurrence.

Rizatriptan, Maxalt. Tabs and oral dissolving wafers. Rapid onset, high 2 hour response rate. Avoid with Propranolol or use 5mg dose.

Sumatriptan, Imigran Tabs, injection, nasal spray.

Zolmitriptan, Zomig. Tabs, oral dissolving tabs and nasal spray. Rapid onset high 2 hours response rate.

Generally these are all one dose immediately then this may be repeated over 2 hours later, no more than 2 doses in 24 hrs. Don't use with Ergotamine, MAOIs, Lithium, avoid in angina, previous M.I. TIAs, or with SSRIs, avoid in focal, hemiplegic migraine etc.

Triptans: 5HT1 Agonists: Act on serotonin receptors in nerve endings and cause cerebral vasoconstriction, also preventing pro inflammatory neuropeptides. Up to 20% patients have chest pain but only a miniscule percentage have significant coronary ischaemia after a dose.

Triptans:	Onset	2 Hr response	Recurrence	
Sumatriptan	30mins	50-60%	45%	Imigran
Rizatriptan	?30mins	67-77%	45%	Maxalt
Zolmitriptan	45mins	65%	22-36%	Zomig
Naratriptan	Slower, longer action than Sumatriptan	17-28%	30%	Naramig
Frovatriptan		37-46%	7%	Migard

A few caveats: Avoid Rizatriptan with Propranolol, if on MAOIs, give Naratriptan, avoid Sumatriptan if on Lithium.

Others: Intravenous magnesium in migraine with aura.

Ergotamine: Cafergot. Tabs 1-2 at onset of attack, 4 in 24 hours. Old fashioned, lots of interactions, same caveats as for the 5HT1 agonists.

Migril is Ergotamine and Cyclizine.

Thus in migraine and tension headache, a reasonable approach would be:
Atenolol/Propranolol or
Amitriptyline initially,
then Valproate or Topiramate
or Gabapentin
and third line
Methysergide.

I personally find the triptans with Domperidone or Metoclopramide and soluble Paracetamol/Codeine, acutely then prophylactic Propranolol and Amitryptyline, swiftly subsituted by

Topiramate (slowly up to 25mg ii BD) and Nortriptyline (slowly up to 20mg bd) usually work.

In acute **severe** migraine IM Pethidine with Cyclizine are effective in most cases.

A new and promising trans dermal gel has been showing some effectiveness in acute and chronic migraine and casts light on a "trigeminal feed forward signalling mechanism" which precedes migraine with and without aura. The gel is applied to various sensitive areas of the scalp and face. It is a form of Ketoprofen and if applied regularly can prevent migraine attacks by reducing "neurogenic inflammation" which is part of the migraine mechanism. I am not clear if this applies to some or all migraineurs. (AAN 67th Annual meeting presentation April 2015).

Melatonin given at night (4mg, 30 minutes before retiring) has been used and found effective at reducing migraine and chronic tension type headache – "primary headache". Melatonin levels rise during headaches apparently.

Migraine in children

Is common, there is usually a family history (ask which parent had bad headaches/abdominal pain as a child?) and the migraine can present confusingly with a periodic syndrome of vomiting and or abdominal pain rather than headache.

Prophylaxis with Pizotifen (Sanomigran) usually works and the acute attack can be treated with nasal Sumatriptan (Imigran).

Status Migrainosus:

>3 days of typical headache or recurring bouts of migraine with <4 hr intervals of relief. Treat with s.c. Sumatriptan (Imigran) and IV Fluids. I assume you have already given rectal domperidone and diclofenac or if necessary IM pethidine and cyclizine (just one dose of these latter two in each attack and only as a last resort as the combination can abort the episode). You may have to explain to the medical registrar what the condition is when you admit the patient, as I have had to on a number of occasions. These days they never seem to have heard of it.

Migraine in pregnancy:

Migraine without aura improves for 70% women after the first three months (especially if it had been "menstrual migraine"). Migraine with aura is more likely to continue in pregnancy and if migraine occurs for the first time in pregnancy it is more likely to be with aura.

Paracetamol is safe, as is Aspirin in the first two trimesters. Up to 600mg/day of Ibuprofen is said to be OK. Buclizine, Chlorpromazine (!) and Prochlorperazine (Stemetil) are safe anti emetics. Domperidone and the other prokinetic, Metoclopramide are probably best avoided during organogenesis in the first trimester.

The safest prophylactics are said to be Propranolol and Amitriptyline. Generally it is advised that the Triptans be avoided if possible.

Medication overuse (Chronic daily) Headache:

This is real, unpleasant, common and deserves your sympathy.

Prophylaxis: Topiramate, Amitriptyline (Initially 10mg), beta blockers, Valproate, Gabapentin.

Cluster Headache:

This is horrible and definitely deserves your sympathy.

Strictly unilateral, with a distinct periodicity and always with autonomic features. It is **severely** painful in a trigeminal and upper cervical distribution with ipsilateral cranial autonomic signs and symptoms. The basic dysfunction is currently thought to originate in the posterior hypothalamus and that is why it can drag-in circadian pathways, autonomic nerves (both parasympathetic – lachrymation and rhinorrhoea, and sympathetic hypofunction-ptosis and miosis) and trigeminovascular involvement.

5M:1F. It commonly starts in the 30's or 40's. A "bout" – the period over which attacks keep recurring, can be months. Attacks are unilateral although sides can alternate. The pain can last 15 minutes to 3 hours. Cluster Headaches come on suddenly and are always associated with

Autonomic symptoms or signs:

Conjunctival injection, lachrymation, miosis, ptosis, oedema of the eyelid, rhinorrhoea, nasal blockage or congestion, facial or forehead sweating, etc.

Some patients experience the nausea and photophobia of migraine but they are more restless and agitated than wanting the peace and solitude of the average migraine sufferer- *generally speaking*. Attacks wear off only to recur with a frequency of up to 6 a day, down to one every other day and bouts going on for a week or so with perhaps a remission of two weeks in between. Annual cluster periods are up to three months perhaps twice a year. The pattern is repeated faithfully in the individual. Some poor individuals develop chronic Cluster Headache with no or very short remissions.

Within the differential diagnosis is Paroxysmal Hemicrania. This is commoner in women with briefer and more frequent attacks and responds to Indomethacin.

Acute treatment: The Imigran group of drugs, including subcutaneous Sumatriptan 6mg, (can use twice daily) or its nasal 20mg counterpart or Nasal Zolmitriptan, Oxygen 100% 7-12 Li/min, covering the facemask apertures, for 15-20 mins. The oxygen must be on high flow.

Nasal lignocaine, Lidocaine Solution, 4-6% as nasal drops 20-60mg can be used as an adjunct to other treatments.

Overall, opiates, NSAIDs, ergotamine etc all have a pretty limited use in CH.

Short term Prevention includes high dose steroids, probably the most effective treatment at bringing a new bout of CH to an end.

Use a big dose of prednisolone. I use the EC tablets with a PPI. I am convinced my patients avoid gastric complications compared with those of my parsimonious non gastric protecting colleagues. 1mg/kg/day (up to 60mg for an adult) daily for 5-7 days then reduce by 10mg every 3days. So 60 60 60 60 60 50 50 50 40 40 40 30 30 30 20 20 20 10 10 10 5 5 and 5mg and stop, – this almost always works but is only temporary, giving you and the patient a valuable breathing space so the preventative treatment you started at the same time (I would normally use Verapamil) has by then started to kick in.

Other advice includes avoiding alcohol, exposure to oil and solvent (etc) fumes and afternoon naps during bouts.

Prophylaxis:

Lithium (better in chronic CH than episodic CH) start, after the usual bloods (see Pathology section) at a dose of 300mg BD then slowly increase the dose to 600-1200mg/day.

Melatonin, steroids, Topiramate, Gabapentin are so far relatively unproven – unlike Verapamil:

The Verapamil Regime in Cluster headache: (both episodic and chronic CH):

The idea is to increase the Verapamil until the cluster stops, the ECG is abnormal or 960mg is reached.

	Morning	Lunchtime	Evening
For 2 weeks take	80mg	80mg	80mg
Then ECG			
For 2 weeks take	80mg	80mg	160mg

Then ECG			
For 2 weeks take	80mg	160mg	160mg
Then ECG			
For 2 weeks take	160mg	160mg	160mg
Then ECG			
For 2 weeks take	160mg	160mg	240mg
Then ECG			
For 2 weeks take	160mg	240mg	240mg
Then ECG			
For 2 weeks take	240mg	240mg	240mg
Then ECG			
For 2 weeks take	240mg	240mg	320mg
Then ECG			
For 2 weeks take	240mg	320mg	320mg
Then ECG			
Thereafter 320mg TDS			

Other prophylactic drugs include: For the short term:

Methysergide, ideal for repeated SHORT bouts of Cluster. 1mg OD initially, increasing by 1mg every 3 days (TDS) up to 5mg a day. Then increase by 1mg every 5 days. Maximum dose is 12mg a day and due to the various fibrotic reactions you need to have a holiday from the drug for 1 month out of every 6.

Ergotamine: 1-2mg orally or rectally 1 hour before the attack is due. You can't also use Sumatriptan and you do need predictable attacks.

There is also a couple of neurological surgical techniques which decompress the Trigeminal Nerve if all else fails and the condition is unilateral.

Cluster Headache: Usual advice:TCAD, Haloperidol, Clomipramine, Lithium, Valproate, Verapamil (Big doses, regular ECGs), Methysergide, Prednisolone. Try Melatonin too.

Breakthrough: Oxygen, Sumatriptan injection, Ergotamine inhaler, Zolmitriptan.

Raised intracranial pressure:

Headache, usually frontal, classically worse after lying down, with coughing, straining, sneezing. Vomiting without nausea, blurred vision, depressed conscious state.

Unilateral or bilateral pupillary dilation. This can be a very sensitive and early indicator of raised ICP if measured accurately – (Neurological pupil index). There is an inverse relationship between decreasing pupil reactivity and increasing ICP.

III and VI nerve palsy (See Cranial Nerves above).

Papilloedema unless RICP is of very recent onset (ie <24 hrs).

Late signs include motor changes, raised BP, widened pulse pressure, bradycardia.

Concussion:

Post concussion:

Symptoms:	Syndrome:
Headache	ICD 10 criteria* (For what this is see below)
Dizziness	History of traumatic blunt injury
Poor attention	+3 or more of the following:
Poor concentration	Headache

Poor memory

Fatigue

Difficulty in processing information

Increased irritability

Word finding difficulty

Increased sensitivity to light and noise

Blurred/double vision

Sleep disturbance

Dizziness

Fatigue

Irritability

Insomnia

Concentration affected

Memory affected

Intolerance of stress, emotion or alcohol

Post Concussion

Most will be recovered in 2-3 weeks.

Severity of traumatic blunt injury is not predictive of recovery and outcome.

Perception of symptoms is a crucial factor in development and maintenance of post-concussion syndrome.

Early brief intervention can be effective.

ICD 9 or 10 means *International Statistical Classifications of Diseases. ICD codes are alphanumeric designations given to every diagnosis, description of symptoms and cause of death attributed to human beings.*

Dementia:

There are 44 million people suffering from dementia worldwide with 50-70% of dementia is due to Alzheimer's dementia. The latest research suggests a link to diabetes and both the use of hypnotic medication and a lack of deep phase sleep as contributing to dementia as well as the benefit of a Mediterranean diet in its prevention. Headlines in August 2015 declared that the seemingly inexorable rise in dementia in the west was however, levelling off. The explanation for this was that vascular dementia was being prevented by the baby boomers' healthy diet, exercise, perhaps statins and lifestyle awareness – even though these laudable changes would have no effect on Alzheimer's dementia incidence.

Ironically however, very low weight in middle age is associated with increased dementia risk and obesity seems to protect against it (Lancet Diabetes and Endocr. Apr 2015). There are 850,000 dementia sufferers in the UK (2015), 15,000 under the age of 65 (Alzheimer's Research Trust).

By 2050 the number of those affected globally will have risen to 115 million according to our best estimates. Dementia is not an inevitable consequence of old age but it is the 6th leading cause of death. Dementia may be a complication of HIV/Aids, CJD, Huntington's Disease, ALS and many other progressive neurological disorders. Currently dementia costs £400Bn or 1% of the world's GDP and some think that it can only increase.

Beta Amyloid is a characteristic pathological finding of Alzheimer's disease. Both Beta Amyloid and Tau proteins accumulate with disrupted deep phase sleep (Brain July 10 2017). It has been postulated that prion infections (BSE, CJD, Scrapie and Kuru) produce proteins similar to proteins produced by our own brain cells. Normally these prion like proteins prevent amyloid fibres developing into plaques and damaging the brain. A lot of Alzheimer's research is currently looking into a the possibility of distorted infecting prion proteins that have folded like hot egg white, are stable and cannot prevent amyloid forming. Tau protein, forming neurofibrillary tangles also is associated specifically with Alzheimer's just as B amyloid plaques are. In fact the cognitive decline is **more** closely associated with the Tau tangles than with the amyloid plaques. In one study on mice genetically engineered to develop Alzheimer's symptoms, an Omega-3 Fatty Acid, DHA, prevented B amyloid plaques from forming (although it had no effect on established plaques). Unfortunately, twenty years of research based on this Amyloid hypothesis, the disease being triggered by the deformed proteins - amyloid and tau, has not produced any effective treatment. It is one of the most disappointing therapeutic areas in the whole of medicine and one of the most urgent. Instead of damaging proteins new research is looking at the primary role of immune microglial cells and the underlying importance of the inflammatory process. It is known that there are at least 20 genes associated with dementia and some of these genes control microglial function. It is possible that something triggers a change in the antigenicity of neural cells and the resulting immune response results in protein deposition in much the same way as post streptococcal nephritis leads to proteinuria. The blame for the prime damaging dysfunction however is now shifting from proteins to immune cells. Other lines of research include the function of cellular microtubules in the dementia metabolic process.

Other Associations:

Low blood levels of Apolipoprotein E are associated with an increased risk of developing dementia. Low blood levels reflect low levels of ApoE in the brain which indicate poor removal of beta amyloid plaques. The accumulation of these plaques is one of the factors causing Alzheimer's. Also linked with the later development of Alzheimer's is a poor adult sense of smell. A worse sense of smell in adulthood is associated with neurodegeneration and elevated cortical amyloid as is a thinner entorrhinal cortex and hippocampus.

Frequent general anaesthesia is not a cause of acute or cumulative cognitive damage (assuming the anaesthetist is competent). Previous concussion and traumatic brain injury are contributory causes of later dementia. Chronic peridontitis is associated with a six fold increase in the rate of cognitive decline. Taking various drugs, possibly including PPIs (via B12 deficiency or amyloid plaque formation?) may contribute to dementia as may various anticholinergic drugs, tricyclic antidepressants, some anti histamines and various anticholinergic treatments for overactive bladder. Benzodiazepines probably do not contribute to dementia development. HRT, surprisingly, reduces grey matter in the Anterior Cingulate Gyrus, Medial Frontal Gyrus, Orbitofrontal Cortex and risks cognitive impairment and dementia in older women (PMID:26974440 PubMed Mar 2016 journal.pone.0150834). Exercise significantly reduces Alzheimer's risk. Progressively deteriorating depression increases dementia incidence in later life more than other patterns of depression.

The baby boomer's healthy diet may have helped reduce vascular dementia but the MIND diet (From the American RUSH University Medical Centre) is one of the best at reducing hypertension, CVD and stroke (Mediterranean Intervention for Neurodegenerative Delay diet), or alternatively it is called the DASH diet: Dietary Approaches to Stop Hypertension but enough with the acronyms. (to misquote Jim Kirk's "Enough with the metaphors".)

The MIND diet has 15 components. 10 brain healthy food groups and 5 unhealthy groups (red meat, butter, margarine, cheese, pastries and sweets etc.) The diet consists of: 3 daily servings of whole grains, a green leafy vegetable plus one other vegetable each day, a glass of wine a day, snack mainly on nuts, have beans every other day, eat poultry and berries twice a week and fish at least once a week. You **must** also limit the intake of unhealthy foods. The results of sticking to this diet are: lowered Alzheimer's risk (by 53% if you are rigid with the diet ! and 35% if you are a bit more flexible) and a slowing of age related cognitive decline. On the other hand:

The odd and rather disappointing association of ischaemic stroke and dementia was demonstrated with diet fizzy drinks in an Online Stroke paper in April 2017. Almost immediately questions were asked whether the association was actually between over-weight hypertensive unhealthy people trying to lose weight via diet drinks and hence CNS disease. I understand that the association was after adjustment for all other risk factors however.

Gout and raised uric acid levels are also inversely associated with dementia risk! A 24% lowered risk for gout sufferers was found and this was published in the Annals of Rheumatic Diseases in a study on 4/3/15. "The Rotterdam study" of 300,000 people showed an inverse relationship between risk of any type of dementia and previous uric acid levels. Living near a busy road was found to increase the risk of dementia in a 2016 Canadian study. A decade long study of 6.6m people (Lancet Dec 2016) attributed 1:10 of dementia cases in people near busy roads to the proximity. Although there was no asso-ciation with M.S. or Parkinson's, there was a 7% higher risk within 50m of the road, a 4% higher risk 50-100m and a 2% higher risk of dementia 100-200m from a major road. After 200m there was no increased risk. Is this due to gaseous or particulate combustion fumes, pollution from brake and clutch linings, rubber tyres, the road surface itself or due to noise, sleep deprivation or psychological factors associated with traffic?

For 50 years Aluminium consumption has been implicated as a cause of dementia. In late onset Alzheimer's brain Aluminium is higher than in control brains. If work or envi-ronmental exposure has occurred and early onset Alzheimer's follows then brain aluminium is even higher. Recent (2017) research has also demonstrated very high aluminium levels in patients who had died of Alzheimer's. Aluminium is, of course in many containers, tap water, vaccines, deodorants, aluminium foil, cans, cook ware and medicines.

In Britain's "Worst mass poisoning", Camelford in Cornwall had its water supply contaminated by the accidental dumping of 20 tonnes of Aluminium Sulphate into a reservoir in 1988. The authorities, despite levels of Aluminium reaching 3000x the accepted maximum safe level failed to announce the event for16 days. Various acute and chronic symptoms are said to be common within the affected population.

Which worried patient has early Alzheimer's?

A poor sense of smell is, like the one leg balance test, (an ability to balance for <20 secs is associated with various brain abnormalities including microstrokes, dementia and an increased mortality) a marker of minor neurodegeneration and a predictor of early Alzheimer's. Those who have a thinner hippocampus (Hippocampal fissure dila-tation has a predictive accuracy for Alzheimer's of 91%) on CT or MRI may be likely to develop Alzheimer's. "Senior moments", inability to recall names or words and temporary forgetfulness are ubiquitous after the age of 40. This may be exacerbated by the ready availability and our willingness to rely on smart phones and Google for data and facts rather than exercising our prefrontal cortices. But all GPs will have to decide when to investigate "normal forgetfulness" in an anxious patient as a possible early symptom of dementia. Loss of memory especially short term memory, planning and executive function (working memory, reasoning, routine itinerary, timetable and schedule planning, problem solving, organisation and "execution") are symptoms of depression and can be treated by antidepressant medication. Early dementia cognitive dysfunction will not respond to SSRIs or TCADs. In the Aging Demographics Study and Alzheimer's Disease Neuroimaging initiative (2015), it was found that declining reconstructive memory (recalling an event by piecing together clues about its meaning) and recollective memory (recalling a word or event exactly) were different in significance. Loss of reconstructive memory implied cognitive impairment (the inability to work things out from clues about its meaning) and thus implied early dementia. Declines in simple recollective memory were a simple consequence of aging and bore no greater significance. Phew.

Mini Mental State Examination: (Folstein et Al) (Can download as a PDF from various internet sources)

Orientation: Get patient to describe where they are, what is the date. Score both out of 5

5

Memory: Name 3 common objects and repeat words* said by the tester, Score out of 3
Attention/Calculation: Take 7 from 100, repeated, spelling 5 letter words backwards. Out of 5
Recall (the words given earlier*) 3
Name a watch, pencil, notepad etc. 2
Repeat a brief phrase ("No ifs ands or buts") 1
Reading and Writing. Show the written: "Close your eyes" etc. and ask to do what it says. 1
Ask to write a short sentence. 1
3 Stage command: i.e. Take this paper, fold it and put it in your pocket/bag 3
Copy two overlapping pentagons. 1

30

Bear in mind the obfuscating factors of hearing, eyesight, illiteracy, physical disability, depression, culture and language.

Normal scores are related to age and years of education. Thus:

Age 60-64	years of education 0-4	abnormal cut off score 19
	13	26
65-69	0-4	18
	13+	27
70-74	0-4	19
	13+	25
75-79	0-4	17
	13+	25
80-84	0-4	16
	13+	25
85+	0-4	14
	13+	24

You can see how remarkably consistent and persistent the beneficial effects of education on cerebral function are.

Diagnosis is based on cognitive impairment, long and short term memory affected, plus at least one cortical cognitive deficit – dysphasia, dyspraxia, agnosia, disturbance in executive functioning, (planning, organising "sequencing"). Also the patient has to have impairment of social and occupational functioning and a significant decline from previous levels.

A score of 20 (or above in the educated) could indicate dementia, acute confusional states, schizophrenia, severe depression.

Dementia: Investigations:

FBC, (RBC), ESR, U and Es, Ca, LFT, B12, Niacin, Ferritin, GGT, TFTs, Gluc, Folate, Syphilis serology-TPHA, VDRL, HIV plus or minus CXR, MSU, ECG, ?? Brain scan, etc

Causes: Various drugs, infections, subdural, (if head injury or headache), hypercalcaemia?, Niacin (Vit B3) deficiency, alcohol, vascular etc.

Drug causes of Alzheimer's?:

A report in 2015 highlighted the increased risk of dementia that **certain common treatments** "Taken by 20% of the adult population" posed: These included:

Anticholinergic drugs (ironic since "anticholinergics" are a treatment class of drug too.)

Antihistamines (Including OTC sleep aids) including Diphenhydramine, Chlorpheniramine,

Oxybutynin, Tolterodine,

TCADs, Doxepin, Amitriptyline, even at low doses. There was a clear Dose: Risk of developing dementia relationship.

(JAMA Internal Medicine Online, 26 Jan 2015) – Other drugs under suspicion are commonly prescribed hypnotic drugs, even for relatively short periods.

Dementia

Treatment   Donepezil, Aricept, reduces disturbed behaviour.
Rivastigmine, Exelon.
Galantamine, Reminyl.
Memantine, Ebixa.

Some studies show alternative treatments such as Vitamin E (2000 IUs/day) and C, Folic Acid, Vitamins B6, B12 and Alpha Lipoic Acid reduce the symptoms of Alzheimer's. Some of these are said to work by reducing homocysteine levels or by reducing B Amyloid.

Solanezumab is said to show very promising results perhaps compatible with stabilising the disease process if taken early? (July 2015).

Vitamin E comes in 8 forms. alpha, beta, gamma and delta tocopherol and tocotrienol. In a 2010 paper (J Alzh Dis 2010:20 (4)) the patients with the highest levels of Vitamin E were found to have the lowest risk of Alzheimer's, 45% lower than those with the lowest levels. If you want to supplement with the vitamin, the delta form has other theoretical neurological benefits protecting against stroke too.

Multi infarct:

Ischaemia score: (Differentiates Vascular Dementia from Alzheimer's):
Abrupt onset 2
Stepwise deterioration 1
Fluctuating course 2
Nocturnal confusion 1
Relative preservation of personality 1

Depression 1
Somatic complaints 1
Emotional incontinence 1
History of hypertension 1
History of strokes 2
Evidence of associated atherosclerosis 1
Focal neurological symptoms 2
Focal neurological signs 2
If total = 6 or more then diagnosis is probably vascular dementia if 4 or less probably Alzheimer's. Some cases are mixed.

In the healthy population "normal" cognitive decline is already apparent by the age of 45. >65 years, 8% have dementia and 1%/year get Alzheimer's. If they have mild cognitive impairment, 12-15%/year develop Alzheimer's. **By 90 years 40% have dementia.** The mean survival is 7 years from diagnosis.

Dementia is a syndrome, there being various causes-Alzheimer's is responsible for 60%, Lewy-Body Dementia 15%. Other diagnoses include: Parkinson's Disease Dementia, Fronto-Temporal Degeneration, Progressive Supranuclear Palsy, Cortico Basal Degeneration, Vascular and so on. Lots of other diseases can cause dementia – Prion diseases, (though some believe that Alzheimer's is a prion disease too), Metabolic Diseases, HIV, Wernicke, Encephalitis etc.

In Alzheimer's:

Dementia is in 2 or more areas of cognition, with progressive worsening of memory and cognition, with no specific detectable cause. There is medial Temporal lobe atrophy, abnormal CSF biomarker, low amyloid B 142, increased TAU, a specific PET Pattern and **Hippocampal atrophy.**(An early CT marker of Alzheimer's). As mentioned, there is a gradual increase in amyloid accumulation in brain and this is probably present 10-20 yrs before the dementia.

Vascular Dementia: Evidence of at least 2 CVAs and probably vastly overdiagnosed. Abrupt, stepwise, personality relatively preserved.

Lewy Body Dementia (D.L.B., dementia with Lewy bodies) and Parkinson's Disease Dementia are the same condition. Lewy Body Dementia shows fluctuating cognition, visual hallucinations, mild Parkinsonism though tremor is rare. Repeated falls, syncope and transient loss of consciousness, neuroleptic sensitivity, systematised delusions. Note Medial Temporal Lobe Atrophy is common in Alzheimer's but not DLB.

In **Fronto – Temporal Lobar Degeneration (Pick's disease)** there is disinhibition, depression, aggression etc. This is rare but instead of the memory going first, as it does in Alzheimer's it is the personality, behaviour, emotions and language that go first with loss of control over a variety of basic functions too.

Treatment of Alzheimer's and other dementias:

Biopsychosocial treatments, Acetylcholinesterase inhibs ACHE I and Memantine: no impact on disease process, cholinergic deficit theory, they increase synaptic acetyl choline. Some cognitive improvement. Now used in mild and moderate AD. Can cause bradycardia, nausea, loss of appetite. The drugs are Donepezil, Rivastigmine, Galantamine, – Memantine has fewer cardiac S/Es. Memantine works differently to Donepezil etc and can be co-prescribed.

Vascular dementia Rx:

Don't use the above drugs unless the patient has AD as well as Vascular Dementia.

Risperidone has a licence for aggressive behaviour in PD and dementias but increased incidence of CVAs – but what else can you practically do???? – Quetiapine?

Haloperidol and Olanzapine have often have to be used as mood stabilisers in disturbed demented patients out of sheer practicality.

Alternative treatments:

B vitamins help improve mild cognitive impairment due to effects of lowering homocysteine levels. So try folic acid, B12 & B6, as these can show a significant improvement in memory at 2 yrs and decline in rate of brain atrophy.

Fish oil has been shown to reduce loss of hippocampal and cerebral cortex grey matter with improved cognitive function. The effect is more pronounced in patients who are not carriers of the apolipoprotein E4 gene which has been linked to Alzheimer's.

Some studies show Alzheimer's dementia is reduced by Vitamins E and C and by reducing Homocysteine as above. Also Alpha Lipoic Acid may reduce amyloid deposits (this is available in food stores and on the Internet). This is an interesting supplement which is said to have multiple beneficial effects, not just in preventing amyloid build up but also in the treatment of MS, ED, Metabolic Syndrome, cardiovascular disease, migraine and so on.

The level of AGEs, – Advanced Glycation End Products in the diet is associated with the development of Alzheimer's Disease.(Journal of Alzheimer's Disease, reporting Mount Sinai research Jan 2015). They bind to the AGE receptor that transports Beta Amyloid through the BBB and contribute to the development of the disease. AGEs are present if food is cooked at high temperatures or stored long periods. The main AGE sources are meat, vegetable oils, cheese and fish. The research seemed to suggest that more undercooked food and soft cheeses (etc) in the diet lower the long term risk of dementia development.

T.I.A./Stroke:

There was a national campaign to encourage patients to seek help soon (FAST) Facial weakness, Arm weakness, Speech, problems, and call (Telephone) 999 in 2013/4.

Various treatable and preventable factors influence stroke risk: Ischaemic stroke can make up as many as 87% of the total and may be thrombotic or embolic but haemorrhagic strokes cause more than 30% of stroke deaths. Haemorrhagic strokes may be subarachnoid or the commoner intracerebral. This latter is usually associated with hypertension. Subarachnoid haemorrhage is associated with a burst aneurysm. This causes the sudden extreme headache symptom.

In terms of risk factors, hypertension is well known, those with blood pressures consistently below 120/80 have the lowest lifetime risk of stroke. Impaired glucose tolerance, increased insulin resistance, low HDL, high triglycerides, raised fibrinogen, raised LDL, arrhythmias, sleep apnoea, migraine, family history, race (Afro Caribbeans), depression, taking NSAIDs and antidepressants together in the first few weeks of combined treatment and a tendency to prolonged sleep, (lying in during the mornings) as well as raised CRP levels may all be associated with or contribute toward stroke. Ischaemic strokes increase when the clocks go forward, (8% higher in the first two days after. Patients with cancer have a 25% increase related to clocks going forward), the risk slightly modified by increasing water, melatonin and magnesium intake. In 2016 reflux medication was implicated: (Am Heart Assn Scientif. Sessions. T Sehested et Al) a Danish nationwide observational study was presented which showed a link between ischaemic stroke and all four PPIs investigated. No association with H2 antagonists was shown. In terms of stroke causation: PPIs affect Nitric Oxide production and thus endothelial function but this was the first study suggesting a link to ischaemic stroke.

In terms of stroke prevention:

Actively managing the blood pressure reduces the stroke risk, giving 800ug Folic Acid daily which reduces Homocysteine levels (optimal is <8umol/li) (the China Stroke Prevention Trial 2008-2013) – lowered the patient's first ischaemic stroke incidence or Vitamin C (haemorrhagic stroke, AAN 66th AGM May 2014), or Omega 3 Fatty Acid, EPA (reduces intracranial haemorrhage), statins, the Mediterranean diet, olive oil, Nattokinase, Carnitine, Vitamin D, flavonoids, increasing dietary magnesium, potassium and calcium all lower stroke risk.

But long working weeks raise stroke risk, an over 55 hour working week increases the risk by 33% compared with a 35-40 hour working week. (it also increases coronary heart disease risk 13%).

TIAs usually resolve within 24 hours but they can presage a damaging stroke and they can have permanent cumulative intellectual and physical effects.

TIA assessment early management and imaging (NICE):

(There is an 80% reduction in stroke if the patient is seen, investigated and treated in 24hrs rather than 4 weeks.)

People with TIA – assessment, early management and imaging

- Start daily aspirin (300 mg) immediately.

- Introduce measures for secondary prevention as soon as the diagnosis is confirmed, including discussion of individual risk factors.

- Assess risk of subsequent stroke as soon as possible using a validated scoring system[a] such as ABCD^2.

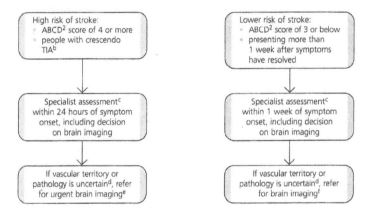

High risk of stroke:
- ABCD^2 score of 4 or more
- people with crescendo TIA[b]

Specialist assessment[c] within 24 hours of symptom onset, including decision on brain imaging

If vascular territory or pathology is uncertain[d], refer for urgent brain imaging[e]

Lower risk of stroke:
- ABCD^2 score of 3 or below
- presenting more than 1 week after symptoms have resolved

Specialist assessment[c] within 1 week of symptom onset, including decision on brain imaging

If vascular territory or pathology is uncertain[d], refer for brain imaging[f]

- Use diffusion-weighted MRI for brain imaging, except where contraindicated. For these people use CT scanning.

---

[a] These scoring systems exclude certain populations that may be at particularly high risk of stroke, such as those with recurrent TIAs and those on anticoagulation treatment, who also need urgent evaluation. They also may not be relevant to patients who present late.
[b] Two or more TIAs in a week.
[c] Specialist assessment includes exclusion of stroke mimics, identification of vascular treatment, identification of likely causes, and appropriate investigation and treatment.
[d] Examples of where brain imaging is helpful in the management of TIA are listed in the NICE guideline (section 1.2.1).
[e] Within 24 hours of symptom onset, in line with the National Stroke Strategy.
[f] Within 1 week of symptom onset, in line with the National Stroke Strategy.

Diagram-NICE Clinical Guideline 68 – People with TIA etc

Unlikely to be a TIA:

Altered consciousness, collapse, seizure, vertigo with no associated neurological features, transient global amnesia.

ABCD2 Score: (A management tool for ? TIA)

Age >60 1 point,

BP >140 and/or >90mm Hg 1 point,

Clinical Features: Unilateral weakness 2 points,

Isolated speech disturbance 1 point,

Duration 60 mins+ 2 points,

10-59 mins 1 point,

Diabetes 1 point,

Score: 1-3 TIA clinic in 7 days, 4-5 TIA Clinic in 24 hrs, 6-7 refer to medic on call to consider admission and TIA clinic next day. If patient has ongoing symptoms admit as a CVA.

Note: TIA Give aspirin 300mg/day (-that is basically everyone) for 2 weeks then 75mg daily. Also +/- dipyridamole 200mg bd. Warfarin (or NOAC) if in AF. If sudden onset of neuro sympts. exclude hypo and image/admit ASAP. (for Alteplase).

Investigation on the day:

CT or MRI Brain, Carotid Dopplers, ECG, CXR, Gluc, lipids, U and Es, creat, FBC clotting, ESR, CRP.

Later:

Ambulatory ECG, ?Echocardiogram, ?Bubble contrast echo in younger patients.

Alternatively: **Investigations for T.I.A.s/C.V.A.s.**

In young adults:

Homocysteine, Cardiolipin antibodies, Lupus anticoagulant, Factor 8 assay, Fibrinogen level, ESR, Glucose, Cholesterol, Tg, Treponema Pallidum serology, ANCA (Antineutrophil Cytoplasmic Antibodies, associated with GPA and MPA rare auto-immune vasculitides).

Emergency Treatment of Acute Stroke (NICE)

Emergency treatment for people with acute stroke

Brain imaging should be performed immediately
for people with acute stroke
if any of the following apply:
indications for thrombolysis or early
anticoagulation treatment
on anticoagulant treatment
a known bleeding tendency
a depressed level of consciousness (Glasgow Coma
Score below 13) unexplained
progressive or fluctuating symptoms
papilloedema, neck stiffness or fever
severe headache at onset of stroke symptoms.

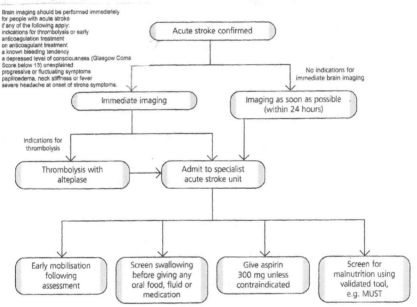

Acute stroke confirmed

No indications for
immediate brain imaging

Immediate imaging

Imaging as soon as possible
(within 24 hours)

Indications for
thrombolysis

Thrombolysis with
alteplase

Admit to specialist
acute stroke unit

Early mobilisation
following
assessment

Screen swallowing
before giving any
oral food, fluid or
medication

Give aspirin
300 mg unless
contraindicated

Screen for
malnutrition using
validated tool,
e.g. MUST

Specialist stroke units

* Admit anyone with a suspected stroke directly to a specialist acute stroke unit[a] after assessment, from either the community or A&E.

[a] An acute stroke unit is a discrete area in the hospital that is staffed by a specialist stroke multidisciplinary team. It has access to equipment for monitoring and rehabilitating patients. Regular multidisciplinary team meetings occur for goal setting.

Diagram NICE Guideline 68

Antiplatelet Therapy:

Aspirin 300mg daily 2 weeks,

Clopidogrel 75mg daily,

NICE: Dipyridamole MR 200mg bd added to low dose aspirin for TIA but not stroke.

Aspirin plus Clopidogrel in severe carotid stenosis.

Warfarin if in A.F. (after stroke, delay for 2 weeks, but give straight away after TIA).
Stop antiplatelet treatment when INR 2.0-2.5.

Thrombolysis in Stroke: (Currently early Aspirin, Alteplase).

Treatment inside 3 hours results in 141 fewer patients/1000 dead or dependent. NNT
per successful outcome: 7.1

Exclude from thrombolysis:

Stroke/head trauma in last 3m.

Major surgery in last 14 days.

Previous intracranial haemorrhage.

Use of anticoagulants.

PT>15 secs, Plats <100x10^3,

Gluc <2.7 or >22.2mmol/li,

SBP>185mm Hg or DBP >110mm Hg.

Spontaneously improving symptoms.

Interleukin 1:

Research shows that this cytokine causes considerable collateral damage around the
primary infarct area once a stroke has happened. It may be that an Interleukin 1 blocker
may be administered to stroke patients in the future to reduce the severity of neurological
damage.

Other considerations: Stroke prophylaxis: As well as aspirin and Clopidogrel:?
Perindopril and Indapamide?

New NICE recommendations (Aug 2016) are for heart attack or stroke patients to
receive Ticagrelor for up to 3 years after their initial 12 month dose.

A Fit, a Faint or a Funny Turn?

These three have always been the "Differential Diagnoses" of a loss of normal awareness
usually leading to some sort of collapse. Funny turns cover everything from panic attacks,
arrhythmias, convulsions and hypotension to behaviour disorders and hypoglycaemic
attacks. We have to clarify all these when patients, especially children, do something
odd with their consciousness that spooks themselves or their parents. Every lecturer on
the subject tries to help us differentiate between the three but given that people who
have simple hypotension, hypoglycaemia or faints frequently have a brief generalised
convulsion, that all sorts of arrhythmias can result in hypoxia and convulsions, it can be
very complicated teasing out what was the chicken and what the egg. Are there absolute
differentiating clues as to a primary cause?

If there is no warning, the cause could be either circulatory or a seizure.

A rapid recovery tends to point to a circulatory cause, patients who have suffered a
seizure take a while to recover.

Incontinence can take place during a faint or a fit.

Faints don't take place lying or sitting (generally).

In paediatric referral clinics for "Syncope" (fits, faints, funny turns, falls), rough outcomes might be:

A quarter have genuine epilepsy (average age at onset 5 yrs).

"Syncope" as defined by a sudden drop in cerebral blood flow or oxygenation, which is often associated with a "reflex anoxic seizure" – make up around 40-45% (median age 9 yrs).

In these cases there are often clues in the history (which is otherwise confusing as the "faint" leads to a "fit"). For instance, there may be a trigger such as injury, pain, thwarting, sudden getting up out of bed. Often in children there may have been some sort of activity, – sometimes even "hair care" surprisingly!, or even standing still for a while, an unexpected shock, surprise, exercise, shocking words or ideas, seeing blood etc.

In "Syncope" (faints) there may be an aura, light headedness, visual disturbance, feeling hot, sweaty, nauseated, flushed and half of children who faint go on to have a "reflex anoxic seizure" which is usually benign. Non epileptic syncope can often be interrupted by a bystander and the EEG is normal. The recovery symptoms are pretty unhelpful in differentiating – just as you may get an aura with the prodrome in epilepsy, hypotension and migraine, children after syncopal episodes not primarily caused by epilepsy may recover immediately or have headache, confusion, drowsiness lasting from minutes to hours. Not very helpful.

About a tenth are "psychological", girls more than boys and a median presenting age of 12.

Other causes in this age group include non epileptic pseudo seizures, day dreams, night terrors, migraine, BPPV, ritualistic movements and parental anxiety.

"Unclassified" make up 15% or thereabouts.

Making an early diagnosis and starting antiepileptic treatment early does not beneficially affect the outcome.

Long QT:

The majority of paediatric syncopal cases are benign but warning signs of a more serious aetiology are: syncope related to: a loud noise or shock, to exercise (check the valves), to lying down (?arrhythmia) and syncope with tonic/clonic movements or a family history of sudden death.

Then you must check the QT – in fact the ECG is the essential investigation in paediatric loss of consciousness or suspected fits – long QT being a relatively frequent cause. Long QT (of which there are at least 15 different genetic types) is associated with ventricular arrhythmias, contact with cold water, a positive family history, exercise related deaths, palpitations. Serum potassium and magnesium must be normalised and it can be treated with beta blockers, an indwelling defibrillator and cervical sympathectomy. It is necessary to avoid competitive sports and the huge number of medicines that affect the QT interval. The ULN QTc is 450mSec. (about 11 small squares). This is measured from the start of the Q to the end of the T.

A third of sudden unexpected deaths in childhood are due to myocarditis.

Adults:

The most dangerous cause of sudden LOC in adults is cardiac syncope with a 1 year mortality of 30%. Try not to miss this.

Various tests can be done by the GP to differentiate some of the common causes:

All the usual haematology and chemistry tests, U and Es, Ca, Glucose, Hb A1C, LFTs,

TFTs etc. ECG of course, (12 lead and a long term portable monitor if available). Tests you can do yourself: Getting the patient to adopt a sudden erect posture after squatting. Spinning the patient then suddenly stopping. Suddenly lying the patient down with the head tilted to one side and holding that position (The Dix Hallpike test). The Valsalva test. Getting the patient to hyperventilate for 1 minute.

-See if any of these trigger the symptoms!

In Epilepsy, clues that help are: Aura/Deja Vu (not light headedness), post episode confusion >2mins, post episode headache, tonic clonic movements, tongue biting, incontinence, head turned to one side during the LOC, unresponsiveness during LOC.

Association with prolonged sitting, standing or sweating before the LOC is more likely to be syncope than epilepsy.

In **Narcolepsy and Catalepsy**, 50% patients have a psychiatric diagnosis, there is no LOC in the latter.

Psychiatric conditions: Syncopal patients often have a psychiatric diagnosis but this may not necessarily be the only cause of the syncope. Depression, panic attacks, severe anxiety are common associations. Beware of labelling the patient though – As already mentioned, I had a sad but likeable female patient in her mid thirties who was a severe alcoholic. She was completely incapable of caring for her much loved 10 year old only daughter who was eventually and rightly removed by Social Services. I attended her regularly at home thereafter and then at Case Conferences where she would histrionically collapse and often bang her head or face violently in the process. She clearly did this once too often. Whether or not she had much control over the episodes became blurred with time as one day I called to attend her and she was confused and drowsy and barely rousable. Not assuming she was just drunk (fortunately for me) I admitted her and she had a large subdural evacuated the same day after a CT scan. After that she had clear episodes of focal fitting and her poor mental state was due to a mixture of previous alcoholic damage, cerebral injury and AED medication. This was a case of syncope that was probably initially "psychological" which eventually acquired multiple aetiologies. At one time or other she had some or all of: true fits, probable vaso vagal faints, "funny turns", syncope, anxiety, depression, cerebral structural damage, cerebral oedema, alcohol toxicity and alcohol withdrawal syndrome, some sort of complex psychogenic fainting akin to hysteria and probably undiagnosed contributory metabolic causes for her losses of consciousness. How do you summarise that to an admitting registrar?

Other causes:

Breath Holding: Only in children. TIA, trauma, toxicity etc. Syncope may be Cardiac, Orthostatic, Reflex (sudden loss of vaso-motor tone) or Metabolic – low calcium, magnesium, sodium and sugar may all cause syncope. Patients with "High Risk Syncope" (using the "San Francisco Rule"*) tend to have either an abnormal ECG, dyspnoea, low systolic BP, low haematocrit, or signs of CCF.

*The San Francisco Rule:

Mnemonic: CHESS:
Congestive heart failure,
Haematocrit <30,
ECG abnormal,
SOB,
Systolic BP<90mm.

One of these criteria,
Test Sensitivity 96%,
Specificity 62% For 30 day mortality.
(Quinn 2004 Ann. Emerg. Med. 43.224-32)

Epilepsy:

1:20 of us have some sort of seizure at some time but after a single generalised seizure only 1:8 have another. 1:50 have epilepsy. 40% of single vehicle accidents are due to seizures and there is a 40% increased risk of fitting while weaning off AED treatment.

The average GP will see 1-2 cases per year, **only 40% of whom will have abnormal EEGs**. 1000 die each year because of epilepsy in the UK. In any "Fits and Faints" clinic 25% are epileptic in origin. In tertiary referral clinics, 25% patients turn out not to have epilepsy. Surgery is a suitable treatment for only 3%.

Seizure Classification:

Partial: Simple   Motor, Sensory, Autonomic, Cognitive/
                              Dysmnestic

            Complex..........Partial

                             +/– Automatism
            Secondarily generalised   Tonic/Clonic. Tonic. Clonic. Atonic.
Generalised ....Absence, Myoclonic, Tonic/Clonic. Tonic. Clonic. Atonic

There are many non epileptic phenomena that mimic epilepsy, even many "Neurological" conditions – Viz: and Psychological conditions:

TIA   Pseudoseizures (normal pupils, plantars and prolactin)
VBI   Panic attacks
Migraine
Transient Global Amnesia
Narcolepsy/cataplexy
Breath holding
Night terrors etc

and Cardiologically, consider: Metabolically exclude:
Vasovagal faint   Hypoglycaemia
Reflex syncope   Hypocalcaemia
Postural hypotension   Hyperventilation
Arrhythmias   Drugs, therapeutic and otherwise.
Cardiac outflow obstruction.

Investigations:

EEG, MRI/CT, (MRI Is more useful), ECG. Blood Screen etc.

If there is an unprovoked LOC you have no choice but to tell the patient to STOP DRIVING until all the investigations are completed and the neurologist has made a recommendation. **The police always seek a custodial sentence for patients who drive against medical advice.** Record what you have said and tell the patient you have done so. 40% of single vehicle accidents are due to seizures. Most people who start anticonvulsants (AEDS, antiepileptic drugs) stay on them until they are too old to drive as they don't want to stop driving for the 6 months after discontinuing treatment. If the patient is keen you can try to wean off after 2-3 years remission. Stop driving immediately and for 6 months after complete cessation of treatment. Breakthrough seizures after changing drugs: stop driving ?1 year D/W DVLA. Stay on the same trade name anticonvulsant as bioavailability can vary 50%.

Higher risk:

Partial seizures; Cerebral lesion (abnormal scan); Later onset (after childhood); Prolonged active epilepsy; Epileptiform EEG.

Epilepsy in pregnancy:

If pregnant, change the patient from Valproate (etc) to Lamotrigine. (Jan 2015 MHRA advice that up to 40 % of babies given Valproate in utero suffered adverse effects). Pre treat with Folic Acid. The patient can breast feed with all AEDs apart from Phenobarbitone. It is generally considered safer to continue on their AED than to stop treatment and risk harming the pregnancy through drug withdrawal and fits. Ideally the pregnancy should be planned and Folic Acid and a phased transition to a drug such as Lamotrigine considered in advance.

1 anticonvulsant increases congenital abnormalities by	2X
2 anticonvulsants	3X
3 anticonvulsants	4X

Anti-epileptic dose frequency/Levels: (Different sources in brackets)

Phenytoin: Half Life Average 24 hrs. (20-40) Toxic >20-30mcg/ml (Therapeutic 10-20mcg/ml) Peak level 3-9 hrs after oral dose. Single or divided doses. Non linear dose response curve, narrow therapeutic index. Do a level 2 weeks after initiation.

Carbamazepine: Half Life 10-26 hrs.(15-40) Toxic >12mcg/ml. Take sample before next dose. Give BD. Linear dose response. Adults: Increase to 200mg BD over 10 days.

Ethosuximide: Half Life 20-60 hrs. (25-70) Toxic >100mcg/ml. Peak levels 2-4 hrs after trough just before next dose. Can be given once daily.

Phenobarbitone: Half Life 1.5-3 days. (Phenobarbital 50-140 hrs adult, 40-70 hrs child). Toxic >40mcg/ml. Trough prior to and peak 4-12 hrs after dose.

Primidone: Half Life 6-12 hrs. (4-12hrs) Toxic >12mcg/ml. (Therapeutic 5-12mcg/ml adult 7-10mcg/ml child). Given as twice daily doses.

Valproic Acid: Half Life 9-18 hrs in adults, 4-14hrs in children (8-15 hrs). Therapeutic Range 40-100mcg/ml. (50-125mcg/ml). Toxic >100mcg/ml. BD, Little practical value in doing level. Valproic Acid (Convulex) and Sodium Valproate have a 1:1 dose equivalence.

Start dose 600mg/day initially (300mg bd). Increase at 200mg per 3 days, max 2.5Gr/day.

Gabapentin: Half life 5-7 hours, inv proportional to creatinine clearance.

Lamotrigine: Half life 26-32 hours, greatly affected by other AEDs (Valproate extends, many other AEDs shorten half life).

Levetiracetam: Rapidly absorbed after oral dose, peak concentration after 1.3 hours, steady state in 24-48 hrs. Half life in adults 6-8 hours, children 5-7 hours.

Vigabatrin: Not significantly metabolised, renal excretion, half life 10.5 hours for adults, 9.5 hours children. Induces CYP2C9 hepatic enzyme.

Anticonvulsant (etc) Therapeutic Levels:

Lithium 0.6-1.6mmol/li 12 hrs after dose.
Phenobarbitone <170umol/li (65-172umol/li).
Primidone 50umol/li (23-55umol/li)
Carbamazepine <24umol/li (17-51umol/li)
Phenytoin<80umol/li (40-79umol/li)
Sodium Valproate 347-693ug/ml (Valproic Acid 347-866umol/li but "Control of symptoms may be improved at Sodium Valproate levels above 350-690umol/L"). Half Life 8-15 hrs (various sources)
Ethosuximide 283-708umol/li
Lamotrigine 4-16 umol/li

Anticonvulsant dose reduction/day/each month:

Phenytoin 50mg
Phenobarbital 15mg
Carbamazepine 100mg
Valproate 200mg
Lamotrigine 25mg
Gabapentin 400mg
Vigabatrin 500mg
Topiramate 25mg
Clonazepam 0.5mg
Clobazam 10mg
Ethosuximide 250mg

Newer Anticonvulsants: AEDs

Gabapentin, Neurontin: Monotherapy or add on therapy in partial seizures with or without secondary generalisation. Titrate up to 1200-2400mg/day.

Lamotrigine, Lamictal: Initially 25mg daily for 2 weeks maintenance dose up to 200mg/day in 1 or 2 doses. Lower starting dose if on Valproate, interacts with COCP (which reduces the effectiveness of Lamotrigine) and is affected by pregnancy. Lamotrigine works in all epilepsies and probably has the fewest overall side effects.

If pregnant, change the patient from Valproate to Lamotrigine. Pre treat with Folic Acid. The patient can probably breast feed with all AEDs apart from Phenobarbitone.

Levetiracetam, Keppra. Monotherapy or adjunct in partial seizures also adjunct in generalised and juvenile myoclonic epilepsy.

Vigabatrin Sabril. Serious adverse effects on mood and visual fields. Infantile spasms and partial seizures, in adults intolerant of other drugs.

Complex partial seizures:

Episodes of impaired consciousness arising from one region of the brain. The patient is unable to communicate, respond or later recall the event. Usually based in the temporal lobe, they may actually arise in any part of the cortex. The episodes may be associated with automatisms (finger or facial movements or even whole limb movements etc) or semi purposeful activity including verbalisation or even speech. There may be a preliminary aura, the nature of which depends on where the lesion is **(Occipital would be a visual aura, Temporal a sense of deja vu or fear, Parietal tingling or numbness etc)**. Next the patient stares, with or without the various bodily movements and then is unaware of the episode or their surroundings for thirty seconds to two or so minutes.

All forms of cerebral damage/inflammation/neonatal damage/neoplastic process or none can cause complex partial seizures. Prolonged febrile convulsions are a risk factor. Some patients may have an episode and appear virtually normal to those around them, simply having lost a few minutes and not knowing how they got from one place to another.

Many patients have temporal lobe epilepsy and "Mesial Temporal Lobe Sclerosis" on MRI. A high proportion actually turn out to have psychogenic (non epileptic) episodes (30%).

Virtually any AED can be tried.

AEDs in pregnancy

Lamotrigine.

There is little teratogenic difference between Valproate, Carbamazepine, Phenobarbitone, Phenytoin, Ethosuximide and Clonazepam although most sources suggest avoiding Valproate in pregnancy. One approach in pregnancy is Carbamazepine with Folic Acid and this is supposed to give the background rate of foetal abnormality.

Typical general epilepsy treatment approaches:

Valproate IS a good first line in most forms of epilepsy, so are Lamotrigine, Carbamazepine in focal epilepsy.

Idiopathic Generalised epilepsies		Localised-related epilepsies	
First line	Valproate Lamotrigine in young women	Carbamazepine Lamotrigine in young women	
Second line (First Rank)	Lamotrigine Topiramate Clonazepam	Topiramate Lamotrigine Levetiracetam	
Second Rank	Clobazam	Clobazam Tiagabine Gabapentin Oxcarbazepine	
Third line	Piracetam	Phenytoin Phenobarbital Acetazolamide Primidone	

or in terms of the epilepsies themselves: (Drs A Sturrock Charles Cockerell, The Prescriber June 2006)

	Generalised Tonic/ Clonic	Absence	Atonic or Tonic	Myoclonic
First Line	Valproate Lamotrigine Topiramate	Ethosuximide Lamotrigine Valproate	Lamotrigine Valproate	Valproate
Second Line	Clobazam	Clobazam	Clobazam	Clobazam

(First rank)	Levetiracetam	Clonazepam Topiramate	Clonazepam Levetiracetam Topiramate	Clonazepam Lamotrigine Levetiracetam Piracetam Topiramate
Second Line (Second rank)	Acetazolamide Clonazepam Phenobarbital Phenytoin		Acetazolamide Phenobarbital Primidone Tonic-Phenytoin	

Latest advice (My thanks to The Prescriber Magazine for permission to reproduce this)

Epilepsy: (2012)

	Focal seizures with or without Secondary generalisation	Myoclonus	Generalised seizures
First line	Carbamazepine Lamotrigine Levetiracetam	Clonazepam Levetiracetam Valproate	Lamotrigine Levetiracetam Valproate
Second Line	Alternative first line therapy or Lacosamide Oxcarbazepine Topiramate Zonisamide	Alternative first line therapy or Lamotrigine Topiramate (avoid Carbamazepine, Gabapentin, Oxcarbazepine Pregabalin)	Alternative first line therapy or Topiramate

Drugs Not to Use

Generalised Tonic/Clonic: Tiagabine, Vigabatrin.

Absences: Carbamazepine, Gabapentin, Oxcarbazepine, Vigabatrin, Tiagabine.

Myoclonic epilepsy: Carbamazepine, Gabapentin, Oxcarbazepine, Pregabalin, Tiagabine, Vigabatrin.

Head Injury:

Refer to hospital if:

Glasgow Coma Score>15; LOC; Focal neurological deficit; Suspected Skull #; Penetrating head injury; Amnesia before or after; Headache or vomiting since injury; Any seizure; Any previous head surgery; High energy injury; Warfarin; Bleeding disorder; Intoxication; NAI; >65yrs; Irritability/altered behaviour; Post traumatic drug prophylaxis with Phenytoin.

Head Injury - Advice for Parents and Carers

This leaflet is to help to advise on how best to care for a child who has a bump / injury to the head. Please use the "Caring for your child at home" advice section (see overleaf) and the traffic light advice below to help you. **Most children can be managed according to the green guidance below especially if they are alert and interacting with you.** It is important to watch the child for the next 2-3 days to ensure that they are responding to you as usual.

Head wounds rarely need stitches and can normally be glued by a health professional. This can be done in Minor Injury Units or Urgent Treatment Centres and some GP practices offer a minor injuries service. To find a local service see overleaf.

Traffic light advice:

Green: Low Risk	Amber: Intermediate Risk	Red: High Risk
If your child:	**If your child:**	**If your child:**
• Cried immediately (after head injury) but returns to their normal behaviour in a short time	• Is under one year old	• Has been involved in a high speed road traffic accident or fallen from a height over 1 metre or been hit by a high speed object or involved in a diving accident
• Is alert and interacts with you	• Has vomited once or twice	• Has been unconscious / "knocked out" at any time
• Has not been unconscious / "knocked out"	• Has a continuous headache	• Is sleepy and you cannot wake them
• Has minor bruising, swelling or cuts to their head	• Has continued irritation or unusual behaviour	• Has a convulsion or a fit
	• Is under the influence of drugs or alcohol	• Has neck pain
	• Has been deliberately harmed and in need of medical attention	• Has difficulty speaking or understanding what you are saying
		• Has weakness in their arms and legs or are losing their balance
		• Cannot remember events around or before the accident
ACTION: If all the above have been met then **manage at home**. Follow the advice overleaf or, if you are concerned, contact your GP when they are open or call 111 when your GP surgery is not open	ACTION: Take your child to the nearest **Hospital Emergency department** if ANY of these features are present	• Has had clear or bloody fluid dribbling from their nose, ears or both since the injury
		• Has 3 or more separate bouts of vomiting
		ACTION: **Phone 999** for an ambulance if ANY of these symptoms are present

Based on: Head Injury - Triage, assessment, investigation and early management of head injury in children, young people and adults. January 2014. NICE clinical guideline 176

Paediatric Head injury Leaflet Insert

Glasgow Coma Score: GCS
(Max 15 is healthy)
Eye opening:
Spontaneously 4
To speech 3
To pain 2
None 1
Verbal response:
Orientated 5
Confused 4
Inappropriate 3
Incomprehensible 2
None 1
Motor Response
Obeys commands 6
Localises to pain 5
Withdraws from pain 4
Flexion to pain 3
Extension to pain 2
None 1
Mild 13-15, Moderate 9-12, Severe 3-8.
Post traumatic amnesia: Generally:
Mild: less than 24 hrs. Moderate: 1-7 days. Severe: 7+ days.

Meningitis:

Acute Bacterial Meningitis: – and see (Infections and Immunisations for greater detail):

Meningococcal Meningitis:

Rx: 50mg/kg Penicillin G (Benzyl Penicillin),

Immediate Rx   >10yrs 1.2Gr Penicillin,

1-10yrs 600mg,

Infant 300mg. All Stat.

If genuinely allergic to penicillin, IV Chloramphenicol can be given. I carry Cefuroxime as the wait to get a purpuric child to hospital for IV second line antibiotics is worth the miniscule risk of allergy to cephalosporins. Of people who think they are allergic to penicillin 10% actually are – and of these, 5-10% have a cross-reaction to cephalosporins. Meningococcal meningitis kills within minutes and whenever I have seen a drowsy or febrile child with a probable purpuric rash I take a sample of blood into a syringe, put the penicillin back through the same needle (or butterfly/venflon) followed by a bolus of Hydrocortisone. After giving the drugs you bend the needle attached to the syringe (if you have used a syringe and IV needle) back on itself using the plastic sheath then push the sheath over the bent needle. Be *very careful* to avoid a needlestick injury while doing this. I have never met a GP who had in-date blood culture bottles in his or her bag – do you? These unfortunate patients die of septicaemia and adrenal shock. The paediatric SHO will put the blood sample into a blood culture bottle from your syringe if he or she knows what they are doing or a sharps bin if they don't. There are plenty of those sort of junior doctors. Dial 999 first, don't bother waiting for the interminable switchboard and registrar to answer the phone before you have transport organised.

Meningococcal prophylactic Antibiotics:

To eradicated nasal carriage of the N Meningitidis, give to all household contacts, family and non family, all people who sleep near the index case (dormitories etc), girl/boy friend (kissing), school children in contact >4 hrs in an enclosed space, healthcare staff who may have had exposure to respiratory droplets, (this is arbitrarily quoted as within 3 feet but would you risk 4 feet or 6 or 10?) Also the index case will need prophylaxis unless already treated with Ceftriaxone (to eradicate nasal carriage). Ceftriaxone has particularly high nasal and saliva penetration and so eradicates the *significant* infection as well as the carriage.

In all groups including the pregnant:

Ciprofloxacin orally: Adults 500mg one dose stat, Children 5-12 yrs 250mg stat, 1month – 4 years 125mg stat.

Alternatively:

Rifampicin orally: Adults 600mg BD 2days, Children 1-12 yrs 10mg/kg (max 600mg) BD 2days, Neonates and infants <1 yr 5mg/kg BD 2days.

Prophylaxis of meningococcal meningitis in pregnant contact: Ceftriaxone 250mg IM stat (one dose) – not licensed so the patient needs to be "counselled".

Things you may have forgotten:

The childhood immunisation regime (which see) now includes vaccination against Haemophilus, 13 serotypes of Pneumococcus, Group B Meningococcus,

Meningococcus C,A,W and Y. Some of these were the scourges that kept we Paediatricians and GPs awake all night in the 70's and 80's and did, with bacterial croup so much harm to children. They have all plummeted in frequency as a consequence of new immunisations and on call GP and Paediatrics is thankfully very different today.

Meningococcal: Under 2 years Group B infections predominate but between 14 and 18 years Group C is more prevalent, occurring in more clusters.

So: Group B is 2/3 of total disease. Group C is 1/3 of the total disease, (school age children, young adults). Group A <2% UK disease. Routine Group A vaccination used not to be generally recommended in the UK because of the strains and low incidence in the at risk age groups. In Africa most Meningococcal Meningitis is Group A. Meningitis vaccinations are all capsular polysaccharide vaccines and all are recommended in Asplenia.

H.Influenzae: There are 6 types but 99% of human disease is B. Of the total infections, 60% were meningitis, 15% were epiglottitis (they *were,* pre vaccination). The vaccine is effective over the age of 2m and after 3 doses. Recommendations: <13 months 3 doses. In Asplenia and 13-48 months, 1 dose.

Pneumococcal: Strep pneumoniae vaccine: Covers 80% UK strains, *relatively* ineffective less than 2 yrs of age, prevents 60-70% pneumococcal pneumonia but less effective against meningitis. 5 yearly vaccination of at risk population.

Haemophilus Influenzae b Meningitis:

Prophylaxis is Ciprofloxacin, Ceftriaxone or Rifampicin (See above):

Pneumococcal Meningitis:

Strep. Pneumoniae is carried nasally in up to 10% of healthy adults and up to 40% of healthy children. Various Co Factors make an aggressive infection more likely: asplenia, HIV, flu, smoking, (in the family), COPD etc. It is second commonest in the UK to meningococcal meningitis. It is vaccinated against as part of the routine childhood vaccination program now.

Treatment: The strep. used always to be penicillin sensitive though this is not now *always* the case. If you don't have time for sensitivities (which presumably, treating suspected meningitis or pneumonia, you won't) try:

Vancomycin and Cephalosporins, Levofloxacin. Possible high dose Penicillin and an Erythromycin group antibiotic (ie a macrolide).

Viral Meningitis:

Viruses are the cause of 75% meningitis.

Mumps 15-50% (epidemics). A leading cause of acquired deafness (Rare in the MMR vaccinated).
Echoviruses 25%,
Coxsackie viruses 35%,
Herpes viruses 5%,
Adenovirus 5%,
Others.

Huntington's Chorea (Disease)

At medical school I learned about Sydenham's chorea (St. Vitus' Dance) which affects some people with Rheumatic fever. The physician it is named after was British: Thomas Sydenham who was born in 1624 – although I thought it was named after the London borough. St Vitus is the patron saint of dancers by the way. Most sufferers who develop this kind of chorea get better. Not so with the far more sinister and progressive Huntington's Chorea, named after an American physician who described it in 1872 – and not the Cambridgeshire town (as I always thought) that sounds like it but has a "d" not a "t".

Huntington's is an Autosomal Dominant condition which, usually presenting in adult life, about 40-50 years of age, is a Damocles sword hanging over members of affected families.

New mutations, where neither parent is affected, are rare.

The underlying problem is an accidental multiple repeat of 3 bases coded for on chromosome 4. This produces the abnormal and neurotoxic protein. The more repeats, the worse the condition.

It affects 1:10,000 people of European Heritage. Some cases present below 20 years with "Juvenile Huntington's Disease".

The first symptoms can be emotional changes or can affect cognition, gait, coordination and then chorea, mental and psychiatric disorders follow. Dysphagia is common, as are speech difficulties. Facial and other movements become more and more uncontrollable and mental function deteriorates unpredictably. Subsequent psychiatric and behavioural problems can be particularly distressing.

There is really only supportive treatment although various new therapies are being assessed. These include gene and stem cell treatments as well as conventional drugs of various kinds. There is gene testing (generally not done under the age of 18 unless the patient is sexually active and "Gillick competent") and antenatal testing.

Most of these unfortunate patients currently live 15-20 years after the onset of the disease symptoms and eventually die of heart failure or pneumonia and possibly, sadly, suicide.

Facial Pain: (See cluster headache)

Trigeminal Neuralgia:

Cervical N2 and the Trigeminal N share sensory innervation of the face, so facial pain can be due to cervical root irritation as much as trigeminal based pain, migraine, atypical facial pain and so on. There are many causes. All unpleasant, some extremely.

Facial pain can be treated by:

Gabapentin (300-1800mg/day), Amitriptyline, Lamotrigine, Pregabalin, (150-600mg/day).

Diabetic neuropathic pain can respond to the above as well as Gamma Linoleic Acid which is supposed to be anti inflammatory and present in various dietary oils. It is unusual amongst the Omega 6 polyunsaturated fatty acids in having an anti cancer effect too. Other treatments include: Mexiletine (an anti arryhthmic), Tramadol and Duloxetine (Cymbalta or Yentreve depending on whether the patient has anxiety or stress incontinence as well as the facial pain!) etc.

Things you may have forgotten:

Upper and lower motor neuron(e) s:

Upper motor neuron(e) s originate in the motor cortex (precentral gyrus), travel into the brainstem, cross to the opposite side in the medulla, then to the lateral corticospinal tract or continue as the anterior corticospinal tract and thence on down to the appropriate spinal nerve root where they synapse with the lower motor neuron(e). Glutamate is the neurotransmitter between the two neuron(e) s.

The Lower motor neuron(e) s connect the UMN synapse which is in the spinal cord ventral horn to the peripheral effector muscle via the peripheral nerve. LMNs are Alpha (standard muscle contraction) or Gamma (part of the proprioception system). Motor control is, of course contralateral.

Motor Neurone Disease: (ALS)

Although rare (3/100,000), with an average age of onset 63, it is probably feared more than cancer by patients for its ability to rob them of independence and dignity and loss of basic bodily functions. It is of course, inevitable fatal. 50% are dead within 2 1/2 years of onset. Stephen Hawkings (diagnosed aged 21 and therefore a sufferer for 50 years) is very rare indeed – though juvenile onset disease does tend to run a slower course. Most people die of respiratory failure as the phrenic nerve becomes involved. Multiple genes have been identified as potentially causing the accumulation of brain proteins that could be the cause of the disease.

Amyotrophic Lateral Sclerosis is the commonest form, having UMN and LMN degeneration together.

Other forms involving UMNs – Primary Lateral Sclerosis,
LMNs-Progressive Muscular Atrophy and
Bulbar muscles-Progressive Bulbar Palsy also exist.

Amyotrophic Lateral Sclerosis ALS:

Progressive painless weakness is the classic presentation but initially at any rate this presentation can be shared by at least thirty or forty diverse and mostly treatable conditions. These include:

Spinal muscular atrophy, Kennedy's disease, Mitochondrial disease, Radiation Myelopathy, thyrotoxicosis, hyperparathyroidism, lead and mercury poisoning, copper deficiency, Polio, Lyme, HIV, Sjogren's, Gluten sensitivity, Myasthenia, polymyositis, spondylotic myelopathy, base of skull and foramen magnum lesions, cord tumours, radiculopathies, lymphoproliferative disease, etc, etc.

Motor Neurone Disease may present:

As generalised weakness affecting the cervical or lumbar spine,
Lower motor neurone type symptoms affecting the limbs,
Focal onset limb syndromes (weakness in a single limb),
Bilateral leg lower motor neurone type lesions,
Bulbar and cortico-bulbar syndromes – this is about a quarter of the total and they go on to get limb symptoms later, – dysarthria generally starts before dysphagia.

Riluzole, Rilutek, started by a specialist has some disease modifying action on the Amyotrophic Lateral Sclerotic form of MND. Prolongs life by 2-3 months only.

Treating symptoms:

Drooling: Amitryptyline, Hyoscine patches.
Cramp: Quinine, Diazepam.
Spasticity: Baclofen, Tizanidine, Zanaflex.
Thick mucus: Carbocysteine.
Urinary disturbance: Oxybutynin, Amitryptyline.
Respiratory distress: Sublingual Lorazepam.
Terminal Dyspnoea: Morphine, Diamorphine.

Extra pyramidal side effects

(Dystonia, akathisia, Parkinsonism, Tardive Dyskinesia, etc).
can be caused by a long list of drugs including:

Fluphenazine	Paroxetine
Flupent(h) ixol	Carbamazepine
Haloperidol	Methyl Dopa
Trifluoperazine	Lithium
Chlorpromazine	
Sulpiride	
Risperidone	
Metoclopramide	
Proclorperazine	
Amitriptyline	

Tardive Dyskinesia: Rx: Tetrabenazine with a small dose of Haloperidol.

Reserpine, Alpha methyl dopa, Ondansetron, Donepezil, Baclofen, Pramipexol and Clonidine are all said to have some effect in certain circumstances.

Neuropathic Pain, Neuralgia: Diabetic Neuropathy, Reflex Sympathetic Dystrophy, Post Herpetic Neuralgia, Trigeminal Neuralgia etc:

Treatment:

Gabapentin, 300mg on first day, increasing to maximum of 800mg TDS. Avoid sudden withdrawal. Pregabalin. Lacosamide, Vimpat. Also Clonazepam, TCAs (Amitriptyline etc.), Paroxetine, Citalopram, Carbamazepine, Phenytoin, Lamotrigine (very slow titration, as with all the anticonvulsants), Epilim, Venlafaxine, Duloxetine (Cymbalta), Topiramate, Mirtazapine, Topical Capsaicin, -Zacin and Axsain cream.

Neuralgia: Post Herpetic Neuralgia etc.

Lidocaine (Lignocaine), Versatis 5% medicated plasters are effective but you apply up to 3 plasters once day for 12 hours and they cost £72 for 30.

Hypnotics (Non Prescription):

Melotonin: Is used for jet lag and also 3-12mg for Children with ADHD.

Nytol is Diphenhydramine and is a sedative OTC antihistamine.

Melatonin is a fascinating substance, – produced by the Pineal Gland, regulating the body's circadian rhythms, it is an anti oxidant, protecting DNA and therefore having anti cancer properties. Secreted at night, it has been discovered that for instance, blind women have a lower incidence of breast cancer – presumably they secrete more.

Shift work is thought to increase the risk of cancer development (WHO 2007) and working in artificial light lowers melatonin levels by interfering with normal circadian rhythms?

Blue light exposure to the retina suppresses melatonin secretion with all the theoretical disadvantages that may accrue. Yellow spectrum light does not do this. It is a powerful antioxidant, protecting against Parkinson's disease, aging, cancers, dementia, SAD and arrhythmias. The level of Melatonin is lower in patients with Autism and administration of Melatonin (it is an effective resynchroniser of the body clock in jet lag) can cause vivid dreams. So Melatonin has been shown to provide clinical benefit in prostate and breast carcinoma, treating menopausal symptoms, in hypertension and in cardioprotection, in treating the symptoms of fibromyalgia (with or without Fluoxetine), in Jet Lag, in treating Autism and as an immune stimulant.

It would be quite natural if you had a degree of scepticism about such a jack of all trades of a hormone but it **does** seem to work in sleep disorders, especially those associated with ADHD, Jet Lag and shift work and its use in cancer seems at worse harmless and at best promising. It's use, especially in the US has increased exponentially over recent years where 3m adults and half a million children have been taking it. The side effects include day time tiredness, bad dreams, interaction with various other medications including antihypertensives, contraceptives and anticonvulsants.

30: Ophthalmology:

THE ANATOMY OF THE EYE

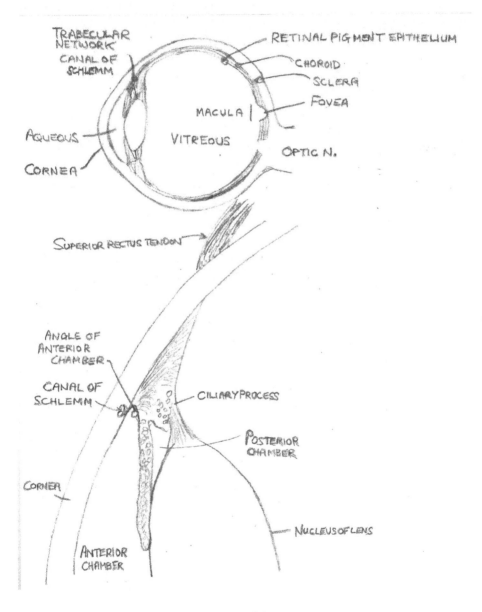

Diagram of the eye.

The Ophthalmoscope:

Stuff you may have forgotten:

The hyperopic (far sighted) eye requires more "plus" black numbers for a clear focus on the retina and the myopic (short sighted) eye requires more "minus" red numbers.

It may be easier to examine a myopic patient with them wearing their glasses.

Use a micro spot aperture if the patient's pupil is constricted and the blue filter if you are using fluorescein.

Commence with a +10 lens as this focuses on the anterior of the lens of the eye. Dial through the lenses towards 0 to bring retina into focus. To check for lens opacities, use a +6 lens and position yourself 6" from the patient.

To find the macula, focus on the disc then move the light 2 disc diameters temporally- or get the patient to look directly at the light. The fovea is in the centre of the macula.

The **Snellen chart**: 6/24 is worse than 6/12 (-you see at 6m what should be clear at 24m).

To elicit the **Red Reflex** (for instance in the newborn) hold the ophthalmoscope 1' away from the eye with a +5 Lens.

Rods and cones: (figures in brackets are from alternative text).

Rods are responsible for low (white) light sensitivity and are more numerous in the retina, at 120m (91m) compared with the 6m (4.5m) colour sensitive cones in the retina. (m=million)

The Macula (the yellow central area) is rich in cones and uncovered by blood vessels – unlike the rest of the retina. The centre of the Macula has the Fovea Centralis which is rod free but packed with cones. Acuity is sharp thanks to these cones but limited to a few degrees either side of the target zone (less than 6^0 away the acuity drops 75%).

Conversely, light sensitivity is much better using the rods surrounding the Fovea and that is why it is better to look to the side of a dim object such as two close stars at night to differentiate them.

The primary colours of pigments (absorbed colours) are red, blue and yellow but cones are sensitive to the "primary colours of light" (discovered by James Clerk Maxwell) which are red, blue and green.

Field Defects:

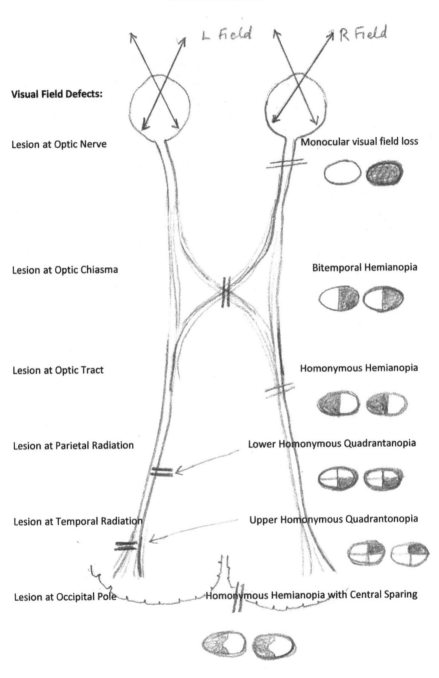

Diagram of Eye and Fields (See Neurology)

Peripheral scotoma (tunnel vision): Retinal disease including retinitis pigmentosa, glaucoma.

Central scotoma: MS, hypertension, drugs, retrobulbar neuritis, (MS), optic atrophy-toxins, B12 deficiency or compression, migraine (scintillating scotomata).

Complete Field loss: Optic N damage.

Homonymous Hemianopia, tract lesions posterior to the chiasma.

Homonymous quadrantonopia: Anteriorly placed lesions in the optic radiation (eg Temporal lobe tumours).

Glaucoma: POAG: Nasal step, arcuate scotoma, general field depression, peripheral field loss before central, tunnel vision, blindness.

Quadrantic hemianopia, temporal lobe lesions. (Parietal = lower quadrantic).

Scintillating scotomata can be benign, associated with migraine, but scotoma may presage preeclampsia or severe hypertension.

Refer to hospital the same day:

Chemical injuries,

Unexplained sudden loss of vision,

Penetrating Injuries,

H. Zoster with Hutchinson's sign – Involvement of the tip of the nose, supposedly indicating a severe eye infection,

Dacrocystitis,

Hyphaema, (blood in the anterior chamber),

Hypopyon, (pus in the anterior chamber),

Keratitis with red eye,

Periorbital inflammation with pain and swelling,

Pulsating proptosis (exclude caroticocavernous fistula, Neurofibromatosis, AV malformation, # orbital roof, arachnoid cyst),

Corneal Foreign Bodies (unless you are skilled at removing them with local anaesthetic drops and a cotton bud or sterile needle tip),

Acute flashes and floaters with tobacco dust (pigment in the anterior vitreous),

Vitreous Haemorrhage,

Central Retinal Artery Occlusion (In 6 hours),

Retinal tears,

Retinal detachment,

Temporal Arteritis (initiate treatment and investigations),

Uveitis,

Wet maculopathy,

Metamorphopsia (distorted vision, wavy horizontal grids and blank areas) usually associated with macular degeneration,

Papilloedema/3rd N palsy (Neurosurgery),

Acute Glaucoma,

New BVs at disc or anywhere else, in diabetes particularly.

Loss of vision:

Sudden loss of vision, causes include:

Glaucoma,

Cataract,

Migraine,
Senile Macular Degeneration,
Retinal detachment,
Giant Cell Arteritis,
MS,
Intracranial neoplasm,
Central retinal artery/vein occlusion,
Malignant hypertension,
Macular haemorrhages,
Carotid artery occlusion,
Methanol consumption,
Hysteria.
All need an acute referral.

Amaurosis fugax:

Painless transient unilateral visual loss. Can be a curtain that descends over the field of vision or any pattern of sight loss affecting one eye. Lasts seconds, up to hours depending on the cause. This symptom may be followed by other neurological stroke related symptoms and can often precede a stroke. Should always be seen straight away and assessed.

Multiple causes:

Carotid or ophthalmic A. atheromata, embolism, vasoconstriction, neuropathy, Giant Cell Arteritis, Angle Closure Glaucoma, raised ICP, compression of the orbit, primary haematological disorders or circulatory problems.

Common in Giant Cell Arteritis – GCA presents with winking vision on and off before the visual loss. The patient can have a very high CRP and N ESR, there is jaw pain and scalp tenderness. 90-97% have raised ESR and 100% have a raised CRP but occasionally raised only a little. In some studies CRP can be raised as little as 5mg/ dL.

So in Amaurosis, assess carotid bruits, ?sinus rhythm, (?AF), exclude valve abnormalities and Atrial Myxoma (?Echo?), check TA pulses, ESR, CRP, cholesterol, BP, BG, AIP (SLE, PAN), blood viscosity, Protein C, Anti Phospholipid, Anti Cardiolipin Abs, Lupus Anticoagulant, Thrombocytosis. Assess the eye itself for local abnormality (inflammation, haemorrhage, vitreous detachment, raised IOP, Optic Neuritis, MS.) etc

Posterior Vitreous Detachment:

Is commoner in the short sighted, as the patient gets older (75% over the age of 65). Causes a "net curtain", flashes, floaters in a temporal ring, **no actual shadow in vision**, settles quickly, generally benign. The risk is of an associated retinal tear or detachment.

Retinal Detachment:

Occasionally preceded by a PVD and retinal tear (a shower of new floaters). Risk factors include AIDs, Cannabis, short sight, eclampsia, trauma and diabetic retinopathy. If a retinal (rather than just a vitreous) detachment is taking place look out for a peripheral shadow moving centrally, a curtain over the field of vision, distortion of straight lines and loss of the central field. Refer to an eye unit if any of these take place.

Horner Syndrome:

Unilateral small pupil miosis, ptosis, diminished facial sweating, anhidrosis. A unilateral sympathetic palsy.

Causes: Carotid A pathology (eg dissecting carotid aneurysm), brachial plexus damage, migraine, cluster headache, brainstem CVA, upper lung infection or tumour (Pancoast tumour), middle cranial fossa tumour.

Glaucoma:

Classically causes "tunnel vision" or a tunnel and an off centre arcuate scotoma with cupping of the disc at the upper and lower temporal edges. If the cup >0.3 of the disc, there is an increased risk of glaucoma. There is also "low tension glaucoma" with normal IOPs but progressive visual damage and treatment needed which lowers the pressure even more. There may be tolerated higher than normal IOPs too, in ocular hypertension.

The various glaucomas: acute closed angle, chronic simple open angle glaucoma, there is also chronic closed angle glaucoma.

The commonest type is open angle glaucoma (chronic). This causes a progressive visual field loss. The visual damage is not directly correlated with pressure. It is commoner in black people and in old age, with a FH, Diabetes, Ocular Hypertension and in systemic hypertension (?2nd to poor arterial perfusion?).

IOP shows a diurnal variation. Highest in morning, it varies with the wearing of a tie and with posture. Use a Goldman tonometer, the puff and Perkins tonometers are not reliable. ULN is 21mm Hg. All pressure measuring instruments are affected by corneal thickness. (Calibrated for standard thickness, so some "Ocular Hypertension" may just be a thick cornea.)

Start treatment at 25mm, lower if there is a positive family hx, target pressure to the mid teens mm Hg, unless the patient is actively losing fields.

Treatment: BBs: Timolol Betoptic, Betaxolol, Carteolol, etc.

Alpha 2 agonists: Brimonidine Alphagan, etc.

Prostaglandin Analogues: Latanoprost, Xalatan. Bimatoprost, Travoprost, etc.

Carbonic Anhydrase Inhibitors: Dorzolamide, Trusopt, Brinzolamide, Azopt etc.

Rarely, Systemic Carbonic Anhydrase Inhibitors: Acetozolamide, Diamox.

Miotics: Pilocarpine.

or combinations of the above.

Surgery: Selective Laser Trabeculoplasty YAG. Trabeculectomy.(c 5FU and mitomycin to stop fibrosis).

Normal Tension Glaucoma:

Check normal thickness cornea, get pressure down even lower and may do well with early surgery.

NOTE:

Acute: Closed angle – the only significant risk with antidepressants.

Cranial Nerves controlling the eyes:

3 Oculomotor: All ocular muscles except Superior Oblique and Lateral Rectus (leaving the eye in the

"Down and out" position when there is a complete 3rd N palsy).

Ciliary muscle, Pupil, Levator Palpebrae.

4 Trochlear: Superior Oblique muscle (gives down and medial gaze).

6 Abducens: Lateral rectus muscle (gives lateral gaze).

Squints:

Cover/Uncover Test: Manifest squint: Look at the eye you are leaving uncovered while covering and uncovering the other.

Alternate cover test: look at the eye being covered while covering and uncovering it (for a latent squint).

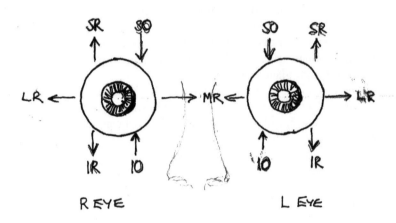

Patient's Abnormal Left Eye

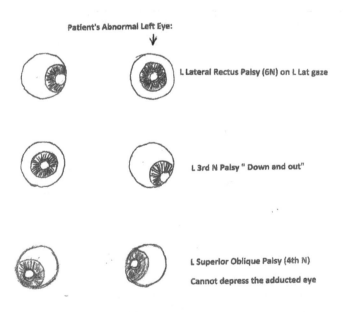

Patient's Abnormal Left Eye:

L Lateral Rectus Palsy (6N) on L Lat gaze

L 3rd N Palsy " Down and out"

L Superior Oblique Palsy (4th N)

Cannot depress the adducted eye

Diagram of eye movements

Conjunctivitis:

Bacterial: Chloramphenicol drops and oint, Azithromycin drops, Bacitracin and Polymyxin oint, Ciprofloxacin drops and oint, Fucidic Acid thick drops, Gentamicin, etc. Bear in mind that Ophthalmia Neonatorum may be chlamydial or gonorrhoeal and that you may catch either quite easily unless your hand washing is scrupulous!

Best guess drops: Sofradex (Dexamethasone, Framycetin, Gramicidin).

Don't forget the possibility of Chlamydial conjunctivitis, not just neonatally, usually a diagnosis (from a swab) of exclusion-which needs oral Doxycycline or Erythromycin (if risk of dental staining).

The TV remote control is the commonest source of family cross infection in persistent conjunctivitis.

Allergic Conjunctivitis:

It is very important not to rub the eyes. Allergic eyes: Good advice at: www.allergyuk.org

The hair is a net that catches pollen on bike rides and on walks in the park and the country and then deposits it on the pillow for you to rub your face in all night. So advise the patient to rinse hair at night before retiring and after washing them, to dry their pillow cases inside the house not on the washing line in the garden. And not to rub their eyes.

Olopatadine (Opatanol) is an antihistamine and mast cell stabiliser, Ketotifen (Zaditen), Nedocromil (Rapitil) are used topically as drops. All are good in allergic eyes.

Blepharitis:

The old advice was: Baby shampoo scrubs to the lid margins, nocturnal chloramphenicol ointment.

Or bd ointment and or oral doxycycline for up to 3 months! These days the advice is warm compresses, lid massage and keep the lids as clean as possible. Avoid make up. If necessary, Doxycycline, Lymecycline orally for 1-3m. Blephasol. Good advice on www.eyebag.co.uk

Uveitis: Inflammation of the iris, ciliary body and choroid (Iridocyclitis):

It can be Anterior (Iridocyclitis and iritis), Intermediate, (Vitritis-the vitreous cavity), Posterior (Chorioretinitis) or Pan uveitis.

Red eye, blurred vision, irregular pupil, photophobia, floaters, HA, eye pain, keratic precipitates, hypopyon etc.

Associated with the HLA B 27 and PTPN 22 genotype, H. Simplex and V. Zoster etc are actually the causes of a lot of what was once called Idiopathic Anterior Uveitis.

Associated with other disease in 1/3 cases, A.S., Juvenile Rh. A., Kawasaki, M.S., P.A.N., S.L.E. etc., Diabetes mellitus, Myxoedema, Sarcoid, Crohn's, Behcet's, Sarcoid, Spondyloarthritis, Infection elsewhere including Brucellosis, Lyme, TB etc., Malignancy-lymphoma etc, etc,

Dry Eyes:

Make sure you exclude ectropion and blepharitis.

A common symptom of the menopause (and improved by HRT) and occasionally of chemotherapy.

Artificial Tears: Most are OTC. I have used Carbomer, Viscotears gel, (Artelan Nightime gel is good). Acetylcysteine, eg: Ilube drops, Carmellose eg: Celluvisc drops, Hypromellose eg: 0.3% 0.35% 0.5% 1% drops (+ Dextran eg: Tears Naturale). Hydroxyethylcellulose drops, eg: Minims Artificial Tears, Paraffins eg: Lacri-Lube Oint. Polyvinyl Alcohol eg: Liquifilm Tears etc.

Hycosan, Systane, Hylotear, Hyloforte-hyaluronic acid drops. VitA POS oint – lasts all night.

If severe, punctal plugging can be considered to occlude tear duct drainage.

Corneal Abrasion/Laceration:

If you have ever scratched your eye by rubbing a piece of blown in grit on to the cornea or had a branch flick into your eye while gardening you will know how intensely painful these common and seemingly trivial lesions are. The cornea has a denser supply of sensory nerve endings than anywhere else in the body and even moving the eye ball against the inside of the abrasive tarsal conjunctiva is then painful. This movement happens involuntarily of course, in REM sleep and the pain can wake patients up for several nights after the injury.

Standard treatment is, it has to be said, fairly poor. Use fluorescein drops to exclude a dendritic ulcer and when the abrasion is confirmed, the usual approach is topical antibiotics (though there isn't much of an evidence base for these as prophylaxis), as drops or ointment. Mydriatic (cycloplegic) drops are supposed to stop painful reflex pupillary contraction and photophobia and these can be used bilaterally. This is as long as you are keeping an eye on the patient (glaucoma) but there isn't much of an evidence base for these either. What does help is topical NSAIDs and strong oral analgesics. The advice on topical anaesthetics is to avoid them as they slow corneal healing and can cause corneal damage. I can only say that the topical anaesthetic from my bag, Amethocaine, used three or four times in the first two days after my last corneal abrasion was the **only thing** that allowed me to work or to function at all. Pressure patches and topical antibiotic ointment are old fashioned and most specialists no longer patch the eye especially if the ulcer is contact lens related.

I put in Amethocaine drops entirely against the standard wisdom and this allowed **me** to work and sleep when nothing else made any difference to the pain at all. As far as I am aware I suffered no residual corneal damage from this.

Macular Degeneration: Age Related Macular Degeneration, Wet and Dry:

Smokers are 8X more likely to get macular degeneration than non smokers (ARMD) – presumably because they are actively damaging their microvasculature throughout their body. Other factors are age and diet (trans fats, and saturated fats), lack of Omega 3 fish oils, (population studies show that diets high in Omega-3 oils and fish are consistently associated with a decreased risk of age related macular degeneration), too much alcohol, lack of exercise, genetics, excessive sunshine, (and ironically, poor vitamin D status), race, (-rare in Afro Caribbeans), short stature, long sightedness. High homocysteine levels may also be a risk factor.

Age Related Macular Degeneration: ARMD: Central scotoma. 15-18% are <45 years 66% are >90 years

Wet ARMD: exudates, clear fluid lifts the pigment epithelium, blindness follows in a few weeks.

Dry ARMD: 85% of total, time to legal blindness (<3/60), 5-10 years. Slow central distortion of vision. Presents with poor vision in dim and in bright light, poor recovery in bright light and poor central vision. There is patchy loss of visual acuity.

Investigations: Fluorescein angiography shows leaks. It is treated with laser if not near the fovea. Investigations include: Optical coherence tomography: Like USS but light used instead of sound.

Treatment can include supplements which help in advanced disease, Zinc, Vitamins A, C, E, Carotenoids, Lutein, Zeaxanthin, (JAMA ophth 2015). Carotenoids are lipid soluble plant pigments in red, orange, yellow and dark green fruit and vegetables. Especially green leafy vegetables like kale, spinach and broccoli. They are also found in corn, (sweet corn), red peppers and eggs. A good diet with a mix of fruit, omega 3 fish oils, nuts and vegetables reduces the incidence and progress of ARMD. VEGF is vascular endothelial growth factor.

Argon laser in Wet Photodynamic therapy, **Anti VEGF** Pegaptanib, Macugen, Ranibizumab, Lucentis and Eylea, Aflibercept injections – all block VEGF

Verteporfin (Visudyne) – the injection is used in combination with photodynamic therapy (-treatment with a laser) to treat abnormal growth of leaky blood vessels in the eye caused by wet ARMD-one form of "**photodynamic therapy**" (which generally uses a dye, light and oxygen to kill malignant or unwanted tissue.)

Note: The various oral treatments are:

Oral Ocuvite (is Vit. C 180mg, Vit. E 30mg, Zinc 15mg, Omega 3 fatty acids 500mg, Lutein (an orange red antioxidant carotenoid which the retina concentrates naturally and absorbs blue light) and Zeaxanthin 2mg (a Lutein related compound).

Lutin and Bilberry extract,

Visionace tabs/caps contain the following active ingredients per tablet: Vitamin A (1000 IU) 300mcg; Vitamin D (100 IU) 2.5mcg; Vitamin E (natural source) 60mg; Vitamin C 150mg; Vitamin B1 12mg, Vitamin B2 4.8mg; Niacin (Vitamin B3) 18mg; Vitamin B6 10mg; Folic acid 400mcg; Vitamin B12 9mcg; Pantothenic Acid 20mg; Iron 6mg; Magnesium 60mg; Zinc 15mg; Iodine 100mcg; Copper 1000mcg; Manganese 4mg; Selenium 150mcg; Chromium 50mcg; Natural mixed Carotenoids 3mg; Citrus Bioflavonoids 15mg; Bilberry extract equivalent to 60mg; Lutein Esters 4mg. The Omega-3 DHA capsule contains 600mg Omega-3 fish oil providing 300mg DHA and 60mg EPA plus 8mg Lutein esters.

Dry ARMD is slowly progressive, but 4%/year convert to the rapidly deteriorating wet type. Here there is active new vessel formation throughout the retina and these blood vessels, a little like diabetic neovascularisation, are leaky. The progression is 4X faster in smokers.

Wet ARMD (this affects the contralateral eye in 90% over 5 years).

Is exudative and consist of 3 main types;

Pigment Epithelium Detachment (PED): Occult CNV type 1: (Choroidal Neovascularisation).

The retina is lifted by leaked fluid forming a dome. Poor prognosis.

Type 2 Occult CNV: New vessel formation, new drug treatments are effective. Usually turns into classic CNV.

Classic CNV-Classic Neovascular ARMD: Some dry types of Macular Degeneration progress to this form of Wet ARMD. Risk factors include: Soft Drusen, raised BP, smoking, lack of exercise and poor diet.

It can take days or weeks to develop and presents with distorted central vision. Treatment with laser (PDT) and the new anti-VEGF drugs – Aflibercept (Eylea),

Pegaptanib (Macugen), Ranibizumab (Lucentis), Verteporfin (Visudyne). The injections are given into the vitreous and are antibodies which block vascular growth factor.

The same injections (or dexamethazone implants) are effective in retinal vein occlusion. In Wet ARMD, 7-8 injections are given in the first year then 4/year or thereabouts afterwards.

Neovascularisation tends to cause visual distortion (bent straight lines and a feeling of looking through water) and is confirmed by fluorescein angiography.

Common confusing ophthalmic terms:

Drusen:

(Something, anything, waste products in the retina, elevating the pigment epithelium). This is a collection of extracellular waste material between Bruch's membrane and the retinal pigment epithelium. A few small hard drusen are normal, especially over the age of 40. It is also seen in early AMD (inspissated material from cone metabolism, dying off cones, pigmentation, etc.) Drusen may predispose to MD later.

Pinguecula:

This is a benign thickening and discolouration of the conjunctiva due to sun exposure. It occurs as a pale yellow area over the medial sclera, usually asymptomatic, although it may sometimes cause irritation or a sense of a foreign body. Lubricant or anti inflammatory drops are sometimes used and occasionally, excision. If it grows as far as the cornea, it becomes redefined as a pterygium.

Pterygium:

Like the pinguecula, the pterygium is a thickening over the medial cornea and is due to UV light exposure and to drying of the eye surface. It looks thicker, more solid, more fleshy more round or oval than pinguecula though. Large ones may even distort the shape of the eye and cause astigmatism. Histologically, pterygia are due to collagen degeneration and thickening.

The eyes can feel dry, itchy or as if there were a FB present. They rarely extend enough to interfere with vision. Treatment includes lubricant drops for dry eyes and occasionally surgery or even radiotherapy.

Recurrence after surgery can be up to 40%.

Coloboma:

This is a gap in some of the structures of the eye, usually due to a developmental fault. It usually affects the inferior structures of the eye, i.e. the lower iris, but the ciliary body, choroid or retina may be affected too.

The commonest appearance is of a keyhole pupil, visible neonatally. The effect of a coloboma varies depending on how far back it extends and how much of the eye is involved. It may simply cause light sensitivity if it only involves the iris or it could significantly affect vision if it involves light sensitive deep structures further back.

Colobomas (?colobomata?) can be associated with more systemic and serious syndromes. (eg "CHARGE" syndrome, strictly CHARGED syndrome) (Coloboma, heart defects, atresia of nasal choanae, retardation of growth, genital/urinary abnormalities, ear abnormalities and deafness).

There may be an increased long term risk of glaucoma. Treatments vary depending on severity but usually start with protection from intense light.

Cataract:

Operations for cataracts were some of the first surgery ever performed and today their "Post code lottery" makes them amongst the most controversial.

It is possible that cataract surgery using sharp knives and gold cannulae was performed by Japanese surgeons 2000 years BC. Babylonians displaced cataracts by squeezing the eye, a risky process which could result in the loss of vision. Couching is dislodging of the lens into the posterior chamber using a blunt or sharp instrument and may have been performed since before 2000 years BC. The first modern European operation was by Daviel in 1748.

A third of people >65 have one or two cataracts. There are nuclear cataracts (which affect colour), cortical (which may present with glare in sunlight) and subcapsular cataracts (which can reduce daylight vision and reading).

Surgery is *appropriate* if vision is worse than 6/12.

Causes: Age, diabetes, injury, steroids, uveitis, UV light, smoking, alcohol, family history.

Symptoms: loss of contrast, cloudy vision, glare, more myopia. Surgery is often *inevitable* when the optician is unable to improve vision with refraction.

The cloudy lens is removed (usually with ultrasound via phacoemulsification or extra capsular cataract extraction) and replaced with a lifelong plastic (acrylic) or silicone lens placed in the remaining lens capsule under a local anaesthetic. (Intraocular lens implant). Only 75% are within +/− 1 D of what you are aiming for. If there are bilateral cataracts, eight weeks are left between operations. There is a risk of endopthalmitis in 0.1%. 90% see better, there is a 1% risk of retinal detachment. High risk surgery: High Myopia, lid infection, patient unable to lie flat.

Minimally Invasive Cataract Surgery (1.8mm incision, small lenses now available), separate phaconeedle and irrigator, only in straight forward cataracts. The accommodative lens is in the pipeline!! So is an injectable transparent polymer. The Symfony lens is in focus from 1m to infinity.

The "Centurion" system vapourises the cataract.

Most people require glasses after surgery or a change in their glasses prescription.

31: Paediatrics:

(See also "Infections/antibiotics and Immunisations/vaccines")

(Some specific conditions are under those systems)

The UK has one of the highest death rates for children under 5 in Western Europe at 4.9/1000 births, more than double that of Singapore which has the lowest in the world. Worldwide deaths in this age group have nearly halved since 1990 (Lancet DOI: 10.1016/ SO140-6736(14) 60497-9).

20% of the average GP's list consists of under 15 year olds and they make up a quarter of consultations. Under 5's see their doctor twice as often as the over 5's. (RCGP Curriculum, Clinical Modules). GPs undertake by far the majority of Paediatric medicine done in the Health Service. Any doctor not confident in identifying a sick baby, infant or child is not fit to practice Family Medicine. Good general Paediatric experience is essential. There is no clear cut off between Paediatric Care and Adult Medicine. Certainly the presence of pubic hair is no proper threshold, but Paediatrics *begins* with Neonatology.

APGAR Score.

Named, surprisingly, after Virginia **Apgar** an American obstetric anaesthetist. Not: after Activity, pulse, grumpiness, appearance and respirations – or any other mnemonic. This is apparently an example of a "Backronym!"-with all sorts of meanings attributed to the word after it had become established. It is fortunate her name wasn't something like Von Recklinghausen.

Assessed at 1 min and 10 mins:
Heart Rate
Respiration
Movement
Irritability
Colour

Limitations:

The American Academy of Paediatrics and College of Obs and Gynae describes the APGAR score as a tool for standardised assessment, a mechanism recording foetal to neonatal transition. They emphasise that it does not predict long term developmental outcomes. In a statement about the score they have said: "Healthy preterm infants may have low scores simply because of prematurity even without asphyxia". The comment goes on: "A 5 minute APGAR of 0 to 3 correlates with neonatal mortality in large populations but does not predict individual future neurological dysfunction".

On the other hand, a bright red screaming, all four limbs moving, wide awake, lusty, ten APGAR baby with a good pulse at one minute, is very reassuring after a difficult delivery and a reasonable indicator that the baby has probably survived intact and hasn't been *significantly* asphyxiated.

Assessing Gestational Age:

	24 weeks	28 weeks	32 weeks	36 weeks	40 weeks	42 weeks
Vernix:	Appears				Decreasing	Gone
Breast Tissue:			1-2mm	4mm	7mm or >	
Nipples:	Barely visible		Well defined flat areola	Raised areola		
Soles:	No creases		Ant transverse	Ant 2/3 Sole	Heel creases from 38 weeks	
Ears:	Flat shapeless		Beginning incurving		Well defined upper pinna incurving from 39 weeks	
Genitalia:	(24 wks Testes undescended.29-35 High in canal. Lower canal from 35 weeks. Usually descended from 38 weeks, scrotum floppy external and soft) (24 wks Labia Majora separated with a prominent clitoris. From 35 weeks the Majora nearly cover the minora. From 38 weeks the minora and clitoris covered.)					

Lanugo: Over entire body from 20 wks, Goes from face 30-36 and from everywhere after.

Tone: Heel to ear: 24 wks no resistance 29 wks slight resistance. Difficult from 34 weeks. Almost impossible from 36 weeks.

Reflexes: **Moro** Barely present from 24 wks. Complete, exhaustible from 27 weeks, Good complete from 31 wks, No adduction from 34 wks, Complete with adduction from 37 wks

Pupils (light): react from 24 wks

Grasp: Weak from 24 wks, fair from 27 wks, strong from 31 wks,

Glabellar tap: Absent at 24 wks. Appears at 29, present from 35 wks.

Turns to light source: Starts to appear at 32 wks.

At Birth Immediate examination:

Length, weight, head circumference.

Appearance, cyanosis, jaundice, anaemia.

Tone, reflexes, grasp, ventrosuspension, spontaneous sounds, activity, reactions, etc.

Limb/neck deformity, (Turner's etc), palmar creases.

Cataract, red reflex,

Fontanelles,

Face: Down's and other Trisomies,

Micropthalmia,

Cleft lip and palate,

Heart sounds (etc).

Full air entry? (diaphragmatic and pulmonary abnormalities).

Single umbilical artery? – This is present in 1% of singleton and 5% of multiple pregnancies. It is associated with no abnormality in 75% babies, but the others are linked with congenital renal, CNS, chromosomal or cardiac abnormalities.

Abdominal mass, hepato-splenomegaly, hernia,

Spina bifida,

Hypospadias,

Imperforate anus,

Descended testes,

CDH,

Talipes,

Femoral Pulses, radio-femoral delay.

By 6 weeks:

Feeding,

Height, weight and head circumference,

Head shape, ears, eyes (red reflex, follows light), palate,

Heart sounds, femoral pulses, liver edge, radio-femoral delay,

Cyanosis, anaemia, jaundice,

Air entry, chest examination,

Abdomen (Liver/spleen/masses),

Hernias,

Genitalia,

Hips,

Tone, reflexes,

Ventrosuspension-head held up, hips extended, pull to sit, less head lag, some head control when held sitting, Stepping reflex disappears 4-5m, still some grasp, smiles, eyes fixate on objects,

Limbs, digits,

Skin.

Neonatal Heel Prick Testing:

800,000 are done in the UK a year, 1,500 a year are positive. Four new tests were officially added in 2015 with an expected pick up rate of an extra 30 cases.

Usually done between day 5 and 8, it includes tests for

Phenyketonuria,

Myxoedema,

Sickle Cell Haemoglobinopathy,

Cystic Fibrosis, (Trypsin),

MCAD, (Medium Chain Acyl CoA Dehydrogenase),

from May 2014 these had been provisionally added:

Maple Syrup Urine Disease,

Homocystinuria,

Glutaric Acidaemia type 1,

Isovaleric Acidaemia.

and

Occasionally these are performed:

Galactosaemia,

Biotinidase deficiency and

CAH, depending on where you are.

also other inborn errors: including

Long chain Hydroxyacyl-CoA dehydrogenase deficiency (LCHADD).

Trisomies:

Trisomy 21 Down's Syndrome:

95% are due to non disjunction of 21, the spare chromosome coming from the mother mostly. These are maternal age related. The remainder are due to translocation of 21, are familial and do not relate to maternal age.

Mental retardation, hypotonia, flat occiput, oblique palpebral fissures, Brushfield spots (grey/brown spots at the edge of the iris), protruding tongue, malformed ears, CHD, cryptorchidism, simian palmar crease, hypoplasia of mid phalanx 5th digit, short neck, intestinal atresia etc.

Trisomy 18 Edward's Syndrome:

Hypertonus, mental retardation, FTT, more females, small features, micrognathia, malformed ears, CHD, diaphragmatic hernia, hernias, horseshoe kidney, rockerbottom feet, cleft lip and palate, simian crease.

Trisomy 13 Patau's Syndrome:

Mental retardation, FTT, haemangiomata, WBC abnormalities, persistent foetal Hb, seizures, apnoea, microcephaly, deafness, CHD, polycystic kidneys, polydactyly, flexion deformity of the fingers, micrognathia, rockerbottom feet, omphalocoel.

Paediatric Cardiology:

In this context CHD is congenital heart disease not coronary heart disease. Most paediatric cardiology is congenital heart disease.

Things you may have forgotten:

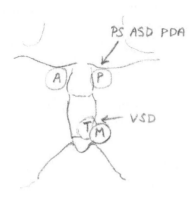

HEART SOUNDS

CLOSURE SOUNDS (First and Second Heart Sounds)

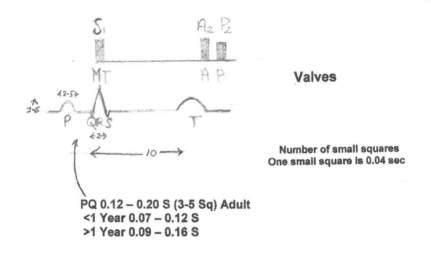

Valves

Number of small squares
One small square is 0.04 sec

PQ 0.12 – 0.20 S (3-5 Sq) Adult
<1 Year 0.07 – 0.12 S
>1 Year 0.09 – 0.16 S

The Heart sounds Diagrams

HEART SOUNDS

Aortic area

-------->Neck in (A)S P2 May be single or reversed

Ejection click if valvular

Pulmonary Area

Second sound split in (P)S
Best area for pulmonary second sound
Loud 2nd sound in pulmonary hypertension
Fixed splitting in ASD, paradoxical in LBBB

(P)S ASD

(P) Apex

(T)Murmur

Fixed split second sound, ASD
An Ostium Primum (low) may involve T and M valves
with an apical pan systolic (M)incomp murmur (rare)

PDA (P)area c thrill. Pulm P2 may be absent

-------VSD Small

Maladie de Roger Tricuspd posn. 4LIS c thrill

Large

P2 Sound may be single 3 Apex (M)flow
in pulmonary area

Tricuspid Area (L sternal edge)

(T)R

VSD

(A)R Austin Flint. Lean forward, hold breath in expiration

(T)S ASD Fixed splitting

Mitral Area

(M)R --------> Axilla

(M)S Carey Coombes-Increased M flow in Rh F. Pre
systolic accentuation unless in AF.

Graham Steell. Early diastolic pulm regurgitant
murmur due to pulmonary hypertension (cor
pulmonale)

A   A2

Fallots Heard in Tricuspid position

Ejection sound Single P2   VSD (P)S

Coarctation Often loudest at back, absent femoral
pulses, associated c PDA, A valve lesions.

[863]

P2 is fixed wide split in ASD, wide split in P stenosis, (P2 soft). The two sounds are close or single in A stenosis and reversed in severe A stenosis.

Murmurs with names: Graham Steell pulmonary regurgitant murmur early diastolic 2 LIS, in pulmonary hypertension e.g. of cor pulmonale.

Austin Flint mid diastolic aortic regurgitant murmur from whatever cause.

Carey Coombes: Short mid diastolic murmur due to "mitral valvitis" in Rheumatic Fever.

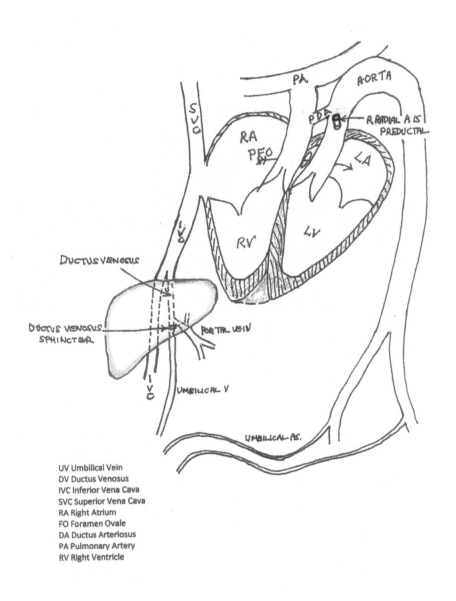

UV Umbilical Vein
DV Ductus Venosus
IVC Inferior Vena Cava
SVC Superior Vena Cava
RA Right Atrium
FO Foramen Ovale
DA Ductus Arteriosus
PA Pulmonary Artery
RV Right Ventricle

The circulation pre birth: Diagram: (Diagram IUFC 1)

Pulmonary vascular resistance doesn't in fact completely drop at the moment of the first breath in a full term infant but drops a varying amount then and progressively over 2-3 months. An absent Ductus Venosus (sometimes screened for antenatally) is associated with a higher foetal mortality, a number of chromosomal abnormalities, Turners Syndrome, Noonan's Syndrome, Pierre Robin, Ebstein's anomaly, Hydrops, Pulmonary Stenosis and etc, but if sequential anomaly scans are normal then, so is the baby. This absence is now screened for at some centres antenatally.

25% of adults are said to retain a PFO. Decompression sickness, cryptogenic stroke and other illnesses including paradoxical embolism (R>L sided embolism) are more common until the foramen is closed.

At the first breath, pulmonary vascular resistance drops, pulmonary blood flow increases as well as pulmonary venous return and L atrial pressure. R heart pressure decreases, L heart pressure increases. The atrial septum primum acts as a one way valve up against the firmer septum secundum and now that the atrial pressures are reversed and the L side greater than the R, it shuts off R atrial to L atrial shunting through the FO. Initially the R ventricle wall is the thicker but by the end of the 1st month the L ventricle wall is thicker.

The PDA constricts in response to aortic PAO2 (at 50mm+ Hg) and via Bradykinin. The Ductus remains open in premature and hypoxic infants. Its persistence increases the risk of IVH. (Intraventricular haemorrhage). Prostaglandin E2 keeps the PDA open and Indomet(h) acin, Ibuprofen, even ?Paracetamol can close it.

Congenital Heart Disease: (and percentage of total CHD):

The commonest congenital heart disease is a Bicuspid Aortic Valve (1:78) Most aetiology is unknown apart from: Congenital Rubella: PDA and VSD, Down's Syndrome: AV Canal defect, PDA, VSD, and Turner's Syndrome; Coarctation.

The examination: Pulse: Feel both arms and one leg. (Reduced in legs = Coarctation, increased Dorsalis Pedis = PDA.)

BP: Use the largest cuff possible (2/3 upper arm, the cuff encircling the arm). Raised in Coarctation, renal disease, RICP, Essential Hypertension. Drops with illness, shock, but varies with respiration, a N. maximum 10mm difference on inspiration, any more means Pulsus Paradoxus – asthma, heart failure, Tamponade, etc.

JVP: Much harder to assess than in adults.

RVH: Parasternal and epigastric heave, LVH: "Lifting" apex.

Types:

Holes:

ASD Primum 3% Endocardial Cushion Defect. ("Atrioventricular Septal Defect") Secundum 7%

ASD: 1/1500 births (Remember the Foramen Ovale shunt and the Septum Primum valve flap in utero) ASDs consist of: Endocardial cushion defects (Ostium Primum defects and persistent AV canal) – low defects. and Ostium Secundum defects.

Ostium Secundum defects are the commonest ASDs and arise from an enlarged Foramen

Ovale. They may involve the M Valve. A patent Foramen Ovale may cause migraine, para-doxical embolism, even decompression sickness later in life. See above:

The murmurs of ASDs are valve flow murmurs through the tricuspid and pulmonary valves: ESM at P area (blowing, 2LIS), a mid diastolic flow murmur (tricuspid) in 4LIS, fixed splitting of S2 at lower L sternal border (accentuated P2). In Ostium Primum defects there is an apical pan systolic murmur of mitral incompetence due to the cleft mitral valve.

ASDs rarely cause problems in children. The ECG shows RBBB in most cases and LAD in Ostium Primum.

VSD 25% 2-6/1,000 births Pan systolic murmur over precordium, 4 LIS, S2 split. If pulmonary hypertension is present, P2 is accentuated and pan systolic murmur quietens. L>R Shunt. Acyanotic until Eisenmenger's syndrome develops. Commonest CHD, medical treatment initially, (includes digoxin, loop diuretics, ACEIs). Up to 3/4 close spontaneously. May cause heart failure in first 18m. ECG RAD.

PDA 15% 2F:1M The duct is usually (often) closed by 1 week in a full term infant. The more premature the baby the longer the duct stays open. No cyanosis until or unless Eisenmenger's Syndrome (pulmonary hypertension and a reversal of the shunt to R>L) develops. Continuous murmur 2 LIS (under L clavicle). Mid diastolic apical flow murmur with big shunts. S2 split P2 accentuated if pulmonary hypertension. Big volume pulses, bounding Dorsalis Pedis pulses. The duct may keep some babies alive (as in Pulmonary Atresia etc) but can cause heart failure.

Narrowed valves:

You should have checked the chests of every child on your list, on the law of averages by the time they are two. When you listen to their lung fields, something you should do with every child who presents with a cough, always take a minute to listen to the heart sounds. It could save a life. (See below)

Pulmonary Stenosis. 5% ESM 2LIS/LSE (harsh), sometimes an ejection click. If severe, only A2 audible (single S2.) Severity of stenosis is proportional to A2 P2 interval (ie how widely split S2 is). Usually presents in older children with murmur, asymptomatic, but can present with cyanosis (R>L shunt through PFO). Can be infundibular, suprav-alvar, a stenotic or abnormal valve. May be associated with various syndromes and other complex heart abnormalities.

ECG: The height of the R waves in V4R and V1 give a good indication of the degree of hypertrophy and stenosis. If severe there is T inversion across the chest. A R ventricular pressure of 60mm Hg is the cut off level for intervention.

Aortic Stenosis 5%. Collapsing episodes or risk of sudden death in older children if not detected. Harsh ESM 2RICS/RSE transmitted to neck with suprasternal thrill. Paradoxically split S2. Sometimes an ejection click.

Tricuspid Atresia 3%. Ejection murmur in 3 LIS (but no murmur in half of patients) S2 single.

Coarctation 5%. M2:1F Common in girls with Turner's syndrome. Soft blowing ESM in 2LIS transmitted to the back. S2 normally split. Delayed weak or absent femoral pulses and arm BP higher than that in the legs (20mm difference). Can develop hyper-tensive encephalopathy. Rib notching in older children on CXR (dilatation of the inter-costal arteries). Infantile is preductal, adult is post ductal. The vast majority have other congenital heart abnormalities as well – PDA, VSD, Aortic valve lesions etc.

Cyanotic lesions:

Fallots Tetralogy: 10%. The commonest cyanotic CHD. A large anterior VSD, Infundibular Pulmonary Stenosis, the severity of which can determine the direction of the shunt. 1/3 have Pulmonary Valve Stenosis too. There are also: R ventricular hypertrophy and the fourth part of the Tetralogy is an overriding aorta which is displaced anteriorly. The condition is usually progressive, the baby being often pink at birth with deteriorating spells of cyanosis. Ejection murmur 3 LIS (harsh). S2 sounds single.

The child can present slightly cyanosed at birth, later with cyanotic attacks and squatting which reduces venous return and oxygen debt after exercise but also reverses the direction of the shunt. Oxygen and B Blockers help. There is an ESM at the L USE and a boot shaped heart on the CXR.

Transposition of the Great Arteries. 10%. Cyanosis from birth. Murmur varies, 1/3 have no murmur. The Foramen Ovale maintains life.

Others:

Total Anomalous Pulmonary Venous Drainage: Cyanosis (in most children), ESM in 3LIS, mid diastolic flow murmur in 4LIS. S2 split. P2 loud. S1 loud. Murmurs depend on the anatomy. The Foramen Ovale maintains life.

Hypoplastic L Heart ? 1 – 1.5% 1:4,400 births. Seasonal variation. Affects the whole of the L half of the heart, the valves and the L Ventricle. Blood shunts from the LA through the PFO to the RA. The commonest form of heart failure in the first few days.

Endocardial Fibroelastosis 1% Most have no murmur, gallop rhythm. Presents as heart failure without cyanosis in an infant. Mumps and Coxsackie are two of many causes.

Eisenmenger's syndrome is when the RA pressure is high enough to reverse the shunt R>L.

Persistent Transitional Circulation Is when there is a persisting foetal direction of flow through a PDA and pulmonary hypertension.

Pulmonary Regurgitation: eg Marfan's. Rare. Can be assoc c VSD, etc.

Ebstein's Anomaly: Approximately 1% CHD. The exact anatomy varies. The posterior and septal leaflets of the tricuspid valve are set low. The anterior leaflet is in the normal place. The valve is misshapen and incompetent. There is a PFO or ASD. There is a muscular infundibulum but the rest of the heart muscle is thin. The RA is dilated with a R>L shunt. There is a split first heart sound (delayed T closure) and often a pansystolic T incompetent murmur.

OR: Looked at another way

Acyanotic: Shunts: VSD ASD PDA Obstruction: AS PS Coarctation.

Cyanotic: Pulmonary oligaemia: Fallots, Tricuspid atresia, Pulmonary atresia.

Neonatal presentation: Transposition, Hypoplastic L heart.

Common mixing situations: TAPVD, Common atrium, Common ventricle, Truncus arteriosus, Endocardial cushion defect.

Diagnosing Congenital Heart Disease on the CXR:

Plethoric CXR: TGA, (If the patient is cyanosed then this is probably the diagnosis)

Truncus Arteriosus,

TAPVR,

Single Ventricle,

Common Atrium,
Hypoplastic L. Heart.
Oligaemic CXR (No pulmonary hypertension) Fallot's,
Tricuspid atresia,
PS and intact septum,
Ebstein's,
Anomalous Systemic Venous Return.
Oligaemic and Pulmonary Hypertension: Eisenmenger.

Other **CXR Signs** are: The egg on a string (Transposition), the Snowman (TAPVR), Scimitar (Partial Anomalous Pulmonary Venous Return), Gooseneck (Endocardial Cushion Defect), Figure of three and reverse figure of three (Coarctation), Boot shaped heart (Fallot's) and box shaped heart (Ebstein's).

Innocent Murmurs:

Most murmurs heard in children are innocent or insignificant. In fact the second sound is probably at least as important in diagnosing significant cardiac abnormalities in childhood as any murmur.

As well as just listening to the heart when you examine a child's cardiovascular system you should do a bit more:

Get a good history and a family history, height, weight, etc. then look for: Whether the child is ill, poorly grown, the respiratory rate, is he or she cyanosed, the peripheral circulation?, sweating?

On examination assess radio-femoral delay, the quality of the pulse pressure and BP (if the child will let you) in an arm and a leg.

Then the murmur itself? Check the following: (Usually benign)

Restricted to systole,

P2 splits normally with respiration in pulmonary area,

Short duration, coarse vibratory quality, etc.

Small area no radiation,

Soft <3/6, low pitched, no thrill, often L LSE.

Increases with heart rate,

Varies with posture and deep respiration,

Free of other significant related symptoms,

Other tests (ECG, CXR) N? Is the child otherwise perfectly well?

Remember;

Straight back syndrome/thin chest/sternal depression/continuous venous hum – continuous, heard in neck, diastolic accentuation (unlike a PDA), disappears on occluding jugular vein, louder on extending the neck, louder on inspiration?

Note that pansystolic murmurs (as opposed to ESMs) are usually organic and due either to a leaking ventricle or regurgitant valve (VSD, M or T regurgitation). Diastolic murmurs are also significant.

Genetic causes of CHD:

Trisomy 21 Down's (non disjunction) 40-50% have CHD. Common AVC, VSD, ASD, Fallot's.

Trisomy 18 Edward's 99% VSD, PDA, Single umb. A, DORV, Coarctation.

Trisomy 15 Patau's 90% VSD, ASD, Single Umb A. Dextrocardia.

Turner's XO 30-40% Coarctation, AS.
Partial deletion of 5 (Cri du chat) 50% have CHD, VSD.
Noonan's, VSD, PS, Cardiomyopathy.
Apert's, VSD.
Carpenter's, PDA, narrow PA, Transposition.
Crouzon's, PDA, Coarctation.
Lawrence Moon Biedl, Tetralogy.
Von Recklinghausen's, PS, Coarctation.
Treacher Collins, VSD, ASD, PDA,
etc etc

Cardiovascular Teratogens:

Rubella 35%, D.M. 5%, S.L.E.?, P.K.U. 25-50%, Alcohol 25%, Phenytoin >2-3%, Lithium 10%, Thalidomide 5-10%, Sex Hormones 2-4%, ?Smoking, ? Various Vitamin deficiencies.

Hypertrophic Obstructive Cardiomyopathy:

One of the causes of young children suddenly and tragically dying without warning. If it has happened to a relative of a patient of yours, make sure your patient is screened (?implantable pacemaker etc). 40% are Aut. Dom. An overgrowth of ventricular muscle with systolic obstruction and Mitral incompetence. Presents with an asymptomatic murmur in children or ischaemia in adults. Occasionally arrhythmias and sudden death. LVH and q waves (septal hypertrophy) on ECG.

David Frost's son Miles apparently died while out jogging because he was unaware that his father who had died of a heart attack two years earlier had this genetic condition.

Heart Failure at different ages:

Premature infant: Large L>R Shunt at ductal level.
Full Term:
First Week: Hypoplastic L heart. Aortic Atresia.
1 week – 1 month: Coarctation (causes severe heart failure) (+ VSD), TAPVC.
Second month: Transposition of the great arteries (with PDA or VSD).
After 3 months: VSD.
After a year: Heart failure due to CHD is rare. Think of the vanishingly unusual SBE or anaemia.

Bacterial Endocarditis:

Never occurs in secundum ASDs but can be due to VSDs, PDAs, Coarctation, A. valve lesions (including bicuspid valves), M valve lesions, Ostium Primum ASD (abnormal M valve) and Fallot's.

In terms of frequency of valve involvement, the Tricuspid is the most commonly involved valve (50%), the Mitral and Aortic are about 20% each, Pulmonary involvement is "rare". (Cardiology Explained NCBI bookshelf).

Rhythm disturbances:

Paroxysmal SVT:

60-70% have N hearts but the remainder have ASD, Ebstein's, or a cardiac muscle defect. Can present with "white attacks" or with polyuria after the attack. HR is regular and between 200 and 300. Sinus arrhythmia is absent in ASDs, heart block (all kinds) can occur.

[869]

Rheumatic Fever:

Is included more as part of a potential differential diagnosis than because you are likely to see a case – unless you work in India or the Middle East. These are now similar to the Victorian and pre-war overcrowded slums of London as far as Rheumatic Fever is concerned.

I have never seen a case (in 6+ years paediatrics and 30+ years of GP etc) but it is the sort of condition, like TB, which may enjoy a resurgence in some of our cities and for the same reasons. There were only 6 deaths in the UK from Rh F in 2010. It is post streptococcal – so compare with glomerulonephritis, scarlet fever, post streptococcal paediatric autoimmune neuropsychiatric disorders, [PANDAS, Paediatric Autoimmune Neuropsychiatric Disorders Associated with Streptococcal Infections], Sydenham's chorea, post streptococcal arthritis, etc. The organism is Strep Pyogenes Lancefield group A, a Beta Haemolytic strep, rare under age 3 and follows a sore throat by 2-3 weeks. Now GPs, anxious to please their local and national super infection police are reducing their prescribing of antibiotics in what seems a fairly indiscriminate way, we may well see a lot more of these old adversaries. Anyway, Rh F is associated with:

Flitting arthritis – the commonest symptom, large joints, bilaterally, Erythema Marginatum, (occasionally Nodosum), 10% of patients have subcutaneous nodules, fever. The carditis affects younger children preferentially – tachycardia, various murmurs (the blowing mitral incompetent murmur and the mitral flow and aortic incompetent (Carey Coombes) murmurs. There is cardiac enlargement, possibly a pericardial friction rub and occasionally cardiac failure. There is scarring and retraction of the valves which leads to the long term heart damage of old.

There is generally a raised ESR, a raised ASOT, (although not all organisms produce this), raised CRP (which is associated with the damage of post streptococcal nephritis, Rh Arthritis and Rh Fever). The ECG shows distinctive changes including prolonged PR and so on.

There may be Chorea (especially in women) – Sydenham's Chorea, "St Vitus' dance" – (The patron saint of dancers and epileptics) involving the hands, face and feet, loss of balance and emotional outbursts, never older than puberty, bag of worms tongue. This usually completely resolves.

The symptoms and signs are defined as major and minor in order to assist diagnosis. Obviously high temperatures, rashes, joint pains and many of the other symptoms are common in a variety of infections in childhood.

Major: Carditis, arthritis, chorea, erythema marginatum, subcutaneous lumps.

Minor: Arthralgia, fever, raised inflammatory markers, arrhythmia or abnormal ECG (prolonged PR), previous episode of Rh F or inactive heart disease.

The diagnosis is inferred if there are 2 major or 2 minor and one major feature.

The basic cause is a co-antigenicity between the strep cell wall and the victim's periarteriolar connective tissue which is damaged by a Type 2 hypersensitivity reaction (see "Allergy"). The Aschoff lesion is the pathological finding in most affected damaged tissues. Prevention of recurrence is achieved by long term penicillin. Acute treatment was always (my paediatric career partly predated the recognition of Reye's Syndrome, which I have never seen a case of either, so the risks are a little hypothetical but must be balanced) with Aspirin or other anti inflammatories or steroids. Steroids are mandatory if there is carditis. Penicillin is given acutely as well as prophylactically.

Mitral stenosis is a potential long term complication and the fatality rate in developed countries (even assuming a correct diagnosis) is about 5%. Recurrences occur with further Step Pyogenes infections and are not prevented by pneumococcal vaccination.

Myocarditis:

Usually viral: Parvovirus B19, Influenza, Adenoviral, Coxsackie B1-5 in infants and A4-5 in adolescents, but can be due to a Streptococcal antigenic confusion and Lyme Disease (Borrelia Burgdorferi), rarely CMV, Rubella, Rubeola, HIV, Hepatitis, Herpes virus. Most children recover with treatment (Immunoglobulin, diuretics, cardiac support, anti coagulants, etc) but a few babies die in the acute stage or develop chronic heart disease. Some auto immune diseases also cause myocarditis in children.

Blood Pressure Measurement:

Sphygmomanometer cuff optimum sizes: in inches

AGE	WIDTH	LENGTH
0-3/12	1	4
3/12-1yr	1 1/2	5
1-3	2	6
3-6	3	6
7	4	7

Odd Paediatric Genetics:

Cystic Fibrosis:

The most common life limiting Autosomal Recessive genetic disease. Both parents must be carriers – as are 5% of the population, (so 1/20 X 1/20 X 1/4 = the incidence of this Aut Rec condition (roughly) of 1:2,000 – 1:2,500 live births), the incidence is lower in non Caucasians. (1:17,000 in Afro-Caribbeans) The fault is on the long arm of chromosome 7, coding for the CFTR (cystic fibrosis transmembrane conductance regulator) controlling the movement of chloride and sodium ions through cell membranes. There are 1900 mutations of this gene now recognised-a deletion of phenylalanine at position 508 is the most common. There are 7,000 patients in the UK with CF.

It presents with meconium ileus, failure to thrive and various congestive respiratory symptoms as various body secretions are excessively viscid (– the basic dysfunction involves sodium and chloride transport across epithelial membranes so mucus, sweat and pancreatic exocrine secretions are abnormal).

There are recurrent chest and later, sinus infections, (Staph and Haemophilus and later Pseudomonas and Aspergillus are the common organisms). Malabsorption, late first meconium, recurrent pancreatitis, steatorrhoea (1/3 of affected children) and rectal prolapse are charactaristic. Nasal polyps and liver disease are other features. Later still, the pancreatic damage overlaps into endocrine territory, causing diabetes although this is not usually severe.

The mainstay of therapy consists of early treatment of chest infections, physiotherapy, treating the pancreatic exocrine deficiency with oral pancreatic enzymes, treating any malabsorption and so on. Infertility may not be accessible to treatment.

There is however a new generation of drugs being produced aimed at specifically restoring the function of the defective CFTR protein. These are:

Agents that promote ribosomal read-through of nonsense mutations eg Ataluren,

CFTR correctors eg Lumacaftor, CFTR potentiators eg Ivacaftor.

In 1938 survival beyond the age of 10 was rare. In 1986 average survival was about 26 yrs. It was 38 yrs in 2008. With gold standard care most of today's young CF patients should make their mid 40's.

Milder forms of CF do exist:

There are some patients who produce enough CFTR protein to maintain lung function but not enough to maintain normal pancreatic function. They develop azospermia and pancreatitis but may have normal sweat tests. They are at risk from chest infections and if detected should be monitored closely regarding lung and liver function.

Diagnosis:

Some areas of the UK screen for CF in the heel prick test (Immunoreactive trypsin) and follow any (two) positive tests with the gold standard sweat test, (raised sweat Cl and Na) – Confirmation of the diagnosis is by finding two CFTR gene mutations.

Follow up of CF patients must include annual FBC, checking Vitamins A, D, E, K (all fat soluble), Mg, Ca, Fe, clotting, LFTs. and stool sample analysis. Annual liver USS (to assess cirrhosis) should also be part of regular follow up.

30% of adult CF patients require insulin so annual OGTTs are necessary as are regular Dexa scans since osteopenia and osteoporosis are common (give Vitamin D supplements).

Obviously, chest infections must be treated vigorously and at length but this can be assisted by nebulised Colomycin/Tobramycin/Pulmozyme (Dornase Alpha). Pseudomonas, Staph and Aspergillus are characteristic and difficult CF pathogens.

85% of CF patients require pancreatic enzyme supplements with all meals.

Holt Oram Syndrome:

Genetic defect that affects arm and heart development, 1:100,000 Aut Dom, 100% penetrance, 85% new mutations, ASDs, VSDs, conduction defects, upper limb deformities.

Ehlers Danlos syndrome

A group of 10 or 11 Dom. and Rec. conditions that affect connective tissue 1:400,000. Now classified as 6 major types since 1997. Classically:

Hypermobility, Loose skin, Weakness, Poor wound healing, Mitral Incompetence, Aneurysm of the sinus of Valsalva (Aortic valve).

But there are many other associated blood, joint, CNS, G.I., skin and other conditions.

Obesity Syndromes in Childhood:

Include:

Frohlich's, Laurence Moon Biedl, Prader Willi, Cushings etc.

Child development and screening: The Health Visitor is said to give advice on these:

The baby's and child's growth and development,

Various medical conditions, allergies and infections,

Breast feeding, bottle feeding and weaning,

Postnatal depression and parents' mental and physical health,

Behaviour issues – sleeping, eating, potty training, tantrums etc.

Support with parenting,

Family planning,

Family health and relationship issues,

Teething,
More serious health concerns,
Health promotion,
Community health and development.

Child Health Surveillance is taking place via the "Healthy Child Programme" currently. This is supposed to have a "greater focus than before" on A/N care, support for both parents, identifying at risk families (if both are unemployed, poor quality housing, no educational achievements, mental health problems, longstanding ill health, low income etc), new vaccination programmes etc. G.Ps do the newborn and the 6-8 week checks.

The best **Screening Ages** are currently said to be:
Week 12 of the pregnancy,
The neonatal examination,
Two week (or thereabouts) new baby review,
6-8 week examination,
1 year,
2 – 2 1/2 years,
At start of education (includes vision and hearing).
Some recommend: Birth, 6 weeks, 6-9m, 18-24m, and 3 – 3 1/2 yrs.

You and I know that whenever a preschool child of any age is brought to us, with any condition, we should have a rough idea of what they should be capable of doing developmentally and have a look over them generally, surreptitiously and ask about:

Talking, hearing, vision, drawing, playing with different toys, crawling, walking, socialising, coordination, vocabulary, sleep, behaviour, anything that seems relevant to the points raised.

Our local Health Authority does screening at 6-9 months, 18-24 months, 3 – 3 1/2 years.

Six week screening examination: (Very basic)
Weight.
Length.
Head circumference (OFC).
Social: Smile.
Hearing.
Vision: Squint, Red reflex (plus 3 lens).
Motor: Grasp reflex, placing, walking.
Movements.
Tone, (support under chest).
Head control.
Attempts to lift head prone.
Physical examination:
Palmar creases.
Facial appearance.
Umbilicus.
Skin etc.
CVS: Pink, heart sounds, radio-femoral delay, liver edge.
RS: Respiratory rate, chest movements, air entry.
GIT. Palate, abdomen, anus.

UGT: External genitals.

Hips: Creases, Ortolanis, Barlows.

Breast Feeding:

Feeding a neonate colostrum reduces the risk of death from subsequent overwhelming infection to 1/3. It reduces gastroenteritis, LRTIs, ear infections and meningitis. There is a 20% lower death rate between 1m and 1 year in breast fed infants, the longer the breast feeding the lower the rate.

It may reduce the rate of some childhood cancers, both adult types of diabetes, inflammatory bowel disease and it reduces adult cholesterol. Breast feeding reduces the incidence of allergic disease in childhood. It improves cognitive development and IQ, reduces childhood obesity and cuts SIDS by a half (exclusive BF at 1m), it lowers rates of maternal post natal depression, ovarian and breast cancer in the mother.

Perinatal Jaundice:(Remember Direct Bilirubin is conjugated, Indirect is unconjugated)

A level of bilirubin >80umol/li gives the baby a jaundiced appearance clinically. Physiological jaundice (unconjugated) occurs in most babies in two phases and can go on for 6 or 8 weeks in breast fed infants.

The pathway is:

Red cells break down>unconjugated bilirubin >via glucuronyl transferase in the liver >conjugated biliribin in bile>gut >intestinal flora>urobilinogen.

Generally there is **liver disease if there is bilirubin in the urine**.

Pathological Jaundice:

Jaundice in first 24 hrs of life.

Total bilirubin >330umol/li,

A more rapid rise in bilirubin than 8.5umol/li/hr or 85umol/li/day,

Direct bilirubin>34umol/li.

Bilirubin causes a number of pathological conditions in babies: Chronic bilirubin encephalopathy, extrapyramidal damage, extra ocular movement abnormalities, high tone hearing loss, (language delay), cognitive defects, damage to dental enamel.

Kernicterus (The Kern is the nuclear region of the brain) is a condition of acute and chronic damage of the basal ganglia, hippocampus, geniculate bodies, various cranial nerve bodies, (oculomotor, vestibular, cochlear) and cerebellum. There are acute and chronic phases and it is (or was) much more likely to affect the premature baby.

Causes of jaundice:

Unconjugated:

Haemolytic:	**Non Haemolytic:**
Spherocytosis, Eliptocytosis.	Cephalohaematoma,
Sepsis, A/V malformation,	Polycythemia,
G6PD Deficiency.	Hypothyroidism,
Pyruvate Kinase Deficiency.	Gilberts – Benign Unconjugated Hyperbilirubin-
Sickle Cell.	aemia).
Thalassaemia.	Crigler-Najjar.
Haemolytic Disease, ABO, Rhesus.	
Breast Milk Jaundice.	

Conjugated:
Hepatitis B.
TORCH infections (Toxo, Other, – Syph, Varicell/Zost, Parvo B19, Rubella, CMV, Herpes).
Galactosaemia.
α1 Antitrypsin Deficiency.
CF.
Drugs.
Total parenteral nutrition.
Biliary Atresia.
Alagille Syndrome   (Aut Dom, inadequate number of bile ducts, cong, heart dis, dysmorphic spine, odd facies, kidneys and CNS affected).

Jaundice Treatment:

Phototherapy
Exchange transfusion if the level of bilirubin exceeds 430umol/li. The risk being kernicterus.

Vitamin K:

This is given to the new born because of the small risk of VKDB (Vitamin K deficiency bleeding, approximate incidence 1 in 10,000). Vitamin K is needed for clotting factors II VII IX and X. This can be early (24 hrs), classic (days 2-7) or late (over 7 days and sometimes up to 26 weeks). There is a higher incidence in breast fed, (20X), sick, jaundiced, premature and babies of mothers on anticonvulsants. The fly in the ointment was a disputed association of Vitamin K (Konakion, given IM) with some childhood cancers from research in the early 90s. Vitamin K is added to formula milk, – it is about the only relative advantage of not breast feeding, so fully formula fed babies only need the neonatal oral dose. Breast fed infants would need this and top ups if the Vitamin K were only administered orally. What happens now (the cancer research was never confirmed) is that IM vitamin K 1mg is given to all babies at birth and this effectively prevents VKDB whatever the mode of feeding. If oral Vitamin K is administered in breast fed infants, a dose at birth, the end of the first week and the first month are necessary. (Alternatively: weekly 1mg 'til 12 weeks or repeating 2mg at week 1 and 4 – Patient.co.uk). Without nationally administered Vitamin K, out of the 800,000 babies born each year, 6 would die from an intracranial bleed and up to 20 would be brain damaged. Subarachnoid haemorrhage is the main risk but subdural, intraventricular, parenchymal and bleeding elsewhere takes place as a result of VKDB – unless prevented.

Other Perinatal/Paediatric Problems:

Cradle cap:

Try: Capasal shampoo, Daktarin Cream, Ceanel Conc (Cetrimide/Undecenoic Acid 1% liqu.) as a shampoo. – antibacterial and antifungal.

Strawberry Naevus:

Capillary haemangioma. Can grow for up to 18m. of age, subsequent involution takes up to 10 years. There are superficial and cavernous (deeper) haemangiomata. "Segmental Haemangiomata" of the face are associated with posterior fossa, cardiac and eye abnormalities. They usually require no treatment but some have applied topical Imiquimod as a last resort and cautiously to shrink them.

Scabies, Head Lice:

Permethrin: Lyclear Dermal Cream, Cream Rinse (Lotion). Apply after a shampoo and leave for 10 minutes then wash out. Two applications a week apart. Scabies, head lice. This is used as an insecticide industrially and I have sprayed the joists in my attic with water soluble Permethrin from a local chemical company to eradicate woodworm. It is toxic to cats and fish but not dogs and hopefully not homeowners.

The wet hair should be checked 2-3 days after the final application with a plastic comb. This, of course is where the expression to search with a fine toothed comb comes from and if there are still adult lice present, try:

Malathion (Includes Derbac-M) Alcoholic Lotion (aqueous in children and asthmatics). Said to be safe in pregnancy although it is associated with aggressive prostate cancer when used as an insecticide agriculturally (Am J Epidemiology 2013). Recommended contact time 12 hours. Scabies and head lice: Other treatments include Phenothrin, Crotamiton, (Eurax lotion), Dimeticone. (-Dimethicone, a silicone used as a hair conditioner which suffocates the lice.) Natural products include aniseed, citronella, coconut, tea tree oil, even warm vinegar under a shower cap although this has to be worn all night.

Avoid swimming pools while treatment is being applied. Derbac-M, Dimeticone and Permethrin are all available OTC.

Undescended testicles:

3% of new born boys, commoner in premature (30%). 2/3 UDTs continue to descend over the first year, but if not yet in the "base" of the scrotum, you need to operate.

Generally speaking, most surgeons operate at 6-12m. I have been to lectures where some surgeons suggested referral at 12-18m, operation at 3-4 years. I would send the child in as soon as you detect the condition, you know how difficult and particular surgeons can be. Currently the median actual age of orchidopexy is about 18 months, it seems.

Foreskins:

50% retract at 1 year
75% by 2 years
90% by 3 years
at 17 years 99% retract without surgery.

Circumcision, neonatal programming, autistic spectrum disorders:

No ethical doctor should be involved in circumcision done for religious or cultural reasons. Performing a surgical procedure that is not correcting an abnormality or preventing harm is clearly unethical, no matter how many people subject their babies to it every year because of tradition. Circumcision causes pain, bleeding, infection, trauma, scarring, many varied morbidities and some mortalities wherever it is practiced. There are no genuine health benefits.

We have evolved no redundant parts of our bodies, save perhaps for the vermiform appendix. Even this organ is now known to act as a reservoir of commensal bacteria during gastro enteritis, helping to maintain the Biome, as well as being a white cell programming and immune centre. Streamlining is what Natural Selection does. It needs no help from us. Whether it is by supernatural design or random luck we are not born with much that we can readily do without. The foreskin serves several important purposes which any adult male who loses it will readily tell you. Otherwise it wouldn't be there. A brief examination of research data in this area shows:

That circumcision, presumably historically performed in hot dry countries which lacked copious supplies of water for washing and to assist in foreskin retraction, was probably originally done for reasons of preventative hygiene which do not apply in the modern world. It then acquired a religious, racial and cultural significance related to the populations that practiced it out of proportion to its ancient, presumably forgotten purpose. Balanitis 2,000+ years ago must have been a major, dangerous and complication prone infection in the Middle East and without effective treatment. Desert communities must have thought circumcision was a sensible prophylactic procedure and the earlier performed the better. Islam followed Judaism in this respect.

It is clear that the procedure has a number of permanent harmful effects even discounting the unnecessary pain, suffering, infection risk, bleeding, scarring, penile damage, surgical complications and occasional death it causes. All Paediatricians, Paediatric Surgeons, Neonatologists and GPs will have seen the misery that this procedure inflicts. The foreskin is the second most sensitive part of a newborn boy's body after the cornea. The vast majority of cultural circumcisions are done with no effective pain relief and the pain persists and recurs at each nappy or dressing change for weeks.

Circumcised boys have their lifelong pain threshold set lower, presumably by virtue of experiencing prolonged surgical and post operative pain within the first few days of life when pain pathways and sensitivity are being centrally programmed. A Univadis article discussed neonates and the effect of unrelieved pain: 20% of perinatal in-patient babies never receive any pain relief *(despite the chest drains, scalp and foot vein drips, the arterial stabs, the arterial and umbilical catheters, the ET tubes and the limb pinioning that is universal in neonatal units* – my italics). To quote the 2015 article "It is quite likely that many neonates have needed pain relief at some point. Experiencing a lot of pain as a newborn may lead to behavioural changes with regard to pain later as an adult and may lead to attention and concentration problems." There is in fact increasing evidence that Asperger spectrum disorders are commoner in circumcised populations than otherwise similar uncircumcised groups.

In a Danish paper which found a link the summary said:

"Given the widespread practice of non-therapeutic circumcision in infancy and childhood around the world, our findings should prompt other researchers to examine the possibility that circumcision trauma in infancy or early childhood might carry an increased risk of serious neurodevelopmental and psychological consequences."

Ritual circumcision and risk of autism spectrum disorder in 0- to 9-year-old boys: national cohort study in Denmark, Journal of the Royal Society of Medicine, doi: 10.1177/0141076814565942

Circumcised adults do not (since the foreskin is heavily endowed with sensory nerves and the glans epithelium undergoes thickening and drying when unprotected) experience the same sensory stimulation during foreplay and therefore do not have the same experience of sex. Young adults who undergo the procedure frequently testify to this change.

Male circumcision in some bizarre way may be also used to justify female genital mutilation. So there are numerous reasons not to remove the foreskins of babies and very few that justify it.

Circumcision is justified when phimosis is causing recurrent balanitis but for not much else.

Inguinal Hernia:

Almost always indirect in children (failure of closure of the internal inguinal ring). 4% boys and 1% girls <1 year old. (But some sources say 9M:1F confusingly) 60% R, 25% L, 15% bilateral. 20% risk of incarceration. 5% of the population.

What you may have forgotten: The anatomy is: Vein Artery Nerve>from medial to lateral. Useful when taking arterial samples in an emergency.

Congenital Hydrocoel:

90% resolve by 18m. If it occurs after the neonatal period or fluctuates then it is due to a persistent Processus Vaginalis. This is a pouch of peritoneum (that is carried into the scrotum by the descent of the testicle and which in the scrotum forms the Tunica Vaginalis) still communicating with the peritoneum. It isn't painful but crying increases intra abdominal pressure and squeezes fluid into the scrotum making the swelling bigger. After 18m a repair of the communicating Processus Vaginalis stops the fluid draining into the scrotum from the peritoneum and solves the problem.

50% of boys are born with some degree of hydrocoel. Like hernias, it is commoner on the R but bilateral in 20%.

Later Hydrocoel

Can be due to other things than draining peritoneal fluid. It can be due to torsion of the testicle or its appendage, orchitis or epididymitis, trauma or very rarely due to tumour.

Synostosis, Craniosynostosis, Plagiocephaly, moulding and the malleable skull:

Synostosis (fusion of two bones)

Posterior plagiocephaly: Non synostostotic skull asymmetry is commoner now everyone puts their babies on their backs to avoid SIDS. The child is generally born looking normal, with the skull flattening slowly developing over 2 months. Thereafter the skull fills out slowly and a normal rounded shape develops over several months or years as sitting, rolling and normal head and body movements follow.

Synostosis occurs in a variety of complex syndromes, the commonest being Apert, Crouzon and Pfeiffer syndromes. It can be recessive or dominant.

When one of the sutures fuses early – and this occurs in about 1:2000 babies, the skull stops growing **at 90 degrees** to the fused suture but continues growing in line with it and therefore becomes lop sided or elongated. The parents will notice the odd shape but generally the baby is unperturbed. It is unusual for generalised or extensive synostosis to cause raised intracranial pressure and symptoms. It can be part of a syndrome or isolated.

The normal time of closure of the sutures is:

Metopic, 3-9 months.

Lambdoid, Coronal, Sagittal, 22-40 months.

Sagittal synostosis is the commonest premature suture fusion not associated with a syndrome.

Scaphocephaly – boat shaped skull, is due to synostosis of the sagittal suture. There is a prominent forehead with frontal bossing and a prominent posterior portion of the skull where compensatory unrestricted growth takes place. This is called Coning, – and not to be confused with the other type of coning, the forcing down of the skull contents through the foramen magnum with raised ICP.

Trigonocephaly is due to metopic synostosis – a narrow forehead and triangular shape to the skull with close set eyes (hypotelorism).

Plagiocephaly – a skew head – anterior plagiocephaly occurs in unilateral coronal synostosis. Posterior plagiocephaly in unilateral lambdoid synostosis.

Brachycephaly (head shortening in the AP plane) can occur in synostosis of both coronal sutures. The skull looks squashed forwards to backwards.

It is rare for the child to present with raised intracranial pressure (headache, vomiting, visual symptoms etc), the usual situation is that comments have been made about the skull shape or the parents have done some Internet research and assumed the worst. In 30 + years of GP and 6 + years of paediatrics I have only had one patient require surgery for synostosis. The worrying symptoms and signs are however: bulging fontanelles, drowsiness, distended superficial scalp veins, irritability and high pitched cry, vomiting or poor feeding, possibly increased head circumference, fits, sunset gaze or inability to look up, bulging eyes, delayed milestones. I would hope we would have picked up the raised ICP before most of these had become apparent however.

Radiography with SXR and CT are the definitive investigations. Surgery if necessary is generally performed between 6 and 12 m.

Helmets which are worn and were thought to aid skull moulding have recently been shown to have no advantage over "No treatment". Where the shape is due to moulding rather than premature fusing, there is a lot that the parents can do themselves: One of our local physiotherapy departments has a hand-out that attributes a variety of exacerbating factors to the pre existing labour-caused head shape. These include tight neck muscles, prematurity, the constant same position in sleep, lack of "tummy time" (Babies should spend at least some time prone while awake every day), car seats which if used a lot prevent free movement and encourage moulding. "Try to restrict use of these only to essential car travel".

My physios suggest encouraging the baby to turn "against the natural roll of the shape of the skull" by changing the position of the cot, putting toys or mobiles where the baby has to roll the head against the camber of the skull, spending time playing with the baby on his/her tummy, encouraging any activity that causes head movement that strengthens weak neck muscles, using a baby sling rather than a car seat when going out as this strengthens neck muscles, feeding the baby with the head turned against the favoured position and so on.

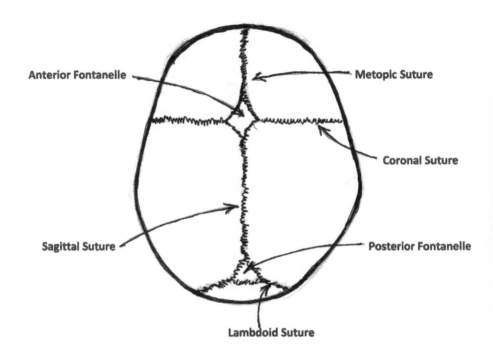

Normal skull of the newborn.

Developmental milestones:

ASQ-3 is the Ages and Stages Questionnaire™ and is available to "Pinpoint developmental progress" between 1m and 5 1/2 years. It is one of a number of developmental assessment tools generally available.

Neonatally: Ventral suspension: Flexed hips, head below plane of the body, limbs hang down. Moro reflex is symmetrical (startle, arms stretched), head lag on pulling to sit. Leg extension in response to pressure, primary walking response, palmar and plantar grasp all present.

Rooting, sucking, swallowing, optical closure to bright light.

1 month: Fanning of digits on limb extension, if corner of mouth touched, turns face to that side. Head lag on pulling to sit, head in line with body on ventrosuspension. Automatic walking movements, stepping if dorsum of foot touched. Turns head to light, briefly follows close slow moving object, follows light with eyes, defensive blink from 6+ weeks. Startle reaction to sudden noise, reacts to soothing voice, vocalises in response to mother's talk. Holds head erect a few seconds.

3 months: Moves hands to mid line in front when lying on back, kicks vigorously, little or no head lag on pulling to sit. Head up on ventrosuspension. Lying prone, lifts head and upper chest clear of the mat, hips and shoulders extended. Taking weight on legs, knees give way. Visually aware, head follows moving objects, watches own hands, clasps and unclasps hands. Palmar grip disappears. May turn to sound and show change in behaviour in anticipation. Gaze fixes on mother's face, pleasure at being handled. Searches for sound with eyes, glances from one object to another, follows person with eyes.

6 months: Lying on back lifts head to examine feet, can grab one, later both feet. Sits with support looking from side to side. Holds arms up in readiness when being lifted, pulls self to sit when hands held. Strong alternating kick, can roll front to back and sometimes back to front. Good head control and straight back on being held in sitting position, sits alone briefly. Lying prone will lift head and chest up on extended arms, if held standing will bounce up and down taking own weight. Binocular vision, no squint, interested and follows activity. Palmar grasp, exchanges from one hand to the other. Out of visual field, things don't exist. Vocalises "tunefully" and turns to mother's voice at several yards. Laughs, giggles, screams appropriately. Responds to hearing tests. Turns head to person talking. Can use a single hand picking up technique (usually double handed scoop though), puts most things in mouth. Passes objects between hands, shakes rattle, usually friendly with new people but becoming a little more suspicious (more so from 7-8m).

9 months: Sits alone, leaning forward or sideways to pick things up. May be beginning to crawl (some babies never even try!) Pulls to stand but can't lower gently back down. Makes stepping movements when held supported. Forward parachute reflex is present (protects against fall damage). Alert and interested in surroundings. Reaches and manipulates (grasp) manipulates two objects at once. Points and jabs with index finger. Scissor grip when pulling string etc. Pincer grip of small objects. Cannot voluntarily release by controlled putting things down but can drop objects. Looks for things fallen out of sight. Shouts to attract attention, "Dad Dad" etc. Babbles, understands "bye bye" etc. Can imitate some simple sounds (unless deaf). Holds and bites biscuits/rusks. Suspicious of strangers. Shakes rattle or bell. Plays "Peep Bo". Can find hidden toy when shown where it has been placed.

One year: Sits well. Gets up to sitting from lying. Crawls or bottom shuffles. Pulls to stand and lets himself down. Cruises furniture. Pincer grip of small objects. Casts toys down and follows where they go. Beginning to have a hand preference, shows interest in pictures. Turns to own name, understands several words and simple instructions, uses a cup with a little help, bell and rattle without. Waves "bye bye" on request, can stand without support (sometimes). Unsteady walk. Creeps upstairs and sometimes backwards downstairs. Tower of two cubes if shown. Interested in pictures, points at desired objects, interested at the world outside the window. Plays pat a cake. Three words with meaning. Retains three cubes.

15 months: Chatters a lot, up to 6 sensible words, knows and points at familiar objects, people etc. Understands simple instructions, "give it to me, wave bye bye" etc, knows and indicates when nappy wet or soiled. More emotional and dependent on reassurance and company. Explores and takes risks. Runs with care in straight lines, climbs stairs holding a hand, creeps backwards downstairs, pushes a trolley or buggy, squats to pick things off the floor.

Places one object on another.

18 months: Fine pincer grip for small objects, palmar or tripod grasp of pencil and makes side to side scribble or dots. Three block tower (after being shown, or on own). Likes pictures in books and turns pages together, with some hand preference. Talks to self while playing. Uses up to 20 words but understands more. Tries to sing. Follows simple instructions, recognises and points to parts of body. Uses spoon to feed and a cup without too much spillage from either. Some have bowel control by now. Can play alone but likes adult company. Alternating dependency and opposition. Runs and can avoid obstacles, squats up and down with ease, pulls larger wheeled toys. Can walk up and often down stairs, can walk backwards. Takes off shoes and socks. Scoots along on a tricycle.

2 years: Retrieves fine objects accurately with delicate grip, eg unwraps a sweet, picks up a small bead or pin. Builds a tower of 6-7 cubes. Holds a pencil nearer the point with two fingers and thumb, can draw circles, copy a vertical straight line and occasionally a "V". Can turn pages in a book. Has a clear hand preference. Can recognise adults (once shown) in photos. Uses 50 words, recognises more, simple sentences, refers to self by name, some monologues while at play. Asking names of objects, follows simple instructions. Uses spoon and cup well, warns need to use the loo, usually dry by day. Unaware of environmental dangers despite curiosity, role play, make believe play. Some tantrums and negativity when thwarted. Plays alongside but not with other children. Cannot defer gratification or satisfaction. Walks up and downstairs holding rail (two feet to a step). Climbs apparatus and runs well, jumps with two feet a short distance. Throws and kicks primitively. Tower of 7 plus. Good eye for details in pictures, hand preference, can draw T and V. Knows four parts of the body and the names of four toys. Copies a horizontal line.

Two and a half years: Uses 200 words. Still shows echolalia while at play. Lots of why, who, where? questions. Remembers some simple nursery rhymes and likes familiar stories. Can be dry at night (lifting helps). Tantrums, likes role play, can use alternate feet going upstairs. Runs around objects, uses pedals on tricycle, can walk on tiptoes, can briefly stand on one foot, can catch a large ball between arms.

3 years: Up to 9 cube tower by 3 1/2 years. Good hand control over pencil which is held near the sharp end in an appropriate grip. Copies various shapes, eg: OVHT etc. Can match a few primary colours, cuts with scissors, knows full name, age, sex. Uses personal pronouns, (I, you, he), plurals and prepositions (on, over, under). Personal monologues and many who, why, where? type questions. Counts to 10, knows several nursery rhymes. Usually dry at night. Helps at home tasks, assists in tidying surroundings, make believe play with other children, floor play with toys, shares, shows affection to younger siblings, beginning to understand present, past and future and waiting for things to happen. One foot to a step on stairs. Climbs ladders and trees, can stand and hop on one foot, bends standing to pick things up. Improving skills with ball and bat.

4 years: Can pick up small things (pins, cotton) with one eye covered. 10 cube tower, can oppose thumb against fingers in turn if shown first. Draws a stick man with arms, head, body and sometimes fingers, draws a house on request, matches 4 basic colours. Good speech, still asking why and where type questions. Good accounts of own recent life events. Likes simple jokes, counts up to 20. Can tell long stories, mixes up fact and imagination. Eats with spoon and fork, brushes teeth, washes and dries hands. Independent, can be quarrelsome, sense of humour. Argues more verbally with peers than physically, needs companion play with peers, takes turns and shares, shows sympathy for unhappy acquaintances. Aware of past present and future. Climbs, slides, swings, skips. Can hop on each foot. Better at various ball games.

5 years: Can build 3 or 4 steps from cubes when shown, threads bigger needles and simple sewing, good drawing and paint brush use. Copies square and at 5 1/2yrs a triangle. Draws a man with features, a house with windows and some architectural features. Better at drawing various subjects, colouring in, counting fingers, matching up to 10 colours, likes listening to stories, Gives names, age, sometimes birthday, address. Curious about abstract words (happy, clever). Uses knife and fork, gets dressed and undressed, becoming more independent, play more constructive, domestically aware of need for tidiness with reminding, cooperates with peers, sense of humour, comforting to peers in distress. Skips on alternate feet.

There is of course a huge variety of normal development within human beings just as there is no standard adult or parent. So much emotional and neurological development depends upon the nurturing, stimulation of and quality of the home environment, particularly how often the parents read and play with the children, ask questions and (from animal studies) how much touching, stroking and physical contact there is in the first few months. From human experience: how much talking to, reading to, how much simple involving conversation during normal family activities, how many books and pictures there are in the house and how RESTRICTED uninformative television and computer games are. Especially how limited is the time that children are left alone in front of TVs and screens of any kind. To this I would add whether growing children eat with and go out on regular trips and walks (etc) with their parents and how limited their access to gaming and harmful social media is later on.

Most concerns and consultations will be on the likelihood of the child being slow due to Cerebral Palsy or Autism or possibly deafness.

There is evidence that the early detection of all these improves the final outcome for function and independence. Apart from severe CP.

Visual Development:

Neonate:
Pupils react to light.
Eyes close to bright light.
Dolls eye reflex.
Head and eyes turn to diffuse light.
Focal length about 12" until 6 weeks.
Briefly follows dangling ball at focal length.
Watches mother's face at 3 weeks during feeds.
Eyes turn to sound reflexly.

1-3 months:
Concentrates on close human face.
Eye convergence for own fingers from 3 months.
Defensive blink from 4-6 weeks (It **is** strange that the eyes are left vulnerable to injury and FB for the first 6 weeks).
Good at following dangling ball 6-10" from face.

4-6 months:
Visually alert (near and distant).
Good eye movements following moving target, all directions.
Looks at small object on surface and reaches towards it.
Reaches for toys (4 1/2m) and looks at them.
Follows moving/falling objects.
Binocular movement of eyes.
Squint now abnormal.

7-12 months:
Finger/thumb grasp for small objects.

Looks for hidden toys (from 9/10 months) if they are hidden while they watch.
Tests with mounted balls at 10'.
Good peripheral vision
1-2 years:
Probable adult acuity.

Visual screening
Is theoretically normally performed (By the GP or HV) at:
Neonatally,
6-8 weeks,
6-9 months,
18-24 months,
3 – 3 1/2 years.

Hearing Assessment and Red Flags:
The risk of deafness is increased in:
FH of sensori-neural hearing loss,
Parental consanguinity,
IU and perinatal infection (CMV, Toxoplasmosis, Rubella, Herpes, Syphilis, etc),
Cranial dysmorphism/anatomical abnormality of the head and neck including Down's
syndrome, cleft palate etc,
SCBU admission lasting more than 72 hours,
Bacterial meningitis/septicaemia,
Neonatal jaundice (Kernicterus),
Head injury, ,
Parental concern about hearing/communication.

Hearing Tests are usually performed at:
(Neonatal at risk policy screening?)
6 weeks,
7-9 months (Distraction test: a pass is 2 out of three tests turning the head in the
direction of the sound),
3 years,
School entry.

Autism (See below)
The Red Flags of Autism are:
Between 1 and 2 years autistic children are less likely to
Show others objects that they are interested in,
Coordinate gaze, gestures, sounds and expressions,
Share interest or enjoyment with others,
Respond to their name,
Share happy facial expressions,
Point out objects they are interested in to others*,
Play with a variety of toys*,
Respond to contextual clues*,
Use consonants in speech*,
Look directly at people.

They are more likely to:
Make repetitive movements with objects,
Make repetitive body movements or body postures (hand flapping etc),
Use odd tones of voice,
* these can also be caused by developmental delay.

Nocturnal Enuresis: (Failure to achieve continence at night by the age of 5 years)

Exclude both types of diabetes from the history, exclude constipation, the commonest association, UTI, stress, abuse, etc.

Check BP, abdomen, spine, neurological examination of legs, gait, anus, genitalia.

Test MSU/dipstix, ?AXR, USS abdomen, urine and plasma osmolality.

Star charts and rewards, "lifting" when the parents go to bed (make sure the child is awake). Reduce caffeine. 5-7 year olds: (7% affected). Star chart, diary, a few cope with an alarm, Desmopressin.

Over 7 year olds: Enuretic clinic if one available? Alarm. Desmopressin.

Commoner in boys. 40% of children of a parent who wetted in childhood and 70+% of children of two parents who wetted in childhood wet themselves at night.

Imipramine 10mg 25mg Tabs, also "Oral solution" 6-8yrs 25mg 8-11yrs 25-50mg over 11 yrs 50-75mg.

Nortriptyline though less sedative may also be used at night – again the data sheet advises against use under age 7 years.

If the problem is "Detrusor Instability" (daytime frequency with a normal USS and MSUs), Oxybutynin 2.5-5mg 2-3X daily can be tried. But make absolutely sure the child is not in retention and overflow and that constipation is treated first.

Reassess Rx at 3m and examine abdomen at each monthly assessment.

Desmopressin: Desmospray and Desmotabs. (etc) Avoid during episodes of diarrhoea and vomiting also avoid fluid overload, excess night time drinking etc as the HPA is switched off by this treatment. 1-2 tabs or 1-2 sprays at bedtime. Stop and review after 3 months.

General advice: Regular micturition, bladder training, avoid infection, unresponsive cases may need urodynamic studies/referral.

Oesophageal Reflux:

If a baby is refluxing and crying (not just ruminating a refluxed feed) it must be assumed that the baby is suffering from oesophagitis due to gastric acid. This is painful and can occur hours after a feed, even shortly before the next feed. Thickening the feed, weaning and sitting the baby up after feeds can help. So can raising the pH of the reflux fluid or trying to tighten up the lower oesophageal sphincter with prokinetic drugs.

SMA Staydown, Aptamil Comfort Milks. Thicken with Carobel Powder (Carob bean gum), or at a push "Multi thick "powder (this is Maize starch) although for some reason they say caution below 1 year?? Also "Thicken Aid" or "Thick and Easy" (both Maltodextrin and Maize Starch).

Gaviscon infant sachets 1/2 – 1 with each feed or mixed with a little boiled water in the breast fed and given after each feed.

Ranitidine (15mg/ml, 300ml bottle) 1m-6m 1-3mg/kg per dose TDS oral solution (10mg/kg/day),

Domperidone (5mg/ml) 1m-12 yrs 400ug/kg 3-4X/daily. These can be used with antacids.

Colic:

The most effective treatment, Dicyclomine elixir, (Merbentyl), was withdrawn in 1985 to the surprise and despair of most of us who were Paediatricians at the time. To quote Consultant Paediatrician Dr Harvey Marcovitch: "In 20 years I have never seen a baby die from the prescription of sedatives for crying but I have seen many killed, blinded or taken into care when crying proved intolerable".*

Hear Hear! I say. – A classic example of the drug regulators being out of contact with clinicians in the trenches and making their decisions based purely on abstract data. What I regard as the institutionalised absence of democracy and consultation in medical policy making.

Simeticone. (Simethicone) Infacol.0.5-1ml before each feed. The same stuff put on hair to suffocate head licebut no real evidence it works in colic. Gaviscon infant sachets.

Colief, Lactase 4 drops with each bottle of feed.

Lactobaciius Reuteri drops given from day 1 may reduce colic. The research paper I read suggested it also reduced "long term visceral hypersensitivity" and "mucosal permeability". The suggestion being that paediatric and adult IBS symptoms would be lessened. Other papers have come out using the same lactobacillus (Pediatrics 2007;119:124-130.) in breast fed infants testing Simeticone against lactobacilli preparations showing a clear advantage of the probiotic in preventing colic.

Probiotics using a daily Lactobacillus products **have** been shown to significantly reduce colic in other studies. In another compelling study (JAMA Paed 2014.168: 228-233) babies were treated in a double blind trial, prophylactically from week one and treated babies cried for half the time that untreated babies did at 1m and 3m.

I have often wondered whether pain suffered in the early perinatal period might programme the patient's pain threshold for life.(There is some evidence for this with peri-natal surgery, circumcision etc) It is an open question whether IBS sufferers are simply more aware of normal gut sensations and interpret them as pain due to programming of pain pathways in the first few months. – in much the same way as fibromyalgia sufferers may over interpret normallish sensory input from the all over the body. Who could say what level of routine subliminal discomfort is acceptable and what constitutes pain?

Cow's Milk Protein Allergy:/Lactose Intolerance:

CMPA Is much rarer than parents and many doctors think and challenge proven milk protein allergy occurs in only 1-3% of children (though some say 2-6%) (It is said to affect about 0.1% of adults) In my experience, far fewer than that. The protein involved is usually alpha S1 casein and this produces a variety of allergic responses in the sensitised, – immediate and delayed, involving skin, respiratory tract or gut etc. Chronic milk allergy may lead to failure to thrive and poor growth. It is IgE (<2 hours, occasionally severe) **or non IgE** 2-72 hours, associated with eczematous rashes and in which IgE based tests, RAST and skin pricks are unhelpful. You can now buy cow's milk from herds genetically bred to produce milk with a different, less allergenic selection of milk proteins. ("A2 instead of A1 protein"). These are less likely to stimulate a negative immune response and the milk, which looks and tastes like normal doorstep milk is available (though much more expensive) from many supermarkets.

Lactose intolerance is a completely different mechanism and due to insufficient brush border lactase to digest the main disaccharide in cow's milk. Lactose intolerance is said to be rare below 5 years. Diarrhoea which responds to a temporary low or no lactose formula is, however pretty common. Genuine lactose intolerence is quite rare.

Rare but certainly not unheard of. Human civilisation began farming 10,000 years ago in the Fertile Crescent (Israel, Lebanon and Syria) of the Middle East. This gave the local tribes the advantage of not having to travel far to their food source and was only efficient in this geographic area due to the relative fecundity of the land. Initially, more effort is needed to farm land than to forage for food. Thus hunter gatherer communities found that they need become only short distance gatherers and with the domestication of animals, dangerous and unreliable hunting could be phased out too. Goats, cattle and sheep were domesticated first in the Middle East 10,000 to 7,500 years ago – although dogs were the first domesticated animals, 12,500 years ago. All the varieties of dog in the world today, from Great Dane to Chihuahua sprang from the Timber Wolf, first domesticated around the camp fires of the stone age. The increase in local populations, the availability of pastures and the withdrawal of glaciers all contributed to fixed farming communities in settled areas. Stone age peoples grew a variety of crops. Recent research into Bronze Age (5-6,000 years ago) skeletons has shown **Lactose Tolerance** was rare then. So our body's ability to handle the milk of another species is a relatively new phenomenon.

Cow's Milk protein intolerance can be demonstrated even by breast fed infants, as small amounts of cow's milk protein are excreted in maternal milk. In these babies, the **mother** needs a rigid cow's milk exclusion diet.

If the baby develops symptoms on a standard formula feed then a soy formula (bearing in mind the warnings regarding possible long term effects) or elemental formula may be substituted. There are also other non animal sources of "milk" substitutes (rice, oat, coconut, hazelnut and almond "milks" which are generally fortified with calcium). Rice milk has low levels of arsenic.

Extensively hydrolysed or amino acid based formulae:
Nutramigen Lipil, >Neocate/Nutramigen AA. Aptamil Pepti is partially hydrolysed but has lactose for palatability. Nearly all hydrolysates are otherwise lactose free.

The symptoms include immediate urticaria, vomiting, rashes, runny nose, cough, colic, reflux and diarrhoea. Delayed symptoms might include diarrhoea, constipation, eczema, respiratory symptoms. Anaphylaxis is rare. These reactions are mediated by IgE.

Diagnosis is by exclusion and cow's milk challenge. RAST, patch testing and skin prick testing to cow's milk are unreliable.

Most children with real allergy start to be able to consume cow's milk during their childhood but a proportion do go on to be asthmatic. It is said that up to 40% with true cow's milk allergy develop soya allergy too. Most early onset Cow's milk allergy has resolved by age 3. Egg allergy persists longer and the later onset tree nut, peanut*, seed, fish and shell fish allergies can persist too.

You can add in normal lactose containing milk 6-8 weeks after resting the brush border in lactose intolerance: Investigations in lactose intolerance: Lactose hydrogen breath test, stool reducing substances, stool pH, trial of lactase supplement.

Food Allergies:

Eight foods account for 90% of food allergies. These are cow's milk, eggs, tree nuts, peanuts (*which are actually ground nuts and legumes), fish, shellfish, soya beans and wheat. These should be avoided before 6 months of age.

The UK is said to be in the top three countries for allergy incidence but we have one allergy consultant per 700,000 sufferers. So proportionately we are probably the worst provided for in terms of allergy services in the world. That means GPs have to be conversant with treating and diagnosing allergic conditions. Hospital admissions of children with various forms of food allergy have increased 7 fold since 1990. The incidence of food allergies in children varies vastly depending on your source and your definition. Some quote an incidence of up to 10%. Various theories have been postulated to explain the apparent increased incidence over recent years: That allergy is related to dietary changes, over cleanliness, use of immunisations and antibiotics (the hygiene theory), early weaning and so on. In my 40 year career I have treated a few cases of what was called "anaphylaxis", many cases or oral allergy syndrome and urticaria, dozens of babies and children whose parents thought they were allergic to various foods and have never seen a really life threatening food allergy.

IgE mediated food allergy usually comes on quickly, non IgE mediated allergy may take hours or days but in some children both mechanisms may co exist.

Specific tests are notoriously unhelpful (skin pricks and RAST tests). Exclusion diets and challenges can be diagnostic. Treatment is avoidance of the allergen if possible, anti histamines in their various forms, possibly bronchodilator sprays where appropriate and if the child has suffered a serious reaction, an adrenaline auto injector. The risk of anaphylaxis is, as I mentioned, vastly exaggerated.

An American study of infant feeding practices, IFPS II, found a food allergy (diagnosed by a doctor) incidence of 6.3% and that it was higher with higher maternal education (!), a higher family income, a family history of food allergy and eczema under 1 year. Strangely, they found that the duration of exclusive breast feeding and the timing of weaning were not related to the development of food allergy.

They also found:

An association between longer exclusive breast feeding periods and lower rates of ear, nose, throat and sinus infections,

A doubling of 6 year old obesity in children who drank sugar sweetened drinks as infants,

An association between longer breast feeding and increased plain water, fruit and vegetable consumption in the diet and less fruit juice and sugary drinks aged 6.

An association between fruit and vegetable consumption in the first year and a continued fruit and vegetable diet aged 6.

So from this study, early feeding practices do not affect allergy but they do affect later diet, infection of the upper respiratory tract and obesity.

Peanut Allergy:

Peanuts are "Ground nuts" a legume, – the other nuts which are all tree nuts seem to be characteristically and antigenically different.

1% are sensitised by age 4. Arachis oil (from peanuts) is in many dermatological preparations and eczema is part of the allergic spectrum. Although the proteins in arachis oil are denatured, putting dermatological creams on eczema may be contributing to peanut sensitivity.-Well it is possible. Anaphylaxis leading to respiratory arrest, despite the ever present anxiety is **exceedingly** rare. A paper in 2002(Arch Dis CH 86: 236-239) stated the risk of a food allergic child dying from a food reaction to be 1 in 800,000 per year, and although 8 children had died of food allergy in the preceding 10 years, no child under 13 had died due to peanut allergy in that decade.

Merbentyl, Dicyclomine, (Dicycloverine is what it is called now) – the syrup can still be used from 6 months onwards – not very useful as colic is less likely then. You may like to remember the quote above* (see Colic) and the tens of thousands of small babies who were treated safely with it before its withdrawal under the age of 6 months. It is an anticholinergic and was used extensively with almost complete success in infantile colic until reports of suspected respiratory distress, seizures and hypotonia appeared about 30 years ago. I remember this well, as it was greeted with disbelief by the whole Paediatric community and reinforced my impression that drug regulating authorities are out of touch with clinicians. No actual causal link was shown with the drug. I had never seen a significant side effect with it as a Paediatrician or GP and none of the alternatives ever worked anything like as well. Consequently mothers, fathers and babies now suffer weeks of sleepless nights and distress before finally growing out of this puzzling and nearly always benign condition (unless it does resolve with a non accidental injury and the child in care). Modern medicine is littered with "you can't be too careful" decisions which leave patients, parents and doctors frustrated, in pain or distress and feeling like unconsulted overprotected idiots.

Teething:

Is painful and distressing in most children until the gum has split and the new tooth erupted. Apart from excessive drooling, the increased saliva that is generated by the gum hyperaemia of teething leads to gastrointestinal hurry, colic, perianal soreness, nappy rash and diarrhoea. The perianal soreness is because the intestinal hurry follows hyperaemia and excessive salivation due to erupting teeth. There is increased peristalsis of the whole GI tract, malabsorption and passage of wet, partially digested stool, full of enzymes, which irritates the nappy area. Hence teething babies DO suffer colic and sore bottoms as well as sore gums. No old wives here, just a lot of young mums. There is great variation in the age at which teeth erupt but a rough guide is:

	Maxillary	Mandibular
Primary, deciduous teeth:		
Central incisors	6-10m	5-8m
Lateral incisors	8-12m	7-10m
Cuspids	16-20m	16-20m
1st molars	11-18m	11-18m
2nd molars	20-30m	20-30m
Secondary, permanent teeth:		
Central incisors	7-8yrs	6-7yrs
Lateral incisors	8-9yrs	7-8yrs
Cuspids	11-12yrs	9-11yrs
First premolars	10-11yrs	10-12yrs
Second premolars	10-12yrs	11-13yrs
First molars	5.5-7yrs	5.5-7yrs
Second molars	12-14yrs	12-13yrs
Third molars	17-30yrs	17-30yrs (Wisdom teeth).

Weaning: In an "Allergic" baby:

If the plan is to try to avoid allergic conditions in the background of an allergic family history, advise exclusive breast feeding for the first 4-6 months of life. If the plan is to maximise IQ, advise 1 year! While breast feeding, the mother should avoid significant family allergens: Cow's milk and dairy products, wheat, eggs, fish, peanuts, citrus fruits if these have sensitised other family members. If breast feeding is impossible then one of the hydrolysed formulae Pepti (hydrolysed whey), Nutramigen (hydrolysed casein), elemental milks, Neocate, Nutramigen, or soya based milks (some reservations under 6months, see relevant section): Infasoy, Prosobee, Wysoy etc can be used.

Solids can start at 4-6months, the later the better, one food at a time. The introduction of new solid foods can be approached as in *food allergy testing* – only if the baby is well, watching and waiting for any adverse reaction. But each food needs to be given for several days and signs of any allergic reaction looked for (usually skin or gut reactions). If there is a significant reaction, exclude this food from the future diet for several months before retrying.

One source suggests an order to try – thus:

Milk free baby rice or gluten free baby cereal (with EBM or appropriate formula), (expressed breast milk)

Pureed root vegetable (potato, carrot, parsnip, swede, turnip),

Pureed fruit (apple, pear, banana) not citrus fruit until the toddler is 9m.

Other vegetables-peas, beans, lentils, broccoli.

Other cereals but not wheat until 8-9 months.

Meats with lamb and turkey first.

Fish at 10 months.

Milk and milk products at 10 months. Yoghurt first, followed by boiled cow's milk etc.

Eggs, hard boiled or well cooked at 1 year.

Any food that seemed to cause a reaction should be excluded then re-challenged about 4-6 months later.

This has been the advice for a potentially allergic baby but the general weaning advice is reasonable for all babies. I wouldn't wait a week in between new foods or leave the cow's milk, wheat and egg so long before giving them but the general order is reasonable.

Assuming the baby has no specific allergies, weaning consists of giving him or her milk and going through baby rice and various pureed vegetables and fruits. The more vegetable tastes the baby experiences early on the more likely he or she will develop a healthy taste for vegetables throughout life. Also the less likely he or she is to become overweight in later childhood and the less likely to develop diabetes later in life.

So about 6m baby rice, carrot puree, pea puree, sweet potato puree, broccoli puree, apple puree etc. might be on the weaning menu. Then baby rice and fruit puree, baby porridge with puree, also a supplement containing Vitamin A, C and D is advised from 6m to 5 years. Now a wider variety of fruit and vegetable purees, with two or three vegetables per meal. Milk is still continuing as the regular main drink. No sugary drinks. Top up drinks during the day should not be fruit juices which are nearly all sugary and risk diarrhoea (see Toddler Diarrhoea etc) and sugar addiction but instead simply water. Now meat, chicken, fish, lamb etc pureed with veg. are added. No processed meats or salty sauces or gravies. Now progress on to mashed and lumpy foods and handling and choosing their own raw foods (as soon as they have enough teeth) such as cut up broccoli, grapes and carrots. Many mums introduce this as soon as solids start at 6 months.

Cot Death, Sudden infant death syndrome SIDS:

When I was registrar in paediatrics I had the frequent and distressing experience of trying to resuscitate collapsed babies who had been found at home by their parents apnoeic and blue. Usually we were too late and any response to our intensive care was short lived or absent. It happened to the baby of a registrar friend of mine while the carry cot was parked in the hall way of a junior doctors' wives coffee morning. I will never forget the anxiety and despair of the baby's mother and the anger and emotional distance of its father. In retrospect it was one of the hardest clinical situations I can imagine for a junior hospital doctor to cope with. The baby had to all intents and purposes died at home and we had only managed to prolong the suffering by keeping it "alive" a little longer.

The parents mentioned, as many in this awful situation did, that the child was well, save for a cold and some mild catarrhal symptoms just beforehand.

I have lived through a number of seeming diagnostic and therapeutic breakthroughs related to this condition over the last 45 years.

The babies typically die in their sleep and by definition, were previously well.

It is known that the babies of mothers who smoke during pregnancy and in the home thereafter and counter intuitively, babies placed on their tummies are more likely to suffer SID. The general advice to put babies down on their backs has significantly reduced the incidence if SID even if it has increased post natal flattening of babies' heads. Males are more affected and in the first month or so after birth SID is less likely than later on.

The age of onset, just like the situation with the specious whooping cough and MMR vaccine "reactions" seems to suggest a late presenting congenital or developmental abnormality, an environmental factor or a developing, slowly deteriorating catastrophe, either not present or not detectable at birth. Or of course, MULTIPLE CAUSES.

SID is associated also with:

Older and teenage mothers independent of smoking,

Low birth weight and prematurity,

Face down sleep position,

which may be linked with the post mortem finding of respiratory debris in some cot death babies, an association with URTIs and new research from America in babies who have suffered previous episodes of ALTEs (Acute life Threatening Events) showing poor control and protection of their upper airways, pauses and gasping respiration. These babies do not clear debris well or coordinate breathing and swallowing effectively. There is said to be poor "Aerodigestive Regulation" after swallowing or refluxing with poor oesophageal peristalsis. Although this makes some logical sense in that babies in utero swallow and "breath" amniotic fluid and they do not have to regulate and separate air and swallowed/refluxed matter until they are aerobic. Why cot deaths are relatively rare in the immediate neonatal period is a puzzle though. If swallowing and breathing coordination were the most crucial issue you would expect this to be its peak incidence.

Overheating (overwrapping) – There was an increase in the number of cot deaths in February 2013. This was a colder than average month and I can imagine mums wrapping up their babies in warm clothing and an extra blanket, perhaps not noticing the URTI, the blocked, runny nose, the baby's temperature going up and up.

Cuddly toys.

Hot environment (overheated rooms: – babies in baby grows can raise their temperature far easier than they can lose it when febrile and overdressed).

2-12 months of age.

Male sex.

Other theories:

Structural brain and cardiac abnormalities, cardiac conduction abnormalities, e.g. Prolonged QT,

overwhelming viral infection, including myocarditis, accidental suffocation in their own bedding or deliberately by the mother. etc.

Child abuse, – although difficult to prove, smothering, suffocation etc, some paediatricians believe this is a cause of a significant percentage of SID, especially when more than one SID happens in the same family. This is said to be far commoner than we naive and trusting doctors think. It is, of course, despite the deliberations and rulings of "distuinguished" judges, impossible to exclude or prove reliably later.

To avoid sudden infant death the mother must have good antenatal care, have the baby in her 20's, not smoke, have a daughter, put the baby down each night on its back, (this advice reduced deaths from cot death in America by 38%), breast feed it, keep the bedroom windows open, have only a few sheets and blankets and make sure the baby is not over dressed. A cold baby cries to be warmed up, a hyperthermic baby is silent.

In 2016 sudden infant deaths were said to be at their lowest level on record in the UK

In 2004 there were 207

In 2013 there were 165

in 2014 there were 128.

Swaddling:

Baby Jesus may have been wrapped in swaddling clothes but I have always imagined this was because the manger (cattle trough) he was laid in was pretty unhygienic and he needed to be immobilised while his primigravida mother, who delivered him unassisted recovered her strength enough to greet the visiting dignitaries. By the way, all that animal dander and dusty stable detritus must have done wonders for his immune system and resistance to infection and allergies. He must have had a great microbiome a few months later.

(Myrrh by the way is an antiseptic and analgesic tree gum with anti cancer properties. Frankincense is likewise a tree resin, the oil of which is said to be calming, antiseptic, antispasmodic, immune stimulating and anti inflammatory as well as having possible anti cancer effects. Gold you will know all about.)

Swaddling is enjoying a popularity again as it is said to improve sleep and to calm fractious babies. It avoids the need for loose blankets in the cot – a SID risk factor. Now wearable blanket suits and snug overalls of fleecy material with velcro fixed limb pouches are available as alternatives to swaddling in blankets or sheets. There are many ways of wrapping a baby's arms and legs to immobilise them, some of which are potentially dangerous. There is some evidence that prolonged immobilisation of the legs (if the swaddling holds the legs firmly together) can cause hip dysplasia. It can cause hyperthermia, something babies seem poorly designed to cope with and recent evidence has shown swaddling the chest too tightly causes tachypnoea. More important, however, are the risks of a loosened blanket or sheet (which starts firmly wrapped around the baby as one swaddling technique) or an ill fitting swaddling suit becoming displaced. If the child is mobile, particularly if he can roll, there is a significant risk of asphyxia. A recent American swaddling study reported on (voluntary feedback) swaddling "incidents". These involved wearable blankets, swaddle wraps and ordinary blankets used to swaddle babies. Altogether there were 22 reported deaths associated with swaddling, mainly from ordinary blankets becoming displaced and the baby's face getting wedged into a position where he/she was asphyxiated. Often the baby had rolled into a dangerous position and became stuck, unable to breathe or extricate himself. **One baby rolled supine to prone at 5 weeks** and died of positional asphyxia in a wearable blanket. Nearly all swaddling deaths involve "sleep environment risks" of some kind. Soft bedding, blankets, pillows, comforters, hyperthermia, cuddly toys, environmental smoke and bed sharing were amongst the various causes.

Loose blankets are dangerous, as are unwrapped swaddling or tight swaddling around a mobile baby. A fleece "Babygro" and a tucked-in sheet or blanket (if the environment is cold) are all that are necessary when "putting a baby down". Certainly, swaddling past 2 months of age when a clever or fidgety baby can roll and get stuck is dangerous. The swaddling then stops the baby pushing himself out of trouble. The advantage of swadding is that babies are not woken by their own REM jerky limb movements so they sleep better and cry less. The risks outside of a tiny perinatal age range exceed the benefits. I am sure Mary would have known that but then baby Jesus wasn't supposed to have cried that much anyway.

Tuberous Sclerosis:(Epiloia)

Autosomal Dominant, 1:7,000 births but most are new mutations. Skin Angiofibromata (especially nasal folds, sparing the upper lip). Facial Adenoma Sebaceum skin rash. Ash leaf or depigmented macules, forehead fibrous plaques, shagreen patches (thickened discoloured skin, usually in the lumbar area), fibromata, (periungual, fingers and toes) and retinal Phakomata, (a retinal Hamartoma). Seizures in 65%, – Infantile spasms, myoclonic seizures, focal or tonic/clonic fits, usually presenting in first year of life, learning disability in 40%. Classic imaging appearances are subependymal glial nodules in the lateral walls of the lateral ventricles and in the third ventricle. Also Calcified Tubers, Giant Cell Astrocytomata and RICP/Hydrocephalus. There is a variety of potential physical, learning and behavioural difficulties. Cardiac Rhabdomyomata, kidney cysts, liver Angiomyolipomata, bone cysts, lung cysts, rectal polyps etc.

The T.S. registry recommends BP and renal function testing annually, a renal USS once, (and every 3-5 years) and annually if lesions are seen or symptoms related to renal damage occur.

Kawasaki disease:

Nothing to do with an obsession with motor bikes but the most common vasculitic disorder of childhood. 80% <5yrs, usually 9-12 months. 24% have coronary artery involvement (aneurysm at 3-6 weeks). Autoimmune medium necrotising vasculitis, 1% mortality (though I have never seen or heard of a child dying of this personally). Think of it if you see a febrile child with a strawberry tongue and cervical nodes even though there may be many other causes of this. Chapped red lips, conjunctivitis, red palms, joint pains,
or at least 5 of:
>5days fever,
Polymorphous rash (maculopapular),
Erythema,
Indurative oedema,

Later hand and feet desquamation,

Oral mucosal changes,

Cervical lymphadenopathy,

Bilateral conjunctival injection,

Cause unknown but possibly a genetic overreaction to a common viral infection – which it frequently follows (as the disease runs in families).

A fifth of sufferers develop coronary arteritis and aneurysm, so admission is advisable.

The treatment may include IV Immunoglobulin and aspirin (despite the age, so vaccinate against Flu and Varicella to avoid Reye's). This and Stills Disease are about the only reasons for giving someone under 16 Aspirin.

?Possibly steroids? Treatment should be started early-certainly within 10 days of the onset of the illness.

Treatment reduces the incidence of coronary aneurysm to 5% (from 20%).

Recently the DMARDs of Rh A and steroid sparing methotrexate etc have been found to be useful.

Differential diagnosis: Enterovirus, Adenovirus, Measles, Parvovirus, Leptospirosis, **Strep**, Staph. Most children do recover fully even without treatment but some do suffer complications if untreated.

Morbilliform Rash in childhood with fever:

A rash that looks like Measles, usually with 2-10mm macules which are pink or red and confluent in places.

Measles,

Rubella,

Parvovirus B19,

HPV6,

Enteroviruses,

Adenoviruses,

E.B.Virus,

C.M.V.,

Streptococcal Infection.

In adults the rash may be due to many causes including the above and:

The commonest type of drug eruption,

Adult T cell leukaemia,

Dengue,

Scrub Typhus,

Typhus fever,

HIV-1 disease,

Infectious Mono,

Secondary Syphilis,

Typhoid fever etc,

Exanthems and other paediatric infections:

Children develop rashes with a large number of infections. Although very few rashes are so characteristic they are instantly recognisable, many infections have clues and viral specific IgM gives the definitive diagnosis if it is needed. It can certainly be useful to differentiate viral exanthems from other significant rashes, Meningococcal disease, Scarlet

Fever, Kawasaki disease, Erythema Multiforme, Systemic Juvenile Rheumatoid Arthritis, allergy, drug eruptions etc. Non specific viral infections are associated with a variety of symptoms from coryza to diarrhoea and vomiting which precede and accompany the rash. There are rarely any specific treatments (you can consider antivirals in chicken pox) but remember meningococcal disease can present with a non specific maculopapular erythematous rash. These children tend to be toxic and have petechiae and or purpura too.

Measles:

Rubeola IP 8-14 days. Infectious 1-2 days before the prodrome. 3-4 days prodrome, fever, coryza, conjunctivitis, cough.

Koplik's spots opposite molars, 1-2 days before the rash. Measles is misery as many of Andrew Wakefield's followers discovered. Red-purple macules on the face, around the hairline, behind the ears and neck, become confluent, spread downward. Complications: O.M. pneumonia, (50% bacterial secondary infection), encephalitis, myocarditis, pericarditis, SSPE (years later).

German Measles:

Rubella called "German" either because it was researchers in Germany who isolated and differentiated the virus from common or garden Measles or because it was first described by German physicians in the mid 1700s. Different sources make different claims.

It is also called 3 day measles. IP 14-21 days. No prodrome, infectious 5-7 days before the rash. Low grade fever, lymphadenopathy-cervical, post auricular, sub occipital. Occasional arthralgia. Fine pink maculopapular rash starts on face and neck, spreads to limbs and trunk. Petechial hard palatal spots (Forscheimer's spots). Complications include peripheral neuritis, encephalitis, thrombocytopenic purpura, 1st trimester foetal injury. The last time I turned off a ventilator on a paediatric ITU sustaining a child (a beautiful black haired 2 year old girl) suffering a "persistent vegetative state" it was after an acute Rubella Encephalopathy. Not such a benign condition after all.

Fifth Disease, (Eythema Infectiosum):

IP 14 days. Parvovirus B19. Younger children, 2-3 days fever then "slapped cheek" appearance of erythematous macules. Can also have a reticulate generalised rash for 7-10 days. Can cause miscarriage or hydrops in pregnancy (1:10 IUD) or an adult Glandular Fever type illness.

Sixth Disease, (Roseola Infantum, Exanthem Subitum):

IP 9 days. Herpes virus 6 and 7. Mainly children 6m-3 yrs, may present with febrile convulsions. Indeed 1/3 of febrile convulsions in 12-15 months old children are due to Human Herpes Virus 6. 3-5 days high fever, suboccipital lymphadenopathy, then morbilliform rash appears and the temperature drops. Rose pink macules start on the trunk and spread.

Infectious Mononucleosis, (Glandular Fever):

IP 4-14 days, E.B. Virus. Fever malaise, generalised lymphadenopathy and often hepatosplenomegaly. Petechial spots at junction of hard and soft palate. 90-100% given Ampicillin will get a rash. "The poor man's Paul Bunnell"

Gianotti-Crosti Syndrome, (Papular Acrodermatitis):

I.P. depends on the trigger. Symmetrical lichenoid skin or copper coloured papules starting on legs and buttocks, then arms and face, sparing trunk. Generalised lymphad-enopathy, age 1-6. This is a non specific response to a variety of viral infections including E.B., Parainfluenza, Coxsackie, Hep B etc. The rash can last 3-6 weeks. Steroid creams can be applied.

Scarlet Fever:

I.P. 2-4 days, B Haemolytic Strep, bright red rash due to fine papules, blanches easily. Presents in axillae and groins, then to limbs and trunk within 24 hrs. Red face, circum oral pallor. Strawberry tongue, white then red Strawberry. Pastia's sign is increased lines of pigmentation in the axillae (petechiae). The erythroderma fades in 2-3 days, followed by generalised desquamation in 7-10 days. The current epidemic which has baffled public health experts (2015-7 etc) is almost certainly due to the failure of my GP colleagues to examine properly, to recognise and be willing to treat significant bacterial throat infections.
See Infection/Antibiotics

Kawasaki Disease, (Mucocutaneous Lymph Node Syndrome, see above):

Cause unknown, large cervical nodes (>1.5cms), red eyes, red mouth, inflamed cracked lips, strawberry tongue, a generalised erythematous rash, swelling, then peeling of the extremities. Treat with IV immunoglobulin as this reduces the risk of coronary aneurysm.

Vesicular Rashes:

Herpes Simplex Virus HSV:

Primary gingivo-stomatitis. IP 2-12 days. Malaise, fever, cervical lymphadenopathy, vesicles of tongue, pharynx and lips. The child may become toxic and dehydrated simply because of the pain of swallowing. Anti-virals are only useful early in the course of the infection. This can be a nasty infection making swallowing even saliva difficult. Regular analgesia is most important and this just prior to the constant (at least 4 hourly) attention to dosing with oral fluids. Occasionally, dehydration intervenes and admission becomes necessary. Since the withdrawal of Adcortyl in Orabase and Bioral Gel (Carbenoxolone Gel), few topically effective treatments for mouth ulcers in children remain. You can try: Corsodyl mouthwash (they don't like the taste), Difflam mouthwash (It stings and tastes odd) and the various forms of Bonjela (Choline salicylate or Lidocaine, both with Cetalkonium) or a few puffs of a steroid inhaler into the mouth 50-100ug twice a day or prednisolone soluble tablets as a mouth wash or application. But don't forget pain relief and in my opinion paracetamol alone is a poor analgesic. You should add an NSAID or (despite official recommendations) some codeine at the very least in the worst cases.

(In apthous ulceration Doxycycline as a mouthwash helps but make sure they don't swallow it if they are still growing).

Varicella Zoster, (Chicken Pox):

10-21 day IP, prodrome 2-3 days of mild fever and malaise. Waves of spots, trunk mainly, dew drop on rose petal. Contagious 1-5 days before spots and until all blisters scab over. Can start as a generalised maculopapular rash, >macule>papule>vesicle>scab. (Takes 3-4 days). Complications include secondary bacterial infection, pneumonitis, encephalitis, cerebellar ataxia, Reye's Syndrome (especially with aspirin). Neonatal Varicella should be treated with anti-virals (risk of disseminated infection). Foetal Varicella affects brain, eye, spinal cord, causes hypoplasia of limbs, motor/sensory deficits, skin damage.

The Vaccine lasts 5 years, there is Anti Varicella Immuno globulin.

Herpes Zoster, (Shingles):

Can develop in any child who has had chicken pox in the past – includes if immuno-compromised, maternal chicken pox in pregnancy, early or sub clinical Chicken Pox. Hyperaesthesia in the nerve root distribution follows, though less so in children than in adults. Vesicular dermatome rash.

Hand, foot and mouth disease:

(Entirely unrelated to the Foot and Mouth scourge of cattle.) IP 3-7 days. Coxsackie infection A16. Low grade fever and headache, vesicular lesions on hands, tongue, lips, feet, occasionally buttocks. The mouth lesions are yellow ulcers with red borders, tongue, lips, gums, buccal mucosa and palate. Lasts 3-10 days. Aseptic Meningitis a rare complication. Otalgia. Caused by enteroviruses, eg Coxsackie A16, Enterovirus 71 etc, Infection from saliva, stool and blister fluid. Enterovirus 71 can cause paralysis, meningo-encephalitis, pulmonary oedema, myocarditis. The Chinese have developed a vaccination against HFM which is a far more serious infection in the Far East. It is 90% effective against Enterovirus 71 but ineffective against Coxsackie A16.

NOTE: **Coxsackie infections** include HFM A16, Cardiomyopathy, M.E., Herpangina group A, Summer Grippe, Pleurodynia-Bornholm Disease, Aseptic Meningitis, severe neonatal infection, etc.

See "**Infections**" section. Coxsackie infections are named after a New York town which itself is named after the local Native American for "Owl's hoot". Coxsackie doesn't sound much like toowit toowoo to me.

Other Infections:

Mumps:

Notifiable, Variable IP 14-24 days, children are excluded from school for 5 days from the onset of parotid swelling. Paramyxovirus. Epidemics at any season, 30 – 40% of infections are sub clinical. Some sources say: Infectious 1 day before until 3 days after the subsidence of the parotitis. Rare prodrome, pain and swelling in one or both (95%) parotids. 30% cases are subclinical. The earlobe is usually displaced and the swelling goes in 3-7 days. Occasional sternal oedema, submandibular glands can also be affected.

Complications: Meningo-encephalitis, orchitis, epididymitis (rare in the prepu-bescent), oophoritis, pancreatitis (5%), deafness (permanent in 1: 15,000), optic neuritis, purpura, possible fibro-elastosis in utero, first trimester miscarriage but not foetal damage if the pregnancy continues.

Confirmation is via IgM, salival culture or a laboratory saliva sponge kit which can be used up to 6 weeks after the onset of symptoms.

The Mumps epidemic of 2003-5 affected predominantly 17-20 year olds.

Pertussis, (Whooping Cough):

Bordetella Pertussis, Gram negative Rod, (but also a parapertussis and adenovirus possible interaction). IP 6-20 days, highly infectious, most deaths <1 year, various stages: Catarrhal, Paroxysmal, 2-4 weeks, – Paroxysmal cough and whoop, Convalescent stage. Marked peripheral leucocytocis. Complications: Pneumonia, bronchiectasis, O.M., S.A.H., I.V.H., hernias, etc Erythromycin can shorten infectivity and can abort the disease if given early enough.

Prophylaxis for Close Contacts:

Treat the Index patient and suspected contacts – unvaccinated, partially vaccinated, under 5yr old children particularly newborn of symptomatic mothers, those with chronic illness including asthma, cong. heart disease, C.F. Immunocompromised, anyone over 5 years of age as well, as immunity wanes with age, in fact everyone with symptoms and anyone in contact APART from fully vaccinated children under 5 years old. Treat with Erythromycin/Clarithromycin: Erythromycin 50mg/kg/day in 3 doses for a child, or 500mg tds for an adult. For 10 days and finish incomplete courses of vaccination.

In other words it seems that the only close contacts of laboratory confirmed pertussis you **don't** treat or give prophylaxis to are children under 5yrs who have been fully immunised.

Macrolides are only of any use in preventing transmission if given within 21 days of exposure so should only be given within that window unless you are treating a secondary infection.

Erythema Multiforme:

Not actually an infection but a "Hypersensitivity" reaction to a variety of stimuli, drugs, infections and illnesses. Common in childhood. Causes: Herpes viruses, Mycoplasma, Coxsackie, Echo and Influenza viruses, Mumps, Salmonella, Diphtheria, Haemolytic Strep, T.B., penicillins, tetracyclines, sulphonamides, barbiturates, aspirin. Paracetamol and NSAIDs rarely, some vaccines, some collagen diseases.

Stevens-Johnson Syndrome is where the skin and two mucous membranes are affected. The rash is symmetrical, crops, mainly limb extensor surfaces, everywhere except the scalp, macular, papular, nodular, vesicular or urticarial. It can be bullous or bizarre urticarial plaques. Intradermal haemorrhage and petechiae are common, iris or target lesions are characteristic, oral lesions in 25% become ulcers, skin lesions crop for up to 3 weeks. The Nikolsky Sign may be positive (the top layer of skin rubs away under an eraser.)

E.M. is often sub divided into E.M. Minor (usually post H Simplex or Mycoplasma) or E.M. Major – Stevens Johnson Syndrome, often a drug S/E.

Treatment, if necessary is directed at the cause and can include steroids.

The" Erythemas"

Erythema Marginatum:
B Haemolytic strep, TB, Leprosy, LGV.
Rheumatic Fever.
Coccidioidomycosis, Histoplasmosis.
Sarcoid,
Drugs: Penicillin, Sulphonamides, the pill,
Barbiturates, anticonvulsants, salicylates,
SLE, vasculitides, U.C, Crohn's.

Erythema Multiforme:
See above
(May include Target or Iris lesions)

Stevens Johnson Syndrome.
Skin lesions which slough but which
may not have E. Multiforme:
Herpes, Coxsackie, Echo, Psittacosis,
Mycoplasma, Histoplasmosis,
Vaccination: (Vaccinia), BCG, Polio,
Reticulosis, Ca, DXT,
Drugs: Antipyretics, Barbiturates,
Phenytoin,
Sulphonamides, Penicillin etc.
No cause 50%.

Erythema Nodosum: (A delayed hypersensitivity to various antigens).

Is a panniculitis (inflammation of subcutaneous fat). Commonly affecting the anterior shins. Occasionally it can affect the thighs or even forearms. Causes include Strep throats, Mycoplasma,

EBV, Cat scratch, Behcet's, NHL, Ca Pancreas, Sarcoid, (with Pulm. Hilar Lymphadenopathy is Lofgren Syndrome). TB, pregnancy or COCP. A variety of drugs, IBD, Leprosy etc. E.N. is usually self limiting. Treatment is of the cause plus or minus steroids and colchicine, potassium iodide.

Other Skin Disorders:

Toxic Epidermal Necrolysis (Lyell Disease):

A hypersensitivity to the same causes as E Multiforme. Up to 25% mortality. Fever, malaise, local erythema and skin tenderness. Bullae and peeling of large sheets. Nikolsky sign. Conjunctivitis and oral symptoms similar to S-J Syndrome.

Staphylococcal Scalded Skin Syndrome (also called Toxic Epidermal Necrolysis, Ritter Disease):

A prodrome then erythema of face, neck, axillae and groins – and wrinkling, bullae, Nikolsky sign. Facial oedema and peri oral crusting. Treatment: The staphylocidal penicillins.

Impetigo:

Commoner in Summer. Erythematous macules >thin walled vesicles and >pustules >honey coloured crusts. Can be circinate, lesions everywhere. Usual cause is Group A βHaemolytic strep with super infection with Staph. Treat with a penicillin/Erythromycin +/– Topical bacteriostatic cream. Isolate patient initially. Recurrent infections may be due to nasal or perineal reservoirs of Staph.

Petechial spots on palate:

Scarlet Fever,
Rubella,
Glandular Fever.

Henoch Schonlein Purpura

First actually described by Heberden of nodes fame not Henoch or Schonlein. The commonest vasculitis in children. Palpable purpura, symmetrical, on buttocks, lower limbs, raised, unusual on the trunk. Hence the importance of stripping ill children off when they consult and not being embarrassed about examining them properly. Often preceded by a variety of non specific rashes, maculopapular, even bullous etc. Diffuse abdominal pain, occasional significant gastrointestinal involvement – vomiting, rectal bleeding, intussus-ception, protein losing enteropathy, pancreatitis etc. Arthralgia and arthritis 80%+. – The presenting symptom in a quarter. Usually large leg joints but rare to have any permanent damage. The renal involvement mimics post streptococcal glomerulonephritis, the studies put this at anything from 12-92%! Probably nearly all patients have renal involvement within 3m. There are haematuria, proteinuria, there can be Nephrotic Syndrome, acute nephritis, renal impairment, hypertension. The renal biopsy shows IgA deposition.
Other rarer features can include orchitis, neurological symptoms, (seizures, mood changes, hyperactivity or apathy), interstitial lung changes etc. Incidence 10-20/100.000. All ages can be affected including adults but 75% are <10 years.

Organisms: 36% Grp. A strep, Hep A, B, CMV, HIV, VZV, Toxoplasma, Adenoviral, Parvovirus B19, Mycoplasma, H Pylori. Some suggest "post immunisation".

Investigations: BP, EMU, Prot/creat ratio. FBC, Coag. U and Es, LFTs, Bone profile, infection screen, ASOT, AIP. F/U if hypertensive, macroscopic haematuria, >++Proteinuria.

Long term morbidity <5%.

In my opinion early steroids avoid much morbidity, especially arthralgia and abdominal and renal complications. Alternatives are cyclophosphamide, methotrexate, mycophenylate, ACEIs.

Prognosis: 33% have some symptom recurrence.

Oral Ulcers:

A common and painful complication of a number of harmless childhood infections (Herpes simplex, Varicella Zoster, HFM, apthous ulceration, etc). It is almost impossible to apply proprietary gels (Dentinox, Calgel, Bonjela, etc) to a fractious child. There are:

Sucralfate mouthwash (Antepsin suspension), Carbomer (Mugard mouthwash), Hyaluronate (Gelclair, Gengigel) because strangely, the previously very useful Adcortyl in orabase and Carbenoxylone Gel (Bioral) have been withdrawn. Carbenoxylone was first produced in tablet form for peptic ulcers but used topically as a gel in the mouth it also healed ulcers there.

Symptoms and signs of specific diseases:

Meningococcal Septicaemia: A sick child with a non blanching rash, purpura >2mm, capillary refill >3 seconds, **possible** neck stiffness, (15-46%), poor response to stimulus. Leg pain is common, abnormal colour, breathing difficulty, cold extremities, 40-70% have a haemorrhagic rash, **Meningitis**: Neck stiffness, possible bulging fontanelle, lowered conscious level and responsiveness, irritability, abnormal tone, sometimes fitting.

Herpes Simplex encephalitis: Focal signs and seizures, reduced conscious level, irritability, headache.

Pneumonia: Tachypnoea: Age up to 5m >60 RR
              12m >50 RR
              >12m >40 RR

(For more detail see page 1097)

Crepitations, nasal flaring, in drawing, sometimes cyanosis, saturations </= 95%.

Urinary tract infection: (>3m) Vomiting, poor feeding, lethargy, irritability, abdo. pain/tenderness, frequency/dysuria, smelly urine, sometimes haematuria.

Younger than 3m do an MSU/clean catch in **any** non specifically unwell, FTT, febrile, non feeding infant.

Septic arthritis/osteomyelitis: Limb or joint swelling, not using the limb, not weight bearing.

Kawasaki Disease: At least a 5 day fever plus 4 of: Bilateral conjunctival injection, upper respiratory mucous membrane signs (pharyngitis, cracked dry lips, strawberry tongue), change in the peripheries (erythema, oedema, desquamation), polymorphous rash and cervical lymphadenopathy.

Sleep related problems:

What you may have forgotten:

Sleep Stages:

Beta wave sleep, while the patient is beginning to drop off, gives way to alpha wave sleep. During this phase the patient may experience hypnagogic hallucinations such as a sensation of falling (unless we **are** actually all fallen angels and only recover our ability to fly temporarily as we drift off to sleep and are levitating temporarily as was suggested in a book I once read!) Myoclonic jerks are common and normal.

Stage 1: Theta wave sleep lasts 5-10 minutes and the sleeper if woken will deny they were asleep.

Stage 2: The EEG in this stage shows "Sleep spindles", the heart rate slows and this phase lasts 20 minutes.

Stage 3: Delta wave sleep, with the depth of sleep getting deeper.

Stage 4: "Delta sleep" which is the deepest level and this is when bed wetting and sleep walking may occur.

Stage 5: Rapid eye movement sleep is when we dream and starts about 90 minutes after beginning sleep. The brain is active but the body very relaxed, almost paralysed.

The sleep sequence may be 1, 2, 3, 4, 3, 2, 5-REM sleep, 2, 3, 4, etc and these cycles are repeated throughout the night, four or five times.

We nearly wake several times in the night and we may be tipped into wakefulness if we are worried, cold, alerted by external sounds or want to empty our bladder. etc. It is certainly easier to wake and to function from a light level of sleep than if we are rudely awakened from deep sleep when we can be confused and disoriented. I remember driving on the wrong side of the road at 3 a.m. many years ago when on night duty. I had been woken from a deep sleep by the phone call, taken the details of the case and their address, got myself dressed, started and driven the car half way out to the house visit, not properly realising what I was doing and without really waking up. It can be hard to wake up or think sensibly when roused in certain phases of sleep. Also it can be quite normal to wake or be aware several times a night and (particularly elderly) patients often need reassurance on this. At least half of our patients will admit to frequent "insomnia" during the previous year. Almost no one it seems is lucky enough to go to bed, lose awareness quickly, sleep without untoward events or awareness of waking and then surface refreshed after eight hours of beauty sleep the next morning.

Sleep disturbance and nocturnal sedation: (When all else fails:)

40% of children between 6m and 5 years are described as having a sleep problem by their parents. Some children (in my experience the ones that will grow into sociable, emotional, popular and extrovert adults) are worse than others at antisocial wakefulness and frequently need nocturnal company.

Sleep is qualitatively different in children than adults: From feeling drowsy, down to stage 4 and back up again takes 90 minutes in an adult but only 50 minutes in the newborn and up to 8 months old. Children sleep lighter more often and are more likely to wake than adults. Sleep disturbance often follows the regular waking that occurs in small children, the parents hearing them and going in to cuddle them or to see what's wrong. This establishes a light sleep-wake-and-need cuddles-before-being-able-to-drop-off pattern. It is learnt behaviour. Similar is the need for a feed which is programmed by feeding a newborn back to sleep each time it wakes.

The GP should always examine the child to exclude asthma, eczema, nasal blockage, constipation, UTI and other causes of sleep interruptions before treating the sleep disturbance as such. Taking the parent seriously and examining the child properly is part of the treatment.

If you need to resort to drugs:

Chloral Hydrate, Welldorm.(The Tabs are 707mg for adults (This is an old fashioned but safe and effective treatment. I have no idea why they have to be this odd strength), Elixir: 2-11 years, 30-50mg/kg. 1 year 300mg, 7 years 600mg, Adult 1.5grm nocte – a single hypnotic dose can be doubled. This nearly always works, gives the beleaguered mother a week of peace and can sometimes "restore a normal sleep pattern". Obviously it can all be much more complicated than just prescribing a sedative but Chloral can preserve relationships, avoid potential NAI, give a parent some hope that there **is** a panic button that can work and avoid an admission. Alternative drugs include the antihistamine, phenothiazine sedatives Promethazine elixir, (Phenergan) and Alimemazine, (Vallergan). Start with a relatively high dose half an hour before bedtime and continue for 2-3 weeks.

I have often gone to talks given by Paediatricians where they have blithely offered the haven of their wards as a place of safety when an insomniac toddler is driving a young mother to distraction.

I was a Paediatric Registrar then a Lecturer before General Practice and I did occasionally do this myself. The change in attitude towards the child shown by non fussing, unindulgent nursing staff can bring about an instant change in the child's nocturnal behaviour and consultants are theoretically "happy to offer this service". But talk to the registrar on call these days and try to get a sleepless but well child onto an acute ward and you soon find out that the junior staff do not share the high ideals of the consultants. In the last 25 years I have never been able to arrange an ungrudging admission for this reason.

What advice can you give a parent?

First of all, acknowledge the problem and sympathise.

Start with a slow and consistent winding down at the end of the day. It is helpful if this is not disrupted by Dad (or Mum) coming home just at this moment and wanting their own quality contact time just before the child is "going down". Stop TV and games sometime before starting the getting ready for bed ritual. Reading a story (not a frightening or overexciting one) has many psychological and practical benefits and is a good way to regularise the bed time routine. Once the child has finished the calm pre-sleep ritual, turn them in to the sleeping position and it may be necessary to stay with them, even talking softly or singing until they are asleep.

If the child is crying: put the child to bed, talking reassuringly and soothingly. Leave when you can. If the child is still crying in 5 minutes, return and without switching on the light or picking the child up, talk reassuringly. If the crying persists, return in 10 minutes and without picking up the child or rewarding them in anyway, be gently reassuring again. Repeat this if the child continues to cry 15 minutes later, – again, no cuddles, picking up, sips of water etc. If the child really needs a drink, do not switch on the light but use a cup already in the room and make it a small drink and over quickly. If the child is moaning or whimpering rather than crying, leave them alone. If they wake in the night do not go to them immediately but when you do the idea is to make them as relaxed as you can as quickly as you can. If they come to your bedroom gently take them back. You can start this regime slightly later than their normal bedtime so that they are tired to start with.

The parent must be resolute and both parents must behave the same way.

Avoid daytime naps or limit the nap to 20 minutes, avoid lying-in the morning after. The regime will need to be restarted if the child subsequently has two bad nights in a row after getting the hang of it.

Older children may respond to small presents for not disturbing the parent all night with a slightly bigger reward for 10 nights (not necessarily successive).

Chloral is sometimes the only alternative. Perhaps junior paediatricians need to do some General Practice as a compulsory part of the course or have a few children themselves? (This should certainly be compulsory for Health Visitors!) Although I recently discovered the statistic that 70% of paediatric junior staff are now female and many units are in crisis because so many of their staff are off on maternity leave, – so it should be something they are already aware of!

Oil of evening Primrose can sometimes aid sleep in the hyperactive child and it goes without saying that "sleep hygiene" – a quiet and consistent run up to lights out, is very important. (In summary: Go to bed at the same time, no exciting TV or bed time stories, regular daytime exercise, no late meals or stimulant drinks, a dark, quiet room that isn't too hot or cold and avoid as much as possible naps in the daytime in older children or at least try to keep them short).

You could also try Melatonin which, of course, is a natural sleep hormone used in children with ADHD and secreted diurnally by the pineal. Use a dose of 3-6mg. This may be more acceptable to the parents than a traditional sleeping pill but all drugs are a final resort.

Nightmares:

May reflect anxiety, for instance after an unpleasant incident, a change of school, an accident or a bereavement. It can take months for these reactive nightmares to settle. While toddlers and some older children are going through the "Why?" stage of development, they are trying to understand how the world works and how they fit in. Common subjects are death and dreams about dying or someone close dying and decomposition and loss are frequent ruminations. Discussing these worries with the child in a simple and reassuring way during the daytime will help solve the nightmares sooner.

The child is easy to wake or wakes them self after a nightmare, remembering some or most of the nightmare itself. These factors differentiate nightmares from night terrors.

Night Terrors:

These occur (unlike nightmares) in deep sleep, (stages 3 and 4). They are arousal disorders, of which there are a few (and include the frightening sleep paralysis) in which not all the brain is aware and awake, some remaining in a sleep state. There is no memory (for the child anyway) the next day. The emotion part of the brain is alert however and the child frequently, after a loud shout or scream, looks very frightened, shaking, sweaty, perhaps garbling some words during the sleep terror. The child is not awake, is hard to wake and should be left to settle-which normally happens after a few minutes.

There is a slight familial tendency, they are commoner in boys and between the ages of 2 and 12 years. They are sometimes worse at periods of stress. Only 5% children suffer from night terrors. Drugs are usually unnecessary but benzodiazepines which paradoxically reduce the time spent in deep sleep, stages 3 and 4 can help if parents are desperate.

Sleepwalking and talking:

Occur in deep sleep (Stages 3 and 4), like night terrors. The part of the brain that is working is the motor cortex (hence complex coordinated movements) but memory and awareness are asleep. There is no purpose to the activity, walking, speech, etc., the patient is unaware and will not remember the event tomorrow. Again, he will be difficult to wake and should be supervised for safety but otherwise not interfered with.

The Acutely Ill child:

The average child can have up to 8 infective episodes in the first 18 months of their life and probably three or four episodes of red ears and earache (depending on sibling and mixing status). Serious infections have been very rare in the past with 100 infants under 12 months dying each year and 30 deaths/year in the age group 1-4 up until recent times. I do not have very recent figures. To put it in perspective, I don't think I lost a single child* to bacterial infection in 30 odd years of General Practice, although of course I saw many die in my six years as a Paediatrician.

There has been great front page national paper concern (see other sections) not only about the number of children dying of "sepsis" with symptoms unrecognised or dismissed by GPs and OOHs doctors but about the "Poor Training" in Paediatrics of many doctors today. There has certainly been an increase in a number of bacterial diseases in the community, the most notorious being Scarlet Fever. This, in the absence of a change in antigenicities can only be due to poor recognition of bacterial infection by doctors, a lack of thoroughness in examination of febrile children or an unwillingness to prescribe antibiotics appropriately. Unfortunately all of these seem to be the case currently (2014-2017). In part due to reduced ward experience (my paediatric career consisted of working weeks 2-3 times as long as the maximum worked today and so I saw at least twice the number of patients in the same number of jobs) and in part due to a misplaced imposed sense of professional guilt about prescribing antibiotics. So I doubt whether my statement above*will be a general experience for today's British Community Physicians if these failings continue.

What follows is a number of ways of assessing sick children:

You could start with a 3 minute assessment,
General behaviour-lively, lethargic, irritable, quiet.
Airway-Stridor, noisy breathing, drooling.
Breathing-Accessory muscles, in drawing etc respiratory rate, auscultation, O2 sats.
Circulation-Peripheral temperature and colour, pulse, capillary refill time, BP.
Disability-Responsive-Alert, voice only, pain only, unresponsive.
ENT-
Temperature.

Pneumonia, Chest Infection, Sepsis:

The two main predictors of a poor prognosis in children presenting with cough to GPs are the
Subjective assessment of **unwellness** by the GP,
The presence of **laboured breathing**.
The former is VERY subjective but very important and depends on experience. The genuinely sick child is very rare in General Practice, fairly obvious and needs to be admitted quickly. Call the ambulance before you call the on call Paediatrician as time may

be of the essence. You might even consider trying to get a venous sample of blood and giving a bolus of IV Penicillin or better still Cefuroxime while you wait for transport and before you scribble a referral letter.

Children who

Do not smile in response to tickling, play, or respond at all to gentle questions, (What's this? – pointing to their umbilicus),

Do not follow visually or take an interest in you, your instruments or their surroundings,

A small baby unwilling to suckle,

Have poor muscular tone and reactions, – are floppy, with few spontaneous movements,

Have poor central capillary return,

Have a pale, grey or patchy peripheral circulation (although this has multiple influences and can be unreliable),

may have a deep rooted infection with or without septicaemia and can be very ill.

Respiratory signs of serious infection include:

Raised respiratory rate, panting, grunting,

Clinical signs in the chest,

Recession (Intercostal, supraclavicular), See Saw,

Cyanosis (tongue) – **Lip circulation is "peripheral"**,

Hyperinflation, accessory muscles in use,

Poor speech, cry etc. etc.

Other factors that determine whether antibiotics (etc) are prescribed in the community may include presence or absence of

Fever,

The trustworthiness of the parents – will they recognise a sick child if things get worse at home later? The expectations, previous use of OOH, or A and E, the medical history (has the child had or have the parents believed him to have suffered a secondary chest infection after a URTI before?), the complaints history of the parents and even the day of the week. – This sounds strange but if you can say "If you have a bad night pop in at eight a.m. before surgery and let me see him again tomorrow" (or call me at home in the old days!) a huge number of pre emptive antibiotics and steroids were avoided. If it is Saturday tomorrow, your normal doctor isn't available and the OOH switchboard is gridlocked from 08.00 til 09.30 then this safety net is not available.

The things that should **not influence** your decision to prescribe antibiotics are national or local antibiotic policies or guidelines. The state of your patient in front of you is a far more important consideration.

Normal Paediatric Respiratory and Pulse Rates:
AGE:

Age	Respiratory	Pulse
0-1 year	30-60	100-160
1-3 years	24-40	90-150
3-6 years	22-34	80-140
6-12 years	18-30	70-120
12-18 years	12-16	60-100

Alternatively: Normal paediatric vital signs:

Age (Years)	BP	RR	HR
<1	70-90	30-40	110-160
1-2	80-95	25-35	100-150
2-5	80-100	25-30	95-140
5-12	90-110	20-25	80-120
>12	100-120	15-20	60-100

1 Degree C raises the pulse by 10b/m and the RR by 10/min

Capillary Refill.

This is a **relatively** new concept in the assessment of paediatric (and adult) illness and circulation – and one "the usefulness of which must be questioned in clinical practice" – in other words **take it with a pinch of salt**. It became popular after 1980 though it was described as early as 1947. It is highly variable between individuals and dependent upon a number of different independent factors. It is supposed to reflect peripheral perfusion, cardiac output, peripheral vascular resistance and therefore how ill the patient is. Some or all of these may be affected by states of infection, shock and fluid loss, skin thickness and many dermatological conditions, the temperature of the patient and the ambient temperature, hydration, medication, the patient's age and so on. It is used as one of the degree of illness parameters in various standard protocols and one of the ways admitting paediatric junior staff (and what, pray, is the child's capillary return time?) like to sound scientific and superior.

In the newborn it is assessed by pressing the sternum. In older patients by lifting the arm so the hand is above heart level and squeezing the finger pad. The toes can be used. The values given as normal usually range between 2 and 3 seconds. Subjective differences between individuals (a mean difference of 0.7 seconds in one study) have been demonstrated as has an effect of simple environmental lighting (not surprisingly).

Debate continues as to how useful it is as a clinical sign. If you look at the literature, there is genuine age and sex difference of the upper limit of normal and a debate about this test's actual usefulness. Adult female and elderly men and women having a longer normal capillary return time and the difference between normal and abnormal being the blink of an eye in a dimly lit bedroom. The median time for children up to 12yrs is 0.8 seconds, ULN 1.9 seconds. Some propose an ULN 4.5 seconds for the elderly. We are talking about fractions of seconds being the difference between normal and abnormal. There are huge relative subjective variations, multiple skin thicknesses, colours and temperatures both of the patient and the room. So the value of the test is, as mentioned elsewhere, mainly to persuade the resistant junior doctor on call who has had less experience than you that he needs to see your patient. They prefer figures and mistrust experience and opinion – the complete opposite to older doctors and patients. Just tell them it was precisely 3.5 seconds.

THE TRAFFIC LIGHT SYSTEM:

NICE have collated their sick child advice into a red amber green chart depending on the degree of unwellness of the child and various local paediatric care organisations have copied their basic approach as follows: (adapted)

"Green Light" Low risk	"Amber Light" Intermediate risk	"Red Light" High risk
Colour: Normal lips skin and tongue	Pallor	Pale/mottled/ashen/blue
Activity: Responsive, awake, smiles, good cry or happy.	Unresponsive, needs extra stimulation to respond, no smile, reduced activity.	No response to stimulus looks unwell, unrousable or drowsy. Unusual, weak or constant irritable cry.
Breathing: Normal Rate (See above) No distress, no stridor/noise	Flaring nostrils, tachypnoea ie: RR>50 aged 6-12m RR>40 aged >12m O2 Sats <95%, audible crackles (crepitations)	Grunting, RR>60 breaths/ min. See saw, intercostal/supraclavicular indrawing other signs of respiratory distress
Hydration: Normal skin, eyes and moist mucous membranes.	Dry mucous membranes, poor infant feeding, capillary refill time >3secs. poor urine output	Reduced skin turgor (very unreliable and subjective sign)
Other:	High temperature 5 days, Swollen limb or joint, Patient sparing a limb, new unexplained lump >2cm	? Under 3m with temp>38C ?3-6m Temp 39C Non blanching rash Bulging fontanelle Stiff neck, Status Epilepticus seizures (I would say NOT just focal) neck stiffness, focal neurology, bile stained vomiting.

There are numerous other worrying situations that require hospital admission and have not been included: extensive soft tissue inflammation, generalised joint swelling with a high temperature, ankle oedema and raised temperature, parental factors and so on and so on...

Some local protocols suggest any "amber" patients under 3m should be sent in for paediatric assessment as should all "red" patients but I would say that this depends on your experience, confidence, the quality of the parents and access to and quality of the local paediatric unit. I personally would not have referred-in all 3m olds with a red throat, a temperature of 38C and good parents who I could trust. I would however have got an opinion on most first convulsions unless they were absolutely 100% right as rain by the time I saw them.

Attached is a number of sick child protocols in use locally which employ a "Traffic Light System" as well as some parent advice sheets:

My thanks to Sussex and Surrey Children and Young People's Urgent Care Network.

Fever Advice Sheet
Advice for parents and carers of children
younger than 5 years

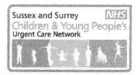
Sussex and Surrey **NHS**
Children & Young People's
Urgent Care Network

Name of Child .... Age .... Date / Time advice given ....

Further advice / Follow up ....

Name of Professional .... Signature of Professional ....

How is your child? (traffic light advice)

Red

If your child:
- becomes difficult to rouse
- becomes pale and floppy
- is finding it hard to breathe
- has a fit
- develops a rash that does not disappear with pressure (see the 'Glass Test' overleaf)
- is under 3 months and has a fever

You need urgent help
please phone 999
or go to the nearest
Hospital Emergency
(A&E) Department

Amber

If your child's:
- health gets worse or if you are worried
- seems dehydrated (dry mouth, sunken eyes, no tears, sunken fontanelle / soft spot on baby's head, drowsy, or passing less urine than normal)
- condition fails to respond to Paracetamol or Ibuprofen
- is 3-6 months old and has a fever

You need to contact a
doctor or nurse today
Please ring your
GP surgery or call
NHS 111 - dial 111

Green

- If none of the above features are present

Self Care
Using the advice overleaf
you can provide the care
your child needs at home

Some useful phone numbers (You may want to add some numbers on here too)

GP Surgery
(make a note of number here)

NHS 111
dial 111
(available 24 hrs -
7 days a week)

Health Visiting Team
(make a note of number here)

For online advice: NHS Choices **www.nhs.uk** (available 24 hrs - 7 days a week)
Family Information Service: Tel: 01243 777807 Website: **www.westsussex.gov.uk/family**

If you need language support or translation please inform the member of staff to whom you are speaking.
For more copies of this document, please email us:
Chichester / Worthing area: contactus.coastal@nhs.net • Crawley area: CCCG Contactus-crawleyccg@nhs.net
Horsham / Mid Sussex area: HSCCG Contactus-horshamandmidsussexccg@nhs.net

Fever Advice Sheet
Advice for parents and carers of children
younger than 5 years

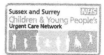

Sussex and Surrey **NHS**
Children & Young People's
Urgent Care Network

Most children with a fever do get better very quickly but some children can get worse. You need to regularly check your child during the day and also through the night and follow the advice given below

Practical things you can do to help your child

- Check your child during the night to see if they are getting better (follow traffic light advice overleaf).

- If a rash appears do "the glass test" (see guidance below).

- If you are concerned that your child is not improving follow the advice on the front of this sheet.

- Children with fever should not be under or over dressed.

- Offer your child regular drinks (where a baby is breastfed the most appropriate fluid is breast milk).

- If your child is due to have immunisations please consult your GP, Practice Nurse or Health Visitor for advice as there may be no need to delay their appointment.

- If you need to keep your child away from nursery or school while they are unwell and have a fever please notify the nursery or school – your Health Visitor, Practice Nurse or GP will be able to advise you if you are unsure.

Using medicines to help

- If your child is distressed or very unwell you may use medicines (Paracetamol or Ibuprofen) to help them feel more comfortable however it is not always necessary.
- Don't give both medicines (Paracetamol and Ibuprofen) at the same time.
- Use one and if your child has not improved 2-3 hours later you may want to try giving the other medicine.
- Please read the instructions on the medicine bottle first for dose and frequency.
- Or you could ask your local community pharmacist for more advice about medicines.
- Aspirin should not be given to children for treatment of pain or a fever.

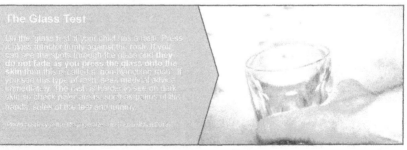

The Glass Test

On the 'glass test' if your child has a rash. Press a glass tumbler firmly against the rash. If you can see the spots through the glass and they do not fade as you press the glass onto the skin then this is called a non-blanching rash. If you see this type of rash, seek medical advice immediately. The rash is harder to see on dark skin so check paler areas such as palms of the hands, soles of the feet and tummy.

First Version: May 2011 • Final Version: Nov 2013 • Review Date: Nov 2015

Based on Feverish illness in children Assessment and initial management in children younger than 5 years 2007 NICE clinical guideline 47 and with consideration to 2013 NICE clinical guideline 160 (May 2013).

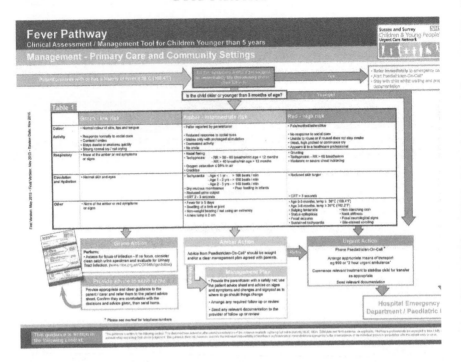

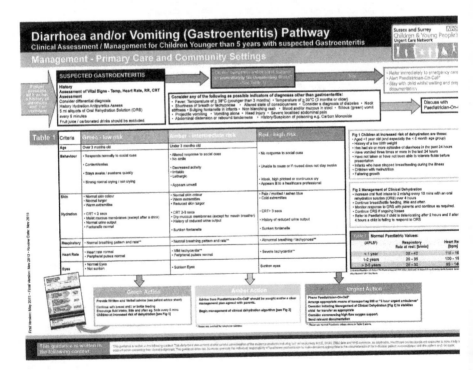

Caring for your child at home & / or on discharge from hospital

- Clean any wound with tap water.
- If the area is swollen or bleeding, apply pressure for 5-10 minutes. If it continues to bleed, keep applying pressure or seek medical advice.
- If in pain give paracetamol or ibuprofen. Always follow the manufacturers' instructions for the correct dose and form.
- Observe your child closely for the next 2-3 days and check that they are behaving normally and they respond to you as usual.
- It is OK to allow your child to sleep, but observe them regularly and check they respond normally to touch and that their breathing and position in bed is normal.
- Give your child plenty of rest, and make sure they avoid any strenuous activity for the next 2-3 days or until their symptoms have settled.
- Following a head injury, do NOT play ANY contact sport (for example football) for at least 3 weeks without talking to your doctor first.
- You know your child best. If you are concerned about them you should seek further advice.

Do not worry unduly - these things are expected after a head injury and may last up to two weeks:

- Intermittent headache especially whilst watching TV or computer games
- Being off their food or feeling sick (without vomiting)
- Tiredness or trouble getting to sleep
- Short periods of irritability, bad temper or poor concentration

Useful numbers

Hospitals with Emergency Departments:

Royal Alexandra Children's Hospital
Eastern Road, Brighton BN2 5BE

Princess Royal Hospital
Lewes Road, Haywards Heath RH16 4EX

Surrey and Sussex Healthcare NHS Trust
East Surrey Hospital, Canada Ave, Redhill, Surrey RH1 5RH

Western Sussex Hospitals NHS Foundation Trust
including:
St Richards Hospital, Spitalfield Lane, Chichester PO19 6SE
Worthing Hospital, Lyndhurst Rd, Worthing BN11 2DH

Minor Injuries Units (MIU) or Urgent Care Centres

Bognor Regis War Memorial Hospital - Minor Injuries Unit, Shripney Road, Bognor Regis, PO22 9PP
Open 9am- 5pm, Monday – Friday (excluding bank holidays)

Crawley Urgent Treatment Centre
Crawley Hospital, West Green Drive, Crawley RH11 7DH
Open 24 hours, 7 days a week

Horsham Minor Injuries Unit
Horsham Hospital, Hurst Rd, Horsham RH12 2DR
Open 9am- 5pm, Monday – Friday (excluding bank holidays)

Queen Victoria Hospital Minor Injuries Unit (MIU), East Grinstead
Holtye Road, East Grinstead RH19 3DZ
Open 8am- 10pm, 7 days a week

West Sussex - Family Information Service
Tel: 01243 777807 www.westsussex.gov.uk/family

For more copies of this document, for more information and to feedback, please email us:
Chichester/Worthing area: contactus.coastal@nhs.net
Crawley area: CCCG.contactus-crawleyccg@nhs.net
Horsham/Mid Sussex area:
HSCCG.contactus-horshamandmidsussexccg@nhs.net

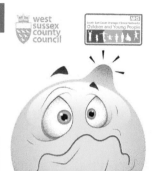

west sussex county council

NHS Children and Young People

Head Injury in Children and Young People

2014 UPDATED Advice for Parents and Carers

Child/Young Person's Name ....

Advice Given By ....

Location of Injury ....

Date .... Time ....

Head Injury - Advice for Parents and Carers

This leaflet is to help to advise on how best to care for a child who has a bump / injury to the head. Please use the "Caring for your child at home" advice section (see overleaf) and the traffic light advice below to help you. **Most children can be managed according to the green guidance below especially if they are alert and interacting with you.** It is important to watch the child for the next 2-3 days to ensure that they are responding to you as usual.

Traffic light advice:

Head wounds rarely need stitches and can normally be glued by a health professional. This can be done in Minor Injury Units or Urgent Treatment Centres and some GP practices offer a minor injuries service. To find a local service see overleaf.

Green: Low Risk	Amber: Intermediate Risk	Red: High Risk
If your child:	**If your child:**	**If your child:**
• Cried immediately (after head injury) but returns to their normal behaviour in a short time	• Is under one year old	• Has been involved in a high speed road traffic accident or fallen from a height over 1 metre or been hit by a high speed object or involved in a diving accident
• Is alert and interacts with you	• Has vomited once or twice	• Has been unconscious / "knocked out" at any time
	• Has a continuous headache	• Is sleepy and you cannot wake them
• Has not been unconscious / "knocked out"	• Has continued irritation or unusual behaviour	• Has a convulsion or a fit
		• Has neck pain
• Has minor bruising, swelling or cuts to their head	• Is under the influence of drugs or alcohol	• Has difficulty speaking or understanding what you are saying
	• Has been deliberately harmed and in need of medical attention	• Has weakness in their arms and legs or are losing their balance
		• Cannot remember events around or before the accident
		• Has had clear or bloody fluid dribbling from their nose, ears or both since the injury
ACTION: If all the above have been met then manage at home. Follow the advice overleaf or, if you are concerned, contact your GP when they are open or call 111 when your GP surgery is not open		• Has 3 or more separate bouts of vomiting
	ACTION: Take your child to the nearest Hospital Emergency department if ANY of these features are present	**ACTION: Phone 999** for an ambulance if ANY of these symptoms are present

Based on: Head Injury - Triage, assessment, investigation and early management of head injury in children, young people and adults. January 2014. NICE clinical guideline 176

Diagrams for Head Injury, Fever Advice Sheet, Fever Pathway, Diarrhoea and or Vomiting (2522 (HI), FAS 0, 1 and 2, DV)

Croup:

Epiglottitis	Laryngo-tracheo bronchitis:
The patient appears systemically ill, quiet.	Patient often noisy and unhappy
Sudden onset.	but loud rather than quiet
High fever.	Flu or cold sympts. come first.
Mainly **inspiratory** stridor.	**Inspiratory and expiratory** stridor

Causes include H. Influenzae (but can be viral, staph or strep etc)

Drooling, swallowing is very painful.	Swallowing is less painful.
	Less drooling
Hoarse and muffled.	Hoarse, barking cough.

Tend to:

Be over 3 years	Less than 3 years.
Rare	Common.
Toxic with the high fever	"Sick but not toxic".
Cannot lie down (saliva pooling)	Less affected by position
Rapid onset	Preceded by a cold.

Respiratory distress, recession, accessory muscle use and cyanosis can occur in both situations and the treatment is basically the same for a sick child with upper respiratory obstruction from whatever cause.

The commonest cause of croup is a viral URTI. Epiglottitis (Haemophilus or other) is very rare since the start of national vaccination but exceedingly rare are: laryngeal Diphtheria, foreign body. (I once fished out ring pull from a croupy child's hypopharynx with a long pair of forceps five minutes into a morning ward round. He had been blue lighted direct to the ward, cyanosed and gasping from home at 9.00 am. This extraction was performed with the help of a brilliant female Australian SHO who held the arms, legs and head (!) of the toddler on the resuscitation trolley at the same time as I laryngoscoped him. The patient was a 2 year old brought in by a 999 ambulance with an instantaneous onset of croup and inspiratory stridor at home. The toddler was without temperature or any signs of being toxic or ill other than the respiratory distress. This had come on suddenly and the clue of the cause was in the history or lack of it.) Other very rare causes are laryngeal trauma, papilloma and angioneurotic oedema.

Epiglottitis which peaks at 6-36m, is rare after 6 but can occur up to adulthood. Between 2 and 5% go to hospital and only 2% of those require intubation. The incidence has diminished since H. Influenzae was included at the 2m, 3m, 4m and 12-13m immunisations. It is still incumbent on GPs to know how to do a tracheostomy and occasionally to be prepared to **accompany the child in the ambulance** to hospital. If you are admitting them then you are worried about obstruction and the riskiest time is when they are furthest from a doctor. Don't send them in by car.

Tongue depressor: Traditionally it is said that a throat examination with a spatula can cause obstruction in epiglottitis. I believe a gentle examination with a bright light and a tongue depressor on the anterior third of the tongue, which often displays a healthy pink epiglottis and a red throat can be very reassuring and instructive.

If, however, you are convinced that the epiglottis is not inflamed then a cold trip in the back of a car with the windows down, a bathroom or kitchen full of cold outside air and steam, some spacered steroid, or preferably nebulised inhaled steroid, (Budesonide, Fluticasone), some nebulised vasoconstictor (I use 1:1 Paediatric Otrivine (Xylometazoline 0.05%)) nose drops in water, (others have use nebulised adrenaline), Oral or I.M. steroids in the form of Dexamethasone 0.6mg/Kg are next. Prednisolone (1mg/kg) is effective but may be associated with a higher early recurrence. I would always give a big dose of a bacteriocidal antibiotic. I use Co Amoxiclav or a cephalosporin if I can – for speed and spectrum.

Whether to admit the child depends as much on the perceived severity of the illness as the reliability of the parents, the time of day (can they call YOU back?) and what the OOH service is like. Hospitals are dangerous places for children unless they really need to be there.

Wheezy Bronchitis/Bronchiolitis/Asthma.

These conditions were once virtually differentiated only by age, with bronchiolitis becoming wheezy bronchitis, becoming asthma as the child grew older. The season of the year (Autumn and Spring), an atopic family history, smoking within the house, damp home conditions, possibly mould and open fires are all factors. Conversely, a history of too little exposure to dirt, having double glazing, the lack of a pet in the home, not growing up on a farm, too much exposure to immunisations and antibiotics, even antibiotics in the last trimester of pregnancy may have also been relevant. Now we know factors such as the microbiome, the actual number of courses of antibiotics (or the respiratory infections for which they are given) and the heat efficiency of the home probably all increase the rates of asthma too – apparently almost proportionately. The greener our home the wheezier our children.

Interestingly, although some reports have linked antibiotic drugs per se to the increased risk of developing asthma (and promulgated an immune mechanism for this) a large study from Sweden which looked into the reasons why the antibiotics **were actually given** to children in early life found something different in 2015. When researchers at the Karolinska Institutet looked at 500,000 children prescribed antibiotics between 2006 and 2010 they found an increased risk of asthma of 28%. The risk of asthma was however much higher if the antibiotics had been given for a respiratory reason rather than, say a UTI or a soft tissue infection. This suggested that the respiratory infection was in fact new *asthma being misdiagnosed*. The respiratory symptoms were actually those of asthma not infection or the respiratory infection itself increased the risk of asthma. The antibiotic was an innocent bystander and not the cause of asthma. Quite reassuring.

The story is often told of the incidence of asthma on the two sides of the Berlin wall. East Berlin, smoky and polluted, with its Trabant cars and diesel trucks pouring out smoke, insufficiently provided with modern western style health care. Fewer antibiotics and childhood immunisations. Cold houses, inadequate insulation and a generally tougher and dirtier upbringing. Which half of Berlin had the higher incidence of asthma? The West of course – by far. It seems that dirt and more infections protect us from asthma (as well as other immune diseases).

In late 2014 a paper was published linking the risk of a child developing asthma directly to the thermal efficiency of their house. Presumably this was because house dust, the associated mites and their faeces, mould spores, air born gases and other debris are not exchanged in greener, hermetically sealed houses and these irritants negatively affect the epithelial lining of developing lungs. After all, we evolved in the open and in smoky caves not in warm hermetically sealed insulated boxes.

Maternal smoking in pregnancy however, increases asthma in offspring, as do a family history of allergy, previous bronchiolitis, other atopic conditions, prematurity or low birth weight. In some children reflux can induce wheezing and high doses of anti reflux medication may be necessary (also the diagnostic pin has to drop first) to relieve the respiratory symptoms.

As mentioned, some new research links the use of antibiotics in infancy with the subsequent development of asthma. (Lancet Resp Med 15 may 2014). If antibiotics are given to babies or small children the risk of developing asthma before six years increases as does the risk of being admitted to hospital. There was a 70% increased risk of asthma after antibiotics and a 164% increased risk of being admitted in a 2014 study. Although the Swedish paper above suggested the antibiotic association with asthma was due to misdiagnosis or the respiratory infection itself causing the increased asthma risk, the alternative view is that antibiotics interfere with normal immune maturation. The theory that bacteria (especially in the gut) are needed to help our immune systems develop and that early antibiotic use harms immune development may not be the whole story however since this study found a slightly different chicken and egg situation. The children who were given antibiotics in infancy had significantly lower levels of cytokines (immune messenger molecules) and had specific genetic markers on Chromosome 17 that indicated an immune deficit. So it is possible that some children are born with impaired antiviral immunity, suffer worse chest infections and asthma. The antibiotics are the medical profession's response to this underlying problem.

So antibiotics may just be innocent bystanders again after all.

It does seem that we need some dirt and mild infections though, to allow our immune system to practice and mature during our formative years. Otherwise it reacts excessively to a variety of non lethal stimulae later in childhood and adult life with asthma, hay fever etc. Children who grow up on farms are 30-50% less likely to have asthma (Ege, NEJM 24.2.2011) and mice exposed to dog dust have less reactive airways (Proc Nat Ac Sc Dec 2013). Children with pets get less allergy. (JAMA Pediatrics, 650,000 children, Nov 2015: Exposure to a dog in the first year of life was linked to a 13% lower risk of asthma later) Undoubtedly some children can develop, as can lab technicians, an allergy to pets, cats, rodents and their epithelial cells and fur but this is a far cry from the advice thirty years ago when I was a young Paediatrician, to remove all pets from asthmatic households. What misery that would have caused if anyone had heeded it.

In terms of triggers for wheezing, the infective stimulae include RSV, Parainfluenzae Type 3, Metapneumovirus, Influenza, Coronavirus, Adenovirus, and Rhinovirus, all potential causes of Bronchiolitis.

Bronchiolitis, Viral Induced Wheeze and Wheezy Bronchitis are interchangeable terms. They describe the dyspnoeic, tachypnoeic, hyper inflated, air trapped, wheezy baby or toddler who has become breathless after a URTI.

There are, on examination signs of respiratory distress with tachypnoea, hyperinflation, accessory muscles in use, prolonged expiration and audible basal crepitations (crackles to newly qualified doctors) and rhonchi (wheezes to the same new comers).

80% have had their infection by 2 years and the autumn, winter and spring months are the commonest. The seasons and the signs coincide with Mycoplasma infection and for that reason I suggest that if an antibiotic is used it should be a reasonable dose of one of the Macrolides, Erythromycin/Clarithromycin.

Interestingly, I got what I feel was some authoritative back up to my 30 year old gut feeling about this when in 2016 (Reuters Health) Dr H Bisgaardof the Copenhagen Prospective Studies of Asthma in Childhood study showed that "preschool viral wheeze" which WAS previously considered to be viral in aetiology and episodes of which were a leading cause of hospital admission in fact responded very well to antibiotics! The antibiotic however which they found to be effective was azithromycin. This antibiotic reduced episodes by 63% when treatment was started before the 6th day of the wheeze. Surely fairly convincing evidence that many childhood wheezy chest infections ARE NOT VIRAL and do require consideration of antibiotic treatment? And this is at the time when large numbers of GPs are withholding antibiotics even from moderately sick children in the name of preventing drug resistance. (See Scarlet Fever etc. comments above and elsewhere)

Breast feeding and avoiding Caesarean Section reduce the incidence of wheeze (both probably via the gut microbiome). Low birth weight, Down's Syndrome, having older sibs, nursery attendance, congenital heart disease, neurological or lung disease all increase it. At many meetings I attend on the subject of "**viral wheeze in childhood**" speakers go to great pains to differentiate asthma from intermittent viral wheeze. This is a new nicety and one which to me has little clinical purpose. It is on the theoretical basis of long term outcome and treatment response. Most current advice is that Montelukast helps viral associated wheeze in children but not much else does. This implies that we should tell the parents of a severely disturbed and worryingly wheezy child to go home or to the hospital, we can't do anything to help them as their wheeze is only "viral". "Viral" means we aren't involved, we can't help, go away we have more important things to deal with.

I think this is utterly wrong. Inhaled anticholinergics, inhaled steroids and in bigger children beta stimulants **can** help improve the symptoms and signs of "Viral wheeze". Oral steroids or in the secondarily-infected child, oral antibiotics can make a difference too. In General Practice, without the benefit of blood gases, chest X Rays, constant oxygen monitoring (even though the value of this in acute bronchiolitis has been questioned) and the paraphernalia of secondary care you have to try everything safe to prevent complications and improve symptoms. You are seeing a sick child for an instant in the course of their illness and you have no ethical right to claim impotence when a variety of medications might well improve their symptoms and outcome. There is no room for rigid protocols and closed minds here – you just have to see what works.

Unfortunately by 2016 there was developing a standard impotent response by many doctors if they started a consultation with the mindset that their patient might be presenting with a "viral illness". This increasingly then excluded a proper examination and assessment and was often dominated by the no antibiotic agenda. Indeed the less the patient is examined, the less likely the doctor is to find justification for active treatment and there is a satisfactory intellectual closed loop of help refusal that goes on, to the dismay of the patient. The doctor usually then offers an information sheet or a web site on viral infection, not having excluded a more serious diagnosis, but providing a small fig leaf of self justification and camouflage and thus dismissing the dissatisfied patient. Result: antibiotic prescribing diminishes, secondary infections, serious complications and deaths increase, patient feedback scores plummet and in the long run the quality of primary care and the GP's self respect deteriorates.

This negative mindset is deplorable. The patient is ignored, feels angry, short changed and let down. Indeed, this is just the lazy response of a medical automaton. But I am told by patients that this is an increasingly frequent standard issue consultation especially in our age of antibiotic paranoia. Especially amongst newly qualified GPs. The doctor doesn't want to prescribe so he doesn't even touch or undress the patient during the "consultation" just in case he finds something to treat. I find this depressing, lazy, dangerous, pointless and unethical. It is the herd response to the national edict against inappropriate antibiotic prescribing. New doctors, GPs particularly, are good at conforming these days and the unfortunate outcome of our compliance has been a vast increase in bacterial infections from Scarlet Fever to Community Acquired Pneumonia, (and soon, no doubt, Rheumatic Fever and Post Streptococcal Glomerulonephritis. All untreated or undetected by doctors who now have a tacit assumption that all seasonal coughs, febrile illnesses and nasty throats are "viral". And viral has nothing to do with us.

Anyway back to bronchiolitis:

Exclude aspiration, pneumothorax, pneumonia, F.B. etc by imaging the chest if you are worried and if you have access. This would be standard practice in the US I am told but depends on where you are in the UK and what is easily available (and the time of day).

The natural history is up to 7-28 days, usually 7-14 days.

Admit the child with bronchiolitis if respiratory rate>70/min, cyanosis, saturation<94%, any possible apnoea, significant respiratory distress, including grunting, see-saw respiration, poor feeds.

Treatment: The studies show that little you can do actually helps a great deal. It is important to exclude the other causes of respiratory distress and in a significantly unwell child an XR needs to be looked at by someone competent straight away.

Nebulised bronchodilators probably don't help much, neither do nebulised or oral steroids. Hypertonic nebulised saline (with or without bronchodilators) and Ribavirin seem to have some effect but these are, of course, hospital treatments.

But quite often there **are** other factors, secondary infections, inflammatory oedema, bronchospasm (If the child is big enough to have smooth muscle in its airways) and I see no harm in giving spacer administered inhaled steroids and either B stimulants to a big child or Ipratropium to any sized child. I would also give oral steroids (Dexamethasone, soluble Prednisolone) and Erythromycin/Clarithromycin to try and avoid admission provided none of the above caveats are present and I can trust the parents to recognise deterioration and call back.

Up to 50% will have recurrent cough or wheeze for some years and it is difficult with an intermittent past history to categorically label a child as a "viral associated wheezer" and destined to grow out of his condition.

A recent report (2015) declared that RSV affected 2/3 of children in their first year, was responsible for 1 in 6 hospital admissions during winter and was particularly harmful to babies who had been born prematurely. In the developing world it is the number two killer after malaria. The first human trials on an RSV vaccine using an attenuated virus were said to be" now under way".

The Journal Pediatrics did an extensive and pretty unhelpful review in 2006 (118.1774) which said oxygen and IV fluids helped in RSV infection but not much else. To summarise their advice:

RSV is an infection, mainly Dec-March, other viruses that cause bronchiolitis are Metapneumovirus, Influenza, Adenovirus and Parainfluenza viruses. As a rough guide **the normal respiratory rates** are

Birth   50
6m   40
1yr   30

Breast feeding probably protects and parental smoking makes bronchiolitis worse. Premature birth and age 6-12 weeks are associated with a worse illness, as are underling CHD, BPD, CF and immune disease. The presence of consolidation or atelectasis on CXR is associated with worse severity. In terms of treatment, most are controversial: For instance: Nebulised Alpha or Beta adrenergic drugs (but if they are helpful Adrenaline might be the best), some patients may respond a little to anticholinergics or oral steroids, Ribavirin, antibiotics, but appropriate oxygenation and hydration are most important.

Palivizumab prophylactically may be useful in premature infants with CLD. (BPD is "Chronic Lung Disease" of prematurity) (Bronchopulmonary Dysplasia).

The use of either intermittent or continuous pulse oximetry makes no difference, transient oxygen desaturation being very common during bronchiolitis (as distinct from persistent significant hypoxia.)

So for the GP it is worth trying all of the above that you have available and if the child is significantly ill or not getting better, admit them for oxygen, observation and fluids.

Recent Treatment Advice for Bronchiolitis:

A MORE recent (Autumn 2014) review from the USA suggested the following treatment approaches:

Humidified oxygen, Attention to hydration, Assisted ventilation if required, Nasal/oral suction, Monitoring for pulse, respiration/apnoea. Temperature control. They said that most medication was ineffective but in selected children the following helped: Alpha/beta agonists, Monoclonal antibodies (Palivizumab), Antibiotics (They suggested Ampicillin, Cefotaxime, Ceftriaxone) I don't think I have ever seen Ampicillin used in the UK, not in the last 35 years anyway. I would add Erythro or Azithromycin. (See earlier). Antiviral agents (Ribavirin), Nasal decongestants (Oxymetazoline), Steroids (Prednisolone, Methylprednisolone). Nebulised hypertonic saline in another study reduced hospital stay by 11 hours (!) and reduced risk of hospitalisation in outpatients by 20%. This is safe especially when administered with a bronchodilator.

The general advice is if the transcutaneous oxygen saturation of a sick child is <92%, they need supplemental oxygen and probably IV fluids.

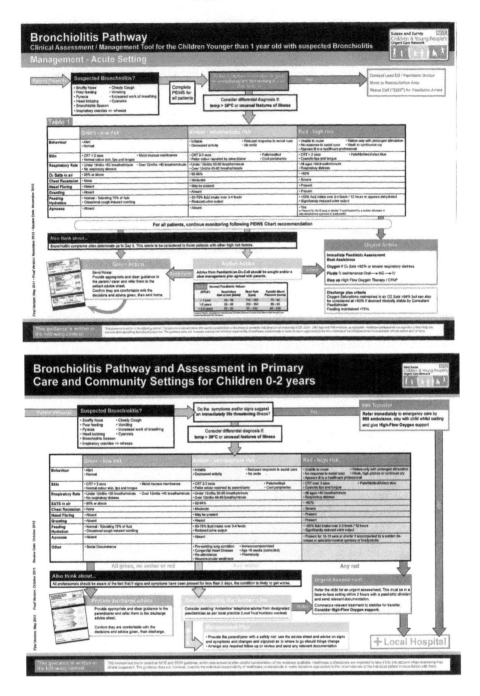

Diagram Bronchiolitis Pathway 1 and 2 (BP1 and 2) The Traffic Light Bronchiolitis Charts.

Acute severe asthma in children:
> Can't complete sentences in one breath
> Pulse>120>5 yrs
> Pulse >130 at 2-5yrs
> Resps. >30 >5yrs
> Resps.>50 at 2-5yrs.

Steroids:

Prednisolone (e.c.) 1-2mg/kg orally/24 hrs for 5-7 days (some say 3 days are enough but if the asthma is associated with a viral chest infection then a longer course will be needed) with or without a stat dose of IV hydrocortisone. Use the bigger dose if already on "maintenance steroids".
> <2yrs 25mg IV hydrocortisone,
> 2-5yrs 50mg,
> 5-12yrs 100mg,
> PLUS
> Nebulised B stimulant and Ipratropium.

Here is a rough guide to healthy, fit, average, mixed sex, "average race" children at different ages in terms of best expected peak flows related to ages and heights. Obviously their best peak flow will depend on how big their chest is, how active they are, whether they are boys or girls, their race, and their technique – but it is something to be getting on with...

Height	Age 50th C (Boys)	Peak Flow
0.9m	2 1/2 yrs	92-95Lmin^{-1}
0.95m	3	104-107
1.0m	4	115-124
1.05m	4 1/2	127-146
1.1m	5	141-169
1.15m	6	157-192
1.2m	7	174-220
1.25m	8	192-247
1.3m	9	212-275
1.35m	10	233-300
1.4m	11	254-325
1.45m	12	276-350
1.5m	12 1/2	299-375
1.55m	13	323-403
1.6m	14	346-430
1.65m	15	370-455
1.7m	16	393-480
1.75m	17	465-505
1.8m	18	488-535

These figures collate a variety of sources which all vary slightly and come from various charts and lists

PAEDIATRIC NORMAL VALUES

PEAK EXPIRATORY FLOW RATE
For use with EU / EN13826 scale PEF meters only

Height (m)	Height (ft)	Predicted EU PEFR (L/min)	Height (m)	Height (ft)	Predicted EU PEFR (L/min)
0.85	2'9"	87	1.30	4'3"	212
0.90	2'11"	95	1.35	4'5"	233
0.95	3'1"	104	1.40	4'7"	254
1.00	3'3"	115	1.45	4'9"	276
1.05	3'5"	127	1.50	4'11	299
1.10	3'7"	141	1.55	5'1	323
1.15	3'9"	157	1.60	5'3"	346
1.20	3'11"	174	1.65	5'5"	370
1.25	4'1"	192	1.70	5'7"	393

Normal PEF values in children correlate best with height; with increasing age, larger differences occur between the sexes. These predicted values are based on the formulae given in Lung Function by J.E. Cotes (Fourth Edition), adapted for EU scale Mini-Wright peak flow meters by Clement Clarke. Date of preparation – 7th October 2004

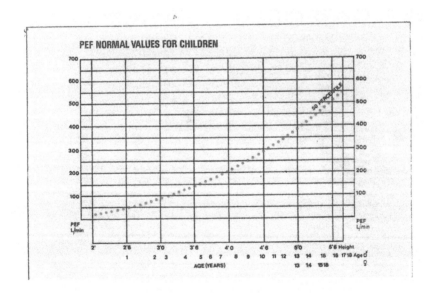

My thanks to Clement Clarke and Allen and Hanburys.

PEAK EXPIRATORY FLOW RATE - NORMAL VALUES
For use with EU/EN13826 scale PEF meters only

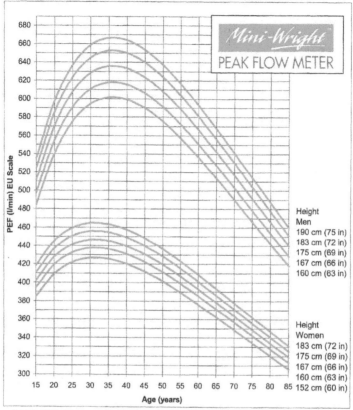

Mini-Wright

PEAK FLOW METER

Height
Men
190 cm (75 in)
183 cm (72 in)
175 cm (69 in)
167 cm (66 in)
160 cm (63 in)

Height
Women
183 cm (72 in)
175 cm (69 in)
167 cm (66 in)
160 cm (63 in)
152 cm (60 in)

Adapted by Clement Clarke for use with EN13826 / EU scale peak flow meters
from Nunn AJ Gregg I, Br Med J 1989:298;1068-70

DIAGRAM (PFV 1, PFV 2, PFV3) (includes adults)

The Hot Child:

One of my colleagues would never prescribe anti-pyretics to any patient because he had read that a group of septicaemic cold blooded (poikilothermic) lizards given paracetamol had all died, but those allowed to become febrile had survived. The assumption was that the temperature was an evolved and crucial defence mechanism against infection. That is as maybe but children, like many adults, feel wretched when very hot. As well as the systemic symptoms of headache, myalgia, rigors, weakness, tremor, myoclonic jerking, etc, there are the central and disturbing symptoms of confusion, hallucinations and if the temperature rises quickly and the child is 1-5 years old, the risk of febrile convulsion(s) despite the rather puzzling NICE assertion that antipyretic agents do **not** prevent febrile convulsions. This is counter intuitive and not my own experience, provided they are started early before the initial sudden rise in temperature at the start of many viral infections.

Although usually benign, these frightening symptoms can be very disturbing for adults and very upsetting for the child.

The rate of temperature rise rather than absolute temperature is said to be the determinant of the fit.

Cooling the child should be done using cool but not cold water (heat is lost from the core through the skin and cold water vasoconstricts turning the skin from a conductor to an insulator), via sponging. The child should be stripped off in a cool but not cold room and a fan used in the room but not directed at the child. All these measures are aimed at allowing core heat to exit via the surface skin without cooling the skin too much. Don't forget babies lose a third of their heat through their scalp so wet the scalp with cool water too.

Elsewhere I quote the high risks of very young febrile children having positive blood cultures and the high percentage who prove in some research to have serious infections. This (see below) is 13% in one study. In GP we see hundreds of hot children each year and we cannot either admit them all, give them all antibiotics or dismiss them as all having a viral infection. We are all fearful of appearing to be thoughtless reflex prescribers of unnecessary antibiotics nowadays. After an era of almost nonexistent post streptococcal glomerulonephritis, scarlet fever, intracranial extension of otitis media, mastoiditis, quinsy, pulmonary abscess, erysipelas and a host of bacterial diseases common decades ago, which then became extinct, we are now seeing the down side of **thoughtless non-prescribing**. These illnesses are becoming common again. Increasing numbers of sick patients who die unnecessarily for the lack of a timely antibiotic. Three such babies were on the cover of the Daily Mail on 27th January 2016. All had been "the victims of NHS staff who had failed to spot the illness ("sepsis") that would kill them." We have to be more diligent in assessing, examining and recognising the signs of significant infection and do what we are supposed to do for a living: Differentiating the ill from the worried well. We do this by staying alert after a dozen hot, lively, well children in evening surgery, by ignoring blanket directives and protocols, by thinking what is best for THIS patient and by thoroughly examining all febrile patients. In 2016 "Sepsis" suddenly became a new killer as far as much of the media was concerned and something we GPs were supposed to be unaware of.

In early 2016 the familiar but still immensely sad story of William Mead came to the public's attention and it summarised all that is wrong in modern Primary Health Care. I do not know the precise details of the consultations William and his mother had with their GP(s) or the exact history and advice exchanged over the 911 phone line but what follows are reasonable assumptions.

It relates to a one year old baby boy who had died the year before and whose articulate mother told the story of his untimely death on the radio and television. Towards the end of the interview she became tearful in telling of his final hours but remained dignified and I thought reasonable and remarkably balanced throughout. All of which added strength to her criticism and dissatisfaction of the "Care" she had received from today's typical NHS. Although journalists love to use any stick they can to beat doctors these days, it isn't difficult for them to find good reason to hit us frequently and mercilessly when stories like William's are told. I do not know whether he saw the same GP each time his mother took him to the local practice or whether they saw, like so many patients, sessional or part time GPs with no past knowledge and familiarity of the family. You would imagine that alarm bells would have rung in the doctor's mind if there had been some personnel continuity or if proper notes about the previous consultations were available. I do not know how long the consultations were or if he was stripped off and thoroughly examined. I do not know whether his chest was checked at the last consultation though it seems unlikely if he died within half a day from septicaemia from what was primarily a chest infection. Presumably he would have had chest signs at that time. Perhaps he was thoroughly examined and this was a case of a fulminant and catastrophic septicaemia in an immunocompromised child. I do not know. Perhaps the GPs were excellent.

He was taken, febrile and unwell to his GP several times in the "weeks" – and I assume days, before he died. I accept that a parent's definition of unwell and ours as GPs are often different but the "several times" should justify a prolonged and thorough examination of any child by the attending doctor. Perhaps the frequency of visits was a factor in the GP not prescribing or perhaps not performing a more extensive examination or refusing an antibiotic? Perhaps he/she thought they were crying wolf again, were frequent attenders. Perhaps personalities were involved – I don't know. This is exactly the sort of situation where sensible and experienced GPs go overboard to exclude serious illness by being thorough and diligent. Even by referral. I do not know. No doctor likes to reward a parent who cries wolf too often. I have no way of knowing why the infection was missed or why an antibiotic was not considered appropriate or what took place between mother and GP. I do not know the dynamics involved but it is the sort of situation I have seen second hand many times. I have often been asked when acting as a "second opinion" on a coughing or wheezy child, the day after seeing another doctor why I want to examine the chest. – "The other doctor didn't need to."

I believe that the final GP consultation was on a Friday afternoon. This time of the week by itself should raise the doctor's index of suspicion of significant illness as it is a time when more short cuts are taken, fewer doctors are available and more mistakes are made by more GPs than any other. In my opinion, no duty GP, covering until the usual 6.30 pm should expect to get home on a Friday until at least 8.00 pm. No reassurance should be given and no dubious telephone advice, no consultation shortened, no visit refused, no social occasion booked, – if getting home promptly is a slightest factor in the decision. When the mother brought William Mead to the GP, was he stripped off and examined fully? Was an MSU requested, were the throat, ears, abdomen, CNS, circulation and degree of hydration assessed? In any febrile child with chest signs I **would** prescribe a decent antibiotic, superbugs or not. The GP, like all GPs would be anxious not to over prescribe antibiotics. This is universal these days. But this pressure from NICE, colleagues, prescribing committees and the Department of Health has led to a culture of not taking febrile illnesses seriously and a tendency to under prescribe antibiotics in **all** sick patients. It is leading to dozens of cases like William and hundreds of near misses. This is completely unacceptable and I feel ashamed that my colleagues are **so rarely** 1) Stripping patients off sufficiently to make a proper examination of febrile patients, 2) Using their stethoscope, auriscope, tongue depressors, urine dipstixes and other aids to properly assess whether an infection is present, 3) Putting the health and comfort of the patient above the theoretical risk of causing a resistant infection, 4) Thinking for themselves instead of happily and blindly acting like a government policy rubber stamp.

Anyway the mum and child were sent home and because he did not improve she called 911 later that night. The call handler used a standard algorithm for febrile children and was not medically trained, something which in my opinion is unacceptable for staff handling emergency medical calls from sick patients. I would hope a doctor or suitably trained nurse would ask open questions and specific enquiries about the liveliness, responses to stimuli, tone, interest, spontaneous activity, thirst, colour, sound of breathing, awareness of the child and so on. These sort of things and this approach were not on the list of questions or job description of the call handler. The parents were again reassured. We had, until a relatively short time ago, a system where all GPs went out to see our own sick patients at night. After that, GP cooperatives were set up, where every call was answered by a local GP. I doubt that today's profession, being mainly part time and female could cope with even the cooperative OOH system now, certainly not proper 24 hour cover as it was. (See the section on feminisation of medicine). In either case the 911 system is a poor substitute and uses non medical personnel who apply rigid medical algorithms to calls but do not themselves have any specific knowledge or flexibility in applying the process. The last few hours of William's life were of the parents checking on him through the night, having been reassured by all the medical consultations that they had received. He died of septicaemia complicating his pneumonia about 5-6 am.

I need hardly say that if the family had had a good relationship with a trusted and familiar family doctor whose partnership offered a 24 hour service and if the family were not frequent misusers of the out of hours service then I don't think the septicaemia would have been missed. The mother clearly knew William was seriously ill and if she had known her GP well and there had been practice continuity (ie few part time doctors) then the doctor on call would know her and have trusted her opinion more. This assumes their GP was not cowed by the current witch hunt against over prescribing of antibiotics and had the basic clinical skills and patience to examine and assess the child properly. In other words if the system was like it was or should have been 20 years ago. Whether the junior paediatrician on call in the hospital (if the GP then chose to admit him), would have managed and treated William appropriately, given the paucity of hours worked today and the reduced total training of all specialist doctors currently, I just don't know (see below). Clearly however, the current doctor-friendly, patient-unfriendly emergency primary and secondary care system that we have is fraught with danger for seriously ill patients of all ages.

All doctors can miss serious illnesses – and septicaemia can kill quickly, out of nowhere. But the fear that some GPs have of prescribing antibiotics, especially to febrile children and the lack of clinical thoroughness of some colleagues (though I repeat, I do not know if that was the case here) are also important issues in many of these sad cases.

The official report criticised

The poor note keeping of the GP,

The failure to recognise William's symptoms as something more serious,

The advice given to his parents about what to do over the weekend if he got worse,

The OOH GP service which had no access to his notes,

The "Pathway Tool" used by NHS111 advisers which had been too crude to pick up "red flag warnings" related to sepsis.

NICE and the Febrile Child:

NICE have several idiosyncratic bits of advice regarding the hot child. Like much of their clinical advice I can only surmise that the relevant committee, like the GMC had few if any experienced GPs on it.

Antipyretics don't stop febrile convulsions: Given early enough (see above) they **may**

well stop FCs and they have other symptomatic advantages as well.

Use electronic axillary thermometers under 4 weeks and tympanic thermometers or axillary chemical dot or axillary electronic thermometers 4 weeks to 5 years: As a busy GP I find my tympanic thermometer requires a supply of membrane covers, is bulky and the batteries are often flat. Despite the health and safety issues the most practical (and accurate) "core temperature" measurement is by using a rectal mercury thermometer in small children. It takes up no space, needs no batteries and is always accurate. Mine is 50 years old and still works perfectly.

A number of studies show that very small hot babies may be harbouring occult bacterial infections, some potentially serious. The problem for me is how often this is the case – given the potential risk of acquiring a new infections by admitting the child (hospitals are dangerous places), the relative lack of diagnostic skills of junior paediatricians these days, highlighted in the press in mid 2013 and since, and the current relatively poor out of hours cover at night and weekends both in GP and hospitals.

In a seminal article "Cold comfort for hot children" in the BMJ, way back in 1983, the recommendation was for admission of virtually all hot children under 12 weeks and for frequent reassessment of those not admitted. They describe one study in which out of 61 under 8 week babies seen at Johns Hopkins Hospital because of fever, 9 had bacteraemia – (this is 15%! – and 2 had meningitis). They also mention a slightly more reassuring Boston study for practical GPs in which only 31 out of 708 feverish babies had bacteraemia at a walk in centre (4%). Do we need to worry about bacteraemia? They quote the risk that a blood culture positive for Strep Pneumoniae gives a roughly 4% risk of subsequent meningitis and the risk of bacteraemia to the patient depends on the organism. The statement is given that doctors should request admission if the child's condition "occasions the slightest concern".

In one American study they used (and were not impressed by) the **"Philadelphia Protocol"** to assess how **ill** children under one month of age presenting at "E.R." with a high temperature actually were. They found some disturbing results. The study assessed more than 250 children with temperatures over 38C at presentation. All babies were screened bacteriologically and given I.V. antibiotics (!) The protocol says if the child appears well at presentation, has normal "lab values" and has no evidence of bacterial infection on examination then they are at low risk of serious bacterial infection. The actual results did not support this but perhaps more surprisingly – and something that goes against my own experience of well-looking hot children, they found 13% did have a serious bacterial infection, mostly UTIs, but others had peritonitis, osteomyelitis, pertussis etc.-all this without obvious outward signs and symptoms other than the temperature.

This puts the GP in a very difficult position given their current antibiotic parsimony, the parlous staffing state of OUR "E.R." departments, the recent public criticisms of the paediatric acumen and experience of junior staff and the traditional unwillingness of S.H.O.s and some registrars to see patients about whom the GP is worried but who don't display simplistic, clear cut and obvious symptoms from their book of standard sick kid protocols.

NICE suggests "Point of Care Testing" of CRP: CRP-POCT to differentiate the febrile child with a bacterial from a "simple viral" infection. And don't prescribe antibiotics if the CRP is<20mg/li. This is not practical for most of us at any time. The commercial testing kits seem straight forward but in real life are complex, fiddly, very time consuming and simply not practical to do half a dozen times between patients in a fraught typically overbooked winter surgery.

The moral is: Take every hot under 1month old and all febrile children with other symptoms and signs seriously. Don't dismiss them as having a viral infection. If you feel justified and concerned and your gut tells you so, learn the techniques to engineer a second opinion in hospital whether the signs are overt or not. But make sure you have fully examined the patient and done all appropriate tests first. AND be prepared to review the child again if the junior paediatrician mistakenly passes them well and sends them home.

Don't forget that Paracetamol elixir begins to have an antipyretic effect one hour after the dose, the maximum effect (reduction of fever by 70%) occurring 1 1/2 to 3 1/2 hours later.

In the sick child: Measure

Temperature,
Respiratory rate,
Heart rate,
Capillary refill time,
Skin turgor,
Temperature and appearance of extremities,
Test urine if possible,
AS WELL AS performing:
Your physical examination: (CVS, RS, Abdo, ENT, UGT, CNS, Skin etc.)

Paediatric bowel problems:

Some children develop a persistent enterocolitis ("Eosinophilic gastroenteropathy") after mesenteric adenitis. This is similar to the adult with persistent IBS symptoms after gastroenteritis. I have seen Sodium Cromoglicate, Nalcrom, Oral Ketotifen, Zaditen or even Mesalazine, Asacol used in this condition with good effect.

Toddler Diarrhoea ("Peas and carrots syndrome"):

The commonest cause of persistent diarrhoea in childhood, commoner in boys, 6m-5yrs. Stools are looser at the end of the day. Generally benign but there is a higher incidence of constipation on F/U and a higher incidence of functional bowel disorders in family members. The child is healthy and growing normally.

Some consider it to be part of the spectrum of childhood functional bowel disorders, which include infantile colic, non specific abdominal pain in childhood, IBS.

The typical sufferer's diet is high roughage, high fluid, high in fruit but particularly high in fruit juices (these contain fructose, sorbitol). The symptoms do improve when fruit, fluid and fruit juice are restricted (also if more fat and possibly probiotics are added to the diet).

At consultation, document the child's growth (height and weight) and velocity and get them back to recheck later.

Must exclude malabsorption and gut and other infections.

Tests*: Ht. Wt.

Possible primary causes:

Motility Disorder: Starch granules in stool and excess bile acids in the colon suggest a rapid transit time and this means increased small bowel motility. Increased dietary fat reduces transit speed and improves symptoms.

Food intolerance; Some have Lactose intolerance especially post gastroenteritis, (+ reducing substances) some have: Cow's Milk or Egg Protein Intolerance (Eosinophilia, High IgE, Low IgA). Perhaps 20% have a food protein allergy. High prostaglandin levels: Prostaglandins are higher in the plasma of TD children and aspirin (etc) does improve symptoms (but beware Reye's Syndrome). Children with TD do not have the normal reduction of motility in response to food. Stress: There are higher levels of family and environmental stress in children c TD. TD children are healthy and growing normally – Check growth and growth velocity. Check FH of functional bowel problems or atopy – perhaps 20% respond to an exclusion diet.

Tests*: Stool Cult and Reducing Substances. MSU. ? FBC (Eosinophils). ?IgE, high. ?IgA low.

Management: Increase fat intake: Low fat diets and high fluid intake contribute to toddler diarrhoea. Any kind of dietary sugar, natural or not may be the culprit. So reduce apple and other fruit juices. Pear, grape and apple juices have all been shown to increase carbohydrate malabsorption and exacerbate non specific diarrhoea. Fructose as well as sorbitol, found in apples, peaches, pears and prunes are associated with diarrhoea in some adults as well. Other dietary content to reduce includes: sugary drinks, fibre and fizzy drinks. There may be some benefit from exclusion diets (milk, egg) in some patients. Try to reduce refined sugars and sweeteners in squashes, chocolate, table sugar added to food and cereals, as well as natural sugars in virtually all pure fruit juices – often considered the healthy option, but can cause diarrhoea. Probably only water and milk are totally innocent and milk only if you can guarantee no lactose intolerance. So slowly dilute the ubiquitous juice more and more. Pure apple juice is probably the worst. Drinks should be restricted between meals and certainly toddlers should not have constant comfort through a continual bottle in their mouth unless it is plain water. Reduce fibre in such things as Weetabix, porridge, grapes, raisins, peas, sweet corn, baked beans etc. A small amount of a high fat food at the end of a meal can reduce toddler diarrhoea. – cheese, yoghurt, ice cream etc.

Only in the very worst cases would drug treatment be considered and virtually all children grow out of the condition in a few years. If dietary manipulation isn't helping then referral to a paediatrician is indicated after a few months.

Treatments:

Sacrosidase (a yeast sucrase supplement), Aspirin (only in extremis, given Reye's risks), Cholestyramine, Loperamide, Alleviate stress.

While we are on the subject, the standard aid in getting patients to precisely describe their stool (not that this actually seems to be of great practical value) is the **Bristol Stool Form Scale** or the **Bristol Stool Chart: (Permission requested from Bristol Paediatric Dept to reproduce)**

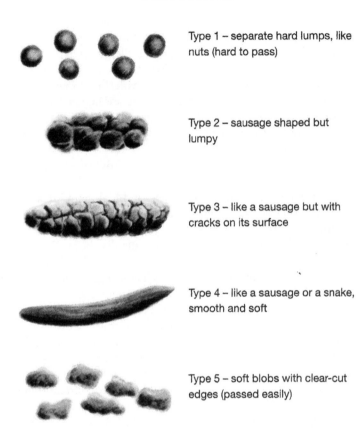

Type 1 – separate hard lumps, like nuts (hard to pass)

Type 2 – sausage shaped but lumpy

Type 3 – like a sausage but with cracks on its surface

Type 4 – like a sausage or a snake, smooth and soft

Type 5 – soft blobs with clear-cut edges (passed easily)

Type 6 – fluffy pieces with ragged edges, a mushy stool

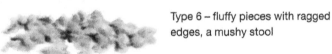

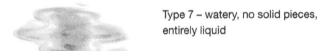

Type 7 – watery, no solid pieces, entirely liquid

ADHD/ADD: (ADD is a term not generally in use now):

Although the guidelines from most PCTs/Health Authorities are that GPs should leave the treatment of these conditions to Paediatricians, Community Paediatricians "with experience" or Adolescent Psychiatrists, I think this can sometimes cause significant harm and delay to the patient and parents. Many of us simply do not have access to a decent adolescent psychiatry unit, even for what we might consider "emergencies" in any reasonable time scale. ADHD and mood disorders, especially depression are amongst the commonest referrals that we make to secondary care. So not only did I have to initiate and supervise treatments for ADHD but for severe depression when our local unit triaged suicidal adolescents, even those who had already attempted overdosing, cutting wrists or wrapping ropes around their neck as "routine". Needs must and the patient comes first.

Its incidence (actually more likely the tendency to be labelled) vary with the country they live in and the era we are considering from 2-15% of school aged children.

Boys are diagnosed far more frequently than girls and the condition can impact severely on a child's social, intellectual and psychological development. They can become not only pariahs in class in terms of learning but also in terms of making friends, joining in and developing normal social networks and groups. They are often socially isolated and some-times the whole family can present very stressed and depressed. This is why, if secondary care is inaccessible or reluctant to help, it may be worth the GP taking on a more decisive role, making their own diagnosis and prescribing decisions.

The symptoms may be
Predominantly Inattentive,
Predominantly Hyperactive-Impulsive,
or
A mixture of the two.
Thus:

Inattentive:

Distractibility, Forgetfulness, Poor focus (butterfly thinking), Inability to process and follow instructions, Easy loss of focus, -not following through to a conclusion, (finishing a story or a TV program), easy boredom. Poorly organised, a tendency to lose things, Daydreaming, Unable to follow instructions, mind seems to be elsewhere.

Hyperactive/Impulsive:

Wriggle/fidgety when seated, Stream of words, Constant movement and touching or moving objects in a room, Unable to settle and be quiet, Impatience, Unrestrained comments and emotions, Can't stand in line or take turns.

A variety of treatments is available including behavioural management, counselling and drugs.

ADHD can be a symptom of or associated with other mental and psychological conditions: Various behaviour disorders, (oppositional, antisocial, temper tantrums etc) borderline personality disorder, depression, anxiety, bipolar disorder etc. Other associations are with enuresis, dyspraxia, etc. Some of the emotional symptoms may be secondary to the social isolation patients suffer due to their antisocial behaviour. A significant number of children with ADHD go on to be adults with a similar set of symptoms.

There was a vogue in the 70's for avoiding various foods, food colourings and additives (**The Feingold diet**) and this can be tried by the GP as an initial approach. At least it is something constructive-and may help. Avoid all food colourings, especially Tartrazine, (E102) as well as 110, 104, 122, 129, and 124, preservatives, e numbers, caffeine, fizzy drinks etc. Probably this will only help a small number of genetically susceptible children and it *is* incredibly fiddly to maintain.

The diet excludes natural salicylates (see the Diet and Allergy sections) and these are present in a huge number of foods – almonds, apples, apricots, peaches, plums, prunes, oranges, tangerines, tomatoes, cucumbers, blackberries, strawberries, raspberries, gooseberries, cherries, currants, grapes, raisins, blueberries etc as well as Monosodium Glutamate, Vanillin, salami, luncheon meat, frankfurters, packet soups, commercial sausages, meat loaf, ham, bacon, barbequed meat, breaded frozen fish, shop bought puddings, ice cream, yoghurt, chocolate, soft drinks, mint, soy sauce, cloves, chilli, crisps (flavoured) coloured sweets and medicines, caramel, coffee, tea, margarine, butter, smoked food.

Drug Treatment: Various forms of Methylphenidate (Ritalin) 5mg OD/BD if >5 yrs. Do initial height and weight. Slow release: Concerta XL 18mg, 27mg, 36mg. Equasym XL 10mg, 20mg, 30mg. Medikinet XL 5mg, 10mg, 20mg, 30mg, 40mg.

Can be used from 4 years, but usually from 6 years.

Dexamphetamine over 3 years (BNF says over 6 years) Lisdexamphetamine (Elvanse) >6 years 30-70mg.

Atomoxetine, Strattera: 10mg, 18mg, 25mg, 40mg, 60mg, 80mg, a NARI.

Other treatments sometimes used include: Combinations with Risperidone, Topiramate, Melatonin, Modafinil, Omega 3 Fish Oils etc depending on the clinical symptoms. Oil of evening Primrose.

One theory is that some children may be deficient in essential fatty acids in their diets. – There are two: Alpha linoleic acid (an omega 3 fatty acid) and Linoleic acid (an omega 6 fatty acid). The body cannot make these. Just as Omega 3 supplementation can be used to treat depression, EFAs are said to improve behaviour in ADHD. They can also improve eczema, asthma and some other allergic symptoms. Their effect (and their conversion to prostaglandins) is helped by zinc, magnesium and Vitamins B3 and C. Apparently boys have bigger requirements than girls, thirst is a sign of deficiency and EFAs are not converted to their many metabolic products if wheat or milk allergies are present.

Melatonin is interesting. It is available OTC in America and is used as a treatment for the sleep confusion of "jet lag". It is thought to have some anti cancer activity (apoptosis and anti angiogenesis) but it is also useful in the sleep disorder associated with ADHD. (For "primary insomnia" it is licensed in the UK as "Circadin").

Depression in ADHD can be treated with Citalopram or Fluoxetine.

Autism: (See above)

Said to be 1-2/1,000 – but this is only the rigid definition of autism and more and more patients, relatives, even colleagues seem to be covered by the ever expanding umbrella term "Autistic Spectrum Disorder". Having trained new doctors, taught medical students at a teaching hospital and appraised GPs, over a total of nearly 40 years, I wonder sometimes whether the selection and training processes for young doctors favour those with a tendency to egocentrism, over intellectualisation, introversion, emotional detachment, an association with computer technology, high intelligence, poor empathy, attachment to rituals and distaste for the expression and experience of emotion (and all that goes with it). In other words autistic spectrum characteristics. Do three or four A stars at A level tend to concentrate applicants who have features of this spectrum ?

One theory of autism is that autistic children tend to be the result of the inter marrying of parents who are "nerds" – who tend to have high intelligence, logical thinking but low emotional and empathy scores. People who are good at designing and using computer software rather than people who are good at listening to and sympathising with other people's feelings.

Autism seems to be a genetic condition but not due to a single gene. There has been a whole variety of environmental causes blamed at various times but none proven. Most notorious was the MMR scandal which has been shown to have no basis in fact but in common with all immunisation scares, combined public ignorance with journalistic irresponsibility. Parents still sometimes allude to the risks of MMR. – As indeed some parents still refer to the potential harm of whooping cough vaccine, not actually knowing the number of innocent unvaccinated children killed and maimed by ignorant parents and reporters.

One of the latest associations mooted is with gestational diabetes diagnosed at 26 weeks (more so than with the presumably better controlled serum glucose of Type 2DM). The theory is that uncontrolled hyperglycaemia during brain development leads to the damage that causes autism.

With the rigid definition of autism, 50% have severe learning difficulties, I.Q.<50.

25% have moderate learning difficulties, I.Q. 50-70. It becomes apparent in the first year of life.

Classically Autism is:

Impaired social interaction, inability to make friends, inability to communicate normally verbally, other communication difficulties, impaired imagination, restricted and repetitive behaviour (ritualistic, repeated, restrictive movements), sometimes self injury, delays in cognitive and language development, eating and other rituals. Few children with full blown autism live independent adult lives. Officially the Autistic Spectrum Disorder is 11/1,000 (and consists of Autism itself, Asperger's syndrome and Pervasive Developmental Disorder).

Asperger's Syndrome:

Abnormalities of gaze, poverty of expression, lack of feelings for others, lack of humour, extreme egocentrism, an idiosyncratic attachment to objects, but intelligence and language are normal.

Milks etc:

Formula Feeding:

A general guide is 150mls/kg/24hrs in 4-6 formula feeds. There are 30mls per fluid oz (actually 28mls) and there are 2.2 lb/kg which is 2.4 oz/lb/24 hrs of feed.

Soya based milks used not to be advised below 6m due to phytoestrogen content (so useful at the menopause) and a theoretical risk to the reproductive health of babies, also the risk of soya allergy developing – this caveat has now been withdrawn to some extent and perinatal soya feeds are deemed safe "at the doctor's discretion" – but only based on clinical need. By the way, rice based drinks are said to have too much arsenic to give to the under 5's. The phytoestrogen concerns were based on studies which included two which found an association between long and painful periods in adult women with being fed soya milks as babies and a change in marmoset testes after they were fed soya based formulae.

NOTE: The background: In March 2003 COT (Committee on Toxicity of Chemicals in Food, Consumer Products and the Environment) published a report on 'Phytoestrogens and Health'. This report reviewed the scientific evidence on phytoestrogens and soya infant formulas and found no evidence to demonstrate that soya infant formulas were unsafe. Overall the COT report was reassuring about the safety of soya infant formulae, but despite a lack of convincing evidence of any short-term or long-term adverse effects in humans they suggested a minor change to the Department of Health advice and to recommend that soya-based infant formulae should only be fed to infants "when indicated clinically". In June 2003 the Paediatric group of the British Dietetic Association issued a position statement on the use of Soya protein for Infants. They recommended that "As a precautionary measure, the use of a soya based infant formula as first line treatment should be discouraged during the first six months of life". However, the BDA acknowledged that there was a clinical need for feeding soya based infant formulae in infants with cows' milk allergy/intolerance who refuse extensively hydrolysed/elemental formulas, vegan mothers and infants with Galactosaemia, as any potential risk as outlined above would be outweighed by the risk of withholding the formula.

Overall the caveats that early exposure to Soya based feeds constitute a long term reproductive or allergic risk to babies seems hypothetical and unproven. Yet again the choice comes down to the doctor's decision and "clinical need".

There are dozens of specialised milks available for different indications: Here is a selection:

Wysoy: Soya based, milk protein free, lactose, sucrose, gluten free too. Nutritionally complete.

Infasoy: Soya based: Lactose, gluten, sucrose and fructose free. Nutritionally complete.

Neocate: An elemental feed, (cow's intolerance etc, some use it in colic). Nutritionally complete.

Nutramigen, Lipil 1 and 2: (Pre and post 6months), Nutritionally complete elemental feeds.

Pregestimil Lipil: Lactose, sucrose, fructose and gluten free. Nutritionally complete.

SMA Staydown: Nutritionally complete, used in reflux.

Omneo comfort milk: Lowish lactose, supposed to help some cases of colic.

SMA LF: Lactose free, gluten free.

Aptamil Comfort: Used in colic, can constipate.

Oral rehydration Fluid: (Dioralyte, Electrolade etc):

In diarrhoea and vomiting, a rough initial guide: You can advise a heaped teaspoon of sugar and a pinch of salt in a standard glass of water as a guestimate to start off with and say: keep offering the child sips. For years doctors have suggested "flat coke". I am not sure why it has to be flat unless the bubbles may make nausea worse. It seems pretty unlikely though. At least one well known anti emetic was marketed for years as a sachet which, when added to water made a weakly effervescent solution (Stemetil) and Lucozade is extremely fizzy and fairly palatable when you are nauseated.

Out of interest, diet coke and diet fizzy drinks wouldn't work as well as the normal sugary drinks because the glucose/sucrose actively increases water absorption across gastric mucosa and is supposed to reduce nausea. But just look at how much sugar there is in these common fizzy drinks:

Coca Cola: 10.6Gr/100mls.

Sainsbury's Lemonade: 4.8Gr/100mls.

Lucozade: 8.72Gr/100mls,

Sainsbury's Taste the difference Spanish Grape and Elderflower Presse 8.36 Gr/100mls. But surprisingly: Pure red grape juice has 16.4Gr/100mls and

Freshly squeezed Orange juice has 9.6Gr/100mls (New Scientist Mar 2017)

This advice comes from various sources but basically you cannot over hydrate a sick child with isotonic fluid as long as they have normally functioning kidneys.

In most children with mild to moderate dehydration, give Oral Rehydration Solution 50-100ml/kg over 3-4 hrs in frequent small amounts, with extra (child <10kg) 60-120ml or (child >10kg) 120-240ml for each extra episode of sickness or diarrhoea.

In my experience few get clinically dehydrated if they continue to (try to) drink despite ongoing symptoms. 5% of the child's body weight lost through dehydration is a significant fluid loss but can sometimes only just be objectively detectable. 10% is a serious situation. For the average child at home with diarrhoea and vomiting: Give at least:

0-6m	150-200mls/kg/day
6-9m	120-150mls/kg/day
12m	90-100mls/kg/day
2yrs	80-90mls/kg/day.

In hospital replacement fluids are calculated thus: Estimated % dehydration X weight of child. (ie 10% X 10Kg = 1000mls deficit) this is extracellular fluid loss and replaced with N Saline IV.

"Maintenance fluids" are given as Dextrose 4%/Saline 0.18%, adding 20mmol K to each 500mls once urine has been passed.

The replacement fluids are usually given over 24 hours unless there is **hypernatraemia** in which case they are given slower, usually over 48 hours and only 3/5 of the first 24 hour's maintenance fluids given in the first day.

The signs of dehydration:

Features	Mild <5%	Moderate 5-10%	Severe>10%
Decreased skin turgor	–	+/–	+++
Tachycardia	–	+/–	+++
Decreased Urine output	+	++	+++
Dry mouth	+/– moist	++ dry	+++ very dry
Sunken eyes	– normal	++ sunken	+++ very sunken and dry
Level of consciousness	– well, alert	+/– restless, irritable	+++ lethargic, floppy, unconscious
Initial oral rehydration treatment	30-50mls/kg	50-100mls/kg	100-150mls/kg or fluid IV treatment over 3-4 hours.

Any child who is symptomatic and in the 10% group should be admitted, preferably with a drip running when the ambulance arrives. All GPs should have Saline or Dextrose/Saline and giving sets in their emergency bags.

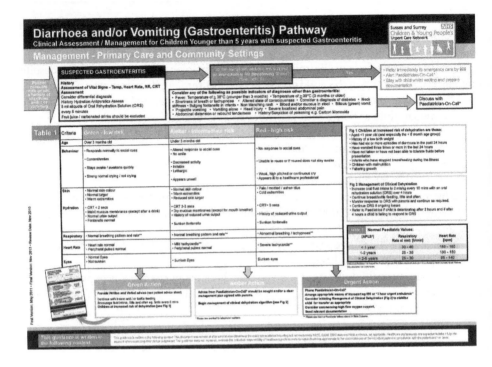

Diagram: WSx (Sussex) DVP Under 5 Diarrhoea-vomiting pathway

Constipation in children:

Lactulose, increase until at least one soft stool a day, or another stool softener,
Docusate paed soln. 12.5-25mg TDS,
plus or minus:
Movicol paediatric sachets from one to eight daily or:
Senna syrup 5-10mls nocte or:
Picolax sachets PRN.

Alternatively:
Lactulose a.m. and Laxoberal p.m.(Sodium picosulphate) or
Disimpaction with Movicol then Lactulose +/– Picolax 2 sachets (stimulant) PRN
or
Movicol 1-2 sachets each afternoon plus eg 6mls Sodium picosulphate soln. PRN for
a 5-6 year old if BNO daily.

Mesenteric Adenitis:

Painful swelling of the mesenteric lymph nodes, clumped around the appendix in the
RIF following gastro enteritis and a variety of systemic infections. The symptoms can
be present from a few days to a surprisingly long and worrying several weeks. Rotavirus,
Norovirus, Salmonella, Staph or Strep infections (Including Strep throats), Yersinia
Enterocolitica, actual appendicitis and rare causes include HIV, TB, lymphoma, Whipple's
Disease, Crohn's, U.C. etc.

The symptoms are a painful and tender R lower abdomen, fever, bloating etc. Obviously it can be a tricky problem differentiating this common (and sometimes recurrent) pain from appendicitis.

Generally in M.A. there is no convincing peritonism, rebound, guarding, or, as my friend and partner showed me, the hopping on the spot test for peritoneal irritation is negative (i.e. It is possible for the patient to hop or jump up and down on the spot 20-30 X in M.A. but very painful in appendicitis with peritonism – Paul Woods). The WBC goes up in M.A. and in appendicitis but sometimes the swollen glands can be seen on USS in the former.

Then of course there is the tricky **"Grumbling Appendix"** which I am convinced is a genuine condition with recurrent R.I.F. pain in a child without other associated symptoms or objective tests for peritonism or inflammation but resolves on removal of the appendix.

Appendicitis in children:

The patient may not be febrile but IS usually tachycardic. As mentioned elsewhere, nausea and vomiting may not necessarily be present and just because you saw them yesterday and they seemed to have gastro enteritis it doesn't mean the diagnosis hasn't changed overnight to an inflamed or burst appendix. I have seen this at least twice.

"Colitis" after Gastro enteritis:

Mesenteric adenitis is the swelling of the glands concentrated around the R.I.F. and which swell in a variety of child hood viral infections. These include gastroenteritis and several upper respiratory and throat infections.

Persisting bloating, loose stools and abdominal discomfort after a gastro-enteritic type infection are common symptoms and often labelled as paediatric post infectious IBS. If you do exclude persistent infection (i.e. Giardia etc) it may be due to Eosinophilic gastroenteropathy. You can try treating it with Nalcrom (Sodium Cromoglicate oral caps), Asacol, Ketotifen (Zaditen) 1mg nocte.

Iron Deficiency in children:

The vast majority are due to diet, but exclude external blood loss, reflux, Coeliac Disease (with folic acid deficiency), various drugs – antacids, tetracyclines, don't forget rare things like haemoglobinopathies, NSAIDs, GI bleeding etc.

Rx Iron eg: Sytron Sodium Feredetate.
Up to 1 yr 2.5ml BD,
1-5yrs 2.5mls TDS,
6-12yrs 5mls TDS,
Adults 5-10mls TDS.

Migraine in children

Is common, there is a family history (ask which parent had bad headaches/abdominal pain as a child?) and the migraine can present confusingly with a periodic syndrome of vomiting and or abdominal pain rather than headache. You must do proper initial and periodic examinations to exclude SOL and other causes of headache and if there isn't a fairly standard clinical picture, consider imaging/referral.

Prophylaxis with Pizotifen (Sanomigran) usually works and the acute attack can be treated with nasal Sumatriptan (Imigran).

Hip conditions:

"Usual" ages at presentation:

CDH: 0-5 years,
Perthe's: 5-10 yrs,
SUFE: 10-15 yrs.

Irritable Hip:

Transient Synovitis/"Observation Hip".
Differential Diagnosis:
Hip sepsis if 2 or more of: Severe spasm, Tenderness, T >38degrees, ESR>20.

Congenital Dislocation of the Hip, C.D.H., Developmental Dysplasia of the Hip, DDH:

A breech delivery increases the incidence 3X, female sex 6-7X, there are twice as many unilateral CDH as bilateral and it is 1.5X more common in the winter than summer. The left hip is affected more often than the right, it is commoner in first born, after a caesarean section, with oligohydramnios and with a positive family history.

Dislocatable hips are much more common, temporarily unstable hips: 1:67 newborn have dislocatable hips. Clicky but stable hips are very common and can be ignored. 1:333 at 3 days. 1.5: 1000 at 3 weeks (True CDH).

If a parent had CDH the risk goes up to 6% in the first child. If that parent had a first child with CDH then the next baby has a 36% risk. The first born overall has a greater risk (? due to an unstretched uterus?) – likewise if there is little amniotic fluid. The dislocation is always posterior at birth.

To investigate, do an USS up to 6m, an XR after. This is of course because the ossification of the femur is present in 90% between 20 and 24 weeks. Most sources say it is present at "4-6 months". Interestingly, a delay in ossification here may be associated with the later development of Perthe's Disease.

Reduced abduction is probably the most subtle but consistent hands-on test and certainly more reliable than Ortolani's or Barlows after 6 weeks. Skin creases are only helpful in high dislocations. The other signs include thigh asymmetry, buttock wasting, limb shortening, odd leg posture and the much more useful limited abduction.

Barlow's and Ortholani's tests are said to have a sensitivity of 66%.

Ortolani's test: Abduction produces the feeling of a mobile clunk in the head of the joint, not just a click which is very common. Occasionally after anterior dislocation, the head will return to the joint on return adduction of the thigh. The movement is one of gentle abduction of the femur while gently pushing the proximal femur anteriorly out of the acetabulum.

Barlow's: Distracting the femoral head in and out of the joint by forwards/backwards movement of the femoral head. Again the movement is felt as a sudden "give" or just the feeling of a floppy, mobile joint. You can stabilise the pelvis by holding the symphysis and sacrum down against the blanket in your other hand while the "leg hand" is telescoping the femur of the examined side.

The most difficult joint to detect is the fixed dislocated joint which if asymmetrical will show asymmetrical creases and limited abduction on the affected side. If bilateral however, there is bilateral limited abduction and you will need a low threshold for USS because there are no other signs.

I find a different technique helpful in C.D.H: This is to gently grasp each thigh between your 2nd and 3rd fingers, curling the second finger over the top of the thigh so that you can push it up and down in a piston movement. Each thumb now curls around the flexed tibia. Then you gently push each side up and down alternately as if there were an invisible see saw between your hands. If the hips are both normal the movement is smooth and symmetrical as the pelvis rocks from side to side. If either or both sides are dislocated then you feel and see a ratchet or cogwheel movement on the affected side.

In early stages the treatment is a Pavlik harness. Later presentation may require a reduction under GA and a spica or surgical reduction, even osteotomy.

Septic Hip: Differentiating it from Transient Synovitis:

Kocher Criteria:

T >38.5C

Cannot Wt bear on affected side,

ESR>40,

WBC>12,000,

Probability:

No factors	<0.2%,
1	3%,
2	40%,
3	up to 93%,
4	59-99+% (depending on source).

Causes of Limp: (Antalgic gait):

Children only develop a "Mature rhythmic gait cycle" after age 7. Two thirds of limping children CAN be managed without referral but if in doubt, bloods, an X Ray or even other forms of imaging etc may be needed.

Causes of Limp By Age:

Up to 3 yrs:

Septic arthritis/osteomyelitis,

Developmental hip dysplasia,

NAI/#,

Transient Synovitis IS RARE at this age.

3-10yrs:

Transient Synovitis (Irritable hip),

Septic Arthritis/osteomyelitis,

Perthe's Disease, typically boys, short hyperactive aged 4-8. May need an MRI or Technetium scan.

or soft tissue injury,

10-15 yrs;

SUFE – younger if obese or sporty. Also called "Slipped Capital Femoral Epiphysis". Ask for a LATERAL X Ray as well as PA, the sufferer tends to be overweight.

Pain can be referred to the tibia. Short, externally rotated leg.

Septic arthritis/osteomyelitis,

Perthe's Disease,

or soft tissue injury.

Other diagnoses: Haematological disorders: Sickle Cell, myositis (including pyomyositis), Rickets, Leukaemia, CP, Muscular Dystrophy, Inflammatory Arthritis etc. These latter diagnoses are rare however, the commonest causes of a child's acute limp being

"Irritable Hip" or Transient Synovitis. "No diagnosis" is the second commonest major group in most studies – so presumably some of these are minor injuries, strains or "post viral synovitis".

Toddler's fracture is a spiral fracture of the tibia which follows trauma and often does not appear on initial X rays. The tibia is usually tender to examination.

Septic arthritis of the hip usually harbours Staph Aureus, occasionally BHS in small babies.

Always examine the spine, hips, knees, ankles, feet, abdomen and check the lower limb neurology as well as external genitals in boys where testicular pain can cause limping.

The **"pGALS"** examination is "paediatric gait arms legs and spine" and involves:

Asking if the child has any pain or stiffness, observing the child walking – on toes and heels, (examining the arms) checking the knees, active and passive, ROMs, effusion etc, hip flexion/rotation/ROM and neurology etc of the leg etc.

Hip examination: Check internal rotation and abduction, the two most sensitive signs of hip pathology.

So: Brief Causes of Limp:

Transient Synovitis: 40% – 90% of irritable hips occur 2 weeks after a URTI and "irritable hip" is the most common cause of a painful limp in children between 2 and 11 years. Most are resolved within 1 week.

Septic arthritis: The child is obviously sick, there is an obvious pyrexia. Up to 6m age Staph Aureus is the usual organism, from then to 5 years it and Haemophilus Influenzae are the common infections.

Haemophilus Immunisation has reduced the incidence.

Trauma: 16%

No Diagnosis: 30%

Perthe's Disease: 2%. 1: 12,000 children. Legg, Calve and Perthes all described the condition at the same time in 1910. It is idiopathic avascular necrosis of the femoral head possibly due to a clotting abnormality. Risk factors: 80% are boys, low birth weight, lower social class, late ossification and passive smoking. It usually presents at 4-10 years with a gradual onset of pain and intermittent limping. The children are often short, with a retarded bone age. It is bilateral in 15%. If so, think of Gaucher's Disease, myxoedema, epiphyseal dysplasia. Presentation after 10 years of age carries a poor prognosis for hip remodelling and recovery. The treatment is an abduction cast and this may need to continue for 18 months. Surgery to the hip gets the patient on their feet quickly but may result in an imperfect femoral head.

Toddler #: 1%.

SUFE: 1% Plump teenagers, a quarter follow a traumatic occurrence of some kind. The epiphysis appears to slide off the back of the femur. 4M:1F. Can be associated with Marfan's, myxoedema, GH therapy, renal disease, Down's syndrome, obesity etc. Pain may develop gradually before becoming severe. The affected leg may be shorter with "out toeing". Investigations: Must do PA and lateral X Rays. The treatment is to fix the epiphysis in position with a screw. Some studies show that half the patients will slip on the opposite side.

Stills Disease:

(Juvenile Idiopathic Arthritis, Juvenile Rheumatoid arthritis – despite some cases having a neg. RhF). Affects about 1:1000 children, usually from about 6 or 7 years to the mid teens.

The condition can present with a systemic fluey illness with swollen joints, large and small as well as spinal joints may be affected.

Extra articular manifestations include anterior uveitis, (various long term complications), growth retardation, osteoporosis and of course, joint damage and deformity.

There is a genetic predisposition, it has a female predominance and is autoimmune.

There are various ways of classifying Stills Disease: Oligoarticular, polyarticular and systemic. OR mine (which may be slightly old fashioned):

	Polyartic, Rh −	Polyart Rh+	Pauciartic 1	Pauciartic 2	Systemic
% JRA	30	10	25	15	20
Sex	90%F	80%F	80%F	90%M	60%M
Age	Throughout CH	Late CH	Early CH	Late CH	Throughout CH
Joints	Any	Any	Large joints Knee ankle elbow	Large joints Hip girdle	Any
Sacroileitis	No	Rare	No	Common	No
Iridocyclitis	Rare	No	50% chronic	10-20% acute	No
RhF	Neg	100%	Neg	Neg	Neg
ANA	25%	75%	60%	Neg	Neg
HLAB27	N/A	N/A	N/A	75%	N/A
Ultimate morbidity:	Severe arthritis 10-15%	Severe arthritis >50%	Ocular damage 10-20%	Subsequent spondylo − arthropathy ?%	Severe arthritis 25%

Treatments include NSAIDs, steroids, systemic and injections, Methotrexate, Etanercept, etc.

The prognosis is highly variable, some patients, perhaps half, developing fairy rapid joint destruction or spondylosis. Other complications, eye disease, amyloid, growth retardation etc may be significant and there are various other complications including some of the treatment such as gut bleeding and osteoporosis.

Children's Feet:

Sever's Disease: Calcaneal Apophysitis:

Age 9-11, due to recurrent impact on the growing heel, boys particularly. The pain is posterior/plantar over the apophysis of the calcaneum. There is a painful squeeze test, no outward signs, and the XR is usually normal. It is worse in over pronaters, commonly bilateral and responds to heel elevation, (ie with a gel heel pad), hamstring and calf stretching exercises, physio, rest.

Freiberg's Disease:

Pain in the 2nd metatarsal head due to epiphysitis, then avascular necrosis followed by damage to the articular surface. This occurs at puberty mainly in girls and the initial treatment is rest, orthoses, sometimes immobilisation, even surgery in extreme cases.

Growing pains: Benign idiopathic nocturnal limb pains of childhood:

The literature describes these as benign pains, poorly localised in the lower limbs, mainly below the knees but in my personal experience they are often in the femurs as well-particularly after a strenuous and busy day. Although this is not always accepted by the text books, I have followed up many of the worst sufferers on my list for decades and they do seem to grow to be pretty tall adults. Rubbing the affected area and paracetamol/ibuprofen relieve the pain. Sometimes it is necessary to give analgesia prophylactically as the pains follow sport and activity. It is important to play the pain down as much as possible talking to the child. The pains are distressing and tend to wake the child (and parents) at night.

Given that a multiplicity of serious conditions could cause limb pain, the basic rules for "growing pains" are that

The child is well, between 3 and 12 years,

There are no significant daytime symptoms,

Sport, play and school performance are normal and unchanged,

The pain is in the lower limbs,

There is no limping,

The pains are not asymmetrical and not limited to joints,

They are not present at the start of the day,

The physical examination (apart from hypermobility) is normal,

-with normal growth-milestones, height and weight.

The child is systemically well otherwise.

Red Flags include:

Fever,

Weight loss,

Anorexia,

Raised inflammatory markers,

Developmental delay or regression,

Impaired function,

Limping,

Morning symptoms,

Upper limb or other pain,

Missing school.

Asymmetry (unilateral limb pain is not a feature of growing pains).

More significant causes of bone pain include:

Bone infection,

NAI/Injury,

Congenital disorders eg hip dysplasia/hip disorders (Perthes/SUFE etc).

CP (Neurological causes) *,

Still's/transient arthritis (regression, stiffness, gelling, difficulty with chairs and stairs),

Inflammatory muscle disease* *ask the child to jump (tends to exclude a proximal muscle weakness),

Leukaemia/Neuroblastoma/malignancy/bone tumour,

Tarsal coalition (congenital fusion of two of the posterior foot bones),

Osteochondritis dissecans.

Other causes include:

Anaemia,

Thyroid disease (especially myxoedema),

Post viral syndromes,

Osteomalacia (ethnic group),

Inflammatory muscle disease,

Still's Disease,

Idiopathic pain syndromes (this can be considered the young person's equivalent of fibromyalgia),

A reasonable GP screen would include FBC, ESR, CRP, CPK, U and Es, Ca++, PO4, LFTs – Alk P'ase, etc TFTs, Vit D, possibly specific (?hip, frog views) X Rays.

Affected children often have flat feet and hypermobility. It may take a few years in some but they do all grow out of growing pains.

Pulled Elbow:

Reduce by pushing and pronating. There is usually a palpable click, a good history and very little force is needed.

Some Paediatric Urology:

Undescended testicles:

Refer 12-18 months. Operate 3-4 years.

Urinary Infections:

10% of girls and 3% boys will have had a UTI by the age of 16. The commonest age is the first year of life. Far more will have bacteriuria (and presumably clear the bacteria spontaneously without help). Infections can lead to renal scarring and can follow on from underlying renal damage so it is important to detect urinary infection, treat it effectively, follow the patient up and exclude damage. A UTI is "bacteriuria in the presence of symptoms" but given the frequency of asymptomatic bacteriuria and the frequency of febrile illness with rigors and so on, it is possible to over diagnose UTI. Better to over than under diagnose however. The strong association between vesico-ureteric REFLUX and post infectious scarring is called reflux nephropathy. Up to 25% of childhood renal failure is due to the combination and if you can detect and treat infections even in the presence of reflux you can prevent damage occurring. Most studies suggest that if the kidneys have not scarred after the first infection then they are not going to.

Remember that babies with urinary infection present with fever, vomiting, lethargy and non specific symptoms. They may not be feeding well, have prolonged jaundice or occasionally if you are lucky they might have more specific symptoms and signs of smelly or bloody urine or dysfunctional voiding (constant dribbling or crying on voiding or holding on to urine etc). Always try to get a urine specimen from a febrile child – unless there is another barn door cause for their temperature or malaise. Just like in the elderly, it is the common deceiver.

Every suspected UTI needs confirmation by an MSU and every unwell child without an obvious diagnosis needs to have UTI excluded with an MSU after 24 hours. **I repeat: Any child with a fever over 24 hours and no good reason for it should have an MSU sent off.** This CAN be done at any age with a willing parent and a clean catch technique. Theoretically.

The general advice (NICE) seems to be to admit children under 3m with a UTI. This depends on the UTI. I have found paediatric staff less than helpful in this and if the parents are trust worthy, the patient well and the antibiotic bacteriocidal and well tolerated, I am not sure that admission into the crowded, septic, noisy, risk filled hospital environment is always justified. Indeed I have never admitted a well child at any age with a UTI and in 40 years no patient in my care with a standard lower urinary infection has suffered adversely because of treatment at home. I do prescribe Co Amoxiclav or Cephalosporins first line, I am personally accessible and get sensitivities as soon as I can and work in a practice with good cover and communication at all times and stable partners.

Strep Faecalis and E.Coli are the common pathogens. Other organisms may point to an abnormal urinary tract.

NICE says:

The risk factors for UTI or serious pathology include:
Poor urine flow,
Previous UTI,
Recurrent PUO,
Antenatally diagnosed renal abnormality,
FH of VU reflux or renal disease,
Constipation,
Dysfunctional voiding,
Enlarged bladder,
Abdominal mass,
Spinal lesion,
Poor growth,
Raised BP.
See below for NICE management of UTI.
Don't give routine prophylaxis after the first UTI.

Urine Testing:

<3m Refer to the Paediatricians. Urgent Urine M C and S.

3m-3yr Urgent Urine M, C and S, specific urinary symptoms: Start antibiotics
and if at high risk refer to Paediatricians.
If at intermediate risk, consider urgent referral but do MSU,
and start antibiotics if MSU pos. or if Nitrite positive.
If at low risk send MSU and start treatment if positive.

What to do before you get the definitive microscopy:

Preliminary microscopy:		Pyuria pos	Pyuria neg
	Bacteriuria pos	UTI	UTI
	Bacteriuria neg	**Start Rx if clinically a UTI**	Not a UTI

>3 yrs: Dipstick leuks and Nit pos: Start antibiotics. If high risk send off sample.-(I would ALWAYS send off a sample especially if you are using one of the* less reliable but cheaper antibiotics encouraged by prescribing committees and bacteriology departments and which are so hit and miss in serious UTIs.)

Leuks neg, Nit pos: Start antibiotics if it was a fresh sample and send sample for culture.

Leuks pos, Nit neg- this result is less reliable than the other way round. Send off sample and only treat if UTI suspected, look for infection elsewhere.

Leuks neg, Nit neg: Don't treat for UTI:NICE Say don't send sample but if the child is unwell, you should be looking for a site of infection and sending a urine sample is essential. These tests are not infallible.

NICE give a list of **Indications for urine spec:**
Diagnosis of upper UTI,
High to intermediate risk of serious illness,
Under 3 years,
A single pos Leuks or Nit on dipstix.
Recurrent UTI,
Infection that does not respond to treatment within 24-48 hours,
Clinical symptoms and dipstick test do not correlate.

I can only say that NICE must have had more accountants on their committee than Paediatricians and GPs on this occasion and certainly very few parents of very small children.

1) NICE Differentiates between an upper and lower UTI quoting symptoms, systemic features, fever, tenderness, loin pain etc. They suggest an USS or DMSA scan to differentiate the two. These two are not available to many GPs. The difference clinically between an upper and a lower UTI in general practice is academic, often clinically indeterminate and not big enough to slip an FP10 in between. Babies and toddlers do not have loin pain, good localising signs or reliable upper tract tenderness. The temperature can be in the higher or lower range whichever part of the urinary tract is infected. 2) What is an intermediate risk? Babies and toddlers with significant urinary tract infections can get systemically unwell and toxic in hours and collapse very quickly so a small baby/toddler/child with a real UTI is at intermediate risk by definition. 3) I can assure the NICE committee that virtually all clean catch specimens on febrile and unwell toddlers are positive for leukocytes whatever is wrong with them. 4) The cheap antibiotics like Amoxicillin and the bacteriostatic antibiotics like Trimethoprim will either not have worked in 24-48 hours or there will as-like-as-not be bacterial resistance to them so they won't work in the quoted time scale. – So proper bacteriology **will** be needed at some time.

So I suggest that if you are at all concerned about the baby/toddler/child's welfare, always send off a sample for microscopy and culture before the first dose of antibiotic (show the mum how a clean catch can be done) and 2) Give a decent dose of a reliable antibiotic from the start.

Acute management (NICE again)

High risk: Urgent referral to Paediatrician

<3m Refer to Paediatrician for IV antibiotics although most of us would dispute the need for this in a well child with good parents, an actively involved lab and a decent antibiotic based on the bacteriology.

>3m with upper UTI: "Consider referral" but give oral Rx 7-10 days "Low resistance antibiotic" or IV antibiotics (Co Amoxiclav or a later generation Cefalosporin). Sometimes start with IV antibiotics but go on for 10 days.

>3m with lower UTI: Oral antibiotics for 3 days, not low resistance antibiotics unless the infection is "complicated". In other words, the usual cheap and cheerful 3 days of Trimethoprim, Nitrofurantoin, Amoxicillin or Cefalosporin. if still unwell after 24-48 hours reassess and send sample for culture- **none of which makes any sense** given the rate of bacterial resistance to common antibiotics, the frequency of structural urinary abnormalities

in UTI (approx 20%), the speed with which small children can "go off" when septic and the caveats outlined above. So send a sample, give a good dose of a decent antibiotic and if the sample is positive get a urinary USS.

Preventing recurrence is helped by treating constipation, not delaying voiding and by encouraging drinking water, not juices (see "Toddler diarrhoea").

NICE Investigations in Paediatric UTI:

Atypical UTI means seriously ill, poor urine flow, abdominal mass, raised creatinine, septicaemia, **failure to respond within 48 hours**, atypical, non E Coli organism, OR recurrent UTI (3 lower UTIs, 2 upper UTIs or 1 upper and 1 lower UTI).

Under 6 months:

	Responds in <48 Hrs	Atypical UTI	Recurrent UTI
USS during acute infection	No	Yes	Yes
USS in 6 weeks	Yes	No	No
DMSA 4-6m after the acute infection	No	Yes	Yes
MCUG	No	Yes	Yes

6 months to 3 years:

	Responds in <48 Hrs	Atypical UTI	Recurrent UTI
USS in acute infection	No	Yes	No
USS within 6 weeks	No	No	Yes
DMSA 4-6m after the acute infection	No	Yes	Yes
MCUG	No	No	No

Over 3 years:

	Responds in <48 Hrs	Atypical UTI	Recurrent UTI
USS during the acute infection	No	Yes	No
USS within 6 weeks	No	No	Yes
DMSA 4-6m after the acute infection	No	No	Yes
MCUG	No	No	No

Investigations of the Urogenital Tract:

DMSA Dimercaptosuccinic Acid Isotope scan: Parenchymal abnormalities in cortices – for scarring. A functional cortical map.

DTPA Diethylene Triamine Pentaacetic Acid: "A glomerular substance giving an excretion picture"

MAG III Isotope Renogram: A dynamic scan, tells about urinary flow out of the kidney and to bladder.

USS: Assesses renal pelvic dilatation, – only 1cm limit being the threshold for investigation in infancy.

Note: Age 4 is the most vulnerable age for infection scarring (excluded by DMSA)

So: A suggested regime of investigations/Management would be:

<1year with UTI,	Micturating Cystogram + USS
1-4 years	Micturating Cystogram or prophylactic antibiotics until out of nappies
>4 years	MAG 111 cystography for vesico-ureteric reflux.

One Suggested Regime of Investigation of UTI in children:

v

Antibiotics (Oral or IV ?5-10 days)

v

Age 0-1yrs prophylaxis	Age 1-4yrs Prophylaxis	Age>4 yrs no prophylaxis?
v	v	v
Renal U/S		
MCU + Abs?	Renal U/S +/- DMSA*	Renal U/S.* DMSA if
DMSA at 9m*	MCU if: Abn DMSA, sympts	recurrent UTI or abn U/S
	of PN, F/H of VUR, RN	? MCU If Abn DMSA
	or recurrent UTIs	
	v	v
	If all normal stop	>If abnormal: Prophylaxis
	prophylaxis	and regular follow up

Note: PN pyelonephritis, VUR vesico ureteric reflux, RN reflux nephropathy.

* Delay DMSA scan until 3m after the infection. Scans should be requested in the order above (unless clinically indicated)

This is somewhat out of date but a little less confusing perhaps than the new NICE protocol.

My approach, which has picked up two children with renal failure, one with hypertension and numerous (approximately 1/5 of those <5 years with UTIs) children with reflux over my 40 years is to send off an MSU on suspicion of a UTI (each occasion), to do an USS after the first proven UTI (I do not differentiate between upper and lower UTI) and to share the follow up of a child with an abnormal urinary tract with a Paediatrician. The DMSA is to assess cortical function in significant reflux and if abnormal they need close follow up, the MCU to assess the severity of functional reflux. If the USS is normal, the child is well and the follow up MSU is negative, I have a low threshold for further urine tests but leave it to the (educated) parents to re-consult.

OR put **very simply:**

infants under 6m USS followed by MCUG in some cases

Atypical infection: USS and DMSA +/– MCUG. Unless >3 yrs in which case just initial USS

Recurrent infections: USS and DMSA at all ages.

Dipstix are reliable over the age of 3 but only if both the Leuks and Nit agree pos or neg.

Non accidental Injury:

The U.K. has the second lowest level in Europe believe it or not. Only in Denmark do they hurt they children less. There are however still 50-70 children killed per year by their carers in the UK.

Convulsions:

Lennox-Gastaut syndrome:

Usual onset age 2-6 with frequently difficult to treat and varying types of seizures. It is often associated with developmental delay, cognitive deficiency, emotional and behavioural problems. Tonic and myoclonic seizures are the commonest, usually at night. A variety of other types of seizure from absences to complex partial, non convulsing status epilepticus, drop attacks with associated injury etc.

The EEG shows slow spike waves between fits. 20% of patients progress from West syndrome* and in most there is an underlying brain pathology, TS, inherited metabolic disorder, previous encephalitis or meningitis, birth hypoxia etc. Only a third are idiopathic with preceding normal development and no structural or historical known cause.

West Syndrome*: Infantile spasms.

1:3,000 children. Presenting around 6 months (Usually 3-12m) A sudden tonic flexion sometimes with a cry, arms sometimes extended, usually symmetrically, usually each "spasm" lasts a couple of seconds and they occur in runs. Also called "jack-knife convulsions" or "Salaam Spasms". Other characteristic convulsions include "lightning" myoclonic convulsions and flexion of the neck, "nodding attacks".

The disorganised EEG is called "Hypsarrythmia". There is an underlying brain pathology in the majority of patients and most have cognitive abnormalities too. It is present in up to 5% Down's Syndrome children. The treatment consists of steroids and anticonvulsants. Half go on to develop Lennox-Gestaut epilepsy.

There is a 5% mortality and a high morbidity (CP, cognitive and learning disability etc) and the prognosis depends on the underling brain disorder.

Paediatric Mistakes:

Missed Diagnoses:
Some of the commonest that lead to litigation are:
Diabetes,
Appendicitis,
Testicular torsion,
Pneumonia/septicaemia,
Slipped upper femoral epiphysis,
and Meningitis.

Paediatric Gynaecology:

The Thelarche (beginning of breast development) and Pubarche (appearance of pubic hair) are usually 1 year before menarche and before 13 yrs.

The mean age for the menarche is 13 years.

In the first 2 years following the Menarche anovulation and cycle irregularity are common.

3 yrs post Menarche 60% cycles are anovulatory and most are 21-34 days.

Just Google **Tanner Stages** if you want to see the normal stages of male and female genital development as well as breast development in girls. (and see below pp961-962)

Diagram

Fused labia: occur in 2-4% of girls and are self limiting. Any condition which predisposes to local inflammation (diarrhoea, trauma, nappy rash, vulvovaginitis) may predispose the child to labial adhesions. These may need surgical division in which case Vaseline may help them stop sticking back again.

Vulvovaginitis: BHS, Haemophilus Infl., threadworms, "non specific vaginitis". Always worth taking a swab, treating with topical anti fungal cream and oral anti helminthic medication.

Blood stained vaginal discharge: Trauma (sexual abuse), foreign body, urethral prolapse, congenital abnormalities of the Mullerian or urinary system, rarely tumours.

Dysmenorrhoea in teenagers: Up to 1/3 of adolescents with pelvic pain may have endometriosis.

COCP Is 90% effective,

NSAIDS 75% effective,

but bizarrely:

Thiamine 100mg/day for 3months can help as can:

Vitamin E 100mg/day for 20 days before each period.

Amenorrhoea:

The four commonest conditions are:

PCOS,

Hypothalamic Amenorrhoea,

Hyperprolactinaemia,

Ovarian Failure.

If the patient has secondary sexual characteristics, refer for an opinion and investigations at age 16. If they have no secondary sexual characteristics, refer earlier at 14 years.

Secondary amenorrhoea is defined as 3 months without periods after previously normal cycles-or nine months amenorrhoea in a background of oligomenorrhoea.

Polycystic ovaries are "Normal" in adolescence and incidence is 40%, 35%, and 33%, 2, 3 and 4 years after the menarche. – 12 or more follicles 2-9mm diameter.

Investigations in Amenorrhoea:

Pregnancy test, LH/FSH, TA U/S (Abdominal USS), Prolactin, TSH/Free T4 Oestradiol, U and Es, SHBG, Androstenedione/testosterone, Karyotype,

Secondary Amenorrhoea:

Uterine (Asherman's syndrome, Cervical stenosis).

Ovarian (PCOS, premature ovarian failure, -genetic, autoimmune, post chemo or radiotherapy, infection etc).

Hypothalamic (weight loss, exercise, chronic illness, stress, idiopathic),

Pituitary (hyperprolactinaemia, hypopituitrism, Sheehan's),

Hypothalamic/pituitary (tumours, irradiation, injuries, sarcoid, TB),

Systemic (chronic illness, Cushing's, thyroid disease etc).

Tanner stages of development:

Boys

Boys: Androgens are manufactured by the adrenals before they come from the testicles (so pubic hair and smelly axillae may precede testicular growth)

Tanner stages are subdivided by reference to various changing parameters:

Stage	Genitals	Testicle Length	Pubic Hair	Annual height velocity	Other
I	Infrequent erections prepubertal	<1.6 cm	Villous hair	5-6 cm	Adrenarche,
II	Skin of scrotum thins and reddens frequent erections	2.5-3.2 cm	Sparse, slightly pigmented (average 12 1/2 yrs)	7-8 cm	Leaner body
III	Lengthening of penis	3.3-4.0 cm	Coarser, darker, curly, (average 14 yrs)	8 cm	Temporary breast swelling, voice breaks
IV	Increased size with growth in breadth of penis and development of glans.	4.1-4.5 cm	Adult in type, limited to pubic area. Average age 15 yrs	10 cm	Testes and scrotum larger, scrotum skin darker
V	Adult genitals	4.5 cm	Adult type, spreading to inner thigh. Average 15 1/2 yrs	Full height 18/19 yrs	Beard, continuing muscle development.

Girls:

Stage			
I	Prepubertal	Velus hair (like abdominal wall)	5-6cm/yr
II	Breast bud stage with elevation of breast and papilla, enlargement of areola.	Sparse slightly pigmented hair along labia	7-8cm/yr
III	Further enlargement of breast and areola, no contour separation	Darker, coarser, curlier hair spreading sparsely over junction of pubes	8cm/yr
IV	Areola and papilla form a secondary mound above level of breast	Hair adult in type, smaller area than in adult, not on inner thighs.	7cm/yr
V	Mature stage: projection of papilla, recession of areola.	Hair adult in type, quantity, feminine horizontal distribution.	Stops at 16 yrs

Tanner stages for breast and external genital development (Thanks to Wikipedia)

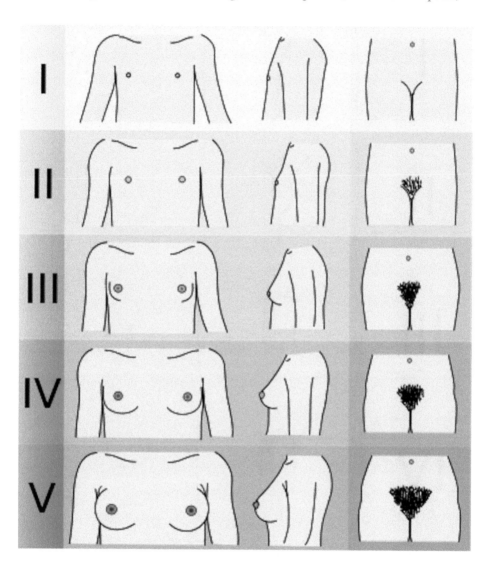

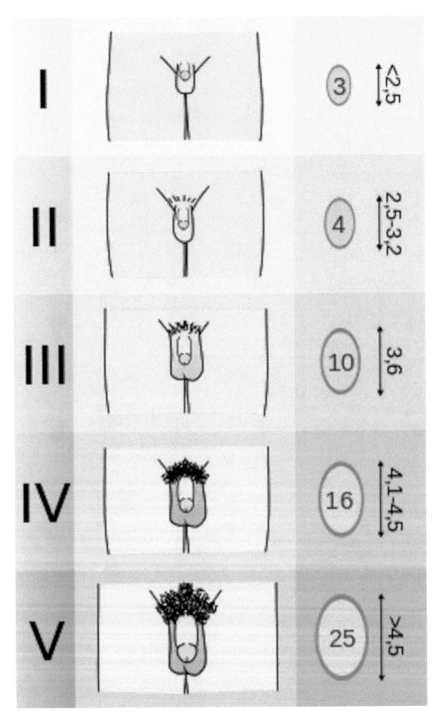

Growth Charts:

These are readily available on line now. The "Red book" actually contains a personal chart that goes up to 20 years for weight and height and 2 years for head circumference. Most parents will hang on to these for years out of shear nostalgia and you can see if the child has lost (or gained) significant amounts of weight over the years to assess investigations.
http://www.rcpch.ac.uk/growthcharts
or in America:
The American "Centers" for Disease Control and Prevention website suggests CDC or WHO charts and provides themwww.cdc.gov/growthcharts
or
Height Weight Charts for your Kids – About.com Pediatrics. As always, the American sites are easier to use and certainly more public friendly.

Testicular pain: The acute scrotum.

The child (or adolescent) with a testicular torsion looks and feels unwell, certainly once he has had it more than an hour or so, with nausea and or vomiting, won't want you to touch the affected testicle which you will have to insist on examining and all of which will be exquisitely tender. There is a number of less serious alternative diagnoses though.

The remnants of the Mullerian Duct – the appendix testis and of the Wolffian Duct and the appendix epididymis can both get twisted and cause acute testicular pain.

The appendix testis is present in over 90% testes (at the superior pole). The appendix epididymis is present in about a quarter of testes usually at the head of the epididymis but its position does vary. Acute testicular pain may be due to epididymitis, but most commonly it is due to torsion of one of the appendices. Up to 3/4 of acute scrotal pain may be due to twisted appendices – which are basically benign situations, the peak age being about 10-11 years and the history being slightly different to the much more serious testicular torsion.

A testicular torsion tends to be of quicker onset than a twisted appendage, the pain can be anything from mild to severe in a twisted appendage and the pain tends to be at a testicular upper pole. With testicular torsion the whole testicle is diffusely painful.

With the appendage there are not usually the systemic symptoms of vomiting and nausea which are seen in testicular torsion.

There are no urinary symptoms – these, dysuria, frequency etc are more common in epididymitis than with any of the torsions.

On examination the cremasteric reflex may be intact in appendix torsion – which is rare in testicular torsion. There is no diffuse general testicular tenderness (**characteristic of whole testicle torsion**). Any tenderness is localised and is usually at the upper pole where there may be para-testicular nodule and a blue dot sign – also the vertical orientation of the testicle is preserved in appendicular torsion.

Taking Blood and Practical Procedures:

The Update Cochrane Review on reducing the distress of blood taking, immunisation and sharps related procedures (39 trials, 3,400 participants) became available in 2014. It showed no evidence for preparation and information, combined CBT, parent coaching, plus distraction, suggestion or virtual reality. The old stand bys of distraction and hypnosis were supported and I would add, topical analgesia, firm and confident, decisive handling of the child and proper assessment of whether the parent is going to assist or obstruct the procedure by their presence. Also, if available, a mature, no nonsense, uniformed assistant.

Fits Faints etc

In paediatric referral clinics for "syncope" (fits, faints, funny turns, falls), rough out comes might be:

15% of children present with one syncopal event before the age of 19.

A quarter of children at syncope clinics have genuine epilepsy (average age at onset 5 yrs).

"Syncope" as defined by a sudden drop in cerebral blood flow or oxygenation, which is often associated with a "reflex anoxic seizure" make up around 40-45% (median age 9 yrs).

In these cases there are often clues in the history (which is otherwise confusing as the "faint" leads to a "fit"). For instance, there may be a trigger such as injury, pain, thwarting, sudden getting up out of bed, often in children there may have been some sort of activity, – sometimes even "hair care" surprisingly!, or even standing still for a while, an unexpected shock, surprise, exercise, shocking words or ideas, seeing blood etc.

In "Syncope" (faints) there may be an aura, light headedness, visual disturbance, feeling hot, sweaty, nauseated, flushed and half of children who faint go on to have a "reflex anoxic seizure" which is usually benign. Non epileptic syncope can often be interrupted by a bystander and the EEG is normal.

The recovery symptoms are pretty unhelpful in differentiating – just as you may get an aura with the prodrome in epilepsy, hypotension and migraine, children after syncopal episodes not primarily caused by epilepsy may recover immediately or have headache, confusion, drowsiness lasting from minutes to hours. Not very helpful.

About a tenth are "psychological", girls more than boys with a median presenting age of 12.

Other causes in this age group include non epileptic pseudo seizures, day dreams, night terrors, migraine, BPPV, ritualistic movements and parental anxiety.

"Unclassified" make up 15% or thereabouts

Making an early diagnosis and starting antiepileptic treatment early does not beneficially affect the outcome.

Long QT:

The majority of paediatric syncopal cases are benign but warning signs are: syncope related to a loud noise or shock (then check the QT – in fact the ECG is the essential investigation in paediatric loss of consciousness or suspected fits – long QT being a relatively frequent cause), to exercise (check the valves), on lying (? arrythmia) and syncope with tonic/clonic movements or a family history of sudden death. Long QT is associated with ventricular arrhythmias, contact with cold water, a positive family history, exercise related deaths, palpitations and can be treated with Beta Blockers, an indwelling defibrillator, cervical sympathectomy and the avoidance of the huge number of medicines that affect the QT interval (See cardiology). The ULN QTc is 450mSec.

A third of sudden unexpected deaths in childhood are due to myocarditis.

Safeguarding:

Learning about, recognising and protecting children from injury is a regular requirement of appraisals and training and an important part of GP life. In my professional life as a paediatrician and GP over 40 years I never saw a child killed by a parent but completely missed a deliberately fractured skull in a 9 month old whose father reported falling forwards onto her while carrying her on the stairs. I believed him completely. He was arrested and subsequently and imprisoned and on his released admitted to me he had caused the injury while "at the end of his tether". He apologised for lying to me.

This was the only serious injury I have seen in 40 years of practice. Some of which was city centre based, in an area of high unemployment and social deprivation.

I also had a patient who was an 11 year old who had been made pregnant by her brother. Both were educationally challenged, their mother had four children by four men, none in evidence at home at any time that I could see, and the family was resentful and angry (and still were ten years later) that I saw fit to involve external agencies, the social services and the police, in their internal affairs.

The pregnancy spontaneously aborted thankfully.

The facts are that 1:4 adults report having been abused as children
1-2 children die each week from abuse or neglect.

1:20 children in the UK are said to have been sexually abused and the average time to disclosure is 3-5 years. 1:3 never disclose what had happened.

90% of abusers are known to them and 40% rape cases are under age 16 years.

Deaths from maltreatment or neglect are commoner than from homicide.

Common associations are previous contact of the family with care organisations, substance abuse, single parents and multiple partners or a partner not the child's father, learning difficulties, physical abuse in the past history of the adults present, unemployment and mental health problems in the protagonists.

Remember that babies too young to crawl are hard put to bruise themselves, that ENT SHOs, Casualty Officers and Orthopaedic Registrars will often see, treat and discharge the condition without thinking how a child has acquired their injury or whether they are at risk. If they haven't done their job, it becomes your job as the GP.

Genital bruising always requires investigation and thought.

You haven't assessed a child properly until you have undressed them fully and examined them from top to toe. The injuries most commonly associated with deliberated abuse (>20%) are rib fractures, intracranial haemorrhage and abdominal trauma. Just over half of all rib fractures under 2 years are due to abuse but a surprisingly low 3.5% of burns in infants under 6 months, only 4.3% of isolated skull fractures and 8.6% of subconjunctival haemorrhages (Pediatrics Lindberg DM et al 2015 136: 831-838.)

Cancer (See Cancer section)

Current cancer cure rate in childhood is 80%. Leukaemia, lymphoma and brain tumours >50%. Some 60% will have a late effect of some kind. 4% will have a second malignancy, usually associated with radiotherapy. There are 35,000 survivors of childhood cancer in the UK currently. 8% of childhood cancers have a genetic predisposition (NEJM Oct 2015). The commonest genes being TP53, APC, BRCA2, NF1, PMS2 and RB1. Non CNS tumours have a 16.7% genetic incidence, CNS tumours 9%, leukaemia 4.4%.

"Aftercure" is a good online support group.

32: PATHOLOGY:

Quick (Everyday) Popular desk top reference values:

Thyroid:	TSH 0.3-3.94
	Free T4 12.3-20.2
	T3 3.5-6.5

		Average patient:
Lipids:	Tot Chol <5.2	<5
	LDL 2-5 (Most people <3)	<3
	HDL M 0.9 – 1.9	>1
	F 1.1 – 2.6	
	VLDL 0.2-1.0	
Ratio:	(Chol/HDL) <5	
	(HDL/Chol) >0.2	
	HDL as % Total	20%
Tg	0.4-1.83	<2

HbA1C Glycosylated Hb
<7% for control of complications in DM (Normal, non diabetic, 3.8-5.5%). Well controlled diabetic: 3.8-7.5%) Some studies suggest much below 7.0 and there is an increase in complications in some diabetics.

Gonadotrophins:	FSH mIU/li	LH mIU/li	17-Beta oestradiol. nmol/li
Normally menstruating women:			
Follicular phase:	4-13	1-18	0.14-0.69
Mid cycle peak:	5-22	24-105	0.34-1.86
Luteal phase:	2-13	1-20	0.18-1.13
Post menopausal:	20-138	15-62	0.00-0.15

LH>FSH with high LH and prolactin in PCO. FSH high in menopause.

Unreliable results:

Lipaemia: Can result in an unanalysable sample or a falsely low amylase level.

Hyperviscosity/paraproteinaemia (myeloma, polycythemia, lymphoma, Waldenstrom's etc):

Can result in an unanalysable sample or pseudo hyponatraemia, false endocrine results for TFTs, RhF, tumour markers, cardiac biomarkers, serum proteins, drugs of abuse, drug monitoring, CRP.

Haemolysis: Increases K, ALT, AST, LDH, Mg, Po4 and Zn.

Icteric serum: Results in decreased creatinine.

Ketoacidosis: Results in increased creatinine.

Renal Failure: Reduces HbA1C by shortening RBC life span (and therefore the time red cell Hb is exposed to glucose).

EDTA contamination: Results in increased K, decreased Ca, Mg, Zn.

Pathology, The Detail:

Investigations appropriate in common specific conditions/situations:

Ambiguous genitalia/Intersex investigations:

Buccal smear, karyotype/chromosomes,

LH FSH testosterone, dihydrotestosterone, HCG stimulation test, (measure testosterone and DHT before and after).

ACTH, 17OH Progesterone, cortisol, androstenedione, DHEAS, aldosterone, 11 deoxycortisol, U and Es, glucose, Pelvic USS, MRI abdo and pelvis,

?laparoscopy/gonadal biopsy etc.

Antenatal blood screening Tests:

FBC. Group.

Rubella, Syphilis, Hepatitis B and C and HIV serology (1 in 4 babies of HIV positive mothers become infected without treatment to both. 1 in 5 HIV infected babies develop AIDS or die in the first year)

In this situation elective LSCS and bottle feeding are recommended.

Others sometimes included are the TORCH blood tests (Toxoplasma, Other {Coxsackie, Syphilis, VZV, and Parvovirus B19 serology} Rubella, CMV, Herpes Simplex Virus: – The TORCH infections cause a syndrome characterized by microcephaly, sensorineural deafness, chorioretinitis, hepatosplenomegaly and thrombocytopenia.)

The usual Down's screening blood test consists of the two pregnancy associated proteins, Papp-A and HCG at 11-13 weeks with the nuchal translucency test. But if missed the" Triple" or "Quadruple test" measuring three or four proteins (obviously) are done between 14 and 20 weeks. These are:

Triple: HCG, AFP, uE3 and

Quadruple: AFP, HCG, uE3 and Inhibin. 15-22 weeks. (Detect up to 75% Downs, with 5% false pos)

Low and high risk for Down's is generally taken to mean below or above 1 in 150.

The Double, Triple and Quadruple tests:

Pregnancy associated plasma protein A (low in Down's syndrome pregnancies)

Beta HCG (raised in Down's syndrome pregnancies)

AFP (low in Down's pregnancies)

Unconjugated Oestriol (uE3) (low in Down's pregnancies)

Inhibin A (raised in Down's pregnancies)

Overall the Down's Syndrome screening has a detection rate of 75% and a false positive rate of 3%.

In 2016 it was proposed that the "Harmony test" (a form of Non invasive prenatal testing, NIPT) which looks for free foetal DNA in maternal serum be introduced nationally. This detects up to 99% of Down's and other trisomies and is usually performed between 10 and 14 weeks. The false positive rate is only 0.1% and this is its advantage. Approximately 2% of women produced no result in the study used to promote the technique.

Blood Group:

Rhesus negative mothers who haven't developed antibodies are given Anti-D injections at 28 and 34 weeks.

C.F.S.(M.E.) Investigations:

There is no characteristic lab test; E.B. virus Abs. B12, Folate and Ferritin.

Actually the list is much longer but will be guided by the patient's history and specific symptoms.

1) VPI Enteroviral specific protein

2) IgM Ab against Enteroviral antigens. Enteroviral serotypes include Echovirus, Coxsackie A and B, Polio etc.

3) E.B. Viral Abs. Our local lab will do EBV Ab and EnteroV Ab and if the latter is pos then they will do the VPI. The basic FBC, ESR, Paul Bunnell and CRP, U and Es, LFTs, Alb, Calcium, CPK, TFTs, Random Gluc, Coeliac Screen, Urinanalysis will have been done by you already.

Coeliac disease:

Gliaden and endomysial antibodies	Positive is >25EU/ml
may indicate Coeliac Disease and Dermatitis Herpetiformis	
(also have reticulin Abs)	90% reliable.
Antigliaden Ab IgG	0-10u/ml
IgA	0-5u/ml
Transglutaminase IgA level	(Neg or pos)

Newest tests include Antigliaden IgG, Tissue transglutaminase IgA Abs. (anti-TTG). Tissue transglutaminase is the antigen recognised by endomysial antibodies (EMA) and will replace EMA as a basic initial screen for Coeliac Disease. Some units perform IgA to endomysial anti EMA if anti-TTG is positive. Antiendomysial Ab IgA is pos or neg and disappears after 3m of a gluten free diet. It is falsely neg in the 2% of patients who are IgA deficient. Endomysial Abs are present in 99% patients with Coeliac Disease. Often there is also a low ferritin, Hb and folate etc.

Patients with IgA deficiency have a 10 fold increased risk of Coeliac Disease.

Connective Tissue Disorders (see other sections:) with Raynauds:

ESR, CRP, LFTs, U and Es, complement. AIP, ANA, cold agglutinins, cryoglobulins, Scleroderma antibodies, double stranded DNA and ribonucleoprotein antibodies, urine for porphyrins, antiphospholipid antibodies etc.

Dementia: Investigations:

FBC, ESR, RBCs, U and Es, Ca, LFTs, B12, Ferritin, GGT, TFTs, Gluc, Folate, Syphilis serology-TPHA, VDRL, HIV plus or minus CXR, MSU, ECG.

Diabetes Investigations: (See Diabetes)

Random venous glucose >11.1mmol/li.

or Fasting plasma glucose (8hrs without calories) >7.0mmol/li (should be 3.5-6mmol/li) OR

Glucose Tolerance Test: after 75gr glucose by mouth. (OGTT)

Abnormal is: >9mmol at 30min,

or 2 hour plasma glucose >11.1mmol/li (2000 criteria).

("Impaired glucose tolerance" is <7-8mmol fasting but 7-11mmol at 2hrs),

non diabetics should be back to N at 2 hours.

"Prediabetes" is fasting plasma glucose 6.1-7.0mmol/li (and OGTT 2 hour level <7.8mmol/li).

Blood Test Levels for Diagnosis of Diabetes and Prediabetes

	A1C (percent)	Fasting Plasma Glucose (mg/dL)	Oral Glucose Tolerance Test (mg/dL)
Diabetes	6.5 or above	126 or above	200 or above
Prediabetes	5.7 to 6.4	100 to 125	140 to 199
Normal	About 5	99 or below	139 or below

Definitions: mg = milligram, dL = deciliter
For all three tests, within the prediabetes range, the higher the test result, the greater the risk of diabetes.

The American Diabetic Definitions:

	2 hour Glucose	Fasting Glucose	HBA1C
Normal	<7.8mmol	<6.1mmol	<6.0
Impaired fasting glycaemia	<7.8mmol	>/= 6.1 and <7.0mmol	6.0-6.4
Impaired glucose tolerance	>/=7.8mmol	<7.0mmol	6.0-6.4
Diabetes	>/=11.1mmol	>/= 7.0mmol	>/= 6.5

Impaired Fasting Glucose: W H O and American Diabetes Association definitions:
WHO criteria: fasting plasma glucose level from 6.1 mmol/l (110 mg/dL) to 6.9 mmol/L (125 mg/dL)
ADA criteria: fasting plasma glucose level from 5.6 mmol/L (100 mg/dL) to 6.9 mmol/L (125 mg/dL)

Micro albumin screening:

	Normal	Microalbumin	Macroalbumin
Urine albumin	<20mg/li	20-200	>200
Albumin/creatinine ratio	<3mg/mmol	3-30	>30

Action: Up to 3X ULN retest in 1yr. 3-10X ULN retest on 2 or more occasions in 6m. >10X ULN + Albustix positive
Treatment: Normoalbuminuria: Treat any BP>130/80, Optimise BG.
Biannual albumen concentration. First voided specimen. Recheck if >20mg/li.
Microalbuminuria: Urinary albumin 2-3X/yr on a timed specimen. Optimise glucose

control, treat BP>130/80. Consider ACEI, avoid excess protein diet.

Macroalbuminuria: (>200mg/li) – Dipstick positive proteinuria, tendency to increased Se creatinine, do quantitative proteinuria 2-4X/yr, Serum U and Es and creatinine 2-4X/yr.

Control BP, restrict protein to 0.7gr/kg body wt.

Refer to nephrologist when creatinine >200umol/li.

End stage renal failure >500umol/li. >Dialysis/Transplantation.

Hypertension Investigations:

Newly diagnosed: FBC, U and Es, LFT, ECG, Gluc, TFTs, Lipids, Urine analysis.

When starting an ACEI: Monitor U and Es at 1 week after starting Rx, with "close monitoring" until stable. Then when stable on ACEI monitor U and Es at least annually.

Hypogonadism Investigations:

Testosterone, FSH, LH, SHBG, Prolactin, digital rectal examination, PSA, Cholesterol, lipids, gluc.

Infertility Investigations: (Trying for 2 years)

Sperm Test

Normal sperm count is	20-200million/ml
Motility	61% 3 hrs
	28% 12hrs
	90% Normal forms
Average volume	3.4mls
pH	7.6 – 8

W.H.O. Guidelines: Vol >2mls. pH 7.2 or more. Sperm concentration 20×10^6/ml. Total sperm numbers 40×10^6 per ejaculation or more. Motility 50% or more with progressive motility. (3 or 4) >25% 4. >15% normal forms.

Some say abnormal forms of 95% are "normal" some say 85%. Liquefaction complete in 1 hr.

Basal temperature chart.

Chlamydia testing, (antibodies) FBC, TFTs.

Rubella screening.

Hormone profile.

(Bloods are done on day 21 of the cycle, day 1 being the first day of the period bleed i.e. post ovulatory)

FSH,	1-4 IU/li
LH	1-15 IU/li

Phase	Day of cycle relative to ovuln.	FSH	LH (iu/li)
Early follicular	– 14 – – 10	2-9	2-7
Late follicular	– 9 – – 4	2-7	2-6
Mid cycle	– 3 – +3	3-13	15-55
Early luteal	+4 – +9	1-5	1-10
Late luteal	+10 – + 14	1-5	1-7
Post menopausal		27-113	15-40

Progesterone

Post ovulatory	6-9 nmol/li
Follicular	1.59-7.6 nmol/li
Periovulatory	1.9 – 21.3 nmol/li
Midluteal	29.3-67.7 nmol/li
Luteal	7.6 – 65.9 nmol/li

Oestradiol

Menopausal	0.01 – 0.4nmol/li
Prolactin	M 78-288 F 72-504mu/li

Prolactin is raised in pregnancy, lactation, pituitary tumour, Cushing's, PCO, hypo-thyroidism, c Metoclopramide, Domperidone, Phenothiazines, some antidepressant Rx, c stress symptoms, galactorrhoea, amenorrhoea, poor libido, E.D., occasionally raised I.C.P.

Miscarriage, recurrent: Investigations:

Anticardiolipin antibodies, thrombophilia screen, AIP, karyotype (both parents), FBC, U and Es, LFTs, TFTs. Pelvic USS (and preliminary bimanual examination).

Myocardial Infarct: Investigations:

There are various cardiac damage markers, some more useful than others.
They include:
Troponins

Troponin T	>1ng/ml
Troponin I	>0.5ng/ml
Creatine Kinase (CK-MB)	>400IU/ml

LDH
AST
Myoglobin
IMA (Ischaemia modified albumin)
Pro brain natriuretic peptide
Glycogen phosphorylase isoenzyme BB

Troponin: (There are three kinds, all found in muscle, Troponin C T and I and they may be elevated in kidney disease, PE, CVA, pre eclampsia, muscle damage etc as well as heart disease)

Troponin I	N	<0.07Ug/li

Serum levels of Troponin T and I increase within 3-12 hours from the onset of chest pain, peak at 24-48 hours and return to the baseline over 5-14 days. Levels **may not** rise for 6 hours and the most sensitive early indicator of MI is Myoglobin.

cTnT Cardiac Troponin T	ULN	14Ng/li 0.014ng/ml

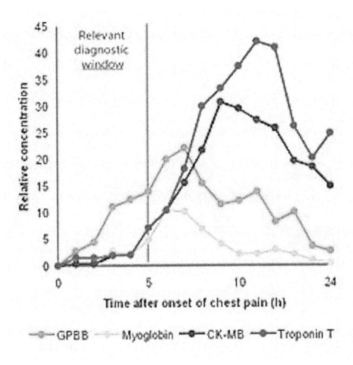

Troponin T is the line above the others on the graph at 12 hr.

GPBB is Glycogen phosphorylase isoenzyme BB. CKMB are two variants of phosphocreatine kinase.

Troponins are more sensitive than CK. An MI has happened if there are definitive ECG changes, Q waves, ST elevation, ischaemic ECG changes, rise or fall in cTnT or cTnI.

Thanks to Wikipedia for the picture.

Body Mass Index

Very obese

Obese

Overweight

Healthy

Underweight

HEIGHT (Feet and Inches)

WEIGHT (Kilograms) / WEIGHT (Stones and Pounds)

```
        4'10" 5'0"  2"   4"   6"   8"  10"  6'0"  2"   4"   6"
126  59 58 56 55 53 52 50 49 48 47 46 45 44 43 42 41 40 39 38 37 36 36 35 34 34 33 32 32   20st
124  58 57 55 54 52 51 50 48 47 46 45 44 43 42 41 40 39 38 37 37 36 35 34 34 33 32 32 31   7lb
122  57 56 54 53 51 50 49 48 47 46 45 44 42 42 41 40 39 38 38 37 36 35 35 34 33 33 32 31 30
120  56 55 53 52 51 49 48 47 46 45 43 43 42 41 40 39 38 37 36 36 35 34 33 33 32 31 31 30   19st
118  55 54 52 51 50 49 47 46 45 44 43 42 41 40 39 38 37 36 36 35 34 33 33 32 31 31 30 30   7lb
116  54 52 52 50 49 48 46 45 44 43 42 41 40 39 38 37 37 36 35 34 34 33 32 31 31 30 30 29
114  54 52 51 49 48 47 46 45 44 43 41 40 39 38 37 36 35 34 34 33 32 32 31 30 30 29 29      18st
112  53 51 50 48 47 46 45 44 43 42 41 40 39 38 37 36 35 35 34 33 32 32 31 30 30 29 29 28   7lb
110  52 50 49 48 46 45 44 43 42 41 40 39 38 37 36 36 35 34 33 33 32 32 31 30 30 29 29 28 27
108  51 49 48 47 46 44 43 42 41 40 39 38 37 37 36 35 34 33 33 32 31 31 30 29 29 28 28 27   17st
106  50 48 47 46 45 44 42 41 40 39 38 38 37 36 35 34 33 33 32 31 31 30 29 29 28 28 27 26
104  49 47 46 45 44 43 42 41 40 39 38 37 36 35 34 34 33 32 31 31 30 29 29 28 28 27 27 26   7lb
102  48 47 45 44 43 42 41 40 39 38 37 36 35 34 34 33 32 31 31 30 29 29 28 28 27 27 26 25   16st
100  47 46 44 43 42 41 40 39 38 37 36 35 35 34 33 32 32 31 30 30 29 28 28 27 27 26 26 25
98   46 45 44 43 41 40 39 38 37 36 36 35 34 33 32 32 31 30 30 29 28 28 27 27 26 26 25 24   7lb
96   45 44 43 42 40 39 38 37 37 36 35 34 33 32 32 31 30 30 29 28 28 27-27 26 26 25 25 24
94   44 43 42 41 40 39 38 37 36 35 34 33 33 32 31 30 30 29 28 28 27 27 26 25 25 24 24 23   15st
92   43 42 41 40 39 38 37 36 35 34 33 33 32 31 30 30 29 28 28 27 27 26 25 25 24 24 23 23   7lb
90   42 41 40 39 38 37 36 35 34 33 33 32 31 30 30 29 28 28 27 27 26 25 25 24 24 23 23 22
88   41 40 39 38 37 36 35 34 34 33 32 31 30 30 29 28 28 27 27 26 25 25 24 24 23 23 22 22   14st
86   40 39 38 37 36 35 34 34 33 32 31 30 30 29 28 28 27 27 26 25 25 24 24 23 23 22 22 21
84   39 38 37 36 35 35 34 33 32 31 30 30 29 28 28 27 27 26 25 25 24 24 23 23 22 22 21 21   7lb
82   38 37 36 35 35 34 33 32 31 30 30 29 28 28 27 26 26 25 25 24 24 23 23 22 22 21 21 20   13st
80   38 37 36 35 34 33 32 31 30 30 29 28 28 27 26 26 25 25 24 24 23 23 22 22 21 21 20 20
78   37 36 35 34 33 32 31 30 30 29 28 28 27 26 26 25 25 24 24 23 23 22 22 21 21 20 20 19   7lb
76   36 35 34 33 32 31 30 30 29 28 28 27 26 26 25 25 24 24 23 23 22 22 21 21 20 20 19 19   12st
74   35 34 33 32 31 30 30 29 28 28 27 26 26 25 24 24 23 23 22 22 21 21 20 20 20 19 19 18
72   34 33 32 31 30 30 29 28 27 27 26 26 25 24 24 23 23 22 22 21 21 20 20 20 19 19 18 18   7lb
70   33 32 31 30 30 29 28 27 27 26 25 25 24 24 23 23 22 22 21 21 20 20 19 19 19 18 18 17
68   32 31 30 29 29 28 27 27 26 25 25 24 24 23 23 22 22 21 21 20 20 19 19 18 18 18 17 17   11st
66   31 30 29 29 28 27 26 26 25 24 24 23 23 22 22 21 21 20 20 19 19 19 18 18 18 17 17 16   7lb
64   30 29 28 28 27 26 26 25 24 24 23 23 22 22 21 21 20 20 19 19 18 18 18 17 17 17 16 16
62   29 28 28 27 26 25 25 24 24 23 22 22 21 21 20 20 19 19 18 18 18 17 17 16 16 16 16 15   10st
60   28 27 27 26 25 25 24 23 23 22 22 21 21 20 20 19 19 19 18 18 17 17 17 16 16 16 15 15   7lb
58   27 26 26 25 24 24 23 23 22 22 21 21 20 20 19 19 18 18 18 17 17 17 16 16 15 15 15 14
56   26 26 25 24 24 23 22 22 21 21 20 20 19 19 18 18 18 17 17 17 16 16 16 15 15 15 15 14 14   9st
54   25 25 24 23 23 22 22 21 21 20 20 19 19 18 18 18 17 17 17 16 16 16 15 15 15 14 14 14 13   7lb
52   24 24 23 23 22 21 21 20 20 19 19 18 18 18 17 17 16 16 16 15 15 15 14 14 14 14 13 13
50   23 23 22 22 21 21 20 20 19 19 18 18 17 17 17 16 16 16 15 15 15 14 14 14 14 13 13 13 12   8st
       1.48  1.52  1.56  1.60  1.64  1.68  1.72  1.76  1.80  1.84  1.88  1.92  1.96  2.00
                                    HEIGHT (Metres)
```

Body Mass Index (The body mass divided by the square of the height) Diagram BMI

Obesity:

BMI	Kg/Sq M
Very severely underweight	BMI <15
Severely underweight	BMI 15-16
Underweight	BMI 16-18.5
Normal	BMI 18.5-25
Overweight	BMI 25-30
Moderately obese	BMI 30-35
Severely obese	BMI 35-40
Very severely obese	BMI >40

Polycystic Ovaries:

Follicular phase bloods (day 5-10) testosterone, androstenedione, LH, FSH, TSH, LH:FSH ratio, Short Synacthen test (Cortisol, 17aOH Progesterone) SHBG

Androstenedione	**2-12 nmol/li**
DHA Sulphate	**0.7 – 11.5 umol/li**
Testosterone	**0.9-2.7 nmol/li**
SHBG Sex Hormone Binding Globulin	**25-100 nmol/li**
Free Androgen Index	**0.5 – 6.5**

Renal Calculus Screen:

24 hr Urine creatinine	7-18mmol/24hr
Urine calcium	2.5-7.5mmol/24hr
Urine phosphate	13-42mmol/24hr
Urine uric acid	1.5-4.4mmol/24hr

The Chemical Pathology of Drugs:

Anticonvulsants: (Old and new units) A.E.D.s

Phenytoin: Half Life average 24 Hrs. Toxic >20-30mcg/ml Peak level 3-9 hrs after oral dose. Single or divided doses. Steady state in 2 weeks. Non linear dose response curve, narrow therapeutic index. Do a level 2 weeks after initiation. Therapeutic 40-80umol/li, <80 umol/li.

Carbamazepine: Half Life 10-26 Hrs. Toxic >12mcg/ml. Take sample before next dose. Give BD. Linear dose response. Adults: Increase to 200mg BD over 10 days. Therapeutic <42 umol/li.

Ethosuximide: Half Life 20-60 Hrs. Toxic >100mcg/ml. Peak levels 2-4 hrs after trough just before next dose. Can be given once daily.

Levetiracetam, Keppra, Therapeutic range 6-20mg/li. Some say 5-30ug/ml.

Phenobarbitone. Half Life 1.5-3 days. Toxic >40mcg/ml. Trough prior to and peak 4-12 hrs after dose.

Therapeutic <170umol/li.

Primidone: Half Life 6-12 Hrs. Toxic >12mcg/ml. Given as twice daily dose. Therapeutic <50umol/li

Generally the therapeutic range is 5-10mg/li (23-46mmol/L).

Valproic Acid: Half Life 9-18 Hrs in adults, 4-14 Hrs in children. Therapeutic Range 40-100mcg/ml.

(Old range 347-693 new range 50-100mg/li).

Toxic>100mcg/ml. BD. Little practical value in doing level. Also quoted are:

Reference Range:
Valproic Acid, Total
  Therapeutic Range: 50-125 µg/mL
  Toxic: Greater than 150 µg/mL
Valproic Acid, Free
  Therapeutic Range: 7-23 µg/mL
  Toxic: Greater than 30 µg/mL
VPA- % Free
  5-18%

Valproic Acid (Convulex) and Sodium Valproate have a 1:1 dose equivalence.

Start dose 600mg/day initially (300mg BD). Increase at 200mg per 3 days, Max 2.5Gr/day.

Clonazepam Half life 12-40 hrs, OD dosing.

Azathioprine: Initially 50-100mg OD maintenance 2 – 2.5mg/kg/day.

Pre-treatment: Do FBC, U and Es, Creat. LFTs, **Consider TPMT testing:** Thiopurine Methyl Transferase genetic testing or the actual enzyme levels. Avoid Rx if TPMT homozygous recessive or low enzyme activity. Immunise against Influenza and give Pneumovax while on Rx. Monitoring: FBC and LFTs weekly for 4 weeks and after dose increase, once all is stable, do 3 monthly U and Es, and creatinine at 1m, 3m, 6m and 12monthly thereafter.

Consultant advice: If WBC >3 then treatment is OK, do FBC, LFTs monthly for 3m then 3 monthly.

For instance: In Ulcerative Colitis, maintenance dose 200mg/day.
If WBC 2.5 – 3.0 then 150mg/day,
If WBC 2.0-2.5 Have a few drug free days, then 100mg/day,
If WBC <2.0 Stop treatment.

Note: 1:300 are homozygous for TPMT absence but low TPMT activity has a 10% prevalence, complete absent activity being 0.3%. These latter are susceptible to bone marrow toxicity with azathioprine, 6-mercaptopurine and other thiopurines.

"Normal level" of TPMT is 25-50 pmol/H/mg/Hb. (Deficit is <10 Carrier is <25.)
68-150mU/L.

Digoxin: Post dose level: 1-2.6 nmol/li or 0.8-2 ng/mL (1.2-2nmol/L). Half Life 36 hrs. So can be given OD. Take blood at minimum level – 6 hrs after last dose. (NICE says 8-12 hrs after dose – minimum level, to monitor toxicity or non compliance). Toxicity more likely above 2ng/mL, or 1.5-3ug/li. Hypokalaemia predisposes to Digoxin toxicity and the antidote is Digoxin Specific Antibody Fragments. DigiFab (1 vial £750!)

Gold I.M. (Sodium Aurothiomalate, Myocrisin) 5-10mg test dose then 10-50mg weekly, maintenance 10-50mg/m. FBC and urine analysis weekly initially then monthly once stabilised.

Hydroxychloroquine:
Plaquenil 200mg od initially, 200-400mg/day maintenance. Also Chloroquine sulph. Nivaquin. 250mg OD initially, 250mg maintenance.

Tests: Baseline and 6 monthly eye checks (retinal damage and corneal opacities.)
Renal function and regular FBCs during treatment.

Lithium: Target range is 0.6-1.6mmol/li. Some authorities say 0.5-0.8mmol/li – it is, basically, fairly safe (blood 12 hrs after dose) but >0.4mmol can be effective. Monitor U and Es, LFTs and TFTS annually, (some say 6 monthly for all), more frequently in the elderly or if levels fluctuate. Initially nocturnal dose, (easier to monitor) use the same trade name drug.

My local prescribing committee advises GPs not to initiate treatment but to supervise it once started by a consultant.

Nonsense.

1) Lithium is one the safest psychiatric treatments available (-compare it with tricyclics or atypical antipsychotic drugs),

2) There are simple and well recognised biochemical tests at recognised intervals and familiar protocols to avoid complications,

3) I don't think in nearly 40 years of initiating and prescribing it I have seen even one case of significant Lithium toxicity or any irreversible S/E,

4) It has a simple dosing regimen, it works and it is free of side effects from the patient point of view.

So why would a competent and diligent GP not initiate and monitor his few bipolar (and other appropriate) patients on lithium? Especially given the frequently sub optimal out-patient psychiatric services available in district general hospitals.

Some say:

Do lithium levels weekly until stable, three monthly thereafter or more frequently if indicated by dose or illness or non compliance. U and Es 6 monthly, eGFR 6 monthly, (3 monthly for the elderly or if other complicating factors), TSH 6 monthly but every 4-6 weeks if TSH raised, BMI 6 monthly. Corrected Ca++ (If raised can indicate hyperparathyroidism) and ECG if appropriate. Lithium toxicity can be due to diuretics, dehydration, alcohol, NSAIDs, also c Fluoxetine, Fluvoxamine, Phenytoin, Carbamazepine, Haloperidol, Metronidazole. Sympts of toxicity: Nausea and vomiting, tremor, muscle weakness, confusion, polyuria, polydipsia.

Methotrexate: 2.5mg-5mg once weekly initially. Maintenance 5-15mg/week. FBC and LFTs monthly for 3m, then 3 monthly. U and Es every 6m. Can co prescribe 5mg Folic Acid daily without compromising effectiveness. All sorts of interactions and S/Es. (Too many to list but go to Drugs.com to see them!)

Penicillamine. 125-250mg daily initially slowly increasing to max 1.5gr/day. FBC and Urine testing monthly. Consider Pyridoxine supplementation as Penicillamine increases its excretion and reduces B6 activity.

Sulfasalazine: Salazopyrin 500mg OD, increase by 500mg/week. Maintenance 2-4 Gr/day.

Tests: FBC and LFTs at 3 weeks, 6 weeks, then 3 monthly.

Tacrolimus: (An immuno-suppressant, used topically for eczema) Level 5-20ng/ml (renal transplant) Clin Biochem 1998 31: 309-316

Theophylline: Therapeutic level 56-111umol/li. Half life varies from 30 hrs in premature babies to 3.5 hrs in children, 5-8 hrs in adults (the lower range is for smokers).

Toxic Levels of Drugs in general Use:

Acetaminophen >250mcg/ml

Amikacin >25mcg/ml

Aminophylline >20mcg/ml

Amitriptyline >500ng/ml
Carbamazepine >12mcg/ml
Chloramphenicol >25mcg/ml
Desipramine >500ng/ml
Digoxin >2.4ng/mL is toxic (N range is 0.5-2.0mcg/li) 6-8 hours after last dose-usually first thing in the morning.
Disopyramide>5mcg/ml
Ethosuximide>100mcg/ml
Flecainide>1mcg/ml
Gentamicin>12mcg/ml
Imipramine >500ng/ml
Kanamycin>35ug/ml
Lignocaine («Lidocaine») >5mcg/ml
Lithium >2mmol/li
Methotrexate >10um/l over 24hrs after last dose
Nortriptyline >500ng/ml
Paracetamol Toxicity depends on the time after the dose was taken and a variety of nomograms are available. Toxicity is likely if the level>1000umol/li at 4 hrs or >500umol/li at 8 hrs or>250umol/li at 12 hrs etc.
Phenobarbitol >40mcg/ml
Phenytoin>30mcg/ml
Primidone>15mcg/ml
Procainamide>16mcg/ml
Propranolol>150ng/ml
Quinidine>10mcg/ml
Salicylate>300mcg/ml
Theophylline>20mcg/ml
Valproic Acid>100mcg/ml

Therapeutic Levels: (other sources)

Drug plasma	half life	time to steady state	ref. range
amiodarone	240 – 2400h	60 – 90d	0.5 – 2.0mg/L
N-desethylamiodarone			0.5 – 2.0mg/L
caffeine (neonates)	40 – 230h		5 – 20mg/L
carbamazepine	8 – 60h	7d	4 – 10mg/L
clobazam	18h	4d	0.1 – 0.4mg/L
clonazepam	18 – 50h	4 – 10d	25 – 85 ug/L
clozapine			350 – 500 ug/L
cyclosporin	8 – 20h	2 – 4d	depends on use ug/L
desmethylclobazam			<2000 ug/L
digoxin	36h	7d	0.8 – 2.0 ug/L
ethanol			Driving limit 800mg/L
ethosuximide	50h	10d	<100mg/L
flecainide	20h	5d	0.15 – 0.90mg/L
gabapentin	6h	2d	</= than 24mg/L

gentamicin (pre + 1h post if on multiple doses)	2h	1d	D/W microbiologist
lamotrigine	24 – 34h	7d	Mono Px </=15mg/li Multi Px 10mg/li
levetiracetam	7h	2d	6 – 20mg/L
lithium – prophylaxis	18-36h		0.4-0.8mmol/li
– acute mania			0.8-1.2mmol/li
mycophenolate	17h	4d	Depends on use
olanzapine			20 – 40 ug/L
oxcarbazepine (monohydroxycarbamazepine)	19hr	4d	15-35mg/L
paracetamol	1-4h		See BNF mg/L
phenobarbitone	Child 70 hr	Child 12 d	Neonate <30mg/L
	Adult 100hr	Adult 20d	Adult <40mg/L
phenytoin	13 – 46h	14d	Neonate 6-14mg/L Adult 10-20mg/L
pregabalin	6h	2d	
primidone	8h	2d	(see phenobarb.) 0 – 11mg/L
sirolimus (rapamycin)	60h	10d	5 – 15mg/L
tacrolimus (FK506)	11h	2d	Depends on use ug/L
theophylline	24hr neonates	5d	10-20mg/L
	4hr children	1-2d	
	9hr non smokers	2d	
	4hr smokers	1-2d	
thioguanine nucleotides	1w	4w	235 – 450 pmol/8x108 cells
thyroxine	7d	5w	TSH in ref. range
tiagabine	8h (3h, enz. induct)	3d	see page on TFTs in text
tobramycin (pre + 1h post if on multiple doses)	2-3hr	1d	D/W Microbiologist
topiramate	20 – 30h	1w	5 – 20mg/L
valproate	12h	3d	50 – 100mg/L
vancomycin (pre)	4 – 11h	3d	D/W microbiologist.
vigabatrin	6 – 8h	10d	5 – 35mg/L
zonisamide	65h	2w	15 – 40mg/L

Apologies for the use of older units for some of the sources above.

The Guthrie Test (heel prick neonatal test) is currently used for Cystic Fibrosis, (Trypsin), PKU, Congenital Hypothyroidism (TSH), Sickle Cell Disease.

It can also be used to screen for: Galactosaemia, MCADD, Biotinidase deficiency, Congenital Adrenal Hyperplasia. See obstetrics section for up to date list.

General Biochemistry: Normal serum levels:

ACE: Angiotensin Converting Enzyme. (Forms angiotensin II from angiotensin I and metabolises bradykinin). Inhibited by ACE Inhibitors. Raised levels in sarcoid, used as a marker of disease activity. Risk of hypoglycaemia. People who produce more ACE tend to have better long distance athletic performance.

Normal   13-25k U/l (some say 8-52)   221-425 uKat/l

Normal Adults have levels below 40 micrograms/L
It may be raised in Hodgkin's Disease
Diabetes
Alcoholic Liver Disease
Chronic Lung Disease (Asthma, cancer, COPD, TB)
Nephrotic Syndrome
MS
Hyperthyroidism
It may be low in:
Chronic Liver disease
Anorexia Nervosa
Steroid therapy
Hypothyroidism
It can also be monitored
in Gaucher's disease and Leprosy,

Acetylcholine receptor antibodies: positive in Myasthenia Gravis

Acid phosphatase: Maximum by some techniques up to 13.4 IU/li but most labs are lower ie

Total acid phosphatase is up to 5.4, prostatic acid phosphatase 1.2 IU/li

Raised in Ca prostate, after rectal examinations, catheterisation.

Tartrate resistant raised in hairy cell leukaemia, HIV encephalopathy, osteoporosis, metabolic bone diseases etc.

Total raised in Paget's, bone secondaries, Gaucher's disease, fracture, leukaemia, hyperparathyroidism, ITP, throboembolism, thrombophlebitis etc.

Albumin:	30-50gr/li
(0-4 days:	28-44 gr/li
14 yrs:	38-54 gr/li
60 yrs:	35-50 gr/li
>60 yrs:	34-48 gr/li)

Albuminuria: is the persistent presence of 30mg albumin/gr creatinine in the urine and is diagnostic of CKD.

Microalbuminuria is 30-299mg/li or 30-299mg/24hrs. (Normal dipstix negative) (But see Diabetes section above – some class >200 as macroalbuminuria).

Alcohol: level Legal driving limits:	80mg % in blood,
	35ug in breath,
	106mg/100mls urine.

Aldosterone:

Adult recumbent	100-500pmol/li
Ambulant	600-1200pmol/li
Alkaline phosphatase: (ALP)	30-125iu/li

It is unusual for alkaline phosphatase alone to be raised in liver disease.

There are bone, liver X2, placental and intestinal isoenzymes. The list of causes of raised ALP is as long as your arm and the likely cause depends on the iso enzyme involved but includes cirrhosis, biliary obstruction, bone cancers, hyperparathyroidism and hyperthyroidism, Paget's, Rickets, pancreatic cancer, splenic infarction, perforated ulcer, steatorrhoea, hepatotoxic drugs, pregnancy, etc, etc

ALP is low in Pernicious anaemia, Coeliac dis., Myxoedema, Vit. D intoxication, various drugs.

Alpha 1 antitrypsin: 1.1-2.1 (1.5-3.5) g/li

Alpha 1 antitrypsin deficiency is a genetic disorder, the gene located on chromosome 14. The Alpha 1 anti trypsin which is normally made in the liver is not released into the circulation and therefore endogenous pulmonary enzymes are not neutralised and emphysema results. These enzymes destroy bacteria and air contaminants. Cirrhosis is the hepatic complication. Approximately 1:4000 people suffer from alpha 1 anti trypsin deficiency in the UK, 1:25 are carriers.

Amylase: 90-300 IU/Li

Raised in pancreatitis, severe uraemia, mumps, cholecystitis, intestinal obstruction and sometimes after Morphine and other opiates due to sphincter of Oddi spasm. Aspirin, COCP, cholinergic drugs, ethacrynic acid, Methyl Dopa, thiazides can all increase amylase levels.

Pancreatic Amylase 28-100 IU/li
(or 23-85U/L and some labs give a range of 40-140U/L)

A.S.O.T: Antistreptolysin O titre ULN 200us/ml

Anti-DNase B 240us/ml
Anti-Hyaluronidase 128us/ml

Anti Phospholipid antibody. IgG. Present in 15-20% of DVTs and 33% of new CVAs in people under 50 years old. They are a major cause of recurrent miscarriage and these complications are preventable.

Anti cardiolipins <13.3U/ml
Anti B2 Glycoprotein-1 antibody level is either pos or neg

In Hughes Syndrome, patients are usually positive anticardiolipin aCL, lupus anticoagulant LA, though some ARE sero-negative.

Antinuclear factor significant level is >1:80

Gastric parietal cell antibodies and intrinsic factor Abs are associated with pernicious anaemia,

Mitochondrial Antibodies are associated with primary biliary cirrhosis,

Smooth muscle antibodies are raised in chronic active hepatitis,

HEp2 test homogenous: Positive if antibodies to DNA, the Hep-2 autoantibody test is the same as the anti nuclear antibody, A.N.A. Positive in SLE, RhA, Sjogren's, Scleroderma, Dermatomyositis, Primary Biliary Cirrhosis, MS etc etc.

Nuclear membrane pattern is positive in systemic rheumatic disease, liver disease, lupoid, chronic active hepatitis,

Nucleolar pattern in scleroderma, SLE, Raynaud's, Sjogren's syndrome,

Centromere pattern in CREST, Raynaud's, primary biliary cirrhosis,

Midbody pattern in Systemic Sclerosis,

Mitotic spindle apparatus MSA in rheumatic disease and SLE,

Centriolar pattern Systemic Sclerosis.

Speckled pattern – an ENA Screen is done.

Proliferating cell nuclear antigen PCNA in SLE.

dsDNA antibodies pos in SLE (<100iu/ml) especially if low C3-good correlation with disease activity.

ENA screen done if ANF pos and Hep2 speckled.

Cardiolipin antibodies in SLE, associated with thrombosis, thrombocytopenia, miscarriages, MI, AIDS.

Cardiolipin antibody   Normal 0-13.3 u/ml

Beta 2 glycoprotein antibodies performed in the evaluation of antiphospholipid syndrome, unexplained thromboses or recurrent miscarriages. Usually negative.

Rheumatoid factor: Rh.F.   <40 iu/ml

This is an auto antibody against IgG. "Rh F" usually detects IgM, ELISA is sensitive to IgG and IgA.

Positive in Sjogren's syndrome, RhA, other connective tissue disorders, 10% of the N population (especially>60 yrs) and with infections.

Anti-CCP1, CCP2 antibodies:

Cyclic citrullinated peptide antibodies. Markers of the erosive potential in Rheumatoid arthritis can be positive 10 years before a clinical diagnosis.

Coeliac disease:

HLA-DQ2 and HLA-DQ8 typing and

Gliaden and   endomysial IgA antibodies   Positive is >25EU/ml

may indicate Coeliac Disease and dermatitis herpetiformis (also have reticulin Abs) 90% reliable.

Antigliaden Ab IgG   0-10u/ml

IgA   0-5u/ml

Transglutaminase IgA level   (neg or pos)

Newest tests include Antigliaden IgG, Tissue transglutaminase IgA Abs. Antiendomysial Ab IgA is pos or neg and disappears after 3m of a gluten free diet. It is falsely neg in the 2% patients who are IgA deficient. Endomysial Abs are present in 99% patients with Coeliac Disease. Often there is also a low ferritin, Hb and folate etc.

Anti neutrophil cytoplasmic antibodies ANCA pos in Wegener's granulomatosis, renal vasculitis, P.A.N.

Bicarbonate: HCO3   24-32mmol/li

Bilirubin: Direct (conjugated) Bilirubin should be less than 10-15% of the total. Generally speaking, in the neonatal period, phototherapy is considered at 200umol/li and exchange Trx at 400 umol/li

B.N.P. Basic natriuretic peptide: If >400pg/ml, (116 pmol/li) arrange a cardiac echo, and if >2000 arrange an urgent echo.

A marker of heart failure.

<100 makes CCF unlikely

>500 on treatment means a poor prognosis and unless you are confident in the

treatment of heart failure, or there are good reasons not too, referral is needed soon.
BBs, ARBs and ACEIs reduce the level.

Generally the advice is for a **specialist referral** if the level is   BNP>400pg/ml
(116pmol/li) or
NTproBNP>2000pg/ml (236pmol/li)

This used to be called Brain natriuretic peptide because it was found in pig brains. It is now called

Basic natriuretic peptide: or B-Type natriuretic peptide. In humans it comes from heart muscle, in response to excessive stretching.

NT pro BNP	0-74yrs.	<125pg/mL
	75-99yrs.	<450pg/mL

C1 Esterase inhibitor C1-INH: Raised in sarcoid. Low in hereditary angio-oedema
N is 16 – 33mg/dl

Caeruloplasmin: The copper carrying blood protein (some is transported by albumen) which also oxidises iron to facilitate its transport on Transferrin. Levels are low in Wilson's Disease (Kayser Fleischer rings) raised in pregnancy, if the patient is on the COCP, in lymphoma and inflammatory states, RhA, angina, Alzheimer's, schizophrenia and OCD (surprisingly).
Normal   0.2-0.6g/li

Calcium: Total 2.1-2.6mmol/li
Ionised   1.25mmol/li
Corrected for low albumen: True Se Ca++ mmol/li= [(40-Serum albumin) X 0.025] + Se Ca++
Treat if se calcium >3.00

The Brit J Cancer published a paper from Bristol and Exeter Universities in 2014 looking into calcium levels. 54,000 patients over 40 years old had calcium levels checked; Mild hypercalcaemia (2.6-2.8mmol/L) was linked in men to an 11.5% **risk of cancer** the next year. (3X higher than in men with normal levels). >2.8mmol/L the risk was 28% and at 3mmol/L the risk rose to 50%. In women these same levels gave risks: 2.6-2.8 of 4.1%, >2.8 of 8.7% and >3mmol/L of 16.7%. Men were more at risk even though hypercalcaemia itself was commoner in women. (hyperparathyroidism is commoner in women). 81% of the hypercalcaemic cancers were lung, prostate, myeloma, colorectal and haematological cancers.

Note: **Parathormone**   Normal   10-65 pg/ml or 10-65 ng/L

Calcitonin: (used to diagnose medullary thyroid cancer) ULN F 5 pg/ml or ng/L
M 12 pg/ml or ng/L
Children <6m   40 pg/ml or ng/L
Calcitonin is stimulated by increased Ca++ levels, as well by as gastrin and penta-gastrin. It lowers blood calcium by inhibiting intestinal calcium absorption, inhibiting bone osteoclastic activity and it inhibits renal tubular absorption of calcium.
It also inhibits renal tubular PO4 reabsorption.

Things you may have forgotten about calcium homeostasis

Parathyroid Glands:

PTH and the kidney
Activates 25 OH Vit D to 1, 25 OH Vit D.
Increases Ca, resorption.
Increases PO4 excretion.
Inhibited by 1, 25 OH Vit D.
Increases Mg resorption.

From the gut:
Increased Calcium absorption.

PTH and bone
Increases Ca and PO4 resorption from bone.

Stimulated by low Ca, high PO4.

1, 25 OH Vit D: (Calcitriol) on the gut
Increases Ca, Mg and PO4 absorption from gut.
Stimulated by PTH, Low Ca, Low PO4.

Calprotectin: (faecal) A marker of inflammation: "Over 50 is significant but probably up to 150 can be considered N in GP ". A neutrophil selective protein in stool, ELISA estimation. Accurately measures the number of neutrophils in the G.I.T. Sensitive marker of untreated inflammatory bowel disease (100%). 90% sensitive for Ca bowel, 50% Colonic polyps.

Normal <50mg/li

If a <than 5 fold increase then likely to have relapse of IBD, UC, Crohn's. Assesses disease activity in Crohn's. Is also raised in Ca Bowel and gastroenteritis.

Cancer/Tumour Markers:

are used for population screening, (though the lack of sensitivity and specificity of all the tests hamper this function), making a cancer diagnosis, assessing prognosis and monitoring response to treatment, recurrence risk etc. No tumour marker is exclusive to cancer cells and two patients with apparently identical cancers can have hugely differing marker levels.

A.F.P. Alpha fetoprotein: 0 – 9 ug/li or <40ug/li (some sources)
Elevated in 80% hepatocellular carcinomas
Is a normal serum glycoprotein and a major component of foetal plasma.

High levels in the foetus, levels are raised in patients with hepatocellular carcinoma, non cancer liver disease, (hepatitis, cirrhosis), pregnancy, testicular tumours, ataxia telangiectasia.

Level above which benign disease is unlikely ">500ng/ml"

Carcino Embryonic Antigen CEA: Normal 2.5ug/li or less (doubled in smoking but <5) may predict cancer relapse.

Raised in bowel tumours, especially on the R side, various other cancers, breast, lung, ovarian, gastric, oesophageal, pancreatic, medullary thyroid, mesothelioma, bony secondaries, non malignant liver disease, CAH, cirrhosis, pancreatitis, CKD, inflammatory bowel disease, IBS, diverticulitis, pneumonia, smoking, old age and atherosclerosis, bladder, head and neck, hepatic cancers, lymphoma, melanomata, etc.

Chromografin A is elevated in phaeochromocytoma, carcinoma of the pancreas and prostate and in carcinoid syndrome. Raised in benign PU, smoking, inflammatory bowel disease, pancreatitis, hypothyroidism, cirrhosis, biliary obstruction etc.

C.E.A. Carcinoembryonic antigen – a complex glycoprotein <2.5, non smokers
The Royal Marsden Normal is   <3.0
                              <0-5 ug/li (ng/ml) smokers
Elevated in less than 25% of early stage colon cancers and 75% late stage colon cancers.
Ca 125 can be raised in non specific inflammation, a non specific   0-35 u/ml
tumour marker, non mucinous ovarian cancer, correlates with response
to treatment. Raised in endometrial ca, pancreatic, lung, breast,
colon cancer. Also raised during menstruation, pregnancy, endometriosis.
Ca125 elevated in 85% of ovarian carcinoma but only 50% of early stage
carcinomas. A large scale UK study in 2015 found that change in the level over time
was a more reliable screening tool than the absolute level.
Ca 15-3   <31 u/ml
Ca 15-3 A tumour marker in breast cancer, predicting adverse outcomes in node negative and positive cancers. Also found in colon, gastric, hepatic, lung, pancreatic, ovarian, prostate cancer.
Also found in benign breast, liver, kidney and ovarian cysts, only found in 5-30% of stage 1 and 2 breast cancer.
Ca 19-9 Gastrointestinal adenocarcinoma, gastric, colonic, pancreatic, biliary tract cancer. differentiates benign from malignant pancreatic disease. Normal is <37 u/ml
Level above which benign disease is unlikely >1000us/ml (elevated in 80-90% of pancreatic cancers and 60% – 70% biliary tract cancers).
Galactosyl Transferase II Raised in a variety of malignancies, particularly GIT tumours. eg: colon and pancreatic cancer.
H.C.G. Human chorionic gonadotrophin.   0-4 iu/li
A glycoprotein normally produced by the placenta, elevated in pregnancy. It is used as a tumour marker in gestational trophoblastic disease where the level correlates with tumour mass and germ cell tumours. Said to be responsible for pregnancy nausea and so hyperemesis is a sign of "effective implantation".
B-HCG can be elevated in gastrointestinal tumours, non seminomatous germ cell tumours, marijuana use, hypogonadal states, gestational trophoblastic tumours.

Immunoglobulins (monoclonal). Paraproteins are produced by Multiple Myeloma and are proportional to tumour volume and response to treatment. They can be of any immunoglobulin subtype.
L.D.H: in N.H.L.
PCA3: Prostate cancer antigen 3. (DD3) A gene expressed in prostatic tissue and over expressed in cancer – so a useful marker.
P.S.A: Prostate specific antigen. Age, race, (higher in black men, lower in Japanese) raised in prostatitis, after vigorous exercise, eating dairy products, cycling, etc
Generally the normal is said to be   0-4 ug/li.
Elevated in more than "75% of organ confined prostate cancers".
but some references: 40-50 yrs   ULN 2.5
                           50-60   3.5
                           60-70   4.5
                           70-80   6.5
Total PSA usually measures protein bound and free PSA. Free PSA is generally

associated with benign conditions, bound PSA with malignancy (see below).

Beware of over interpreting the results and remember the generally benign nature of 90% prostate cancers as well as the morbidity of every type of treatment. **If a patient's PSA is <0.5 aged 40 then the risk of ever getting prostate cancer is very low.** The usual advice is: If at 40 yrs the PSA is >1 (but not significantly raised) then repeat the test annually. If <0.65, repeat the test when the patient reaches 55-65 years. **If the PSA is <1 at 60 then the patient is very unlikely ever to get prostate cancer.**

Even watchful waiting or "Active Surveillance" can lead to the unnecessary anxiety of screening the well patient. Undoubtedly there are a few highly aggressive prostate cancers in which early detection can save lives. Blanket PSA screening however probably (?) seems to cause more harm than good. The American Preventive Services Task Force study on PSA screening (2012) suggested 1:1000 derived a benefit from random PSA testing and 100 will have false positives. Many will go on to have (painful) biopsies and related complications. The same study found that 90% of men would then have radiotherapy or surgery for cancers that would never become life threatening and 5% would die within a month of the treatment! In my experience this is a vast exaggeration. On the other hand more recent American data have shown – and in distinction to breast mammogram screening, that since large scale PSA screening began, deaths from prostatic cancer presenting with metastatic disease have fallen significantly whereas breast cancer presenting with metastatic disease has not.(See urology section)

Also, in Europe, after 9 years of follow up the ERSPC concluded that PSA screening did reduce prostate cancer deaths by 20% between 55 and 69 years (but 1410 men need to be screened and 48 additional cases of prostate cancer need to be treated to avoid one death). Neither were glowing endorsements in their populations of random prostate screening.

So just as in most things, it is up to the GP to take the responsibility as to whether to offer the test (which you probably **should do** in any man over 40 with lower urinary tract symptoms or who actually asks for the test) or to unreasonably refuse the only screening test other than testicular examination available to men.

All sorts of lifestyle changes can reduce the risk of prostate cancer, especially, thoughtful sexual behaviour, a vegetarian based diet with plenty of tomatoes (Lycopene), pomegranates, more vegetable fat and reduced meat and dairy products. Regular sex with the same partner seems important.

PSA, the antigen itself, inhibits angiogenesis and as such is actually part of the body's own defence mechanism against tumour formation. A level of

4-10ng/ml can be due to BPH but at

4-10ng/ml the risk of carcinoma is still   15-25%.

>10ng/ml   it is   60-67% but at

>4ng/ml 75% do not have cancer.

Free PSA: The higher the free to total PSA ratio the less likely there is to be cancer. The cut off is   15% or 0.15

Some references say <20% or even 25% may be indicative of cancer, it may depend on the local lab.

The flies in the ointment are that 5-10% prostate tumours are very aggressive and there are no reliable biochemical markers of these tumours as yet, (see below) that 2/3 of men with raised PSAs do not have biopsy positive prostate cancer, that 15% men with a normal

PSA do have prostate cancer and that many biopsies miss anterior placed cancers anyway. But one of the main difficulties in decision making is that even when a high Gleason graded prostate cancer is detected it is not possible as yet to predict and segregate the highly aggressive tumours from the indolent ones. The ones you die of from the ones you die with – and that is why PSA testing has a chequered history and a battered reputation.

Before the test the patient should avoid vigorous exercise and ejaculation for 2 days, not have had a DRE in the last week, a prostate biopsy in the last six weeks and there should be no UTI (which can raise the PSA for months.) Personal experience suggests that any raised PSA should be repeated after a course of a proper antibiotic. (I use Co Amoxiclav or Norfloxacin). For all these reasons and for the relatively common obfuscating and difficult to diagnose prostatitis.

Alternative tests to PSA for investigating prostate pathology are:

Prostate cancer 3 PCA3,

Human kallikrein 2 HK2,

Early prostate cancer antigen 2 EPCA2,

Genetic markers: like 2+Edel, which has distinguished between aggressive and non aggressive tumours in some studies.

In a 2015 Swedish study to improve the selectivity of blood testing for prostate cancer, the Stockholm 3 (STHLM3) study, Various other prostate tests were included with the PSA. These were the biomarkers PSA, Free PSA, intact PSA, hK2, MSMB, MIC1 and genetic polymorphisms (232 SNPs). They performed better than PSA alone in detecting Gleason 7+ cancers. This combination reduced biopsies and benign biopsies by 32% and 44%.(2015)

Neuron Specific Enolase is a marker for various CNS tumours including neuroblastomas.

Cancer marker hormones:

Insulin: Islet cell tumours.

Calcitonin: Medullary thyroid carcinoma.

Catecholamines: Phaeochromocytoma.

Ectopic ADH, ACTH in Lung Cancer.

HCG: Trophoblastic disease, Germ cell tumours, goes up in pregnancy from 5-426 at 4 weeks to 7650-230,000 at 8 weeks. 25,700-288,000 at 12 weeks etc. Higher levels in multiple pregnancy and molar pregnancy. Back to normal 4 weeks after loss of pregnancy. If >1500-2000mIU/ml and no pregnancy on USS, then an ectopic is likely.

CDT Carbohydrate Deficient Transferrin:

M 8-17mg/ml. Alcohol abuse: 9-136mg/ml

F 11-22mg/ml. Alcohol abuse 13-60mg/ml

A sensitive indicator of alcohol abuse, raised within a week of increased consumption, drops within 2 weeks, can be slightly raised in liver disease.

Carboxyhaemoglobin:

CoHb (EDTA Bottle, full):

Normal level up to: (in a non smoker)	1.5%
In a smoker up to	6%
Chloride:	**95-105mmol/li**
Cholesterol: (etc)	

Familial Hypercholesterolaemia is marked by LDL >75th C. Generally total Chol >7.5 and LDLC >4.9.

The national guidance is to keep:

Total Cholesterol	<5mmol/li
LDL	<3mmol/
HDL	M 0.9 – 1.9 >1
	F 1.1 – 2.6
VLDL	0.2-1.0
Ratio: (Chol/HDL)	<5
(HDL/Chol)	>0.2
HDL as % Total	20%
Tg	0.4-1.83 <2

For high risk patients:

Total cholesterol	<4mmol/li
LDL	<2mmol/li

Chromium (see Cobalt too):

Normal	<134nmol/li

(Metal on metal joint replacements)

Clotting studies: see Thrombophilia screen and chapter 8, Anticoagulants/Clotting.

Prothrombin time. P.T.   12-16secs

A measure of the extrinsic clotting pathway. The INR is derived from this. The reference range for prothrombin time is usually around 12-16 seconds and the

INR in the absence of anticoagulation therapy is   0.8-1.2. See below

Note: Rapid Warfarinisation:

10mg, 10mg, 5mg on successive days and the fourth day request an INR with an urgent result (Warfarin 3-9mg/day usually maintains the INR in the desired range).

I N R International Normalised Ratio: (similar to the old B.C.R., it is the ratio of the patient's prothrombin time and that of a "normal patient")   aim for 2 – 3.75

in most anti-coagulated patients. (See section on anti-coagulants)

Normal INR	0.8-1.2
DVT prophylaxis for general surgery:	2-2.5
Prophylaxis after hip surgery, M.I.	2-3
P.E., T.I.A.	2-3
Treatment of venous thrombo-embolism, DVT	2-3
In VTE the lowest VTE and bleeding rates are at 2.5	
In PE with a mechanical heart valve	3-4.5
In non-Rheumatic A.F	2.0 may suffice
(but most authorities say non valvular AF, to reduce stroke, >2)	
A.F. If previous cerebral ischaemia	2-3.9

Activated partial thromboplastin time (A.P.T.T.)   29-37 secs

A measure of the intrinsic pathway.

D-Dimer: Dd – A measure of fibrin turnover. Can be raised in atrial fibrillation. A risk marker with

t-PA, tissue plasminogen activator. A specific derivative of fibrin, produced when the fibrin clot is degraded by plasmin. Raised in VTE, malignancy, pregnancy, surgery.
Has good negative predictability only.

Normal	<0.5ug FEU/ml

aPTT is a *rough* guide to the effect of Dabigatran (Pradaxa)   No more than 80 secs.
CNP: see C-type natriuretic peptide
Cobalt: (See Chromium)

Normal	<119nmol/li

(Metal on metal joint replacements):
Cold agglutinins:
Ig M antibodies against RBCs, monoclonal or polyclonal, primary idiopathic or associated with infections, – Mycoplasma, HIV, Infectious Mono. or with leukaemia or lymphoma.

Complement proteins:

C3	0.8-1.5 g/li
C4	0.2 – 0.5 g/li

C3 is raised in inflammatory conditions, C3 and C4 decreased in active S.L.E.

Copper: 16-31 umol/li
In Wilson's Disease (Autosomal recessive, Hepatolenticular Degeneration) copper accumulates in various tissues. (The brain and liver etc, Kayser-Fleisher rings at the outer edge of the iris). The copper transport protein **Ceruloplasmin level is low (<0.2gr/li)**
   Normal Ceruloplasmin in serum (Adult)   14-40mg/dl 0.93-2.65umol/L
unless acute inflammation drags the level up.
Serum copper is also low in Wilson's Disease but urine copper is raised.
   Urine copper >1.6umol/24 hr confirms Wilson's disease. Other conditions which involve high urine copper level are various forms of cholestasis and some forms of hepatitis.
Cortisol:
Peak plasma levels normally occur at 8-10 am.

Cortisol 8-10 am	5-28 ug/dl	(138-773 nmol/li)
4-6 pm	2-14	55-386
8 pm	<50% of the morning level.	

From another source:

24.00 Hrs	200 nmol/li
09.00	138-717 nmol/li
17.00	55-497 nmol/li

Urinary Cortisol Adult	10-100ug/day (27-276 nmol/day)
Child	2-27ug 5-75nmol in 24hr urine

Dexamethasone suppression test:
Overnight suppression after Rx 1mg or 2mg of Dexamethasone the night before and do a morning cortisol. Then Full Dexamethasone suppression test consists of 48 hours of low dose then high dose (8mg/day) for 48 hrs – reliable.
   Normal: 24 hr urines should be <50% baseline, Plasma cortisol <5ug/dl, Urinary free cortisol <25ug/24 hrs, Urine 17-OHCS 4ug/24 hrs.

   Short synacthen test: 250ug of the injection (not depot) then cortisol at 0, 30 and 60 minutes. In Addison's, N, Base>250, Rise >550

(Also Urine 17-OHCS increased 2-4X between the first and second 24 hr collection.) – Diagnostic of Addison's Disease.

Most patients with Cushing's Syndrome have a pituitary tumour (80%), so are ACTH dependent. "Ectopic" ACTH or CRH (Corticotropin-releasing hormone) in 15%. (eg Small cell lung tumour)

If available you can measure late night salivary cortisol. The Dexamethasone suppression test or 24 hour urinary Cortisol are equally sensitive. 9am plasma Cortisol is not very helpful.

24 Hr Urinary Free Cortisol	25-280nmol
Creatinine:	60-120umol/li

Creatinine clearance: Collect urine in a plain bottle for 24 hrs and serum creatinine at the end of the period.

Normal 24 hr urine creatinine output	7-17mmol/24hrs
Creatinine clearance test	97-130ml/min
Other source: (M 97-137, F 88-128ml/min)	

BUN and creatinine are not raised until 60% total kidney function is gone.

See GFR, eGFR

Creatinine phosphokinase, Creatine kinase, phosphokinase, CPK, CK:

Male 38-174 IU/li Fem 26-140IU/li

Stop statin Rx if level is >5X ULN.

CK or CPK is a good early indicator of heart damage within 6 hrs of the event. Isoenzymes are MM (Skeletal muscle) MB (Heart) BB (Brain). Raised in newborn, parturition, MI, muscular dystrophy, muscle injury, (statins etc), surgery, exertion, myxoedema.

C Reactive Protein C.R.P:

Goes up in a variety of states: Tumours, pregnancy, infection and inflammation etc.

Has a half life of 18 hours and binds to the surface of dead cells facilitating phagocytosis.

An acute phase protein released by the liver. Raised in tissue damage, MI, (not angina), after surgery by up to 10X, inflammatory bowel disease, rheumatic disease, infection. Often used as an indicator of active but occult infection in neonates. "Acute phase proteins" include CRP, haptoglobin, alpha-1-acid glycoprotein, haemopexin, macroglobulin, thiostatin etc.

C.R.P. N   0-10mg/li

NICE have suggested using **Point of Care Testing (POCT) for CRP** to guide the use of antibiotics in patients with symptoms of lower respiratory tract infection in the primary care setting. Their guidance is:

Do not prescribe antibiotics if the CRP is <20mg/litre

For CRP values of 20-100mg/litre provide a prescription to be used if symptoms worsen

For CRP >100mg/litre prescribe antibiotics

this strategy is supported by a randomised controlled trial by Cals JW et al (Ann Fam Med. 2010 Mar-Apr;8(2):124-33)

Newer evidence ("Straight to the point") suggested in July 2015 that GPs measure CRP using "point of care testing" in the newly extended acronymed CRP-POCT. This is to try to differentiate viral from significant bacterial upper respiratory infections. How reliable, available and effective is this likely to become across the surgeries of Britain? A Cochrane review of CRP-POCT in six randomised trials led to a reduction of 41% in the amount of antibiotics prescribed. How much longer did these collected patients suffer unpleasant symptoms I wonder, or serious complications, (the ever increasing variety of septic complications) or go to A and E or the OOH Service for the antibiotics anyway, and will the GP ever realise? This technique can result in a defendable 5 minute decision as to whether antibiotics are appropriate (In case of complaint or litigation). However, I suspect the newly qualified dogmatic doctor who ignores thick sputum, pus on the tonsils, cervical lymphadenopathy, past patient experience and an ill, septic patient is still pretty unreasonable, uncaring and silly. In which case it is pronounced CRAP POCT. We know that practices and doctors who prioritise biochemistry results, ignoring the symptoms, history and clinical state of their patients risk missing serious early sepsis, divert precious clinical patient contact time to fiddling with the testing apparatus and process, are responsible for the exponential rise in Scarlet Fever, purulent tonsillitis and other infections including life threatening community acquired pneumonia, paediatric sepsis etc, lose the confidence and trust of patients as reflected in patient feedback and often adopt a mindset where a proper clinical assessment of the patient including a full examination is dispensed with as unnecessary.

C-Type natriuretic peptide CNP:
Occurs naturally in the body, acts as an anti inflammatory, regulates vascular tone and repairs damaged tissue. Renal production increases in renal failure, levels go up in heart failure and cirrhosis.

D-Dimer: Dd – A measure of fibrin turnover. Raised in pulmonary embolus, can be raised in atrial fibrillation. A risk marker with

t-PA, Tissue plasminogen activator. A specific derivative of fibrin, produced when the fibrin clot is degraded by plasmin. Raised in VTE, malignancy, pregnancy, surgery.

Has good negative predictability only.

Normal	<230ng/ml	<0.5ug FEU/ml
Normal D Dimer	<230ng/ml	< 0.5ug FEU/ml
Normal t-PA antigen	1-20ng/ml	
Normal t-PA activity	0.2-2 IU/ml	

eGFR
>90 Normal
60-89 MAY not be abnormal in the absence of a structural or functional abnormality,
30-59 Moderate GFR impairment,
15-29 Severe GFR impairment,
<15 established CKD.
For Afro-caribbeans multiply the result by 1.212.

Not reliable in Acute Renal Failure, <18 years age, pregnancy (increased), oedema states, muscle wasting, amputees, malnourished. May be raised in early kidney damage (e.g. in diabetes.)

Alternatively:
CKD Staging: >90 stage 1
60-90 stage 2
30-60 stage 3

15-30 stage 4
<15 stage 5

60-90ml/min Normal unless proteinuria, haematuria, diabetes with microalbuminuria or PCO or reflux nephropathy.

<60ml/min: Assess rate of deterioration, medication, test for prot (+>do urine prot/creat ratio) and blood. Assess clinically, BP, CCF
repeat eGFR etc.

REFER if stage 1 or 2 with malign. hypertension, K>7mmol/L, Nephrotic Syndrome, proteinuria +/− haematuria, diabetic
proteinuria, macroscopic haematuria, rapid fall in eGFR
or recurrent pulm. oedema.
If stage 3 with above plus microscopic haematuria,
proteinuria, anaemia, abn. electrolytes, other disease
(SLE, vasculitis, myeloma) severe hypertension,
If stage 4 or 5 without terminal illness.

Management: All stages: BP, eGFR, Prot/Creat ratio, annually. Cardiovascular prophylaxis (aspirin, statins). Meticulous BP management and Rx, (esp ACEI, ARB if DM or proteinuria), check for RAS*, stop NSAIDS, salt, K retaining diuretics, ACEIs and ARBs if raised K.

Stage 3: Do Hb, K, Ca++, PO4, six monthly. Refer for I.V. Fe if Hb low. Renal USS. Review drugs. Check Pth.

Stages 4 and 5: Check HCO3 and Pth three monthly. Diet, Hep B imm, referral re Parathyroid, acidosis, treatment options, ??dialysis etc.

*Renal Artery Stenosis

Estradiol see under the correct spelling, oestradiol:

Ferritin (See haematinics) and iron: M 18-270 ng/mL (mcg/li)
F 18-160 ng/mL
(Also 30-400ug/li or our local lab 15-150ug/li)

If Ferritin is raised due to tissue damage or as an acute phase reaction it can be differentiated from iron loading by measuring the fasting **Transferrin Saturation:**
In tissue damage or as an acute phase reaction it is usually less than 50%,
In iron loading it is usually over 50%.

Ferritin is the major iron storage protein and is present in virtually all cells. It is not the transport protein of iron (which is Transferrin). Ferritin can be raised with the ESR as an "acute phase reactant". It can be raised by chemotherapy and is concentrated in various cells, for instance: macrophages, hepatocytes and erythroblasts.

(Other source: >70ng/ml for optimum hair growth. "Normal" is 30-400ug/li.

A low serum Ferritin is only seen in an iron deficient state but there are several causes for a raised Ferritin.

For instance Ferritin goes up if Ferritin containing tissues are damaged (liver, bone marrow), with inflammation or infection, (Ferritin is an acute phase protein), genetic iron loading conditions, secondary iron loading conditions, (transfusions, haemosiderosis), chronic anaemias caused by ineffective haematapoesis – thalassaemias etc.

It is part of the routine screen in Coeliac Disease and alopecia. If anyone over 50 presents with iron deficiency anaemia, they need an upper and lower GI Endoscopy. G.I. cancers are a common cause. You can temporise by doing 3 occult bloods. The government believes in them even if my local biochemist says the test is no better than tossing a coin in excluding GI bleeding. Over my 30+ years in GP these simple tests have picked up at least 3 G.I. cancers and missed none that I am aware of in my patients by simply doing screening OBs as an investigation in patients with abdominal symptoms, tiredness or iron deficiency.

Other iron studies:

See IRON

Note: in **Haemochromatosis**: Ferritin is increased.

Aut recessive, 1:300 northern Europeans. Genes H282Y and C63D 9M:1F, (men don't menstruate). Rapid gut iron absorption and accumulation in various tissues. Causes cirrhosis, liver cancer, cardiomyopathy, diabetes, joint problems and pigmentation. Hence "Bronze Diabetes".

Bloods: HFE C282Y gene, iron studies, ferritin raised, (but this is raised in many conditions, see above). Transferrin index (saturation is >50%), (>55% M, >50% premeno-pausal F). Serum Ferritin only rises after liver stores are full. Liver biopsy?

1:4 sibs are affected. Rx Venesection. Deferoxamine SC, Deferasirox orally.

Folate (Red cell):	149-645ug/li
Folic Acid (See haematinics):	14-34 nmol/li 3.1-12.4ug/li
FSH – See gonadotrophins:	

Fructosamine:

Gives an impression of the blood glucose average for the last 2-3 weeks.
Normal level   3.8-6.0%

Full blood count/film:

Burr Cells – ("Echinocytosis") indicate a number of things: storage changes, uraemia, Pyruvate Kinase deficiency, transfusion.

Giant platelets-"excitable bone marrow" – L shifted megakaryocytes, not significant.

Platelets		$150\text{-}425 \times 10^3$/cu.mm
W.B.C.s		$5\text{-}10 \times 10^3$/cu.mm
Neutrophils		2500-5800/cu.mm
Lymphocytes		1500-3500/cu.mm
Monocytes		200-500/cu.mm
Eosinophils		40-250/cu.mm
Basophils		15-50/cu.mm
Red blood cells	M	5.4×10^6
	F	4.8×10^6
Haematocrit (Same as **PCV**, M 40-54, F 35-46)		0.42-0.5
Polycythaemia (erythrocytosis) *		PCV >56

Haematocrit can be affected by tourniquet, exercise, anxiety, hypertension, alcohol, smoking, obesity.

Haemoglobin	M	14-17 g/dl
	F	12-15 g/dl

Polycythaemia*   Hb>19g/dl
Mean corpuscular volume MCV   78-93fl
Mean corpuscular haemoglobin MCH   27.3-31 pg, 1.7-1.9 fmol
Mean corpuscular haemoglobin concentration MCHC 33-38% (gr/dl) 20-24mmol/li

In **pregnancy** you want MCV>80 MCHC>30. Some ANCs give iron if booking Hb<11 or if MCV <83fl later in pregnancy. But it is safe to leave if Hb is 10g, as long as MCV and MCHC are OK. There is a lot of haemodilution in pregnancy.

MCV is an unreliable indicator of alcohol consumption if B12 and folate levels are abnormal.

RDW Red cell distribution width (The range of *variation* of red cell volume)
                                                            11.5-16.5%
Reticulocyte count. <2% red cells: Absolute reticulocyte count   25-85x10⁹/li
Reticulocyte count   18-158x10⁹/li

There is a reticulocyte response within 2-3 days of a significant haemorrhage, maximum in 6-10 days.

Reticulocyte Index (corrected reticulocyte count) which compensates 1-2% in healthy individuals in anaemia, as the reticulocyte count is a percentage of a depleted total number of red cells.

Erythrocyte sedimentation rate ESR   **0-8mm/hr**

Neutrophil Counts at various ages:

Age Birth	Median Neutrophil Count	7,750
6 hrs		12,500
12hrs		12,500
18hrs		11,000
24hrs		9,100
36hrs		7,200
48hrs		5,800
3days		4,800
4days		4,250
5days		3,850
7days		3,400
10days		3,250
2weeks		3,200
3-4weeks		3,100

Blood Gases
PCO2   34-45mm Hg 4.5-6.0 KPa
PO2   110mm Hg 12-14.6 KPa

Glandular Fever. Monospot. Heterophil Antibody and Paul Bunnell Tests:
When patients develop Glandular Fever their antibodies to the EB Virus agent happen to agglutinate red cells from many different animal species. This is why they are called Heterophil (they like different things). The PB test uses sheep red cells, the Monospot uses horse red cells. The tests are not positive in the incubation period and are only useful during the active illness and shortly after (up to 3months – so they are of limited value in CFS.) The virus is, of course a persistent one, staying alive in the body despite the

improvement in symptoms. Burkitts and Hodgkin's Lymphoma, nasopharyngeal cancer and various HIV associated infections are caused by the infection long term but there is a number of other infections that can cause a Glandular Fever like illness.

To differentiate GF from other infections, the antibody (an IgM) is put up against Ox erythrocytes which absorb it but Guinea Pig kidney cells do not.

The test is specific and sensitive but can be falsely positive in Toxoplasmosis, Rubella (two of the conditions which, with CMV simulate GF) as well as leukaemias and lymphoma.

Epstein and Barr were both British but Paul and Bunnell are the sir names of the two American doctors who have to be admired for working out how the test would work. Not as I have imagined for 4 decades just one person.

The EB virus is a Herpes Virus, which causes Glandular Fever in half the teenagers that it infects. Neonates and the new born have maternal humeral immunity to protect them for up to six months and nearly all adults have antibodies.

Glomerular Filtration Rate: Urine concentration X Urine flow

$$\text{-----------------}$$

Plasma concentration

GFR is usually estimated using creatinine clearance (which is an overestimate of GFR due to active secretion of creatinine by peritubular capillaries.) You can estimate the normal creatinine clearance via "140 – age".

>90 is Normal
60-90 May not be abnormal –"in the presence of a structural or functional abnormality"
30-60 Moderate GFR impairment
15-30 Severe GFR impairment
<15 Established CKD.

Glucose:
In **Diabetes** (See diabetes section):-
Random venous glucose >11.1mmol/li.
or Fasting plasma glucose (8hrs without calories) >7.0mmol/li (N should be 3.5-6mmol/li) OR
Glucose Tolerance Test: after 75gr glucose by mouth. (OGTT)
Abnormal is:
>9mmol at 30min
or 2 hour plasma glucose >11.1mmol/li (new 2000 criteria)
("Impaired glucose tolerance" is <7-8mmol fasting but 7-11mmol at 2hrs)
-non diabetics should be back to N at 2 hours.
"Prediabetes" is fasting plasma glucose 6.1-7.0mmol/li (and OGTT 2 hour level <7.8mmol/li).
"Lucozade test"
3.2-7.8mmol/li
Lucozade™ (original flavour only) 73 kcal/100ml
Other flavours of Lucozade, Lucozade Light and Lucozade Sport Isotonic drinks contain different amounts of glucose so use the "original" only. The volume of Lucozade required for adults is **394ml**. (To avoid excessive fizziness, open the bottle 30 mins before

the test begins). The patient must consume the whole drink as quickly as possible and in no more than 5 minutes. Time '0' minutes is when the patient begins the drink.

Interpretation (WHO criteria) (Alternative source)
Venous Plasma Glucose mmol/L

	Normal	Diabetes Mellitus	Diabetes Mellitus ("Provisional")	Impaired Glucose Tolerance	Impaired fasting glycaemia
Fasting	6.0 and below	7.0 and above	7.0 and above	Below 7.0	6.1 – 6.9
	and	and	or	and	and
2 hour	7.7 and below	11.1 and above	11.1 and above	7.8 – 11.0	7.7 and below
			Note: If at least one other abnormal level on another occasion, then diagnosis of DM can be made		

Glucose-6-Phosphate Dehydrogenase Deficiency in RBCs:
Haemolysis of Red Cells takes place in children treated with
Aspirin, Chloroquine, Chloramphenicol, Dichloralphenazone, Dimercaprol, Mepacrine, Methyline Blue, Napthalene, Nalidixic Acid, Nitrofurantoin, PAS, Phenacetin, Phenazone, Primaquine, Probenecid, Quinidine, Sulphones, Vit C, Vit K1, Fava beans etc.

Glutamic Acid Decarboxylase (GAD) antibodies tests.
Anti GAD Anti IA2 etc help make the early diagnosis of Type 1 DM, GAD Ab tests are used to differentiate between LADA (latent auto immune diabetes of adulthood) and Type 2 DM, the differential diagnosis of gestational diabetes, risk prediction in family members of Type 1 diabetics and to monitor the progress of type 1.

Gonadotrophins:	FSH miU/li	LH miU/li	17-Beta oestradiol. nmol/li
Normally menstruating women:			
Follicular phase:	4-13	1-18	0.14-0.69
Mid cycle peak:	5-22	24-105	0.34-1.86
Luteal phase:	2-13	1-20	0.18-1.13
Post menopausal:	20-138	15-62	0.00-0.15

LH>FSH with high LH and prolactin in PCO. FSH high in menopause.

FSH: If >30iu and the patient is >50 years then you can stop POP or other contraception. Pregnancy is extremely unlikely.

The three gonadotrophins used to be known as LH, LTH (luteotropic hormone) and FSH. LTH is now more often known as prolactin or luteotropin.

LTH, prolactin:
Prolactin   102-496MU/li
Other sources: Hyperprolactinaemia >580miu/li in women and >450miu/li in men

It causes lactation, irregular periods in women, E.D. hypogonadism, infertility in men.

Raised with a Prolactinoma, Acromegaly, Cushings, hypothyroidism, Sarcoid, CRF, PCO and post epileptic seizures.

Drugs and hyperprolactinaemia: – More likely with the DRD2A1 allele and higher in women and in antipsychotic treatment for instance with Risperidone. Less with "Typical" antipsychotics – Haloperidol and with Olanzapine. Least with Clozapine and Quetiapine of the atypicals.

Many other drugs raise prolactin levels apart from major tranquillisers:

Metoclopramide, Domperidone, TCAs, Reserpine, Minoxidil, Benzodiazepines, Buspirone, MAOIs, SSRIs, Methyl Dopa, Oral Contraceptives, Sumatriptan, Valproic Acid, Verapamil, Atenolol, Cannabis, Ergotamine and occasionally some PPIs, H2 antagonists and Bendrofluazide.

Levels are lowered by Cabergoline, Bromocryptine, Quinagolide.

Growth Hormone:

Random Growth Hormone levels: Men: <5 ng/mL (<226pmol/L)
                                    Women: <10ng/mL (<452pmol/L)
                                    Children 0-20 ng/mL (0-904pmol/L)

Haematinics:

Ferritin   M 18-270 ng/mL (mcg/li)
                                    F 18-160 ng/mL
                                    (Also 30-400ug/li or our local lab 15-150ug/li)

and see Ferritin in section F above

Vitamin B9 (Folic Acid)   4.6-18.7ug/li

Vitamin B12   147-590 pmol/li 179-1132 ng/li

Other references: N 200-1100pg/ml 147-810 pmol/L 191-663ng/li 243-894ng/li

There seems to be no absolute **agreed** normal range of B12 – but you get the idea.

Raised Vitamin B12 levels may indicate a significant underlying disorder if levels exceed 660pmol/L or 900 pg/ml. Leukaemias, myeloproliferative disorders, hypereosinophilic syndromes, hepatoma, cirrhosis, hepatitis and so on can cause these raised levels.

Haemoglobin electrophoresis:

Thalassaemia: Autosomal recessive haemoglobinopathies which confer an advantage against malaria. They result in haemolytic anaemia, hypochromic anaemia with a N iron. There is a low MCHC as well as Target Cells.

Alpha Thalassaemia results in inadequate Alpha Hb production with excess beta chains.

Beta Thalassaemia affects Beta haemoglobin production.

(Note: Hb-A2 2.2-3.7% and Hb-F 0.2-1.0%.)

In Thalassaemia Major (Homozygous Beta chain Thalassaemia) there is lowered HbA and an increased level of HbF and HbA2.

Thalassaemia Minor is heterozygous Beta Thalassaemia. Hypochromic anaemia with N iron, Target cells, increased Hb A2.

In the Haemoglobinopathies, the haemoglobins are:

Thalassaemia Major: Hb A, F, A2

Minor: Hb A, (F), A2

Sickle Cell Thalassaemia: S, (A), F2
Haemoglobin C Thalassaemia: C, (A), F
    D   D, (A), F
    E   E, (A), F
Sickle Cell anaemia   S, F
Sickle cell haemoglobin C S, C (F)
Sickle Cell Trait   A, S
etc.

Sickle Cell Anaemia: Again, there is a mild advantage in malarial areas. No Hb A in the RBCs. It is replaced by HbS and HbF. Homozygous is the disease, heterozygous the trait. Chronic anaemia, haemolysis, vascular complications, childhood splenomegaly, osteomyelitis, African, Caribbean, Middle Eastern, Eastern Mediterranean and Asian populations.

Sickle Cell Trait: 10-20% black people. Usually asymptomatic until a hypoxic stress then Sickling can occur. Sickle Cell Screen; Hb F increases in pregnancy. Heel prick screening.

HbA1C: Glycoslated (glycated) haemoglobin:
Gives the glucose history over the past 2-3m (Fructosamine is 2-3 weeks).

Glycosylated Haemoglobin gradually increases over 120 days of exposure of the Hb molecule to 4 months of glucose and is a reflection of glucose control. There are HbA1a, HbA1b and HbA1c (the largest proportion). This doesn't work in chronic renal failure due to shortened erythrocyte life span.

The normal range is 20-40mmol/mol (4%-5.9%). It used to be suggested that:
A well controlled diabetic would have a level of 48-59mmol/mol (6.5%-7.5%)
Non diabetic   20-42mmol/mol
Recent research suggests 53mmol/mol (7%) is more appropriate as a target for managing most diabetics – as aiming lower may introduce a high risk of hypos.

A level less than 48mmol (6.5%) in diabetic patients has been associated with a higher mortality.

Also the diagnosis of diabetes can now be made on the HbA1C not the OGTT so:
HbA1C 6.5% and symptomatic – treat
6.5% and asymptomatic repeat in due course
6 – 6.5% give "lifestyle advice" and review ("Δ Prediabetes".)
Note: that Sickle Cell anaemia and G6PD deficiency give a falsely low HbA1C – and B12, iron and folate deficiency give falsely elevated levels. Fructosamine (but this reflects a shorter "window of observation") may be used in these cases. The level is unreliable in kidney disease (shortened red cell life span). Other situations that affect HbA1C are Erythropoietin treatment, alcoholism, splenectomy, RhA, antiretroviral Rx, aspirin, opiates, hyperbilirubinaemia, etc.

So roughly speaking:
An HbA1C of 5% (31mmol/mol) suggests an average blood glucose around 5.5mmol/li

6	42	7
7	53	8.5
8	64	10.2
9	75	12
10	86	13.5
11	97	15 etc

HbA1C ("DCCT" – Diabetes Control and Complications trial") is now being translated to mmols/mol (IFCC – International Federation of Clinical Chemistry)

So: HbA1C 5% = IFCC 31mmol/mol

6%   42mmol/mol

7%   53

8%   64

9%   75

10% 86

11% 97

12% 108

H.C.G. Human chorionic gonadotrophin:

H.C.G.   Normal values Urine HCG 0-24 IU/l

Serum HCG 0-4 IU/l

No ectopic if <50Us

Pregnancy >50 Us

Homocysteine:

High levels can lead to cardiovascular disease. Taking vitamins B12, B6 and B9 (**Folic Acid**) reduce levels. Levels are raised in excess alcohol intake, homocysteinuria, PCOS.

Therapeutic target   <6.3umol/L

Some consider the range 4-15umol/L acceptable depending on age and <12umol/L a good target

I have also read that optimal is <8umol/li for stroke prevention (If taking, for instance, prophylactic folic acid supplements (See section on strokes))

Human chorionic gonadotrophin:

Raised in trophoblastic disease, germ cell tumours, also goes up in pregnancy from 5-426 at 4 weeks to 7,650-230,000 at 8 weeks. 25,700-288,000 at 12 weeks etc. Higher levels in multiple pregnancy and molar pregnancy. Back to normal 4 weeks after loss of pregnancy.

If >1500-2000mIU/ml and no pregnancy on USS, then an ectopic is likely.

Immunoglobulins:

IgG   7.2-15 Gr/li (100mg=1U)

IgA   0.9-3.25 Gr/li

IgM   0.45-1.7 Gr/li

IgE (Routine investigation with RAST in asthma and allergies)   0 – 41 U/li

Iron:

Plasma levels undergo day to day and circadian variations of up to 30%, it can be increased by inflammation, oral iron, ineffective erythropoiesis.

Total Iron binding capacity   44.8-74.3 umol/li

Decreased in cirrhosis, haemochromatosis, haemorrhage, hypothyroidism, microcytic (I don't know why the same source says it can go up or down in microcytic anaemia, you would expect it to go up.) and pernicious anaemia, thalassaemia, various drugs etc. Increased in hepatitis, microcytic anaemia and pregnancy.

Iron

Adult male   50-160ug/dl 8.8-28.7umol/li (Different source: 9-26.9 umol/li)

Adult female   40-150ug/dl 7.2-26.9umol/li

Transferrin (The transport protein) saturation (with the iron it carries) has a diurnal pattern with a morning peak. It decreases in malnutrition like many plasma proteins. It also fluctuates with inflammation, malignancy, liver disease and malnutrition and is increased in pregnancy and on oral contraceptives.

Adult Transferrin	200-400mg/dl 2-4 g/L
Maternal	305mg/dl 3g/L
Newborn	130-275mmg/dl 1.3-2.8 g/L

TIBC is the maximum amount of iron that can be bound to Transferrin. It is increased in anaemia but normal in chronic inflammation.

Haemochromatosis:

Transferrin >55% (M)

      >50% (Premenopausal F)

Transferrin Saturation	Fem 12-45% Male 15-50%
Ferritin (correlates to body stores)	M 18-270 ng/mL (mcg/li)
	F 18-160 ng/mL

                            (Also 30-400ug/li or our local lab 15-150ug/li)

(Other source:) Ferritin must be >70ng/ml for optimum hair growth.

-can be raised with the ESR as an "acute phase reactant". It can be raised by acute and chronic inflammation, in hepatitis, haemochromatosis, porphyria, thalassaemia, haemolytic anaemia, cirrhosis, hyperthyroidism, MM, leukaemia, chemotherapy and also in certain other cancers: GIT, lymphoma, Hodgkins etc. Interestingly Ferritin may stimulate breast cancer and some cancer cells are known to manufacture isoferritins so the relationship is complicated.

Low levels usually indicate iron deficiency. Ferritin is a routine screen in Coeliac Disease and alopecia. Ferritin is not a transport protein but the plasma concentration is proportional to the body's total iron.

Transferrin is a glycoprotein iron transport protein that carries more than its own weight in iron.

Traditionally serum iron and TIBC and the % saturation (an indirect measurement of Transferrin) have been used to determine iron status. Although as you will be gathering by now iron levels and their measurement can be pretty hard to assess if the patient has started taking iron, has something else wrong with them, is pregnant, on the pill, has inflammation, cancer, or is on chemotherapy etc etc !

Fe Concn. = Transferrin saturation (Usually 20-50%).

TIBC

Iron deficiency tests: Low Fe, High TIBC, Low Transferrin Satn.

Serum Ferritin:	<Normal range	= Iron deficiency, "High degree of confidence".
	<40ug/l	=Possible Fe def – Lesser degree of confidence.
	<70ug/l	=Fe def in pts c inflammn. – "Moderate degree of confidence".

Serum iron decreased)   = Iron deficiency "Moderate degree of confidence".

TIBC elevated   )

TIBC normal   = "Results are inconclusive".

Iron overload: Haemochromatosis, Iron treatment, Raised Fe, TIBC N or low, transferrin saturation raised.

Serum Ferritin Increased levels: = reflect increased body stores.

Serum iron increased   )   = Increased stores but changes are not proportional
TIBC decreased or normal)   to the degree of overload. >60% M >50% F.
% saturation increased   )

Raised TIBC or raised transferrin is usually iron deficiency.

Low TIBC or low transferrin can be haemochromatosis, nephrotic syndrome, inflammation, malnutrition, liver disease.

If anyone over 50 presents with iron deficiency anaemia, they need an upper and lower GI Endoscopy. G.I. cancers are a common cause. You can temporise by doing 3 occult bloods, the government believes in them even if my local biochemist says the test is no better than tossing a coin. Over my 30 plus years of GP, doing these tests has picked up at least 3 G.I. cancers and missed none that I am aware of in my patients.

Other iron studies:

See Ferritin

Note: **Haemochromatosis**: Ferritin is increased

Aut recessive, 1:300 northern Europeans. Genes H282Y and C63D 9M:1F, rapid gut iron absorption and accumulation in various tissues. Causes cirrhosis, liver cancer, cardiomyopathy, impotence, diabetes, joint problems and pigmentation. Hence Bronze Diabetes.

Bloods: HFE C282Y gene, iron studies, ferritin raised, (but this is raised in many conditions). Transferrin index (saturation is >50%), (>55% M, >50% premenopausal F). Serum ferritin only rises after liver stores full. If the Ferritin is raised due to tissue damage or an acute phase response (ie not iron overload Haemochromatosis) then the fasting Transferrin saturation will be <50%. Liver biopsy? Rx Venesection.

1:4 sibs are affected.

Can be secondary as well, (haemolysis, Thalassaemia etc.)

Transferrin saturation is the percentage of Transferrin iron biding sites actually bound to iron.

The normal ranges are:

Serum iron   60-170ug/dl (10-30umol/li)
TIBC   240-450 ug/dl
Transferrin saturation   Fem 12-45% Male 15-50%

Transferrin is an acute phase protein and goes up non specifically in inflammation/ tissue damage. So if the saturation is <50% but transferrin is raised then the cause is inflammation not iron overload.

Iron Kinetics:

1-2mg of iron is lost in skin and shed mucosal cells each day and absorbed from the gut. Only a small fraction of the body's 4 gr of iron circulates as transferrin at any given time. Most iron is in haemoglobin and ferritin (2.7gr and 1gr)

Suggested Management Nomogram:
Iron Deficiency Anaemia:
Upper GI Symptoms?>>>>>>>>>>>>>>>>>>>Yes>>>>>>>>>>>2WR Upper GI Referral
v
v
No
v
v
Hb<10 g/dl (F)
or <11g/dl (M) >>>>>>>>>>>>>>>>>>>>>>Yes>>>>>>>>>>>>>2WR Lower GI referral
or lower GI symptoms
v
v
No
v
v
Male>>>>>>>>>>>>>>>>>>>>>>>>>>>>>>>>Yes>>>>>>>>>>>>>Urgent GI Referral
Female Age >50years/post menopausal>>>Yes>>>>>>>>>>>>Urgent GI Referral
v
v
No
Test for Coeliac antibodies, treat with Iron. Refer to GI Team if recurrent.

Lead: (Various sources) Children	<1.8umol/li (<1.21)	
Adults	0.3-2.0umol/li (<1.93)	
	Toxic concentration>4.8 umol/li	

LH, see Gonadotrophins:

Lipids:
The usual advice is to fast for 14 hours: But everything to do with lipid levels and appropriate treatments are goal posts that keep moving. Falsely elevated levels if the patient is on ascorbic acid, chlorpromazine, steroids, Vitamin A. Falsely low levels if the patient is on nitrates, nitrites, propythiouracil.
Generally:

Cholesterol (total)	3.5-5.2mmol/li (3.6-6.5)
Triglycerides	0.8-1.8mmol/li
H.D.L. High density lipoprotein	>0.9mmol/li
HDL/Cholesterol ratio	>0.2
Chol/HDL ratio	<5.0

But on the basis of Chol 3.5-7.2 and HDL 0.9-1.45, Normal HDL: Chol ratio 2.4-7.2.
LDL cholesterol   <5mmol/li
Primary prevention 5.5, secondary prevention 4.9-5.2
Alternatively: One teaching hospital says Tot Chol <5.2 desirable, >7.8 abnormal.
Tgs 0.8-2.0.
HDL (M) 0.9-1.9 (F) 1.1-2.6 LDL 0.0-4.9

In the US currently (2016) A "desirable cholesterol level" is
<5.17mmol/L >6.21 is considered high

HDL is considered acceptable	between 1.04 and 1.56mmol/L
HDL	is unacceptable below 1.04mmol/L
Triglycerides	should be below 1.69mmol/L
LDL	optimal is less than 2.6mmol/L

In Diabetis: Lipids:
Aim for Tot chol <5mmol/li   LDL <3mmol/li   HDL >1.2mmol/li   Tg <1.7mmol/li

Liver function tests:

If <3XULN can repeat in 2-3m if otherwise well. Commonest causes are fatty liver and statin treatment. The other two common causes in the UK are alcohol and Hep C.

Transaminases: A.L.T. A.S.T. Elevated:

Minor (<100iu/li) by chronic hepatitis B and C, Haemochromatosis, and the *commonest* cause is probably fatty liver ("hepatic steatosis", NAFLD)

Moderate (100-300 iu/li) as above plus alcoholic hepatitis, non alcoholic steatohepatitis, auto immune hepatitis, Wilson's disease.

Major (>1000 iu/li) Drugs, especially paracetamol, acute viral hepatitis, auto immune hepatitis, ischaemic liver.

Alkaline phosphatase   30-125iu/li

It is unusual for alkaline phosphatase **alone** to be raised in liver disease.

Gamma G T   M<0-50iU/li F 0-35iU/li

Can indicate alcohol consumption within a few weeks, also liver and pancreatic disease, various medications, anticonvulsants, etc. An isolated raised GTT with a N albumin and PTT and an absence of signs of liver disease may not require investigation. (JRCP 2002)

If raised GGT assoc with macrocytosis then 95% are assoc with alcohol consumption. Without macrocytosis, 25% assoc with alcohol.

Lactate Dehydrogenase LDH   266-500 IU/li

There are 5 isoenzymes

LDH-1 is found primarily in heart muscle and red blood cells.

LDH-2 is concentrated in white blood cells.

LDH-3 is highest in the lung.

LDH-4 is highest in the kidney, placenta and pancreas.

LDH-5 is highest in the liver and skeletal muscle.

LDH levels are used to differentiate an exudate from a transudate (eg pleural or pericardial). If the LDH in the aspirated fluid is >2/3 the ULN of serum LDH (200-300 IU/L) then the fluid is an exudate, less then it is a transudate.

Various drugs increase LDH levels and these include Aspirin, anaesthetic agents, fibrates, Mithramycin, narcotic analgesics and Procainamide etc.

Transaminases:

SGOT (AST) Aspartate-aminotransferase, Aspartate transaminase, Glutamic oxaloacetic transaminase   10-26 iU/li

Can be raised in liver and non liver damage. Slow rise after liver damage-from microsomes.

Raised slightly in new born. Glandular Fever, IM injections, pancreatitis, intestinal injury, liver diseases, musculoskeletal disease, toxic shock etc etc.

SGPT (ALT) Alanine aminotransferase, Alanine transaminase, Glutamic pyruvic transaminase   7-46iU/li

A more sensitive indicator of liver damage. Raised in liver disease, Glandular Fever, CVA, brain tumours, CCF, DTs, dermatomyositis, IM injections, MI, obesity, pancreatitis, post op, pulmonary infarction, P.E. Reye's Syndrome, rhabdomyolysis, various drugs.

5-Nucleotidase: 1.5-17IU/Li

If raised with Alkaline Phosphatase helps differentiate liver disorders from bone conditions (where it remains normal.)

Luteinising Hormone: 6-18iU/L
See gonadotrophins

Metals:

Cadmium	smokers	5.3-34.7nmol/li
	non smokers	2.7-10.7nmol/li
	toxic	0.9-26.7umol/li
Chromium		
Normal		<134nmol/li
(Metal on metal joint replacements)		
Cobalt		
Normal		<119nmol/li
(Metal on metal joint replacements)		
Copper		11-22umol/li
Lead		<1.93umol/li
Mercury		3-294nmol/li
	non fish eaters	<25nmol/li

Magnesium Normal Above 0.7mmol/li. Test Mg level in patients on long term PPIs, (which reduce absorption) on Citalopram (arrythmia), especially if on thiazide or loop diuretics, cortisone, aminoglycosides, amphotericin, cisplatin, cyclosporin(e) etc. Increased excretion in alcohol abuse, laxative abuse, diuretics, digitalis, malabsorption, excess sweating. Some evidence suggests Mg is needed as well as Calcium to prevent osteoporosis.

Low magnesium increases ischaemic and fatal ischaemic heart disease, arrhythmias, sudden cardiac death, causes Raynaud's. Magnesium inhibits platelet aggregation, lowers diabetes risk and enhances Nitric Oxide synthesis.

Normal   0.7-1.2mmol/li
See **Minerals** in Diet section
Zinc   10.7-23umol/li

Deficiency occurs in coeliacs, breast milk in the preterm may be deficient in copper and zinc (one of the very few disadvantages of breast milk made very slightly worse by pasteurising). One symptom of Zn deficiency is alopecia.

Oestradiol:

Early cycle	20-170pg/ml	73-626pmol/li
Mid	70-500	258-1840
Late	45-340	166-1250
Post menopausal	15-18	18.4-66
On OCP	12-50	44-184

(Plasma) Osmolality: (with an L it is per Kg, with and R it is per litre)
278-290m.osmol/kg
Plasma osmolality=2(Na+K) + Gluc + Cl mmol   (Generally: Osmolarity = 2Na+2K+gluc+Urea)

Parathormone:	Normal	10-65 pg/ml or 10-65 ng/L
pH of whole blood:		7.36-7.42. 36-42nmol/Li

Phosphorous inorganic PO4: 0.8-1.5mmol/li

Low Phosphate: Phosphate <0.9mmol/L. Ethanol?, time of day, ketoacidosis, post CHO-rich meal, glucose iv, exogenous insulin, malnutrition, malabsorption, Vit D deficiency, hyperparathyroidism, severe hypercalcaemia, renal tubular defects, hypomagnesaemia, osteomalacia, Rickets, dialysis, gout. Suggests need to check urea, creat, K, Na, urate, Ca, PO4, PTH & Vit D.

High Phosphate: Phosphate >1.5mmol/L. ?Old sample CRF, ARF, bone neoplasia, Vit D toxicity. Acromegaly, hyperthyroidism, hypoparathyroidism, leukaemia, sarcoid, uraemia, healing fractures, magnesium deficiency. Suggest assays of urea, creat., K, Na, Mg, urate, Ca, PO4, PTH, Vit. D & IGF1.

Potassium: 3.5-5.0mmol/li

After decades of prescribing sodium restriction to hypertensive patients, there is now some evidence that salt restriction may lead to increased Renin secretion which contributes to hypertension. An alternative is to tell the patient to supplement potassium. Increasing oral intake of potassium lowers blood pressure without affecting renal function. The "highest intake of 4700mg/day was associated with the largest SBP reduction" (Medline March 2015).

Potassium is found in high concentration in

Figs, molasses, seaweed, dates, prunes, tree nuts (ie not peanuts), avocado, bran, wheat germ and lima beans. Traditional sources are oranges and their juice as well as bananas.

High potassium

Potassium >5.5mmol/L. ? K-EDTA contamination from FBC tube haemolysis heelprick ++ fist clenching. High platelet/wbc count, drugs eg. ACEIs, ARBs & NSAIDs ?GFR, ivi, acidaemia. Addison's. Check urea, creat., K, Na, bicarb., glucose, FBC, cortisol, renin & aldosterone if cause unclear.

Low potassium

Potassium <2.5mmol/L. ? drugs eg. diuretics, insulin & salbutamol ivi. ?intake ?losses mineralocorticoid excess, renal dysfunction, liquorice (Na retention), alkalaemia, hypomagnesaemia. Suggest assay of: urea, K, Na, bicarb., glucose, Mg, Ca, PO4, aldosterone & renin, if cause is unclear.

Procalcitonin PCT:

A prohormone, 116 AAs, the cleavage of the molecule yields Calcitonin. Procalcitonin has a different biological activity to that of calcium homeostasis, levels rising within 4-6 hours of bacterial, fungal or malarial but not viral infection. In critical care septicaemic situations:

A maximum PCT level of 1-5ng/ml correlates with a mortality of 11%
51-100ng/ml   90 day mortality of 42%.

Progesterone (See Sex hormones):

Male 0.1-5.3 nmol/li (alt source: <2nmol/L) 0.3-1.2ng/ml (Alt source 0.1-0.3ng/ml)
Female follicular phase   0-5 nmol/li
Luteal phase   3.5-67 nmol/li
Post menopausal   0-4.4 nmol/li

Prolactin: 102-496MU/li
Other sources: Hyperprolactinaemia >580miu/li in women and >450miu/li in men
It causes lactation, irregular periods in women, E.D., hypogonadism, infertility in men.
Raised with a prolactinoma, acromegaly, Cushings, hypothyroidism, Sarcoid, CRF, PCO, and post epileptic seizures.
Drugs and hyperprolactinaemia: – More likely with the DRD2A1 allele and higher in women and in antipsychotic treatment for instance with Risperidone. Less with "Typical" antipsychotics – Haloperidol and with Olanzapine. Least with Clozapine and Quetiapine of the atypicals.
Many other drugs raise prolactin levels apart from major tranquillisers:
Metoclopramide, Domperidone, TCAs, Reserpine, Minoxidil, Benzodiazepines, Buspirone, MAOIs, SSRIs, Methyl Dopa, Oral Contraceptives, Sumatriptan, Valproic Acid, Verapamil, Atenolol, Cannabis, Ergotamine and occasionally some PPIs, H2 antagonists and bendroflu(meth) azide.
Levels are lowered by Cabergoline, Bromocryptine, Quinagolide.
Prostate Specific Antigen: (See Urology)
P.S.A. Prostate specific antigen. Varies with age, race, prostatitis, vigorous exercise, etc
                                           0-4 ug/li
Beware over interpreting the results and remember the generally benign nature of 90% prostate "cancers" (Gleason 6 and less, certainly) as well as the morbidity of virtually every type of treatment.
Even watchful waiting can lead to the unnecessary anxiety of screening.
On the other hand, up to 15% men with a level <4ng/ml have cancer positive biopsies. But then again,
4-10ng/ml can be due to BPH
4-10ng/ml the risk of carcinoma is 15-25%
>10ng/ml   the risk is   60-67% but
>4ng/ml 75% do not have cancer.
There are many confusing and conflicting statistics about PSA and whether they have any relevance to the health of the **individual** man attached to the result.
Free PSA: The higher the free to total PSA ratio the less likely there is to be cancer. The cut off is   15% or 0.15 (or 20% or even 25% depending on local lab).

If a man's PSA is <than 0.5 aged 40 his chances of getting Ca prostate at any age are very low.
PSA testing: a contemporary American view:
The American National Comprehensive Cancer Network has updated its screening advice, seeking a "Middle ground" approach.(2014)
They suggest routine screening on all healthy men from 45-70 years.
The American Urology Association suggests routine screening 55-69 years of age.
On the other hand,

The US Preventative Services Task Force recommends not testing PSAs in healthy men.

The ANCC has, despite casting its testing net further, supported conservative, active surveillance rather than definitive treatment in "early, low risk disease" (Half of PSA detected cancers they say are low risk).

European studies have looked at regular screening from the age of 55, not 45 but there was also a large Swedish study which did *one test before around 45yrs* and used the result to predict the next 30 years cancer risk. This baseline PSA result is more significant than family history or ethnicity in giving prostate prognosis. If this first test is "below the median" you do another aged 50 but you do 6 monthly or annual testing for those above the median.

The median PSAs are 0.7ng/ml between 40-49 yrs
and   0.9ng/ml between 50 and 59 yrs.
At least annual tests are done for everyone with a result >1.0ng/ml.

This is controversial as these levels are pretty low and a lot of young men are going to be worried and biopsied unnecessarily. Also, we don't know whether it makes any difference to the outcome, detecting and treating what may be fairly benign cancers five years later – (50 rather than 45)

Also when do you stop PSA testing?

PSA testing should only be offered to men with a life expectancy >10 years. The American Urology Association doesn't think screening >70 years is sensible, but the NCCN suggests we stop screening at 69 or continue screening to 74yrs but biopsying only if the PSA is >3ng/ml !! This is an excessively low level to biopsy at any age in my opinion and I tend to agree with the American Urologists (who presumably have to do the biopsies and deal with the frequent complications thereof) who suggest a biopsy threshold of 10ng/ml.

Even the experts do not have an agreed approach to dealing with the pesky PSA. Which is why its discoverer, Richard J Ablin, calls it "persistent stress and anxiety" (American National Comprehensive Cancer Network 19th Annual Conference 14/3/14).

Just to add to the mix however, the death rate in America from prostate cancer presenting as secondary disease has fallen significantly in the years since large scale PSA screening began-whereas the death rate from breast cancer presenting as secondary disease has not. Mammograms have been a national screening campaign in the US for about the same length of time as PSA testing. One saves lives apparently and one doesn't (– but it isn't the one you might have thought.)

Blood Proteins:

What you might have forgotten: Whole blood consists of red cells, white cells, platelets and plasma (plasma is 55% of the volume of whole blood). The Plasma is the intravascular fluid of the extracellular fluid compartment. The **Serum is the blood less the cells and clotting factors**-it includes the non clotting proteins, all the electrolytes, antibodies, antigens, hormones and any foreign agents (drugs, infectious organisms etc). Plasma is 95% water with dissolved proteins (albumin, globulins, fibrinogen), clotting factors as well as electrolytes, glucose, hormones and so on. Serum is just plasma without the clotting factors. Fresh frozen plasma may be separated from the RBCs and then the serum saved in order to be transfused to a sick recipient in need of volume replacement. Plasma factors are used in plasma transfusions, plasmapheresis, and components are used in Rhesus disease, Haemophilia etc. The main plasma components used therapeutically are human albumin, clotting factors and normal human immunoglobulin.

Cryoprecipitate from spun frozen plasma contains various clotting factors, Fibrinogen, Factor 8, Von Willebrand Factor, Factor XIII and is used in a variety of bleeding disorders.

Total protein	60-80gr/li
Albumin	30-50gr/li
CDT Carbohydrate deficient Transferrin	M 8-17mg/ml. Alcohol abuse: 9-136mg/ml
	F 11-22mg/ml. Alcohol abuse 13-60mg/ml

A sensitive indicator of alcohol abuse, raised within a week of increased consumption, drops within 2 weeks, can be slightly raised in liver disease.

Protein electrophoresis:
Plasma has these plasma proteins plus fibrinogen:
Albumin: α1 globulins, mainly α1 antitrypsin,
            α2 globulins, macroglobulin, haptoglobulin,
α2 are acute phase proteins (recent infection, after a few days and are actually anti-inflammatory),
            β globulins, transferrin and C3 complement.
Gamma globulins all immunoglobulins, reflect infection/inflammation.
Changes: Parallel changes in all fractions in malnutrition, haemoconcentration/dilution.
Acute phase pattern: α1 and 2 are up in acute inflammation, gammaglobulins go up in chronic inflammation.
Cirrhosis: Albumin and α1 reduced, gammaglobulin raised with fusion of β and gamma bands because of increased IgA.
Nephrotic syndrome: Low albumin, α1 and gammaglobulin, increased α2. Gammaglobulin may be raised if due to SLE.
α 1 antitrypsin deficiency: Reduced or absent α1 band (obviously).

α 1 antitrypsin	1.1-2.1 g/li

Produced by the liver, enters the circulation and travels to the lungs to bind with endogenous pulmonary enzymes designed to promote lysis of dead white cells and bacteria. Deficiency causes emphysema and cirrhosis.

Red Cell Folate	149-645ug/li

Renin: 0.5-3.1ng/ml/hr Levels raised in Addison's, cirrhosis, essential hypertension, haemorrhage, (renal compensation) hypokalaemia, renovascular or malignant hypertension, etc.
Low levels in primary hyperaldosteronism, ADH or steroid therapy.
If raised, you can try treating slowly with an A2RB or BB, if low or normal, Spironolactone or Amiloride.
More precisely: Adult recumbent: 0.5 – 2.2nmol/hr/li ambulant: 1.2 – 4.4 nmol/hr/li

Rheumatoid factor: Rh.F.	<40 iu/ml

This is an auto antibody against the Fc portion of IgG. "Rh F" is usually an IgM but it can be Ig A, G, M, E or D.
Positive in Sjogren's syndrome, RhA, in other connective tissue disorders, in 10% of the N population (especially >60 yrs) and with infections (EB, Parvovirus etc).

Sex Hormones:

Progesterone	Male 0.1-5, 3nmol/li
Female follicular phase	0-5nmol/li
Luteal phase	3.5-67nmol/li
Post menopausal	0-4.4nmol/li
Prolactin	102-496MU/li
Female:	
S.H.B.G.	26-110nmol/li
DHEAS	1-11.2umol/li
Testosterone (female)	0.2-2.9nmol/li
Free androgen Index	0.5-6.5

Sodium: 135-145mmol/li

Hyponatraemia can be caused by over hydration especially in the elderly, SIADH, – syndrome of inappropriate antidiuretic hormone (lung tumours, some brain tumours, ACTH deficiency, drugs etc) causing excess urinary sodium loss. Drugs which cause low sodium include: Thiazide and Loop diuretics, SSRIs (Citalopram etc), Venlafaxine, Moclobemide, Carbamazepine, Phenytoin, Sodium Valproate, ACEIs, Celecoxib, Desmopressin, Oxytocin, Cytotoxics (Vincristine, Vinblastine, Carboplatin, Cisplatin, Cyclophosphamide), Temazepam, opiates, Metoclopramide, Prochlorperazine, and some antipsychotics.

Hyponatraemia can be antagonised by the Vasopressin antagonists Demeclocycline/Tolvaptan (if due to SIADH).

Trimethoprim also causes hyponatraemia but with hypovolaemia (unlike SIADH) and needs treatment with sodium supplementation.

High Sodium

Sodium >150mmol/L. ? Fluid & elec. balance, renal function, ivi, drugs. If cause unclear, *clinically assess ECF vol.* & relate the physiological aims predicted from this to osmo. and Na conc. in spot urine.

Low Sodium

Sodium <125mmol/L. ? fluid & elec. balance, ivi, renal function, Addison's drugs, water retaining states eg. post-op., oedema, ascites, SIADH. If cause is unclear, *clinically assess ECF vol.* & relate the physiological aims predicted from this to osmo and Na conc. in spot urine.

T score:

Bone mineral density Negative values:

0 to − 1 are normal,

-1 to − 2.5 are osteopoenia,

Less than − 2.5 are osteoporosis.

Testosterone: Low is defined as <10nmol/li and Normal M 8.4-28.7 nmol/li

Free (blood)   M 174-729 pmol/li   >0.25 nmol/li

                                 F 3.5-29.5 pmol/li

        Percentage of total testosterone: 1-2.7%

        Total (blood)   Low level is <8 nmol/li M 10.4-41.6 nmol/li

                                          F 1.0-3.3 nmol/li

Male Hypogonadism if two separate tests before 10 am are <10-12 nmol/li. Do the sample at 09.00 hrs. Lower levels in February and October!

Hypogonadism: Testosterone, Free androgen Index? FSH, LH, SHBG, prolactin, digital rectal examination, PSA, cholesterol, lipids, gluc.

Thrombophilia screen:

Prothrombin time, Partial thromboplastin time, Thrombin time, FBC, Homocysteine level, Protein C, Protein S, Thrombin 3, Factor V Leiden and Prothrombin gene variant, Lupus (anti) coagulant, Anti cardiolipin antibodies, Anti B2 glycoprotein1 antibody, Activated protein C resistance, Fibrinogen tests, etc.

Thyroid Function Tests:

Can be affected by heterophilic antibodies, which alter TSH and T4 results. Low TSH in patients with non thyroidal illness, on glucocorticoids, dopamine.

TSH   Adults   3.0 – 20mU/li 0.35-5.5uU/li
           >age 60   F 2-17mU/li 2-17uU/ml   M 2-7.3mU/li 2-7.3 uU/ml
           Newborn   3-20mU/L 3-20uU/ml

T3 Tri-iodothyronine (Free)	3.5-6.5 pmol/li
Free (active) T4 Thyroxine	11.5-22.7 pmol/li
Total T4 Thyroxine	51-141 nmol/li
Thyroid antibodies Anti TPO Ref range	ELISA <155 IU/ml
Some say (anti) thyroid peroxidase (effectively the same as above)	0-35 IU/ml

Present in Sjogren's syndrome, Pernicious Anaemia, Addison's Disease, Myasthenia Gravis, Diabetes Mellitus and the healthy.

Toxoplasma Dye Test:

0-6 months any level reflects maternal antibodies.

6m-10 yrs 1-10% Positive at 1/16, rising steeply with age.

11-40 yrs 10-40% positive at 1/16 or more.

Adults: 1% have a titre of 1/256. Only rising titres indicate current or recent infection.

In ocular Toxoplasmosis, the majority show "Normal Titres" of 1/8 – 1/128. Negative results are rare and therefore helpful in excluding the disease.

The Toxoplasma Immunofluorescence serology is Norm: IgM titre <1:64 IgG <1: 1024
Indirect haemagglutination, No previous infection   titre <1:4
                              Probable past infection   1:4 – 1: 256
                              Recent infection   >1: 256.

Transferrin: (See Ferritin and Iron above):

CDT Carbohydrate deficient Transferrin: M 8-17mg/ml. Alcohol abuse: 9-136mg/ml
                                 F 11-22mg/ml. Alcohol abuse 13-60mg/ml

A sensitive indicator of alcohol abuse, raised within a week of increased consumption, drops within 2 weeks, can be slightly raised in liver disease.

Tryptase (Mast cell tryptase):

A marker of Mast Cell activation in systemic anaphylaxis and in anaphylactoid reactions. Less likely in food allergic reactions. Raised in Mastocytosis.

                                N 0-13.5 ug/li (ng/ml)

Urea:	2.8-6.6-7.7mmol/li
Blood Urea Nitrogen:	1.6-3.3mmol/li

Zinc: 8-23umol/li

Uric Acid: Aim to get level of Uric Acid as near as possible to 300umol/li (300-360) when treating gout with allopurinol etc. Certainly, less than 360umol/li.

If the average level is 300, there is a 10% risk of acute gout over 1 year. If average level is 600 then the risk is 87%

One regime is:

2 Gout flares per year:

V

Acute Rx: Colchicine, NSAID, steroid, diet

V

Wait two weeks or until asymptomatic
Aim for Uric Acid level 360 umol/li Rx Allopurinol (Start with 100mg) or Febuxostat 80mg
(Adenuric) – if intolerant to Allopurinol, mild/moderate renal failure, or patients on Warfarin.

V

Initially check 3 monthly uric acid levels then annually after first year, titrate Allopurinol
by 100mg (BNF Max dose in an adult is 900mg. Doses over 300mg in divided doses) until ULN
dose range or Uric Acid level <360 umol/li
With Febuxostat administer prophylactic NSAID (non salicylate) for 6 months after starting therapy
to avoid an acute attack.

Uric Acid Normal levels: M 202-417 umol/li
                                                  F 143-339 umol/li

Vitamins:

Vitamin A: 0.5-2.1 umol/li

Vitamin B9 (Folic Acid):   4.6-18.7ug/li

Vitamin B12 (see haematinics):   147-590 pmol/li 179-1132 ng/li

Other references: 243-894ng/li

The normal supplemental dose is 50-150ug/day as Cyanocobalamin.

Vitamin D (See Diet, vitamins and nutrition section):
Severe deficiency: <25nmol/li,
Insufficient Vitamin D: 25-50nmol/li – secondary hyperparathyroidism likely,
50-75 nmol/li replete but secondary hyperparathyroidism possible,
75-200 nmol/li optimum Vit D concentration.
Some texts will quote the "normal level" as seasonal, 1, 25 dihydroxy cholecalciferol (vitamin D3)

for instance in serum being   60-108 nmol/li
but in plasma in the summer   37-200 nmol/li
and in the plasma in the winter   35-105 nmo/li

Vitamin D toxicity is over 250-375nmol/li if sustained.

In terms of oral doses, 10mcg= 400IU.Supplements should be Vitamin D3 cholecalciferol not D2 ergocalciferol.

I don't know whether "normal" vitamin D levels are different in different racial groups but there is an American Vitamin manufacturer that says:

(this is according to GenSpec), one of the "targeted nutrient" pills contains more vitamin D for African-Americans and Hispanics because darker skin reduces the amount of vitamin D their bodies can take from the sun.

It is a good idea to correct the patient's Vitamin D level if it is abnormal in asthma and multiple other clinical situations.(See diet section for details)

Vitamin D supplementation has all sorts of proven health benefits: Seemingly legitimate studies show reductions in various cancers (colon, prostate, breast*), possible beneficial effects on Alzheimers, cardiovascular disease, respiratory disease, the immune system, infections, diabetes, metabolic syndrome, even on balance, – reducing falls and so on.

Raising 25(OH) Vit D from 30 to 40 ng/ml reduces breast, bowel and lung cancer 80% (Lappe et al*). Vitamin D does not overcome the negative effects of heavy smoking however. But probably "no one should run a level less than 30 ng/ml 25(OH) D" and President Obama was supplemented when his level was found to be 22.9ng/ml (2014.) New research however, shows that at high serum levels there is an increased mortality risk (J Endocr and Metab Mar 2015) so it is not QUITE the panacea some of my colleagues might have perceived it as. For its multiple other benefits see diet section p15.

Urine normal values:

Specific Gravity. S.G.	1.015-1.025
pH	4.8 – 8.5
Volume	600-2500mls/day
Creatine	<75mmol/day
Creatinine	0.13-0.22mmol/kg/day
	M 13-18 F 7-13mmol/TV
Urinary creatinine	7 – 17.7mmol/24hrs
Creatinine clearance	1.7-2.1mls/sec
	75-125mls/min
	150-180li/day

5 Hydroxyindole acetic acid 5HIAA (Carcinoid)	10-47 umol/day
Vanillyl mandelic acid VMA (Neuroblastoma, Phaeochromocytoma etc)	
	up to 45 umol/day
Normetanephrine	<2.2 umol/TV
Metanephrine	<1.3 umol/TV
3 Methoxytyramine	<2.0 umol/TV

24 hour VMA**, catecholamines, 5HIAA, Ca and PO4 are done in acid free containers but avoid bananas, plums, walnuts, ice cream and >4 cups of coffee for 3 days beforehand.

For the 5HIAA test avoid avocado, banana, pineapples, plums, walnuts, tomatoes, kiwi, aubergine, health food supplements, paracetamol, caffeine, ephedrine, diazepam, Nicotine, cough medicines, phenobarbital, aspirin, alcohol, imipramine, levodopa, MAOIs, heparin, isoniazid, me.dopa, TCAs.

V.M.A. Screen **

VMA	**<4.0mmol/mol creatinine**
	35-45 umol/day
Urine Nor Adrenaline	<500 nmol/24hr
Urine Adrenaline	<100 nmol/24hr
Urine Dopamine	<3000 nmol/24hr
24 hr urine protein	up to 0.2G/24hrs

More precisely:

Always quantify proteinuria with a urinary albumin/creatinine ratio (first morning sample)

Microalbuminuria is Albumin: Creatinine ratio >2.5mg/mmol (men) or >3.5mg/mmol (women) or Albumin concentration of >20mg/li.

Proteinuria is Albumin: Creatinine ratio >30mg/mmol or Albumin concentration >200mg/li

in other words:

Proteinuria: Significance (ie in Diabetes Mellitus)

	Spot Albumin mg/l	Albumin excretion mg/24hrs	ACR* mg/mmol
Normal	<30	<30	<2.5 (M)
			<3.5 (F)
Microalbuminuria	30-300	30-300	2.5-30 (M)
			3.5-30 (F)
Clinical proteinuria	>300	>300	>30
(macroalbuminuria)			

*Albumin creatinine ratio

Renal Calculus Screen:

24 hr Urine creatinine	7-18mmol/24hr
Urine calcium	2.5-7.5mmol/24hr
Urine phosphate	13-42mmol/24hr
Urine uric acid	1.5-4.4mmol/24hr

Stool:

Calprotectin (Faecal) A marker of inflammation: "*Over 50 is significant but **probably up to 150 can** be considered N in GP*" (?!). A neutrophil selective protein in stool, ELISA estimation. Accurately measures the number of neutrophils in the G.I.T. Sensitive marker of untreated inflammatory bowel disease (100%). 90% sensitive to Ca bowel, 50% Colonic polyps.

| Normal | <50mg/li |

If a <than 5 fold increase then likely to have relapse of IBD, UC, Crohn's. Assesses disease activity in Crohn's. Is also raised in Ca bowel and gastroenteritis.

Other source: Age:	2-9 years ULN Calprotectin	166 ug/g faeces
	10-59	51
	>60	112

Occult Blood (Faecal):

Some Trust departments have withdrawn the test as unreliable despite its "negative usefulness" to GPs and the national value as a screening test. Very puzzling.

According to NICE, referral to a GI Specialist should be based on Hb, gender, age and clinical details so these would not have helped my 25 year old female, with menorrhagia, with no bowel symptoms but with a R sided colonic cancer and a Hb of 7.0.

Wet faeces are unstable (false neg) (faeces on card is better). Vitamin C must not be taken beforehand as it gives a false neg.

The patient should be advised to avoid

Underdone red meat for 3 days, Horseradish, Turnip, Radish, Parsnips, Cauliflower, Broccoli, Melon, Vitamin C, Aspirin, NSAIDs, steroids, Iron.

Avoid while menstruating, suffering bleeding from piles, bleeding into the mouth (dentistry), diarrhoea, constipation, haematuria.

FIT:

Faecal Immunochemical Testing has an overall accuracy for detection of CRC (Colorectal Cancer) of 95% and 79% sensitivity, 94% specificity (Lee et Al 2016) FIT has been shown to have a greater sensitivity in detecting advanced adenomata and CRC than standard guaiac-based faecal occult blood testing (gFOBT).

Normal Adults usually show less than 2-3mg Hb/gm stool and lose 0.5 – 1.5mls blood into the bowel/day.

Faecal Elastase:(Stool elastase, Pancreatic elastase):

Elastase originates from the pancreas and remains intact as it passes through the gut. It indicates pancreatic exocrine function.

Faecal Elastase 1 is a highly sensitive and specific pancreatic exocrine function test. It is a good way of assessing (chronic) pancreatitis, Cystic Fibrosis, chronic inflammatory bowel disease, cancer of the pancreas and situations with abnormal pancreatic exocrine function.

Values   200ug/gr stool indicates normal pancreatic exocrine function

<200ug/gr stool indicates exocrine pancreatic insufficiency

In Cystic Fibrosis it tends to be <130ug/gr often <20ug/gr.

33: Obstetrics/Gynaecology/Pregnancy/Contraception:

These days a woman with an uncomplicated pregnancy is managed in the community by a midwife with or without the GP. Because we don't share in the routine clinical reassurance of normal women with normal pregnancies now I think we as GPs have "sleep walked" into giving up something which is rather important to our role as family doctors. Although most GPs would probably say they have enough to do today without managing the antenatal care of healthy women, as I and my colleagues all did from the start of the NHS til about 2005, there were some real benefits to this community role. Seeing a list of generally healthy, optimistic and happy women and (usually) confirming their normal pregnancies was a positive, cheerful and life affirming task for me which I looked forward to every week. I got to know my patients better, I had the pleasure of visiting happy whole families at home the day after the birth for no real clinical reason other than to check mum and baby were well. But this also had the effect of befriending me with the extended family, letting me assess their home environment legitimately and associating me with the positive feelings which were abroad at the time. It also cemented my role as the **family physician** to them all – birth to death, crying to dying, nappy to inco-pad. It was the only time I actually saw happy healthy people who were as pleased to see me as I was to see them. Obstetricians only became involved when additional care was needed.

After first contact (ideally at or around 10 weeks) there are generally 10 appointments for a nullip, 7 for a parous patient. The exact number of appointments will depend on the "risk" of the current and previous pregnancies (see below).

The benchmark manpower provision is supposed to be one midwife per 28 hospital births and 35 births in a midwife led hospital unit or at home. (RCM 2011). In 2013 there was 1 MW per 29.5 births.

The Mat B1:

Enables pregnant women to claim Statutory Maternity Pay or Maternity Allowance. Certificates must not be issued more than 20 weeks before the date of confinement. The EDD is put in part A.

SMP or MA is paid for a maximum of 39 weeks starting, at the earliest, 11 weeks before the EDD and at the latest, the day after the baby's birth.

Information for mothers:

Any woman thinking of getting pregnant should take 400mcg Folic Acid daily for the whole of the first 12 weeks of the pregnancy and for every day while trying to get pregnant. If they are planning a pregnancy I think they should be advised to take this from about three months before stopping precautions. They should try to avoid any alcohol, certainly drunkenness, and most medication.

Diet: Pregnant women in the top 25% of diet quality have a lower risk of having babies with certain heart defects-Fallots and ASDs than those in the bottom quartile. This is irrespective of folic acid intake or smoking.

The first midwife appointment should be 6-8 weeks after the first day of the LMP. At this the FW8 form (free prescriptions and dental treatment until the baby is 1 year old) is completed, the place of delivery, the scans (at 11+ – 13+ weeks, the nuchal scan – part of the combined screening test and the 20-22 weeks, the anomaly scan) and the blood tests that will be offered are all discussed.

After 20 weeks, the midwife will give the Mat B1 form, used to claim maternity pay or benefits. A Sure Start maternity grant and Healthy Start vouchers are available to those on low income later in the pregnancy.

The routine bloods in pregnancy are: FBC, BG and Rhesus, Rubella Abs, Syphilis serology, HIV, Hep B, Thalassaemia and HbS.

The "**Combined Test**" to exclude Down's syndrome is done around 11 weeks and consists of two blood tests:

Pregnancy associated Plasma Protein A (PAPP-A)

Free B-human Chorionic Gonadotrophin (Free B-hCG)

and the Ultrasound Nuchal Translucency test.

Nuchal scanning discloses not only increased Downs and other trisomy risks, but various chromosomal disorders, foetal malformations, genetic syndromes and congenital heart disease risks.

Major cardiac defects are

5/1000 when NT (**nuchal translucency**) thickness is below the median,

8.7/1000 when NT thickness between median and <95th C,

18.2/1000 when NT thickness 95th-99thC.

Thicker nuchal translucency is seen in a variety of foetal defects including:

Turner's syndrome,

Trisomy 18,

Trisomy 13,

Triploidy.

Nuchal thickness

up to 2.9mm Normal Karyotype:	96%
3.4mm	86%
4.4mm	71%
>4.4mm	38%.

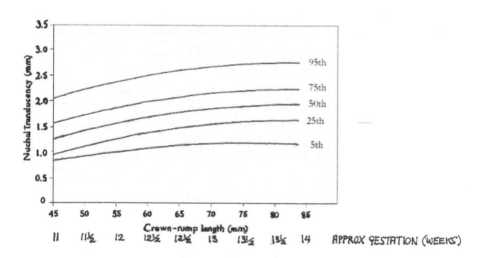

Diagram CRL NTD

Non Invasive Prenatal Testing, (NIPT) for aneuploidy (abnormal number of chromosomes) using cell free DNA in maternal plasma with whole genome sequencing can detect all three major trisomies and other genetic abnormalities via whole genome or targeted sequencing. It is not yet (2017) cost effective as a genetic screening tool.

This is also called **Harmony** testing, can be done from 10 weeks and is due to be introduced (according to a report in the Guardian in 2016) sometime in 2018 nationally. This detects up to 99% of Down's Syndrome pregnancies and has a relative lack of false positive results.

Things you may have forgotten:

Diploid cells are most specialised bodily cells – liver, muscle, skin etc. and contain two complete sets of chromosomes. They reproduce by mitosis to make exact replicas of themselves. Haploid cells have half the diploid number of chromosomes and are the result of meiosis, the formation of a germ cell. At fertilisation two haploid gamete cells (sperm and ova cells) will merge to form a diploid zygote. Normal human cells have 23 pairs of chromosomes, 46 in all in normal diploid cells. 22 pairs, autosomes, are the same in males and females, the other two are the X and Y.

Down's Screening USS tests include:

Nuchal Translucency: Average nuchal thickness at 12 weeks is 2.18mm.
At the end of the second trimester the nuchal fold is measured.
Invisible/visible nasal bone.

Ductus Venosus doppler:

This is normal when the "a" wave is positive, abnormal when the "a" wave is absent or reversed.

In one study, a reversed a-wave was observed in 3.2% of the euploid (normal number of chromosomes) foetuses and in 66.4%, 58.3%, 55.0% and 75.0% of foetuses with trisomies 21, 18 and 13 and Turner syndrome, respectively. Inclusion of ductus venosus flow scan in all pregnancies would detect 96%, 92%, 100% and 100% of trisomies 21, 18 and 13 and Turner syndrome, respectively, at a false-positive rate of 3%. It is also an independent predictor of congenital heart defects (eg PS) and a number of chromosomal abnormalities.

Intrauterine Foetal Circulation: See Diagram Paediatrics Chapter, page 864.
Movements:

First movements are felt by the mother from 16-20 weeks gestation (later in first pregnancies). Babies tend to be more active in the afternoon and evening. The number of movements felt increases up to 32 weeks then stays static. If the pregnant woman lies on her left side and is unable to feel ten separate movements in 2 hours, she should seek medical assessment. What assessment this is depends on the gestation. Lack of foetal movements or a sudden diminution in them is a warning sign of foetal distress and can be an early warning sign of risk of impending IUD.

Low Risk Ante-Natal Care appointments:

Pre booking 6-8 weeks: With M/W or GP at the surgery.
Before 11 weeks: Full booking appointment with M/W and bloods at hospital.
11+-13+ weeks: Combined screening blood and nuchal scan tests at hospital.
16-18 weeks: M/W appointment to review bloods and USS.
20-22 weeks: Anomaly USS.

25 weeks: First baby only: M/W appointment. Mat B1 can be issued.

28 weeks: Repeat bloods at hospital plus Anti-D if Rhesus Neg plus M/W appointment (Mat B1).

31 weeks: First baby only: M/W (Review 28 week bloods).

34 weeks: M/W Review 28 week bloods plus 2nd Anti-D if required.

36 weeks: M/W Confirm presentation.

38 weeks: M/W.

40 weeks: M/W Membrane sweep offered if first baby.

41 weeks: Post dates appointment (membrane sweep offered to all women and appointment made for induction of labour at T+12).

High Risk Ante-Natal Care Appointments:

Early booking 6-8 weeks: Pre booking appointment with Midwife or GP at GP surgery.

Before 11 weeks: Full booking appointment with M/W plus booking bloods.

11+-13+ weeks: Combined screening test &/or nuchal scan at hospital.

16-18 weeks: M/W appointment to review bloods and USS/or see obstetrician at hospital.

20-22 weeks: Anomaly USS.

24 weeks: M/W at surgery (Mat B1).

28 weeks: Further bloods, (Anti D injection if Rh Neg) M/W appointment or obstetrician OPA.

30 weeks: M/W or Obstetrician (to review bloods).

32 weeks: M/W or Obstetrician.

34 weeks: M/W.

36 weeks: M/W or Obstetrician to confirm presentation and mode of delivery.

37, 38, 39, 40 weeks: M/W or Obstetrician.

41 weeks: Post dates appointment at the hospital.

Refer patient to the first available A/N appointment:

Cardiac history including murmur,
Blood disorders,
Chronic renal disease,
Epilepsy,
Skeletal abnormalities: Scoliosis, #pelvis,
Diabetes,
Significant respiratory problems,
History of VTE or FH of VTE,
Haemoglobinopathy,
Autoimmune disease,
Malignancy.

Other early referrals:

Cone biopsy, diabetes in previous pregnancy, contact with infectious disease, cervical incompetence, Rhesus Antibodies, previous PET, IUGR, large baby, previous 3rd degree tear, shoulder dystocia, preterm labour, PPH, traumatic delivery, LSCS where appropriate, anaemia, obesity, fibroids, multiple pregnancy, "lifestyle", the very young and old, essential hypertension, recurrent UTI, significant other infections etc.

Although only 1:1000 births go "seriously wrong" in 2013 1/5 of the budget was spent on compensation claims and now according to The Telegraph (13/7/17) the amount spent on negligence claims has doubled since 2011 to £1.7Bn. This largely being perceived as negligence in the management and or supervision of labour and delivery. Errors during birth account for half of the total compensation payouts made by the NHS every year. This anachronism is dealt with elsewhere but briefly, is due to compensation levels set by the courts at the start of the NHS, ignoring that a cost free NHS does the lion's share of the caring for disabled babies and children. The courts assume all care will be privately funded. Penal compensation awards have never been shown in any country to improve standards or services. Compensation was designed in 1945 when the NHS was very different. For every multimillion handout the available funding for services and staff is subsequently reduced so that the likelihood of fewer on call obstetricians, available theatres and adequate midwife numbers in the future is increased. Undoubtedly, seriously damaged babies have an added practical day to day cost but this is nothing like the amount usually paid out and not the punitive purpose and sums of "compensation". The more compensation claims paid out the more disasters will happen. This is not, of course, how the lawyers see it. In 2016 they took home a staggering £500,000,000 in costs, 19% of the total compensation. If front line soldiers are (2016) to be exempt from vexatious lawyers and their self financing claims, should not front line doctors, who fight the enemies: infection, thrombosis, occult infarction, injury, asphyxia, inadequate staffing and facilities be protected when working in good faith too?

The Risk of getting pregnant:

Is 8% every time a normal couple has unprotected sex. 2% after PC4, 1% best risk after POEC (Progesterone only emergency contraceptive).

Sex ratios and recurrent miscarriage:

Male and female babies are equal in number at conception*. More male embryos are genetically abnormal however, so more male embryos are lost in the first few weeks after conception. Then in the next ten to fifteen weeks female embryo mortalities exceed male mortalities and this continues until the end of pregnancy with a final male preponderance. Overall (in 2014) the global sex ratio bias at birth was estimated at 107 boys to 100 girls (934 girls per 1000 boys).

You can try HCG 5000us Choragon injection weekly from week 6-12. It is unlikely that this treatment will preserve a genetically abnormal foetus but it may help support a weak corpus luteum until the pregnancy becomes self sufficient. But then again:

Sex ratio of foetuses: (alternative source):

At conception boy and girl foetuses are equal in number*. This is assessed by adding up embryos derived from all forms of assisted reproductive technology (3-6 days old). Then by one to two weeks after conception embryos with faulty sex chromosomes or 15th and 17th chromosomes are spontaneously aborted. Details from medically induced abortions and CVS shows that these faults are largely in males so slightly fewer than 50% of foetuses are male between 0 and 13 weeks. Subsequently a rise in the number of deaths of female babies due to developmental abnormalities in one of the two X chromosomes occurs throughout the second trimester. Here male foetuses outnumber female. At 38 weeks boys reach their birth critical weight triggering labour so the ratio by the 39th and 40th weeks is slightly female like it was in the first trimester. (The Vicissitudes of Sex, Scientific American, Oct 2015).

Miscarriage Risks:

Last pregnancy miscarried	19%,
Only miscarriages in the past	24%,
Last pregnancy successful	5%,
All pregnancies successful	4%,
Only pregnancy successful	5%,
Previous TOP	6%,
Primip	5%,
3 previous miscarriages	40-50%.

Dilatation and curettage increases preterm birth in subsequent pregnancies – as you might expect from instrumentation and dilatation of the cervix. M Lemmers et al Hum Reprod 2016: 31 (1) 34-35.

Although most web sites try to be reassuring about previous TOPs, they probably have a bit of an axe to grind and any instrumentation of the cervix increases the risk of subsequent miscarriage or premature labour. The more times the cervix is manipulated the more likely its competence is to be compromised. The figures above ignore early miscarriages which are extremely common. 50% of early pregnancies are aborted in total, 35% of recognised early pregnancies are lost early, 80% of miscarriages happening within the first three months (Web M.D. 23/7/17) and these are more likely after the cervical manipulation of abortion.

Investigations in recurrent miscarriage:

Chromosomes,
Rubella status,
Serology,
Anticardiolipin Abs,
Lupus anticoagulants,
Screening for Toxo, CMV etc.

I.V.F.

In vitro fertilisation: (Edwards and Steptoe the pioneers, – Louise Brown born in July 1978 was the first "test tube baby" and 17,000 UK patients are conceived per year now with these techniques. This is from 48,000 women having 62,000 cycles of treatment). In 2010 Edwards (who was non medical) was awarded the Nobel Prize, Steptoe died in 1988. Four million people have been conceived through IVF worldwide (2014).

Chances of a live birth:

32%	under 35,
28%	35-37,
21%	38-39,
14%	40-42,
5%	43-44,
2%	>44.

Flying:

The RCOG Guidelines (which contain lots of useful information on all aspects of pregnancy) advise no flying after 37 weeks in an uncomplicated singleton pregnancy and after 32 weeks in twin and multiple pregnancies.

To minimise the risks of DVT on flights of over 4 hours, they suggest graduated elastic compression stockings and Low Molecular Weight Heparin (LMWH) (Air Travel and Pregnancy, Scientific Impact Paper No 1).

Immunoglobulins and Infections in pregnancy:

Note: IgM goes up acutely, IgG later after infections. So a current or recent infection is usually indicated by a specific IgM. But IgG crosses the Placenta not IgM. Easy to remember, GPs help the mum and baby. MGs go fast.

Chickenpox/Varicella: A higher risk of pneumonia and encephalitis/hepatitis to the mother during pregnancy.

The baby may be born with Foetal Varicella Syndrome, if acquired before 28 weeks and may show:

Hypoplasia or loss of a limb,

Hypotonia,

Cicatricial (scarred) lesions in a dermatome distribution,

-Segmental areas of skin loss,

Hydrocephalus,

Microcephaly,

Horner's syndrome,

Cataracts,

Chorioretinitis,

Micropthalmia,

Growth retardation,

GI structural defects,

GU structural defects,

or develop shingles (28-36 weeks), or may be born with chicken pox (>36 weeks) or Genital Herpes.

Risks of Foetal Varicella are:

0.5% at 2-12 weeks,

1.4% at 12-26 weeks,

0% >28 weeks.

(DTB Dec 05).

Management of chicken pox contact in pregnancy:

If a woman who is pregnant has a past history of Chicken Pox and or has the typical scars she can be reassured. 90% of the UK born adult population is immune but caution is suggested with immigrants. In many other countries Varicella may have been rarer. If concerned, ask for booking blood to be checked for VZV IgG.

First there must have been SIGNIFICANT EXPOSURE ie: Face to face conversation or being in the same room at least 15 minutes. The infectious period begins 48 hours after the onset of the rash. The window for giving VZIG is 10 days after first exposure. This may not prevent but should attenuate the disease. Usually the bacteriologist on call will supply the VZIG on confirmation of negative serology.

German Measles/Rubella: Contracted in the first three months of pregnancy may result in miscarriage or the baby suffering: (The risk drops between 12 and 20 weeks):

Congenital Rubella Syndrome which Includes:

Cataracts, micropthalmia, glaucoma,

Deafness,

Pneumonia,

PDA, Pulmonary A. stenosis and other congenital heart defects,

Microcephaly, intellectual delay, motor disability, micrognathia,

Hepatosplenomegaly,

Blood (thrombocytopoenia) and

Bone disorders,

Inner ear disorders etc.

Group B Strep: Which can cause septicaemia, pneumonia and meningitis in the neonate. 30% carriage, 1:1000 babies a year get neonatal disease, need prophylactic IV antibiotics pre-delivery. Do treat Strep UTIs in pregnancy. Increased risk if premature ROMs >18 hrs. If a carrier, the risk to the baby is 1:300. Oral antibiotics don't eradicate infection/carrier state. IV antibiotics are now given at the onset of labour and four hourly thereafter.

Hepatitis B: Vertical transmission occurs in 90% where the mother is Hep B e Ag pos and 10% where mothers are surface Ag pos e Ag neg. 90% of infected infants become chronic carriers. Infants are vaccinated and given Hep B immunoglobulin at birth, reducing the transmission by 90%. Possibly this can be further improved by giving the mother Lamivudine in the last month of pregnancy.

Breast feeding has no negative effect on the risk.

Hepatitis C: Transmission to the baby is less if the mother is HIV negative and has not abused IV drugs or had blood transfused (<18%). Transmission is higher if the Hep C RNA Titre >1million/ml and transmission doesn't happen if the levels are undetectable. There is no current prevention treatment given.

HIV/Aids: Only 2% mother to child transmission of HIV occurs in pregnancy. The rest happens during blood transfer at delivery or during breast feeding.

1 in 450 pregnant UK mothers are HIV pos.

Mother to child transmission more likely in:

Higher levels of maternal viraemia,

HIV Core Ags.

Lower maternal CD4,

If the primary infection had taken place in the pregnancy,

Chorioamnionitis,

Other STDs or Malaria co existing,

Instrumental procedures around delivery,

ROM >4 hrs,

Vaginal delivery,

Preterm Birth,

Female babies,

Older mother,

First Twin.

Less likely if:

High levels of HIV Neutralising Ab.

Elective LSCS,

Zidovudine (etc) treatment,

No instrumental delivery.

Drugs:

Three antiviral combination treatment from 20-28 weeks unless needed earlier for maternal reasons. ZDV is given to the baby for 4-6 weeks.

A planned vaginal delivery may be offered to women on high dose combination anti retroviral treatment with low viral loads.

Breast feeding increases mother to child transmission 15% and should be avoided. With a combination of all these treatments the risk can be as low as 1%.

Genital Herpes: If there are no symptoms of an impending outbreak then a vaginal delivery may still be possible. Most gynaecologists would offer antiviral therapy from 36 weeks. However if a genital infection has been acquired late in the pregnancy or there are warning symptoms of a new eruption (with viral shedding) an elective LSCS will be offered. If there are no maternal antibodies to be acquired by the foetus (i.e. a new infection), the risk of transmission is up to 50% via vaginal delivery.

Listeria: Usually a D and V type illness, it can cause meningitis and a more severe generalised infection. Pregnant women are 20X more likely than the general population to get Listerial infections. Killed by proper cooking, the organism can be present in soft cheeses, (unpasteurised), blue veined cheese, luncheon meat, pates and meat spreads, smoked salmon, pre packed sandwiches etc. If acquired in pregnancy the maternal illness is usually mild with flu like symptoms, rarely it can cause serious CNS complications. It is more dangerous to the baby however – causing miscarriage, neonatal pneumonia, meningitis, septicaemia, micro-abscesses, with a mortality of 25%. Ampicillin and Erythromycin are effective.

Food etc to avoid:

All pregnant women should avoid raw and undercooked meats, sausages, handling minced meat, poultry, pate, (all types, including vegetable pate), probably Salami, Chorizo, Pepperoni, Parma Ham (Toxoplasmosis), raw eggs, mayonnaise, Brie, Camembert, mould ripened soft cheese made with goats milk, Danish Blue, Gorgonzola, Roquefort, unpasteurised milk, pregnant animals, cats and their faecal matter, sheep during lambing, more than a unit of alcohol a day (and preferably not that), liver products – pate and sausage, Vitamin A supplements (ie too much Vitamin A), raw shellfish, shark, and they should try to reduce caffeine. It is probably wise to avoid canned tuna because of the mercury and the FDA in America has sounded alarm bells regarding this. There are other restrictions – I would add horse riding, skiing, contact sports, water skiing, climbing, but not 90% of normal work. The government has also recently (2013) advised avoiding canned foods and plastic bottled liquids especially if they may have been allowed to get warm. The ubiquitous and totally unnecessary contemporary habit of carrying bottles of water everywhere (especially it seems by girls) may be hiding a health risk in the same way as some canned foods do. Traces of hydrocarbons from the plastics leach out over time, accelerated by freezing and by warmth or by microwaving plastic containers and these seem to be cumulatively carcinogenic, oestrogenic and may cause birth defects. Bisphenol A, Epoxy resins, DEHA, and various other compounds could be involved.

There is still an active debate about all this. Good foods to eat, other than a healthy mixed diet with plenty of green vegetables, folic acid and iron might include omega 3 fish oils in the last three months of pregnancy as this has been shown to reduce asthma and allergic respiratory symptoms in the first six months in the baby.

Vitamins:

Multivitamins were declared "a waste of money" by researchers in DATB in July 2016.

They did however support the taking of prophylactic Folic Acid and Vitamin D as well as eating a well balanced diet.

Fifth Disease: (Slapped Cheek) Parvovirus B19 can cause foetal death, hydrops (in 5% of infected pregnancies) due to anaemia. This is worse in patients with Spherocytosis and Sickle Cell Disease necessitating an intrauterine transfusion. There is only a 1% chance of a non immune exposed mother passing the infection onto her baby. Neither the cheek nor lacey general rashes in adults are always typical so any fluey illness with joint pains should raise your suspicion and prompt a blood test in pregnancy.

Swine Flu: (H1N1) Causes a 5X increase in miscarriage, spontaneous abortion or perinatal death due to congenital defects. Premature labour is more common. It can be vaccinated against and this is recommended for all pregnant women. If infected, antivirals, Zanamivir, Relenza or Olseltamivir, Tamiflu can be given for what they are worth. (See "Bad Pharma" which suggests these antivirals are pretty ineffective and much of the trial data which showed this was not made available).

Toxoplasmosis: Women and their pregnancies are safe if they have antibodies at the onset of pregnancy – however this is not routinely tested for in the UK. The convention in France is to test at the first visit and to keep testing the non immune throughout the pregnancy. This is because early treatment leads to improved foetal and infant outcome in terms of mortality and severe sequelae in later life (F Martin 2000 Trinity student medical journal).

The infection is spread via cat faeces, cat litter and food contaminated by cats, undercooked meat and poultry, unwashed fruit and vegetables. Most infected patients are asymptomatic, 1:10 feel fluey with pyrexia, lymphadenopathy, headache, myalgia and sore throat. Some develop encephalitis or even chorioretinitis. There is even a suspected link to some cases of schizophrenia.

Treatment: Azithromycin, Clindamycin, Spiramycin, Prednisolone, Sulfadiazine, Pyrimethamine, Folinic Acid. If a pregnant patient becomes fluey, it might be sensible to check this as well as the various other titres.

Tell pregnant patients to wash hands, surfaces and utensils etc. after handling raw meat and fruit/vegetables, to cook meat thoroughly, to avoid goats milk, to wear rubber gloves if handling cat litter and clear it daily, to cover children's sand pits to keep cats out and to avoid sheep at lambing time.

If an infection is demonstrated during the pregnancy (eg from maternal blood or a foetal cord blood sample after 20 weeks) detailed U/S scans are done and antibiotic treatment given before deciding on the next option.

Toxoplasmosis and CMV in pregnancy are very similar: In both, the mother can have a flu – like illness, a glandular fever type illness or be asymptomatic. Infection is transmitted to the foetus in 50% of maternal Toxoplasmosis and 40% of maternal CMV, both infections may result in abortion. For severely affected babies there are distinct syndromes:

Congenital Cytomegalic Inclusion Disease: Blood dyscrasias, Low BW, chorioretinitis.

Congenital Toxoplasmosis: Hydrocephalus, intracerebral calcification and chorioretinitis.

With both there may be jaundice, hepatosplenomegaly, oedema and haemorrhagic rashes, microcephaly, mental and physical retardation. The overall percentage and severity of those affected is worse with Toxoplasmosis than CMV.

Telling the patient how to avoid
Toxoplasmosis:
Don't clean cat litter trays (or do it daily wearing gloves),
Wash hands after gardening and after contact with sand pits, play areas, etc,
Wash vegetables,
Do not eat undercooked meat,
Wash hands after handling raw or undercooked meat,
Avoid unpasteurised milk.
and CMV:
Wash hands after touching wet nappies,
Keep baby and toddler fingers away from your mouth,
Avoid kissing babies and toddlers on the mouth.

Rashes in pregnancy include:
Rubella, Parvovirus 19 (Hydrops), Chicken Pox (20 weeks), all potentially dangerous.

Pregnancy and lambing. Potential infections:
Ovine chlamydiosis,
Toxoplasmosis,
Listeriosis.

B Haemolytic strep:
Can be up to 30% carriage in mothers, 1:1,000 babies/year get neonatal disease. GBS is a cause of severe early life threatening disease in the new born. DO treat strep UTIs in pregnancy. There is an increased risk if PROM>18 hrs. If the mother is a carrier, the risk to the baby is 1:300 but oral antibiotics don't eradicate the infection or carrier state.

There has been a debate as to whether to screen and treat the mother as they do in some other countries. (US, Australia and Canada). Intrapartum antibiotic prophylaxis (IAP) IS suggested for all women who have had a previous baby with neonatal GBS disease and who have GBS bacteriuria in the current pregnancy but until recently not for those in whom GBS is detected incidentally antenatally.

IAP should also be considered if there is: Intrapartum pyrexia (>38C) prolonged ROM, (>18 hr), at term, prematurity, (<37 weeks). IAP Is not needed after LSCS if there was no labour. The chemoprophylaxis is IV penicillin or Clindamycin IV/orally.

In many NHS hospitals now (2017) an incidental finding of BHS in the mother is a reason to get her in at the first sign of labour and commence 4hrly systemic Penicillin. Culture is by Enriched Culture Medium (ECM) swab, (low vagina or rectum), Rapid Test PCR or MSU. IV antibiotics reduce the baby's risk from 1:300 to 1:6,000.

Some hospitals use this check list:
Antibiotic prophylaxis in labour if:
Previous baby infected with BHS*
Positive MSU during pregnancy for BHS*
A temperature in labour of 37.5C or above or other signs of chorioamnionitis*
A positive vaginal or rectal swab this pregnancy*
Labour starting or ruptured membranes before 37 weeks
Ruptured membranes >18hrs before delivery.
The RCOG indicators for offering antibiotics are*.

See Fundal Height Diagram below.

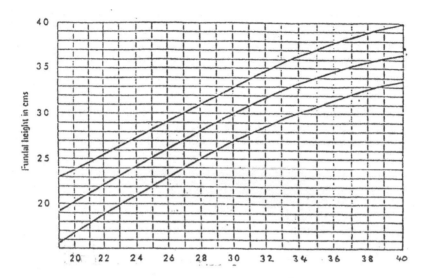

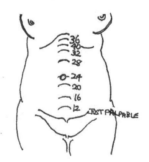

Fundal height measured in inches.

Normal Weight Gain in pregnancy is
10-12.5kg (just under 2 stone, or 24lb) – most after 20 weeks. The average baby is 3.3kg, 7.3lb. The placenta is 600gr. Breasts increase by up to 400gr. and the blood increases in weight by 1.2kg.

37-42 weeks gestation is generally considered "Term".

The growth of the foetus at different gestations:

Crown to Rump:
4 weeks: a poppy seed size (1mm).

8 weeks: (1.6cms) has eye lids, knee joints.

12 weeks: (5.4cms) eye lids, ears, recognisable arms legs hands and feet.

16 weeks: (10cms) now a small baby looking baby with a relatively big head and skinny limbs.

Crown to heel:
20 weeks: (26cms) a small baby, all organs formed, limbs skinny, big head and body. Now has vernix, is swallowing more and making meconium in lumen of large bowel.
24 weeks: Weighs 600g, (30cms) has taste buds and fingerprints.
28 weeks: About 1kg, (38cms) has eye lashes, turns head and blinks in utero.
32weeks: 1.7kg, (42cms) some hair, practices breathing, boys have descended testes.
36 weeks: 2.7kg (47cms).

Vaccinations in pregnancy:

Currently Flu and Pertussis vaccinations are recommended in the UK. The latter is to protect the baby prior to its own first Pertussis vaccine at 2 months and this now only comes as a combined vaccine (with Dip Tet and Polio) (28-38 weeks changed to 16 weeks in 2016).

The former is to avoid pneumonia in the mother and perinatally in the baby and to reduce the miscarriage risk.

Antenatal Screening:

U.S.S: Usually 2 in pregnancy, "8-14"weeks*, the dating (nuchal scan) and 18-21 weeks, the anomaly scan.

Nuchal Translucency:

This isn't actually a measure of "translucency" but a measure of the thickness of the neck translucence on ultrasound. The thicker the neck, the more oedema, the more likely there is a degree of heart failure and Trisomy. 3mm is the ULN at 10-13 weeks. There is a 5-20% false positive rate depending on the thickness chosen.

The best gestation to do this is 12 1/2 weeks but it can be done between 11 weeks 2 days and 14 weeks 1 day*. (Usually coinciding with the dating scan). The oedema and thickness of the neck of the foetus can be related to the presence of a genetic abnormality – particularly a Trisomy for some reason, or of congenital heart disease. The translucency is measured at the end of the first trimester and the nuchal fold thickness measured at the end of the second trimester. These results are taken with the Triple (blood) test (perhaps soon with the Harmony Test) to improve reliability. If the tests are positive, CVS is offered (If <13 weeks) or amniocentesis (>15 weeks). Both these are invasive and have a 1% (Amnio.) or 1-2% (CVS) miscarriage risk.

Antenatal Blood Screening Tests in detail:

Blood group: Rhesus negative mothers who haven't developed antibodies are given Anti-D injections at 28 and 34 weeks.

FBC, group.

Rubella, Syphilis, Hepatitis B and C and HIV serology (1 in 4 babies of HIV positive mothers become infected without treatment to both. 1 in 5 HIV infected babies develop AIDS or die in the first year).

In this situation Elective LSCS and bottle feeding are recommended.

Others are The TORCH blood tests (Toxoplasma, Other {Coxsackie, Syphilis, VZV, and Parvovirus B19 serology}, Rubella, CMV, Herpes Simplex Virus: – The TORCH infections cause a syndrome characterized by microcephaly, sensorineural deafness, chorioretinitis, hepatosplenomegaly and thrombocytopenia.

The usual Down's screening blood test consists of the two pregnancy associated proteins, Papp-A and HCG at 11-13 weeks with the nuchal translucency test. But if missed the" Triple" or "Quadruple test" measuring three or four proteins (obviously) are done between 14 and 20 weeks. These are:

Triple: HCG, AFP, uE3 and

Quadruple: AFP, HCG, uE3 and Inhibin. 15-22 weeks. These detect up to 75% Downs, with 5% false pos.

Low and high risk for Down's is generally taken to mean below or above 1 in 150.

The Double, Triple and Quadruple tests may include:

Pregnancy associated plasma protein A (low in Down's syndrome pregnancies),

Beta hCG (raised in Down's syndrome pregnancies),

AFP (low in Down's pregnancies),

Unconjugated Oestriol (uE3) (low in Down's pregnancies),

Inhibin A (raised in Down's pregnancies).

Overall the Down's Syndrome screening has a detection rate of 75% and a false positive rate of 3%.

The Triple test is unreliable in Diabetes.

Foetal Nasal Bone:

The absence of the nasal bone is a good predictor of Down's Syndrome and can be looked for at the same gestation as nuchal translucency.

Amniocentesis and Chorionic Villous Sampling:

Amniocentesis is the aspiration of amniotic fluid using ultrasound guidance, (no local anaesthetic is used for some reason), the cells in the fluid being examined for chromosome analysis. Generally the miscarriage risk is between 0.5 and 1%.

Chorionic Villous Sampling can be utilised earlier than an amnio to get cells for chromosome analysis (11 weeks onwards). Again a small needle is used, this time to biopsy part of the placenta (which is foetal tissue chromosomally). This time a local anaesthetic will be used. About 1% risk of miscarriage.

Down's Syndrome risks by age: (Overall 1:1000)

1:1900	age 20,
1:900	age 30,
1:340	age 35,
1:100-300	age 40 (various sources),
1:30	age 45.

The Crown Rump Length:

is useful in assessing gestational age at USS. It is accurate to within +/– half a week in early pregnancy, less so later on. The umbilical cord length = the CRL throughout pregnancy.

Thus: CRL at

6.1 weeks is 0.4cms,

7.2 weeks is 1cms,

9.2 weeks is 2.5cms,

10.9 weeks 4.9cms,

12.1 weeks 5.5cms,

13.2 weeks 7.0cms,

14 weeks is 8.0cms etc.

Anti – D

Is not needed if the bleeding, pregnant, RH neg. patient is less than 12 weeks gestation and is having a painless non surgical spontaneous miscarriage.

Folic Acid

Suggestion: All women 0.4mg/day OTC from stopping contraception to 12th week of pregnancy,

Women with a family history of neural tube defect 5mg/day (POM-prescription only).

Women who are epileptic 5mg/day. Folic acid may reduce facial clefts too.

Folic Acid 0.4mg was the recommended dose to prevent NTD given before pregnancy and 4 or 5mg/day to prevent recurrence. 5mg/day is the dose during Carbamazepine treatment in pregnancy. Naturally occurring folates are in green vegetables, liver, breakfast cereals, kidneys, yeast, beef extracts, Marmite, Bovril, sprouts, cauliflower, green beans, spinach, orange juice, milk, fortified corn flakes and bread. The *average* daily intake is 200ug/person. Doses >500ug "need a prescription" although 360 X 500ug tablets are actually cheap and readily available on the Internet. Water soluble, it is not overdosable. Doses >5mg/day may cause SACD (Sub-acute combined degeneration of the spinal cord) in the B12 deficient however. This is a condition I have often read and lectured about but have never seen. Preparations: 5mg Tabs, 2.5mg/5ml susp. Lexpec etc.

Pre-eclampsia, Toxaemia, significant hypertension:

This is commoner in the obese, the first time mother with a family history of PET, those with a history of hypertension and those with multiple pregnancies. It affects up to 8% of all deliveries.

If the patient's diastolic blood pressure increases above 90mm as well as >20mm from the 12-16 week baseline, this is suggestive of developing pre eclampsia. If with + proteinuria, then the patient's safety cannot be guaranteed for 24 hrs and they should be admitted. Oedema is not necessary for the diagnosis.

The treatment is aspirin, delivery, (post partum pre eclampsia can occur), anti hyper-tensives, IV magnesium sulphate.

In idiopathic hypertension:

You can try aspirin prophylaxis from 12 weeks. Methyldopa causes maternal S/Es in 15%. There are reputedly no foetal effects. Beta Blockers: proven: Atenolol, Labetalol, Oxprenolol all safe. Modified release Nifedipine is effective, Hydrallazine proven but weak, or give in emergency (I.V.). ACEIs are contraindicated.-? Prazosin Hypovase?

Diabetes in pregnancy:

Pre existing IDDM: Important to keep good blood glucose control before conception (4-6mmol/li pre meals.) Take Folate preconception, 0.4mg/day for 3m preconception and for the first 12 weeks of pregnancy. Shared care with Obstetrician and Diabetologist. The triple test is unreliable in Diabetes. Serial USS from 26 weeks, shared care plan from 36 weeks. Pre term Labour: Aim for BG of 4-6mmol/li. Normal management of planned labour involves admission the day before, IV short acting insulin and Dextrose, hourly blood sugar monitoring. Again the aim is a BG 4-6mmol/li. The IV soluble insulin is stopped at delivery.

Gestational diabetes:

At the first A/N visit, a BG>6mmol indicates the need for an OGTT (more than 2 hrs from the last meal means 6mmol is abnormal).

Any random glycosuria at each clinic visit prompts a lab glucose.

At 28 weeks a random glucose is performed.

If any of these risk factors is present then do a 75gr OGTT at 28 weeks:

>25 years,

Random gluc >6mmol/li,

Glycosuria more than twice,

BMI>27,

Diabetes in 1st degree relative,

Previous baby >4kg,

Previous unexplained SB,

Previous non chromosomal structural congenital abnormality,

Previous history of gestational diabetes,

Pregnancy hypertension.

A previous History of gestational diabetes requires a OGTT at booking, 28 and 34 weeks.

Note:

75gr Glucose or 375mls Lucozade **OGTT:**

Time mins	Normal mmol	Impaired	Diabetic
0	<6	6-8	>8
120	<9	9-11	>11

Women with gestational diabetes should be seen in the next joint Diabetes/Obstetric OP. If insulin is commenced in pregnancy it can usually be stopped at delivery but a 2 hr 75 gr. OGTT is done at 6 weeks post-natally.

Gestational Diabetes is commoner in women with central obesity and excess visceral fat. 3% of British pregnancies are affected. Gestational diabetes increases the risk of pre-eclampsia and hypertension during the pregnancy. After delivery there is a long term increased risk of Type 2 DM, CVD and Metabolic Syndrome. (Waist circ is a surrogate for visceral fat – apple shaped people not pear shaped).

Which women with GDM develop Diabetes? About a fifth over a period of 10 years. A higher risk is associated with older mothers, higher fasting glucose levels and 2hr level s on GTT, higher Tgs, higher BP and bigger waists, BMI>30 and lower HDL levels. I suppose most of those are just different ways of saying overweight, negative lipids, insulin resistance – ie metabolic syndrome. The need for insulin in pregnancy is also a risk factor.

The theory is that the metabolic stress of pregnancy unmasks a pre existing tendency to develop diabetes temporarily which improves once the baby is born, only to return in those women who don't look after themselves and develop or already have developing metabolic syndrome.

In a 2016 study (Zhang, BMJ Jan 2016) following 22,000 pregnancies over 10 years, there was a 27% increase in GD in the (nurses) who ate 2-4 servings of potatoes a week. Over 5 portions a week and the risk went up 50%. Chips, boiled, mashed, any kind of potato exacerbated risk but other vegetables and whole grains reduced it. Much as you would expect in fact. My experience of nurses in hospital restaurants is that they have at least one helping of potatoes a day – and a disproportionate number of them, now they have cut out smoking, are overweight.

Hyperemesis:

"Morning sickness" (actually a complete misnomer) affects 60-85% of pregnant women. 5/1000 have "Hyperemesis" in which there is significant weight loss. I would put the incidence at much higher than this, it isn't only wives of heirs to the throne. Overall, women with significant pregnancy sickness have a lower rate of miscarriages. So sickness really is a sign of foetal well being – this isn't just an old midwives' tale.

Vomiting in pregnancy: Try small high carbohydrate meals or sugary, fizzy drinks every few hours. Note that Thalidomide was a treatment for pregnancy sickness and only treat with drugs if absolutely necessary.

MOST of the drugs used are covered by caveats in their data sheets so only use them if you consider the benefits outweigh the risks and you have tried to temporise. Fluid replacement is paramount of course but IV fluid replacement is only very rarely necessary. Commonly used drugs are Promethazine, (25mg tds MIMS Mag 1/5/91), Prochlorperazine, Cyclizine and even Metoclopramide – which actually has the safest review in some write-ups.

There is a web site: Safe fetus.com (sorry about the American spelling) which gives a traffic light safety rating for drugs in breast feeding and pregnancy and Metoclopramide seems to be suggested as first line in pregnancy.

Unfortunately, Domperidone which also usefully comes in suppository form (although this is now very hard to get hold of) is said by some authorities to be contraindicated in pregnancy. However it has been used for a number of years in pregnancy without being recognised as causing any foetal harm or abnormalities. (Pregnancy Sickness Support online.) Both it and Metoclopramide do stimulate milk production though.

Ginger in various forms is as effective as Dimenhydrinate and Pyridoxine if you want a safe and alternative treatment but does actually affect bleeding. Not that many pregnant women are on anticoagulants but if they are on aspirin and ginger beware of the extra increased bleeding risk. The dose is 250mg (it comes in capsules) TDS (Summary of Evidence in Medscape Family Medicine Jan 2014).

If other treatments fail, Ondansetron, Zofran and even Prednisolone can be used (Monitor Weekly 18/1/95).

Other illnesses in pregnancy:

Depression in pregnancy:

Has been treated in various ways: Obviously there are risks associated with stopping pre existing drug treatment. CBT etc if available carries no teratogenic risk. Drug risks are generally small too. Various treatments are routinely used by obstetricians and these include Amitripyline and Fluvoxamine. Both are Class C according to "Safe fetus.com" (-"Studies on animals show adverse effects on foetus, no adequate studies on humans, only give drug if the benefit outweighs the risk" etc) It is probably best to avoid Venlafaxine and Paroxetine although the relative risk to the foetus is small even with these drugs.

A 2015 study on depression in pregnancy showed (Alan Brown):

Preterm birth is reduced 16% by antidepressants,

Very early preterm birth is reduced 50%,

Depressed women not on medication had a higher LSCS rate (26.5%),

compared with non depressed or treated depressed women (17%).

Depressed women had a very slightly increased risk of perinatal bleeding (3.5%) compared with non depressed and treated women (both 3%).

Antidepressant treatment did increase the risk of neonatal complications:

SSRIs increased "breathing issues" in babies leading to longer hospital stays.

DVT in Pregnancy:

Enoxaparin (Clexane) 40mg daily SC or Dalteparin (Fragmin) 5000IU SC OD – Pregnancy DVT prophylaxis. In suspected DVT, Clexane 1.5mg/kg/24hrs for 6 weeks.

Urinary Tract Infection:

Avoid Trimethoprim in first Trimester and Nitrofurantoin at Term.

Epilepsy in pregnancy:

If pregnant, change the patient from Valproate to Lamotrigine. Pre treat with Folic Acid. The patient can breast feed with all AEDs apart from Phenobarbitone. It is generally considered safer to continue on their AED than to stop treatment and risk harming the pregnancy through drug withdrawal and fits. Ideally the pregnancy should be planned and Folic Acid and a phased transition to a drug such as Lamotrigine considered in advance.

As a rough rule of thumb:

1 anticonvulsant increases congenital abnormalities by	2X
2	3X
3	4X.

Drug safety in pregnancy:

The organs vary in their gestational sensitivity to teratogens. There are critical post conceptual gestations at which harm can take place. Although damage can happen at any gestation, particular vulnerability to the:

CNS is at 3-5 weeks,

The eye is at 3 1/2 – 6 1/2 weeks,

The palate 10 weeks,

Dental lamina 6 1/2 weeks,

Lower limb bud just over 4 weeks,

Upper limb bud 4 1/3 weeks,

Gonadal differentiation 6 1/2 weeks,

External genitalia differentiation 9 weeks,

Excretory system 4-9 weeks,

The ear 5 1/2 to 7 1/2 weeks,

The nose 4 1/2 to 24 weeks,

Upper lip 6 1/2 weeks,

Heart 3-6 1/2 weeks.

Some well known Teratogenic agents:

Drugs account for only 1-5% of severe malformations.

The main teratogenic risk period is the first trimester but drugs given later can cause growth disorders particularly affecting the brain and eye. Genetic factors may determine some susceptibility to drug teratogenesis.

ACEIs ARBs   Oligohydramnios, renal damage and skull malformation (hypocalvaria) pulmonary hypoplasia, PDA, IUGR.

Alcohol   Abortion, growth retardation, minor effects on intellectual function and IQ, Foetal Alcohol Syndrome – craniofacial abnormalities, mental retardation, various major malformations, impaired growth.

Antidepressants Withdrawal symptoms. Some evidence that women who take SSRIs may have increased risk of autistic offspring. This happens, however, in women who are severely depressed on no treatment. In a 2015 study of SSRIs there were no birth defects linked to Citalopram, Escitalopram and Sertraline but there were defects linked to Fluoxetine (heart wall defects and craniosynostosis) and Paroxetine (heart defects, anencephaly and abdominal wall defects.) RVOTO is commoner with both drugs. Defects associated with both drugs were 2-3.5X more common in women taking the drugs in early pregnancy. (8/7/15 BMJ online) Again, in a more recent summary of SSRIs (Nov 2015) the risks of teratogenicity with the class were low but the two worst agents were found to be **Fluoxetine** and **Paroxetine.**

Antineoplastic drugs/antimetabolites. Particularly Folic Acid antagonists. Spontaneous abortion. CNS, limb and kidney deformities. Also included are colchicine, podophylotoxin, azathioprine which are teratogenic in animals.

Antipsychotics   Withdrawal symptoms.

Anxiolytics/Lithium Withdrawal symptoms, hypotonia.

Benzodiazepines   IUGR, characteristic facies: slanted eyes, short retroussé nose, epicanthic folds, dysplastic ears, lack of expression, high arched palate, webbed neck, wide nipples, mental retardation, choreoathetosis, muscle weakness, cranial N dysfunction. At lower doses functional rather than structural neurological abnormalities (hypotonia, delayed coordination, motor and intellectual development) are more common.

Beta Blockers   IUGR, bradycardia, hypoglycaemia.

Cytotoxics   IUGR, stillbirth.

NSAIDs   Closure of PDA, pulmonary hypertension.

Older antiepileptics Impaired neurodevelopment. The incidence of congenital abnormality is 2-3X higher in mother taking AEDs For instance: Foetal Phenytoin syndrome (Hydantoin) includes microcephaly and craniofacial defects etc. Carbamazepine affects foetal head growth, Valproate causes a number of congenital abnormalities including spina bifida.

Foetal Valproate Syndrome: Craniofacial abnormalities – epicanthic folds, flat nasal bridge, shallow philtrum, thin upper lip, thick lower lip, anteverted nostrils. Trigonocephaly, skull defects, facial hypoplasia, narrow forehead, low set ears with deformed lobes, infraorbital eye creases, carp mouth, inguinal hernias, polydactyly, deformed thumbs, spina bifida, VSD, PDA, coarctation, hypospadias, cryporchidism, retarded growth, developmental delay, various neurological abnormalities etc.

Most epileptic mothers taking prophylaxis do have normal babies though and it has to be remembered that there is a considerable risk to the baby of an uncontrolled epileptic. Minimise the number of drugs, give Folic Acid early.

Opioids   Withdrawal, respiratory depression.
Retinoids   CNS dysfunction.
Salicylates   Foetal/neonatal haemorrhage.
Sex hormones   Masculinisation/feminisation of the foetus (this includes Norethisterone). Any risk to the foetus of the COCP being taken at conception (or immediately before) is very small but some studies have shown negative effects including a small risk of Down's Syndrome if conception takes place within 1m of taking the pill.
Steroids   Cleft palate, cataract.
Sulphonamides   Jaundice, kernicterus.
Tetracyclines   Staining of teeth, impaired bone growth.
Valproate   Autism, Foetal Valproate Syndrome (See below).
Warfarin/coumarins* Foetal haemorrhage, CNS abnormalities. Foetal Warfarin Syndrome – nasal hypoplasia, chondrodysplasia punctata, optic atrophy, microcephaly, mental retardation. Switch to Heparin (long term use of which can cause osteoporosis.)

Triptans in pregnancy have been found to be remarkably safe: A registry of major birth defects covering 16 years and 680 pregnant women with 689 children, published in September 2014, found major birth defects at a rate of 4.2%. This is the same as the background (non drug) rate. This applied to Sumatriptan and Naratriptan taken in the first trimester.

Anticoagulants and pregnancy:*

Heparin in first 6-9 weeks then oral anticoagulants 16th-36th week then heparin again. Heparin throughout can cause osteoporosis. Anticoagulation in some studies caused (in 7%) congenital abnormalities, S.B. or abortion, in 16% if oral treatment continued throughout pregnancy.

Warfarin if given perinatally can cause CNS defects, spontaneous abortion, SB, prematurity and haemorrhage. Ocular defects may occur if given anytime during pregnancy. There is a foetal Warfarin syndrome if given in the first trimester. (Nasal hypoplasia, hypoplasia of the extremities, developmental retardation etc). Most of these effects are dose dependent, especially >5mg/day.

Epiphyseal stippling is seen on X Ray. 2/3 of foetuses exposed to Warfarin in pregnancy are born normal and breast fed babies of mothers taking Warfarin are generally considered safe.(Drugs. com)

Caesarean Section:

The more evidence gathered about this surgical form of delivery, the less healthy it sees to become. In the US between a quarter and a third of babies are born this way (having gone up 5X in 20 years). It is the most common surgical procedure done in the US, at 32.9% (2010) of deliveries. It is one in four deliveries over here. When I trained it was more like 5%. There is now evidence that babies born by section become fatter children and suffer a variety of other subtle long term side effects-including those related to a deprived gastrointestinal microbiome. *Arch Dis Child doi:10.1136/archdischild-2011-301141.*

The complications of Caesarean Section are:
For the mother:
Infection of wound,

Endometritis,

UTI,

DVT,

Ileus,

Adhesions,

Anaesthetic complications,

Surgical complications (urological and gynaecological),

Possible emergency hysterectomy,

Pain,

Bleeding,

Possible further operative deliveries,

Slightly increased risk of subsequent placenta praevia and placental implantation that may be too deep,

1:200 uterine rupture in future labour,

Longer total recovery time,

Medication adverse reactions,

Slightly higher maternal mortality,

Bonding issues/attachment/breastfeeding difficulties,

Endometriosis is commoner,

Infertility,

Future prematurity and LBW/SB?,

Appendicitis, stroke and gallstones are commoner in the following year,

For the baby:

Resuscitation procedures (oropharyngeal suction etc) discourage breast feeding,

Adverse maternal drug reactions in foetus,

Less and delayed skin to skin contact time,

Calculating the correct gestation problematic if the LSCS is elective (increased risk of prematurity),

Foetal tachypnoea,

Prematurity complications,

Increased admission to SCBU,

Delayed breast feeding,

Childhood asthma,

Death perinatally,

Low APGARS (Anaesthesia, lack of the normal preparation associated with a normal labour),

Possible surgical injury,

Microbiome disruption of the neonate and subsequent complications related to that.

Perinatal Injury/Stillbirth/Prematurity:

Worldwide, prematurity kills more children than the traditional, historic, developing-world killers, accidents and infectious diseases. That amounts to 1m deaths a year with the complications of childbirth leading to a further 720,000 deaths a year. In the UK approximately 1400 babies die directly from *prematurity* annually. One in every eight babies in the UK is born premature. That is 80,000 babies every year. Air pollution levels (of particulates) increase the rate of premature birth especially if the mother is exposed in the third trimester.

In 2014, the RCOG announced a 5 year plan* to halve the number of stillbirths, newborn deaths and brain injuries in the UK. 500 British babies each year are severely disabled or die from *labour complications.* Smoking increases the risk significantly of "birth complications". Obesity increases stillbirths: 17.3 stillborn/1000 being the incidence in the severely obese mother (BMI>or= 35) The incidence for "lean" (BMI <or= 25) being 7.7/1000. The hazard ratios for stillbirth are:

BMI 25-30   1.1-1.8
BMI 30-35   1.3-2.4
BMI >35   1.5-2.8

In the UK there are 4,000 stillbirths and 40,000 miscarriages a year resulting in hospital admission. (The total of 3286 SBs was quoted in a radio programme on SB in January 2016 – "More than Cot deaths and more than deaths between the age of 1 and 5"). Higher incidences of SBs are seen in the obese, smokers, drinkers, ethnic minorities. I would estimate that of those who come to my attention as a GP I only refer between a quarter and a third of symptomatic miscarriages during or after the event. Most settle without treatment at home so the real number, even excluding "early miscarriages" is therefore much higher. SANDS, a stillborn and neonatal death charity, says 60% of term pregnancies ending in stillbirth could be prevented by applying the minimum standards of antenatal care and guidance for mothers and babies. According to NHS choices, 10% of stillbirths have a birth defect linked to their death while half are related to placental complications. If all women had placental dopplers, 1,500 babies a year could be saved (Prof Kypros Nicolaides 2014).

The current initiative* is called "Each baby counts" – a rather pointless, trendy, obvious, Royal College of Midwives focus group type of statement, you might think. You can't imagine a "Call the Midwife" era midwife bothering to say something as bland and obvious as this.

As well as smoking, pre term delivery, low birth weight, various "life style factors" can cause foetal damage around delivery. Smoking alone causes 2,200 preterm births, 5,000 miscarriages and 300 perinatal deaths per year in the UK. Maternal smoking even directly reduces the rate of foetal cell division.

New evidence suggests that being born pre term or low birth weight (<32 weeks or <1.5Kg) may affect the baby's brain development and long term personality.(Arch Dis Ch Fet and Neonat Ed, Univadis 31/Jul/2015) with a socially withdrawn personality, autistic features, neuroticism, introversion and decreased risk taking being commoner as the child becomes an adult).

As if we needed more evidence that prematurity caused long term harm, a study in Arch Dis Ch(2014-308059) blamed it, congenital abnormalities and untreated infections for the double preschool death rate in the UK compared with Sweden. At the time, Sweden spent 8% of GDP on healthcare, just as we did. The paper raised questions about the **paediatric training and competence of UK GPs**-something I allude to elsewhere. I think it should be a compulsory part of all GP rotations. Our death rate between 2006 and 2008 of under 5's was 614/100,000 compared with 328 in Sweden.

Our main causes of death under age 5 were problems associated with premature birth, congenital abnormalities and infections. In Sweden the three commonest causes of death were congenital abnormalities, complications of pregnancy and labour and infections. The incidences of the latter were 64 and 35/100,000 in UK and Sweden respectively which must reflect the quality of paediatric skills of GPs or relative access to early paediatric services in the two countries. The current obsession with withholding antibiotics in the UK can surely only make things worse (?)

The death rate from premature birth was 13x higher in the UK and the rate of prematurity in the UK is still rising. This poor outcome was said to be due to adverse social determinants rather than poor neonatal intensive care. On the other hand where medical care was at fault was:

Treatable infections, pneumonia, meningitis and septicaemia in neonates and young children were treated late and poorly and had higher mortality rates in the UK (P<0.001). The authors comment that the **main determinant is the lack of paediatric experience of British doctors** compared with their Swedish counterparts. Amen to that.

In a slightly different study which looked at single normal babies carried to term but stillborn in 2013 (133 in the study in total) it was stated that there were 1000 of these babies in the UK per year. The notes of the mothers were examined and it was found that:

2/3 of mothers with a risk factor of developing diabetes were not offered testing,

2/3 did not have the growth of their baby monitored as set out in national guidance (unbelievable).

Half of the women had contacted the maternity unit concerned that the baby's movements had slowed, changed or stopped. The study noted half these cases had missed opportunities to save the baby which included misinterpretation of the foetal heart trace.

Only a quarter of cases were followed by an internal review and the reviews that did happen were of very variable quality.

These reviews, and not suing the doctors, are the only things that have been shown to improve the quality of care in any medical environment all over the world and it is hard for me to believe that these departmental (once weekly) meetings don't happen everywhere. They were the focus of my week as an obstetric and neonatal SHO and registrar **35 years ago.**

The report suggested a post mortem and follow up for all parents of stillborn babies with the consultant, specifically to discuss future risks. Surely though, all this is obvious and mandatory in any ethical unit?(Harris Birthright Centre).

Perinatal Mortality Rates in the UK:

(Perinatal mortality is the number of stillbirths and deaths in the first week of life, Infant mortality is the first year, neonatal mortality is the first 28 days.)

In 2011 the infant mortality rate was 4.1 deaths per 1,000 live births, the lowest ever recorded for England and Wales.

Infant mortality rates were highest among babies of mothers aged under 20 years and 40 years and over at 5.4 deaths per 1,000 live births, much as you would expect.

Perinatal mortality rates were also higher for mothers in the 'under 20' and '40 and over' age groups, at 9.2 and 11.2 deaths per 1,000 live births respectively.

Very low birth weight babies (under 1,500 grams) had the highest infant and perinatal mortality rates, at 172.1 and 260.8 deaths per 1,000 live births respectively.

Infant mortality rates were highest for babies registered solely by their mother and those registered jointly by parents living at different addresses, at 5.7 and 5.4 deaths per 1,000 live births respectively.

Girls

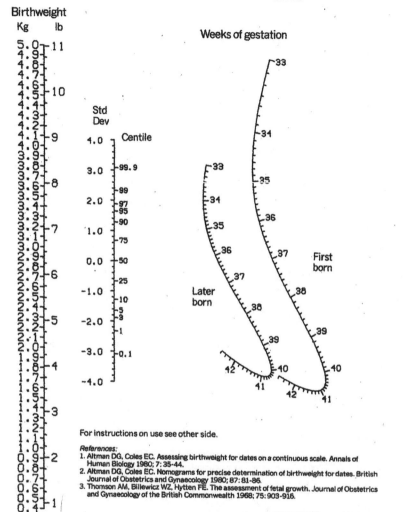

Birthweight
Kg   lb

Weeks of gestation

Std Dev

Centile

For instructions on use see other side.

References:
1. Altman DG, Coles EC. Assessing birthweight for dates on a continuous scale. Annals of Human Biology 1980; 7: 35-44.
2. Altman DG, Coles EC. Nomograms for precise determination of birthweight for dates. British Journal of Obstetrics and Gynaecology 1980; 87: 81-86.
3. Thomson AM, Billewicz WZ, Hytten FE. The assessment of fetal growth. Journal of Obstetrics and Gynaecology of the British Commonwealth 1968; 75: 903-916.

Boys

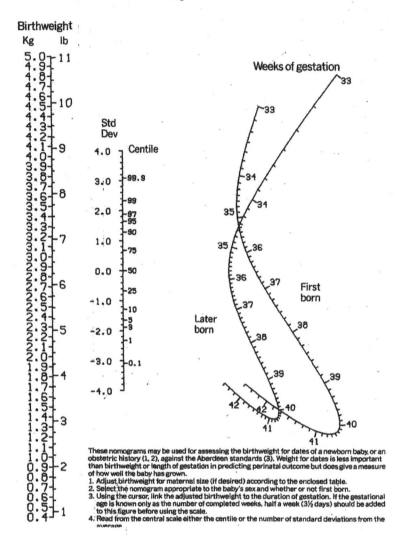

Birth weight for Dates: Nomograms Diagrams (BWD No 1 and 2):

Post Natal Depression:

Prophylaxis: Medroxyprogesterone injection, Depo-Provera at delivery, followed by Dydrogesterone (If you can get it) 10mg BD or Cyclogest pessaries bd until the first period.

Tricyclic antidepressants are said to be excreted in only tiny amounts in breast milk. Of the SSRIs Paroxetine and Sertraline are usually said to be safe.

Dysmenorrhoea:

GTN Patches can help if cyclical progesterone, NSAIDs, alverine, COCP, etc. are all ineffective.

Suppression of Lactation:

Cabergoline (Dostinex) 0.5mg (a treatment for hyperprolactinaemia). For suppression of lactation: 1mg as a single dose on day 1. To suppress established lactation: 0.25mg BD for 2 days.

Breast Milk:

Has many advantages over formula from the very first "milk", **Colostrum,** which is full of antibodies and leukocytes, – the IgA being absorbed across intestinal mucosa into the baby's circulation. There are also other immune protective and priming molecules, lacto-ferrin, lysozyme, complement, various growth factors and vitamins contained as well. This complex soup primes, protects and stimulates the sleeping sterile new born gut.

We all know that a probiotic is a supplement which contains beneficial live micro organisms but a prebiotic is a food that beneficial gut bacteria thrive on. Breast milk is full of this, encouraging Bifidobacteria, Lactobacilli and other useful gut organisms. Breast milk contains antibodies, immune factors, enzymes, cytokines, white cells, iron transport proteins and so on so that breast fed babies develop fewer gut infections, allergies, asthma, eczema and atopic conditions generally than formula fed infants. Breast feeding more than six months reduces childhood lymphoma and leukaemia between 36% and 50%, it reduces SIDS, as well as the later incidence of Crohn's, IBS, even Type 2 DM (though this may be because formula fed infants are fatter).

There is an interaction between the bacterial insemination that the previously sterile gut gets during a vaginal delivery and subsequent breast feeding that programmes the baby's gut "Biome", so crucial for the normal development of many body systems. This is slower and obviously different after a Caesarean. Babies born by Caesarean section have completely different gut flora to those "contaminated" by the commensals of their mothers' genital tracts during vaginal delivery. Indeed, the process of **vaginal seeding** – using wet swabs removed from the mother's vagina to wipe around the new born baby's mouth, eyes and facial skin is now popular in some countries in order to kick start a more normal microbiome.

Drugs in breast milk: A rough guide; (and see Safefetus.com)

Avoid:

Anti inflammatories/analgesics: Indomet(h) acin, Phenyl butazone, Gold.

Antibiotics: Chloramphenicol, Nalidixic Acid, Tetracyclines.

Anticoagulants/CVS Drugs: Phenindione.

CNS Drugs: Lithium.

Endocrine treatments: Iodides, higher dose oestrogens.

Other drugs: Anticancer drugs, Atropine, Ergot derivatives, higher dose Vitamin A and D.

May be safe if monitored:

Anti inflammatories/analgesics: Salicylates.

Antibiotics: Aminoglycosides, antimalarials, Co Trimoxazole, Ethambutol, Isoniazid, Sulphonamides (In G6PD deficiency).

Anticoagulants/CVS drugs: Beta Blockers, Clonidine, Diuretics, Nicoulmalone, Reserpine, Warfarin.

CNS drugs: Higher dose Barbiturates and Benzodiazepines, possibly Carbamazepine, Chloral, Dichloralphenazone, MAO inhibitors, Meprobamate, higher dose Phenothiazines, Phenytoin, Primidone, Valproate.

Endocrine drugs: Carbimazole, high dose steroids, oral hypoglycaemics, low dose oestrogens, Thiouracils, Thyroxine.

Other drugs: Bronchodilators, Danthron, Probantheline, Theophylline.

Should be safe:

Some anti inflammatories/analgesics: Codeine, Dextropropoxyphene, Fluphenic Acid, Ibuprofen, Ketoprofen, Mefenamic Acid, Paracetamol, Pentazocine, Pethidine, low dose salicylates.

Antibiotics: Cephalosporins, Clindamycin, Erythromycin, Lincomycin, Metronidazole, Nitrofurantoin (G6PD deficiency), Penicillins, Rifampicin.

Anticoagulants/CVS drugs: Digoxin, Heparin, Methyl Dopa.

CNS Drugs: Low dose barbiturates, benzodiazepines and phenothiazines, TCAs.

Endocrine drugs: Low dose steroids. Insulins, progestogens.

Others: Antacids, antihistamines, Bisacodyl, bulk laxatives, Folic Acid, Iron, Cromoglicate, Vitamins B and C and low dose A and D.

Hydatidiform Mole: (Molar pregnancy)

A Trophoblastic Tumour. Interestingly there are different kinds: If a single sperm combines with a nucleus free egg, the sperm duplicating its DNA, this is a "Complete Mole". A "Partial Mole" is when an egg is fertilised by two sperm or a sperm duplicates itself. The Complete Mole is more likely to become a Choriocarcinoma. As soon as the diagnosis is made, molar pregnancies (if single) are evacuated. Occasionally they can become (10-15%) invasive moles or (2-3%) Choriocarcinoma with a good prognosis and a good response to Methotrexate.

Monitor Serum HCG levels (which are raised in molar pregnancies) 2 weekly until normal levels obtained, then urine 4 weekly until 1 year post evacuation then 3 monthly for another year. Follow up 6m-2 years after evacuation.

H.C.G. Normal values Urine HCG 0-24 IU/l
　　　　　　　　　　Serum HCG 0-4 IU/l.

IUCDs/IUS

There are currently 18 intra-uterine devices available in the UK, three release a progestogen. (2016) Previous ectopic pregnancy, tubal infection or surgery, PID, nulliparity and endometriosis are all contraindications. Antibiotic prophylaxis is needed with a valvular heart disease and it is essential to exclude pregnancy before inserting.

Most are copper with a silver or plastic core. Some have an 8 year life, a 0.1% pregnancy rate and the progesterone releasing IUS systems are said to protect against PID. (ie: Mirena, which releases Levonorgestrel). This lasts 3 years. It is supposed to be safe with a past history of venous thrombosis.

Copper bearing IUCDs are said to have no risk of PID when introduced by a "Safe operator". IUCDs have lower mortality rates than OCs, barrier methods or planned pregnancies.

Other intra uterine progesterone containing devices currently listed in MIMS include

Jaydess and Levosert. There are 15 plain copper coils (including Copper T380A, Flexi T 380, Load 375, Multi-safe 375, Novaplus T 380 Cu and so on).

If an IUCD is fitted >age 40 years it may be left until 1 year after the last period. When removal is necessary you can give HRT for 1 month and remove at the withdrawal bleed.

IUCDs work by thickening cervical mucus, changing the endometrium and acting as a mechanical barrier. The progestogen in the IUS also prevents cyclical endometrial hypertrophy, cutting down menstrual loss.

Progestogen Only Contraceptives and the risk of VTE:

Basically the few studies done are inadequate and slightly confusing but the consensus is and most people stick to:

Mirena type coils do not increase the risk of VTE.

Progestogen only pills MAY increase the risk slightly especially if Co-Risks (obesity, immobility, surgery etc) are present.

Depoprovera type injectable progestogens do slightly increase the risk of VTE.

PEARL INDEX:

The number of unintended pregnancies per 100 woman years.
for instance: Typical values: (Just put % after the figure):
No Contraception: 85,
Withdrawal: 35,
Vaginal sponge 28,
Spermicide alone 21,
Rhythm: 14-40,
The Cervical Cap: 4-20,
Diaphragm with spermicide: 2-3,
Condom: 3-12,
Female condom: 1-5,
Injection: 0.03-2,
IUCD: 0.1-1.5,
Hormonal IUCD: 0.05-0.1,
COCP: 0.1 – 1.0,
Sterilisation: 0.1-0.4 !
Implant: 0 ??

Normal **conception** Rates:
50% normal couples at 2 months,
85% at 1 year,
90% at 2 years.

Abnormal uterine bleeding:

The mean menstrual loss is "normally" 36mls, (2-80mls range), 70% in first 2 days. Menorrhagia is >80mls/cycle.

Exclude: Fibroids, polyps, adenomyosis, PID, coagulation disorders (including Von Willebrand's), POP, IUCD, drugs, thyroid abnormality.

Cancer: risk factors include PCOs, obesity, diabetes, previous Tamoxifen and family history.

Do an USS, endometrial biopsy if >40 yrs and a risk of cancer or medical treatment has failed. Then can refer for O.P. hysteroscopy.

Treatments: Progestogens, (Norethisterone, Depo provera) NSAIDs, Mefenamic Acid, Tranexamic Acid, Mirena, IUS.

COCP may be helpful but Qlaira (Oestradiol and Dienogestrel) reduces blood loss 88% after 6m.

Endometrial ablation using: Rollerball, TCRE, Hydrothermal ablation, Thermachoice balloon, Laser, Microwave, Novasure (Radiofrequency endometrial ablation) etc.

A useful algorithm is:

Abnormal Uterine Bleeding by Age:

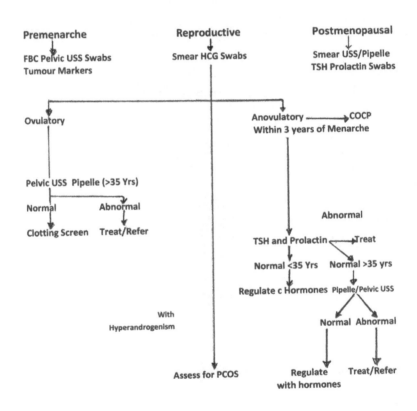

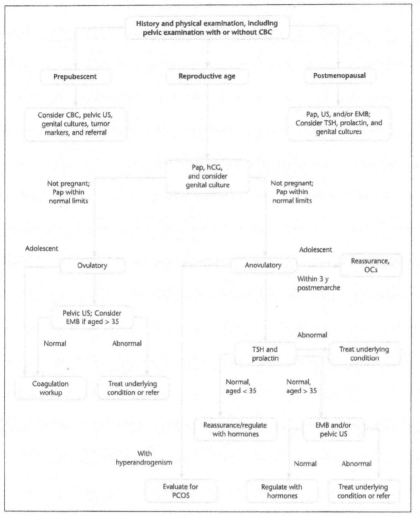

FIGURE. Initial approach to abnormal uterine bleeding.

CBC = complete blood cell count; US = ultrasonography; Pap = Papanicolaou test; hCG = human chorionic gonadotropin; TSH = thyroid-stimulating hormone; OCs = oral contraceptives; EMB = endometrial biopsy; PCOS = polycystic ovary syndrome.

CBC is the American for FBC and stands for Complete Blood Count.

MOST LIKELY DIFFERENTIAL FOR AUB BY AGE:

	Pre-pubescent	Reproductive age	Post-Menopausal
Pelvic pathology	Malignancy, trauma, infection, urethral-prolapse, foreign body.	Endometriosis, ovarian tumour, fibroids, polyps, adenomyosis, PID, hyperplasia, cancer	Malignancy, atrophy, polyps.
Pregnancy		Ectopic, abortion, placenta praevia, abruption, GTD -Gestational Trophoblastic Disease (but GTD also means Genetically Transmitted Disease and Gonadotrophin Deficiency!)	
Systemic	Coagulation disorder precocious puberty.	Thyroid disorder, prolactinoma, Lupus, liver and renal disorders, coagulation disorders, hypothalamic disorder	
Iatrogenic		Anticoagulants, antidepressants, antipsychotics, steroids, hormones, herbal medication.	
Dysfunctional uterine bleeding		PCOs Polycystic ovaries.	

Screen for thyroid disorders, Herbs: Garlic, gingko, gingseng, soy, St John's Wort.
My thanks to Dr J Keehbauch.

Abnormal Vaginal/uterinebleeding: See Diagrams AUB 1-3

Vaginal examination

Peri and post menopausal bleeding

FAST TRACK
Recurrent heavy bleeding
Recurrent PCB >35 years
Still bleeding 1m after stopping HRT
Suspicious lesion on VE

No HRT

On HRT
Breakthrough bleeding over 6m
on CCHRT
Irregular bleeding on cyclical HRT

T.V. USS

Endometrial thickness
<8mm no focal lesion

Refer 1) Thickness >8mm
    2) Focal lesion, ie fibroid, polyp

Pipelle

If under 5mm thickness and refuses pipelle,
OK to reassure.

Alternatively: The management of Abnormal Uterine Bleeding

By Age:

See Diagrams (AUB 1 and 2). My thanks to Drs Keehbauch and Nystrom for permission to reproduce their Clinical Flow Chart.

Cervical Smears

Who currently has them?

Since 2003:

Age <25 years: "No screening unless clinically indicated": Although what is "clinically indicated?" – This has been the subject of many distressing news stories over the last few years with younger and younger girls developing cervical cancer and some dying after their GPs refused a simple cervical smear at the age of 18 or 19. I would advise you never to refuse a direct colposcopy and a smear on any patient if they are worried that they may have a gynaecological cancer. This is the least you owe them. It takes 5 minutes to look and 5 minutes to do the smear. A normal cervix is obvious and simple reassurance is all the patient wants. I despair at GPs who apply rigid rules like this as if the patients were there to serve the algorithms rather than the other way round.-Or could this be related to the fear modern GPs have of performing intimate examinations on their female patients without a time consuming, inconvenient and in reality, unnecessary chaperone? It is now a major hassle, stopping a busy surgery to find a completely pointless chaperone to stand outside the curtains while the patient wonders whether you are perhaps a weirdo who needs an eye kept on him where women are concerned. Perhaps what used to be no more significant than taking a blood pressure has become such a major inconvenience that the GP often can't be bothered and blames the algorithm for not doing it. The net result is bad medicine, lazy practice, a good excuse to avoid an appropriate examination of the patient and so the patient suffers. It used to be a quick, gentle and professional colposcopy. Now it's an often hopeful unjustified reassurance and dismissal. Unforgivable.

Think of you denying your 19 year old patient her smear like this: Her father is in his mid 50's. He has paid his taxes since he left school at the age of 16. The NHS costs each tax payer £1900 a year, so the father has paid £76,000 in tax solely towards the NHS in his lifetime. His wife has worked for 20 of her adult years and has paid £38,000 towards the NHS. Together this is a total of £114,000 in tax *specifically towards the NHS*. Their daughter could be about to die (like the teenager in the paper this week, March 2014) for the want of "Being checked properly" (To quote the parents of Sophie Jones). Marie Stopes International perform smears for £79 and the NHS cost is about the same. So given the amount that these parents have already paid into the NHS, a thousand smear's worth, who's side are you on? If they are really worried, **Just do it.**

Anyway back to smears:

Currently the NHS Smear regime is:

25-49 years 3 yearly,
50-64 years 5 yearly,
>65 years only if not screened since 50 or if one of the last three tests abnormal.
Thereafter if "clinically indicated".

By the way, I would always write on the form "irregular vaginal bleeding" or the officious histopathology technician or secretary – who have never had a tearful patient pleading with them in their lives, will just deny the patient their smear without a second thought.

You can do a smear in the mid trimester of **pregnancy** if necessary. Although I have always tried, at least for the last 30 years to avoid this because of the inevitable bleeding and worry this causes. The 6 week post natal smears always seem to need repeating due to inflammation, leukocytes and contamination. So these are best delayed if at all possible too.

Cervical smears are now tested for HPV (from July 2012) if they show borderline changes or worse. A positive test reduces the interval for follow up after treatment for CIN.

New evidence suggests that smears may be superseded by **urine HPV DNA**, so close is the association between abnormal smears and infection with Human Papilloma Virus.

Urine testing correctly identifies 87% of positive and 94% of negative HPV cases. The test's accuracy is improved by using the first urine of the day.

Post Hysterectomy: If the hysterectomy was because of cancer then do 2 vault smears- at 6m and 1 year if CIN completely removed. If in doubt about removal then continue 3 yearly screening.

These are the official guidelines but I have never been rigid in applying them to the patient who is worried with any reasonable justification at all (previous STDs, multiple partners, odd discharge, irregular bleeding or any gynaecological symptom at all really) – If in doubt, do smears until you are absolutely sure their cervix cannot be unhealthy. The cervix can become dysplastic very quickly, the last smear may have been inadequate and anyway, within reason, they pay your wages and a smear a bit more frequently than the guidelines has been known to save a life.

Cervical smears detect Cervical intraepithelial neoplasia or CIN (caused by HPV usually). The sample may be smeared onto a microscope slide and fixed or washed off a cervical brush into a bottle of preservative in the liquid based system – the sample being centrifuged at the lab before examination.

Smear tests are still recommended after HPV vaccination since the vaccines do not cover all the Papilloma viruses and sexual contact may have taken place pre-vaccination.

I didn't do anything like 200 tests a year but it would apparently take that many per week in a professional lifetime to save one life from cancer of the cervix. There would be 1 death from cancer of the cervix despite screening during those 38 years for the same practitioner statistically.

Abnormal results: 1:10 – 1:20 smears are abnormal officially. My experience is it is about 1:3 or 1:4.

Borderline, low grade dyskaryosis or CIN 1......Colposcopy, rescreen 6m X3 or 3-5 years if HPV negative. If resmearing is still abnormal then colposcopy.

Moderate, severe (high grade) Dyskaryosis: CIN 2 CIN 3............Colposcopy and resmear in 6 months.

NHS Cervical Screening Programme

HPV Triage and Test of Cure Protocol

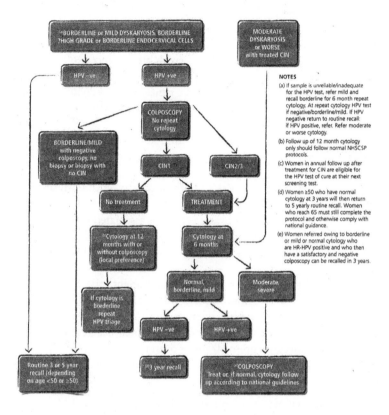

NOTES

(a) If sample is unreliable/inadequate for the HPV test, refer mild and recall borderline for 6 month repeat cytology. At repeat cytology HPV test if negative/borderline/mild. If HPV negative return to routine recall: if HPV positive, refer. Refer moderate or worse cytology.

(b) Follow up of 12 month cytology only should follow normal NHSCSP protocols.

(c) Women in annual follow up after treatment for CIN are eligible for the HPV test of cure at their next screening test.

(d) Women ≥50 who have normal cytology at 3 years will then return to 5 yearly routine recall. Women who reach 65 must still complete the protocol and otherwise comply with national guidance.

(e) Women referred owing to borderline or mild or normal cytology who are HR-HPV positive and who then have a satisfactory and negative colposcopy can be recalled in 3 years.

HPV Triage and Management

Cytology Result (1st Occurrence)	Current Management	HPV Triage Management	
		HPV −ve	HPV +ve
Borderline	Repeat in 6 months	Routine recall	Colposcopy referral
Mild dyskaryosis	Colposcopy referral	Routine recall	Colposcopy referral

Diagrams (HPV triage) (Diagram HPV T1A and B). HPV Triage and test for cure protocol (2 diagrams)

Ovarian Cancer:

Genetics:

Families with high risk of ovarian cancer:

Families with two or more individuals with ovarian cancer at any age who are first degree relatives of each other,

One with ovarian cancer at any age and one with breast cancer <50 years who are first degree relatives of each other,

One with ovarian cancer at any age and two with breast cancer <60 years who are first degree relatives of each other,

One individual with known ovarian cancer genes, three individuals with colorectal cancer, at least one having been diagnosed <50 years and one with ovarian cancer who are first degree relatives.

Genes that predispose to both breast and ovarian cancer are BRCA1 and BRCA2 autosomal dominant, maternal or paternal inheritance – Screening via USS and CA125 from 35 years.

Note: BRCA genes: Increase the risk of both breast cancer in both sexes and ovarian cancer in women.

The likelihood that a breast and/or ovarian cancer is associated with a harmful mutation in *BRCA1* or *BRCA2* is highest in families with a history of multiple cases of breast cancer, cases of both breast and ovarian cancer, one or more family members with two different primary cancers.

Harmful *BRCA1* mutations may increase a female patient's risk of cancer of the cervix, uterus and pancreas as well as colon. *BRCA2* mutations may also increase the risk of pancreatic, stomach, gallbladder and bile duct cancers as well as melanoma.

In the normal population, 12% or thereabouts of women will get breast cancer. With a BRCA 1 or 2 mutation this goes up to 60%. For ovarian cancer, 1 1/2% of women will get ovarian cancer. This shoots up to between 15% and 40% with a harmful BRCA mutation.

Menorrhagia:

1:5 women have heavy menstrual bleeding. 80mls is the normal blood loss or 1 doz sanitary towels/period. Clots mean a heavy period.

40% women with menorrhagia think there is no treatment for it.

60% with heavy menstrual bleeding have painful cramps.

50% are depressed, moody or irritable during menstruation.

47% have bloating and fatigue.

44% have headaches.

33% have frequent bleeding.

20% are anaemic.

Fibroids

20-40% of women will get fibroids at sometime. More if they are Afro Caribbean, hypertensive, overweight, nulliparous, or have PCO or DM.

The symptoms largely depend upon the size, number and position of these mainly benign tumours.

Symptoms include abnormal bleeding, iron deficiency, bloating, constipation, discomfort with defaecation, backache, urinary symptoms – which can be due to hydro-nephrosis, occasionally infertility, miscarriage and very rarely malignant change to a leiomyosarcoma.

Fibroids can be on the outside surface of the uterus-subserosal, in the wall – intramural and on the inside – submucosal.

Investigations include vaginal examination, USS, MRI etc.

Treatment:

There were 75,000 related interventions as an in-patient in 2009-10.

Basically the treatments are numerous: NSAIDs and others agents to reduce bleeding and anti oestrogens or anti progestogens. Also the various surgical and local procedures.

Thus: **Drug treatment:** NSAIDs, The bizarrely spelt: Cyklokapron 500mg 2 tds (Tranexamic Acid), Dicynene 500mg qds (Etamsylate), Mefenamic Acid 250mg-500mg TDS, Cyclical Progestogens, Norethisterone, Depo provera injection,

Norethisterone doesn't work unless you use 5mg TDS from day 5-25.

IUD – Hormone releasing: up to 50% have the Mirena removed because of S/Es at 5 years. It works in 40% of patients. The Mirena lasts 4 years and works by reducing menstrual flow.

Cabergoline (Dostinex), Danazol.

Ulipristal acetate, Esmya, a Selective Progesterone Receptor Modulator, SPRM. Causes cell apoptosis. Given 5mg daily for 3m – £342. The patients need effective contraception during treatment. Mifepristone.

Myosure is an intrauterine submucous hysteroscope fibroid excision device.

Goserelin, Zoladex. GnRH analogues, can be used to make the fibroids less vascular pre myomectomy.

Endometrial ablation – Microwave, hydrothermal balloon, heated saline, etc.

Novasure takes 90 seconds, high radio frequency current endometrial ablation. This effects amenorrhoea in 75%.

Hysterectomy – Retaining the cervix (if normal) to preserve bladder and sexual function.

Uterine artery ablation, myomectomy etc.

Mastalgia/Breast Pain

Multiple treatment approaches:

Pyridoxine: 100mg OD.

Oil of Evening Primrose: 160mg BD (Efamol) with or without Vitamin C.

Danazol: 300mg reducing to 100mg over 3 months. Multiple side effects that limit its usefulness including amenorrhoea and weight gain.

Bromocriptine: 1mg OD to 2.5mg BD. Suppression of lactation 2.5mg OD then BD for 2 weeks.

Tamoxifen: 10mg BD for 3m.

Goserelin (Zoladex).

Ibuprofen gel topically!

Endometriosis:

Endometriosis treatment:

GnRH analogues: (Luteinising hormone releasing hormone agonists, LHRH agonists) Buserelin, Gosarelin, Luprorelin, Nararelin, Triptorelin.

Danazol, Gestrinone, Dydrogesterone, Medroxyprogesterone, Nor ethisterone, COCP

+/– analgesics
Common treatment: Zoladex (Goserelin) and Tibolone (Livial).
Progesterone receptor modulator Ulipristal (Esmya) 2 tabs £114.
Progestogens: Norethisterone, (Primolut N), Medroxyprogesterone (Provera).

Medroxyprogesterone Acetate, Provera. (5mg and 10mg) 10mg TDS for 3 months. This is also used in **opposing Oestrogen HRT treatment**: 10mg daily for last 14 days of each 28day cycle.

Also used in **"Cycle Dysfunction"** to regularise the cycle, 2.5mg-10mg from day 16-21 for 3 cycles. (or something similar) and in **Secondary Amenorrhoea** 2.5mg-10mg daily from day 16-21 for 3 cycles.

Norethisterone:
Can be used for similar indications to medroxyprogesterone but also for putting off periods and PMS, thus:
Endometriosis: 10-25mg daily for 4-6m.
Dysfunctional bleeding/menorrhagia: 5mg TDS for 10 days to arrest bleeding. 5mg BD from day 19-26 to regularise periods.
Dysmenorrhoea: 5mg TDS day 5-24 for 3-4 cycles.
Premenstrual Syndrome: 5mg TDS day 19-26 for 3 cycles.
Putting off a period: 5mg TDS from 3 days before the expected period. The "period" then usually happens 3-4 days after stopping treatment.

Delaying periods:

Can also be done using Provera, Medroxyprogesterone Acetate 5mg OD from 2 days before the period was due.

Infections:

Bacterial Vaginosis:

Generally due to **Gardnerella Vaginalis.** Fishy smell, relative alkalinity (pH >4.5), **Clue Cells** on microscopy. Must be differentiated from Thrush and Trichomonas as well as other causes of discharge (a proper speculum VE and pelvic assessment are essential – how often have these patients forgotten a lost tampon?)

Treatment: Metronidazole, orally and/or topically as vaginal gel (Zidoval) 1 applicatorful nocte X5. Tinidazole (Fasigyn, 4 stat then 2 daily for 5 days). Clindamycin orally or cream (Dalacin Cr. 1 applicatorful nocte X7, Clindamycin 2% Cream).

Trichomonas: A protozoan infection with 70% of patients unaware of their infection. I.P usually 1-4 weeks, but can be longer. Urethritis in both sexes, vaginitis, with a long term increased risk of cancer – both of the cervix and prostate, (many cancers throughout the body are due to chronic inflammation) white, yellow or green discharge, which, like GV, is fishy. *It may be fishy to the sufferer but the cause is straight forward, – sex.* TV is an STD. TV can prompt premature labour, increase the risk of other STDs like HIV and although half of men expel the infection spontaneously. Women do not.

Treatment: Metronidazole, oral, 2000mg once ! or topically (Zidoval vaginal gel) or Tinidazole. Must treat both partners.

Clue Cells:

are present in mild bacterial vaginosis, but may be normal.

Pelvic Inflammatory Disease:

Chlamydia: Asymptomatic in 90% women 50% men.
Azithromycin 1 gr Stat.
Gonococcal: Ciprofloxacin 500mg Stat. (Based on sensitivities.)
Unknown: Ofloxacin and Metronidazole 7 days.
"Uncomplicated" Doxycycline 100mg Bd 7 days or Azithromycin 1 Gr stat.
Alternative treatments abound and include Minocycline, Lymecycline, Ofloxacin and Amoxycillin/Erythromycin in pregnancy.

Implants:

Implanon/now the Nexplanon: 68mg Etonorgestrel contraceptive implant. Lasts 3 years. Prevents ovulation. (Note: The **Mirena** lasts 5 years). Note also: The contraceptive effect is gone 3 days after its removal and but sperm are viable for 7 days.

Antibiotics in Pregnancy

Antibiotics taken during pregnancy account for only 1% of congenital malformations. Virtually every data sheet for them has the unhelpful caveat that benefits and risks must be balanced. How do you do that when two reports of malformations in pregnant rats followed the intraperitoneal instillation of huge doses of Metronidazole in the first trimester of the rat pregnancy but your patient is 32 weeks, human and has a horrible Trichomonal or Gardnerella discharge? – Give them the Metronidazole most of the time I imagine.

Categories:

In America, and since most of the information is indirect, from animal studies and probably overcautious, they use 5 categories of risk:

- Category A: Studies in pregnant women do not demonstrate any risks to the mother or foetus.

- Category B: While animal studies show no risk, human studies are inadequate or animal toxicity has been noted, but the studies on humans show no risk.

- Category C: Animal studies indicate toxicity but studies in humans are inadequate.

- Category D: There is evidence of human risk.

- Category X: There have been reported foetal abnormalities in humans.

Obviously, in all classes of drugs, the benefits of antibiotic use must always outweigh the risks.

Commonly used antibiotics

- Penicillins (Category B) All the penicillins **including Co Amoxiclav** are said to be safe throughout pregnancy though you may need to use higher doses due to the larger extra cellular fluid volume.

- Cephalosporins (Category B): This group has not been well studied in the first trimester and should therefore not be considered the first line of treatment in this stage of pregnancy. Generally, these drugs are considered safe though.

- Sulfonamides (Category C): Can cause hyperbilirubinaemia in the newborn perinatally if given in the 3rd trimester. Can cause Haemolysis in G6PD deficiency. Co Trimoxazole should be avoided in the first trimester as it has been associated with foetal cardiovascular defects.

- Tetracyclines (Category D): Tetracyclines can harm the mother and foetus: The pregnant mother can develop liver fatty necrosis, pancreatitis, kidney damage. Tetracyclines can adversely affect foetal growth, discolour and damage dental enamel (and colour bones). Deciduous teeth are affected unless the antibiotic is given near term when the crowns of the permanent teeth are affected.

- Aminoglycosides (Category D): Aminoglycosides if used in the presence of low Mg, Ca or with CCB treatment may result in neuromuscular blockade. Streptomycin and Kanamycin can cause foetal deafness. Gentamicin appears not to do this (Category C).

- Nitrofurantoin (Category B): Safe except in G6PD deficiency.

- Quinolones (Category C): Possible first trimester administration problems, ?? – Spina bifida, limb defects, hypospadias, inguinal hernias, eye, ear, skeletal and cardiac defects. Higher incidence of LCCS for foetal distress. Cartilage damage of weight bearing joints in animals. No human studies and no human teratogenicity. High affinity for bone and cartilage.

- Metronidazole (Category B) Although it is recommended to avoid this during the first trimester, (Possible mutagen – this is controversial) there is no known association with foetal damage.

- Macrolides (Category B): These agents, including azithromycin, have not been associated with birth defects and are considered safe for use in pregnancy.

- Clindamycin (Category B): This drug has not been associated with birth defects.

- Vancomycin (Category C): No congenital abnormalities have been attributed to use of vancomycin – based on limited data.

Oral Contraceptives and our teenage birth rate:

Bear in mind that in the UK, theoretically, sex under 16 years old is illegal and a girl having sex under 13 has been raped. You have to involve Social Services.

The now famous Gillick case deliberation:

(1985: "The Department of Health and Social Security issued a circular to area health authorities containing, inter alia (among other things), advice to the effect that a doctor consulted at a family planning clinic or in the GP surgery by a girl under 16 would not be acting unlawfully if he prescribed contraceptives for the girl, so long as in doing so he was acting in good faith to protect her against the harmful effects of sexual intercourse. The circular further stated that, although a doctor should proceed on the assumption that advice and treatment on contraception should not be given to a girl under 16 without parental consent and that he should try to persuade the girl to involve her parents in the matter, nevertheless the principle of confidentiality between doctor and patient applied to a girl under 16 seeking contraceptives and therefore in

exceptional cases the doctor could prescribe contraceptives without consulting the girl's parents or obtaining their consent if in the doctor's clinical judgment it was desirable to prescribe contraceptives.")

-was supposed to have settled the rights of the underage child (under 16) to have access to contraception and to have clarified the doctor's role and responsibilities when making contraceptive decisions in the surgery. The DoH guidance based on the full ruling finally came out in 2004.

We had the worst teenage pregnancy rates in Europe for decades and 200,000 abortions a year were and are the norm. All this despite free and readily available contraception from GPs and anonymous clinics, sex education at every school and post coital contraception over the counter or free from GPs. By 2015 the huge number of abortions on request and the message that single parenthood wasn't necessarily a shining, care free existence were making significant inroads into the pregnancy mountain with a mere 26,000 babies born to mothers under 20. This was actually the lowest figure since the war.

Although we did have the highest teenage pregnancy and abortion rates in Europe, the UK birth rate had fallen by 32.3% since 2004 compared with 15.6% in the rest of Europe and by 2015 we were at last beginning to be in line with Europe in this statistic by virtue of our dizzying number of abortions.

The birth rate is now 23.3/1000 aged 15-17 This is "more in line with the rest of Europe". 185,000 abortions were still being done in the UK in 2014. A staggering number. The birth rate overall is 1.9 births per woman in the UK.

Fraser Guidelines and Gillick Competence:

Lord Fraser gave these guidelines in his judgement of the Gillick Case in 1985:

"...a doctor could proceed to give advice and treatment provided he is satisfied in the following criteria:

1) that the girl (although under the age of 16 years of age) will understand his advice;

2) that he cannot persuade her to inform her parents or to allow him to inform the parents that she is seeking contraceptive advice;

3) that she is very likely to continue having sexual intercourse with or without contraceptive treatment;

4) that unless she receives contraceptive advice or treatment her physical or mental health or both are likely to suffer;

5) that her best interests require him to give her contraceptive advice, treatment or both without the parental consent."

Gillick Competence:

Lord Scarman's comments in his judgement of the Gillick case in the House of Lords (1985) are often referred to as the test of "Gillick competency": Although if you find these words helpful in the surgery you are more of a lawyer than a doctor:

"...it is not enough that she should understand the nature of the advice which is being given: he (she) must also have a sufficient maturity to understand what is involved."

He also commented more generally on parents' versus children's rights:

"Parental right yields to the child's right to make his (her) own decisions when he (she) reaches a sufficient understanding and intelligence to be capable of making up his (her) own mind on the matter requiring decision."

Now then – did that clarify whether a thirteen year old, who just comes in wanting the pill is sensible enough to know what having condomless sex with her sixteen year old, feckless, sleazy boyfriend means for her moral, physical, emotional and educational future? Of course not. Can you hear the scraping sound of a buck being passed and the wheezy breathlessness of the judge? That is because he has slipped out the back door as fast as he can. He will never have to sit down here in the messy real world with us doctors in a packed surgery of in your face consequences. He or she has just crawled up to the neat, quiet and tidy moral high ground where such messy decisions are left to others.

The Gillick case related to the provision of contraception to the under 16 year old child. Another, related challenge came from Sue Axon, a mother of 5 children who wanted to be told if a doctor were planning to treat STDs or offer an abortion to an underage girl. In 2006 The High Court decided that the Gillick Competency rules applied to children seeking abortions and treatment for sexual infections too. The last paragraph applies – only twice as much.

So if British children of 13, 14 and 15 can now have sex without their parents even knowing (thanks to the **legal profession and politicians**),

with the tacit approval of the establishment and our prescriptions (you and me, the **medical profession**),

and there is precious little effective teaching about the value of closeness, commitment, relationships and "morality" (**the priesthood and the teaching profession**),

and are immersed in an over sexualised culture which surrounds them in teenage films, television, music, video, the internet, and teen fiction (**the artistic, cultural and media professions**),

and there are seemingly no consequences,

no wonder we have the highest teenage pregnancy and STD rates in Europe.

It seems **all** the old and new professions have all failed them and are saying just get on with it we don't care..

Anyway, in the real world there is:

The Oral Contraceptive Pill

Venous thrombo-embolism risk:
Normal women   5-10/100,000
COCP containing Levonorgestrel (2nd Gen progestogen)   15-20/100,000
COCP containing Desogestrel/Gestodene (3rd Gen progestogen) 25-40/100,000
Pregnancy   60/100,000.

Advice for Missed pills:
If less than 12 hours late, take pill and continue as normal.
If more than 12 hours late:
In first week of pack take last missed pill continue as normal, use barrier 7 days.
– But
if has had SI in last 7 days, ?PCP (post coital pill).

In second week of pack take missed pill. If >4pills missed, use barrier 7 days.
In 3rd week of pack, take missed pill, at end of pack continue new pack without a break.

Combined Oral Contraceptives:

The general advice is avoid combined (oestrogen containing) OCPs in over 50 year olds although I would say this is far too old having lost two patients from P.E. in their late 30's, both on 30ug pills for no reason other than the husband's fear of vasectomy. I feel that every couple should have made its mind up about having children by the age of 35 and that the pill is a potentially risky form of REVERSIBLE contraception. After 35 and possibly younger in smokers you should encourage patients on to safer forms of contraception, avoiding oestrogens if possible. The combined pill is contraindicated in the overweight (avoid in BMI 35kg/m2.) Other contraindications include diabetes with complications, significant hypertension, migraine, pre-existing or new after starting the pill.

In single older women who are overweight and not in a stable relationship, the rules are different, they need the reliability of a combined pill until they settle down.

Combined OCP:

Fixed Combination (Monophasic) (Historic)

21 or 28 Pills
Ethinylestradiol 20ug Desogestrel 150ug Gedarel 20/150
Mercilon
Munalea 20/150
Lestramyl 20/150
,, Gestodene 75ug Femodette
Millinette 20/75
Sunya 20/75
Aidulan
,, Norethisterone 1mg Loestrin 20

Ethinylestradiol 30ug Desogestrel 150ug Gedarel 30/150
Marvelon
Munalea 30/150
Alenvona
Bimizza
Cimizt
Lestramyl 30/150
,, Drospirenone 3mg Yasmin, Lucette
Acondro Dretine
Cleosensa
Eloine Yacella
,, Gestodene 75ug Femodene
(Femodene ED with 7 dummy pills)
Katya 30/75
Femodette
Millinette 30/75
Aidulan
Levonorgestrel 150ug Levest Elevin
Rigevidon
Microgynon30
Erlibelle Maexeni
(Microgynon 30 ED with 7 dummy pills)

Ovranette
Rigevidon
Norethisterone 1.5mg Loestrin30
Ethinylestradiol 35ug Norgestimate 250ug Cilest Lizinna
Norethisterone 500ug Brevinor
Ovysmen
Estradiol 1.5mg   Nomegestrol 2.5mg Zoely
Ethinyl Estradiol 35mcg Norethisterone 1mg Norimin
Mestranol 50ug   Norethisterone 1mg Norinyl-1

Variable Combination ("Phasic")
Ethinylestradiol 30/40/30ug Gestodene 50/70/100ug Triadene
,,   Levonorgestrel 50/75/125ug Logynon
TriRegol
Ethinylestradiol 35ug Norethisterone 500ug/1mg BiNovum
Ethinylestradiol 35ug Norethisterone 500ug/1mg/500ug Synphase
,,   Norethisterone 500ug/750ug/1mg TriNovum
Ethinylestradiol 30/40/30ug Levonorgestrel 50/75/125ug Logynon ED
(with 7 dummy pills)
Estradiol 3mg/2mg/2mg/1mg Dienogest 2mg/3mg   Qlaira
(with 2 dummy pills)

Progestogens:

NOTE: Gestodene and Desogestrel constitute a higher risk of venous thromboembolism. Qlaira is said to cause less bleeding during and at withdrawal, less effect on metabolism and is "better for older women".

Discussion: If thrombosis a risk, avoid the COCP or, at a push, use LNG or NET. If arterial circulation is a risk factor use a pill with DSG or GSD (GTD). If there is any one arterial or venous risk factor plus age>35 then this is an absolute C/I to the COCP.

In young first time pill users a LNG or NET pill is probably the first choice.

(I TRY to stick to the rule that there has to be a very good reason to prescribe synthetic oestrogens to women over 35 unless they have exceptional social or personal circumstances. Is it unreasonable to expect this to be the age at which most women in stable relationships should be envisaging their final families? They should have decided by now how many children to have and so avoid the risks either of taking hormones or of the higher risk pregnancies in their later 30's by arranging permanent (safe) contraception? This often means a discussion about vasectomy with the husband but there are always **two** people involved in the decision – excluding you, the catalyst.

If you happen to have a female patient with **Tuberous Sclerosis**, remember that the COCP can cause pulmonary Lymphangioleiomyomatosis. Always consider this in a woman with TS who is pregnant or on the pill.

Obesity: (A healthy BMI is 18.5-25) Obese is>30

Childhood obesity is linked to early menarche. Women who had their first period aged 13 have the lowest risk of heart disease in later life. But the earlier the menarche, the higher the risk of later hospitalisation and heart related death. Those who start periods before the age of 10 or after 17 are 27% more likely to be hospitalised or die due to heart disease in later life. They are also 16% more likely to be hospitalised or die from stroke and 20% more likely to be hospitalised or die from the complications of later hypertension. These risks are independent of the adult's later weight, smoking or income status.

Late starting periods can be due to dozens of systemic causes ranging from "constitutional" causes, athleticism, chronic illness, anorexia, diseases of the HPA, CF, endocrine disorders, including CAH, hypothyroidism and some tumours etc. These can either raise or lower BMI.

The definition of a late Menarche is: no breast development by the age of 13 or no periods three years after breast development or by 16.

Increasing BMI decreases fertility among women (and men). Obesity causes E.D., reduced number of motile sperm, disorders of sex hormone secretion and metabolism, hyperandrogenism in women, reduced testosterone in men. Obesity increases the pregnancy risk of developing DM, hypertension, preeclampsia, VTE, LSCS, stillbirth.

OCs are less forgiving of "imperfect use" among very heavy and obese women in terms of pregnancy risk. There is also, of course, an increased VTE risk in very heavy women on oestrogen pills.

Post coital contraception is very patient-weight dependent, losing efficacy as low as 75-80kg for levonorgestrel containing oral PCCs. IUCDs are more effective.

After bariatric surgery hormones are not absorbed properly so IUDs are likewise more effective contraceptives than OCPs.

Cerazette – If woman weighs >100kg consider a double dose and if the patient is seriously obese, you may need to change her Nexplanon early.

Progesterone only pills ("Mini pills")

Desogestrel 75ug	Cerazette
Etynodiol 500 ug	Femulen
Norethisterone 350ug	Micronor, Noriday
Levonorgestrel 30ug	Norgeston.

Cerazette inhibits ovulation.

Depoprovera: Medroxyprogesterone acetate:

An extremely useful once three monthly injection for the large number of women who forget the pill, want reliable contraception, are active, perhaps recently or currently breast feeding and so on.

There is a risk of osteoporosis in long term use. I have never seen this become of clinical significance and indeed lowered bone mineral density seems to be one of those surrogate trial outcomes that are of little real-world significance.

There may be a new depot available in the UK (I believe it is in use in the USA) – Depo SubQ Provera. It is a lower dose than normal depot, given subcut. and with an applicator such that patients could administer themselves. The osteoporosis problem may not be such an issue – despite there being warnings about it all over the related literature.

Other injectable hormones include:

Norethisterone Noristerat. Lasts 8 weeks may be repeated once,
Etonogestrel Nexplanon Sub dermal implant. "Remove within 3 years",

Medroxyprogesterone Sayana press injection. Repeat 13 weekly – patients may "self inject".

Other uses of the COCP:

Dianette (Co-Cyprindiol), Cyproterone plus 35ug Ethinylo estrodiol used in severe acne, idiopathic hirsuitism. Withdraw 3-4 cycles after condition resolved.

"Emergency contraceptives"***:

(although this is stretching the definition of an "emergency" a bit far don't you think?- "A sudden state of danger, something dangerous or serious such as an accident that happens suddenly and unexpectedly and needs immediate action to avoid harmful results" to use this terminology to apply to the ending of a normal, natural, inevitable and predictable process – *a potential pregnancy* – which these days is so easy to avoid in the first place.-**but a sudden state of danger** to end a simple, potential but easily preventable pregnancy - **an emergency, –** *really* ?)

Levonelle 1500: Levonorgestrel 1500mcg 12-72 hrs after unprotected intercourse. Repeat if vomiting in <3 hrs.

Average pregnancy risk is 10% per cycle. Levonelle gives 75% protection. Avoid if previous focal migraine, DVT/PE.

Proportion of pregnancies prevented if given in:

<24 hrs 95%,

25-48 hrs 85%,

49-72 hrs 58%,

Ectopics are a small risk, so review if no period follows.

In the past "Levonelle 2" was mimicked by giving Levonorgestrel 25 tablets of 30mcg (ie Norgeston)

twice, twelve hours apart. This was said to be 98-99% effective. Up to **3 days** after unprotected intercourse.

The Local "Patient Group Directive" for Levonelle obtained OTC from pharmacies includes the following rules: it must be within 72 hours of unprotected sex or contraceptive failure, for patients between 13 and 19 (the under 16s must be "Gillick competent"), the "treatment" (?) must be for themselves, the patient must not want medical contraceptive advice as well, or if they have vomited within 3 hours of the first dose they are coming back for some more.

There is a whole list of impractical exclusions which include ectopic pregnancy, pelvic infection, irregularly menstruating, under 16 and not Gillick competent, uncertainty (or dishonesty) about date and time of sex, the possibility of other unprotected sex in the same cycle, abnormal vaginal bleeding, fallopian surgery, cardiovascular history, diabetes and now the patient's weight etc etc.

I wonder how often this Gold Standard is actually put into practice on the floor or in the flimsy plasterboard side-rooms of the average packed, noisy retail pharmacist or with the final add-on 6th extra "emergency" GP patient at 7pm on Friday evening?

Ellaone (pronounced:"Ellawun") – Ulipristal 1 tab up to **5 days (120 hrs)** after unprotected sexual intercourse. A progesterone receptor modulator, inhibits ovulation and changes the endometrium. It is prescription only whereas the levonorgestrel compounds are OTC in many European countries. Avoid breast feeding for 36 hours.

The European Medicines Agency recently (2014) put out a warning on the ineffectiveness of Emergency Contraception in overweight patients.

This was in reference to women over 75kg: The warning related to the progestogen containing: (Levonorgestrel) Norlevo, Levonelle/Postinor and Levodonna as well as EllaOne which contains Ulipristal acetate.

The EMA warning said that high body weight could impair the effectiveness of emergency contraceptives. In Sweden the Medicines Regulation Agency warns about levonorgestrel containing emergency contraception and the risks at 75Kg body weight and lack of effect at 80kg.

The IUCD as an emergency contraceptive:

No more than 19 days after the last period. This is probably the safest emergency contraceptive with a BMI>25 (*"Bedsiderinsider"*). Up to 5 days after unprotected SI or within 5 days of the earliest date of possible ovulation. Not within 28 days of delivery. Review needed 3-4 weeks later to check position etc.

Levonorgestrel and enzyme inducing drugs:***

It was reported in 2016 that there had been at least 400 pregnancies since the 1970s due to interactions between a variety of liver enzyme inducing drugs and levonorgestrel contraceptives. At the same time the MHRA advised that women taking these enzyme inducing drugs should be given double dose LNG post coital contraceptives. Interactions are likely with St John's Wort, anti epileptic agents including Carbamazepine, anti fungal agents and drugs used in HIV and TB infection. (Rifampicin, Griseofulvin) etc.

Ullipristal is also less effective. In America The faculty of Family Planning suggests 3mg Levonorgestrel as the dose of PCC.

Polycystic Ovaries PCO:

5-18% women in reproductive age

(but in the younger group: 40% 2 years post menarche, 35% 3 years post menarche, 33% 4 years post menarche according to some figures.)

Not all women with PCOS (syndrome) have polycystic ovaries. Not all women with polycystic ovaries on USS have symptoms.

Anovulation,

Irregular menstruation,

Infertility,

Acne,

+/– Masculinisation (androgen excess),

Hirsuitism,

Also associated:

Insulin resistance,

Diabetes,

Obesity,

Metabolic Syndrome,

Late sequelae: Diabetes, dyslipidaemia, hypertension, CVS disease, endometrial Ca., breast disease.

Biochemistry:

Raised serum Insulin, raised serum Insulin resistance, raised Homocysteine, raised Androstenedione, raised Testosterone (especially Free Testosterone), raised LH, normal

FSH, (LH>FSH), lowered SHBG, raised Free Androgen Index, raised Oestradiol, raised Oestrone and Prolactin.

Also check OGTT (impaired in 30% women with PCOS), fasting lipids, TSH.

Treatment

If overweight: Diet – Low CHO or low glycaemic index and regular exercise restores menstruation. It needs to be at least 30 minutes of sweaty exercise a day though.

Metformin (If BMI>25) which reduces androgens and works even up to a BMI of 37. (Safe in first trimester, don't give if eGFR <30-40) and Glitazones which improve insulin sensitivity.

Reduction of unsaturated trans fats reduces infertility. So increase polyunsaturated and monounsaturated fats.

Cardiovascular risk is related to hypertension, lipids, weight, snoring.

Ovulation can be encouraged initially with Clomiphene and Metformin.

For thin women, Clomiphene and FSH injections, IVF, ovarian drilling/diathermy. Ovulation can be induced by Tamoxifen or Clomiphene or if resistant, ovarian surgery, gonadotrophins.

The pill may improve the associated hirsuitism and acne (lipid friendly if possible), Dianette*, Yasmin*, Cilest, Spironolactone*, Vaniqa, (Eflornithine) cream. Bromocriptine. Flutamide*, Finasteride* (* in hyperandrogenism).

If amenorrhoeic, protect the endometrium with some form of progesterone supplementation.

eg Duphaston (as Norethisterone is too androgenic) – cyclically to induce a withdrawal bleed. Give the patient 3-4 periods a year so they avoid endometrial hyperplasia and cancer of the endometrium (a much higher incidence later in life if they are not made to ovulate).

The "Alternative" treatment, Resveratrol, improves some symptoms of PCOS.

Polycystic Ovarian Syndrome:	Exclude: Thyroid disorders,
Weight gain,	Congenital adrenal hyperplasia,
Obesity,	Hyperprolactinaemia,
Hirsuitism,	Androgen secreting tumours,
Virilising symptoms,	Cushings.
Oligomenorrhoea,	
Infertility.	

Problems include: Ovulatory failure, infertility, hyperandrogenism, hirsuitism, obesity, impaired glucose tolerance, Type 2 DM, sleep apnoea, adverse CVS risk profile, hypertension, dyslipidaemia, visceral obesity.

Treatments:

Oligomenorrhoea: Give a withdrawal bleed: OCP, or progesterone withdrawal 3-4 periods/year, or Mirena, if no withdrawal bleed refer for investigations.

Obesity: Encourage at least 30 minutes of sweaty exercise a day (this improves fertility, reduces risk of DM, increases ovulation).

Metformin can be taken with Clomiphene-11% reduction in androgens. Bariatric surgery.

There is a 10-20% risk of DM In middle age in PCOS.

Treat hypertension and hyperlipidaemia.

Anovulation: Clomiphene +/– Metformin then if this fails GnRH treatment or laparoscopic ovarian drilling.

Hirsuitism: Vaniqa, Cyproterone acetate, Spironolactone, Flutamide, Finasteride.

Vaginal Lubricants:

Replens, Sylk, Hyalofemme, Repadina, topical oestrogens.

The Vulva

Lichen Sclerosis (LS):

Use Dermovate oint once nightly for a month then alternate nights 1m then 2x/wk 1m then prn after 3m, use a small blob of ointment each time so a 30g tube should last six months.

Warn patient that the label says not for use on genital area etc. but GPs take precedence over data sheets.

LS does not affect the vagina just the vulva (unlike Lichen Planus).

Lichen Planus (LP):

May be vaginal, oral or vulval, more destructive with greater loss of skin architecture than LS.

Vulvodynia:

5% lidocaine oint. Apply at night for 6 weeks or can use as a small plug on a piece of cotton wool at introitus.

Abortion, Termination of Pregnancy:

Is legal up to 24 weeks even though at this gestation 18% of babies survive a normal birth. The Hippocratic Oath includes the following: I will not give a lethal drug to anyone if I am asked, nor will I advise such a plan: and similarly I will not give a woman a pessary *to cause an abortion*. Under the current (40 year old) abortion on demand act 200,000 abortions per year are performed despite this ancient undertaking that we are all supposed to give lip service to. A third of women having abortions are back for their second or subsequent time – some women seemingly taking advantage of abortion on demand as a form of lazy birth control. In the legal section, I discuss abortion and how it slipped into law as a way of saving the lives of women having back street abortions. It turns out that the statistics show only a tiny number have been saved by the abortion act since the act came in. No one dreamt we would be doing this number of abortions for the reasons we are now nor with the consequences to society. Could it be time to debate abortion on demand as we now have it, honestly and objectively? *That's all of us involved* this time, – the politicians, the doctors, the parents groups, the teachers, the religious leaders, the pro choice and pro life interest groups?

In Northern Ireland abortion (2016) is still illegal but an estimated 1000 Ulsterwomen travel to the mainland for terminations and an average of 30-40 have terminations on the NHS in their homeland annually.

Infertility: (Trying for 2 years) 1 in 8 women.

Pathway:
In brief:
Sperm Test,
Chlamydia testing,

Rubella screening,

Hormone profile/other bloods,

BMI (19-29 currently funded 2013, Contact your local CCG for up to date information.)

Laparoscopy/hystero-salpingogram (HSG.)

If endometriosis with open tubes >Clomid>Intrauterine insemination I.U.I.

blocked tubes, >I.U.I.

No endometriosis I.U.I. possibly I.V.F. or I.C.S.I. – usually below age 40. 3 cycles (2013) restricted and varied geographically (2016).

To elaborate:

With regular sex and patients who are healthy, not heavy drinkers, smokers, overweight and no confounding past history,

84% conceive in one year,

92% in 2 years, and even

35% aged 35 after trying for 3 years.

At age 30, 75% will have a live birth after 1 year of trying, 91% after 4 years.

At age 40, 44% will have a live birth after 1 year and 64% after 4 years.

In their early 20s healthy women have a 25% chance every month of conceiving if having regular unprotected intercourse.

Failure to conceive and when to investigate will depend on past history – chemotherapy, tubal surgery, chronic amenorrhoea, undescended testicles, viral hepatitis, >35 years, PID etc. It is usually said to be 1/3 due to male factors, 1/3 female and 1/3 both.

It is worth advising the couple on healthy life styles and prescribing Folic Acid (0.4mg daily or 5mg if there has been a previous baby with a NTD to the prospective mother).

Male:

Take a full history and do a proper examination.(Including external genitals.) I get the two partners together for an initial double appointment obtaining the histories and doing his examination then, asking the wife (?) to return for a V/E at a separate appointment.

Semen should be

2ml+

Liquefaction time within 60 mins,

pH 7.2 or more,

Concentration 20m/ml or more,

Average volume 3.4mls,

Motility 50% or >motile or

        25% with progressive motility within 60 mins.

75% or >live,

<1m/ml WBCs.

Normal morphology 15 or 30% (depends on how assessed).

Then if appropriate:

Testicular surgery, IUI (X6?), IVF.

Female:

Take a full history (-including drugs, prescribed and illegal) and do a proper examination including a pelvic examination.

Bloods: Serum progesterone in the midluteal phase (day 21/28 up to 28/35 depending on the length of the cycle etc) which confirms ovulation. FSH/LH.

Although NICE says don't worry about TSH or prolactin in the average patient, I don't see the logic of this. Why not exclude potential causes and get all the pieces of the jigsaw on the table at the start? I do a sperm test, take a few months waking, morning temperature, (It has to be after at least 3 hours of uninterrupted sleep), day 21 hormones, chlamydia testing, (antibodies), FBC, U and Es, LFTs, TFTs, cortisol, progesterone, oestradiol, prolactin, gonadotrophins, (FSH and LH) and Rubella screening. You could add in others if you think appropriate.

Bloods are done on day 21 of the cycle, day 1 being the first day of the period bleed – i.e. post ovulatory.

Tubal blockage?

Female investigations then move on to Hystero-salpingogram, Laparoscopy and Dye (or equivalent assessment of tubal patency).

The treatment if blockage is confirmed (assuming you have already done chlamydial studies) is tubal surgery, adhesiolysis, cystectomy of endometrial cysts, IUI.

With no blockage it is Clomiphene, IUI or fallopian tube sperm perfusion.

Ovulatory disorder

Ovulation disorders constitute 21% of female infertility problems, for instance: Hypothalamic-Pituitary Failure/Hypothalamic Pituitary Dysfunction (ie PCO).

The treatment depends on the precise problem: Gonadotrophins, Clomiphene or Tamoxifen +/– IUI +/– Metformin, hMG, uFSH, rFSH, Ovarian drilling (-less likely to produce multiple pregnancies) +/– Bromocriptine if hyperprolactinaemic.

In vitro fertilisation:

2 embryos each cycle, progesterone luteal support, prior salpingectomy if there are hydrosalpinges. This is tried currently on the NHS in azoospermia, bilateral tubal obstruction, or after 3 years of infertility. It is at this stage that NICE suggests hepatitis and HIV screening. I hope you will have done these already – after appropriate counselling.

Intracytoplasmic sperm injection:

Is offered with very poor semen quality or poor IVF response.

Donor Insemination:

In poor or absent semen, rhesus iso immunisation, infectious or genetic diseases in the man.

Oocyte donation:

Ovarian failure, Turners syndrome (etc), oophorectomy, post chemo or radiotherapy, inherited genetic disorders etc.

You will get to know your infertile couples quite well as you will need to see a fair amount of them. You should tell them that you are going to do every test right at the beginning and what the tests are (-I have a hand out) before referring to the infertility clinic. This is a good way of assessing their commitment to each other, to the process, offering (as I do) to prescribe at least SOME of the drugs on the NHS if they are going privately (they will be grateful and never forget this) and checking their progress.

The NHS system is often an unpredictable and unfair lottery. Well established and stable couples committed through marriage don't necessarily get priority in the system despite the statistical likelihood of their staying together and their children being better cared for. There is little else in the way of assessing who will make good parents or stable committed couples before offering them the chance of children funded by the tax payer.

There is after all no fairness or logic to who finds themselves to be infertile. It isn't just a punishment for STDs contracted in a misspent youth, or an unexpected nasty reward for a woman who prioritised her early career and income over a family. Women are at their most fertile in their teens and early twenties. We all suppose we have a right to healthy children when we choose and being deprived of that potential future can be worse for some couples than a serious illness or disabling injury.

HRT and the menopause:

"Estrogen deficient women are nothing but the walking dead." Marie Hoag The average age is around 53 years and 99% have gone through the change by 55 years. – Theoretically. My patients seem to hang on to their periods much longer than this these days for some reason.Over the age of 50 if a women in the menopause needs contraception, give it for 1 year, if under 50 years, give it for 2 years. Often recommended >55 years are Livial or continuous combined therapy.

Some also use Testogel or even Sustanon or Zyban for poor libido. You can combine these with Replens or Sylk if the patient has a particularly dry vagina.

Surgical Menopause hastens cognitive decline in a variety of areas, only partially reversed by HRT.

But if HRT is initiated within 5 years of surgical menopause and continued for at least 10 years then there is a decreased slope of decline in global cognition and less decline in episodic memory, semantic memory and visuospatial ability.

Duration of HRT use was associated with "more gentle slopes" of decline in episodic memory, visuospatial memory and perceptual speed but not an *abolition of the decline* in a number of studies of HRT and cognition.

34: PSYCHIATRY:

Man does not strive for happiness: only the Englishman does that – *Nietzsche*

Inpatient Psychiatry:

In 1948 half the NHS' beds were for psychiatric patients-peaking at 150,000 in 1955. Hard to believe isn't it? We now have a shrinking just under 150,000 {130,000, 2017 (NHS England)} hospital beds **in total**. In 1966 there were133,000 psychiatric beds, dropping to 39,000 in 1995, by 2007 there were only 28,000. The projections for psychiatric beds in 2020 are 17,200. So in less than the lifetime of the NHS, psychiatric in patient provision will have been reduced to one tenth of its original size.

Clearly, from the point of view of we GPs, the patients, relatives, psychiatric staff and the innocent man and women (I say innocent because they often **are** the innocent *victims of this policy*) in the street, psychiatric provision in the NHS has been pretty inadequate for a long time and things have now (since about 2000 – 2016) gone too far. By "things" I mean the off loading of inpatient psychiatry into an unwelcoming, unprepared "Community" and the decimation of secondary care psychiatry. (Decimation is used in the colloquial sense of being completely ruined not just reduced by one tenth.)

The huge distance that many patients and relatives have to travel simply to access an inpatient NHS psychiatric department with a bed has been a secret disgrace for decades. The latest of many public enquiries (2016) was a Royal College of Psychiatrists Commission under Lord Crisp. This found that many units had beds "blocked" because there was nowhere for patients to be discharged to. OR, having been discharged home to unsuitable unsupported housing were bouncing back (Marjorie Wallace Chief executive of Sane) into secondary care. Some politicians appeared to be taking a genuine interest at long last in early 2016. By why shouldn't they? The situation had been a scandal for years. Why should mental health patients be treated so poorly? Half of us will be one at some time, some data says a quarter of us have a mental health problem every year – and we all vote. In 2016 an independent task force promised a billion pounds extra annually within 4-5 years. Sounds a lots but it is only a paltry 1% of the NHS budget.

The trouble is that we, the public, still half believe that, even if you smoke forty cigarettes a day and get lung cancer or COPD or are obese and get breast cancer or are promiscuous and get an AIDs related cancer or drink heavily and find your liver fails, these are acts of God. After all, lots of people do those things and live to a ripe old age. On the other hand schizophrenia, hypomania, suicidal depression are somehow partly a choice, a lack of self control, a question of individual backbone. Could that be why we deprive psychiatry of the funding it desperately needs and deserves? We think the patients are undeserving, chose to get ill, could get better if they really wanted to?

The Occupancy of psychiatric Units in some inner city areas is 120% according to some independent surveys and my personal experience is that trying to get a sick patient admitted to a psychiatric place of safety is a long, tortuous, GP unfriendly, final resort. If it is possible at all, it follows many hours of fraught negotiation, multiple refusals and confusion and then your patient is found a bed several miles, sometimes several counties away. In 2013 the situation was described as being in crisis by the Head of The South London and Maudsley Trust after 1700 beds disappeared in 2 years (9% of the total) and London patients were being forced into beds in Somerset as there were none in the capital. At the end of 2014 it was announced that seven patients had killed themselves in the preceding 2 years while waiting for mental health beds. Surely there were more than that who had reached breaking point I thought? There are Eastern European and developing countries where this level of routine, daily mental health chaos doesn't happen. I was a medical student in the early 70's when a depressed man jumped off a roof in Oxford Street in London not far from my hall of residence. He survived the fall but killed the woman he landed on. Approximately two people a week are murdered by disturbed psychotic patients. You would think that even if the Government had to withdraw funding from, say, self induced cancer patients they would continue funding treatments that so clearly saved the lives of so many totally innocent people as well as the sufferers.

By 2015 the CQC said that acute mental health patients got more help from GPs, ambulance crews and police officers than casualty staff and acute psychiatric services. Only a third of patients felt emergency care was adequate and 42% who experienced out of hours psychiatric support said it had not helped to resolve their crisis. I am not surprised by this at all. I was a psychiatric registrar in a big city and I have been a GP for over 30 years in the sticks. You will have gathered from my comments in the Emergency, Psychiatry and Therapeutics sections of the book, as well as the parts relating to consultations, language skills of doctors and appraisal that Psychiatry demands a highly specialised, dedicated and particularly skilled doctor. If you have a general and unbiased experience of the NHS outside big city teaching hospitals, you will know that many average DGH psychiatry units give a pretty inadequate service to their patients, young and adult. There were in 2014 70,000 acute mental health admissions.

Considering the burden of psychiatric illness in the community it is truly shocking that the secondary care mental health services and bed availability have been progressively denuded of resources for decades and continue to be so. Why on earth is this? Add to this the off loading of psychiatry into the community in the name of political cost cutting, ("Care in the community" didn't fool anyone), the chaos in casualty, the predictable rejection of psychiatric patients by the community, (yes I am afraid that IS what happens to the majority – there is precious little "Care" in the real community), and the poor GP out of hours cover and we now see the result. The self destructive patient is a far greater danger to them self and the dangerous patient a far greater danger to the rest of us than ever before in the history of the NHS. There are at least two murders plus all the suicides by uncared for psychiatric patients unsupervised and at liberty amongst us each week now. **There were 573 homicides in the UK in the last year for which we have figures (2015) so approximately a tenth to a fifth of the murders committed in the UK are because of uncontrolled, unsupervised or poorly treated mental health patients.** This figure is disputed by various mental health charities who argue about what constitutes a mental health patient and how much worse alcohol is as a factor in violent death than mental illness. Indeed, there are web sites defending mental patients' rights not to be incarcerated. They argue that we have to accept this sort of thing will happen from time to time in a liberal country that respects human rights. I disagree. Given that some Trusts are far worse than others, the conclusion is obvious. Birmingham and Solihull Mental Health NHS Trust patients killed 13 people between 2010 and 2012 and was probably the worst in the country (The Times, 5/10/2013). Clearly the **murder rate of a group of mental health patients is related directly to their lack of supervision, the lack of available inpatient facilities, the quality of supervising staff, appropriate medical management and reluctance to use compulsory inpatient care for dangerous patients.** – in some units. Then surely the safety of the public depends more on the number of beds, the wording and spirit of the actual Mental Health Act itself in any given country, the number and abilities of the available staff, the willingness of individual psychiatrists to use compulsion and their common sense and worldliness. These then, are the main determinants of public risk.

25 "mental health patients" commit suicide each week. These are patients under medical care for their mental health condition at the time of their suicide. Although you could argue that all suicidal patients are mentally disordered at the moment they commit the self destructive act, by definition. **This is 1300 out of the total of 6,233 suicides/year (2013) – a quarter to a fifth** – roughly the same percentage as the number of mental health related homicides.

So of this group of avoidable early violent deaths – suicides and murders in the UK, diagnosed mental illness is responsible for a large proportion: or more accurately poor mental health services – perhaps as much as *a fifth.*

One of the saddest and most disturbingly unjust cases of murder by an unsupervised psychotic patient that I can remember took place on a leafy London street in December 2015. The Sunday Times and the BBC reported some of the case during the second week of October 2016. It demonstrates the utter failure of many of our national agencies, now after decades of human rights brow beating by politicians and lawyers, impotent and incompetent. It shows how the human rights of potentially violent and dangerous patients trump the safety of us all. The victim, Dr Jeroen Ensink had popped out of his flat in North London to post some cards telling his relatives of the birth of his second child. He was attacked and murdered without warning by a paranoid psychotic Nigerian student, Femi Nandap who believed himself to be "The Black Messiah". He had a history of violence, carrying knives (when he had previously been arrested) and breaching bail conditions. He had been arrested for an assault on a police officer which the CPS did not pursue despite knowing the student's carrying of knives, his violent and disturbed history. He was ordered to stay in the UK by the court but left, going to Nigeria, before returning again. His mental health team were clearly not supervising or treating him adequately if at all. If they were he would have been assessed and sectioned. He was not charged with a breach of bail conditions or arrested, the CPS dropping the case against him for lack of evidence despite the three knives on him when arrested, the violence against the policeman and his serious mental health history. So we have a murderer wandering the streets thanks to the politicians who framed the current ineffectual Mental Health Act and fail to provide enough secure units for dangerous patients, we have a total failure of the mental health team to supervise, assess and treat a dangerously psychotic and violent patient, a failure of the Immigration Service who let him out, then back in to the country unquestioned, an incomprehensible failure of the CPS who, with a plethora of evidence, failed to act and charge him, the Police who failed to arrest him for assault and carrying dangerous weapons, – no wonder he thought he had special powers. Any agency on this list might have done their job and saved the young father's life. But they didn't. The failings however all began with the impotent current Mental Health Act and the ineffectual nature of the Mental Health Team.

As I have said, it is clear that patients with overt mental illness are not tolerated, welcomed or supported well by the community at large. Patients with longstanding psychiatric symptoms who are living with us often barely cope socially, being isolated, shunned and alienated by their neighbours and the population as a whole. There is a huge iceberg of difficulty and distress caused by "Care in the community" that is indicated by the 90% loss of in-patient psychiatry beds over my life time and the failure to provide the compensating but incredibly expensive hospital – equivalent 24 hour community support services at home. Most of my chronic schizophrenic, psychotic, severely personality disordered, Asperger spectrum or bipolar patients have few contacts and friends around them and do not mix well. They are isolated, bored, ostracised, ignored, even under constant suspicion by their neighbours and certainly not integrated or cared for.

All hospital psychiatric units used to have locked doors. Today's regimes are much freer and very few patients are considered suitable for a secure, locked unit at any age now. One of the obvious results of "this open doors psychiatry" of the last few decades, apart from the regular murders by dangerous patients, has been the suicides by patients who had "left psychiatric wards without permission" – for instance: 470 suicides between '97 and '06. You can make up your own mind whether a truly humane society would treat more patients in genuinely secure places of safety and only discharge them once a better threshold of security for themselves and others had been reached.

Perhaps this is yet another way that soft politics by way of human rights trumps patients rights and kills vulnerable patients. All we need to do is offer a routine locked door on psychiatric wards. But clearly if your beds already have 120% occupancy you are far less likely to compel a patient to remain an in-patient despite being unsure of his or her outcome. Your safety threshold shifts when you need the bed for several others.

We need more psychiatric in-patient beds, more long stay units, places where the patients feel life is safer – as well as making life safer for you and me, for our children and neighbours. We need better laws that balance the human rights of the average member of society against those of the psychiatrically unwell patient and are willing to protect the patient from them self. We also need more assertive, worldly wise psychiatrists. We need politicians that are a bit less hopeful and naive and a bit more experienced in the real world of the dangers of the street, of the risks of untreated psychiatric patients and not just human rights theory. We actually need MORE psychiatrists who are accessible, who care (or seem to) and who have access to a local place of safety. And as I have said many times, psychiatrists who are culturally, verbally and communicatively able to connect with the average sick British patient.

The average GP with 2,200 patients will see about:

500 patients with significant psychiatric conditions a year.

20-30 patients with severe depression (of which he will try to admit perhaps one or two.) This applies to those who have attempted suicide I imagine, as many patients find psychiatric units themselves very depressing.

Marital or personal relationship crises 20-30 a year. (Surely this is per fortnight!).

Suicide attempts about 3 a year, 75% of adult suicides are male.

Alcohol crises 2-3 a year. I describe home detoxification in this section.

Compulsory psychiatric hospital admissions 2-3 a year.

Suicide: this is said to be about one every 5 years but I have had two in 30+ years – both without any warning of psychiatric illness. In fact without any previous contact with me at all for months or years.

Acute mania one every 5 – 7 years.

About one in ten of the adult population of the UK is said to be on antidepressants (National press Jan 2015). This makes us the third or fourth saddest nation in the EU and the third of the fourth worst provided with alternative treatments for depression.

The 2009 British Mental Health Survey (which is performed every 7 years) showed:

Depression	2.6 in 100 people
Anxiety	4.7 in 100 people
Mixed anxiety and depression	9.7 in 100 people
Phobias	2.6 in 100 people
OCD	1.3 in 100 people
Panic disorder	1.2 in 100 people
Post traumatic stress disorder	3.0 in 100 people
Eating disorders	1.6 in 100 people

were suffering from these conditions that year. Are a total of over a quarter of the population really suffering from a diagnosable, referable and treatable mental health disorder (?!) – Possibly of course many of the same people are suffering multiple diagnoses simultaneously.

This is from the Mind website.

The Mental Health Act 1983:

The books say one in two hundred of the mental health patients who present to a GP require In – patient treatment, that half the adult population will suffer a significant episode of depression/anxiety/or emotional problems in their lifetime and that 90% of patients who do go in, go in voluntarily.

My experience has been slightly different in that the lack of beds, the poor, over-stretched local psychiatric services and over latter years a complete disappearance of a practice CPN have meant that referral to secondary care has, for me and my practice been an extremely rare, difficult and often relatively unproductive process. A bed, when one is eventually found, tends to be out of the region, so visits by relatives are impossible. Also the conditions on many in-patient units are fairly uncontrolled and chaotic and many patients who were hoping for a place of calm and sanctuary find themselves almost literally in Bedlam. This can be particularly true for adolescents who are often taken from a caring family at the end of its tether and thrown together with chaotic, threatening, substance abusing, fellow patients. These can be self harming, often highly disturbed and aggressive, powerful, controlling, frightening and intimidating influences on them and 75% of adult mental health problems do begin in childhood.

Summary:

1983 Act section No:	Purpose	Duration	Application for admission	Medical recommendations:
2	Assessment	28 days	Approved SW or nearest relative	2 Drs incl. one approved under sect 12 and with knowledge of patient
3	Treatment	6 months	Approved SW or nearest relative	"
4	Emergency Ass't	72 Hours	Approved SW or nearest relative	1 Dr, preferably with knowledge of pt.

Compulsory Section:

Section 4: Emergency 72 Hrs: Used in exceptional circumstances, the GP alone recommending the detention using pink forms 5 and 7. Used when there is not time to obtain a second medical opinion and there is real danger to the patient or others. In the absence of the approved S/W only the nearest relative can make the application. The patient must then be reassessed by a section 12 approved doctor in hospital to reassess the length of the detention.

Form 7: The medical recommendation to be completed by a doctor with previous knowledge of the patient or one approved as having special experience (GPs should always carry a copy of this.)

Form 5: The Application to be completed by the nearest relative:

GPs should have a copy of this too.

Form 6: The application to be completed by an approved Social Worker when no nearest relative can be found, or refuses to fill in Form 5.

Section 2: Non emergency 28 days: The duty psychiatrist or other Section 12 approved doctor with another doctor, preferably the GP (with prior knowledge of the patient). No more than 5 days must pass between the two examinations. The Consultant, GP and Approved S/W all have an equal voice and the S/W provides the actual forms.

Form 3: The medical recommendation to be completed by both a doctor with a previous knowledge of the patient and an approved doctor with special experience, (GPs should always carry a copy).

Form 1: The application to be completed by the nearest relative.

Form 2: To be completed by an approved Social worker.

D.S.M. (IV) The diagnostic and statistical manual of mental disorders.

This is the American Psychiatric Association's publication and carries a list of 347 separate psychiatric diagnoses. The 5th edition came out in 2013. These include all the "real psychiatry" plus such things as: pica, encopresis, (is soiling a psychiatric diagnosis?), body dysmorphic disorder, adult antisocial behaviour, sibling relational problem etc, etc. – The book is the list of diagnoses and criteria which in the U.S.A. clarify what is a formal recognised psychiatric condition so that American psychiatrists can be paid. The problem is that some conditions which many regard as a variant of normal (which could include severe grief reaction, adolescent oppositional behaviour, pathological shyness, separation anxiety disorder, female hypoactive sexual desire, etc.) are being given a label, a treatment and therefore being "medicalised".

See if you can come up with more than 20 real psychiatric diagnoses from your own experience – it is pretty hard. The plethora of diagnoses and psychiatric conditions can be blamed on the way American psychiatry is funded. If a British GP isn't paid per diagnosis, he or she is unlikely to label someone as pathologically shy requiring treatment and if we think a relative is undergoing an excessive grief reaction I assume we would treat the symptoms with drugs and counselling (and with "ourselves") without giving them a new and significant diagnosis. Over here we tend to rely on the slightly more prosaic and down to earth I.C.D. system The International Classification of Diseases.

Interestingly, even the American National Institute for Mental Health is now thinking twice about the expansion of psychiatrisation of our behaviour and feelings and has revolutionised the diagnostic basis and categorisation of mental illness.

In Psychology Today in May 2013, an article stated the following:

"In a humiliating blow to the American Psychiatric Association, Thomas R. Insel, M.D., Director of the NIMH, made clear the agency would no longer fund research projects that rely exclusively on *DSM* criteria. Henceforth, the NIMH, which had thrown its weight and funding behind earlier editions of the manual, would be "re-orient(at) ing its research away from *DSM* categories." "The weakness" of the manual was, he explained in a sharply worded statement, "is its lack of validity." "Unlike our definitions of ischemic heart disease, lymphoma, or AIDS, the *DSM* diagnoses are based on a consensus about clusters of clinical symptoms, not any objective laboratory measure."

Despite this demand for some scientific objectivity, we are stuck for now just with symptoms. We can only objectively measure brain function poorly and cannot do assays of brain stem Serotonin, Dopamine or Acetyl Choline or assay a patient's paranoia or mood level.

In an article on "an obsolete DSM" and the problem of psychiatric diagnoses being "studies of disorders not the underlying systems" even New Scientist ran a two page spread on the new initiative to reclassify psychiatric disorders by cause rather than symptoms in May 2014 ("Psychiatry: The reboot starts here"). NIMH have now published 23 core brain functions with associated circuitry, transmitters and genes as well as the behaviour and emotions that go with them. They come under the five main headings: Negative Systems, Positive Systems, Cognitive Systems, Social Systems, and Modulatory Systems. There is no clear overlap between current clinical disorders and these brain systems. (For instance memory in the cognitive section is affected in depression, anxiety, bipolar disorder, schizophrenia etc.)

A full list of the brain's systems identified by NIMH are at bit.ly/1iGuqTz

This is adapted from New Scientist 10/5/2014:

The mind's 23 building blocks

These are the brain systems the NIMH has identified. They are grouped into five categories:

Negative systems

Acute threat – also known as our fear circuitry. Active when we sense danger

Potential threat – active, not in presence of a threat, but when we know the risk of danger is higher than normal. Associated with a sense of unease or anxiety

Sustained threat – negative emotional state caused by prolonged exposure to unpleasant conditions. Can cause loss of enjoyment in usually pleasurable activities

Loss – circuits active during permanent or sustained loss of a loved one, or emotionally significant objects or situation, such as shelter or status.

Frustration non-reward – reactions to lack of reward after sustained efforts. Can involve aggressive behaviour

Positive systems

Approach motivation – circuits that control our efforts to obtain a reward, such as sex or food

Initial responsiveness to reward – feelings of pleasure on obtaining a reward. Involves opioid and endocannabinoid receptors, those activated by morphine and cannabis

Sustained responsiveness to reward – mechanisms that terminate reward-seeking behaviour, such as satiety, the feeling that enough food has been eaten

Reward learning – processes by which we acquire information to predict rewards and learn to repeat the positive experience

Habit – repetitive behaviours that, once started, can be done unconsciously. Habits can free up cognitive resources

Cognitive systems

Attention – a range of processes that regulate access to awareness and higher cognitive systems

Perception – the processes that take sensory data and transform it into representations of the environment

Working memory – the system that can hold and manipulate many items of information on a temporary basis

Declarative memory – the encoding, storage and retrieval of representations of facts and events on a long-term basis

Language behaviour – systems that allow production and comprehension of words, sentences, and coherent communication

Cognitive control – systems that modulate the operation of other cognitive and emotional circuits. Can involve inhibition of behaviour or selection of best response from competing alternatives

Social systems

Attachment – systems for bonding with friends and family. Involves hormones such as oxytocin and vasopressin

Social communication – processes involved in exchange of socially relevant information, such as speech and body language

Perception of self – circuits involved in understanding ownership of one's own body or actions

Perception of others – processes involved in being aware of and reasoning about other animate entities, such as our "theory of mind" networks, which allow us to understand that other people can have different beliefs to our own

Modulatory systems

Arousal – a spectrum of sensitivity to stimuli, from coma and unconsciousness, through anaesthesia and sleep to full consciousness

Circadian rhythms – self-sustaining oscillations that organise the timing of biological systems

Sleep-wake cycle – recurring behavioural states that reflect coordinated changes in the brain. Regulated by physiological and circadian processes

Thanks for permission to use this from New Scientist.

There is quite a serious point here: My definition of depression may not be the same as yours-or your threshold for prescribing an antidepressant or an anxiolytic may be vastly different from mine. It is important for all doctors to agree what symptoms constitute a specific illness, what causes it and what the treatment is. Otherwise we would have no consensus or therapeutic uniformity at all. Agreed, many patients have bizarre health beliefs and there are many current applicable treatments (for instance certain foods in certain cancers) which might work but may not yet be generally accepted to do so. I have seen patients from France treated with Warfarin for post viral malaise and I was the subject of a protracted complaint from a Spanish air stewardess whose own doctor at home insisted that she needed six months of high dose penicillin and steroids for what seemed to me to be work related neck and shoulder pain complicated by depression-and so on. The Spanish doctor's diagnosis was persistent streptococcal asthenia and it needed these powerful treatments as far as he (and the patient) were concerned. (All my blood investigations, including ASOT, ESR, CRP etc. were, by the way normal).

Indeed, my own definition of depression is probably a lot looser than that of many doctors and I am sure my threshold for prescribing antidepressants consequently sometimes lower. On the other hand I can introduce you to dozens of patients whose lives have been transformed for the better and whose families are genuinely closer and happier as a result of TCADS and SSRIs. Is "depression just" any presenting complaint that improves with an antidepressant? When does grieving become "pathological" and justify medication? When do the "normal" effects of the break-up of a relationship become so upsetting as to justify giving a drug to the patient to help them cope? So much of General Practice psychiatry depends on the personality, feelings, beliefs, personal experience and sensitivities of *the doctor*. As well of course as the relationship between the doctor and that particular patient at that particular time. The same is far less true in other areas of treatment and prescribing.

Medically Unexplained Symptoms:

It is a most extraordinary thing, but I never read a patent medicine advertisement without being impelled to the conclusion that I am suffering from the particular disease therein dealt with in its most virulent form.

Jerome K Jerome

This heading includes somatisation disorder and conversion disorder – which used to be known as Hysteria.

Somatisation disorder consists of 6 or more symptoms in at least 2 physical groups (gastrointestinal, cardiovascular, genitourinary and skin or pain areas). The patient is more concerned with the symptoms than the underlying disease.

Conversion disorder is a disturbance of bodily function that does not conform to known anatomy or physiology of the central and peripheral nervous system. Typically it occurs in a distressful patient setting. Chronic conversion disorders can have the effect of stabilising a dysfunctional family unit or situation and take the form of motor, sensory or visceral symptoms. It therefore becomes established as it provides some sort of feedback "gain".

Hypochondriasis is a preoccupation with the fear of developing a serious disease (or the fear that the patient has one already). In this, the male and female incidence is equal. There is more concern with disease than symptoms.

There are also body dysmorphic disorder, factitious disorder (Munchausen's) and chronic pain disorder.

My own worse patient with factitious disorder was a pleasant lady in her thirties married to a police officer. She also had what seemed to be a genuine severe migraine with cyclical vomiting as well as her "invented" symptoms. This fact complicated her management somewhat as her synthesised symptoms were of abdominal pain and vomiting. These initially convinced me and then, in sequence: my practice colleagues, the out of hours doctors, multiple 999 ambulance crews and finally A and E doctors. She managed to systematically visit every A and E unit in four counties over a two year period, driving to hospitals up to 3 hours away saying she had become ill while visiting friends and giving a false name and address. She was admitted to at least two ITUs, had CVP lines sited (which she removed herself in the patient's toilet a day or so later before taking her own discharge unannounced – her car would have been left parked outside). She obtained a large number of controlled drug doses from a variety of doctors. All were convinced that she was worryingly ill and indeed significantly dehydrated though this wasn't ever confirmed biochemically. She also persuaded her children's school teachers that one of her children had cancer and that she had (convincingly) witnessed him to have a series of focal fits. Eventually she managed without my knowledge to arrange respite care for the child in a children's hospice and support at home from a network of neighbours. Thus she was demonstrating Munchausen's by proxy. As with so many other bizarre physical and psychiatric conditions which have an emotional or psychological basis, this patient disproved many of my preconceptions. She, her husband and her two children looked, acted and socialised in a pleasant and friendly way. She had a self deprecating sense of humour and constantly promised that she was trying to control her "attention seeking" behaviour". She was a pleasure to consult and we got on well despite her husband being at his wits end. She seemed to be a genuine victim of her own behaviour. *The NHS was entirely unable to make her better.* She was not "sectionable", antidepressants were ineffective, I went to and spoke with the psychiatrist who saw her but who gave up fairly quickly, counselling and psychotherapy were not available for her – I checked and enquired everywhere I could. The psychiatrists were singularly unhelpful. We had a case conference and Social Services did not feel that they had anything to contribute either. They felt the children were at no serious risk. My making myself available to see her immediately at the surgery at the onset of the vomiting and pain simply transferred the development of symptoms to the out of hours period. Thus, so as far as I know she is still arranging her own admission to A and E units, hundreds of miles away, where her reputation hasn't yet preceded her. The cost ? I cannot imagine.

Clearly there was something seriously wrong with her, it was complicated, had a deep rooted emotional cause, part of which was under her control and neither the psychiatric or physical NHS services were any use at all in making her better.

Interestingly it is more expensive to prove someone has "nothing medically wrong" with them than it is to "prove" that they have. The costs are on average is around £1000 per referral.

Simple things you can do to try and stop your patient having MUS:

1) Do advise a set of blood tests as a safety net but explain to the patient at the time of the test that you expect them to be negative, (so they are not concerned when they are), also don't get drawn into discussing what you are testing for as this plants a seed of doubt in the patient's mind. Keep it vague-avoid specific diagnoses.

2) Just reassuring the patient that nothing is wrong doesn't work and generally only lasts as far as the door of the surgery. It is better to give a physiological explanation of their symptoms and then discuss the effect of anxiety, the sympathetic nervous system and adrenaline on the body.

3) Some counselling services have a specific MUS service.

Common "Functional" symptoms and syndromes: The Frequent attender, the "Heart – Sink" patient etc.

These symptoms make up the arsenal of complaints of many "frequent attenders":
Muscle and joint pains (including Fibromyalgia),
Low back pain,
Tension headache,
Atypical facial pain,
Chronic fatigue syndrome,
Non cardiac chest pain,
Palpitations,
Non ulcer dyspepsia,
Irritable bowel,
Dizziness,
Insomnia.
-but any symptom can be complained of.
The more somatic symptoms that a patient has, the less likely it is that they represent a diagnosable disease – other than depression and or anxiety.

Trying to help:
Look at the 3 p's: Precipitating factors, predisposing factors, perpetuating factors.

The management consists of a good history (a psychiatric assessment is part of this – what are the specific concerns, reaction to coping with symptoms and so on), a proper examination, agree a limited number of investigations and tell the patient that if these are normal we won't need to do any others before starting treatment. Give a sympathetic rational explanation. It helps to explain the symptoms are real and familiar to the doctor. Give a positive summary linking the symptoms with behavioural, emotional and psychological factors and explain how the body reflects conflict or "stress". Offer the chance to discuss the patient's own or family anxieties. Encourage working through the symptoms and leading as normal a life as possible. Treat anxiety/depression, have a treatment and follow up plan and agree it with the patient.

Suggest a behavioural plan, antidepressants (which help *even in the absence of "depression"*), CBT, a graded return to normal activities (and work), a rehabilitation programme if one is available and appropriate.

"Chronic multiple Functional Symptoms" (CMFS), – rather than isolated or few complaints, are demonstrated by the heart sink, fat files, frequent attenders who make up 4% of the population. Each GP is said to have at least 10-15 such patients. (Although if this percentage is correct the number is more like 100). This group tends to consist of women, with chronic depression, problems with their personal relationships, occasionally misusing drink or drugs. Their childhood was often emotionally deprived and they may have been abused physically or sexually.

In various studies, patients defined as frequent attenders are those who have 10-13 consultations per year. So those who see the GP 3-5X the average rate and are: Female, (80-90%), tend to be divorced or widowed, or a single parent who used to have a partner, (social isolation and relative poverty are factors), have children under 5, are unemployed, from lower social classes, renting their accommodation and often the South Asian or Afro-Caribbean ethnic group. They receive prescriptions for more therapeutic groups of drugs and have 5X the average number of prescriptions overall. Patients living close to the practice tend to over consult more than those living far away. They not surprisingly but nevertheless disappointingly have 5X the average number of referrals to secondary care. Most have a "chronic health problem" which includes a mental health diagnosis, mainly depression and most score highly on depression scales.

How should we handle them?

They should be seen by one partner only and a proper review of their history made once this diagnosis is settled on. I find it helpful to do a (time consuming) summary and have this readily accessible in the notes so that you don't repeat referrals, or investigations or try unsuccessful past treatments. Start with a long appointment and an explanation and agreement about what further tests and future treatments are appropriate. Regular appointments and the avoidance of any extra or emergency appointments should be agreed on. It can be helpful to discuss the patient with a partner but some authors suggest the GP should seek ongoing psychological support for themselves. *This isn't practical or available* or usually necessary in my experience. Don't expect a cure – simply damage limitation and an agreed understanding of what can be expected by the patient and what they usually have to do. I have said this many times in various sections in this book: Effective management depends on being registered with a full time committed named GP. But the good management of difficult clinical situations is becoming increasingly impractical due to the discontinuity of modern Family Medicine. The above gold standard is impossible if the patient has a GP who is part time or is not actually even registered with a named doctor as is commonly the case in industrial practices, large practices, the "*You see who you get practices*" or practices which depend on many sessional or locum doctors.

Associated factors:

Depression, anxiety or panic disorder,

Chronic family or marital disharmony,

Dependent or avoidant personality traits,

Work stress,

Abnormal illness beliefs,

Tendency to somatisation,

Litigation pending,

Iatrogenic factors,

"I'm a doctor Jim, not a social worker"

– Bones, Star Trek

The reason they cause our hearts to sink is that most of the causes and effects of their problems are outside our ability to cure and not part of our bailiwick.

Grief, The phases:

Shock and numbness,

Yearning and searching,

Disorganisation and despair,

Reorganisation.

Alternatively some describe stages of:

Denial and Isolation,

Anger,

Bargaining,

Depression,
Acceptance.

This description seems realistic and natural, the disbelief and questioning – if the death were unexpected which is often accompanied by a feeling that the dead relative is still present. I remember hearing my father in the bathroom and even catching a glimpse of him in the back garden as I got up early one morning in the week after his sudden death. The reaction is different if the death is long and slow, – I always say to relatives that a sudden death is easier for the patient, far harder for the bereaved. It sounds glib now I read it written down. That's not all I say, obviously. A long terminal illness can be the other way round, – hard for everyone but it does give the relative time to prepare for loss and to emotionally say goodbye, to prepare. Grieving after a year or two of a loved one's cancer is completely different from that of an unexpected coronary or an accidental death on the way to work.

Death can bring out guilt and resentment, occasionally misdirected at the doctor by relatives. Why didn't you act sooner, why didn't you refer us to a different hospital, give us stronger drugs, keep her alive longer, let us have food supplements on the NHS, visit more? etc.

There is, despite grief being a natural and inevitable part of human life, sometimes a place for medication though. Grief can become obsessional and persistent, leading to withdrawal and depression and although it is said that some SSRIs cause dissociation from feelings, I believe that a brief respite from the unmanageable intensity of grief may sometimes be necessary to allow a relative to achieve a degree of perspective and to begin the process of renewing their life. Antidepressants and a short period of hypnotics can be a great help in certain situations and this can be one of them.

While we are on the subject of grief and how people cope with it, a word of warning: Most doctors are powerfully affected by the abundance of *feelings* that they have to deal with every day. The vast majority of it, now we have dispensed with antenatal clinics, post natal visits and many pastoral house calls is negative and depressing emotion. This accumulates the longer you are a doctor and obviously some specialities are worse than others. What is worse, the GMC and various recent studies looking at doctors undergoing complaints and investigations suggest the profession has progressively lost its previous thick skin. Whether this is in part due to the feminisation of medicine, the complaints readiness of patients today, the less challenging, gentler and more sociable training of junior doctors or the personal over sensitivity of very bright people it is hard to say. I believe that for some of us in GP, feeling little more than data input technicians and protocol administrators has reduced some of our professional independence, pride, decision making and emotional pleasure at the job. Our previous self determination and **control** which contributed to the GP's identity has been lost. So our feelings can become blunted, dysfunctional, protective, distorted, withdrawn. We work in an emotionally difficult world which many of us seem peculiarly unsuited for and find we have forgotten how you are supposed to respond to the constant outrageous fortune. This can be particularly true regarding our emotional response to **personal** bereavement. GPs have, thanks to the "burden of work" stopped seeing the most innocently happy, healthy and undemanding patients on our lists – our antenatal patients, some years ago. These cheerful mums and young children, who we then see with their brand new tiny babies in tow used to more than make up for all the miserable elderly, the worn out, the unhappy, those in pain or dying, the depressed majority. But no longer. We have given up our ante natal contact with these human antidepressants. No wonder many of us eventually become distant, cynical, negative and depressive – a defence mechanism against all the emotional drain on us. But a situation where many of us become divorced from our own feelings and natural emotions for fear of being overloaded by them. Unfortunately we often then find that we have forgotten how emotions are supposed work when we do need them. This applies to both positive and negative situations with our own families and friends.

Some doctors deal with even more sadness and emotion than the rest of us. One kind and caring Paediatric Oncologist I worked for thirty years ago killed himself without warning. He was loved and respected by everyone who worked with him. Perhaps he cared too much. I suppose that is possible. But the average oncologist in my experience becomes either

1) Hopelessly and unrealistically optimistic with their patients (-and this is just as damaging as being permanently negative and pessimistic) after a decade or two in their career.

or

2) Unwilling to share eye contact, to empathise or be warm and open with their patients.

Both are the defence mechanisms. One lies and one hides but both are a result of the repeated losses they suffer as an inevitable part of their job.

In some ways, the doctor, particularly the managing consultant who is over positive and unrealistically optimistic up to the day of the patient's death is harder for the GP to cope with. I have known and worked with both types.

I had just moved in to a new house and only superficially knew my neighbours when the husband rushed round one weekend saying his wife had collapsed. I knew she had been receiving treatment for breast cancer but my brief and directed questions as I grabbed my bag and hurried with him to his kitchen were answered with how well she had been doing and although her "lungs and bones were involved", the consultant had told them yesterday she would almost certainly get better. The poor woman was dead on the kitchen floor when I arrived, cachectic and clearly at the end of a long struggle with her illness. I took the decision not to attempt resuscitation although this was before DNAR forms existed. I simply confirmed death and stayed with him for a while to help out. The husband subsequently became a good friend over the years and never forgave the (private) consultant for her withholding the truth about his wife's illness. He never had the chance "to say goodbye" to her properly or to have the conversations that he felt in retrospect she and he would have wanted had they known the truth about how ill she was. (See section on Atul Gawande and Terminal Care).

The best and most committed psychiatrist we ever had at our local hospital gave up and left to everyone's huge disappointment, burnt out after five years in post. Twenty five years later we still talk about how good she was. Others, less effective and caring, less liked and committed have carried on since then. Most doctors need some sort of an emotional flak jacket. For some it is just not caring that much about patients to start off with. There was a long running local joke that one GP in my town who never seemed to have much empathy with most of his patients had bolted the patients' chairs to the floor on the opposite side of his desk, so they couldn't pull them closer towards the desk for a more intimate consultation. One patient with multiple problems including long running depression tried to register with him. Halfway through her initial consultation she was just into her history of IBS and was told "I had better stop you there, I really think you would be better off with another doctor, I don't have the time for those kind of psychological consultations". There are, I'm sure, times when we would like to say that to some patients. For others it is doing our best to "care" but developing a protective inner insensitivity that shields us from the suffering, the demands and the unreasonableness of many patients.

So most of us **are** affected by our patients. Well, I think we **are** if we are any good at our jobs, if we give *of ourselves* anyway. I have known GPs and other doctors who worked for 30 – 35 years, remaining emotionally just as positive and sure of themselves afterwards as before they started. BUT they were all pretty uninvolved, inaccessible doctors and all had well defined boundaries of what doctors should give to their patients. – And for their patients who wanted a little more than prescriptions and referrals, there wasn't much available.

If you aren't THAT kind of doctor, ungiving, wrapped up and thick skinned, If you are accessible and appropriately vulnerable your patients will benefit hugely. However you must be aware that the long term effect of caring for and losing hundreds of patients over three or four decades of a working life is to make your own loss and grieving mechanism harder, slower and less responsive than that of most people. Also, to make things worse for you, your own relatives will place far more responsibility and faith in you at times of family loss than is fair or reasonable. You **will** have slightly blunted, confused and unpredictable emotions but your relatives will sometimes think you don't have any at all. *"Let xxx sort out the funeral, he's a doctor, he's used to death, undertakers and hospitals, he can cope".*

While we are on the subject,

(Terminal Care:)

Terminal care is the discipline that rewards the GP the most for his or her caring and input, it separates the sheep from the goats in our profession. Give a little extra and you get great self justification and pleasure from the job and you are appreciated and rewarded for it. I always give my home phone number to the relatives and call in at weekends, on the way in and on the way home from the surgery. I carry Diamorphine, without which proper terminal caring is impossible. Shipman or no Shipman. Being available and accessible makes an immense difference to the management, quality, appreciation of the patient's care and to your relationship with the family, community, your reputation and your own self esteem. It makes the job a way of life and a vocation. Compared with good terminal care everything else can seem boring, routine and repetitive.

Terminal care gives us a time to make choices and to consider how we wish to work: Such things as quality of life as opposed to length of existence, the dividing line between professional and personal, looking after and caring, pastoral and hands on rather than just managing a death, getting involved and whether giving is actually its own reward. Indeed, what Primary Care, General Practice, Family Medicine actually *means*. Sorry, I didn't mean to be profound, I am not terribly religious and death can be a messy, smelly, practical, unspiritual thing but it will happen to us all and it is very easy to do badly. Hospital nurses in some infamous units, academic doctors designing standard care pathways and one GP psychopath have destroyed the confidence that patients once had of a painless and supported death. We GPs have also given up the high ground by being unwilling to carry Diamorphine and other effective controlled pain killers in our bags and to be available 24 hours a day to the few terminal patients on our list. I feel it is the issue that each of us has to be prepared to be judged on. Especially since the patient's best interests may be opposed by all around, – the family – with the wrong priorities, rigid medical and nursing "pathways", local and national nursing protocols, "Gold Standards" of Care, vindictive lawyers, Health Authority and PCT (CCG) administrators, most of whom, just like virtually all the current members of the GMC have no experience of General Practice and terminal care at home. – which is, after all, where most of us want it. Add to this Controlled Drug regulations, the Media, relatives' expectations, the 9 to 5 ethos of this generation of doctors, the poor out of hours services and there is one inevitable outcome:

All these factors ensure that rapid, flexible, *responsive* decision making, 24 hours day, putting the patient's interests first, is impossible and the patient suffers. You as the GP have to overrule **all** these factors and make executive decisions with the patient's interests paramount, sometimes shortening their life but improving their care and their quality of life.

I would go further than that: When I read about "GP Leaders", "Prominent GPs", "Leading GPs", "Keynote GP Speakers", "Prize winning GP practices" and so on, I always wonder what gives them the right to be called notable figures in the profession? Did their patients spontaneously assemble and throw flowers, cheer them to heaven outside their practices, carry them on their shoulders through the streets? No, – I often find that they have gained their kudos for all the *wrong reasons*. For instance: Firstly they are usually well known in GP politics or administration and so have reduced their patient contact or given up seeing patients altogether. That in itself is suspect. Secondly they will be have gained fame not for love of their patients or dedicated work, but for organisational or administrative changes, usually involving cost saving that can be quantified and published. For instance: A blanket reduction of antibiotic prescribing, large numbers of telephone consultations, low prescribing costs or high generic percentage, high turnover of patients seen, all sorts of measurable and publishable administrative changes. The *real things of value* to patients are never assessed by this journalistic hall of fame, – perhaps they are too hard to quantify: Objective patient satisfaction, the sense of overall patient well being, personal accessibility, doctor friendliness, mutual loyalty, overall health of the list, feeling of mutual trust, some measure of morbidity, the strength of the Doctor/patient bond, the number of visits to lonely or isolated patients, the willingness of patients to wait to see their own doctor, the willingness of the doctor to see distressed patients who may not be "emergencies", mutual confidence between doctor and his patients etc. One of the ways I assess a first class practice or GP is: Do(es) the partner (s) carry emergency drugs in their bags including Diamorphine and do the partners give their home phone numbers to the families of dying patients, Do they go out in the night when needed to supervise terminal care of their patients?

There is, from the point of view of families, no better way of assessing a good GP.

Post Traumatic Stress Disorder:

A pathological response to any significant trauma that the sufferer has been personally involved in. The symptoms may sometimes take weeks or months to develop and have previously been called shell shock, battle fatigue and so on in the case of service men at war.

The normal emotional response to significant trauma tends to improve with time. In the case of PTSD it often worsens and the memory and its associated feelings are disconnected, often being stimulated by a sensory link or trigger to the event.

The main symptoms are increased anxiety, the re-experiencing of memories of the trauma (flashbacks, nightmares, intrusive memories) and distress when reminded of the event, – also trying to avoid reminders of the event.

The avoidance of memories, places and things connected with the trauma, emotional detachment and insensitivity.

Poor sleep, emotional lability, irritability, poor concentration.

Other symptoms of depression, guilt, as well as drug and alcohol abuse can be present.

In children, developmental regression, separation anxiety, sleep problems, aggression and "acting out" may occur. Personal assault or injury seem to be worse than complete accidents in the causation of PTSD and risk factors include previous significant trauma, a history of physical or sexual abuse, substance abuse, a family history of depression etc.

The basic problem seems to be the compartmentalisation of and failure to emotionally deal with the trauma of the unpleasant event. All treatments attempt to enable the patient to safely think about, re experience and process the feelings caused by the event in a healthier way. They include

Trauma focussed CBT,

Family Therapy,

Anti depressants and

Eye movement desensitisation and reprocessing. EMDR (rapid sideways eye movements are supposed to unlock the information processing system of the brain while the patient is asked to recall the distressing event). Following the therapist's gestures by the eye movements of the patient allows a dissociation of painful thoughts and reactions and then a reconnection of less painful feelings with a recalled memory of the traumatic event. With each session a new goal may be set and intercurrent auto relaxation therapy can be used. It is not yet know whether it is the recollection and desensitisation by exposure or the "bilateral stimulation" (which can be occasioned by a number of different sensory stimuli not just eye movements) that is the therapeutic agent. Or indeed a bit of both.

Useful Psychiatric Drugs:

Bipolar Disorder: (Bipolar mood disorder):

Lithium and Valproate are anti manic mood stabilisers.

Lamotrigine has a similar effect and is an antidepressant mood stabiliser.

Olanzapine reduces manic mood switching and bipolar relapse.

So:

Lithium (avoid sodium excretion): monitor Lithium level and U and Es, creatinine 3 monthly, TFTs 6 monthly. This is much safer than its reputation would have you think.

Others: SSRI and Quetiapine or combinations of Fluoxetine, Sertraline, Mirtazepine, Venlafaxine, Quetiapine, Other treatments include Pramipexole, Carbamazepine.

Acute relapses: Antipsychotic or Vaproate or Lithium or combinations. Consider short term benzodiazepine e.g. Clonazepam 500ug nocte or BD if patient already on prophylaxis. Check levels (Lithium, Carbamazepine, Valproate etc.)

Lithium: Target range is 0.6 – 1.6mmol/li (blood 12 hrs after dose) But >4mmol can be effective. Monitor U and Es and TFTS annually, more frequently in the elderly or if levels fluctuate. Initially nocturnal dose, (easier to monitor) use the same trade name preparation.

Do levels weekly 'til stable, three monthly thereafter or if toxic (which I have never seen) or non compliant. Lithium toxicity can be due to diuretics, esp thiazides, dehydration, alcohol, NSAIDs, also c Fluoxetine, Fluvoxamine, Phenytoin, Carbamazepine, Haloperidol, Metronidazole. Sympts. of toxicity: Nausea and vomiting, tremor, muscle weakness, confusion, polyuria, polydipsia.

The Madness of King George:
By the way, it seems likely that bipolar disorder was George III's diagnosis and not porphyria as was long suspected. Apparently his odd coloured urine was a common side effect of some of the medication he was given.

Narcolepsy: Modafinil, Provigil 100-400mg mane and at lunchtime, can also be used for tiredness due to obstructive sleep apnoea. Has been abused by students cramming for exams to stay awake.

Panic Disorder: Imipramine 25mg Tabs. Clomipramine (Anafranil): 10mg 25mg 50mg 75mg SR-"The most powerful antidepressant ever", an SSRI as well as a TCAD. Citalopram with or without Diazepam.

Disruptive behaviour: Short term with no alternative (as is so often the case), agitation and confusion: Haloperidol 0.5-2mg BD. Injection, 2-10mg IM. Risperidone 0.5-2mg BD. Olanzapine 5-10mg OD.

Note: **Citalopram** a useful SSRI with comparatively few S/Es, it can be used for depression with or without panic, with or without Diazepam, also for agoraphobia, pathological crying and depression after stoke.

St. John's Wort: (Hypericum perforatum)
"The poor man's Prozac." It acts as an SSRI via the active agents: Hyperforin and Hypericin.

Trials conflict but it does seem to have some antidepressant activity.

It also has many potential interactions:
HIV Protease Inhibitors,
other HIV treatments,
Warfarin,
Ciclosporin,
OCPs,
Anticonvulsants,
Theophylline,
Digoxin,
Triptans,
SSRIS.

Flupent(h)ixol. Fluanxol, Depixol. A Thioxanthene antipsychotic with antidepressant properties at low doses. Fluanxol is useful in mixed anxiety/depression (500ug-3mg daily) and Depixol is an oily depot injection given every 2-4 weeks in schizophrenia and other psychoses.

Anxiolytics:
Generalised Anxiety Disorder: All sorts of drugs of many classes have been recommended at various times:
Pregabalin (150-600mg/day in 2 doses), Paroxetine, Sertraline, Escitalopram (long

term), Venlafaxine, Duloxetine (Cymbalta) Quetiapine, Amisulpiride, Risperidone.

Note: Benzodiazepine antagonist: Flumazenil. Anexate 200ug IV then further doses every minute. In a hospital setting usually.

Midazolam, Hypnovel Injection 10mg in 2ml. This is sedative, tranquilising and amnesic as anyone who has opted for "the injection" rather than the inhumane "spray" before an endoscopy will attest.

Hydroxyzine, Atarax, 50-100mg QDS: Anxiolytic and antipruritic.

Alprazolam Xanax 250ug and 500ug. Rapid onset anxiolytic, hypnotic, sedative and anti nauseant. Has to be on a private prescription. Although disinhibition IS quoted as a possible side effect, I find of the available benzodiazepines it is the quickest onset and safest to prescribe for fear of flying. It is also the least likely benzodiazepine to cause the patient to jump up and head for the exit mid flight, having become disinhibited.

Buspirone, 5mg, 10mg, 2-3x daily. May take weeks to work, interacts with grapefruit juice, vertigo the commonest S/E. Short acting, 2-3 hour half life.

Clobazam, Frisium, 10mg. Is an effective benzodiazepine tranquiliser which can be given at night and works all day. It is now only available for the treatment of epilepsy on the NHS, marked "SLS". (Selected List Scheme).

Chlordiazepoxide, Librium. 5mg and 10mg Caps and Tabs. Useful in a detox. regime in alcohol withdrawal as well as short term treatment of anxiety.

Other treatments in Anxiety: Amisulpride, Solian, 25mg BD and increase, an atypical antipsychotic. Much bigger doses used in schizophrenia.

Schizophrenia, Psychoses, Antipsychotics: And anti inflammatories?

Core features:

Hallucinations,

Delusions,

Disorganised or strange speech,

Agitated or bizarre behaviour,

Negativity (flatness, poor motivation),

Extreme or labile emotional state,

Withdrawal from friends and work,

Change in behaviour/personality that affects daily life,

Cognitive disturbance,

A split personality doesn't usually figure at all.

Causes: High levels of C Reactive protein in pregnancy are associated with a 60% increase in the development of schizophrenia in offspring. (Sept 2014 Am J Psych.) A growing body of evidence suggests that infection and immune activation play a role in the aetiology of schizophrenia. Various studies have shown epidemiological evidence relating maternal antibodies to Influenza, Rubella, Toxoplasma and H Simplex Type 2 and the subsequent development of the condition.

For every increase of 1mg/L of maternal CRP, the risk of schizophrenia in offspring increases 28%.

Interestingly, the same Finnish research group that published this finding in 2014 previously noted an association between raised maternal CRP and childhood Autism. Some new research suggests that Omega 3 supplementation in adolescence reduces the later risk of schizophrenia in high risk groups (by reducing dopamine levels or via their anti inflammatory effect?) Research published in October 2015 highlighted the role of the brain's own "over active immune system" in causing damage, documented via microglial cell activity. These are over active in those at risk of and patients suffering from schizophrenia and are quantified by specific labelling techniques. It is suggested that anti inflammatories may be useful in the treatment of schizophrenia but if that is the case, why do steroids sometimes trigger psychoses?

Various genes are known to be associated with schizophrenia. Four central nervous system signalling genes are recognised, being involved in the growth and regulation of nerve circuits. One gene, – PTPRG causes early onset severe psychosis. The SLC39A13 gene causes early onset schizophrenia, disrupted cognition, severe psychopathology and frequent suicide attempts. ARMS/KIDINS220 causes a late cognitive decline as of a degenerative process. TGM5 causes ADD and a less severe disorder.

If rapid tranquillisation is required:

Oral preparation first and then I.M: Lorazepam, Haloperidol, Olanzapine (long acting, very expensive, improved cognition, less restlessness but causes weight gain.) Can use Lorazepam and Haloperidol together. May need anticholinergics with Haloperidol.

Alternative Drugs in Schizophrenia:

Clonazepam, Pramipexole, (Mirapexin)

Typical Drugs:

Old fashioned:

Pimozide, (Orap),

Sulpiride, (Dolmatil),

Benperidol, (Anquil),

Chlorpromazine, (Largactil),

Fluphenazine, (Modecate),

Levomepromazine, (Nozinan), which is also an analgesic and anti emetic.

Trifluoperazine, Stelazine. For severe agitation, anxiety, schizophrenia, for anxiety 1-2mg tds etc. can be co-prescribed with SSRIs.

Promazine: 25mg tab, 25mg and 50mg per 5mls soln. Use in agitation and restlessness qds.

Haloperidol, Haldol, Serenace, caps 500ug, tabs 1.5mg, 5mg, 10mg, 20mg, Injection 5mg/ml (useful in the acutely disturbed or agitated out of hours patient). The decanoate injection is 50mg and 100mg/ml, given four weekly in schizophrenia etc.

Used as an adjunct to the short term management of anxiety as well as childhood behavioural disorders, in bigger doses in mania, hypomania, organic psychoses and so on.

Dose varies a great deal: In adults, 1.5-20mg/day (maximum dose 200mg!!)

So in anxiety start with 0.5mg BD/TDS and increase, in aggression and agitation try 3-5mg TDS and reduce when possible.

High doses of B vitamins (B6, B8 and B12) can reduce the symptoms of schizophrenia (Psychological Medicine 2017.)

The "Atypical Antipsychotics"

Clozapine, (Clozaril) – Risk of myocarditis and cardiomyopathy (look for tachycardia). Used in "treatment resistant schizophrenia". Watch WBC (neutropoenia) also rarely, convulsions, hyper salivation, drowsiness, generally less tardive dyskinesia.

Risperidone, (Risperdal) – 2mg on first day, 4mg on second day. For acute (probably the best treatment) and chronic schizophrenia. Occasionally used in children for oppositionality and aggressive behaviour. 1/2mg-5mg/day.

Quetiapine, (Seroqual).

Olanzapine, (Zyprexa) 10mg nocte, good at treating negative symptoms, low incidence of extrapyramidal S/Es.

Amisulpride (Solian).

Aripiprazole (Abilify). Mania, Hypomania 15mg/day, Schizophrenia 10-30mg/day. Long term mood stabiliser. Can increase risk of CVA in dementia.

Paliperadone (Invega, Xepilon).

ADD OTHERS HERE:

Smoking, cannabis and schizophrenia:

Research published in 2015 (Lancet Psychiatry 10 July) Suggested that not only do schizophrenics smoke more but smokers were more likely to develop schizophrenia. 57% of patients having a first episode of psychosis are smokers, >3X the general population. In daily smokers the onset is on average a year earlier. Smoking cannabis with tobacco in the words of the study could give you "a double whammy" for schizophrenia, as cannabis use is known to be associated with first episodes of psychosis in the young.

Even worse: in male adolescents with a high risk of schizophrenia (polygenic risk score) there is a negative correlation between cannabis use and cortical thickness. This is not the case for females or low risk males.

Alcohol: See Later in section: ***

Alcohol withdrawal:

Diazepam, Lorazepam, Chlordiazepoxide, can be used at home in a slowly reducing regime. Plus or minus anti psychotics such as Haloperidol or Olanzapine if necessary. Sometimes you can be reluctantly forced into supervising an alcohol withdrawal at home as the least worst option in someone who convinces you they are now motivated to change, refuses to engage with secondary care and (most importantly) has a sensible and caring person living at home with them. Chloral Hydrate reduces some life threatening side effects, Carbamazepine or Topiramate can be used as anti convulsants. Chlormethiazole (Heminevrin) is still helpful as an adjunct sedative with or instead of benzodiazepines.

Other alternatives are Gabapentin and Baclofen (the latter in a highly variable dosage regime with very variable side effects and response rates).

I use Chlorpromazine or Chlordiazepoxide over 7-10 days. Stop all alcohol on the first day.

Thus:

Chlordiazepoxide 5-10mg (up to 15-20mg) 3-4X daily, slowly reducing.

Community detoxification should last 7-10 days and preferably be supervised by a motivated friend, partner, loved one, as well as by you. You don't have to visit them every day but they do need someone else in attendance or close at hand who is sober of habit as well as sober – and you should probably phone daily at first and see them again at least on the last day (as well as a few weeks after).

There is, of course, a small risk of Wernicke's Encephalopathy (the triad of ophthalmoplegia, ataxia, and confusion and usually asthenia as well) +/-Korsakoff psychosis which can be prevented by supplementing Vitamin B1. Oral absorption is unpredictable so give big doses of B1 systemically, other B vitamins and Vitamin C, preferably a few days before detox begins. **Ideally** the B1 should be given **IM** as 250mg Thiamine daily 3-5 days before or during the process.

Treat other symptoms of withdrawal, anxiety, hallucinations, confusion, diarrhoea, hyperthermia, nausea, headache, palpitations, tachycardia, tremors, paranoia, with haloperidol, heminevrin, lomotil, beta blockers, increased doses of benzodiazepines etc.

Wernicke's Encephalopathy may prompt Korsakoff's Syndrome: poor memory, confabulation, confusion and change in personality.

By the way, Wernicke's Encephalopathy may follow bariatric surgery if vomiting is treated with glucose/electrolyte infusion without Thiamine. Thiamine is one of the many deficiencies that can occur after bariatric surgery.

Maintaining abstinence:

Antabuse: Disulfiram. An Aldehyde dehydrogenase inhibitor: 200mg tabs. Initially 4 stat, then 3 on second day, 2, 2, then 1 daily, review regularly especially after 6 months. Any alcohol drunk is metabolised to acetaldehyde which causes the unpleasant symptoms. Flushing, tachycardia, hypotension, headache, dyspnoea, vomiting. Starts in 10 mins, lasts for hours. Avoid in pregnancy and avoid with Metronidazole. Avoid alcohol for 2 weeks after stopping medication. Up to 50% users remain abstinent. All sorts of contraindications. Liver disease, renal failure, epilepsy, D.M. CHD, heart failure, hypertension, psychosis, personality disorder, the suicidal, porphyria, breast feeding etc.

Acamprosate, Campral. A Centrally acting stimulator of GABA receptors and a modifier of glutamate levels, (which surge in level within the brain on alcohol withdrawal), this reduces the adverse effects of alcohol withdrawal and abstinence.

Also **Adepend Naltrexone***in alcohol dependence.

Opioid Dependency:

Sublingual Buprenorphine Subutex. in Opioid dependancy.

Also in Opiate withdrawal: Lofexidine, Britlofex. Alpha adrenergic agonist, takes 7-10 days, 0.2mg BD gradually increasing, maximum 12 daily, slightly sedative.

Naltrexone* Nalorex Opizone, Heroin dependence. Adepend *Alcohol dependence.

Smoking Cessation:

NRT: Nicotine Replacement Therapy.
A bewildering number of treatments:

Nicorette:	Tabs 2mg,
	Chewing Gum 2mg various flavours.
	Lozenges 2mg,
	Patches 5mg, 10mg, 15mg, also "Invisi patches",
	Oral spray,
	Nasal spray,
	Inhalator,
Nicotinell:	Gum 2mg, 4mg,
	Lozenges 1mg, 2mg,

TTS Patches. ("10" "20" and "30", which I take to be roughly equivalent to the number of cigarettes previously consumed in 24 hrs that they should substitute for). The 24 hour patches do cause dreams but prevent the morning craving as it takes an hour or two for Nicotine levels to rise when a patch is applied. The whole point of *smoking* a drug is that the "hit" is as quick as an IV dose.

Niquitin: Gum 2mg, 4mg.

Lozenges 1.5mg.

Patches, 7mg, 14mg, 21mg.

Electronic Cigarettes: E-cigarettes: Vaping: These are miniature battery driven vapourisers which look like cigarettes, – well actually they don't. They are much bigger and look like smoking penny whistles you suck. They usually appear to "smoke", produce inhalable flavoured vapour with or without Nicotine and without tar, carbon monoxide and the hundreds of inhalable toxic organic carcinogens of burning tobacco smoke. The liquid contains propylene glycol, glycerin, Nicotine and flavouring generally. They are clearly safer than real cigarettes and they do **seem** to help people quit smoking the real thing. They are potentially addictive – since Nicotine is addictive, they are currently unregulated and there is precious little reliable trial evidence as to their efficacy and safety as yet. Political concern has been expressed about them becoming part of youth culture-in much the same way as real cigarettes did for their parents' generation. There is also some concern that they may be a way young people are introduced to the pleasures of smoking and that the flavours, (8000 in all!) including menthol, bubble gum, cherry (the most irritating to the airways apparently), various fruits and so on may be specifically designed for children.

2.8 million people used them in the UK in mid 2015, 9 million Americans.

Antismoking Drugs:

Bupropion, Zyban. 150mg OD for 7days then BD 7-9 weeks. Set the stop day around day 8. Taper off after the end of the course. Avoid in a history of psychiatric illness.

Varenicline, Champix. 500ug OD for 3 days then BD for 4 days, then 1mg BD for 11 weeks. Stop smoking at 2 weeks. Review and possibly repeat at 12 weeks £55/m. Probably the most reliable current available treatment.

Smoking and the psychiatric patient:

If you have worked in a psychiatric ward you will know how important the anxiolytic Nicotine is to many patients. On psychiatric wards and occasionally with disturbed patients at home I have seen and used the calming pharmacological and social effect of a cigarette on a disturbed patient. Virtually all psychiatric in-patients seemed to smoke heavily when I was a registrar, as did the nurses – if not the doctors. A quarter of those patients who smoke in mental health units took up smoking in hospital and mental health patients are three times more likely than the general population to smoke. Perhaps the reasons for so much self destructive smoking behaviour are the combined pharmacological effects of Nicotine, the peer group pressure, boredom, the reward ethic, trying to give the day some sort of punctuation and structure or simply addiction or self harm in a group prone to addictive and self harming behaviour.

Either way I doubt whether the psychiatric unit is a good place to try and ban smoking inside despite the general health benefits.

THE SAMARITANS: Phone no. 116 123.

Depression:

The prevalence of depression in the developed world is 18%. It is 9.4% in the developing world. There are 800,000 suicides per year worldwide. In the UK, 500 under 25 year olds kill themselves a year, 25% after a bereavement. 1:9 under 20 year olds who commit suicide do so following a friend's suicide. A half of fatal suicides in the young are preceded by an episode of non fatal self harm- so regularly dismissed by mental health services (Today Programme 13/7/17). The lifetime prevalence of mood disorders in the US is 20%. I am amazed I found any reference that put it this low. Over a half of American depression is classed as severe or very severe. Three quarters of depressed adults have other mental health diagnoses and 40% of substance misusers have a mood disorder too. There are 87,000 depressed children in the UK (Today program April 2016).

I suppose that, by definition, all "suicides" must have suffered a degree of depression although I can imagine situations where drug reactions, personality disorders, manipulative behaviour taken accidentally to extremes, inappropriate overreaction to emotional stimuli, even extreme sexual game playing could lead to accidental suicide. Apparently 2007 saw the lowest suicide numbers recorded in the UK but 3/4 were, as usual, men. Rates peaked in 2014 according to Paul Farmer, Chief Executive of Mind. Interesting that his name should be Paul Farmer. Amongst occupations, farmers have one of the highest incidences of suicide for a variety of reasons, as do a number of other specific professions (see the Work chapter). Significantly for doctors, the number of us killing ourselves while we are being the subject of a GMC investigation, a complaint or without *any obvious* trigger factor has increased over the last couple of decades. These are mainly women. This is while huge changes have taken place in the demography of the profession, its working conditions and training – which have become, by any standards, **easier** over the same period. Suicide is the leading cause of death among boys and men aged 15-49. In 2015/6, 122 people killed themselves with men 3X as likely as women to "die at their own hand". One in five mothers are said to suffer mental health problems during pregnancy or in the first year of their child's life but from my experience of the last 40 years this is either a vast over estimate or a very elastic definition of "mental health problems."

Concussion triples the long term suicide risk of the sufferer even though clinically fully recovered.

Depression in the young, as measured by the prescription of antidepressants is definitely increasing throughout the west. Admissions of under 13 year olds for self harm in the ten years up to 2015 increased in boys from 235 to 277 and in girls from 489 to 708.

In mid 2016 a study noted 17 gene sites associated with increased risk of depression. Given the social withdrawal, sleep disturbance, poor eating and self harm that go with it, it is hard to see why evolution has tolerated any genetic residue of depression. Unless, partially expressed, depression genes confer caution and further consideration in dangerous environments when the more confident and cheerful get eaten by predators, fall off precipices, drown or starve because they were over optimistic about their chances of success.

In under 18 year olds between 2005 and 2012 one study saw a rise of 54% of antidepressant prescribing in the UK. This was unsurprising as it coincided with an almost complete absence of talking treatments outside teaching hospitals and a few University hubs – and so what most GPs had to offer was ten minutes with themselves each appointment and the doctor-in-a-pill, in the form of an antidepressant or tranquilliser. There wasn't much else.

The same seems to have been true throughout Europe: Denmark saw an even greater increase in antidepressant prescribing-of 60%, Germany of 49%, the US of 26% and the Netherlands of 17% over the same timescale. In a separate study (Swansea Univ, of 360,000 children) between 2003 and 2013 there was an increase of 30% of antidepressant use recorded. Fluoxetine 20mg capsules are £1 a month for 28. They are the only SSRI recommended for children and young adolescents (although NOT the only anti depressant that works). Perhaps this explains the reason why drug treatments were popular in the cash strapped NHS instead of expensive talking therapists.

All sorts of activities and occupations are associated with depression: (See **Work section**). In a study published in the Mayo Clin Proc in 2015:90 (2) 184-93, it turned out that two of the things most of us spend a huge part of our lives doing are associated with an increased risk of developing depression. Namely watching TV and driving. – and it seems you don't have to do much of either. In a study involving 5000 patients, people who spent >9hours/week in a car had a 28% greater risk of developing depression than those who spent <5 hours. That is a Monday to Friday commute of only 55 minutes each way – assuming you keep away from the car at weekends or a half hour commute with two hours in the car each weekend day. Those who watched >10 hours of TV a week had a 52% greater risk of depression than those who watched TV for <5 hours.

Those spending >19 hours a week in a combination of TV and driving had a 74% increased risk of depression compared with those under 12 hours. Physical activity mitigated these risks.

Certain sub cultural groups have a high incidence of depression. Goths, the youth group typified by leather clothing, black nail varnish, heavy make-up, multiple drug use, morbid mood and music, but who are probably non violent and hold apolitical beliefs, have 5x the average level of self harm and 3x the age matched level of depression. In one Scottish study, 7 out of 15 Goths studied had attempted suicide. Do you become attracted to the negativism of Goth culture because you are chronically depressed and feel alienated from your peers or do you become depressed because you are so heavily invested in a self destructive and suicide obsessed identity cult? My gut feeling is that it is the former.

If we suffer depression, of course, it influences everything we do – so it adversely affects control of such conditions as diabetes that require our attention, awareness, thought and supervision. One survey (The National Survey on Drug Use and Health) found a prevalence of suicidal ideation amongst adults with depression of 26.3%. It is, like hypertension and probably most conditions, under recognised and under treated, patients don't cash in their prescriptions and don't comply with or fully understand their treatment instructions. So they tend not to take their treatment properly either. In one Dutch survey, moderate and severely depressed hospital patients were under treated in 43% cases (how did they assess this?) In general Practice cases the figure was 73% (but by whose standards?)

Newer research relates markers of inflammation such as CRP with depression severity and higher levels of CRP result in poorer antidepressant response (Escitalopram and Nortriptyline). Other inflammation markers associated with poor SSRI and TCA response are Migration Inhibitory Factor and Interleukin-1beta. Supplementing Omega 3 or oily fish (which are known to be anti inflammatory), on the other hand, improves response to SSRI treatment. Treatment resistant depression is being treated in some units with supplementary anti inflammatory drugs.

Even changing the clocks increases depression. When the clocks go back in autumn one study saw an 11% increase in unipolar depression in 185,400 hospital contacts. The effect dissipated over the following 10 weeks. Bipolar disorder was unaffected by either forward or backward clock resetting.

Antidepressants:

There are various ways of approaching the prescribing of antidepressants – for instance you could say if the patient is:

You should prescribe:

	Lethargic:	Anxious:
and **Male:**	Reboxetine	Paroxetine
	Lofepramine	Dosulepin
	Moclobemide	
	Imipramine	
	or with **physical symptoms,**	Duloxetine
and **Female**	Fluoxetine	Paroxetine
	Lofepramine	Dosulepin
	Imipramine	
	Reboxetine	

in **breast feeding and pregnancy** Fluoxetine and Dosulepin if **psychotic symptoms** add Olanzapine.

A review in 2014

Recommended SSRIs such as Citalopram, Escitalopram, Sertraline in **depression with anxiety.**

Venlafaxine should be avoided in patients with **depression and anxiety.**

Depression and fatigue responds better to a NA/Dopamine reuptake inhibitor – Bupropion, or Venlafaxine or Fluoxetine.

Depression with insomnia is best treated with Mirtazepine or Nefazodone.

Depression with pain responds to Tricyclics or Duloxetine.

Other specific antidepressants:

TCADs: Tricyclics have a 3 ringed molecular structure, each ring having six sides. 27 are listed in the literature. They and Venlafaxine are said to be better at major depression but worse, obviously, in overdose. They have Alpha 1 and H1 blocking effects.

Amitriptyline: 10mg-150mg can be used in neuropathic pain, IBS Fibromyalgia etc.

Nortriptyline: Allegron can be used for neuropathic pain and migraine. 10mg TDS to a max of 150mg daily, NARI, stimulant, least postural hypotension, less sedative.

Imipramine: Tofranil, used in nocturnal enuresis, 25-75mg Nocte.

Clomipramine: Anafranil (Obsessive/compulsive Disorders), 10-150mg daily especially potent with lithium.

Trimipramine: Surmontil. A sedative TCA.

Dosulepin: 25mg – 75mg Nocte. A reasonable substitute for benzodiazepines in the chronic insomniac, increases seizures, toxic in overdose.

SSRIs:

Safer in overdose than TCADs and though *they can* make migraine worse (though this isn't my patients' experience-actually the reverse) they are said to be less likely to cause mania in Bipolar disorder. You can of course prescribe the two, SSRIs and TCADs, together.

Fluvoxamine: Faverin: 50-100mg nocte initially. Good in the young, obsessional and children, quite sedating. Low concentration in breast milk. Anxiolytic, nausea, convulsions.

Fluoxetine: Prozac. 20-60/80mg daily. The most famous and therefore most controversial anti depressant. Give a bigger dose in eating disorders and in the obsessional. Long half life, (of Fluoxetine 2-4 days and its metabolite, Norfluoxetine 7-15 days) – avoid in epilepsy and in diabetics. The wash out period is 5 weeks before giving eg MAOIs/ sumatriptan with potential interactions: (Serotoninergic Syndrome). One current controversy (-and since "Prozac Nation" there has been a constant public debate about Fluoxetine) is whether it works. Apparently the initial trial data wasn't retained and was destroyed so that it is no longer available for reanalysis. I can categorically say that Fluoxetine lifts depression in the majority of withdrawn and symptomatically retarded depressed patients and has helped the recovery of dozens of my own patients. I can introduce anyone who doubts it to at least twenty individuals whose lives were transformed by Prozac. I would tend to avoid it in agitated, insomniac anxious depression or use it along with other medications because other SSRIs may be better at anxiolysis. It is particularly helpful in teenage depression.

Sertraline: Lustral, 50-200mg daily. Licensed for long term use, can co prescribe with Lithium, sedative. Need high doses.

Paroxetine: Seroxat, 20-40mg Half life 21 hours. Good in panic disorder, obsessive/ compulsive, the least bad in epilepsy. Possible discontinuation reactions, (tail off slowly) If no response at 20mg, you often need a **big** dose.

Paroxetine has an interesting history. I find it the most helpful calming SSRI and have never had a serious problem tailing it off in patients who were previously well. The "Discontinuation Syndrome" can be a convenient label for unresolved pre existing psychiatric morbidity, it being easy to blame the drug (or the doctor) for how unsettled you still feel. There was however concern that information regarding teenage suicide risk may have been played down and later that payments to generic drug companies to delay production were made by the manufacturer. GSK was fined £38m in 2016 for "bribing" generic manufacturers not to make Paroxetine when Seroxat came off licence.

-You pay your money. I find it safe and effective.

Paroxetine and Fluoxetine reduce the beneficial effects of Tamoxifen in breast cancer by inhibiting the enzyme CYP2D6 that activates it.

Citalopram: Cipramil. 20-60mg: For depression and panic disorder with or without agoraphobia, also for pathological crying and depression after stroke. Low seizure propensity. Few side effects but often relatively ineffective. May affect QT, – this or Escitalopram, Cipralex, (left enantiomer of Citalopram) is probably one of the first to try in the young with depression or generalised anxiety disorder.

NOTE: Stop the SSRI 2 weeks before commencing an MAOI. Any interaction, hyperthermia, rigidity, myoclonus, autonomic instability, delirium, coma, treat with Cyproheptadine, Dantrolene.

Avoid interactions by:

Starting MAOI:
>1 week after Sertraline,
>2 weeks after Fluvoxamine/Paroxetine,
>5 weeks after Fluoxetine.

SSRIs are potent P450-2D6 inhibitors, particularly Paroxetine. Fluvoxamine is probably the least. – hence a variety of potential drug interactions.

Tetracyclics, as you would expect, consist of four rings of six sides stuck together forming a molecule. They include: Amoxapine, Mianserin, Mirtazepine. Tryptophan and Maprotiline are similar but don't quite make the four rings. Flupentixol (Flupent(h) ixol – Depixol, is an anti psychotic depot and at a lower dose Fluanxol – an anti depressant) has four similar rings.

Others:

Venlafaxine: Ef(f) exor. An SNRI, a TCA without Histamine or Adrenoceptor blockade. Anxiolytic. Quick onset. Does not impair psychomotor function. Possible withdrawal reactions. Used in generalised anxiety disorder as well as depression. Avoid with SSRIs (Serotonin(ergic) Syndrome). Need >300mg in major depression. Not for the agitated, insomniac, anxious or panicky. Sexual dysfunction and insomnia are S/Es.

Mirtazepine: Zispin. (NaSSA) 15-45mg: Nocte. No sexual dysfuction, an anxiolytic antidepressant. Can be used in OCD and migraine. May have a discontinuation syndrome. Sedating. Good for the anxious insomniac and panicky. Racemic. L and R hand versions are effective.

Reboxetine: Edronax. Selective NARI. Used in depression – restores "motivation", in panic and ADHD. 8-12mg daily. Various drug interactions. Non sedating. Having said all that some studies say it is no better than placebo (Bad Pharma, Ben Goldacre).

Moclobemide: Manerix. 300-600mg/day Reversible MAOI, RIMA. Good in Chronic Fatigue Syndrome, (M.E.) with Amitriptyline (with care) and phobic/anxiety disorders. No significant hypertensive reaction with Tyramine unlike the non selective irreversible MAOIs. Improves most aspects of sexual function.

Stop SSRI for 4-5 half lives before starting. A washout period is not necessary after Moclobemide however, as MAOI inhibition is back to normal after 24 hours. Wait 2 weeks after stopping Paroxetine despite its apparent half life of 21 hours!

Agomelatine: Valdoxan is a Melatonergic agonist and 5HT 2c antagonist. Its use and experience is currently limited to adults with major depressive illness. It has a positive effect on sleep without daytime drowsiness as you would expect from the receptors it stimulates but is currently regarded as a drug to use when others have not worked. Watch transaminases. Various drug interactions, Cytochrome P450 metabolism.

Nefazodone: Dutonin, Good for anxious agitated insomniacs, helps in migraine, fewer sexual S/Es, REM sleep and appetite side effects. Rare serious liver dysfunction.

Antidepressants increase the risk of dental implants failing. This may be via osteoporosis, bruxism, dry mouth and akathisia but the net result is an increased failure rate of 4X. AADR Meeting 2016.

Depression in young patients:

There is supposed to have been a 70% increase in teenage depression in the UK over the last decade or so. Adolescence is clearly a time of rapid change: Think of the growing challenges of independence and the daily confusion related to identity, sexual awareness, appearance, competition, personal success or failure, planning the future, the development of individual confidence and separateness, the world of work. Never mind the difficulties intrinsic to social media and electronic communication. All are competing with the daily need to perform academically, be popular with one's peer group, the challenges of navigating relationships and surviving. The wish to be different but conform socially and at a time when peer group and sexual pressures are at their most exacting. Who would want to be a teenager again ?(-unless you were in the tiny minority of clever, good looking, successful and popular teenagers). Cyber bullying, sexting, chat room predators, grooming, face book peer group pressure, on line mob cruelty – all things that did not exist even ten to twenty years ago are now major factors in the self worth and security of young people at school. Especially it seems, young girls.

1:10 school children have some sort of significant mental health condition during their school careers. According to the Sunday Times in several articles on the young person's mental health crisis in March 2015, 17,000 young people were admitted as emergencies with mental health crises the year before. I am amazed they were found beds. Teenage mental health service provision has been a scandal for at least ten years and was taken up as a political issue just before the 2015 election. The same paper had two distressing stories of mentally ill teenagers: One was about parents needing to take out a second mortgage to fund the private care for their self harming and anorexic daughter ("We all know she could die") and another about the independent educational sector providing its own mental health services for its pressurised distressed students. The first family made two significant comments (Their words): *"An Indian trained consultant said he had patients DYING on other wards – of course he had someone dying in Jenny's room too but he didn't see it that way"* – This brought home to me the importance of foreign trained doctors being culturally aware of today's British attitudes, illnesses and values. This was exactly the issue raised by the case brought against the RCGP by the British Association of Doctors of Indian Origin who are demanding a "culturally neutral" MRCGP because so many of their members are failing it. There is no such thing as a culturally neutral patient or consultation. Also the article quoted: *"The GP said that further treatment was up to CAMHS but CAMHS had disappeared "*. *When they were available, they never returned phone calls (which they don't to GPs either by the way) and they did not seem to provide any effective care, treatment or even place of safety at any time to a child who was seriously ill.* **Unfortunately this is the experience of many if not the majority of parents and patients using many CAMHS units.**

The factors quoted for the rise in childhood and adolescent mental health morbidity were middle class "forcing" of academic expectations, early age exam pressures, parental divorce, on line manipulation by peer groups, cultural, family, life and career expectations as well as the individual's personal value often being assessed by academic success. Children from well off families are twice as likely to suffer depression and anxiety as the poor. Presumably because of inflated life expectations.

Anorexia has a 20% death rate in the young. As I mention time and time again, in my neck of the woods, GPs have had to be their own CAMHS because the local unit has long been inaccessible, ineffective and not fit for purpose. It has had a high turnover of staff, did not return calls, had no beds, no way of seeing urgent cases quickly and functioned in an isolated world of its own. Inaccessible to both relatives and GPs. If CCGs ever now genuinely put GPs in control of what secondary care services they buy and what services they close, our local CAMHs would be the first department that I would close.

It is thought that some SSRIs may increase the risk of teenage suicide (for instance Paroxetine) but good quality counselling is thin on the ground and antidepressants prescribed and supervised by the GP are the mainstay of treatment for most depressed teenagers and young patients. Basically, practical treatment often comes down to the GP and a handful of carefully chosen drugs – and, as I will mention elsewhere, regular follow up.

Fluoxetine is still the most effective antidepressant in teenagers and older children even though the name "Prozac" still has unhelpful associations of "happy pills" and a sort of therapeutic self indulgence for some parents. When they ask you what the risk or side effects of treating their child or themselves with antidepressants are, make sure you tell them the difference between antidepressants and tranquillisers (ie not addictive), the risks of not treating in terms of high teenage suicide rates and the subtle adverse effects of depression such as:

social withdrawal or rejection,

loss of a normal peer group interaction and experience,

academic failure,

loss of self esteem which can change their whole future, social and academic,

-this is an important age to develop normal social connections and self image,

(There are no data sheet inserts for the side effects of not treating – and antidepressant patient information leaflets are frightening)

and make sure you tell them that all drugs have SOME side effects but that these quickly wear off

For instance:

Fluoxetine works well but takes two weeks and sometimes you need to add something else to temporarily help sleep – Dosulepin or even Amitriptyline.

Sertraline which is also helpful with obsessional symptoms is somewhat sedating.

Citalopram is slower acting, generally free from side effects.

Of course make it clear that these drugs take 10 days to 2 weeks or more to work and you may well need to increase the dose when you **review them at 2 weeks**.

Pregnancy and depression:

These drugs have been used and are relatively low risk: Bear in mind that depression has a significant morbidity itself in pregnancy.

Amitriptyline,

Imipramine,

Nortriptyline,

Fluoxetine.

Depression and breast feeding:

Paroxetine and Sertraline have shorter half lives and more data. If given during pregnancy, don't change after delivery. See safe fetus.com, – Sertraline and Fluoxetine have a slight edge over Paroxetine.

Carers and depression:

There are said to be 7m carers in the UK. In 2013 the RCGP suggested that they should be screened for depression as up to 1/3 would suffer from a depressive illness. Also, practices were encouraged to create carers registers, give appointments at convenient times and have a practice carer's champion.

Treatment-Resistant Depression:

Causes included thyroid disease, taking CCBs, occult cancer, alcoholism, relatively minor head injury: Treatment: Add Lithium to TCAD or SSRI, or try Quetiapine, added to standard antidepressant treatment, 50mg increasing to 300mg a day.

Or try an MAOI or Venlafaxine or an anti inflammatory.

Antidepressants and Sexual Dysfunction:

Nearly all antidepressants in all classes adversely affect sex in one way or another. SSRIs are particularly well known for this but TCADs, MAOIs, SNRIs all have sexual side effects, especially at initiation of treatment.

Loss of libido,

ED,

Dysorgasmia,

and problems with "arousal or satisfaction" are common.

There are said to be significantly lower rates of sexual dysfunction though with Bupropion and Nefazodone.

CBT:

CBT was found to be moderately more effective in primary care depression than "Standard care without talking therapies" in a study of 5160 patients published in 2015.

In 30 RCTs assessed and results published in Oct 2015, there was more benefit from face to face CBT than from "standard care without talking therapies" but face to face problem solving therapy, interpersonal psychotherapy and "other psychological interventions" also achieved better results than "usual care". CBT with a remote therapist (over the phone) was also better then "standard care".

-A few points: This was a German study where they spend at least 3X as much per patient as we do here and I have never in my 3+ decades of General Practice had **reliable, consistent** access to any of these talking therapies: one to one counselling, psychotherapy, psychoanalysis, CBT, mindfulness or any of the 153 psychological therapy types listed in Wikipedia. Attack therapy, Dreamwork, Guide Affective Imagery, Holotropic Breathwork, Nude Psychotherapy, Psychedelic Therapy, Rebirthing Breathwork, Sandplay Therapy and Wilderness Therapy all sound particularly interesting but weren't available on the NHS in my part of the world – more's the pity. If standard care doesn't include the GP doing a LOT of assessing, supporting, counselling and so TALKING to the patient then he isn't a proper doctor doing a proper job in primary care in the first place. Seeing the GP **IS** a talking therapy or should be. If he or she is a genuinely concerned and interested doctor anyway.

Obsessive compulsive disorder: OCD

There are significant overlaps between the various psychiatric conditions. It isn't surprising that many patients with schizophrenic or obsessive compulsive symptoms become depressed or that paranoid or delusional patients develop anxiety about their suffering. In fact it is probably true to say that since many conditions are descriptions of symptoms (anxiety, depression, social phobia, paranoia etc) rather than diagnoses and many symptoms are upsetting, disturbing, inexplicable or frightening that there is no single pure psychiatric condition as such. Most schizophrenics are depressed a lot of the time, most depressive are anxious as well.

There was a large Danish study published in September 2014 which looked at 3 million patients between 1995 and 2012 and showed that OCD patients had a higher risk of developing other psychiatric conditions, not just sharing symptoms. There was a 7 fold greater risk of OCD patients developing schizophrenia and a 6 fold increased risk of "schizophrenia spectrum disorder". The children of OCD patients were also at higher risk. Overall, nearly 3% of those patients developing schizophrenia had a previous diagnosis of OCD. I suspect OCD patients are also at greater long term risk of depression, chronic anxiety and so on – and how many phobic and severely anxious patients don't eventually get depressed?

OCD treatments:

Cognitive behaviour therapy.

Rx: SSRIs in biggish doses (Fluoxetine),

Clomipramine or SSRI +/– an atypical antipsychotic if severe (Risperidone/ Olanzapine/Quetiapine).

Effective Psychiatric Combination Treatments: (eg for severe depression etc).

Fluoxetine and Trimipramine,

Fluoxetine and Dosulepin,

An SSRI and Mirtazepine,

An antidepressant plus a mood stabiliser:

Lamotrigine,

Valproate,

Quetiapine,

or plus CBT.

Half Lives of Antidepressants: (Vis a vis withdrawal symptoms, "Discontinuation Syndrome" etc)

Fluvoxamine 17-22 hrs,

Fluoxetine 4-16 days. 99% gone in 25 days,

Sertraline 22-36 hrs. 99% gone in 5.4 days,

Paroxetine 21 hrs Variable. 99% gone in 4.4 days,

Venlafaxine 5-11 hrs. 99% gone in 1 day,

Citalopram 1.5 days. 99% gone in 7.3 days,

Escitalopram 30 hrs. 99% gone in 6.1 days,

Nefazodone up to 24 hrs.

The shorter the half life, the commoner the withdrawal effects.

The worst include Venlafaxine, Sertraline, Paroxetine and Citalopram. These effects can be reduced by a very slow withdrawal or by substituting the longer half life Fluoxetine and slowly withdrawing that.

MAOIs:

Before starting Moclobemide wait 4-5X the half life of the SSRI you have stopped (5 weeks with fluoxetine). No treatment free period is required after Moclobemide as it has a short duration of action. The half life generally stated as 2-4 hours.

Stop standard MAOIs 2 weeks before starting SSRI or a TCAD, (3 weeks with Clomipramine/Imipramine).

An MAOI should not be started until 1-2 weeks after a TCAD, (3 weeks with Clomipramine/Imipramine) has been stopped.

Psychiatric Screening Tools:

Edinburgh maternal depression screen (10 items) or
Edinburgh Postnatal Depression Scale EPDS.
PHQ-9. Depression, 9 Items.
PHQ-2. The first two PHQ-9 items (a rough screening test).
PHQ-A. Adolescent anxiety, eating, mood, substance abuse problems.
MacMaster General Function Scale. Family Function.
PSI. Parents stress Index. (Parent/children issues) Parental pressure as well as units of tyre pressure in pounds per square inch!
SIPA: Stress Index for parents – of Adolescents.
PDS: Post Traumatic Stress scale.
BIS: Brief Impairment Scale: Adolescent interpersonal relationships.
Beck Depression Inventory: 21 items.
Scared (!) Self report for childhood anxiety related emotional disorders – 41 items.
GHQ 12 HADS anxiety and depression scale (14 items).
Geriatric Depression Scale (GDS).
GAD-7 Anxiety rating scale.
Zung self rating scale for depression.
Screening for depression questionnaire SDS.
Carroll Self Rating Scale (depression).
Inventory for diagnosing depression (IDD).
Hospital anxiety depression scale (HAD).

A brief trawl online and you will find dozens of psychiatric scales, some copyrighted, some not. You can download nearly all of them it seems. You can make up some clever acronyms, like the "scared" scale above.

How about a parents scoring system for relating to coping with difficult teenagers-

The **P**ersonal **I**nventory of **S**pecific **S**elective **E**pisodic **D**epression **O**n **F**amily **F**riction.-The PISSEDOFF Scale ?

Various screening "Tools" are available on the net under licence from Pfizer at: www.phqscreeners.com

PHQ-9: (Copyright Pfizer Spitzer, Williams, Kroenke et al, no permission needed to reproduce.)

Over the last 2 weeks have you experienced?:
Not at all 0. Several days 1. More than half the days 2. Nearly every day 3.
1) Little interest or pleasure in doing things.
2) Feeling down, depressed or hopeless.
3) Trouble falling asleep or sleeping too much.
4) Feeling tired or having little energy.
5) Poor appetite or overeating.
6) Feeling bad about yourself, feeling a failure or thinking you have let yourself or your family down.
7) Trouble concentrating on things (reading papers or watching TV etc).
8) Moving or speaking slow enough for others to notice or being fidgety and restless.
9) Thoughts you would be better dead or hurting yourself.
Accessory question:

10) If you have felt any of these problems, how difficult has it made it to work, look after things at home or to get on with people? Not difficult at all, somewhat difficult, very difficult, extremely difficult.

Interpretation and one local suggested management regime:

5-9: Minimal symptoms. Support, return if worse and in 1 month.

10-14: Minor depression. Support, "watchful waiting".

Dysthymia ("Neurotic Depression") i.e. Symptoms most days for at least 2 years, never better for more than 2 months, but no major depressive, manic, cyclothymic or psychotic symptoms, and not due to drugs or illness. Try antidepressants or psychotherapy. What many of us would explain as "Serotonin Deficiency" and often present for many years or even the patient's whole life. (Churchill, Hitler and Stalin*?) Mild major depression. Try antidepressants or psychotherapy.

15-19 Major depression, moderately severe. Antidepressants or psychotherapy.

>/= 20. Major depression, severe. Antidepressants and psychotherapy, especially INB on monotherapy.

*The second world war and its 70 million dead were in large part due to the unavailability of antidepressants in the 1930s. Stalin, Hitler and Churchill all had dysfunctional family upbringings, poor relationships with their parents and symptoms of depression throughout their lives. Churchill had his "Black Dog", a strong family history of mental illness (his father had lifelong psychotic symptoms and his daughter had severe depression and eventually committed suicide). Hitler is said to have had manic depression and various drug addictions including cocaine and Stalin had a drunken abusive father and probably suffered from manic depression too. (Political psychology14.4(1993):607-625.)

So we have been born into an era of fortunate therapeutic largess as far as psychiatry is concerned-certainly if you think what can happen when psychiatrically unwell but powerful men vent their depressive feelings on others in our planet's recent history.

These screening tools are only guidelines. I am willing to treat relatively mild depression early and to use more than one drug. As I mentioned, any type of Psychotherapy has been effectively unavailable for decades to many of us and even now there is a one type fits all cheap and cheerful service whose initial and sometimes subsequent contacts can be just by phone. YOU and the drugs you prescribe are what get 95%+ of your patients better.

Generalised Anxiety Disorder Questionnaire

GAD-7: (Copyright Pfizer Spitzer, Williams, Kroenke et al, no permission needed to reproduce.)

Feeling nervous, anxious or on edge,

Not being able to stop or control worrying,

Worrying too much about different things,

Trouble relaxing,

So restless it is hard to sit still,

Becoming easily annoyed and irritable,

Feeling afraid as if something awful might happen,

In the last 2 weeks:

Not at all 0/Several days 1/>Half the days 2/Nearly every day 3. Out of a maximum of 21.

Autism

There are various tests of empathy to assess autism or degrees within the autistic spectrum. Simon Baron-Cohen, who's cousin is a comedian, is a controversial psychologist at Cambridge University who has devised a questionnaire which assesses the degree of an individual's empathy. This is available with various others online. He has also postulated an interesting theory and one borne out by the experience of most GPs that "Geeks" (people who are good at maths, science and technology skills) might be marrying each other and giving their children a double dose of introversion and emotional unintelligence, thus having children with the genes for autism.

The experience of many GPs is that patients who are good at computers, logical intellectual pursuits, mathematics and various related technical skills are often poor at expressing emotions or empathising with others. They deal with depression and anxiety in themselves and others very poorly. One of his other postulates is that autism is the result of an over masculinised brain as male brains are programmed to systematise and female brains to empathise. So the theory goes.

Autism has also been associated with severely depressed mothers, a raised CRP in pregnancy, the taking of Valproate, SSRIs and TCAs in pregnancy, exposure to various toxins, especially heavy metals, mercury, lead, manganese and some organic compounds as well as diesel fumes during pregnancy and in early life. There is also some evidence that autistic spectrum disorders may be commoner in low birth weight and pre term babies and in circumcised boys. New research has linked a lack of carnitine, in the foetuses of vegetarian and vegan mothers to autism in their children via a gene mutation (Vytas A, Bankaitis et al Jan 2016 J. Celrep. 2016.01.004). Carnitine is present in red meat and milk.

Some have erroneously blamed vaccination (eg MMR) but recent evidence in the USA suggests that the rise in autism in the first decade of the third millennium is wholly due to reclassification of children with "neurodevelopmental disorders". (Am J Med Genetic Aug 2015.) The prevalence of diagnosed autism had gone from 1:150 to (2002) to 1:68 (2012). Children enrolled in the USA for special education total about 6.2m. annually. Those classified as Autistic went from 94,000 to 420,000 over the 10 years to 2010. There was a compensating decline in the number of children defined as having "Intellectual Disability" sufficient to account for 2/3 of this increase.

By the way, if GPs recognise geeky programmers and systems analyst patients as being poor communicators, perhaps somewhere on the autistic spectrum, then patients most definitely frequently identify their technologically gifted, computer savvy GPs as not having much in the way of personal empathy or communication skills and way too much display screen eye contact too.

Fibromyalgia

I am still not sure if this condition should be in the psychiatry, neurology or subjective symptoms with no physical cause section. FM can be due to abnormalities in several different neurotransmitter systems regulating pain perception, sleep, mood and alertness. Drug and non drug therapies should be used together. You can try treating the pain with Duloxetine, Pregabalin, Gabapentin or Amitriptyline and the underlying cause(s) with TCAs SSRIs, SNRIs. Second tier treatments include high dose sertraline, paroxetine, fluoxetine, low dose naltrexone, cannabinoids, gamma hydroxybutyrate. Other treatments include acupuncture, yoga and psychotherapy, "education", exercise and CBT.

Newer research says the most effective treatment must include aerobic exercise (Winfried Hauser, European League against Rheumatism Congress 2014).

M.E. C.F.S CFS Chronic Fatigue Syndrome

I am putting this in the psychiatry section rather than the infectious diseases or the musculoskeletal or gastroenterology sections. The condition was not recognised when I trained in the early 70's, being called "Royal Free Disease" and lumped together with other forms of psychosomatic illness. It was thought to be a form of mass hysteria or group neurosis especially amongst young women living or working together, like student nurses or schoolgirls. Most doctors now believe some sort of infection or probably many different types of infection can trigger a susceptible individual into an illness leading to a post viral malaise/tiredness/weakness/depression. In these susceptible patients the symptoms persist for a variable period. It may be because they have an immune deficit, a pre existing propensity to depression, their personality, upbringing or various environmental reasons, a tendency to slow recovery or for some other as yet unknown reason. So I have put this condition in the psychiatry section because of the effective treatments, the likely underling personality types and their families and because of 40 years experience treating CFS. Psychological factors certainly exacerbate and prolong the symptoms even if they don't always trigger them.

Current thinking:

65% are triggered by enteroviruses but not by mouse retrovirus XMRV which was thought at first to be a major breakthrough when published in 2009. Some cases follow Glandular Fever which certainly made me feel exhausted for six months after my own infection in my mid twenties. (Mind you I was a Registrar Paediatrician doing on call weekends of 80 hours and a one in three rota – and we had young children at home who didn't sleep well.) But exclude: Adrenal insufficiency, anaemia, chronic infections, Coeliac Disease, immunodeficiency, malignancy, anxiety, depression, M.S., myasthenia, primary sleep disorders, rheumatic disorders, somatisation disorder (this must be the most difficult to exclude), thyroid disease.

The latest review I read (2015, Medscape) summarised the situation like this: "Experts in the field conceptualise ME/CFS as an abnormal immune system response to any of a number of infectious or environmental triggers resulting in a chronic state of inflammation, autonomic dysfunction, impaired HPA axis function and neuro-endocrine dysregulation".

So now it is thought of as a spectrum of diseases, immune related, with subsets that are auto immune, subsets that are virally triggered, or a chronic viral infection and perhaps other triggers and stressors. It hasn't been decided whether to regard it as a chronic infection or an auto immune condition with a variable psychological overlay.

The hallmarks are severe fatigue – for 6 months in adults and 3 months in children, malaise, following physical or mental exertion, unrefreshing sleep and cognitive dysfunction. Chronic pain is common and many patients also have the features of Fibromyalgia. Co existing symptoms include orthostatic intolerance (positive tilt test), IBS, heat or cold intolerence, migraine. There can also be reduced exercise oxygen consumption in the peripheral tissues, altered natural killer cell activity and increased proinflammatory cytokines etc.

Tests:

1) VPI Enteroviral specific protein,

2) IgM Ab against enteroviral antigens. Enteroviral serotypes include Echovirus, Coxsackie A and B, polio etc.

Our local lab will do EBV Ab and EnteroV Ab and if the latter is pos then they will do the VPI.

The basic FBC, ESR and CRP, U and Es, LFTs, Alb, Calcium, CPK, TFTs, random Gluc, coeliac screen and urinanalysis will have been done by you already.

Treatment: Try large doses of Multivitamins, and/or Imipramine, or Sertraline+/-Trimipramine+/-Amitriptyline, or an SSRI or Neuro Linguistic Programming, (The Lightning Process) or MOAIs. It remains to be seen if anti retroviral treatment helps.

The literature talks of graded exercise and goal setting, "pacing" with or without CBT. 1:50 children are said to have CFS and in a report published in 2016, internet CBT was said to help 63% recover or nearly fully recover.

Patterns of illness: Boom and bust – Exercise followed by exhaustion – in response to the symptoms – a self perpetuating cycle which leads to a repetition of the behaviour which brought on the tiredness.

Rest must start by being routine, regular and consistent – for instance 30 minutes 3-4 times a day but the aim of treatment must be to plan a recovery and a normal return to engagement in work and life. Not, as so many CFS therapists and campaigners seem to lobby for:-the provision of statutory and financial protection, state benefits and no involvement in a recovery plan or a personal physical or emotional commitment to improvement. In other words, a perpetual supported withdrawal from normal life with no challenges. This to me seems exactly the wrong approach.

Anorexia/Bulimia

Some patients who present binge eating respond to exclusion diets removing wheat, dairy products, refined sugars, potatoes. Why? I have no idea.

Patients suffering severe weight loss have a high mortality and morbidity and should be detained under the MHA. If the BMI is 13-14 plus continuing weight loss, the patient is usually admitted, the hospital usually aims for 1kg gain/week and a BMI of 19 before discharge. Anorexia has existed for centuries but has increased with the explosion in social networking sites and modern concepts of the body beautiful being one with a low BMI. Ironic considering the Western World's epidemic of obesity and Type2DM.

A higher rate of childhood abuse has been suffered by patients who present with this condition. Most patients are female (Nearly 10:1) and have a distorted body image.

Associated psychological features are withdrawal, depression and obsessive compulsive disorder. The serum potassium and sodium drop, the periods stop and there are several complicating secondary symptoms related to malnourishment or induced vomiting etc. These include growth and bone restriction, fatty liver damage, arrhythmias, convulsions and it is a condition with one of the highest of the psychiatric mortality rates.

The patient often abuses purgatives or induces emesis. When self induced vomiting is a major and regular part of the condition it is Bulimia Nervosa.

Drug treatment includes high dose Fluoxetine, Olanzapine, Mirtazepine – and interestingly, Zinc supplementation and Omega 3 fatty acids. Then there are CBT, psychotherapy and family therapy. Anorexia remains one of the most dangerous, inexplicable, frustrating and difficult psychiatric conditions to treat.

Personality Types:

Type A
Ambitious Aggressive, competitive, driven, impatient. Initially thought to be at CVS risk. The impatient self perpetuating hypertensive who complains about you being 15 minutes late when they come in to the consulting room-and so there is almost no point in doing their blood pressure. He is probably Type A

Type B
Relaxed, easy going, takes life more slowly. Probably late for his appointment and kept **you** waiting so don't do your own blood pressure. You don't want him or her as a work partner. They will always be running late and the receptionists will always be asking you to see a few of their extras before you start visits.

Type C
Cancer prone, responds to stress with depression and hopelessness. Introverted, eager to please, respectful, conforming.

Type D
Distressed. Negative emotions. Socially inhibited, depressed mood, anxiety, anger, hostile emotions, 3X higher risk of CVS death.

Personality Disorders:

Suspicious:	Emotional and Impulsive:	Anxious:
Paranoid	Borderline	Avoidant
Schizoid	Histrionic	Dependent
Schizotypal	Narcissistic	Obsessive compulsive
Antisocial		

One person may fall into more than one group, having a mixture of characteristics. There are various other definitions of different personality disorders. The obsessive compulsive type is also called anankastic and these people have a significant lack of adaptability to new situations.

Although "personality disorders" are not strictly mental conditions, some aspects of them *can* be treated. For instance with SSRIs, Lithium, Valproate, Lamotrigine, for impulsive, suicidal or aggressive behaviour.

Out of hours psychiatry:

If the patient seems likely from the first contact to be at risk of harming themselves or others, phone the police and ask for them to accompany you on the visit if you are alone.

If the patient is liable to self harm and there is no one else available, it may be necessary to remain with the patient until help arrives from Social Services, the duty Psychiatrist or PSW. The mental health assessment should normally be carried out by the visiting GP.

Out of hours psychiatric calls can be unpredictable and time consuming. You may not be available to cover other emergencies or you may need to make some difficult distance triage decisions. Given how hard it is to access psychiatric beds within commuting distance you may decide to be kind to the family and to the patient at a time of extreme distress. If there is a suitable and motivated relative it might be less disruptive to initiate a one dose systemic treatment (a depot or antipsychotic) followed up by clear instructions, oral treatment and strict supervision. This is assuming the relatives have access to you or a partner in an emergency out of hours.

Substance Misuse:

Although illegal drug misuse has diminished in the UK over recent years (Home Office July 2017) 10 people per day still die of the effects of illegal drugs and we use 3X as much heroin, ecstasy and amphetamines as the rest of Europe per person. Our death rate being 60.3/m (Today Programme 14/7/17).

Classes of drugs legally: (and see below)

Class A drugs: Cocaine, Crack, Crystal Meth, Ecstasy, Heroin, LSD, magic mushrooms
Penalties up to 7 years in jail for possession and life imprisonment for supply.

Cocaine, Class A: Sniffed, smoked or injected. A short acting stimulant which improves confidence, relaxation and self importance. Highly addictive, causes local mucosal damage and occasionally acute respiratory or cardiovascular collapse. There is a withdrawal after taking cocaine which causes tiredness, depression and paranoia. Crack cocaine leads to a more severe withdrawal which can be violent. Massive rise in BP with a 23X increase in MI risk in the hour after use. Regular use vastly increases atheroma build up.

Crack Cocaine: is made from Cocaine and baking powder. It is smoked or injected. A quicker more intense high than Cocaine, it is very addictive causing severe mood swings, insomnia and paranoid delusions. Can cause hyperthermia and apnoea. Smokers and injectors may need to use it up to 20X a day due to its short duration and "crash" withdrawal. Smoked or injected with heroin it is known as "snowballing" or "speedballing".

Cocaine use has increased in the UK. The British Crime Survey statistics show that the percentage of 16-59 year olds admitting using it in their lifetime has increased from 3.1% in1996 to 9.4% in 2008.

Ecstasy, Class A: MDMA: A stimulant, intensifying feelings and stamina. Usually to prolong and intensify dancing. It can cause panic, anxiety, confusion, tachycardia, arrythmias, acute anuria, fluid overload.

A new type of Ecstasy, **"PMA"** became available in 2013. It was slower onset but more powerful and so users tended to take more expecting a quicker "hit" and 20 deaths were recorded by half way through the year.

Class B drugs: "Speed" etc. (Class A if injectable)
Cannabis. Up to 5 years for possession, 14 years for supply. Unless you live in Holland, Uruguay, Washington State or Colorado. In Colorado there are reports of more frequent ER room visits and various increased morbidities of individuals who had recently used Cannabis. There is also a seemingly endless debate concerning the therapeutic use of Cannabis for muscle spasm and pain relief in certain neurological as well as terminal illnesses.

Traditional cannabis produced THC around 3%. Modern"Skunk" (selectively bred for concentrated drug yield*) can produce 15-20% and is far more hallucinogenic and psychoactive/damaging.

The effects of cannabis are tachycardia, hypotension, increased appetite (the munchies), hallucinations, time distortion, memory loss and poor attention, disinhibition and exacerbation of any pre-existing mental health condition:-anxiety, panic, paranoia and the triggering of psychoses. It is licensed for AIDs associated anorexia in the US and for chemotherapy nausea. Nabilone is a synthetic form of THC and used as an anti emetic and analgesic in neuropathic pain. Sativex is a natural cannabis extract used as an oromucosal spray in MS spasticity. Cannabis has been used in MS for ataxia, tremors and spasticity. It may be neuroprotective and can be opioid sparing.

(A Green et Al. The Pharmaceutical Journal Nov 2012.)

More on Cannabis:

Hash, weed, skunk, grass. Eaten or smoked. Effect: Initially cheerful and relaxed, can enhance perception of colours and sounds. Long term use causes poor memory and concentration as well as demotivation. MI 4X higher rate in the hour after use, a cause of coronary syndromes, arrhythmias, peripheral and cerebral artery "events" but not exclusively in the young. A doubling of psychotic illness associated with use as well as structural brain changes similar to those in schizophrenia. More carcinogenic than tobacco. Can increase anxiety, paranoia and acute psychoses (X2). One of the commonest causes for acute psychoses in the young. Linked to structural brain changes – including of the nucleus accumbens, amygdala, etc (grey matter density and shape) in the key areas affecting motivation, emotion and reward. These effects occur even in occasional (once or twice weekly) and new "recreational" cannabis users. The changes last for at least "years after cessation of use."

Skunk is a potent and artificially modified form of cannabis containing a higher concentration of THC, the stimulant.*

In an article on cannabis on Radio 4's World Tonight, Nov 17th 2016, the risks of addiction to cannabis were stated as follows: In adult users 9%. In teenage users 17% become addicted.

Class C drugs: Anabolic steroids, Growth Hormone, Ketamine,

Illegal possession of prescription drugs such as tranquillisers. Two years in jail for possession, up to 14 years for supply.

Solvents: Gas lighter fluid, hair spray, volatile glues, solvents etc. When inhaled can cause a feeling of disinhibition, impetuousness and drunkenness. Can cause sudden death by arrhythmia, fitting, respiratory obstruction, choking etc. The only drugs where girls exceed boys – usually around age 13. 7% of secondary school children will have tried inhaling solvents once.

GHB, Gammahydroxybutyrate: (and GBL): Class C. Capsules, liquid or powder. Causes euphoria, disinhibition, loss of consciousness, can be fatal with other drugs, has been used as a DATE RAPE drug. Can be used in narcolepsy or to remove superglue or paint.

Heroin, Diamorphine: Powder, Smoked, snorted, heated and inhaled – as in Opium dens, in the days of Sherlock Holmes "chasing the dragon" or injected. It gives an initial "rush" and feeling of calmness, dissociation and freedom from pain anxiety and stress. Overdose causes sedation, unconsciousness, coma and apnoea. It is highly addictive physically and emotionally, causing withdrawal symptoms, tremors, cramp, insomnia, paranoia etc. Bigger doses are required to achieve the same effect due to tachyphylaxis.

Fentanyl: A synthetic opioid 100x stronger than morphine and the cause of "Prince's" death. Available in various forms, tablets, lollipops and patches it is increasingly "cut" with other drugs to enhance their effect. The US and Canada are seeing an epidemic of addiction and deaths and in the UK deaths have risen 8x in seven years. 88 have died in ten months of 2017 (Times Oct 21 2017)

LSD. Lysergic Acid Diethylamide. Small squares of paper into which the LSD is impregnated. A hallucinatory: Sounds, sights and colours become more intense, appearances of objects are distorted. A bad trip is like a living nightmare and some people suffer flash backs months later. Can cause panic attacks or uncover mental illness. Can cause the individual to kill them self deliberately or accidentally (Nick Cave's son Arthur who fell from a cliff in Ovingdean), occasionally to act aggressively to others.

Ketamine Class C (B): A white powder or tablet. It is used as an anaesthetic agent. Causes dissociation and hallucinations for up to 3 hours. Causes anaesthesia and immobility, panic, depression, dyspnoea, heart failure etc. Can exacerbate pre existing depression/paranoia etc., 2013 reclassified as Class B, partly due to its pernicious effect on the bladder. Some regular users having had bladder excision to cope with the damage.

Magic Mushrooms: Psilocybin: Class A. (Includes Liberty Cap.) Drug harm experts rank alcohol as the most harmful drug and magic mushrooms as the least harmful. Sense of feeling "high", relaxed and pleasant feeling, hallucinogenic, shorter and milder effect than LSD. Nevertheless causes nausea, flash backs and bad trips.

Methadone: A heroin substitute, a long acting synthetic opioid analgesic which can be used as a cough suppressant as well as a potent long acting analgesic.

Meth(yl) amphetamine-Crystal meth: Class A: Tablet, powder or crystals. A stimulant with an "intense rush" lasting 4-12 hours. Very addictive, damaging the teeth and gums and causing nausea, diarrhoea and vomiting. Causes skin damage through self harm and irresponsible sexual behaviour.

Speed – Amphetamines, stimulants: Class B. Causes alertness, enhanced energy, suppresses hunger, keeps you awake. Snorted, injected or swallowed. It can cause anxiety, irritability, aggression, tachycardia and withdrawal symptoms.

Controlled Drug Classification: (CDs)
Misuse of Drugs Act 1971;

Categorises Drugs in Classes and Schedules:
There are 3 drug classes:
Class A:
Cocaine, Crack, Ecstasy, Diamorphine, Dipipanone, LSD, Methadone, Pethidine, Psilocybin, mushrooms.
Class B:
Amphetamines, Barbiturates, Cannabis, Codeine, Pentazocine, Pholcodine, Methyphenidate.
Any class B drug that is prepared as an injectable becomes a Class A drug.
Class C:
Amphetamine related drugs, Ketamine, Buprenorphine, Diethylpropion, Meprobamate, Benzodiazepines, HCG, Anabolic steroids, etc.
There are 5 schedules:
Schedule 1: LSD, Ecstasy, Cannabis.
Schedule 2: Opiates, Diamorphine, Pethidine, Methadone, Fentanyl, Oxycodone, amphetamines, Methylphenidate, Quinalbarbitone, Lisdexamphetamine.
Schedule 3: Minor stimulants, Benzphetamine, Midazolam, Temazepam, Buprenorphine, Flunitrazepam, Phenobarbitone, Midazolam, Tramadol.
Schedule 4: Most benzodiazepines, most anabolic steroids and androgenic steroids.

Zopiclone and Zaleplon.

Schedule 5: Low strength Codeine, Pholcodine, Cocaine, Morphine.

There are various constraints on the prescription and use of schedule 2 drugs: The prescription must show full details with the total quantity in words and figures, the form and the strength. It must be signed in the prescriber's own handwriting, in indelible ink. It must specify the prescriber's address, it must specify the name and address of the patient and age if under 12 years, the name and form of the drug even if only one form exists, the strength of the preparation, the dose, the total quantity, the number of dose units in words and figures (except for Temazepam). All details except the signature can be printed and because of Shipman the total prescription will be for no more than 1 month's supply, it will be valid for no more than 28 days and the person collecting the scrip will have to prove their identity.

The prescriber must guard against the risk of the patient becoming addicted to the drug and must avoid supplying addicts. Controlled drugs held by the doctor must be double locked in a secure safety cabinet and recorded on a CD register. Their use must be monitored and recorded and their disposal witnessed and all recorded in ink in a CD register.

Methadone:

Class A Schedule 2

This is an analgesic, invented in pre-war Germany, although its main pharmacological use these days is as a morphine/heroin substitute. It comes as a linctus, tablets and injection (Physeptone). It can be used as an effective cough suppressant and analgesic, including in neuropathic pain.

It has a long half life which can be hugely variable and ranges from 4-200 hours, usually 8-60 hours. It is said to be less harmful to the foetus than the natural opiates. It is one of the very best cough suppressants in everything from TB to Pertussis.

Legal Highs:

These are various synthetic substances which are taken by users for some sort of psycho active effect, stimulant, hypnotic, sedative or hallucinatory but which have not yet been investigated, classified and registered harmful and therefore illegal. About one new such substance becomes available across the EU every week. They are often sold as plant food or some other household product as they cannot be marketed "for human consumption". They might be taken by any route, including by injection.

In 2012 68 people died taking these perfectly legal and readily available "legal highs" and a Home Office review of the situation was launched in 2013. 1600 died from overall drug abuse that year. By Oct 2014 there was talk of these agents being banned in the UK like they were in Ireland in 2010.

In May 2016 a blanket ban on "Legal Highs" came into force in the UK with the "New Psychoactive Substances Act" making it illegal to supply ANY "Legal Highs" for human consumption. It is now an offence to sell or to give such substances away, – even to friends. In the UK, 113 died from "Legal Highs" in 2013 and 67 in 2014.

Other drugs subject to misuse and dependence include Gabapentin and Pregabalin. Both can cause significant euphoria and there is, apparently, a growing illegal market for both drugs. Bear this in mind if one of your patients keeps losing prescriptions.

Drug Driving:

A new offence, The Drug Driving Law, came in to being in 2015. The police are now able to perform roadside tests on saliva to assess whether a driver has a number of psycho-active drugs affecting his ability to drive safely.

There are two groups of medications covered by the new offence – licensed medications and recreational drugs. Common recreational drugs covered by the legislation include Cannabis, Cocaine, MDMA, LSD, Ketamine, Heroin/Diamorphine metabolite and Methylamphetamine. The limits for these recreational drugs have been set at a low level.

The second group are mainly licensed medications, for which higher limits are acceptable in the bloodstream. They include benzodiazepines (Clonazepam, Oxazepam, Diazepam, Lorazepam, Temazepam), Methadone and Morphine. Amphetamine may be added to the regulations at a later date.

Opiate Withdrawal:

Symptoms within 12 hours, peaking at 72 hours, the worst symptoms lasting 1 week. Methadone has a longer half life than Diamorphine (Heroin).

Withdrawal signs/symptoms mimic sympathetic over activity:
Dilated pupils,
Runny nose,
Nausea,
Vomiting,
Abdominal pain,
Diarrhoea,
Muscle pain,
Anxiety,
Tachycardia etc.

Treatment: Metoclopramide, Lomotil, Mebeverine, occasionally Diazepam for anxiety, muscle pain. (Not if Benzodiazepine overuse is also part of the problem). Chlorpromazine unless the patient is also alcohol dependent.

Methadone on an exponential withdrawal plan can be used. Buprenorphine, Subutex, Suboxone (with Naloxone) and Naltrexone are alternative drugs in short term and maintenance use.

Naltrexone*: Is an extremely interesting drug which is used in low doses to reduce the risks of cancer recurrence (various cancers). Some studies suggest that up to 60% of cancer patients with a variety of tumours may benefit. The mechanisms may be via adrenal endorphin production, by altering opiate receptors on tumour membranes or by stimulating NK (natural killer cell) numbers.

Lofexidine BritLofex: A centrally acting Alpha 2 adrenergic agonist, not a CD, not if on more than 30mg Methadone, 7-10 days, slightly sedative.

Naltrexone*: Nalorex, Opizone Can be used to reduce relapse in opioid and alcohol dependent abstaining patients.

Alcohol:***See previous item in Psychiatry section:

1967 Drink driving Act:
Legal Limit:

80mg alcohol per 100mls blood. Now In Scotland	50mg
35ug alcohol per 100mls breath	22ug
107mg alcohol per 100mls urine	67mg.

Alcohol withdrawal:

Diazepam, Lorazepam, Chlordiazepoxide, can be used at home in a slowly reducing regime. Plus or minus anti-psychotics such as Haloperidol or Olanzapine if necessary. Sometimes you can be reluctantly forced into supervising an alcohol withdrawal at home as the least worst option in someone who convinces you they are now motivated to change, refuses to engage with secondary care and (most importantly) has a sensible and caring person living at home with them. Chloral Hydrate reduces some life threatening side effects, Carbamazepine or Topiramate can be used as anti-convulsants. Chlormethiazole, – Heminevrin is still helpful as an adjunct with or instead of benzodiazepines.

I use Chlorpromazine or Chlordiazepoxide over 7-10 days. Stop all alcohol on the first day.

Thus:

Chlordiazepoxide 5-10mg (up to 15-20mg) 3-4X daily, slowly reducing.

Community detoxification should last 7-10 days and, preferably, be supervised by a motivated friend, partner, loved one, as well as you.

There is, of course, a small risk of Wernicke's Encephalopathy (+/- Korsakoff psychosis) which can be prevented by supplementing Vitamin B1. Oral absorption is unpredictable so give big doses of B1, other B vitamins and vitamin C, preferably a few days before the detox begins. **Ideally** the B1 should be given **IM** 250mg Thiamine daily 3-5 days before or during the process.

Treat other symptoms of withdrawal: anxiety, hallucinations, confusion, diarrhoea, hyperthermia, nausea, headache, palpitations, tachycardia, tremors, paranoia, with Haloperidol, Heminevrin, Lomotil, beta blockers, increased doses of benzodiazepines etc.

Maintaining abstinence:

Antabuse: Disulfiram 200mg tabs. Initially 4 stat, then 3 on second day, 2, 2, then 1 daily, review regularly especially after 6 months. Any alcohol is metabolised to acetaldehyde which causes the unpleasant symptoms. Avoid in pregnancy and avoid with Metronidazole. Up to 50% users remain abstinent.

Acamprosate, Campral. A Centrally acting stimulator of GABA receptors and a modifier of Glutamate levels, this reduces the adverse effects of alcohol withdrawal and abstinence.

New Middle age Drug and alcohol Misuse:

The European Centre for Drugs and Drug Addiction has estimated that the number of people needing treatment for drug problems over 65 in Europe will have doubled between 2001 and 2020. This is supposed to be because of the disreputable lifestyle of baby boomers continuing. They also say that 1.4 million people over 65 exceed recommended safe drinking limits. Between 2002 and 2010 alcohol related hospital admissions for men >65 had risen by 136% and for women 132%. The Office for National Statistics shows that alcohol related deaths among over 75s are at their highest level now since records began in 1991.

Overall the number of people in treatment for drug abuse is declining – except those over 40 and those over 40 who are starting drug use. These are mainly using heroin but another growing problem in middle age is cannabis abuse. The cannabis available today is a whole different kettle of fish from the pot available to students in the 60's.

35: RESPIRATORY:

Sudden Severe breathlessness:
Acute LVF,
Acute asthma and
Bronchitis are the three commonest causes.
Rarer are:
Spontaneous pneumothorax,
Pulmonary embolus
and Hyperventilation according to the books. But in young girls and women with no preceding history, hyperventilation is probably the commonest cause, certainly if they are not taking thrombogenic hormones.

Normal respiratory rates: 90th C

Age:	Rate:
0-2	40
2-4	30
4-7	28
7-14	25.

Asthma: Objective measurements: The basics you may have forgotten;

β receptors
B2 receptors are mainly in the airways (these seem to be dependent on size and weight i.e. they are not present at birth and nebulised salbutamol (B stimulants) etc do not work in small babies but start to work in bigger babies at the turn of the first year. These receptors are also in the uterus, liver, skeletal muscle, peripheral vascular bed and the R atrium. Stimulation leads to bronchodilatation, dilation of the muscular blood vessels, glycolysis and glycogenolysis. Beta blockers antagonise this action.

Peak Flow variations of 15-20% indicate asthma. FEV1 variability of 15% indicates? Asthma. An American expert I heard lecturing said a variability of 12% with reversibility in the FEV1 was asthma but then the Americans have a slight tendency to over medicalise natural variability in many things. The obstruction is to expiration, hence the lungs look and feel hyper inflated. There is often a biphasic bronchospastic response to any antigenic challenge (for instance at <1 hr and at 4 hrs) so beware nebulising the patient, then giving steroids and thinking the crisis is over at 2-3 hours.

Asthma appears to have increased in incidence in the USA (is this due to cleanliness, more immunisation and antibiotic use in children and a consequent failure of immature immune systems to develop and operate properly?) Conversely, asthma seems to have dropped in incidence over the 40 years since I have been a paediatrician/GP in the UK (Is this due to universal prophylactic steroid inhaler use?)

The "Great Smog" took place over 5 days in early December 1952 in London. Warm air settled over the city, trapping cold air underneath it. The inhabitants burnt more coal to keep warm, the extra smoke becoming trapped at ground level due to the "Shell" of warm air above it. Here it mixed with heavy fog. In places visibility contracted to 12". Buses, taxis and aeroplanes stopped functioning. 100,000 were treated for pneumonia and bronchitis and undertakers ran out of coffins. There were 3-4,000 extra deaths during the smog and 8,000 extra deaths after the smog were attributed to its effects. The Great Smog was one of the major triggers for the Clean Air Acts (1956 and 1968).

Infants who were in utero between 1945 and 1955 in London (during the era of "Pea souper" smogs) have a 20% increase in later life asthma. People who were exposed to the Great Smog during the first year of life were 4-5X more likely to develop asthma as a child and 3X more likely than others to have asthma as an adult.

Asthma research is now suggesting that it is several different diseases. Type 2 immunity is involved, it is a lymphocyte modulated disease with remodelling of small airways over time caused by inflammation. Starting with reversibility, the airways eventually become relatively fixed. There is an asthma gene, which works through interleukin 13 and an enzyme called chitinase. 20% of asthmatics are worse than all the others, however. These patients are the hardest to treat and take most of the resources. Most GPs will be able to identify these, the small number of unpredictable and worrying asthmatics of all ages on their lists who **they** will know and always be willing to see immediately as an emergency. At least I would hope so.

There is a very useful free peak flow value converter from Wright-McKerrow (which unbeknown to me I have been using for 4 decades quite happily) to EU 9EN 13826. – "Wright to EU". This is at http://www.peakflow.com/peakflow.zip. I assume the relentless medical obsession with standardisation (bendrofluMEthazide, fUROsemide, amoxIcillin, beclomeTasone, cromoglIcate, HbA1C units etc etc) will extend to PEFR measurements soon too.

Wright/EU
104 = 101
200= 165
304= 250
400=344
504= 462
600= 584
704= 730
800= 877 etc

SO:(Various sources)

Peak Flow: when to worry:

80% of best score indicates the need to increase/double dose of inhaled steroids.

60% of best score give oral steroids.

Some references say your Respiratory Nurse should refer to the Doctor if PEFR is 30%-40% of best ever. This is after the horse has bolted and is gone as far as I am concerned. Anything approaching 66% – 75% of best ever is worrying and deserves the doctor's attention I believe.

Asthma severity:

Acute PEFR 33% of best **is life threatening**.

33-50% is acute severe asthma.

50-75% is a moderate exacerbation.

So you should have a record of every asthmatic's **Best Ever Peak Flow** recording prominently displayed and accessible in the notes for all doctors/nurses.

Objective diagnosis of Asthma:
Reversibility with nebuliser,
(2.5mg Salbutamol or 4 puffs from an MDI and spacer),
If PEFR varies >20% over 3 days,
FEV1 >15% (and 200ml),
are indicative of asthma.
Obstructive spirometry pattern (see below).

Asthma: The under treated grey area:

In 2015 NICE made things unnecessarily complicated by saying that asthma was over diagnosed in some and unrecognised in other patients. No surprise there, we GPs work in a world of grey areas and asthma is like hypertension, CFS, PMS, depression, "predia-betes", ADHD, fibromyalgia, peripheral arterial disease, alcohol and substance misuse and dozens of other partially subjective conditions. But to make the diagnosis, NICE said it was no longer enough to rely on spirometry, reversibility, peak flows, subjective improvement or years of experience. These would be good enough for any reasonable doctor and given the safety of today's inhalers, the majority of patients. After all, most patients do stop using their medications, including inhalers when they stop being symptomatic-whether you have asked them to or not. Indeed the problem is usually that of keeping patients with obvious asthma from becoming lazy and omitting essential prophylaxis, not that of well patients taking unnecessary inhalers.

NICE now recommends that we do a fractional exhaled nitric oxide concentration, – FeNO test (NIOX MINO, NIOX VERO, NObreath) if patients have "an intermediate probability" of having asthma. Nitric oxide is a marker of airway inflammation, particu-larly if the inflammation is associated with eosinophils rather than neutrophils. Negative tests do not rule out asthma and NO is increased by URTIs, airway "acidity", exacerba-tions of COPD and brochiectasis.

If still unsure you should consider a bronchial challenge. My problem with all this is that asthma is an intermittent condition in which the airway inflammation may well have settled by the time you see and test the patient. Their asthma may be secondary to acute bacterial infections, not immune mediated (presumably this is neutrophilic?), the NO test is far from specific and you are, as in so many conditions in General Practice, treating the patient's symptoms as much as the degree of bronchial oedema. If an inhaler improves his or her exercise performance to "normal", stops them waking at night coughing and reduces their cough and wheeze with hay fever and colds then they need an inhaler, for a while, surely? But basically, asthma is a paroxysmal and unpredictable condition and doctors are INCREASINGLY UNAVAILABLE in our community at short notice. This is all given the current chaos in GP out of hours and reduced in hours accessibility of many practices. Surely we want the bottom line to be the patient having their own treatment stability, treatment autonomy and **safety**?

A confidential report published in 2014 reviewing the 200 asthma deaths between 2012 and 2013 found half the deaths occurred before admission to hospital. This is why GPs have to be:

A) Available to respond to and see emergencies at short notice either at home or at the surgery.

B) Do enough surgery sessions to know their own lists properly and recognise the unstable patients on their lists who can "Go off" quickly.

C) Preferable have their OWN lists and be full time or almost. (Infrequent sessional and very part time doctors cannot possibly know which patients who phone to say their child has a tight chest really need to be seen soon and who do not).

D) Be familiar with the recognition of and emergency treatment of seriously ill children. All GPs should have done a paediatric "SHO" job (ST 1, 2, 3).

E) All GPs should carry Ambubags or similar equipment for adults and children, Guedel's Airways and if they feel confident, ET Tubes. I have used this endotracheal emergency respiratory equipment approximately once every 6 or 7 years on house calls over my career.

Many of the deaths were related to inadequate steroid treatment. I accept that some patients become blasé about their own condition and don't consult when things are clearly getting dire. But given these facts, national guidelines recommend that all patients over five years old with severe asthma exacerbations should be given IV or oral steroids within one hour by the doctors they see. Apparently they often aren't. I of course, extend this to all patients under five as well. The recommended doses and treatments are: 20mg prednisolone for 2-5 year olds, 30-40mg prednisolone for over 5 year olds and 40-50mg for adults. Children and adolescents should have this for three days, adults for 5 days – although I fail to see why a young child should have a shorter and presumably less safe course of steroids than a slightly older child. This just reflects the all pervading paediatric treatment parsimony that applies to analgesics, antibiotics and steroids and often under treats young children.

The doses for smaller children are 1-2mg/kg orally and either IV (Hydrocortisone up to 4mg/kg IV) or soluble prednisolone.

See Diagram Peak Flow (Diagram PF V1, 2, 3) in Paediatrics pages 920, 921.

Acute severe asthma in children:

Can't complete sentences in one breath.
Pulse>120>5 yrs,
Pulse >130 at 2-5yrs,
Resps. >30 >5yrs,
Resps.>50 at 2-5yrs.

Steroids:

Prednisolone (etc) 1-2mg/kg orally/24 hrs for 5-7 days with or without a stat dose of IV hydrocortisone, (up to 4mg/kg IV, max 100mg).
<2yrs 25mg IV hydrocortisone,
2-5yrs 50mg,
5-12yrs 100mg.
PLUS
Nebulised B stimulant and Ipratropium.

Severity can also be assessed by:

Ability to complete full sentences,
Pulse>110,
PEFR <50% of Best, or predicted.
Respiratory rate>25,
TCO2 (unreliable except perhaps as a trend),

Accessory muscle use,
Pursing of lips (and blowing expiration),
Altered inspiratory/expiratory ratio,
Difficulty eating/drinking,
Auscultation (poor air entry),
Subjective distress or rate of deterioration,
Patient's own experience of their pattern of disease. Although some patients, including children do become blasé sometimes and underplay their distress. These patients need to be recognised as they won't come back to you when they are getting tired and acidotic.

Life threatening Asthma
Silent chest,
Cyanosis,
Bradycardia,
PEFR <33%-50% of best or predicted.

Asthma Symptoms:
Wheeze, breathlessness, chest tightness and cough.
Symptoms worse at night and early morning,
Symptoms worse after exercise, allergens, cold air, or after
Aspirin, Beta Blockers,
History of atopic disorder,
With:
Widespread rhonchi (wheeze) on auscultation of chest,   ,
Low FEV1 or PEFR,
Eosinophilia.
10-15% asthma in adults is due to work factors.

Less likely to be Asthma:
Prominent dizziness, light headedness,
Parasthesiae,
Chronic productive cough without wheeze or dyspnoea,
Normal on examination of chest when symptomatic, voice disturbance,
Symptoms only with colds,
Significant smoking history,
Cardiac disease,
Normal PEFR or spirometry when symptomatic.

Asthma Inhalers:
Bronchodilator, Short Acting: Blue.
Salbutamol, Includes Ventolin Evohaler. Airomir Autohaler. Asmasal Clickhaler. Easyhaler Salbutamol 100ug/200ug. Ventolin Accuhaler 200ug. Salamol Easibreathe. Terbutyline. Bricanyl Turbohaler (0.5mg).

Bronchodilator, Long Acting: Green (Greeny/blue)
Formoterol. Includes Atimos Modulite MDI. Oxis Turbohaler (6ug, 12ug). Foradil Inhaler, grey coloured, (Dry powder 12ug). Formoterol Easihaler (12ug).
Indacaterol, 150ug, 300ug. White/blue breath actuated, dry powder, Onbrez.
Salmeterol. Serevent, dry powder, breath actuated Accuhaler 50ug. Diskhaler 50ug.

Neovent and Serevent Evohaler are Salmeterol MDI 25ug.

Steroids: Brown or Buff coloured, Pink, Red, Orange
Beclometasone: MDIs: **Clenil Modulite** 50ug (buff), 100ug (brown), 200ug (pink), 250ug (red): (CFC Free) and **QVAR** 50ug (pink), 100ug (red): (CFC Free).
Clenil is the equivalent dose to Betametasone inh. Qvar is more potent dose for dose.
Also Asmabec Clickhaler:100ug, 250ug (White). Becodisks: 100ug, 200ug, 400ug (in buff, brown and pink boxes). Also Easihaler Beclometasone: 200ug, QVAR Autohaler: (50, 100), QVAR Easibreathe: (50, 100) etc.
Budesonide: Easyhalers: (200, 400ug), Pulmicort: 200, 400ug.
Also Ciclesonide: 80, 160ug. Alvesco.
Fluticasone, Flixotide. Evohaler (50, 125, 250ug), Accuhaler, (50, 100, 250, 500ug) (shades of orange).
Also Mometasone, Asmanex (200, 400ug), "Twisthaler" (shades of pink.)
Don't forget: In children >400mcg ICS (Inhaled Corticosteroid) can cause 1cm growth suppression.

Non steroidal preventers (Mast cell stabilisers):
Sodium Cromoglicate 5mg MDI, Intal. Nedocromil 2mg MDI Tilade.

Long acting Relievers and Preventers, including combinations:
Fostair, Formoterol 6mg and Beclometasone 100ug. MDI (pinky-red.)
Symbicort.(Budesonide and Formoterol.) Turbohaler 100/6, 200/6, 400/12ug. White and red, breath actuated.
Symbicort (Budesonide and Formoterol 100/6 and 200/6) can be used as a preventer and reliever as the "SMART" system 1-2 bd up to 4 puffs bd.
Seretide MDI: 50, 125, 250. Salmeterol 25ug and Fluticasone of varying dose, – 50, 125, 250 ug.
Seretide Accuhaler: 100, 250, 500. Salmeterol 50ug and Fluticasone of varying dose, 100, 250 and 500ug.
Fluticasone and Formoterol – Flutiform etc See MIMS for updates.

Anticholinergics:
Always worth trying early in children with "bronchiolitis/wheezy bronchitis", intransigent asthmatics as well as the elderly with COPD who can all surprise you with their response.
Ipratropium, Atrovent 20ug MDI.
Tiotropium, Spiriva 18ug Handihaler (capsules) and 2.5ug breath actuated/Respimat the same time once every day.
Tiotropium and Olodaterol (a LABA). Spiolto used in COPD.
Umeclidinium, Incruse (Ellipta inhaler is with Vilanterol a long acting B2agonist).
Aclidinium, Eklira. Glycopyrronium, Seebri are other long acting anticholinergics. The latter is an interesting and flexible drug of course and used as an anticholinergic in injection form as a premed and in terminal care. (Robinul).

Spacers:
At the younger and older age range, a well fitting spacer, with the time devoted to explaining how it is used is essential. Then get the patient/parent back with the spacer and ask them to demonstrate it (even if their chest is better). You will be amazed how much of

your adequate, patient, simple explanation has been ignored, misunderstood or forgotten but the second time you go over it, it **should** sink in.

For instance:

Name	Type	use with
Ablespacer,	Small volume device,	Any pressurised aerosol inhaler
Babyhaler	Paediatric device	Becotide and Ventolin
E-Z Spacer	Large volume, collapsible	Any pressurised aerosol
Haleraid		Used with standard inhalers to increase pressure on inhaler mechanism
Nebuhaler	Larger 750ml plastic cone	Bricanyl, Pulmicort.
Nebuchamber		Pulmicort
Volumatic	Larger 750ml reservoir	All GSK MDIs (Evo) Inhalers – Ventolin, Serevent, Clenil, Flixotide

as well as:

Aerochambers, (with adult, child and infant masks) These are simple to use, inconspicuous to carry and fit most MDIs.-Airomir, Atrovent, Qvar, Alvesco, Ventolin, Becotide, etc etc

Pocket Chamber, various masks, Vortex,

Optichamber Advantage etc.etc

Summary of stepwise management of children under 5 years:

Step 1 Inhaled short acting B2 agonist as required,

Step 2 plus 200-400ug corticosteroid/day,

or Leukotriene receptor antagonist* if inhaled steroid cannot be used,

Step 3 In those children taking inhaled steroids 200-400mcg/day consider adding an LRA*. In those on an LRA alone reconsider adding a steroid.

Step 4. Under 2 years refer to a paediatrician.

Summary of stepwise management of children aged 5-12 years:

Step 1 Inhaled short acting B2 agonist as required,

Step 2 Add inhaled corticosteroid 200-400ug/day,

Step 3 Add LABA, (long acting B agonist) adjust steroid (400ug), LRA and or theophylline etc.

Step 4 Increase steroid to 800mcg/day, consider referral.

Step 5 Lowest maintenance daily steroid 800mcg/day, refer.

Summary of stepwise management in adults:

Step 1: Inhaled PRN B2 agonists:

Step2: Inhaled 200-400ug/day corticosteroid.

Step 3: Add LABA and assess control. May need to increase to 800 ug steroid, or add LRA (Leukotreine receptor agonists), SR Theophylline, etc.

Step 4: Consider a trial of 2000ug inhaled steroid or 4 separate agents simultaneously (-LRA, SR Theophylline, B2 agonist orally and steroid tablet).

Step 5: Daily low dose oral steroid. While maintaining inhaled oral steroids at high dose (2000ug). Refer to specialist if you think there is anything else you haven't thought of.

LABAs alone increase the CVS risk.

Give the patient a steroid card if they have the equivalent of >800ug/day inhaled beclomethasone. Tail it off if they are on 1000ug/day.

Practical problems with asthmatic patients:

I remember asking a new, dismissive elderly patient, not on my list, to show me her inhaler technique a few years ago. Her daughter was with her and they both said she knew what she was doing, having used the inhaler for twenty years. Her own doctor trusted her so why was I wasting their time? Her problem was that she "obviously needed a stronger inhaler". She then removed one inhaler from her bag and puffed it into her open mouth, taking a gentle breath outwards a couple of seconds later. As I resigned myself to a difficult ten minutes of basic inhaler technique education with precious time I didn't have, I saw that she hadn't removed the mouthpiece from the inhaler either. The inside of this was coated with a thick layer of white active drug when I final managed to pull it off.

Always check the patient's inhaler technique every so often, even if you have a nurse who runs your asthma follow up clinic.

I find that my brilliant nurse and I frequently disagree on doses and drugs, even how long to hold your breath after the puff and inspiratory gasp.

In late 2014 Asthma UK disclosed the obvious fact that many patients were on stronger than necessary inhalers due to poor technique and many were not **ever** taught how to use their devices. This is unforgivable. They also said that patients struggle with auto Injectors which they have been prescribed for allergic emergencies. There is a recent US study which shows only 16% of patients in America use Adrenaline auto injectors properly. Common mistakes are not holding the injector in the thigh muscle for 10 seconds after activating it and not pushing the plunger hard enough. As someone who accidentally injected his own thigh through his trousers, while demonstrating an Epipen to a patient (I thought the injector had already been triggered), I sympathise. It is quite difficult to sign prescriptions with adrenaline shaking hands though the overall systemic results were nothing like as severe as I expected. In the same study only 7% of asthma patients used their inhalers properly. Allergy UK does a leaflet on the proper use of inhalers and auto injectors by the way.

Giving Up smoking: (and see psychiatry section:)

"**More doctors smoke Camels than any other cigarette**"

1940's advertising slogan

Who actually smokes?
Male Bangladeshis 44%,
Polish 40%,
Male Irish 39%,
Transgender people 39%,
Homosexuals 37%,
Black males 35%,
Lesbians 28%,
General adult population: (46% 1974) 19% in 2016 (HSCIC) >17%
Teenagers (2016): 18% of secondary school "children" say they have "ever tried a cigarette" – the lowest since records began in 1982 (when it was 50%).

Of the average British population only 17% were said to smoke by September 2016. The lowest level "ever" and this was at least in part "attributed to e Cigarettes".

Nearly all COPD is due to and proportionate to the amount of smoking and the number of the patient's "Pack years". Presumably before Raleigh and the discovery of Virginia there was virtually no COPD. (20 cigarettes a day for 10 years is 10 pack years). Currently 1 in 5 UK adults smoke in 2016 (It was 82% men and 41% women in 1948) and 120,000 die a year as a result. Only 2% smokers who try to quit without help are successful.

Aids to smoking cessation:

Nicotine gum is available GSL (General Sales List) from pharmacies (2 or 4mg) as are a large number of other forms of Nicotine replacement and there is an NHS smoking Helpline 0800 022 4332 (QUIT is 0800 002200).

Electronic Cigarettes, e cigarettes, were courting controversy from the outset. (2014) They vapourise Nicotine or non Nicotine containing flavoured solution (and this contains such solvents as propylene glycol and polyethylene glycol) and some look like cigarettes. They come in flavours such as bubble gum, cherry, various fruit flavours and chocolate. They are as or slightly more effective than patches and some other forms of NRT in getting patients off cigarettes (which isn't saying much). They are currently unregulated and some authorities think that a teenage interest in them may be an entry into real smoking with tobacco. The e cigarette Nicotine solution can be toxic, even transdermally, especially in children. The Welsh Parliament is considering banning them in public places and so not everyone sees them as helpful and harmless weapons in the battle to get more people off cigarettes. A puff from an e cigarette with a "high Nicotine "content generally contains only a fifth of a normal cigarette's Nicotine and there is a poor correlation between the dose stated and that delivered.

The E cigarette does however have none of the combustible poisons that burnt tobacco smoke is full of. Tobacco smoke contains 4,000 chemicals including 43 carcinogens, 400 known toxins, tar, carbon monoxide, formaldehyde, ammonia, hydrogen cyanide, arsenic, DDT and many more. It was estimated in September 2014 that if all 9 million UK smokers took up E Cigarettes, about 54,000 of the 60,000 premature deaths due to smoking would be prevented. By mid 2015 2.6million Britons were using E Cigarettes. Indeed a sea change in official attitudes seemed to be taking place by August 2015 when Public Health England suggested that E Cigarettes might even become prescribable as they were "95% less harmful than cigarettes" and did not lead to real smoking.

A slight swing of the attitudinal pendulum began taking place by December 2016, however, when the American Surgeon General warned that they were at least as dangerous as real cigarettes and the vapour contained harmful ultrafine particulates and damaging vapour. These included carcinogenic carbonyls and some nitrosamines. Also some flavourings though safe swallowed are harmful inhaled -Diacetyl etc.

Bupropion: Zyban (an antidepressant). Can lower seizure threshold. Avoid in eating disorders, bipolar disorders, diabetes, history of head Injury, alcohol or benzodiazepine withdrawal. Avoid in pregnancy.

Start treatment 1-2 weeks before a chosen cessation date. 150mg OD for 6 days then 150mg BD 7-9 weeks. Adverse reactions: Insomnia, dizziness, tremor, depression, anxiety, urticaria, chest pain – most of which can be S/Es of giving up smoking! Avoid in a history of seizures, eating disorders, head trauma, treatment with antidepressants, antipsychotics, theophylline, systemic steroids. All sorts of potential drug interactions. I have never seen any of significance.

The worst case of severe agitated depression I have seen in a previously well man of

60 with absolutely no other trigger or psychiatric history was when he decided to stop smoking 20 cigarettes a day after 50 years. This went on despite combination treatments and psychiatric support for three to four months. He then presented with shoulder pain and haemoptysis and had an underling bronchial tumour from which the poor chap quickly died. Sudden spontaneous distaste for cigarettes is of course a presenting symptom of lung (and other) cancer. If you want to see how people can become severely addicted to simple tobacco and how they can suffer when something (In this case love of a good woman) makes them decide to go "cold turkey" read the brilliant "The Moonstone" by Wilkie Collins. In those days, GPs gave controlled drugs (laudanum) to patients without their knowledge or consent as a plot device as well as a treatment for Nicotine withdrawal. No GMC then!

Vareniclene: Champix. Can be associated with agitation, depression, even suicidal thoughts so monitor closely all those with a history of psychiatric illness. Avoid in pregnancy.

Start treatment 1-2 weeks before smoking cessation date. Then 500ug daily for 3days, then 500ug bd for 4 days, then 1mg bd for 11 weeks. The starter pack has the first 3 weeks worth of treatment. (Wouldn't four weeks have been more logical?)

NRT: Nicotine Replacement Therapy:
A bewildering number of treatments:

Nicorette: Tabs 2mg,
Chewing Gum 2mg various flavours,
Lozenges 2mg,
Patches 5mg, 10mg, 15mg, also "Invisi patches",
Oral spray,
Nasal spray,
Inhalator.

Nicotinell: Gum 2mg, 4mg,
Lozenge 1mg, 2mg,
TTS Patches. ("10", "20" and "30", which I take to be roughly equivalent to the number of cigarettes previously consumed in 24 hrs-that they should substitute for). The 24 hour patches cause dreams but they do avoid the morning craving as it takes an hour or two for Nicotine levels to rise when the patch is applied. The whole point of smoking a drug is that the "hit" is almost as quick as an IV dose.

Niquitin: Gum 2mg, 4mg.
Lozenges 1.5mg.
Patches, 7mg, 14mg, 21mg.

Recent (2014) studies show that "Pill and patch replacement therapy" is more successful at producing a smoke free patient at 26 weeks (49% vs 33%) and with better short and long term outcomes generally.

Smoking offers few non psychological benefits and a panoply of harmful side effects. These are not limited to the smoker him or herself: Children whose parents smoke are more likely to develop bronchitis and pneumonia, are at increased risk of SIDS, asthma, middle ear infections and meningitis. (New Scientist Feb 2014 p7.)

Research published in 2015(Lancet Psychiatry 10 July) suggested that not only do schizophrenics smoke more but smokers were more likely to develop schizophrenia. 57% of patients having a first episode of psychosis are smokers, 3X the general population. In daily smokers the onset of schizophrenia is on average a year earlier. Smoking cannabis with tobacco in the words of the study could give you "a double whammy" for schizophrenia.

Smoking offers few reliable significant health benefits that I am aware of. There is some evidence that it can reduce some symptoms of inflammatory bowel disease. (-as suggested by Hugh Laurie to a patient in an episode of "House"). There is also some data to suggest that smokers suffer less from fibroids U.C., Sarcoid, Kaposi's Sarcoma and possibly breast cancer in some women with the BRCA gene. How and why I cannot guess.

Stopping smoking:

Is generally a good idea but it can have some negative adverse effects: Stopping smoking can cause severe depression and anxiety, exacerbate Ulcerative Colitis and, presumably via a similar mechanism may cause acute episodes of apthous oral ulceration. Nicotine patches are used by some as a treatment. As previously mentioned, if you want to see what a really extreme case of Nicotine withdrawal can do to *almost* ruin a man's whole life, read the brilliant Moonstone – reputedly the first detective novel, by Wilkie Collins – with Inspector Cuff predating that more famous product of a failed GP's imagination, Sherlock Holmes.

Cough: When to worry and do an X Ray:

Duration >3 weeks in an OLDER patient.

(Persistent cough is common in the younger patient with post nasal drip, cough variant asthma, reflux etc).

Haemoptysis (always),

Chest or shoulder pain,

Dyspnoea,

Weight loss,

Chest Signs (especially a unilateral monophonic exp rhonchus) – (this is a wheeze to younger doctors).

Hoarseness,

Finger clubbing,

Signs of secondaries,

Neck or supraclavicular lymphadenopathy.

Persistent cough in a healthy person:

The well child can cough up to at least 30X a day. Stand in an assembly or sit watching a PG film in a cinema and you know how ubiquitous both dry and wet coughs are.

Many children develop a prolonged post viral wheeze and cough after trivial chest infections and these can respond to inhalers, including Ipratropium, Cromoglicate, inhaled steroids or even Monteleukast.

Cough variant asthma:

requires a longish course of inhaled steroids to diagnose and to treat, B stimulants often don't help much. It is a persistent cough (usually 6-8 weeks) without the other symptoms of asthma, the cough being worse on exercise, on exposure to cold air or allergens. Occasionally beta blockers or aspirin sensitivity may be the trigger.

Some physicians use spirometry or a Methacholine challenge to confirm the diagnosis. Having excluded TB, post nasal drip, reflux, chronic infection, COPD, drug S/E, CF, bronchiectasis, cancer, sarcoid and FB (in a child), I would always treat this sort of cough AS ASTHMA and just see if it gets better.

An acute wheezy cough below the age of two responds frequently, despite our current apparent phobia of prescribing antibiotics to almost any patient, to Macrolide group antibiotics.

Post nasal drip requires topical nasal steroids or anticholinergic drops.

Oesophageal reflux is of fluid, not necessarily acid, so treatment requires a prokinetic to stop "non acid fluid reflux" as well as Anti Acid drug Rx.eg Domperidone/Metoclopramide as well as a PPI.

– and **always** consider a drug side effect (ACEI, BB etc.)

Post infectious (many viruses and other infections – Mycoplasma, Pertussis etc).

In **chronic cough** unresponsive to anything else, try Mucodyne and Montelkast.

BUT EXCLUDE PERTUSSIS FIRST.

Should you worry about the risks of doing Chest X Rays? – Assuming you have access to them.

X Ray doses compared with ambient exposure to radiation:

CT Abdomen and pelvis	3 yrs
CT Abdomen and pelvis with and without contrast	7 yrs
CT Colonography	3 yrs
IVP	1 yr
X Ray Spine	6 m
X Ray extremity	3 hrs
CT Head	6 m
CT Head with and without contrast	16 m
CXR	**10 d**

CT and PET scans (**see "miscellaneous"**) are slightly different to basic XRs as can be seen. A typical PET scan involves 5-7mSv radiation. Often PET and CT scans are done together and these may add up to 25mSv. Compare this with the "classification" level for radiation workers of 7mSv, the 2.2mSv average annual UK background radiation, 0.02mSv for a CXR, 7-8mSv for a chest CT and 4-9mSv for annual aircrew exposure.

Spirometry/Respiratory function:

Of no value unless the patient puts in their maximum effort (on full expiration and peak flow).

FEV1: The Forced Expiratory Volume in 1 second. Reduced in obstructive conditions.

Classically, COPD is diagnosed when FEV1 is <80% of predicted and FEV1/FVC is <70% predicted.

Asthma may show the same spirometry pattern as COPD.

FVC: Forced Vital Capacity. The total volume that can be forcible exhaled in one breath. Reduced in restrictive lung conditions.

FEV1/FVC: The ratio as a percentage.

Thus: An average normal ratio is 75%, <75% Obstructive?, >75% Restrictive Airways Disease**?

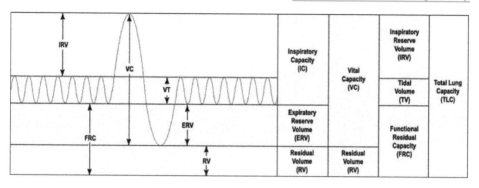

Diagram of spirometry – basic physiology you have forgotten: Block diagram of TLC, VC, RV etc. etc.

So:

Tidal Volume: Vt	500ml Quiet Breathing
Inspiratory Reserve:	2500ml Forced Inspiration
Expiratory Reserve:	1000ml Forced Expiration
Vital Capacity:	4000ml (Insp. Reserve + T.V. + Exp. Reserve)
FRC:	Functional Residual Capacity: The volume in the lungs at End Expiratory Volume.

Forced Vital Capacity: The Vital Capacity from a maximum Forced Expiratory Effort.

Residual Volume:	1000ml Always left in the lungs
Total Lung Capacity:	5000ml

The normal FEV1/FVC ratio is 75-80%**. In obstructive airways disease (asthma, COPD, emphysema, chronic bronchitis) the FEV1 is disproportionately diminished. Significant airflow obstruction is <70%.

Very severe COPD shows a below 30% FEV1:FVC ratio or FEV1 <50% with respiratory failure. In restrictive lung disease (pulmonary fibrosis) both FEV1 and FVC are affected and the ratio may be normal or even increased.

Forced expiratory flow FEF is usually assessed at different fractions of expiration. For instance at 25%, 50% and 75% of the Forced Vital Capacity. FEF at 25-75% or 25-50% may be more sensitive than peak flow at detecting small airways disease.

MMEF or FEF 25-75%: The maximum mid expiratory flow is the average expiratory flow over the middle half of the FVC.

PEAK EXPIRATORY FLOW RATE IN CHILDREN

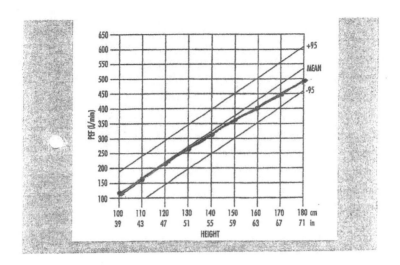

There are several Peak Flow charts for children: The dark slightly bent line amalgamates scores from other commonly used charts.

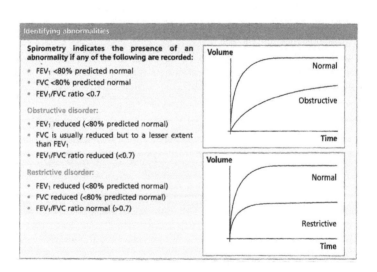

Diagram "Identifying abnormalities"

COPD or Asthma?

	COPD	Asthma
Smoker or Ex smoker	Nearly all	Possibly
Symptoms <35 yrs age	Unlikely	Common
Chronic productive cough	Common	Uncommon
Nocturnal dyspnoea/wheeze	Rare	Common
Dyspnoea	Persistent	Fluctuates
Significant diurnal or day to day variability	Uncommon	Common
Response to Beta stimulants	None or partial	None, partial or significant.

Note that a poor response to some bronchodilators does not necessarily suggest a poor response to long acting B agonists or anticholinergics.

Don't forget the HYPOXIC DRIVE that maintains respiration in patients with COPD and avoid giving too much oxygen in the ambulance (ie use a Venturi mask at 24-28%).

Remember that COPD severity and prognosis are related to "Pack years" (the number of packs of 20 cigarettes smoked each day for how many years). In the UK there are probably 2 million undiagnosed patients with COPD.

Regular exercise of 2 hours of walking or cycling a week reduces admission and respiratory mortality in COPD by 30-40%. (-like it seems to do in nearly every condition, cardiovascular, neoplastic, psychological etc).

The MRC Dyspnoea Scale:

1) Not breathless unless strenuously exercising.

2) S.O.B. when hurrying or walking up a slight hill.

3) Walks slower than peer group on the flat because of dyspnoea or has to stop for breath when walking at own pace.

4) Stops for breath after 100m or after a few minutes on level ground.

5) Too dyspnoeic to leave the house or breathless on dressing/undressing.

Before referral/diagnosis, always consider;

Recent history of infection, (Pertussis in adults for instance),

Their smoking history,

Bird ownership (Parrots, Budgerigars, Cockatiels, Pigeons etc-Psittacosis),

Drug history (ACEI, BB etc),

Work (soldering, farms, wood workers, attic and house dust, paint sprayers, bakers, nurses, chemical workers, animal handlers, laboratory workers – nearly all of whom develop skin and or respiratory allergy to rat epithelium and urine protein after a decade in post, etc).

This is interesting since children brought up on a farm (Respirology Oct 2007, NEJM Feb 24 2011) or with dogs have less asthma – so age at exposure as well as the actual animal antigen are both important.

Over 10% asthma is occupational:

Common work allergens are isocyanates, flour and grain dust, colophony, fluxes, latex, laboratory and other animal fur and skin, aldehydes, wood dust especially MDF, epoxies, resins, chromium, chromates (cement), aromatic amines, etc. There are 3,000 agents known to cause contact dermatitis. There is no reason to think there are that many fewer that could cause respiratory sensitisation too.

Symptom variability/progression.

Chronic Obstructive Pulmonary Disease:

(Chronic bronchitis, Emphysema, C.O.P.D.)

Classically the "blue bloaters" with chronic inflammation of the bronchi, a wet mucoid productive cough but also the patients with predominantly emphysematous lung changes. Classic signs include hyper inflation, prolonged expiration (pursed lips giving a positive end expiratory pressure and prevent collapse of airways), cyanosis, clubbing and later signs of R heart failure. Smoking, occupational exposure to air borne irritants and atmospheric pollution are the main aetiological factors. Alpha 1 antitrypsin deficiency is a rare genetic cause.

Spirometry In COPD:

$FEV1 < 80\%$ predicted,

$FEV1/FVC$ ratio $< 70\%$ (0.7),

COPD is not present if FEV1 and ratio return to N with bronchodilators. (Asthma if >400ml response to bronchodilators, serial PEFRs show diurnal or day to day variability, >400ml response to 30mg prednisolone daily for 2 weeks).

Severity of COPD (GOLD scale)	FEV_1 % predicted
Mild (GOLD 1)	≥80
Moderate (GOLD 2)	50–79
Severe (GOLD 3)	30–49
Very severe (GOLD 4)	<30 or chronic respiratory failure symptoms

GOLD-is the Global Initiative for Chronic Lung Disease

Don't forget the hypoxic Drive:

Although this may often be exaggerated, the average chronic COPD patient may be surviving on a hypoxic rather than hypercapnic respiratory stimulus and over oxygenating them may reduce their saturations and prognosis. Anything over 24-28% oxygen by mask and 4 li/minute flow at the supply may result in respiratory depression, respiratory acidosis and $CO2$ retention.

Treatment: Suggested Adult NHS COPD Management:

In recurrent or persistent dyspnoea:

Step 1A PRN Short acting B2 Agonist* +/– PRN Short Acting Muscarinic Antagonist**
Use a spacer and MDI

Step 1B   Regular SABA*   +/–   Regular SAMA**
Use a spacer and MDI

Step 2   FEV1>50%   FEV1<50%
LAMA (Tiotropium, Spiriva) for 4 week trial   LABA plus inhaled steroid or
**   LABA plus LAMA**

LABA (Salmeterol, Serevent/Formoterol, Foradil)   or LAMA alone.
Olodaterol-Striverdi for 4 week trial

Step 3 LABA Plus ICS or LABA plus LAMA   LAMA plus LABA plus ICS

Step 4 ,,   ,,   ,,   **Refer to chest physician.**
                                                For diagnosis, deterioration, severity, other
                                                conditions, heart failure etc.etc
NOTE:
ICS Inhaled Corticosteroid.
LAMA Long acting Muscarinic Receptor Antagonist.
S/LABA Short/Long Acting B2 Adrenergic Receptor Agonist.

Doesn't this sort of guideline make your head spin with its abbreviations, compliant patients who always return for review, collect and use their prescriptions properly, give up smoking and all fit in with your 7-10 minute GP appointments?

Who designs this sort of algorithm? Our hospital respiratory specialist nurse is a great resource but is spread very thin and always hard to find and there is the usual long Out Patient wait for the Respiratory Consultants. How many weeks do you spend working your way down to the more effective (and if you are experienced in dealing with COPD patients) more logical polypharmacy at the bottom of the chart?

I will personally prescribe anything that improves the patient's respiratory function, subjective sense of well being, exercise capacity and improves their quality of life from the start so I would basically start with a higher strength combination LABA and inhaled steroid through a spacer, (taking time to make sure they know how to use it) and almost immediately add in a SAMA (Atrovent through a spacer ii qds) or once settled, a LAMA (Spiriva – again, making sure they can use it properly). Since Spiriva is given once a day at the same time of day I slightly prefer the scattergun of four puffs of a shorter acting Atrovent through a spacer assuming that if you get most of the dose, most of the time, even if it is short acting, is better than sometimes getting none of a longer lasting treatment).

Many chest physicians I know think that anticholinergics are more effective than B stimulants in COPD anyway and use them far earlier. I have a low threshold for oral steroids and broad spectrum antibiotics in big doses. It seems illogical to believe that a patient receiving their 30th course of Amoxicillin in 10 years and who is unwell should respond to yet another course of Amoxicillin.

Purulent sputum **IS** a good indicator of likely response to antibiotics by the way. But vary the antibiotic. Forty years ago the colour of the sputum was said to be a good indicator of whether the chest was *bacterially* infected or not. But as we know asthma and viral infections can generate catarrh from watery to yellow, grey and brown, so this pointer rather fell into disrepute. There is however increasing evidence that a change in the thickness and volume but particularly the colour of phlegm **is** associated with genuine bacterial lower respiratory infections thus indicating the need for antibiotics. Like hemlines on a catwalk, attitudes to phlegm come and go and come back again.

Other drugs:

Leukotriene antagonists: Montelukast, Singulair, Zafirlukast, Accolate. Leukotrienes are immune system inflammatory mediators. They are released by Mast Cells or Eosinophils and cause bronchospasm. This sounds analogous to the activity of Cromoglicate and presumably works with all the other inhalers synergistically, if a little unpredictably and ineffectively.

PDE4 Inhibitors: This relates to phosphodiesterase no 4, – there being various sub classes of phosphodiesterase inhibitors. Caffeine is one, Viagra is a PDE5 inhibitor and Diazepam is a PDE4 inhibitor. Cilostazol, Pletal, is a PDE3 inhibitor, (used in claudication). Roflumilast, Daxas is a PDE4 inhibitor and has anti inflammatory effects. It can be used in asthma and COPD (if FEV1<50%) but does cause nausea, diarrhoea and headache.

Mucolytics:

Carboci(y) steine: Mucodyne. 375mg caps (2-3 bd) and syrup 250mg/5mls. Effective in Cystic Fibrosis, some COPD and Glue Ear etc, as well as many clinical situations where thick mucus is a problem. The other mucolytics, Mecysteine, Visclair and Erdocysteine, Erdotin, no doubt help patients with viscid mucus and intractable hacking coughs too.

Lobelia extract/tablets are said to have a similar effect on catarrh. I cannot personally vouch for this.

Omalizumab: Xolair injection is an IgG monoclonal antibody that binds with the patient's IgE. (It actually blocks receptors on mast cells and basophils to which the IgE/Ag complex would have attached). It is used in uncontrolled severe persistent allergic asthma. It isn't easy to determine which asthmatics it is going to help however and it does need 2-4 weekly expensive injections. It seems to be good in chronic idiopathic urticaria though.

Oxygen Supply:

Since February 2006 when a simple prescription prompted the provision of bottled oxygen to the patient's home and a phone call to the local branch of Boots secured its delivery within hours, things got much harder for GPs and patients with the awarding of the oxygen supply contract to a national specialist respiratory organisation – at least in my neck of the woods.

The HOOF form (Home Oxygen Order Form) is the prerequisite, unintuitive form that has now to be faxed to the company's anonymous, distant customer services department and must be filled in to the call handler's total satisfaction. This usually involves completing the request form at least twice and more often than not a back up phone call explaining the details all over again.

Requesting life saving oxygen is an excellent example of how today's NHS has made the simple fuss-less processes of the past complex, bureaucratic and stroke-inducingly frustrating. Before the change of supplier, we had a seamless system that worked 100% of the time with a phone call and a prescription and no Kafkaesque forms or bureaucrats. We got to know our local pharmacy supplier personally and they us. It pretty much worked 24/7 and the patients just took the oxygen turning up for granted. Part of your anger and disbelief today is that the person at the other end of the phone seems intent on preventing you from helping a real patient who has a real illness. Patients are the people who pay for everything, whom we are here to serve. Not only that but like all the other myriad health administrators on the phone, the oxygen controller usually sounds like so many powerful, obstructive NHS, faceless paper shufflers today, about sixteen years old and like he or she has had to pause his play station just as he was about to go up a level. Restrictive and obstructive simultaneously without knowing the clinical significance of either term.

The qualifications to do this job, based on endless strained phone calls regarding what is, after all, a simple but urgent request on behalf of a sick patient, seem to be ignorance of respiratory physiology, complete anonymity, an obsessional focus on form filling and a desire to be as awkward as possible.

To successfully fill a HOOF form,
You have to remember that: Venturi valve colour:
2 li/min flow rate is 24% blue,
4 li/min flow rate is 28% white,
6 li/min flow rate is 35% yellow,
8 li/min flow rate is 40% red,
12 li/min flow rate is 60% green.

The new system requires precise statements of the concentration, flow, rate and details of the patient.

The truth is that most oxygen administration is not as scientific as this and provided you don't forget the hypoxic drive of patients with COPD, the precise percentage administered is not as crucial as the HOOF form and its bureaucrats think.

These days the request form usually needs to be corrected and re-faxed no matter how accurate it was the first time and I fail to see why the old system, which worked extremely well and was far more patient centred was so suddenly dropped **without any consultation** with GPs or patients.

Bronchiectasis: Much commoner than you think.

1:1000 adults, Female 70%

A thickening and dilatation of the medium sized peripheral airways leading to chronic cough, excessive mucus production, frequent infections, haemoptysis, dyspnoea with a very variable clinical course. Bronchiectasis usually affects the lung bases but can be more localised or generalised. There is a vicious circle of infection, failure to clear infected mucous, local tissue damage with airway dilatation, further infection in the residual sputum and more damage to the lung etc.

Localised or focal bronchiectasis may be due to local compression or obstruction (FB, tumour, nodes) or from a previous local chest infection. This may have been decades before.

Generalised (diffuse) bronchiectasis can be secondary to:
Pertussis,
Measles,
other forms of pneumonia,
Rh A,
ABPA,
HIV or immune deficiency,
CF,
Primary Ciliary Dyskinesia,
Inflammatory Bowel Disease,
Aspiration damage (G.I. reflux),
α1 Antitrypsin Deficiency,
Marfan's and Young's Syndromes.

About half of UK patients have no obvious cause, 30% follow a significant childhood chest infection, 8% have an immune defect, 7% have ABPA and the rest are divided amongst the other causes listed above.

The prognosis varies widely and depends upon the extent, the stage at diagnosis, the intensity of treatment, the frequency of exacerbations, the presence of an underlying cause, smoking, infection with Pseudomonas. Complications are R heart failure, infection, respiratory failure, chronic ill health etc.

Many general Respiratory Physicians are not, it has to be said, good at managing or in my experience even diagnosing bronchiectasis. Bronchiectasis often co exists with asthma and COPD. Some consultants, especially these days, will ration the screening tests on the grounds of cost. This is unforgivable, given the irreversible damage that can be occurring with every missed infection. If you, as a GP suspect bronchiectasis (In adults: persistent coarse crepitations on early inspiration and productive cough, dyspnoea, occasional haemoptysis, a third have wheeze. In children: FTT, recurrent LRTI, dyspnoea, wheeze, occasional haemoptysis, inspiratory crackles that don't go away with treatment, also a suspicion of background CF) then see if there is a local Respiratory Physician who specialises in bronchiectasis.

The CXR is abnormal in 90% but it is more to exclude other diagnoses and of course you should have done a spirometry and proper chest work up etc before referral, -preferably with a trial of treatment or treatments already. A better test than CXR is a high resolution CT which, as GPs don't have access to this will be the consultant's job. As will be a sweat test (even in adults), Immunoglobulins, Alpha 1 Antitrypsin screening, Aspergillus precipitins and so on.

The treatments are chest physio, (taught to the patient), active cycle breathing techniques, postural drainage, breathing devices that produce gentle internal expiratory vibrations (Acapella, RC Cornet etc), stop smoking, exercise as much as possible, a low threshold for high dose broad spectrum antibiotics or specific antibiotics based on sputum culture, nebulised therapy if it helps, including (after a hospital trial) hypertonic saline and inhaled steroids if symptomatically useful, nebulised anticholinergics and B stimulants, oral steroids likewise, if effective.

Antibiotics can be given orally for 14 days, usually after a sputum culture. They can be used prophylactically or by nebuliser. Mucolytics and Leukotriene receptor antagonists are sometimes helpful.

Very occasionally a lobectomy of a particularly damaged lung, acting as a sump, may be considered.

In Bronchiectasis:

Antibiotics: All 14 days	First line	Second line
Sputum positive for:		
Strep Pneumoniae	Amoxicillin 500mg tds	Clarithromycin 500mg bd
Haemoph Infl B lact Neg	Amoxicillin	Clarithromycin or Ciprofloxacin 500mg bd
Haemoph Infl B lact Pos	Co Amox 625mg tds	Clarithrom or Ciprofloxacin
Moraxella catarrhalis	Co Amox	Ciprofloxacin
Staph Aureus (MSSA)	Fluclox 500mg qds	Clarithromycin
Staph Aureus (MRSA)	Rifampicin +Trimethoprim 200mg bd	Rifampicin + Doxycycline 100mg bd
Coliforms (Klebsiella, Enterobacter)	Ciproflox	IV antibiotics
Pseudomonas Aeruginosa	Ciproflox	IV antibiotics

Chest Infection:

The decision whether to start treatment in someone presenting to the doctor with a possible chest infection can be a complicated one, based on symptoms, the patient's past history of respiratory illness, co existing other illnesses, the doctor's perception of the recent course of the illness, the likely pathogen(s), some objective findings, -respiratory rate, tachycardia, cyanosis, ability to speak, in drawing, recession, accessory muscle use, etc, transcutaneous oxygen level (although this was found to be unhelpful in the latest American Bronchiolitis guidelines), auscultatory clinical chest signs, even the time at which the patient presents. Increasingly too, external pressure from local prescribing committees, dire warnings about drug resistance from the Department of Health and expert Public Health commentators have led to a therapeutic nihilism and even a reluctance amongst some GPs to properly examine, look for or recognise the signs of infection in many sick patients.

We are consequently seeing an increase in Scarlet Fever, other Post Streptococcal Illnesses, community Acquired Pneumonia and deaths from Paediatric "Sepsis". We are also seeing an increase in prizes, awards, congratulations and plaudits to practices and many individual doctors for a blanket reduction of their antibiotic prescribing. There are current epidemics of treatable and previously treated serious bacterial infection. Clearly there is a current (2014-2017) professional mismatch between the large number of patients presenting with respiratory symptoms to primary care and the thoroughness with which some PCPs (Primary Care Physicians) assess, manage, prescribe for and arrange follow up of the patients with respiratory infection. It is of course impossible to appropriately manage any patient with a respiratory infection without a thorough examination.

Community acquired pneumonia:

The common organisms are: only established in 1/3 cases but of those isolated, Strep. Pneumoniae, Haemophilus Influenzae, Moraxella Catarrhalis, make up 50%. Mycoplasma Pneumoniae, Chlamydophila, Pneumoniae, Chlamydophila Psittaci Psittaci, Coxiella Burnetti and Legionella Pneumophilia make up 15%. Influenza A and Rhinoviruses constitute up to 30%. Staph Aureus is a rare cause.

Assessing severity can be done by **"CURB-65 Score"**

CURB-65 Score	Severity	Management
Confusion of new onset Abbreviated mental test score </= 8	Score 0-1 Low 30 day mortality <3%	Manage in the community
Urea >/= 7mmol Respiratory rate >/= 30/min BP <90 syst or 60 diast	Score 2 Moderate 30 day mortality 9%	Consider hospital admission
Age >/= 65	Score 3-5 High 30 day mortality 15-40%	Hospital ITU/High dependency

Treatments:
Amoxicillin, Co Amoxiclav, Clarithromycin or Doxycycline – or combinations thereof.

Legionnaires' Disease: (Notifiable) Legionella Pneumophila.

First described in 1976 when an outbreak occurred at a meeting of the "American Legion" in Philadelphia.

Begins with flu symptoms, headache, myalgia, sometimes confusion, dyspnoea, cough and chest pain. Ataxia, confusion, haemoptysis and bradycardia are also common. IP highly variable, 2-19 days. Legionella bacteria thrive in warm fresh water supplies in buildings, (symbiotic with amoebae) such as air conditioning systems, showers, sprinkler systems, hot tubs, fresh water ponds. Aerosol/droplet spread. Urine antigen and mucus/sputum culture diagnostic tests.

Patients tend to be or have been smokers, drinkers, have co existing other diseases (Diabetes, chronic pulmonary disease, renal disease), to be over age 50, or have an immune deficit. No person to person spread. Treatment is with Erythromycin/Clarithromycin/tetracyclines/quinolones.

What is Mycoplasma Pneumoniae? The smallest free living organism, unusual in our host of bacterial adversaries in lacking a cell wall.

It is an organism that causes Atypical Pneumonia. Other causes are Psittacosis, Q Fever and Legionella. A different Mycoplasma can cause Pelvic Inflammatory Disease. Interestingly it may cause carcinogenic chromosomal transformation of cells. It used to be called the pleuro-pneumonia like organism. Mycoplasma causes 7-10% of community acquired pneumonia and occurs in epidemics every 3-4 years.

It commonly affects children and young adults, in autumn and spring. The infection is slow in onset, a hacking cough developing with flu like symptoms, contagious for 10 days or more, IP 14-21 days, up to 28 days and it lasts from a few days to 3-4 weeks. On examination focal crepitations (crackles for younger readers) are common; patients can also have a red throat and cervical lymphadenopathy. There is a lot of variability. It can mimic bronchiolitis in small children which is why wheezy toddlers should usually be given Macrolides not Amoxicillin or other classes of antibiotics. There is a dry cough, often a wheeze and 10% develop frank secondary pneumonia. Complications include otitis media, haemolytic anaemia, pneumonia, rashes.

Erythromycin, Clarithromycin, Azithromycin all work if you need to treat it, penicillins etc don't work as the organism has no cell wall.

CXR is usually worse than the clinical symptoms suggest, with such things as bronchopneumonia, plate like atelectasis, effusions and lower lobe infiltrates. Patchy changes.

Cold agglutinins are positive in 50-70%. As a bedside test: Put a few drops of blood in the citrate of a prothrombin tube then put the tube in a fridge for 10 minutes: Cold agglutinins show as a coarse granular appearance that clears on warming in the grip of your palm – but there are more specific CFT and immuno assays etc. WBC is usually N.

CRP-POCT

NICE has suggested using **Point of Care Testing (POCT) for CRP** to guide the use of antibiotics in patients with symptoms of lower respiratory tract infection in the primary care setting. The motivation is, of course, to reduce the thoughtless blanket over prescription of antibiotics for all seasonal infections. Unfortunately, as is typical of my profession, many of us have gone from an over readiness to prescribe inappropriately to an unwillingness to prescribe at all. Anything to save the doctor from spending time clerking and properly examining, – that is: doing our job properly with the patient. The epidemic of small children on the front pages of newspapers who have recently started dying of "Sepsis" over 2015-17 may be evidence of this. I wonder what the general (elderly, frail, COPD), mortality rates have shown over the same period of antibiotic rationing?

NICE guidance is:

Do not prescribe antibiotics if the CRP is <20mg/litre,

For CRP values of 20-100mg/litre provide a prescription to be used if symptoms worsen,

For CRP >100mg/litre prescribe antibiotics.

This strategy is supported by a randomised controlled trial by Cals JW et al (Ann Fam Med. 2010 Mar-Apr;8(2):124-33.)

Various GP practices have won awards and been praised for reducing their antibiotic prescribing by using CRP as a quick way of differentiating bacterial from viral infections. I will leave aside that these practices gain universally worse patient approval scores than those whose doctors spend TIME examining their patients properly and discussing what treatment decision to make with their patients*, AND ARE FLEXIBLE, but I would love to know:

1) How reliable CRP is in **EARLY** community acquired pneumonia, quinsy, OM, sinus infection etc. and how many bacterial infections it misses at the start of a **progressive** infection? After all, most infections do have a deteriorating course. Do the patients just have to keep coming back to be retested every day? I myself have been admitted dehydrated, after vomiting for over a week on three separate occasions with maxillary sinusitis. I then responded to IV antibiotics and fluids. Each infection began with a viral URTI but I knew instantly when the secondary infection had taken hold and I am pretty sure I would have known well before my CRP was >100mg/li. And what about the dozens of other causes of a raised CRP?, -exercise, IUCDs, atheroma, cancers, pregnancy, the pill, IBD, SLE , Rh. A, simple obesity and then all the inflammatory conditions and so on.

2) How reliable is POCT-CRP in predicting secondary infections in patients with known **risk factors** such as bronchiectasis, immune deficits and COPD (who often present early, knowing the course of their disease better than a nurse and a blood test) ? This question is a little facetious but it does make the point that in susceptible patients, prevention is better than cure. Especially if they and we know their past typical clinical course and history.

3) What are these prize winning practices' morbidity, mortality and duration of illness statistics? Patients and illnesses are never standardised and I would have thought the new NHS had learnt by now that applying a simple one size fits all box-ticking approach to the infinite variability of patients, doctors, nurses and illness leads nowhere but to disaster.

Practices that place too much emphasis on "objective tests" in clinical decision making, such as point of care testing, tend to use them as a substitute for spending doctor/patient assessment time together. If the patient isn't seen by a doctor, examined thoroughly, counselled appropriately and given an opportunity to be part of the treatment decision, then they are being short changed. Patients are not stupid. No wonder extremist low antibiotic prescribers are given poor scores by their patients. Generally the doctors are also poor examiners of chests, throats, glands and ears and very poor communicators. Or even worse, the offload their face to face duties on to a nurse practitioner. They are not using CRP-POCT and other POCTs as a way of improving care or preventing MRSA but of avoiding dealing with endless patients with flu and colds, a proportion of whom are quite ill and will take a lot of effort, experience, skill and patience to find and treat.

"And aren't surgeries during flu epidemics tiresome? Let's get the nurse practitioner to do them for us with a simple blood test to back her up just in case one of them is actually ill. That will cover

us medico-legally in case one of the children dies from septicaemic shock or develops Scarlet Fever. We can concentrate on the other more interesting patients..

You see that is the problem, right there, with General Practice. GPs **have** to deal with all the endless repetition of the viral hoards while keeping a high index of suspicion for the occasional genuinely seriously ill patient. It's not easy BUT THAT IS THE JOB. It is often very hard to stay interested, friendly and alert in interminably repetitive surgeries so no wonder some clever GPs would rather have a nurse practitioner, an algorithm and a questionable blood test take their place and no wonder the patients can see through their little game.

Cystic Fibrosis:

It is possible that Cystic Fibrosis persists because the Heterozgous state confers some protection against infections of various kinds. It was once postulated that Typhoid infection was less likely in this situation. See Paediatrics.

Asbestos:

3000 deaths a year in Britain – Lung cancer, cancer of the pleural lining – Mesothelioma, and Asbestosis (the scarring of parenchymal lung tissue). A pernicious and untreatable set of conditions. The straight (Amphibole) asbestos fibres are inert and cause a marked inflammatory and fibrotic reaction with much lung damage and scarring.

There are various types of asbestos. Chrysotile (serpentine or curved fibred) white asbestos still in use at the end of the 90s, is slightly less carcinogenic than the long straight (Amphibole) fibres of Amosite or Brown asbestos or Crocidolite, (Blue) asbestos. Asbestosis occurs with all types of asbestos but it is much less likely to occur in the future due to today's exposure limits.

Chrysotile is less likely than Amphiboles to cause mesolthelioma. There is also an Amphibole preponderance in asbestos related lung cancers.

NOTE: **The RESPIRABLE PARTICLE SIZE:** (Important in places of work and in therapy of inhaled dry powders) is probably about 5um (microns). Some authorities use 10 microns as the boundary. "Dust" is from size 1 micron – 1mm, anything larger is grit and too big to stay suspended in the air! The size determines how far down the respiratory tract the various atmospheric contaminants will travel.

To compare:
Mould spores are 1-100 um
Pollen is 10-100 um
House dust mite allergens are 0.1-10 um
Viruses are <0.01-0.1 um
Tobacco smoke is 0.01-1 um
Bacteria are <1-10 um

Flying:

The cabin pressure of commercial aircraft is set at 2000-2500m height. Here water boils at 93 degrees C. That is why you don't get proper coffee or tea in planes.
Mt Blanc is 4807m,
Everest 8848m.

Lung Cancer: (see cancer):

Is the commonest cause of cancer death. It kills more in the UK (still) than breast, bowel and prostate cancers. The totals for 2010 were 34,859 (19,410 (56%) men and 15,449 (44%) women). But in comparison there are 900,000 COPD sufferers.

Carbon Monoxide Poisoning:

Headache is the commonest symptom but very many others – nausea, drowsiness, dyspnoea, abdominal symptoms, chest etc. pain will vary with place. Migraine, depression. Shared symptoms with other family members.

Ask whether new double glazing has been fitted, a new gas appliance, are the gas appliances all serviced? Soot stains around appliances or increased condensation, yellow rather than blue flames, exhaust exposure at work or in their own car.

Diagnosis can be made via breath test for exhaled CO or COHb (heparinised venous sample) but CO has a 6hr half life.

If worried contact the Local Health Protection Unit. Make sure the suspect appliances are turned off and windows are all opened before permitting exposure. Tell them to get a meter.

I had a whole family brought in dead except for one severely brain damaged child one winter in the 1970's while I was a Paediatric SHO. They all had the cherry red lip discolouration and the diagnosis was obvious. Their gas boiler had never been serviced.

36: Sex and Sexually Transmitted Infections:

Sex:

No child under 13 can consent to sex and legally, sexual intercourse at or below this age is considered rape. A "competent" 13 year old can however consent to an (intimate) physical examination and to treatment irrespective of its parents' wishes so you might want to discuss with a colleague what is in a child's best interests as the law in this area has done what it always does. Passes the buck and sits back waiting to apportion blame. There aren't many, but this is one area where, should you need to perform a personal examination, it would probably be appropriate to have a nurse as a chaperone.

As many as one in six children are said to suffer sexual abuse from an adult (usually someone they know) although other estimates vary. In 2016 a campaign group put the incidence at 1:10 girls and another web site said one in six boys. Another reported 1 in 6 boys and 1 in 4 girls before the age of 18 had suffered some form of sexual abuse.

Sexual abuse is a broad term and includes physical contact and even non touching abuse. For instance:

Touching a child's genitals for sexual pleasure,

making a child touch someone else's genitals, play sexual games or have sex putting objects or body parts inside the vagina, in the mouth or in the anus of a child for sexual pleasure,

showing pornography to a child,

deliberately exposing an adult's genitals to a child,

photographing a child in sexual poses,

encouraging a child to watch or hear sexual acts,

inappropriately watching a child undress or use the bathroom.

The National Child Abuse and Neglect Data System (NCANDS) has surprisingly, reflected a true decline in prevalence since the 1990's.

If a child comes to you requesting contraception and she is not yet thirteen then obviously she is thinking about having intercourse, planning for it, trying to avoid at least some of its consequences – so you could argue – is that girl willingly planning her own rape? On the other hand, is she worldly wise enough to know what she is letting herself in for and by the time she changes her mind will things have gone beyond her control? Is this where you as a parent substitute (half the time) and a moral guide (?) take the opportunity to clarify what she really wants? Is that how you see the role of a GP?

What about the learning disabled girl who functions at a 9 or 10 year intellectual level but is a chronological teenager and on the pill because of heavy periods or is in an arranged marriage ? You know she has an older "boyfriend" or husband who comes with her to consultations and that he is using her for sex, something you judge her unfit to fully understand. Perhaps there are sensitive cultural issues involved. Would you call in social services? Life as a GP is complicated. Where is the line between social responsibility and meddling interference?

What about the lonely, emotionally disturbed child in the dysfunctional family who behaves in a sexually precocious way and appears far more mature than you judge her to really be?

These are situations like dozens of others where you will have to make snap decisions based on what you perceive to be the patient's best interests, without moralising, making personal judgements and with almost no real information. Decisions and situations you may well be called upon to justify to the patients' irate relatives (and this applies whether you agree and condone questionable sexual relationships or refuse and put the child at risk of possible abuse and unwanted pregnancy). This is something no judge has ever had to do, – make a real time decision in 10 minutes with real life people and real life consequences with almost no evidence. In short, to take intelligent risks with serious implications at crucial times in people's lives on the evidence of little more than a history from a child.

Homosexual men make up 1.5 – 6% of the male population depending on the source you believe.

Some sources say the Gay Gene is XQ28. Many people believe that homosexual behaviour is not all genetic but powerfully influenced by the relative quality of relationships with each parent growing up and the type of sexual role models you receive in your formative adolescent years.

70 year old men have sex 4X a month on average.

A recent survey of sexual behaviour – The National Survey of Sexual Attitudes and Lifestyles was published in 2013. (NATSAL).

Previous surveys were carried out in 1990-91 and 1999-2001. Various changes in behaviour and attitudes were charted.

The main changes are in the number of sexual partners that women have, the younger age at onset of sexual activity, the later age that sex continues. It is now well into the 70's that people continue having sex and almost a third of 16 year olds are having or have had sex. There is a reduced frequency of sex, a growing intolerance of infidelity but growing acceptance of same sex relationships.

There is still a high risk of HPV and chlamydia suggesting that barrier methods are not being widely used (and adding further support to those that demand an end to sexism in HPV vaccination) but HIV and Gonorrhoea are "restricted to those with high risk factors".

1:6 pregnancies are unplanned. 1:60 women in the UK have an unplanned pregnancy in any year.

"Four out of ten" men and women have "had a recent sexual problem". Lack of interest in sex affected 15% of men but women were twice as likely to report this "as an issue".

10% of women and 1:70 men reported sex against their will although this was not defined as rape in a radio interview with one of the main research coordinators. Fewer than half of either sex had mentioned their "Non volitional" sex to anyone and only 13% women and 8% men had reported it to the police.

Some changes over the years: Same sex experience:

		1990-91	1999-2001	2010-2012
Male	Any same sex experience	6%	8%	7%
	Involving genital contact	4%	5%	5%
Female	Any same sex experience	4%	10%	16%
	Involving genital contact	2%	5%	8%

Percentage who had had sexual intercourse with someone of the opposite sex before age 16:

Male	Age at interview	Female
31%	16-24	29%
26%	25-34	25%
27%	35-44	18%
27%	45-54	15%
17%	55-64	10%
15%	65-74	4%

Average number of sexual partners:	Male	Female
1990-91	8.6	3.7
1999-2001	12.6	6.5
2010-2012	11.7	7.7

Other statistics:

70% of 16-24 year olds had given or received oral sex in the last year (same for males and females). The figure for 65-74 year olds was 30% men and 20% women. 18% of both males and females had been involved in anal sex in the previous year and a quarter of both men and women do not share the same level of interest in sex as their partner.

There was a clear relationship between the number of partners and the risk of STD infections.

Given this information, – the frequency of unwanted and unexpected pregnancies, of STDs related to unprotected sex and the greater number of sexual contacts, the "serious" STDS being the result of higher risk taking behaviour, the nearly 1/5 of men and women having anal intercourse, the almost a third who have had sex below the age of 16, you have to wonder whether our current national regime of sexual education and family planning is having any influence at all on the behaviour of young (and not so young) people in our society. Is it time to rethink the availability and influence of the endless sexual propaganda in films, pop songs, lyrics, videos and on television? What is the difference between societies where teenage pregnancy is low and where, like the UK, it is high? Is it the strength and influence of "The Family"? The 2014 figures made us the 4th worst in the 15-19 year old European age group – **better than just Bulgaria, Romania and Slovakia**. With 20 live births/1000 women in the age group we are 4x worse than Denmark, Slovenia, Netherlands, and Sweden. We are 25th in the European 28. What makes the UK so sexually irresponsible?

4 out of 5 women between 15 and 44 in the UK use some form of contraception. We had 48,000 pregnancies in 2012 – 3 out of every 100 girls between 15 and 19 years in the UK give birth annually. In France the rate was 0.9. In Germany 1.1 and Japan 0.4. So whatever the cause, it isn't through ignorance about contraception. 7 out of 10 UK girls know that the morning after pill works *after* 24 hours so the endless mantra that **we need more education is not true**. A survey by The Prince's Trust suggested that many teenage girls **assume pregnancy offers financial benefits** and separate council accommodation and this is a way of escaping their parents' home and their boring and hopeless existence. It seems likely that the only real way then to address this meaningfully is for councils not to re-house single parents but to provide them with long term supported but managed accommodation – such as a room in a social service run hostel. Here the

well being of both mother and baby could be supervised but social, sexual and personal freedoms restricted. Too illiberal? But aren't we at the bottom of the sexual, pregnancy and family cohesion league tables because of decades of liberal and generous social and medical policies? We have had 40 years of sex education, free family planning, all confidential, given the weight of law so that even children can access it, everywhere, at almost any hour, multiple contraceptive alternatives, education about reproduction and loss of any residual innocence at a younger and younger age, over the counter morning after pills, condoms in pub toilets, free terminations, – **200,000 a year of them to all comers**, making the original intention of the abortion act a bit of a farce and we are still fourth from bottom in the league tables. One of only 3 rich nations with a teenage pregnancy rate of >30/1000. We have one of the highest alcohol abuse rates by young people and children and our children are far less happy than those in The Netherlands, Norway, Iceland, Finland, Sweden, Germany etc (Though they **are** happier than the US, Spain, Italy Austria, and Canada apparently (2016).)

And we are in the bottom third of the infant mortality league tables, – all in all, a pretty unimpressive set of statistics to show for four decades of state tolerance, understanding, largess and the NHS.

Perhaps after all the endless contraception carrots we need to try the pregnancy "you are stuck with the consequences of your behaviour" stick now?

While we are in the general area of "morality" – this and taking a stance on it is something that modern GPs, of course, fall over themselves to avoid. 40-50 years ago we were not so mealy mouthed about what was good for patients. Regulating authorities believe that even the consideration of the concept of judgement or of right and wrong is now irrelevant to our job. When I qualified 40 years ago we were far more judgemental, I assure you. AND it might be worth remembering something: If you think child welfare is an important issue, remember that one half of unmarried, co – habiting couples split up before their child is 5 years old. The figure for married couples is 1 in 12. Should this fact influence us when we are requested by two people who happen to be living together and sharing a bed and want to be referred for infertility treatment – or is it **really** none of our business? (Mail online Nov 27 2013.) Most CCGs restrict secondary services on the basis of cost, some are restricting treatments on grounds of obesity, smoking and other sabotaging factors. Drug treatments are effectively rationed on a cost basis, even life saving anti cancer drugs have their cost effectiveness reviewed by NICE. It seems a given that co-habiting couples offer a bad long term financial investment.

Sexual Infection:

Although Gonorrhoea and HIV AIDs are said to be "largely restricted" to the "at risk communities" the huge increase in oral sex (given Michael Douglas' very public confession of his misdiagnosed throat cancer and its likely cause) will almost certainly become more common and spread to involve large numbers of non drug abusing, heterosexual adults who's only risk factors had been several sexual partners and a taste for oral sex.

In 2003 a House of Commons Select Committee described the sexual health situation in the UK as a "Public Health Emergency". Between 2008 and 2010 there were 420,000 new diagnoses.

The commonest "GP STIs" are Chlamydia, Gonorrhoea, Genital Warts, Genital Herpes and Trichomonas.

Chlamydia:

Between age 16 and 24 1:10 young people have Chlamydia. A shocking statistic for anyone with teenage children. The end result can be salpingitis, tubal obstruction, ectopic pregnancy and infertility in women and girls as well as urethritis, epididymitis and sterility in young men. It also assists the transmission of HIV.

Treatments include:

Azithromycin 1gr stat (>95% effective) said to be safe in pregnancy,

Doxycycline 100mg BD 7days (>95% effective),

Erythromycin 500mg qds 7 days (77-95% effective),

Ofloxacin 400mg OD 7 days (95% effective).

The "Target Chlamydia" initiative

-For the 16-25 year olds, despite irresponsible older "I don't need a condom" age groups being a rapidly growing set of STD generations. It consists of a postal male urine and female HVS swab service. The result is within a few days and very reliable.

Target Chlamydia is the government's screening campaign for young people, providing swabs for girls and urine specimen pots for boys. These are included with freepost and packaging and the patient is phoned or texted with their result with a few days. Generally it works very well. It has found a staggering 8% of the young people who did the test to be positive.

Chlamydia can be transmitted by oral as well as conventional sex. It can infect the rectum as well. The trouble is that 70% of infected women and 50% of infected men have no symptoms.

The symptoms when present are dysuria, urethral or vaginal discharge, pelvic inflammatory disease, epididymo-orchitis, rectal discharge or bleeding, irregular vaginal bleeding. 2% develop arthritis.

Investigations are a first catch urine in men and a vulvo vaginal or endocervical swab in women. Symptomatic women should be tested for Gonorrhoea too.

There is a 10% risk of infertility in women after the first infection, 20% after the second, 40% after the third. Don't forget Opthalmia Neonatorum and pneumonia in the babies of infected mothers – so a test for cure after treatment is essential in pregnancy.

Gonorrhoea:

Neisseria Gonorrhoeae is the second commonest STD in the UK. Commoner in homosexuals and in black ethnic groups. The complications are epididymitis, prostatitis, P.I.D. and "Disseminated Gonococcal Infection". A Co-infection with Chlamydia is common.

Treatment: **Ceftriaxone 500mg IM and Azithromycin 1gr stat – 99% effective** * Or Cefixime 400mg stat plus Azithromycin 1gr stat. Make sure you contact-trace as many partners as you can. An outbreak of Azithromycin-resistant gonorrhoea in mid 2015 changed this standard treatment advice. These cases were in Leeds, Oldham, Macclesfield and Scunthorpe. The organism was still treatable with second and third line (microbiologist guided) antibiotics.

*This was available by booking at "Superdrug" in 2016 for £45.00 – although they mention that 30-40% of women with gonorrhoea have chlamydia as well, the dual treatment, swabs and sensitivities did not seem to be mentioned as part of the service in their accompanying literature.

Between 2000 and 2011 GPs diagnosed Chlamydia in 193,000 patients and Gonorrhoea in 17,000.

(These were 9-16% cases of all Chlamydia cases and 6-9% of all English Gonorrhoea cases.) In terms of incidence, there was a significant increase over this period from 22.8/100,000 in 2000 to 29.3/100,000 in 2011. The proportion treated by GPs rose from 60% to 80%. In contrast, the number of Gonorrhoea cases varied between 3.2 >2.4/100,000 and the number treated by GPs ranged from 33% to 54%. National guidance is that patients with Gonorrhoea be referred to specialist centres for resistance testing but many GPs were still using relatively ineffective Ciprofloxacin, in 2011.

It became clear in July 2017 that New Zealand patients previously immunised (2004-2006) against Meningococcal meningitis had some cross resistance (31%) to that other Neisseria organism, Gonorrhoea. This is the first partially effective Gonorrhoeal vaccine.

Syphilis:

Treponema Pallidum. High rates in "men who have sex with men". Four stages: Primary, secondary, latent and tertiary. From 9 to 90 day IP. A painless primary chancre (genital or anal). Secondary Syphilis 4-8 weeks later. Flu like symptoms, diffuse rash, lymphadenopathy, general malaise. Long term neurological and cardiovascular complications as well as the skin granulomata, and the gummata (tertiary).

Treatment: Penicillin followed by a VDRL to check effectiveness. Alternatively Ceftriaxone, Doxycycline or Azithromycin.

Genital warts:

Caused by the human Papilloma virus of which there are more than 100 genotypes. Some (16 and 18) have the greatest neoplastic risk.

Treatment: Cryotherapy, Podophyllotoxin 0.15% cream (Warticon, recurrence 50-80%), or solution – both C/I in pregnancy. Imiquimod 5% cream (Aldara, recurrence 50-60%) or excision.

Genital Herpes:

HSV types 1 and 2, like other STDs, increases the risk of HIV transmission. Primary attacks can be very painful, recurrent attacks can be asymptomatic. Topical Instillagel (Lidocaine 2%) helps. Valaciclovir works quickly (primary attacks respond quicker) and the three effective oral antivirals are Aciclovir 200mg 5x daily for 5 days, Famciclovir 250mg TDS 5 days, Valaciclovir 500mg BD 5 days. Suppressive treatment (daily antivirals for up to a year) may be appropriate in frequent attacks. (eg >6 episodes a year).

HIV/Aids:

Human immunodeficiency virus. A retro virus generally spread during the exchange of body fluids, causing immune damage and a variety of neoplastic diseases. Macrophages, dendritic cells, "CD4+" TCells (Helper T cells) and other immune cells are invaded and damaged, reducing cell mediated immunity. After infection the viral RNA genome is copied once, migrates to the cell nucleus where it can lie dormant or be copied into new viral RNA. Then new HIV virions are finally assembled at the cell membrane. Two specific sub types of HIV exist, the common, worldwide more virulent HIV – 1 and the less infectious HIV-2, restricted to Africa.

The HIV virus was first described in homosexual men and drug abusers in the early 80's in the US but sporadic cases probably presented as early as the 50's. Relatively unusual infections including Pneumocystis Carinii and tumours – Kaposi's sarcoma were found to be more common in these groups. 25% of infected patients do not know they have the infection. It takes up to 3m for antibodies to appear after infection occurs. – So it is sensible to delay doing blood tests immediately after presumed contact.

In 2010 70% HIV patients were male, 54% white, 33% Afro Caribbean, 12% "Not stated".

46% had acquired the infection by being "MSM" (men who have sex with men"- presumably code for homosexual). A WHO report in 2014 stated that men who have sex with men are 19 times more likely to have HIV than the general population. 46% were heterosexual, 8% not stated (? IV drug abusers?).

5% had been tested at A/N clinics, 54% at GUM clinics, 10% by GPs, 15% as in-patients or during acute admissions, 7% in OP.

In the UK in 2014, the year with the most recent available statistics, 6,100 people were diagnosed with HIV, 40% late, after they should have started treatment.

1 in 20 of all UK men who have sex with other men has HIV.

3,360 MSM were diagnosed with HIV in 2014, the highest level yet.

MSM are 55% of people diagnosed with HIV.

Black African people are 1.8% of the UK population but 29% of those with HIV.

There were 2,650 Black Caribbean people in the UK with HIV in 2014.

Those patients over 55 years make up 15% of the total.

(National AIDS Trust).

Trichomonas vaginalis

Commonly co exists as a me-too STD. Like many other STDs it is associated with HIV transmission and its presence should trigger a full STD screen. It can cause premature labour and even low birth weight in babies of women sufferers, prostatitis in men.

The treatment is metronidazole (2gr single dose, avoid this regime in pregnancy) or 400mg BD 7 days (OK in pregnancy). Tinidazole can be used (2 gr stat) in metronidazole treatment failure.

Gardenerella Vaginalis

(Fish odour) is one of the bacterial vaginoses characterised by Clue Cells on microscopy.

Bacterial vaginosis

in pregnant women may indicate iron deficiency. In fact it has also been shown to be partially caused by psychological stress. It is associated with a relatively alkaline pH of the vagina (higher than 4.5) and on microscopy the presence of Clue Cells. By definition, Candida (fungal) and Trichomonas (protozoan) are not bacterial vaginoses.

The discharge is thin and yellowy, fishy smelling, >pH 4.5 with Clue Cells on microscopy.

Gardenerella or organisms called Mobiluncus are the usual infecting agents.

Just like Trichomonas, it can cause increased risk of HIV infection, premature labour etc.

Treatment is Metronidazole or Clindamycin orally or topically. The treatment of partners of affected women **is not** now considered essential.

Non gonococcal urethritis: (NGU, NSU etc)

Usually due to Chlamydia. 80,000 cases a year in the UK. Chlamydia cause up to 40% but other organisms include Mycoplasma genitalium, Ureaplasma urealyticum, Trichomonas, UTI, Neisseria Meningitidis (!), H.Simplex, Adenoviruses, Thrush, etc.

If a first catch urine (FCU) is Pos 3+ Leucocyte Esterase on dipstix then treatment is indicated – Ofloxacin 200mg BD 7 days (treats UTI and NGU) alternatively treat as for Chlamydial urethritis alone with Azithromycin 1gr stat or Doxycycline 100mg BD 1 week.

In June 2015 a "Sharp rise in syphilis and gonorrhoea" was reported by Public Health England. They said a major rise in the numbers of these two STDs were due to men who had sex with men and the numbers had gone up by nearly half in the case of syphilis (2375>3477) and a third in the case of gonorrhoea (13,629>18,029) in 2013-4.

Annual data showed 440,000 STDs reported overall, a small (0.3%) drop in the total. Chlamydia was the commonest infection, making up nearly half the cases (206,000) followed by genital warts (70,000). The authors wrote that the increases in gonorrhoea and syphilis were mainly due to condomless sex in HIV positive men. "we are particularly concerned about the large rise in diagnoses in gay men" said the head of STI surveillance at Public Health England. She also noted how gonorrhoea was becoming more difficult to treat because of antibiotic resistance. They recommended three monthly STI screening of homosexuals not using condoms and involved in casual sex. They also recommend that sexually active young people should be screened for Chlamydia annually and on changing partners. Now how on earth are they going to organise that?

37: Sleep: (and see paediatrics)

"When people see you lying down with your eyes closed they ask are you asleep? "No I'm training to die"

– James Haarsma (?)

"Sleep that knits up the ravelled sleeve of care (Macbeth). Not poppy, nor mandragora*, nor all the drowsy syrups of the world shall ever medicine thee to that sweet sleep which thou owedst yesterday (Othello). To die, to sleep, to sleep perchance to dream: Ay there's the rub. For in that sleep of death – what dreams may come?"

– Hamlet

*Mandrake extract has been used medicinally over the centuries for a variety of purposes. Containing many alkaloids, including Atropine, Hyoscine etc it can be poisonous but has been used as a sedative.

The diurnal cycle is complex and functions via the integrated working of environmental light, the retina, the suprachiasmic nucleus, which controls various hormone and bioneurological pathways, temperature control, activating systems and melatonin. Melatonin released from the pineal, via the action of the SCN, regulates sleep and has a multitude of other bodily effects. Bright light, even artificial light, inhibits pineal melatonin release and this is why shift workers suffer a number of adverse effects from low melatonin levels. These include increased rates of various cancers. See below**

We spend about a third of our lives asleep. It was once said that sleep's only purpose was to be a cure for sleeplessness but given how much time vertebrates waste doing it and how vulnerable it makes us to predators, it must have some completely irreplaceable and vital survival roles. Otherwise we would have worked out how to do them all while we were awake. Sleep then, a bit more than just "training to die".

In recent years the true value of sleep and the harm caused by its deprivation have become more of a contentious area than ever to doctors and other employees. (See first two chapters.) These issues came to the fore particularly during the junior doctors' strike in 2015-16. This was an industrial campaign in the NHS partly regarding night duties and extending normal working back to seven days a week. – Many of the striking doctors used the perceived risks of long hours, sleeplessness and shift work on the health of workers as a justification for not wanting to return to a 24 hour, 7 day NHS. They said that tired doctors made more mistakes. In fact several conflicting papers are available that fail to clarify the argument regarding sleep and decision making in doctors. Some studies show that sleep deprivation results in poorer decision making, but some definitely do not*.

*Postgrad Med J 2002 78:85-87 (SHOs performed better than house officers and length of continuous sleep not related to appropriateness of confidence-junior doctors: "Can still monitor their performance and retain insight into their own ability when sleep deprived" etc.etc.

Is it better to have no doctor or a tired doctor? How much of your day to day work do you do on "Autopilot?" This 'how much sleep is essential?' is a serious question. Restricting the hours of young doctors to 48 a week has meant less experience, less competence, cumulatively less skill and proposed even longer consultant training. I clearly remember falling asleep standing at the side of an incubator while preparing to put up a drip on a 26 week neonate. This was after 60 hours of continuous work on SCBU punctuated by two hours sleep one Sunday evening in the 80's. It was during a weekend between two hectic one in 3 working weeks. (1 in 2-3 rotas could be up to 140 hours a week and weekends of 80 hours of continuous duty.) But the nurse woke me and I then got the drip in first time as I had done a hundred such procedures before and could almost literally do them "in my sleep".

While I was writing this and feeling rather guilty about accusing my contemporary colleagues of a lack of personal and professional determination ("emotional resilience" to quote the GMC) and listening to the "Not safe, Not fair" refrain of the strikers on TV, I was surprised at something that started happening. This was the number of self employed workers, professional patients and friends who I met who volunteered in passing that a 12 hour day, a 48 hour week and a starting GP salary of 100K with immediate parity was something most professionals looked at with green envy. And anyway most young professionals work far more hours than that at the start of their career and doing without sleep when you are young whether through working your way up a greasy pole or surviving young children was what every young person did every-where. – And that the junior doctors were symptomatic of a wider malaise in today's society that seems to assume good things should come to us all without self sacrifice. The Working Time Directive today limits the working week (dynamised) to 48 hours, *one third* of the one in two rotas done by the author and his peer group for decades after qualifying. This has now led to clinical discontinuity, poor or sometimes no proper hand over, reduced competence, poorer training and poor experience – which is as worrying or worse for patients than those of tired doctors a few decades ago. This is because the end result is less safe doctors due to inexperience rather than tiredness. Which doctor is the safer? What is worse, I believe that the new family friendly and predictable office hours rotas have also produced something surreptitious and harmful in the attitude of many young doctors. This is an unwillingness to put themselves out and stay late to learn something new, to see a new type of case, or to be inconvenienced by staying for an unusual condition or to visit a dying patient they know at home or do all the standard extra duties which were part of our open ended apprenticeships a few decades ago. If it means being home late. Anyway back to the subject of Sleep:

It is clear that sleep deprivation **can** cause depression and anxiety in some individuals as well as triggering mental health disorders in those with an inherent tendency to mental illness. Time off for mental illness, stress and depression are far commoner in junior doctors today than ever before, despite the at least halving of their duty hours. So there must be **personal susceptibility factors involved** (see "Emotional Resilience" in other chapters) and the morale, attitudes and toughness of doctors in the last two to three decades **have** changed dramatically. I believe this is due to current medical school selection processes. The typical medical student is now young, female, highly intelligent, disproportionately from an ethnic minority background, privately educated or highly coached, ambitious and focussed on a medical career for a long time. Initially very optimistic but without life experience and with a naive idea of the personal stresses and unpleasantness inherent in a medical career. Panglossian indeed. What medicine really needs are not these intel-lectual, emotionally vulnerable, Asperger Spectrum, naive, over supported and protected individuals but thick skinned, optimistic, communicative but tough cynics and in my day, cynics who could smile and function for three days with almost no sleep. And probably *young men* who prioritise their jobs at the start of their careers. I doubt that there are any newly qualified doctors who would be capable of working the rotas we did in the 70's and 80's. (See "Who are we?")

But lack of sleep is only a small part of the challenges of a medical career. Why do we need all this sleep?

We now know that restorative sleep is needed for the function of the immune system, proper hormone balance, emotional and psychiatric health, the laying down of memory and learning and through altered blood flow to enable waste products and toxins to be cleared from the brain.

Every psychiatric condition is associated with and exacerbated by insomnia and abnormal sleep patterns. Classically, depression can present with early morning waking but then so can anxiety and hypomania. Schizophrenia may result in insomnia or excessive sleeping. Sleep disturbances (disruption in the normal circadian rhythm) can predict and induce manic episodes in Bipolar Disorder. Insomnia is said to be the commonest reported "mental health complaint" and results in sleepiness, poor concentration, memory loss, depression, fatigue, immune depression and loss of energy during the daylight hours.

It isn't just mental conditions that disturb sleep: Many physical illnesses directly affect sleep: Any condition which causes difficulty breathing, intermittent pain or an awareness of a bodily function – OSA, (Obstructive Sleep Apnoea), sore throat, quinsy, croup, asthma, COPD, LVF, CCF, palpitations, crescendo angina, ascites, pregnancy, physical pain or discomfort – terminal illness, arthritis, BPH, various chronic conditions and disabilities may all affect our ability to sleep comfortably or cause us to wake early.

Immunity:

In a 2003 study, a group of American students were given Hep A vaccine and half were prevented from sleeping the night of the immunisation. The antibody response at 4 weeks was 97% greater in the group which was allowed to sleep normally.

In another study the standard three doses of Hep B were given and average sleep recorded each night in the week after the first immunisation. Then the antibody levels after the second dose were checked and it was found that the antibody levels increased 56% for every extra hour of sleep in that first week. After the third and final dose, those who had had less than 6 hours of sleep a night back in the first week after the primary dose were seven times more likely to have insignificant antibodies.

Hormones:

In a studies looking at the effect of insulin and sleep deprivation it has been found that in healthy young men given only 4 hours of sleep a night for 5 nights, their endogenous insulin was 40% less effective at reducing blood sugar. Also in sleep deprivation studies, Ghrelin, an appetite stimulating hormone increases 28% and Leptin which limits hunger, decreases. Dozens of studies have subsequently confirmed the effect of sleep deprivation causing weight gain. Children from 6 to 9 years of age who get less than 10 hours of sleep are twice as likely to be obese. Adults who get less than 6 hours sleep are 50% more likely to be obese. Shift workers eat more at night and metabolise sugar less well. They also tend to snack rather than eat healthily, as I certainly did if I could find biscuits or chocolates on the wards at night or fast food, chocolate and fizzy drinks machines in the corridors in the early hours. Comfort eating I suppose.

Memory and Depression:

Various studies have shown how important sleep is for the laying down of memories.

Sleep deprivation however seems to selectively reduce our ability to lay down positive or neutral memories. We continue to remember negative events though. Perhaps this is why sleep deprivation leads to depression.

Taking Hypnotics adversely affects the laying down of memories:

In one recent study, the taking of either of two different Z drugs on retiring negatively affected declarative and procedural memory the following day. If the drug were taken in the middle of the night however, it had no effect. So don't cram the night before an exam, get over tired and take a sleeping pill. You won't remember a thing you learnt the day before.

Many studies on sleep apnoea, which does of course lead to sleep deprivation, have shown a strong association with depression. It too negatively affects memory. Men and women with sleep apnoea are 2.4 and 5.2 x more likely to have major depression. CPAP, by the way, reduces depression by a quarter in sleep apnoea.

Treatment of apnoea in children with ADHD symptoms improves their hyperactivity symptoms more than standard medication.

During sleep the brain processes information and consolidates memory which helps us to learn and function normally when we wake. It strengthens, tidies and organises memories, helping us with new insights and creative ideas.

Animals use sleep in different ways: dolphins sleep using one half of their brain at a time. Hibernating animals stop hibernating to sleep, then wake in order to re-hibernate (which is not the same process as sleep). Dolphins, ducks and Frigate birds use unihemispheric slow wave sleep, keeping one eye open at a time and allowing half the brain to sleep. The dolphin carries on swimming. The Frigate bird, thanks to research with a tiny portable 10 day Max Plank Institute EEG, can fly nonstop for 10 days and during this marathon from the Galapagos Islands they were found to be able to go to sleep completely and fly with both hemispheres switched off. They even had brief periods of REM sleep when their heads drooped while flying but they didn't fall out of the sky!

Cleansing the brain:

Finally, the space between brain cells gets bigger during sleep and injected beta amyloid is cleared at twice the rate during sleep as it is while awake. Research is taking place as to whether the increased clearance is restricted in patients with Alzheimer's. Do people who get Alzheimer's sleep differently to those who don't? There is some research that suggests that long term taking of drugs with sedative side effects (antihistamines, anticholinergics, benzodiazepines, hypnotics) may increase the risk of Alzheimer's.

The sleep pattern:

New born babies have no circadian rhythm but sleep several times a day. The circadian rhythm in adults is controlled by the suprachiasmatic nucleus (which is light sensitive) producing Melatonin (See above).

Sleeping Pills:

Insomnia is, apparently, the third most common reason that Americans see their doctors (after colds and headaches). About one third of patients will complain of significant regular sleep disturbance if you ask them and given that Nicotine, (and Nicotine withdrawal), caffeine and alcohol all adversely affect sleep, this is not surprising.

The commonest sleep disorders are "insomnia", sleep apnoea, restless leg syndrome and narcolepsy.

Although alcohol enhances the ability to initiate sleep it also disrupts the normal sleep pattern a few hours later. Early morning waking is a common symptom not just of depression but of drinking too much the previous evening too. Alcohol disrupts non REM stage 3 sleep as well as REM sleep and these are "restorative" sleep stages. Alcohol also increases nocturnal disturbance via urination and upper airway obstruction, snoring and obstructive apnoea.

Various other medications may adversely affect sleep and these include SSRIs, (which may cause restless legs, insomnia, poor sleep quality), TCAs, steroids, statins (vivid dreams), decongestants and vasoconstrictors via stimulant effects, ACEIs, (via cough), CCBs (Itchy legs) etc.

People at all ages consult about sleeplessness and parents ask regularly about their sleepless children. They all deserve a sympathetic hearing and a decent history to exclude the rare physical cause but then the conversation inevitably moves on to whether or not it is reasonable to prescribe something to help the patient sleep. This is where you ask about their own preconceptions, lay down a few rules and limits and discuss all the alternatives to a pharmacological sleep (see below).

No one in their right mind would use Laudanum or anything like it nowadays – which is Opium mixture and was available from many retail outlets OTC until 1868 and then freely available from chemists. It was taken regularly in Victorian England for sleep and various other reasons. Many Victorian artists and their muses were addicted to it – Coleridge, Byron's daughter, (Ada Lovelace), Elizabeth Siddal (Ophelia in the famous Millais painting), D.G. Rossetti and probably Wilkie Collins who wrote the first detective novel, "The Moonstone". This is partly based on a Laudanum fugue state induced in its lead character by a mischievous GP ostensibly treating Nicotine withdrawal! It was even given to babies with colic and irregular sleep patterns. None of us would prescribe Barbiturates either, which were routinely used earlier in the 20th century to promote sleep in insomniac patients. Barbiturates were the overdose cause of "accidental" death in many famous people of the last several decades including, Marilyn Monroe, Judy Garland, Jimi Hendrix, Kenneth Williams, Tony Hancock and the visionary folk singer Nick Drake. They have a very narrow therapeutic range. The sedative side effects of benzodiazepines, Benadryl and other antihistamines, Sinemet, Pramipexole, tricyclic antidepressants, Depakote (Valproic Acid) and other anticonvulsants have all been used to help patients go to and stay asleep. All via their sedative and central side effects.

There are various OTC preparations today: For instance, Nytol is Diphenhydramine and is a sedative OTC antihistamine. In any given individual, it either works or it doesn't. Many will have tried it before seeing you and it turns out that it may be a contributory factor in some cases of dementia in the chronic user. Other drugs implicated include Benadryl, (Acrivastine), Piriton, (Chlorphen(ir) amine) and so on.

There are also many herbal preparations said to promote sleep: Lavender and Sandalwood oils, Chamomile, Valerian, cherry concentrate, magnesium oil, rescue remedy, lemon balm etc. Most of them at least smell nice. Kiwi fruit contains serotonin and promotes sleep.

The disturbed sleep caused by many Beta Blockers (including vivid dreams) is counteracted by Melatonin by the way.

**Indeed, Melatonin is a fascinating substance, – produced by the Pineal Gland, regulating the body's circadian rhythms, it is anti oxidant, protecting DNA and therefore having anti cancer properties. Secreted at night, it has been discovered that for instance, blind women have a lower incidence of breast cancer – presumably because they secrete more. It is supposed to lower the rate of all cancers when supplemented orally.

Shift work is suspected to increase the risk of cancer development (WHO 2007) and working in artificial light lowers melatonin levels – by interfering with normal circadian rhythms? Long haul air travel increases breast cancer in air hostesses, night shift work triples prostate cancer in men, increases bladder cancer, it doubles the rate of bowel cancer and increases lung cancer by 79% (Night shift working and higher risk of cancer in men: Univ Quebec, Cancer Active). Blue light exposure to the retina suppresses melatonin secretion with all the theoretical disadvantages that may accrue. Melatonin is a powerful antioxidant, protecting against Parkinson's disease, aging, cancers, dementia, SAD and arrhythmias. The level of Melatonin is lower in patients with Autism and giving Melatonin (it is an effective re-synchroniser of the body clock in jet lag) can cause vivid dreams. (Although this has not been my experience).

It would be quite natural if you had a degree of scepticism about such a jack-of-all-trades hormone but it does seem to work in some sleep disorders, especially those associated with ADHD, Jet Lag and shift work and its use in cancer seems at worst harmless and at best promising.

Many doctors have reservations about prescribing nocturnal sedatives for patients as these tend to become repeat prescriptions very readily. Chronic, regular poor sleep however is a cause of, or associated with depression, suicide, aggressive and impulsive behaviour, poor memory, poor work performance, poor concentration and bad executive decision making. So insomnia from whatever cause may affect all areas of a patient's life, health and performance and lead to long term and complicated negative consequences. I remember doing locum GP sessions in inner city practices thirty years ago where elderly patients I saw were regularly kept awake by neighbour's loud music and parties. Sometimes night after night and all night. Occasionally, after a few months, the temporary neighbours would be moved on by the council to be replaced others, just as bad or worse. Apart from the obvious advice and help with phoning Environmental Health, a month's supply of hypnotics were sometimes what kept that old person sane and the only real practical help I could give.

I have to admit I have a lower threshold than some GPs for prescribing nocturnal sedatives to patients I know and trust. I understand that some jobs and therefore some lives can be punctuated by regular periods of stress and insomnia and the tricyclics (Amitriptyline or Dosulepin) favoured by some colleagues may not be appropriate short term remedies.

As long as I am sure the insomnia is not a symptom of depression or physical illness, I would be happy to offer a short supply of conditional nocturnal sedatives after a proper discussion.

The Z drugs are now thought to have the same problems of habituation and withdrawal as the benzodiazepines although I am really unable to remember a single patient over the last 35 years in whom a dependency on hypnotics has become a difficulty that required dedicated treatment.

If you have no worry about costs (and I accept these days this is unlikely) Lormetazepam, a middle half life Benzodiazepine, seems a rational choice. Warn the patient about driving and concentration the next morning however.

Lormetazepam has a half life of about 10 hours.

Nitrazepam, the commonest hypnotic when I qualified has a half life of 15-35 hours and

Temazepam, probably the commonest current benzodiazepine is 8-22 hours.

Triazolam which has been used as a "date rape drug" has a half life of 30mins – 2 hours. Zopiclone on the other hand which causes similar alterations to sleep architecture and EEGs to the benzodiazepines and also reduces REM sleep and Delta waves has a half life of 4-7 hours.

All sleeping pills, however, can cause an increased risk of death (up to 5X higher) and as mentioned, affect the nocturnal organisation of memories and mood. They are associated with higher rates of various cancers, of falls, possibly sleep apnoea, suicide, car crashes, arrhythmias etc. Possibly, of course, some of these may not be due to the hypnotic but associated with other factors that caused the insomnia in the first place. The most important thing for the GP is to make it clear that simple hypnotics are not for regular or long term use and the **GP MUST review** all repeat prescriptions regularly. A metallic after taste and a metallic halitosis are particular side effects of the Z drugs.

Again, Melatonin may be an alternative for some patients if you really are concerned about dependency. It is prescribable (Circadin) in certain situations, presumably not physically addictive, and to the motivated patient or the traveller, it is OTC in America or obtainable as a dietary supplement on the Internet from legal American sources. Oddly, it doesn't cause day time drowsiness if accidentally taken in the daytime when you want to stay awake. Supposedly.

Failing drug treatment, it is important to have covered "**Sleep hygiene**" techniques:
Fixed bed times,
Relaxing before turning in,
A comfortable sleep environment (not hot, cold, noisy or bright),
No daytime naps, certainly nothing more than one nap of no more than 20 minutes (longer affects quality of night time sleep).
No caffeine, Nicotine or alcohol within 6 hours of bed,
Exercise in the day but not within 4 hours of going to bed,
Avoid a heavy evening meal,
Don't clock watch at anytime in the night,
Keep the bedroom for sleep (and sex) only,
and some even use CBT – which has been shown to be better overall in some trials than the Z drugs.

Obstructive sleep apnoea:

(Any cessation of breathing that exceeds 10 seconds during sleep). Up to 60% of people over 65 have OSE. Periods of inspiratory obstruction due to glottal/upper respiratory laxity and upper respiratory blockage. This causes 20-40 seconds of apnoea, followed by a noisy inspiratory gasp only to be repeated over and over again while the patient is asleep. The sufferer may be completely unaware of the condition but it causes alarm in partners and observers. OSA is associated with loud snoring. Both are due to upper respiratory obstruction.

Temporary respiratory obstruction due to tonsillitis, glandular fever or the muscle relaxant effect of sedative drugs or alcohol may cause OSA. Obesity is a common factor. It is commoner in men, in smokers, in some (thin) children and in women during pregnancy.

The daytime complications of the poor sleep quality consequent upon OSA are headaches, fatigue, forgetfulness, depression, hypertension, weight gain and reflux. Other associations are Type 2 diabetes, hypertension, reflux and occasionally depression. Weight gain may be a cause or a result of OSA. Localised and specific cerebral damage (to the hippocampus and R frontal cortex, associated with certain aspects of memory restriction) can result.

Long term the cardiac complications include an increased risk of infarct, hypertension, stroke as well as Cor Pulmonale and pulmonary hypertension. Sleep apnoea worsens the prognosis of malignant melanoma, managing and improving sleep apnoea helps improve blood pressure control, as well as reducing AF recurrence rate.

Once the earlier stages of sleep have been traversed and paralytic (REM) sleep reached, the upper respiratory obstruction in a susceptible individual takes place. This is associated with increasing inspiratory effort, negative intrathoracic pressures, hypoxia, hypercapnia and when these mechanisms reach an arousal level, "neurological arousal" takes place and the patient suddenly awakes with a gasp. Sleep is regularly interrupted and the quality of sleep reduced.

Treatments include weight loss, stopping sedative medication, avoiding evening alcohol and smoking, using mandibular advancement devices and CPAP. Generally these are assisted by an assessment by an ENT or sleep clinic referral. Topical nasal steroids are a good starting point and trying to get the patient not to sleep on their back and to sleep tilted slightly head up.

There are various forms of upper airway reduction surgery (uvulopalatopharyngoplasty or Ts and As in children etc) that may be tried.

Snoring

37% UK adults snore. 2M:1F. Shorter, wider necks, smoking, nasal congestion and drinking alcohol in the evening make it worse. The first approach, as in OSA is weight loss, reduced alcohol consumption, stop smoking, topical nasal steroids and ask the dentist about mandibular advancement prosthetics before contemplating ENT surgery.

Restless legs/Periodic limb movement syndromes

RLS can happen with the patient both awake and asleep and is a voluntary movement in response to an unpleasant leg sensation. PLMS is when asleep (periodic limb movements in sleep or nocturnal myoclonus). RLS and PLMS are common in pregnancy, iron deficiency, renal failure and myxoedema. Treatment is Iron if appropriate, avoid caffeine.

PLMS do not occur during REM sleep (when muscles are atonic), it results in poor sleep quality and daytime tiredness. Narcolepsy, Parkinson's, benzodiazepine withdrawal, stress, obstructive sleep apnoea etc are causes. PLMS can be treated with anti-convulsants, Parkinson drugs, benzodiazepines (including Clonazepam). Avoid antidepressants.

Other drug treatments include: Ropinirole, opiates, Codeine (!), Tramadol (!), Dopamine receptor agonists (Anti Parkinson drugs).

The Epworth Sleepiness Scale:

Measures daytime somnolence as an aid to sleep disorders or conditions which affect sleep (narcolepsy, obstructive sleep apnoea etc).

It was invented by Dr Murray Johns and is named after his hospital in Melbourne.

It records how likely you are to actually doze off rather than just feel tired in these situations: this refers to your usual way of life recently. Even if this hasn't happened recently try to work out how they would have affected *you*:

Situation/Chance of dozing:	Never:	Slight chance:	Moderate chance:	High chance:
Sitting and reading	0	1	2	3
Watching TV	0	1	2	3
Sitting in a public place ie a theatre/meeting	0	1	2	3
As a car passenger for an hour without a break	0	1	2	3
Lying down to rest in the afternoon when circumstances permit	0	1	2	3
Sitting and talking to someone	0	1	2	3
Sitting quietly after lunch without alcohol	0	1	2	3
In a car while stopped for a few minutes in traffic	0	1	2	3

Total score 0-10 normal. 11-14 mild. 15-18 moderate. 19-24 severe.

According to the BMA junior doctors still complain about their hours. But with the working time directive junior doctors conditions have improved beyond recognition. I and my SHO colleagues would regularly fall asleep at dinner tables and meetings thirty years ago and I would routinely have worked 100+ hours a week and scored 19.

There is a "Stop Bang" sleep apnoea questionnaire which is copyrighted which is readily available on the Internet and predicts obstructive sleep apnoea based on daytime tiredness, snoring, BP, sex, BMI, neck circumference, age and whether someone has seen the patient stop breathing in their sleep. There are also examples from the OHIO Sleep Medicine Institute Center of Sleep Medicine Excellence/The British Snoring and Sleep Apnoea Association etc.

The Stages of sleep:

Waking: Relaxed wakefulness, muscles tense and eyes moving erratically initially, slowly slowing and relaxing.

Non REM sleep: lasts 90-120 minutes, each stage being 5-15 minutes.

Non REM sleep: is 75% of the night.

Stage 1: Drowsiness, 50% reduction of "polysomnograph" activity. Eyes closed but patient will not feel rested or that they have slept if woken.

Stage 2: Light sleep, spontaneous periods of muscle tone mixed with periods of relaxation. Heart rate slows and body temperature drops. Body preparing to enter deep sleep.

Stages 3 and 4: Both are deep sleep stages. Slow wave sleep (Delta waves, slow, high amplitude waves, are seen on the EEG or EMG). The most restorative stages of sleep. Tissue growth and repair, the release of Growth Hormone in the young.

REM Sleep: (Stage 5): Occurs about 90 minutes after sleep onset, repeated roughly every 90 minutes. Melatonin is at its lowest. Dreams occur, body paralysis. Five or so times a night on average. "Encephalitic excitement" but muscular relaxation (to stop acting out the movement of dreams). Only eyes and the diaphragm are spared. Rapid eye movements begin. The EEG shows a pattern similar to stage 1. HR and RR speed up and there is twitching of face, fingers and limbs. Most muscles are paralysed despite dreams taking place in this phase. REM sleep periods vary through the night. The first is the shortest at about 10 minutes, the last one the longest at about an hour. As you get older you spend less time in REM sleep and most older people complain they do indeed awake easily. The purpose of REM sleep is supposed to be to allow your muscles to relax and your brain to organise and review the day's events, to consolidate memories and to connect new and old experiences. It is the brain's housekeeping and thought re-organisation period. The average young adult spends 96 minutes a night in REM sleep and infants up to half their night in REM sleep. This time reduces progressively with age.

GABA helps your brain to "wind down" and calm active thinking as a prelude to deep sleep. Research shows many patients with disordered sleep patterns have lower GABA levels and deficiency interferes with "deep delta sleep".

Sleep Duration

In an interesting study published in 2013 on 230,000 nurses (Gangwisch et al "Results from nurses' health study", Am J Hypertens 2013 Jul 26(7) 903-11) It was discovered that 5 hours of sleep time or more (not just time in bed) were a critical protective factor against hypertension and independent of all other variables. So shift work, stress, family history, menopause and other factors (except perhaps obesity) were all counteracted by five hours or more of regular decent sleep.

In another (2015) study, sleep duration was also found to be important in warding off colds. After adjusting for lifestyle factors, researchers found those who slept less than 6 hours a night were 4X more likely to catch cold from a nasal infusion of cold virus than those who had 7 hours sleep. Those who slept five or fewer hours were 4.4X more likely to catch a cold. So amongst its other functions, sleep maintains immunity.

In a 2015 study of three "primitive" societies, The Hadza, The San and The Tsimane, – groups of indigenous peoples were monitored for sleep patterns away from the modern distractions of artificial light, heat and noise.

The three groups (two in Africa, one in South America) gave similar sleep results: Average sleep duration was 6 hours 25 minutes, with the individuals almost never taking daytime naps. They did not wake in the middle of the night or sleep in two shifts as some had previously thought was normal. Natural light had less influence than was previously thought with most people falling asleep 3.3 hours after sunset. Temperature however was important with people falling asleep when the temperature drops and when it reaches the lowest, they awaken. Traditional societies sleep less than the American "National Sleep Foundation's" recommended 7-9 hours a night – indeed, only six and a half hours being sufficient. And they had no insomnia and were never tired during the daytime.

Causes of Sleep disorders in older people include:

Pain,
Heart Failure/Dyspnoea,
Nocturia,
Reflux,
Drugs: BBs, Theophyline, (etc.)
Stress/anxiety,
Dementia,
Personality disorders,
Sleep apnoea,

Restless leg syndrome,

Periodic limb movement disorder,

Alcohol,

Excessive daytime sleeping and circadian rhythm confusion. – Perhaps this is the ideal situation for the natural (non addictive and anticancer) sleep hormone, Melatonin.

Sleep deprivation, poor sleep and sleep paralysis:

Is a temporary inability to move on waking (hypnopompic) or occasionally on drifting off to sleep (hypnagogic). Sometimes associated with hallucinations, often frightening and due to disrupted REM sleep. It could be regarded as awake REM sleep or overlapping sleep phases and is a "Parasomnia". This can happen frequently in some people or can be associated with other conditions, Narcolepsy, migraine, anxiety, obstructive sleep apnoea. It is also commoner in people who work shifts, who are sleep deprived.

Short episodes lasting up to one minute are common but longer, recurrent isolated sleep paralysis episodes can last for up to an hour or can take place one after another.

The episodes can be associated with hallucinations. These are often frightening and sometimes associated with a sensation of suffocation or strangulation. The only episode I ever experienced was on a sunny Sunday afternoon, waking after a snooze in the garden. I couldn't move at all. I just remember wondering how I could breath if I couldn't move and wracking my brain to remember my neurology and anatomy as to whether it could be Temporal Lobe Epilepsy, a spinal CVA, Guillain Barre, Polio, Acute Myasthenia or what else. I imagine I gradually returned to normal after about 2 minutes but was totally paralysed except my diaphragm and external ocular muscles for all that time. I didn't hallucinate anything frightening but I did think I was suffering a catastrophic bilateral CVA or demyelination or something similar for the duration of the whole experience.

The treatment is to get enough sleep, avoid caffeine and Nicotine, avoid alcohol before retiring, try Clomipramine, SSRIs, and not to sleep on your back.

Another "parasomnia" is:

Night Terrors:

In children they start as early as 3 years of age, wearing off in teenage. 18% of children suffer but only 2.2% of adults. In adults they occur in the twenties. The sufferer appears fearful, sweaty, panicky, but is unrousable and inaccessible. They do not recognise family and may lash out if woken. Sleep walking may be a feature, as is next day amnesia. There is high delta activity on the EEG.

Night terrors may be linked in some adults to TLE and some psychiatric conditions (PTSD, anxiety etc) but in children it is more benign.

It can be treated with rectal diazepam, or oral diazepam on retiring or even Midazolam (Buccolam). Sometimes waking the patient before the usual time of their terror reduces their frequency.

Narcolepsy:

Onset is usually in adolescence and with an incidence about 1:2000. So you should theoretically have at least one on your list. It often takes years to recognise an excessively tired teenager as having a diagnosable (and treatable) condition though.

The main characteristic is severe sleepiness during the day. This is another condition in which the brain fails to organise sleep/wake cycles normally. REM sleep occurs very quickly (5 minutes) on falling asleep instead of the usual hour and a half after drifting off.

Narcolepsy can be associated with:

Cataplexy – a sudden complete muscle weakness sometimes after an emotional trigger, sleep paralysis (usually on waking), hypnagogic hallucinations (when half asleep, usually falling asleep), sometimes automatic behaviours with no subsequent recollection of the action.

Narcoleptics are constantly tired, fall asleep without being able to resists and experience vivid dreams on doing so. At night their sleep is broken and of poor quality. 0.045% of the population.

Various REM sleep characteristics are therefore happening out of synch and while the patient is awake: There are paralysis, dreams while the patient is aware and so on.

Treatments: Modafinil, Armodafinil, Dexamphetamine, Sodium Oxybate (Xyrem), Methylphenidate, Atomoxetine, (and oddly, Clarithromycin!):

Hypersomnia:

People with hypersomnia complain that they are not fully awake until sometime after getting up.

Not just all teenagers, 0.3% of the population.

Talking about the stages of sleep occurring out of synch. and too soon, there are neurological disorders in which fragments of REM sleep intrude into wakefulness. – with sudden sleepiness and vivid dreams at sleep onset and also when half asleep (hypnagogic hallucinations – falling asleep/hypnopompic – on waking). The brain takes short cuts straight to REM sleep within minutes of closing the eyes without the usual intervening phases (which usually take an hour not 5 minutes).

These patients also can also suffer cataplexy – a sudden loss of muscle tone during which wakefulness is preserved. The cataplexy responds to TCADs, SSRIs, Modafinil (Provigil), they also suffer poor, broken sleep and daytime sleepiness.

Shift work and health:

The number of UK shift workers is increasing. It was 3.2m by 2015 according to the TUC. This is a rise of 6.9% since 2007 while the labour force increased by only 4.6%. Men are more likely to work nights than women (15% vs 10%) even though the largest number of workers are "care" workers – including nurses and midwives.

Shift work and "insufficient sleep" increases diabetes, obesity, heart disease, mental health problems including depression and various cancers.

Breast cancer is increased 50% in female night workers and 70% in flight personnel.

The mechanisms for increased cancers in people who are awake at night are:

The usual nocturnal production of melatonin is prevented by light. Melatonin has direct and indirect anticancer effects.

Sleep disruption causes the HPA to produce steroids which suppress immune function.

A "phase shift," in which the peripheral rhythms of functions such as digestion are out of phase with central sleep and wake rhythms takes place. This may result in changes in the control of cell and tissue proliferation.

A reduction in Vitamin D production/activation.

Increased eating/smoking/drinking etc due to social/stress factors are related to nocturnal working. It makes sense to offer night workers melatonin to help them sleep in the day and protect them against cancer although I am unaware of any GPs who are currently doing that.

For daytime workers:

A 2015 study (Medscape) found that patients who took daytime naps had 24 hour ambulatory systolic blood pressures 5% (6mm Hg) lower than those who worked on all day without a snooze. More than 20 minutes asleep however would disrupt their nocturnal sleep pattern.

Doctors, sleep and shift work:

As I mention elsewhere, my first medical jobs included one in twos and one in three rotas, both involving continuous duty weekend sessions of 80 hours. There were NO regular sleep sessions pencilled in and I remember at least a couple of weekends, one as a neonatal SHO and one as a Paediatric lecturer, that each involved three days without any sleep.

My busy weeks on duty in my one in two jobs were 136 hours of on call. This was three times the current Working Time Directive averaged limit of 48 hours. Some current articles on medical shift work and sleep deprivation emphasise the dangers to health and safety of tiredness both to the doctors and patients of, presumably, 12 hours sleep deprivation and up to 24 hours of being on duty. This finding is not, however, universal. Despite what we know regarding how shift work can affect our long term health, the profession WAS made of sterner stuff then – absenteeism due to sickness was a third of current levels and I don't remember any of my colleagues who considered their on-call "unacceptable" forty and thirty years ago. One of the many contradictory and puzzling facts about today's work force that I can only explain by citing its new feminisation is the apparent lack of vocational dedication, by which I mean a willingness for some degree of personal suffering to benefit both the patient and one's long term career. This may also be due to the intellectualisation and new emotional sensitivity of the profession, the pervasive societal sense of human rights, at least in the west and the relative indulgence and softness of training today. In an article in the Royal College of Physician's Commentary magazine in October 2015,

It said that doctors should have two full night's sleep before doing a night on call and a 2 hour nap the afternoon before the session. A two hour "nap" enables a full cycle of deep and dreaming sleep although there is the penalty of temporary "sleep inertia" on waking. The suggestion was they should start their duty without a "sleep debt".

It quotes these facts: It says as little as 2 hours lost sleep decreases cognitive performance. Being awake 24 hours can reduce cognitive performance 70% and clinical performance by 85% and that this gets worse with more complex tasks. Once you are tired due to sleep debt, the more complex the task the worse the performance.

Tiredness increases negative mood and this is associated with more errors and burn out. Depressed doctors make more mistakes.

If shift patterns allow circadian sleep then 30% fewer mistakes are made. If shifts are limited to 16 hours then 36% fewer serious medical errors are made and (you can guess this:) physicians report many more fatigue related errors with increased work hours and extended shift frequency.

So you should have two decent night's sleep before a night on call, a long lie in (til lunch time the day before) or a 2 hour afternoon nap before the duty starts. (Naps are better recumbent or lying than sitting up – in a cool darkened room with an eye mask and ear plugs if practical.) Once the night session starts, keep well hydrated and eat a light meal mid way through.(Complex carbohydrates are best in order to prolong absorption) and try to consume caffeine every 2 hours.

During the night duty, strategic naps, regular caffeine and exposure to bright light, (though this is hard to avoid in most hospital environments at night anyway) are said to keep one alert. Blue enriched light – high CCT, 5,000-8,000K is more alerting than lower CCT light. Decide whether you can stay awake and how to cope with the post doze confusion if you are woken to work from a deep sleep. I personally think that the severity of this dysphoria is dependent upon how long you have been asleep what part of the sleep cycle you are woken from. This is called "Sleep Inertia" and is confusion, inability to think straight or recall simple facts or even how to do procedures. It can feel like drunkenness and so you must decide whether you are actually going to try to sleep on duty. This confusion usually lasts 30-40 minutes after arousal, apparently. I well remember driving on the wrong side of the empty road at four am on a night GP call ten years ago before really shaking myself properly awake. This must have been twenty minutes after taking the call, getting dressed and into the car.

Between 03.00 and 06.00 the body circadian clock most demands that we sleep. This is the best time for a "power nap". To avoid clinical mistakes, some commentators suggest that you repeat any communication back to the speaker in a "Copy that" military radio "Received and understood" type acknowledgement.

After on call, on the way home, don't wear blue sunglasses, try not to wear sunglasses at all. Stay in bright light as much as possible, stay relatively cold, or use a taxi or public transport. Then try to sleep, use ear plugs, switch off your phone and don't have caffeine at home. The more night shifts the greater your cumulative sleep debt.

All this will seem totally bizarre and, well, indulgent to doctors who qualified in the seventies, eighties, nineties and so on.

We did our eighty hours, drove home, in my case over thirty miles, to a house with two small children who had missed their dad, wanted to be read to and played with and often had disturbed nights, there too. Then got up at 6.30 for the return journey for the next 32 hour stint without sleep. I am not saying it did us no harm but I do believe we accepted the hard life of the medical apprenticeship as a means of learning our craft and getting competent.

Jet Lag, light and sleep:

Westward Travel may be better tolerated than Eastward travel as staying awake longer then sleeping is easier than going to bed wide awake but problems do occur in both directions. It is certainly very hard sleeping when the daylight is pouring in around your curtains. (See "Insomnia" with Al Pacino and Robin Williams). Symptoms include sleep disturbance, loss of appetite, nausea, occasionally vomiting, bowel changes, – especially constipation, malaise, tiredness, poor concentration. There is a 24 hour cerebral clock which controls a number of bodily cycles and is mediated through the hormone Melatonin, normally released cyclically in response to cyclical changes in light.

Caffeine and hang-overs make jet lag worse. Taking a sedative/hypnotic on the flight can reduce the effects of jet lag. Unlike Melatonin (OTC in the USA and Hong Kong, available from various internet sites in UK) they do not speed up time zone adjustment and need to be taken for several nights. Melatonin is said to resynchronise the circadian rhythm and help the brain get day and night reorganised quicker than the Z drugs or Temazepam.

Circadian Rhythm: One of the most ancient bodily systems, having connections with virtually all body functions. The genes and proteins of the circadian rhythm are those that were produced by primitive life to protect vulnerable DNA from UV light. 12-14 key genes are involved and this periodicity is possessed by every living cell. The length of the endogenous cycle automatically adjusts with the shortening/lengthening of the daytime with seasons. The supra chiasmatic nuclei in the hypothalamus (50,000 cells) provides the pacemaker control for our 24 hour clock. It is informed by neither rods nor cones but by specialist retinal sensors – 1 in 100 of the total, using melanopsin. Totally blind people have no connection between the light/dark cycle and their own endogenous cycle. There are some completely blind people who still have these specific light sensitive retinal cells however and who retain a 24 hour circadian rhythm.

Caffeine and exercise affect circadian rhythm but not as much as light.

Sleep Hygiene:

Avoid caffeine, alcohol and Nicotine. Advise the patient to have a light snack before retiring rather than going to sleep hungry. Rice and oats contain Melatonin which aid sleep. Dairy products contain tryptophan which is a melatonin precursor and may help sleep too.

Avoid food with colouring, additives and preservative as well as refined sugar and caffeine. No arguments before retiring (American Assocn Retired People), no pets, phones or electronic gadgets in bedroom.

Various psychological approaches including CBT are effective in most cases of "primary insomnia".

38: TRAVEL:

(and see Infections/Immunisations/Vaccines Sections).

I have refrained from printing FULL vaccine and immunisation advice to every destination as these will be out of date very quickly and can easily be obtained from a variety of
sources. I have included various of the best Internet sources and a brief summary of travel
vaccines and prophylaxis.

Full and updated travel advice – You can input complicated requirements such as "travelling with children" "chronic disease" and "extended" stay" into the US CDC website at:
http://www.cdc.gov/
Alternatively: The NHS Fitfortravel.nhs.uk (NHS Scotland) is almost as good.

**The UK MASTA (Medical Advisory Service for Travellers Abroad), was estab-
lished 30 years ago and operates the largest network of private travel clinics in the UK.
Many of your patients will just go and get their advice and treatment direct from them.
Also* ** and see the Malaria section.**

Many **pharmacies** can provide to patients for a fee:
Hepatitis A Vaccine,
Hepatitis A Booster,
Hepatitis A & Typhoid Vaccine,
Hepatitis B Vaccine,
Hepatitis B Booster,
Typhoid Vaccine,
Rabies Vaccine,
Rabies Booster,
Diphtheria, Polio & Tetanus Booster,
Meningitis ACWY Vaccine,
Japanese Encephalitis Vaccine,
Japanese Encephalitis Booster.
Yellow fever vaccination is of course only available from specific centres. These are
usually £55-£65 (2016 prices).

Many patients will ask for antibiotics to take with them on exotic or unusual trips
abroad. I rarely refuse these if they are back packing or trekking in the wilderness or the
third world. Especially if they are doing anything loosely associated with raising money
for a charity. I give clear instructions about when to take them and what the pros and cons
of broad spectrum antibiotics are.

I am slightly indulgent when young people I know are travelling abroad and they ask
for my help. Not everywhere has accessible and competent health care and a different
culture speaking a strange language can be a frightening place when you are ill.

One of my daughter's friends cycled from London to Berlin for GOS and his own
curmudgeonly London GP refused even to discuss the poor young man's concerns about
recurrent saddle sores. This was a constant problem. I prescribed him some Daktacort as
a T/R and this made the whole trip possible as it turned out. This is not strictly Travel
Medicine but why are Family Physicians (PCPs as we are known in the US, Primary Care
Physicians) sometimes so unlikable, so rigid, narrow minded and unempathetic? How
much effort did that take?

I take the opportunity to discuss Tetanus and other immunisations and refer them to my travel nurse and to the above web sites. I suggest Dioralyte, Imodium, or similar preparations. Also topical antiseptics and sterile dressings, insect repellents, mosquito precautions, water sterilising tablets and similar precautions at the same time.

The letter I give to trekers with their Ciprofloxacin:

Dear...................

Thank you for your request for a prescription for antibiotics. This is enclosed although I am not completely sanguine about giving this for several reasons.

I would like to make sure that these are not used unless there is no alternative. Many infections are made worse by antibiotics. Diarrhoea can sometimes be worsened, sore throats likewise and most infections you may pick up travelling will not respond to any antimicrobial treatment. –The only problem is that some serious infections (bloody diarrhoea, tonsillitis, pneumonia etc) *might* need them.

Please try alternative treatments first, -fluids, analgesics etc and only take these antibiotics if you feel significantly ill for more than a few days. There are many other issues of resistance, allergy etc which I won't go into but antibiotics are a final resort.

I don't want to cause more trouble than I cure!

I enclose the scrip which I hope and expect you won't need. Have a good trip.

Best Wishes,

Travellers' diarrhoea:

Usually due to E Coli but can be caused by Campylobacter, Salmonella or Shigella.

Treatments include: Ciprofloxacin 500-750mg as a single dose for travellers to remote areas given clear instructions or 500mg BD 3-4 days and then Metronidazole 800mg TDS INB – but only if no support is available.

Alternatively: Rifaximin-a (Xifaxanta) a non absorbed antibiotic 200mg TDS for 3days. It can be used in non bloody, <8 stools in 24 hours, no systemic symptoms, Travellers' Diarrhoea.

Tropical Sprue is the end result of an acute bout of travel diarrhoea and is a chronic diarrhoeal illness with malabsorption, steatorrhoea and deficiencies of Vitamins A, B12, D, K, also of Calcium and Folic Acid. It is treated with Folic Acid, Co Trimoxazole and Doxycycline. (See "Microbiome").

Insect Repellents:

"Walkabout", Citronella, "Incognito" and others must be backed up by common sense advice about nets, avoiding risk areas and times of day etc.

*Malaria: (See Immunisation/vaccines section)

Malaria imported to the UK increased 9% in 2013 (1501 cases vs 1378 in 2012) Falciparum cases increased to 79%, the proportion of Vivax cases falling.

The highest proportion of patients developing Malaria are those not born in the UK, travelling to their country of origin to visit their family (PHE 2014). The biggest risk groups being of black African ethnicity.

For up to date chemoprophylaxis, Google Malaria chemoprophylaxis and go to the Health Protection Agency, travellers from the UK website or use the printable update on the MIMS website advice or at the back of the printed MIMS.

There are four parasite species that cause malaria in humans:

- *Plasmodium falciparum*

- *Plasmodium vivax*

- *Plasmodium malariae*

- *Plasmodium ovale.*

Plasmodium Falciparum and Vivax are the most common, Falciparum is the most lethal.

Prophylaxis:

Malarone is Atovaquone. 250mg and Proguanil 100mg. Dose: 1 a day from the day before until 7 days after leaving the area. For up to 3 months. Protects against benign malaria (the blood forms of P Vivax and Ovale). It does not eliminate the hypnozoites from the liver. Absorption is reduced by tetracycline. Avoid in pregnancy and BF. 95-100% effective.

Chloroquine: Avloclor/Nivaquine. 2 tabs, (150mg base) once weekly. Try a trial course to predict side effects but initiate a week before departure anyway. Safe in pregnancy, not safe in OD.

Proguanil: Paludrine. 200mg daily. One or two doses before leaving, then while away and for 4 weeks after return. Give folic acid if taken in pregnancy.

Doxycycline: Vibramycin. 100mg daily from 1 day to 1 week before to 4 weeks after leaving the area. Can cause photosensitivity and there is the risk of an oesophageal ulcer if the capsule breaks in the gullet so lots of fluid with each dose. Avoid in pregnancy, BF and under 12 years, various interactions, with anticonvulsants, the pill etc. >90% effective.

Mefloquine, Lariam: 250mg weekly from 1-3 weeks before to 4 weeks after (three weeks before if the patient has never previously taken it). Can cause hangover the day after (some people take half the dose twice weekly), vivid dreams and rare psychiatric reactions. Avoid in epilepsy or with a first degree relative with epilepsy and with a significant psychiatric history. Various cardiac drug interactions. Avoid in first trimester. >90% effective.

A controversial drug. The RCGP "Chair" thinks GPs "steer clear" of Mefloquine although this is not what all the GPs I have ever met do or have ever been advised to do. (Clare Gerada). Various serving soldiers have been guilty of homicides at home and abroad which have been blamed on drug adverse effects. These include one US Special Forces soldier who killed 16 Afghan civilians, 4 US soldiers at Fort Bragg who killed their wives and Canadian peace keepers who killed Somalian teenagers. The effects of PTSD and the emotional trauma of active service must make diagnosing a violent drug side effect very difficult in these circumstances. However, the French military do not prescribe Mefloquine and it is NOW third line in the US military. According to UK parliamentary questions 14% of UK military personnel had sought treatment for side effects (Johnny Mercer MP) and since 2008 994 service personnel had been treated at psychiatric clinics for side effects.

200 soldiers are seeking compensation for side effects and Lord Dannatt, ex Head of the Army added to the controversy by saying in august 2016 that he hadn't taken it as he believed that his son had suffered mental side effects from it.

Doxycycline and Malarone (Atovaquone/Proguanil) are said to be a safer alternative. No British soldier has died from Malaria for 20 years. (The Pharmaceutical Journal 12 Nov 2015). I have never had a patient have a significant side effect from Mefloquine, having prescribed it several dozen times.

What SHOULD replace mefloquine if you really don't want to prescribe it as first line prophylaxis in locations where chloroquine resistant Pl. Falciparum exists? Doxycycline. As the monohydrate, not hyclate. Marketed in the UK as Efracea, it has fewer S/Es than the hyclate.

Childhood doses:

	<6kg	<10Kg	<16Kg	<25Kg	<45Kg	>45Kg
Chloroquine tabs	1/4	1/2	3/4	1	1 1/2	2
Proguanil	1/4	1/2	3/4	1	1 1/2	2
Mefloquine	N/R	1/4	1/4	1/2	3/4	1
Doxycycline					100mg from 12 yrs	

Malarone	<11kg	<21Kg	<31Kg	<40kg	>40kg
	NR	1 Paed tab	2 Paed tabs	3 paed tabs	1 Adult tab

	<4.5Kg	<8Kg	<11Kg	<15Kg	<17Kg
Chloroquine Syrup:	2.5ml	5ml	7.5ml	10ml	12.5ml

**There are many websites and guides on line and elsewhere regarding Malaria Prophylaxis. I like the CDC Malaria prevention web site with maps and countries in alphabetical order, drugs and general advice to travellers etc.
www.cdc.gov/malaria/travelers/drugs.html

Good Travel advice handouts:
www.travax.nhs.uk
www.fitfortravel.scot.nhs.uk
National Travel Health Network and Centre or the excellent American:
http://wwwnc.cdc.gov/travel

The following travel vaccinations are usually available free on the NHS:
Diphtheria, polio and tetanus (combined booster),
Typhoid,
the first dose of Hepatitis A,
Cholera.
These vaccines are usually free because they protect against diseases thought to represent the greatest risk to public health if they were brought into the country.
Many GPs do not charge for the second (booster) dose of Hepatitis A or the combined Hepatitis A and Hepatitis B vaccine.

Most patients pay privately for:
Hepatitis B,
Japanese encephalitis and tick-borne encephalitis,
Meningococcal meningitis,
Rabies,
Tuberculosis,
Yellow fever,
Yellow Fever vaccines are only available from designated centres. The NaTHNaC website lists these.
The cost of travel vaccines at private clinics will vary, but most charges are around £50-£60 for each dose of a vaccine.

Vaccinations usually recommended for travellers:

These are on the various travel web sites, updated and frequently revised. The, advice is too complicated to include fully but briefly:

Where	Course	Lasts	Min. age
Cholera: Wherever endemic.	2 doses oral vaccine a week apart Booster at 2 years	2 years	Two years
European tick borne encephalitis Central Europe, Russia	3 IM Injs – stat, 1-3m later and 5-12m after that- then 3 yearly booster	3 yrs	none
Hepatitis A, where there is poor sanitation	2 IM Injs. – Stat and then 6-12m	Up to 10 yrs if booster but 6m-1yr after first dose	None but not usually <1 yr
Hepatitis B Endemic countries	3 injs at 0, 1 and 2 or 0, 1 and 6 months	Can be for life	Birth
Japanese B encephalitis Areas of SE Asia, India, China	injs stat, 1m and 1-2 yrs booster for longer protection.	1-4 yrs	None
Meningococcal. Sub-Saharan Africa, Brazil, parts of middle and East Asia	1 sc inj (infants may need 2)	3yrs	2m
Polio. Everywhere	3 oral doses each a month apart	5-10yrs	none
Rabies. Endemic countries	Doses on days 0, 7, 21 and 28 booster at 1 yr and 3-5 yrs for longer protection.	5yrs	1yr
Tetanus. Everywhere.	3 sc injs, 4-6 weeks apart	10yrs	none
Typhoid. Where sanitation is poor	One stat inj or oral capsule days 1, 3, 5,	Booster every 3 yrs Annual booster	1yr
Yellow Fever. Central Africa, Parts of South and Central America.	1 sc inj	Valid from 10d-10yr	6m

Insect Repellents:

Permethrin (as used against woodworm, scabies and head lice) can be used on fomites.

DEET 30% concentration lasts about 6 hours. Safe in children 2m and older (10-30% DEET)
      20-24% lasts 4-5 hours   Avoid hands and around eyes.
      6-10% lasts 1-3 hours.

Picaridin   20% lasts 7 hours   Not under 6m
           10% lasts up to 5 hours
IR 3535   7.5% 10-60 minutes   2 months and older
Lemon Eucalyptus oil Up to 2 hours   No younger than 3 years

39: UROLOGY:

A bladder regularly passing less than 100mls is one that is not emptying properly or not filling properly and "irritable" or possibly indicates the presence of significant bladder pathology. Approximately 2 – 2.5 li urine is normally passed by a 70kg man in 24 hrs although this depends on many "normal" variables. 300-350mls is an average output per voiding, -"bursting" is 500mls. Most people suddenly want to go as soon as they arrive home at their own front door even if the bladder is at a fraction of this capacity.

"Urgent" Urological referrals:
Macroscopic haematuria in adults.
Microscopic haematuria in adults over 50 years.
Swellings in the body of the testis.
Palpable renal masses.
Solid renal masses on imaging.
Elevated PSA in men with a >10 year life expectancy. (But try repeating the PSA after a course of antibiotics).
A High (>20ng/ml) PSA in men with a clinically malignant prostate or bone pain.
Any suspected penile cancer.

Various Urological Infections:
Haematuria:
In haematuria with a positive MSU, treat the infection, but wait 4 weeks for the inflammation and haematuria to settle before rechecking for ?persistent haematuria.
Only 3% of patients >50 years old with haematuria have a "significant" abnormality.
Post vasectomy soft tissue Infection: Rx Cefradine and Metronidazole are the most effective antibacterial combination, I find.
Urinary Infections: Nitrofurantoin 50-100mg QDS. Not <3m age. Long term suppression 50-100mg Nocte. Child: Acute UTI 3mg/kg/day as a qds dose for 7days. Suppressive therapy 1mg/kg/day as a once daily dose (>10 years same as adult). Safe in pregnancy except at term (haemolysis in G6PD deficient babies). The kidney is its main route of excretion/ metabolism. 25 million prescriptions written annually. Generally considered bacteriostatic, but is concentrated in urine and reaches bacteriocidal concentrations.
Recurrent UTIs in women: Try Cranberry juice 30mls nocte (not shown to be double blind cross over proven but many patients do find it oddly effective as a preventative for some reason and one or two studies have shown AN effect) with 50mg nitrofurantoin nocte plus probiotics during the daytime. – All a little bit alternative, I agree – but some women are plagued by this and all the double micturition, emptying the bladder immediately after sex, loose cotton underwear, no tights, no bubble baths, etc. etc. just serve to make them feel unfeminine as well as constantly dysuric. So why not try?

Dipstix testing:
Leukocyte esterase test: Sensitivity for pyuria 80-90%. Specificity for pyuria 95-98% but to diagnose a UTI you need "symptoms" too. Without symptoms there can be up to 50% overtreatment. UTIs can exist with a negative leukocyte esterase. Symptoms of urethritis, vaginitis, or STD can exist without a UTI and with a neg leucocyte esterase test.

Pyuria: Less likely in a neutropoenic patient with a UTI. Oliguric and anuric patient may have pyuria without UTI. Patients with haematuria are pyuric, as are catheterised patients, those with ARF, STDs and non infectious cystitis.

"Nitrates": (Actually Nitrites) (Bacteria convert non ionic nitrate into nitrite) Urine nitrites alone are not enough to indicate a UTI. "Nitrates" indicate bacteriuria but this is not necessarily a UTI. You need other symptoms and signs of a UTI.

A negative leukocyte esterase and a negative urine nitrate largely rule out UTI in the pregnant, elderly, in Family Practice and urology. (88% negative predictive value 95% confidence int.).

If Leuk Est and Nit are both pos the sensitivity for bacteriuria is only 48% in elderly NH residents. Indicating the need to correlate these to symptoms.

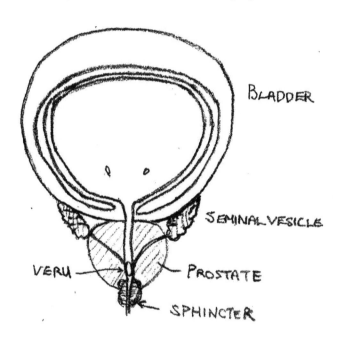

Diagram Urol A1 (Male bladder/prostate anatomy)

Prostatic Hypertrophy: BPH

"As much a part of aging as grey hair" – with 90% of men between 50 and 60 suffering. Medical treatments include:

Alpha blockers:

Prazosin: Hypovase eg 2mg BD, Alfuzosin: Xatral, 2.5mg TDS (SR 5mg BD) a uro-selective apha blocker.

Tamsulosin: Flomax 0.4mg OD, (Flomaxtra XL is same dose, slow release) can try withdrawing after 18 months treatment.

Also Doxazosin, Indoramin, Terazosin (Hytrin starter pack >maintenance 5-10mg Nocte).

Dutasteride: Avodart, halves the PSA. Works in 1m-4 years!

Tamsulosin: (an Alpha 1 adrenoceptor antagonist) also comes with Dutasteride, – a 5 Alpha reductase inhibitor (which improves male pattern baldness) in the combined "Combodart".

Tamsulosin also comes combined with Solifenacin (competitive, selective muscarinic receptor antagonist) in "Vesomni".

Another 5 alpha reductase inhibitor is Finasteride: Proscar. This reduces PSA, the patient should take contraceptive measures if fertile. 5mg daily for 6m. Must do initial and follow up DREs.

Many consultants start with alpha blockers and Finasteride in combination. Beware however: blocking the production of testosterone does not protect against prostate cancer development.

TURP

TUR can be monopolar, bipolar, hot loop, laser, holmium, or green light. BPH can be treated with a simple bladder neck incision too – though this, like TURP risks retrograde ejaculation. Other complications, ED, operative fluid overload, incontinence etc, are rare. Even retrograde ejaculation, common immediately after TURP may improve and resolve as time passes.

A new alternative to TURP is the Prostatic Urethral Lift procedure (UroLift System) which consists of the retraction of the obstructing urethral lobes by the introduction of a patent anterior channel in the prostatic urethra. This is done trans urethrally, 3-5 UroLift implants being inserted through a urethral needle. This can be done under a spinal or even topical anaesthetic.

International Prostate Symptom Score:

	Not at all	Less than 1 time in 5	Less than half the time	About half the time	More than half the time	Almost always
1) Over the last month how often have you felt you haven't completely emptied your bladder on urinating?	0	1	2	3	4	5
2) Over the last month how often have you had to urinate again less than 2 hours after you finished urinating?						
3) Over the past month how often have you stopped and started again several times while urinating?						
4) Over the last month how often have you found it hard to postpone urinating?						

5) Over the last month how often have had a weak stream?

6) Over the last month how often have you had to push or strain to begin urination?

7) Over the last month how often did you have to get up at night to urinate on average?

Add the scores from 1) to 7) to find the IPSS score

Quality of Life due to urinary symptoms:

	Delighted	Pleased	Mostly satisfied	Mixed, about equally satisfied and satisfied	Mostly dissatisfied	Unhappy	Terrible
If you were to spend the rest of your life with your urinary symptoms unchanged, you would feel:	0	1	2	3	4	5	6

Sexual Health Inventory: (For men, to identify E.D.)

In the last 6m

How do you rate your confidence that you could get and keep an erection?
Very low 1, Low 2, Moderate 3, High 4, Very high 5

When you have had erections with sexual simulation, how often were they hard enough for penetration?

No sexual activity	Almost never or never	A few times – much less than half the time	Sometimes – about half the time	Most times – much more than half the time	Always or almost always
0	1	2	3	4	5

During S.I. how often were you able to maintain the erection after penetration?

Did not try	Almost never or never	A few times (<half)	About half the time	Most times	Always or almost always
0	1	2	3	4	5

During SI how difficult is it to maintain the erection to completion?

Did not try SI	Extremely difficult	Very difficult	Difficult	Slightly difficult	Not difficult
0	1	2	3	4	5

When you tried SI how often was it satisfactory for you?

Did not try or never	Almost never (much<half)	A few times almost	About half the time	More than half the time	Always or almost always
0	1	2	3	4	5

The Erectile Dysfunction is 1-7 severe, 8-11 moderate, 12-16 mild to moderate, 17-21 mild E.D.

All men should get 40-50 minutes of a sleep erection each night which improves oxygenation of the penis. Erections are important to maintain the structure and function of the penis and are a marker of good cardiovascular health. You can try the postage stamp test – getting the patient or his friend to wrap a strip of second class stamps around the limp member as he goes to sleep and sticking the last on top of the first. When he gets the unconscious early morning priapism, the stamps should tear, hopefully at the perforations so they can be reused ligitimately. Then you know the vascularity and neurology are probably capable of normal function. And stamps are so expensive these days, it would be a shame to waste them.

Lower urinary tract symptoms (LUTS) are associated with ED and with BPH and 70% of men with LUTS/BPH in fact also have ED. Tadalafil (5mg) can be used as a regular prophylactic daily dose to improve most of these connected symptoms.

Loss of Libido:

A systematic review of 15,000 men published in early 2015 found that the average flaccid penis was 9.16cm and erect penis 13.12cm (5 1/4") long.

Libido and what that actually means for any given person at any particular time of life is a difficult topic. What is normal? I had a (professional) partner who treated most patients, including women, with depot testosterone at the drop of a hat. He didn't seem to have an upper age limit but I do admit to having some distaste at the thought of prescribing hormones and PDE5 Inhibitors to patients much past the mid 70s of age. I am however inclined to agree that might be not only ageist but utterly unreasonable given the active and full lives many fit 70 – 80 year olds can live. So when is your libido supposed to wane?, what if the spouse isn't quite as keen on sex as the patient? Here is a typical example where a quick prescription can let everyone down and a good GP should talk to and get to know both partners before offering a quick fix and a short appointment.

On the other hand, some relationships place a higher value on sex than others and the figures show that the AVERAGE 70 year old couple is having sex once a week....

In America half the female population is now said to suffer from "Female sexual arousal disorder." Somehow here it does seem that a normal state is being medicalised and innocent people made to feel guilty. Perhaps this is just the sort of thing that has driven the D.S.M. IV into disrepute. (Diagnostic and Statistical Manual No 4).

In women as well as men, loss of interest in sex and diminishing "lust" is normal for many, probably most of us as we go through middle age and older. Depression, alcohol and drug abuse, anaemia, other systemic illnesses, diabetes, myxoedema, some prescribed drugs (e.g. diuretics, BBs, sedatives, SSRIs, Cimetidine, Finasteride, Cyproterone), can affect sex drive, hyperprolactinaemia, tiredness for all reasons, a new baby, work stress, some conditions, a poor relationship with your partner, (– of course), previous sexual abuse, previous sexual difficulty (and consequent performance anxiety), guilt and all sorts of varied emotions and worries can affect sexual interest and performance.

A few tests may be in order, FBC, fasting glucose, electrolytes, Testosterone, Prolactin, Gonadotrophins and so on.

You can suggest Intrinsa (testosterone in a patch form) for women but some virilising side effects may be irreversible or you can even try Sustanon in the short term. PDE5 inhibitors have been tried in women but it is hard to see how vasodilating the vagina improves a woman's sexual interest in an otherwise undesirable male partner. Less dramatic treatments include Venlafaxine and Trazadone, Mianserin, Imipramine, Trimipramine. The bottom line is that the couple may need to see a relationship (or sex) therapist. These exotic things are few and far between on the NHS and you could argue anyway that this is a classic example of where the NHS is overreaching its original intentions. Warn the patient that they may need to be prepared to fund the therapy privately.

Erectile Dysfunction:

The stuff you may have forgotten:

Apparently 52% men between the ages of 40 and 70 have erectile dysfunction. If this is so then the vast majority keep quiet about it and of those that come to their GP (I would like to do an audit of the percentages who consult male vs female GPs!) most will not qualify for PDE5 Inhibitors on the NHS. Some drugs in the group are just now becoming generic however so costs of private prescriptions are a little less than they were. - And now a private prescription can be obtained via various pharmacy chains without a face to face consultation.

Erection occurs when sexual stimulation increases parasympathetic nervous system activity causing vasodilatation, increased blood flow through the Cavernous and Helicine Arteries. The veno occlusive mechanism maintains the venous pressure.

Detumescence: Increased sympathetic activity increases tone of Helicine Arteries and stimulates contraction of trabecular smooth muscle >encourages outflow from Corpora Cavernosa and Corpus Spongiosum.

Neurology: Sacral Plexus: S2-S4 is part of a reflex arc, involving down coming spinal and incoming messages from penile stimulation. The presence of local stimulation and a foreskin assists in this.

Causes of erectile dysfunction: 51-80% are "Organic", (different authoritative sources) – often a marker for peripheral arterial disease. 20% may be due to low testosterone (<12 or <8 nmol/li – different sources) in which case PDE5 inhibitors don't usually work. 18% are "Psychological" (although in my experience "psychological factors" come in to play in most cases) and most urologists agree.

30% or so are "Mixed" – ie "Organic and Psychological."

Don't forget ED as a drug side effect, of antihypertensives, (most of them!) particularly diuretics, BBs, Verapamil, Nifedipine, ACEIs, Spironolactone, of histamine receptor antagonists (H1 and H2), anti-Parkinson drugs, anti depressants, anxiolytics, anticonvulsants, chemotherapy agents, anti-prostate and muscle relaxant drugs, of tobacco, alcohol, analgesics as well as cardiovascular disease, diabetes, prostate cancer and prostatic surgery.

BUT caffeine (85-170mg a day, 2-3 cups), protects against ED compared with men who drink no caffeine at all or more than this. The risk being reduced by 42%. This protective effect holds for the hypertensive and obese but not diabetics. Less or more coffee than 2-3 cups a day are not as effective. (Univ of Texas. Web MD May 21 2015.)

Investigations:

A morning testosterone will help identify pituitary adenoma or occult hypogonadism Free Testosterone or Androgen Index, dipstick urine analysis, LH/FSH (if testosterone low), prolactin (if testosterone low or lack of libido), U and Es, creat, haemoglobinopathy screen (HbS), LFTs, (abnormal LFTs are linked with ED).

"Organic" Causes of Erectile Dysfunction:

Diabetes,
Hypo/hyperthyroidism,
Hypogonadism,
Hyperprolactinaemia,
Cushings,
Cardiovascular Disease, (Peripheral Vascular Disease, Hypertension),
CVA,
Spinal cord/bladder/prostate rectal injury/surgery,
Urological Surgery,
M.S.
Peyronie's/Priapism,
Renal Disease,
Depression/Anxiety/Stress,
Alcohol/Drug Abuse,
Smoking,
NSAIDS,
etc.

Another list of Drugs that cause E.D: (and see above)

H2 Receptor antagonists (Ranitidine, Cimetidine etc),/Metoclopramide/etc,
Alcohol, Barbiturates, hypnotics, sedatives,
Narcotics, Heroin, etc.
Anti psychotics,
Butyrophenones-Haloperidol,
Antidepressants: MAOIs, TCAS?, SSRIs,

Lithium,

Stimulants etc, Amphetamines, Cocaine, Cannabis,

Hormones, Oestrogenic drugs, corticosteroids, Cyproterone,

Antihypertensives, Centrally acting: Me Dopa, Diuretics, Spironolactone, BBs,

Anticholinergics,

Disulfiram,

etc.

The list of drugs that affect a "man's sexual arousal and performance" in *MedlinePlus* is over 100 long and consists of virtually every common drug except antibiotics.

Who can be prescribed PDE5 Inhibitors on the NHS?

Patients with:

Diabetes,

Renal Failure on Dialysis,

Post Renal transplant,

MS,

Parkinson's,

Polio,

Ca Prostate,

TUR and other prostatectomy,

Radical Pelvic surgery,

Severe pelvic injury,

Single gene neurological conditions,

Spinal cord injury,

Spina Bifida.

Or if a consultant believes the ED is causing "*Severe distress.*"

-Now here we enter one of medicine today's many ivory tower abstractions and you wonder who the people who think these rules up **are**, who chose **them** and whether they spend much time awake in the same world as you and me.

"*Severe erectile dysfunction related distress*" is a situation assessed by a consultant and involves: *Significant disruption to normal social and occupational activities*, (occupational?) – Does this mean a man is missing sex so much he cannot work? I thought that footballers were told to deny themselves sex the night before the cup final because they performed **better**. – Or does it mean that he normally works in the sex industry? *A marked effect on mood, behaviour, social and environmental awareness*, what has environmental awareness got to do with erectile function? The patient is so distressed about his poor erections that he doesn't know if it's raining or sunny outside? Again, what does all that actually mean and who drafts together all this PC stuff? *and a marked effect on interpersonal relationships* – I understand that bit.

and men already receiving ED treatment on 14/9/1998.

PDE5 inhibitors: (Selective inhibitors of Phosphodiesterase 5:) Tonight Josephine?

ED occurs in 52% of men surveyed over age 40 years. (Mass. male aging study) and is associated with hypertension, DM and several medication classes. In the first 7 years of availability (since 1998) Sildenafil was prescribed to more than 23m men worldwide, one of the most popular ever drugs.

PDE5 inhibitors work in 80% men with a prostate, 45% men who have had a radical prostatectomy. (This is the official wisdom but my experience is that virtually all my patients who have had a radical prostatectomy get some benefit if they continue taking a PDE5 inhibitor for several months).

Note there is potential hypotension with alpha blockers and interactions with CYP3A4 inhibitors including Grapefruit juice – Only Tadalafil, Cialis doesn't seem to do this.

Sildenafil: Viagra, 25mg, 50mg, 100mg 1 hour before sex. Half life 3-5 hrs. Onset 30mins. The FDA in America apparently wrote to Pfizer regarding visual side effects (distortions) with Viagra. I have not seen this but bear it in mind. Rhinitis, flushing and headache are common. Many non responders need 100mg.

Tadalafil: Cialis 2.5mg, 5mg, 10mg, 20mg. Rapid onset, (25mins), half life 4.2 hrs. Long duration of action: 24-36 hours. This means it can be taken as a low "maintenance" daily dose daily, or PRN. The low daily dose is used for lower urinary tract symptoms in men with BPH. Available also as Tadalafil Mylan.(Generic bioequivalent of Cialis tablets.) Headache, flushing, dyspepsia, rhinitis, backache the S/Es. The only PDE5I not affected by a fatty meal.

Vardenafil: Levitra, 5mg, 10mg, 20mg. 30-60 minutes before sex. Peak response though is said to be 10 minutes.

All can cause flushing and headache. Rare risk of retinal vascular occlusion and hypotension.

Opiates including Dihydrocodeine can prolong the erection even causing priapism.

Avanafil: 50mg, 100mg, 200mg tabs. With or without food and with "up to 3 alcoholic beverages" Can be used as little as 15 minutes before sex.

Apomorphine: Uprima which has been used to treat homosexuality, heroin addiction, Parkinson's Disease and Alzheimer's and was available, briefly, for E.D. but withdrawn in 2006.

Other E. D Treatments:

Alprostadil, Caverject and Muse. Intracavernosal injection or intraurethral pellet administration. Then there is a number of different pumps and rings under the heading of "Appliances" which are prescribable.

Alprostadil is now available as a topical cream as well. (June 2014)

Invicorp, (Aug 2016). Intracavernosal injection containing Aviptadil and the non selective alpha blocker phentolamine.

Premature Ejaculation:

Treatment:

Lidocaine/Prilocaine cream/spray applied to glans. (Side effects include female anorgasmia).

SS cream applied an hour before and washed off immediately before sex.

SSRIs of which Paroxetine seems the most effective and Clomipramine. They take two weeks to work.

Dapoxetine: Priligy, made appropriately by Menarini is a PRN on demand SSRI for PE. And available on line (18 tablets X 60mg £169!)

Prostate Cancer: see cancer section and PSA (in Pathology) sections

40,000 diagnosed a year, 12,000 die in UK. 1/4 men present with metastatic disease. The younger the cancer, the more aggressive – generally speaking. However, unlike the mammography screening campaign in America which began at the same time as the large scale and somewhat confusing to interpret PSA screening, deaths from prostate cancer presenting with metastases have dropped significantly. The same cannot be said for advanced presentation of breast cancer. Most tumours begin in the periphery, tend not to present with flow symptoms and by the time men are 80 years old, nearly all will have prostate cancer. ("80% of 80 year olds have prostate cancer but only 3% of men die of prostate cancer"). When PSA is screened, there is one life saved for every 1410 men screened and for every 48 "treatments". If the PSA is <than 1 at 40 or 60 years then the chances of ever getting prostate cancer are negligible. Our local (trusted) urologist investigates, offers radical treatments to patients with a raised PSA and a life expectancy over 10 years (below the age 70-75).

The prostate produces 30% of seminal fluid which neutralises vaginal pH and provides an antibiotic and nutrient function. Most of the rest comes from the seminal vesicles which are unfortunately removed at radical prostatectomy.

Although Charles Huggins gained a Nobel prize for discovering that castration slowed the progress of prostate cancer, the assumption that this was due to lowered testosterone is now debated. Orchidectomy also lowers oestrogen and prostate cancer is now known to be as oestrogen sensitive as breast cancer. Indeed, testosterone has been shown to reduce prostate cancer growth in laboratory animals. All very counter intuitive. Oestrogens are becoming ubiquitous in the environment thanks to female contraceptive and menopausal therapeutic hormones. These are excreted in urine and present in the water supply as a quick examination of the genitals of fresh water amphibians will disclose (and by the way have a molecular similarity to many plastics and plastic related chemicals).

Certain pesticides are associated with an increase in prostate cancer, these include Aldrin, Fonofos, Terbufos and Malathion. The latter is of course used therapeutically to treat head lice in children. BPA, found in plastic bottles, the lining of metal cans, till receipts and so on are mutagens to prostate tissue also.

Men with large waist circumferences (ie fat men) are more likely to get prostate cancer. A 4" larger waistline increases prostate cancer risk by 13% (Study 140,000 European men from 8 countries, pres 2016 Eur Obesity Summit Gothenburg). The higher the waist circumference the more aggressive and higher grade the cancer. There is also a greater risk of dying from the cancer, the bigger the waist size. At 37" the risk of having an aggressive prostate cancer was found to be 13% higher than at 33".

Genes:

There is a family history in 10%, (the BRCA1 (twice the normal risk) and BRCA2 (eight times the normal risk) genes are associated. There are however now 100 common genetic variants linked to prostate cancer and testing for them can identify the 1% of men of European ancestry whose risk is 6X higher than the population average or the 10% whose risk is 3X higher.

Diet:

There is some evidence that deep fried foods increase the risk but cooked tomatoes, ketchup, Lycopene, Saw Palmetto, pomegranate, selenium (possibly), vegetable fat and a vegetarian diet – well at least: eating less red meat may all reduce symptoms and or risk. Low vitamin D levels are associated with an increased risk of prostate cancer. But then low vitamin D is associated with an increased risk of most illnesses it would seem. Multiple sexual partners and early sexual activity, obesity and some sexual infections are also risk factors. Omega three fish oils either lower the risk, slightly increase it or have no effect: – the studies are a bit confusing. Low ejaculation frequency may increase the risk.

Being black increases the incidence 3x, (one in four black men gets prostate cancer), being oriental gives you the lowest racial incidence.

The main risk factor is, of course, age, and the normal range of PSA goes up with age. (See pathology section).

If affected relatives:

1 first degree relative <70 yrs,   RR X2.
2 FDRs (one <65yrs)   RR X4
3 or more relatives   RR x7-10

Chronic prostatitis increases the risk 4X. Regular ejaculation reduces the risk; Prostate cancer risk is 20% less in the unlikely event of ejaculating 20X a month compared with 4-7x per month.

A third of impalpable tumours have already spread.

The lower the Gleason grade the less likely the patient will die of prostate cancer.

Diagnosis of prostatic cancer is by PSA (often misleading), digital rectal examination (which is not reliable alone), the painful ultrasound guided trans-rectal prostate biopsy and template trans perineal biopsy. Two thirds of biopsied men have normal histology but the trans rectal biopsy often misses the anterior part of the gland or apex where many tumours lurk. A template biopsy is (thankfully) done under GA and is transperineal, ultra-sound guided and with 32 core samples (sometimes more) – this may be more common in the future. There is a greater chance of finding a small tumour with this "saturation" biopsy. Whatever the patient literature says, these biopsies are not without morbidity. Even ignoring the post operative urinary infection, prostatitis and bleeding, most men if you ask them will experience persistent urge, frequency and other lower urinary tract symptoms after their prostate has been shot full of holes via the rectum or perineum and left to heal by scarring. These injuries and symptoms are something a prostate has not evolved to deal with and some can be lifelong.

The NICE Guidance suggests (2014) – and it seems that most urologists agree, that an MRI should be done as part of the initial work up of suspected prostate cancer. Logically this should be before biopsy as it will help reduce biopsy misses. The preliminary MPMRI (multiparametric MRI) is more humane than the transrectal biopsy being done blind. It is becoming more available and is good at finding masses that random biopsy might miss. It can still (2016) occasionally misinterpret inflammation for tumour however and is at a relatively early stage of development/image interpretation.

DRE:

The digital rectal examination is only as good as the examiner. Not even as good as them. It is of course, only a superficial feel of the back of the prostate and misses hard lumps in the body or front of the gland as well as softer lesions at the back. Many hard lumps are calcification and not cancer. A third of cancers are missed by DRE and by biopsies (trans rectal biopsies are done from behind and often miss anterior tumours) and that is why many units are offering MRIs as part of the work up of a raised PSA, before the TRUS biopsy is done. The DRE will pick up rectal tumours and a fixed prostate if the cancer has spread outside the capsule. It will also demonstrate the tenderness of prostatitis.

If the PSA is normal and the DRE abnormal, only a third of suspect cases turn out to have cancer. Palpation is not a good way of diagnosing early disease compared with, say trans-rectal ultrasound or mpMRI.

Gleason Scoring:

A biopsy of the prostate is done, the two most common histological types looked for and graded. The most common tissue in the microscope field is listed first. These two tissues are graded from 1 to 5, 1 being the most benign (normal prostate), 5 the most aggressive (poorly differentiated tumour). (This is the Gleason Grade.)

Then the two scores are given in the report – for instance "3+4"

A "Gleason Score" of 3+4 (total 7) Is not as bad as 4+3 as the commonest tissue (4) in the latter is more aggressive then the commonest tissue (3) in the former.

Many urologists say a score of 6 or less is not really cancer. Gleason 6 has the propensity for local growth and extension but rarely for metastasis. The problem is however, that you can only really confidently exclude the higher scores elsewhere in a Gleason 6 biopsy positive prostate by examining the whole (excised) gland after prostatectomy. Gleason 6 often co exists with other undetected higher grade cancers if you look closely enough. Increasingly, biopsy is now targeted at areas suggested by the MPMRI rather than randomly throughout the gland as now.

PIN Prostatic Intraepithelial Neoplasia, needs follow up. ASAP, Atypical Small Acinar Proliferation suggests possible cancer and the need (unfortunately) for another biopsy.

So the higher the **Gleason Score** the worse the prognosis.
Thus:

4-5 mean survival	20 years
6	16
7	10
8-10	5

There is now a supposedly easier prognostic system that groups Gleason scores into **Prognostic Grade Groups** thus:

Gleason 1, 2, 3, 4, 5 and 6 become Prognostic Grade Group (PGG I)
Gleason 3+4 = 7 (PGG II)
Gleason 4+3 = 7 (PGG III)
Gleason 4+4 = 8 (PGG IV)
Gleason 9-10 (PGG V)

Gleason score		Proportion metastasising each year
2-4	Grade low	2%
5-7	medium	5%
8-10	high	13%.

Staging:

T1 in the prostate gland
T2 still in gland T2a only in 1/2 of 1 lobe
   T2b >1/2 of 1 lobe
   T2c in both lobes

T3 tumours are outside the "capsule" (although the prostate, strictly, does not have a capsule)

T3a through the capsule
T3b into seminal vesicles
T4 local spread e.g. to rectum or bladder or pelvic muscles-locally advanced.

Nodes:	Metastases:
Nx Nodes not checked	M0 No cancer outside the pelvis
N0 No local nodes affected	M1 Cancer outside pelvis
N1 Tumour in nodes	M1A Cancer in nodes outside pelvis
	M1B Cancer in bone
	M1C Cancer elsewhere.

The UCSF-CAPRA Score (Cancer of the prostate risk assessment score:)

Is an extremely useful way of calculating a man's risk of metastases, overall mortality and cancer specific mortality. It is a tool which may help reduce the negative effects of treatment on those who would never have died from their (relatively) benign screen detected cancer.

It rates age at diagnosis, PSA at diagnosis, Gleason score (primary/secondary), T stage and percent of cores positive for cancer.

It then gives a percentage risk which helps greatly in making an informed decision about (eg) declining or choosing prostatectomy or brachytherapy etc.

This can be accessed easily on the Internet just by Googling UCST-Capra (University of California San Francisco)

The Roach Formula is used to calculate the risk of pelvic node metastases

[2/3 X PSA + (Gleason Score – -6) X 10] This appears to over-estimate risk by 2-5X

Risk of local spread:

Go to the RADONC toolbox website and with the Pretreatment PSA and Gleason Score you get an estimate of **Extracapsular extension risk,** (3/2 X PSA) +[(GS-3) X 10]

Risk of **Seminal vesicle involvement** PSA +[(GS-6) X 10]

and **Lymph node involvement** (2/3*PSA) +[(GS-6) X 10] all calculated for you.

Multiparametric MRI **MPMRI** staging (using a "3 Tesla magnet") gives highly detailed prostate pictures, may soon give non invasive detailed prostate staging and gives good negative predictive value in lower Gleason Score disease (eg 4-6.) The lumbar spine is often visualised at the same time to exclude metastases.

There is growing evidence that the dangerous sub group of biopsy detected Gleason 6 tumours which are the therapeutic grey areas today do have unique genetic and biochemical signatures. Once these markers are simple requestable tests we will be able to differen-tiate the patients with genuine benign "prostate cancer" from those with cancer that will suddenly and unpredictably go wrong and clinically deteriorate.

Metabolism: Metabolic Syndrome is associated with low testosterone. Erectile function is a marker of cardiovascular health. LUTS (lower urinary tract symptoms) and ED are associated with DM, hypertension, metabolic syndrome and dyslipidaemia. Male visceral fat (like female buttock and thigh fat – brown fat) causes insulin resistance, hypertension, LUTS and other features of metabolic syndrome, being metabolically active converting testosterone to oestrogen and metabolising angiotensinogen.

Standard comparisons of the size of the prostate:

Most are Walnut sized 25-30mls but
A ping pong ball would be 33mls,
A golf ball 40mls,
An average Clementine 65mls,
and a tennis ball 130mls.

Drugs:

GnRH Analogues: {(**Things you may have forgotten:** Gonadotropin-releasing hormone analogues or agonists are synthetic types of hypothalamic gonadotropin releasing hormone that stimulate the release of FSH and LH. Usually after a hyper stimulation, there is a reduction in output of these hormones for as long as the analogue is given). Note: Gonadotropin-releasing hormone **antagonists** reduce LH and FSH levels and are used in IVF to stop endogenous ovulation}.

Most hormone dependent cancers become resistant to hormonal manipulation within 3 years.

Goserelin, Zoladex. 3.6mg and 10.8mg Depot (monthly or 3 monthly). LHRH analogue (also used in endometriosis and breast cancer. May need to use the anti androgen Cyproterone Acetate for 3 days before and 3 weeks after commencing treatment (Initial rise in testosterone and oestradiol). Average response 2 years.

Leuprorelin, Prostap 3.75 and 11.25mg depot (also in endometriosis and fibroids). Benefit is to all three stages of prostate cancer.

Flutamide is a potent anti-androgen used in advanced prostate cancer.

Bicalutamide, Casodex, adjuvant anti-androgen in advanced prostate cancer.

Also in some circumstances Stilboestrol, corticosteroids.

Abiraterone seems to have significant beneficial effects in advanced but also in early prostate cancer.

Management:

Watchful waiting. Slow progressing tumours, follow up in primary care. This is suitable for men likely to die but not from the prostate cancer. Palliative treatment is offered only if symptoms of prostate cancer develop.

Active surveillance, or active monitoring, watching PSA and symptoms in men with low risk cancer then re-biopsying and reassessing, avoids the problems and side effects of treatment in situations where the treatment itself may be worse than the condition. MPMRI is done at the start, the prostate is biopsied at 1 year and PSAs/PSA kinetics and DREs regularly performed. There is a NICE proforma. The follow up is by a urologist or oncologist. Usually younger patients with less aggressive cancers. About 40% of men with low risk cancer choose active surveillance. This can be typically 6 monthly PSAs, annual biopsy and a 2 yearly MRI. One third of these patients require treatment later and the risk is that the disease spreads, particularly locally. However if the disease progresses, the intention is to offer "radical treatment with curative intent". Patients have to have a confident and fatalistic mind set as they often lose their confidence and just want to "get rid of it" mid way through apparently. I can understand this.

Brachytherapy/Radiotherapy:

In organ confined disease, low to medium risk cancer, volume <60ccs, PSA <20, no obstruction, no previous TURP but it can cause a lot of urgency and frequency at first.

Seed implantation involves placing 50 – 100 tiny low dose radioactive seeds in the prostate. These are the width of a standard sewing needle (0.8mm) and 4.4mm long – so they are pretty small. They are canisters of Titanium containing radioactive Iodine 125. The half life of radioactive iodine is 60 days. Most of the radioactivity is released in 3 months but they are biologically active for a total of 9 months. This technique has been in use (2015) for up to 15 years. The seeds remain in the prostate and release radiation over a few months. They are effectively inactive between 4 and 6 months after insertion. Medium risk patients have the option of high dose rate brachytherapy which involves placing radioactive rods for a predetermined time in the prostate then removing them (all under one GA).

Minimum side effect profile. So Low dose brachytherapy – LDR is the permanent implantation of small radioactive seeds in the prostate, High dose brachytherapy, HDR is the insertion of catheters into the prostate through which the radioactive source is temporarily placed. This technique is used for less than Gleason Grade 7 tumours. An initial assessment by trans rectal USS is performed, a three dimensional computer model of the prostate and tumour is built up and the seeds inserted transperineally under GA. 80-120 seeds are usually implanted. 5% patients have acute retention shortly after insertion of the seeds. Most patients are given an Alpha blocker, an anti inflammatory and antibiotics after the procedure. 25% patients can experience ED subsequently. PSA is usually checked 3 monthly for a year, then 6 monthly. The PSA often bounces up between 6 months to 2 years.

Initially it is usually advised not to sleep with pregnant women, to use a condom (the first 3-4 times) just in case a seed is expelled (-a radioactive one), to avoid sitting next to pregnant women and to avoid sitting small children on your lap. In the event of cancer recurrence, a radical prostatectomy, cryotherapy, HIFU etc are all possible after brachytherapy treatment.

Urinary incontinence is a less than 1% complication, ED is less than with surgery or external beam DXT. Urinary symptoms do deteriorate for 6 months after treatment though. The seeds are titanium made radioactive with isotopes of palladium, Iodine, thulium (which gives Euro bank notes blue fluorescence in UV light) or iridium.

External Radiotherapy:

Radiotherapy aims to be a cure. Short term and long term side effects include bowel, bladder and sexual complications. Not usually recommended for patients with less than 10 years life expectancy. +/– hormones for locally advanced disease. eg 20-30mins, 5 days a week for 6-7 weeks. Neoadjuvant (preliminary) 6m then adjuvant (additional to the primary treatment) for 2 years. Pelvic DXT if >15% pelvic lymph node involvement risk. (See Roach formula.)

Focal Therapies:

(Which may be the middle ground between "Active surveillance" and Radical Prostatectomy) include:

High Intensity Focussed Ultrasound "HIFU" – Heating the prostate up, -fewer long term adverse effects it is said, but a bit early to give a definitive outlook on.

Focal Brachytherapy,

Focal Photodynamic Therapy,

Focal Electroporation,

Cryotherapy – Freezing the prostate.

Adjuvant therapy:

Used with radiotherapy for localised disease, in metastases and in the watchful waiting regime for men who develop symptoms of active disease: LHRH analogues, anti-androgens, etc.

Vascular Targeted photodynamic therapy (VTPD)

Came to public knowledge when a trial was announced in the national press as a breakthrough in prostate cancer therapy in December 2016. The treatment used a light activated "Free radical" toxin WST11, given intravenously. This was found in underwater bacteria that live in eternal darkness and then in the trial, lasers were introduced into the prostate to activate the toxin.

Unfortunately, the therapy left half the treated population with residual cancer and a quarter progressed within 2 years. 30% had a serious adverse event (19% in the control group) and a third experience ED. So at first sight not as clean and effective as the news reports were suggesting?

Surgery:

Robotic Da Vinci surgery:

Less blood loss and transfusion and ?**possibly** better oncological and functional results.

It is now thought that specialists need to have done at least 200 robotic prostatectomies to have gained adequate competence in the technique and the *reliability* of an open prostatectomy.

Radical Prostatectomy

Best for the young patient with a big prostate, a fast growing tumour, marked symptoms, possible previous TURP, low grade, low PSA. It involves removal of the prostate and seminal vesicles. Over half have ED (**far** fewer in some hands). 20% go on to have disease recurrence.

All ejaculate is lost though patients do continue to have orgasms during S/I.

	Watchful waiting	Active surveillance
No initial treatment	Yes	Yes
No treatment morbidity		
Ideal patient with localised disease	Unsuitable for curative treatment: elderly, unfit	Suitable for curative treatment, younger, fit
Treatment intention	Palliative	Curative
Typical F/U protocol	6 monthly clinical/PSA bone scans etc as requ'd	3 monthly PSA with kinetics, 6 monthly clinical review
Repeat prostate biopsy	No	Yes every 1-2 years and if indicated

Active surveillance follow up studies show death rates from prostate cancer at the 0-1% level.

So how do you advise your anxious patient with relatively localised prostate cancer?

Long term studies comparing radical surgery and radiotherapy haven't yet produced results. There is always "watchful waiting" although most patients interpret that as doing nothing. The NICE guidelines may be helpful and the wish to conceive may be relevant. Historically, now is not the best time to get prostate cancer as we simply don't yet have the data for best treatment option advice for all given stages, histologies, ages and patients. This is not true of, say, breast cancer or lung cancer.

The best you can do is offer the risks of each treatment and try and think what you would do in each situation. This is the classic well what would you do if you were me doctor? situation. The first two GP patients of mine with early prostate cancer I detected by high routine PSA screening opted for radical prostatectomy. But I am not sure everyone would want the potential complications of these procedures even with the promise of a probable complete cure. The last GP patient I had with a Gleason 3+4 (asymptomatic, PSA10) went for brachytherapy.

They all tell me they are very happy with the result.

PDE5 inhibitors work in 80% men with prostates but only 45% men who have had a radical prostatectomy.

Daily Tadalafil (Cialis) reaches a steady state in 4-5 days.

Metastatic Ca prostate:

LHRH, Intermittent androgen withdrawal, Casodex if men want to continue sex but need to use vacuum device and PDE5 tablets. Gynaecomastia and slightly lower survival rates.

Orchidectomy:

Chemotherapy with Docetaxel androgen withdrawal, steroids, Abiraterone, immuno-therapy, bisphosphonates.

So Possible options:

if in 60's, lots of symptoms, adv radical surgery?
No symptoms, adv brachytherapy.
In 70's with lots of symptoms adv DXT,
No symptoms adv brachytherapy.

Side effect risks of treatment:

Risks:	Incontinence,	Impotence.
Brachytherapy	<1%	10-50%
DXT	5%	30-60%
Surgery	2-12%	30-70%.

There are 15,000 new cases of prostate cancer a year in the UK (cf Breast 30,000, Cervix 3,000, Lung 45,500) Median survival with secondaries is 5 years.

The Difficult PSA Test:

The PSA is described as "**Persistent Stress and Anxiety**" by its discoverer (1970), Richard Ablin and "A profit driven public health disaster". Indeed, he actually co-wrote a book entitled "The Great Prostate Hoax: How big Medicine hijacked the PSA test and caused a public health disaster." He is against routine PSA testing and feels the American FDA should have resisted the test as a screening procedure. His four concerns (New Scientist February 2014) about PSA testing are: To quote him:

1) PSA is not "Cancer specific".
2) 4ng/ml or higher, the "worrying level" is arbitrary – as PSA is not cancer specific,

no level is "diagnostic".

3) Prostate cancer can be aggressive or, more often, very slow growing. We can't tell which is either clinically or from the PSA.

4) Many men will develop prostate cancer by age 70. If an older man has a PSA level that prompts a biopsy, it is likely you will find cancer. If you can't tell if its aggressive, many men will be treated unnecessarily and risk life altering side effects."

The facts: 1 in 26 (3.8%) men in England and Wales will die of prostate cancer but the incidence of prostate cancer is much higher at:

Age	20-29	30-39	40-49	50-59	60-69	70-79
Autopsy + prostate cancer	8%	28%	39%	53%	66%	80%

Prostate cancer incidence has shot up since the late 80's but the death rate has remained the same until recently. Meaning PSA is being used to present large numbers of "innocent" and "harmless" prostate cancers early which would in all likelihood not have killed the patient.

Even though it is the only public health screening test for the individual specifically available to men, the P.S.A. is not a reliable screening test. (See above and below). As you will see even the experts vary in their attitude to PSA testing on populations if not symptomatic individuals. Notwithstanding the current confusion surrounding interpretation of results, I offer testing to any male over 50 who requests it and to those younger with prostatic symptoms – but only after a lot of discussion. I then fervently hope it comes back low. Indeed you need to factor in the age, race and watch the trend, do total and free PSA, perform a digital rectal examination (obviously, even though this is unreliable) and do an MSU at the same time. It is possible that just **doing** a PSA might be the worst thing you could do for an asymptomatic patient as a raised level causes great anxiety in the doctor and patient and demands action. Having said that, numerous patients including three local doctors, patients of mine in their 50's, think I gave them retirements *above ground* by suggesting we check their PSA and finding their early cancers. This view is shared by many including the actor Ben Stiller who at 50 years old had a raised PSA (the test was done at his doctor's suggestion) and opted for a radical prostatectomy (The i 5/10/2016). Many raised PSAs are benign, many tumours being indolent and many investigations and treatments have a high morbidity. Undoubtedly though, some tests do pick up malignant tumours early.

One large study showed that screening via PSA did save lives but you had to screen 1,410 men to prevent 1 death from prostate cancer, that 48 men needed to be treated to prevent 1 death, there was a high rate of over diagnosis and 3 out of 4 biopsies were negative. Many feel the morbidly of screening, biopsying and treating healthy asymptomatic men outweighs the benefits. On the other hand, the death rate of prostate cancer presenting with advanced disease* (metastatic disease) has dropped since wide spread PSA testing has been performed in the USA. This is in the same time scale as mammography screening has been in use nationally. No comparable drop in the death rate of breast cancer presenting with advanced disease has occurred. But there is no clamour to save money by stopping mammography screening.

The new American Urology Association Guidelines Are:

No PSA screening under age 40.

No routine screening for average risk men 40-54 yrs old.

Between 55 and 69 years make a shared decision on whether to do a blood test.

No routine screening over age 70 or on any man with less than 10-15 years life expectancy.

In the UK the advice seems to be: do the first PSA around 45 unless there is a strong FH.

If PSA >1.0, then regularly screen til age 70 (above average risk.)

if PSA <1.0, then repeat PSA in early 50s and at age 60 and do no other tests.

By the way: A single PSA <1 in a man's 60s largely rules out **clinically significant** prostate cancer ever.

STOP PRESS:* In November 2015 the beleaguered PSA was given a boost by the NEJM which looked at metastatic breast and prostate cancer incidence following widespread use of mammography since 1985 and PSA testing since the 1990's. It turns out that prostate metastatic disease had dropped 50% within 7 years of the start of PSA screening but breast metastatic disease had not been affected by mammography.

As you can see it is a very difficult area generally and one that demands a good familiar, open, informal doctor/patient relationship, a fair bit of thought and time. Also and I hardly dare I say it, from my own and other doctors' patient feedback, I believe it is one of the situations that sometimes benefits from the ability of the patient to talk to a *male* GP. It is impossible, of course, to refuse a worried patient a PSA test and stupid to refuse a symptomatic patient one. Before over-reacting to a raised PSA, however, my experience suggests trying a prostate – effective antibiotic (Norfloxacin, Co Amoxiclav Doxycycline) for at least 10 days, probably up to 4 weeks and waiting another 1-2 weeks before repeating the PSA. This is because prostatitis (interestingly the spell checker wants this to be corrected to "prostitutes"!) is a common cause of a raised PSA, lower urinary tract and prostate symptoms, AND (transrectal) prostate biopsy is **very** unpleasant and sometimes permanently damages the prostate.

More on PSA:

A (August 2014) major study on PSA was not very helpful in clarifying this conundrum either:

Published in the Lancet, it concerned 162,000 European men studied for 13 years and it found that screening saved one life per 781 men regularly screened over this time The writers said that the risks of treatment side effects and over diagnosis outweighed the benefits of mass screening though.

The European Randomised Study of Screening for Prostate Cancer recruited men aged 50-74 and they either had 4 yearly PSA screening or not. They were biopsied at over 3 ng/ml PSA. After 13 years there were 13,500 cancers. Screened men had a 27% lower risk of dying from prostate cancer than the control group. Screened men were less likely to develop advanced prostate cancer. The screening reduced deaths from prostate cancer at a level similar to that of breast cancer screening however there was an over diagnosis of 40%. I can't help wondering whether there is a degree of sexism in the decision not to screen men using PSA and to let *them* make the decision about treatment especially since the rate of death reduction **in this study** was similar to that other controversial, national but female, breast cancer screening campaign.

Indeed by May 2015 the American Urological Association was saying it disagreed with the US preventative Services Task Force's new advice against widespread screening as there had been a potential increase in aggressive cancers as a consequence.

STOP STOP PRESS:

In July 2015 in an article on line in the American Journal of Clinical Oncology, Jonathan Shoag et Al from NY Presb Hosp also argue that the evidence now shows that PSA testing does reduce prostate cancer mortality and they call for a return to screening, albeit not a population-wide annual PSA testing. Instead, they proposed that all men should undergo at least baseline PSA testing in their 40s or early 50s (except for individuals with a limited life expectancy). Subsequent screening after that would be tailored to individualized risk according "to schedules put forth in newer screening guidelines." "The rapid uptake of PSA screening followed by its equally rapid decline in the United States has been analogized to a pendulum swinging back and forth," they comment. They warn that "reversion back to the pre-PSA era in recent years will translate into more prostate cancer deaths in the United States."

Yet more PSA background:

The American National Comprehensive Cancer Network had updated its screening advice, seeking a middle ground approach (2014) before the American Urological Association expressed concern about an increase in aggressive cancer rates (2015).

They proposed routine screening on all healthy men from 45-70 years.

The American Urology Association had suggested routine screening 55-69 years of age.

On the other hand,

The US Preventative Services Task Force recommended not testing PSAs in healthy men.

The ANCC has, despite casting its testing net further, supported conservative, active surveillance rather than definitive treatment in "early, low risk disease" (half of PSA detected cancers they say are low risk).

European studies looked at regular screening from the age of 55, not 45 but there was also a large Swedish study which did one test before around 45 and used the result to predict the next 30 years cancer risk. This baseline PSA result is more significant than family history or ethnicity in giving prostate prognosis. If the first test is "below the median" you do another aged 50 but you do 6 monthly or annual testing for those above the median.

The median PSAs are 0.7ng/ml between 40-49 yrs
and   0.9ng/ml between 50 and 59 yrs.
At least annual tests are done for everyone with a result >**1.0ng/ml.**

This is controversial as these levels are pretty low and a lot of young men are going to be worried and biopsied unnecessarily. Also, we don't know whether it makes any difference to the outcome, detecting and treating what may be fairly benign cancers five years later – (50 rather than 45)

Also when do you stop PSA testing?

PSA testing should only be offered to men with a life expectancy >10 years. The American Urology Association doesn't think screening >70 years is sensible, but the NCCN suggests we stop screening at 69 or continue screening to 74yrs but biopsying only if the PSA is >3ng/ml !!

This is an excessively low level to biopsy at any age in my opinion and I tend to agree with the American Urologists (who presumably have to do the biopsies and deal with the frequent complications) who suggest a biopsy threshold of 10ng/ml.

So as you can see even the experts are far from agreed on a uniform approach to dealing with the pesky PSA.

(American National Comprehensive Cancer Network 19th Annual Conference 14/3/14)

The Contemporary Australian View (2014):

The most up to date Australian advice on repeating (and repeated) PSA testing is that between age 50 and 69, after discussion, you should do the test two yearly. If the patient is black or has a positive family history start testing age 45, don't routinely do a DRE as part of your initial assessment (!) if the patient has no symptoms. The DRE is reserved for urologists pre-biopsy. The Prostate Cancer Foundation of Australia also says that the first PSA should not be used as a comparison (or baseline) for subsequent tests. Each test should be seen in isolation (unless there is a clear cut unremitting and progressive rise I assume). So much for the PSA trends of previous guidelines.

So what to do about PSA screening in the real world?

If the patient is asymptomatic, don't do it. Between the ages of 55 and 70, screening would pick up cancer in 1.7%. There is no potential benefit and considerable harm. 90% of the cancers detected would not have caused any harm anyway.

On the other hand if a patient presents with lower urinary tract symptoms **or they ask you**, it is wise to check the PSA. A DRE and PSA are said to pick up 75% of prostatic cancers and what other public health screening do men get?

Less screening in the real world has seen an initial "lower incidence" (lower detection rate) of prostate cancer, followed subsequently by an increase in secondaries and deaths from prostate cancer. Exactly what you would expect if mass PSA screening **were saving a significant number of lives** irrespective of the collateral damage it may cause.

The transrectal prostate biopsy

This consists of a transrectal examination, (TRUS), the introduction of an ultrasound probe and a long needle per rectum for the local anaesthetic. The prostate "capsule" is VERY pain sensitive and the whole procedure can be very unpleasant. The infiltration of the local and biopsy are through the anterior rectal wall and the prostate pseudo-capsule and it hurts. Then a biopsy gun is introduced, which fires off at least a dozen times, reaming out cores of prostate and rectal wall and each time it fires it is more anticipated by the patient and painful than the last. This is all done in the X Ray department as it needs to be under ultrasound control (so the gun misses the prostatic urethra). I think it is all pretty barbaric. Many of my patients expressed their dislike to me (which would no doubt be dismissed out of hand were it to be expressed to the hospital) that it was performed by a young female radiologist. There are portable ultrasound probes which could be used in theatre and I have myself given many safe, short anaesthetics to patients undergoing procedures in the X Ray department. A general anaesthetic would seem to be safe and far more humane. I was told a prostate biopsy couldn't be done under a G.A. because it needed to be in X Ray and was safer done under hit and miss local anaesthetic. Rubbish.

The imaging technique, the multiparametric (mp) MRI should help find any tumour and localise it prior to biopsy. It is increasingly available in the UK. A third of TRUS detected cancer is currently misclassified and up to 30% missed altogether. Up to 6% of victims of biopsy get a serious urinary infection. The PROMIS trial is currently assessing mpMRI and any technique that rationalises, focuses and reduces unnecessary biopsies has to be welcomed.

The diet, supplements and prostate cancer and alternative treatments:

At the AGM of The American Society of Clinical Oncology in 2013 the results of a placebo controlled, double blinded trial of "natural compounds" in the treatment of refractory prostate cancer patients was presented. A supplement containing pomegranate seed, broccoli, green tea and turmeric (the active agent is curcumin), all of which are believed to have significant anti inflammatory, antioxidant and anti cancer effects, resulted in a 64% mean reduction in PSA levels in these patients. This is better than almost any published conventional treatment. Never dismiss the alternative treatments your cancer patients will probably ALL be taking. They want to take any chance however slim. None of them will be telling their trial doctors that they are taking Curcumin, Vitamin D, Metformin, Vitamin K, lycopene, Omega 3, Selenium, Boron, and so on. They don't want to be excluded from the conventional trials. Many of my patients go to alternative treatment centres which administer high dose Vitamin C, hyperthermia, low dose Naltrexone, Minocycline, Metformin or other retasked prescription drugs etc. They are run by ex London teaching hospital trialist oncologists who just tell the patients not to mention their alternative treatments to other doctors. Their focus is the patient's survival, the trial doctor's focus are the trial statistics.

In another study, patients in between transrectal biopsy and radical prostatectomy (based on the biopsy result) were placed on "large doses" (10,000 Us) of Vitamin D. The vitamin D prevented clinical deterioration of the cancers and reduced Gleason scores.

PSA from various sources:

P.S.A. can be confusing:
PSA >4.0, 75% patients do not have ca prostate,
PSA 4.0, misses 15% cancers,
PSA 4-10, Ca risk is 22%,
PSA >10, Ca risk 67%,
Put another way:

PSA <0.	6.6% prostate cancer risk (!),
0.6-1.0	10.1%,
1.1-2.0	17.0%,
2.1-3.0	23.9%,
3.1-4.0	26.9%,
Age	Range "ULN"
40-49	2.5ng/ml,
50-59	3.5ng/ml,
60-69	4.5ng/ml,
70-79	6.5ng/ml.

Free and bound PSA: In BPH free PSA goes up. In prostate Ca, bound PSA goes up.
So Free/Total: >0.25 low probability of cancer,
<0.15 greater possibility of cancer.
The ratio is usually used to determine the need for a second biopsy if the first was negative and the PSA is creeping up.

Overactive bladder

(L.U.T.S., Lower urinary Tract Symptoms – Detrusor Instability, Urge incontinence etc).

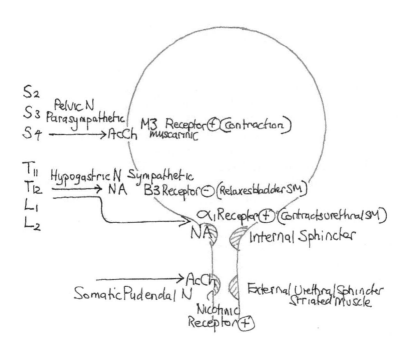

Diagram (IOB 1): (Bladder Innervation/Receptors).

There is a huge number of treatments for OAB but remember to exclude bladder outflow tract obstruction as a cause of frequency in men, – as anticholinergic drugs may precipitate acute retention. Always document an abdominal examination (noting an absent bladder fundus) and exclude UTI. In children make sure you are not missing constipation, UTI or a neurological cause (check the lumbo-sacral spine and legs neurologically etc).

When the bladder is full, the detrusor generally contracts for *only* 40 seconds although it may **feel** like a lot longer when the bladder is at capacity. The detrusor relaxation period then varies depending on the severity of the OAB and also the rate of the bladder filling. Mild OAB patients can put off a voiding contraction for 15 – 30 minutes. In more severe OAB it can be only a few minutes and these patients will need medication.

Treatments include:

Oxybutynin, Cystrin, Ditropan, Lyrinel XL etc. 2.5-5mg BD/TDS (in children>5yrs, try stopping medication every 4 months).

Kentera is an Oxybutynin patch which lasts 3-4days.

Darifenecin, Emselex 7.5-15mg OD.

Propiverine, Detrunorm 15mg BD. TDS. (Calcium antagonist and anticholinergic).

Tolterodine, Detrusitol 1-2mg BD. 4mg XL OD, Mariosea, Santizor, Neditol.

Trospium, Regurin 20mg BD, (Flotros etc). This is generally the one I try first.
Fesoterodine, Toviaz. 4-8mg OD.
Solifenacin, Vesicare. Anticholinergic, avoid in outflow tract obstruction 5-10mg OD.

Distigmine, Ubretid is used for post op retention and neurological bladder only. (An anticholinesterase, a parasympathomimetic, stimulating detrusor contraction to empty the bladder. So the opposite of the above drugs which are anticholinergic and reduce bladder detrusor activity.)

Duloxetine: An SNRI (This comes as Yentreve 40mg BD for stress incontinence and Cymbalta 30-120mg OD for anxiety/Depression). Improves the strength of the urethral sphincter.
CCBs,
TCAs,
Mirabegron, Betmiga. B3 adrenoceptor agonist (relaxation stimulator – reduces detrusor activity) can be co-prescribed c anticholinergics.

NICE currently recommend:

Diagram OAB 2

Adapted from NICE Guidelines 2015

Tolterodine or Oxybutynin (not in the frail elderly woman)   If anti muscarinics are C/I
immediate release tabs or transcutaneous Oxybutynin
patches

If not tolerated or ineffective

Tolterodine MR   If patient not willing to
Trospium MR   take another
Fesoterodine MR   antimuscarinic
Darifenacin

Review after 6 months

Mirabegron MR Tabs

"Solifenacin not recommended"

(Diagram OAB 2)

Investigations of the urogenital Tract:
DMSA Isotope scan: Parenchymal abnormalities in cortices – for scarring.
MAG III Isotope Renogram: A dynamic scan, tells about urinary flow out of the kidney and to the bladder.
USS assesses renal pelvic dilatation, – only 1cm limit being the threshold for investigation in infancy.

Note: Age 4 is the most vulnerable age for infection scarring (excluded by DMSA).
So: A suggested regime of investigations/management would be:
<1 year with UTI, Micturating cystogram + USS.
1-4 years   Micturating cystogram or prophylactic antibiotics until out of nappies
>4 years   MAG 111 cystography for vesico-ureteric reflux.

Peyronie's Disease:

Up to 10% men apparently (?) plaques of thickening in the Tunica Albuginea, the surrounding membrane of the Corpora Cavernosa, resulting in a bent erect penis. There are associated connective tissue disorders and these may involve the hands or feet.

Avoid BBs and CCBs as Peyronie's may be caused or exacerbated by these. Various treatments: Traction, Viagra, Co Enzyme Q10, "High dose anti oxidants" (?) Vitamin E, Tamoxifen and NSAIDs have been tried. In more persistent cases, Nesbit's operation or laceration of the plaque (Leriche Technique) can help.

Foreskins in adults:

At the age of 17, 99% can retract.
(50% by 1 year, 75% by 2 years, 90% by 3 years).

Balanitis Xerotica Obliterans

BXO-The epidermis of the foreskin atrophies with areas of hyperkeratosis. The foreskin becomes non retractile and erections are painful. White scarring of the foreskin CAN be premalignant in adults.

A paraphimosis is when a retracted foreskin gets stuck. The longer it is left, the more oedema and the more likely a reduction under a short GA will be needed.

Circumcision:

The vast majority of circumcisions performed in the world have no medical justification. Prophylactic circumcision is never justified given the increasingly apparent harm that the procedure seems to cause. Infection, scarring, bleeding and surgical complication are obvious and often immediate. But not invariably so. Research over a number of years has also linked circumcision to

1) A life-long reduction in pain threshold. Individual pain level settings are adjusted early on in life and adapted to what the developing brain receives as early sensory input. For hundreds of thousands of boys circumcision will be the first and only seriously painful experience in their early years and given the rich sensory nerve supply of the foreskin, an agonising one which continues for several days or weeks. Anyone who has nursed a child who has undergone a therapeutic circumcision knows what the post operative pain can be like for several weeks as nappies or dressings are removed or changed.

2) Linked to this is a study that relates circumcision to autism (ASD). (M. Frisch, Aalborg Univ doi: 10. 1177/0141076814565942 JRSM). This is not the first time a link has been queried but in Jan 2015 a paper looking at 340,000 Danish children who had been circumcised was published. The risk of developing Autistic Spectrum Disorder before the age of 10 years was doubled by the procedure. Perhaps the inflicting of severe pain at such a vulnerable early stage of emotional and neurological development not only affects the pain threshold but causes some boys to resort to a degree of reactionary permanent emotional withdrawal. There is a relationship between a country's level of circumcision and the level of Autistic spectrum disorder, as well as animal studies which link painful

early injuries to lifelong deficits in stress response. This was according to the authors (J of RSM). It would be interesting to see if perinatal painful accidents and injuries have the same lifelong sequelae.

3) The neonatal foreskin is supplied with, except for the cornea, the most dense and sensitive sensory nerve endings in the body. Its job is to protect the prepuce and prevent that delicate surface drying, thickening and becoming insensitive. It also acts as a main sensory input for the male during sexual foreplay. This isn't possible if it has been cut off and sexual pleasure (if adults who have undergone circumcision are to be believed) is nowhere near as stimulating.

What does circumcision benefit the recipient? Presumably large scale male circumcision, which was first recorded over 4000 years ago in desert communities of the middle east was to prevent balanitis in the absence of running water and easily accessible hygiene. I imagine a chronic preputial infection in the ancient Middle East would have been a bit of a disaster – so a simple prophylactic surgical procedure at birth must have started amongst the communities living there. Then it was adopted by Judaism and Islam both of which incorporated it into ritual and still practice it. I understand that newborn Jewish baby boys whose two brothers have already died due to the process are exempted. Presumably because of haemophilia or a similar bleeding disorder. The health benefits often quoted of reduced infections and penile cancer would only apply in the presence of a tight phimosis, the absence of retractable foreskins and the absence of running water.

A judge in the first Female Genital Mutilation case in the UK (Jan 2015) said any form of FGM amounts to "serious harm" for the purpose of care proceedings. Later it was officially described as a form of "Child Abuse". Many think the same applies to male circumcision – which is more invasive than type 4 FGM. For a care order to be made however, the local council must prove that the harm is attributable to parental care that is **not what a parent would be reasonably expected to give.**(Judge James Munby 2015.) So male circumcision is child abuse but if you come from a community that habitually does it – then it isn't. If that makes rational sense then you are a lawyer not a doctor. This ruling also clearly contradicts the High Court's ruling on Good Practice in Medicine. You may remember (See legal section) that twenty years ago we all used to rely upon the Bolam defence that if we gave advice or treatment that harmed a patient but it was what most doctors in the same situation would do then we were protected by the law?

Then the High Court changed that general rule and made it a "Best Interest of the patient rule".(Commonly held and *responsible*) Well surely circumcision, whether or not it is normally done by a parent within a particular community is never in the best interests of the patient? Shouldn't the same rule apply?

Prostatitis – a common cause of a raised PSA

Acute Prostatitis:

Not usually sexually transmitted. Dysuria, frequency, urgency, low back and suprapubic pain. Very tender prostate PR.

The MSU often shows the organism. Treatment a quinoline antibiotic, broad spectrum penicillin (Co Amoxiclav) or combination treatment or trimethoprim for a month.

Chronic Prostatitis:

Causes chronic pelvic pain, (CPP Syndrome) affects erectile function can present as "recurrent UTIs" and other urinary symptoms. Rx Alpha blockers eg: Tamsulosin,

NSAIDs, Quinolines, (Ciprofloxacin, Norfloxacin) given for 2-4 weeks, sometimes for a further 2-4 weeks. With or without alpha blockers or anti inflammatories. This duration of broad spectrum antibiotic treatment upsets the gut "Biome" for months.

Use of 5-alpha reductase inhibitors and phosphodiesterase type 5 inhibitors, such as tadalafil, have been proposed, but there is no evidence base for these at present.

If the pain is neuropathic, try Gabapentin, Amitriptyline, Duloxetine.

Prostatitis is the commonest urological diagnosis in men. (15% lifelong prevalence – some articles say 30-50% lifelong prevalence).

Some urologists define three types of prostatitis:

Type 1: Acute Bacterial. Gram Negative (may need admission for treatment, – quinolines, Co Amoxiclav).

Type 2: Chronic Bacterial: Recurrent UTIs associated. Needs 4 weeks treatment.

Type 3: Chronic pelvic pain syndrome: The commonest reason for a young man to see a urologist. Not chlamydial, not bacterial (Is this ureaplasma?) Either way it is an inflammatory reaction, a type IV hypersensitivity reaction. All men apparently reflux urine into the prostate and the chronic inflammation that this can cause may over time lead to neoplastic change.

Rye pollen extract can be tried or alternatively Quercetin, a flavonoid in plums, capers, dill and watercress etc which is said via its anti inflammatory effects to improve chronic prostatitis. You can buy supplements of this anti oxidant, anti inflammatory and it is said like many other flavonoids to have multiple health benefits. I cannot vouch for the prostate claims of these alternative treatments.

Chronic Kidney Disease:

This is a new concept, "invented" in 2002 in America. The arbitrary eGFR of 60 results in defining 1:8 adults as having chronic kidney disease. A Norwegian study showed fewer than 1% of people with Stage 3a CKD actually had end stage renal failure after 8 years.

eGFR:

CKD Staging: >90 stage 1
60-90 stage 2
30-60 stage 3
15-30 stage 4
<15 stage 5

60-90ml/min Normal unless proteinuria, haematuria, diabetes with microalbuminuria or PCO or reflux nephropathy.

<60ml/min Assess rate of deterioration, medication, test for prot (+>do urine prot/creat ratio) and blood. Assess clinically, BP, CCF repeat eGFR etc.

REFER if stage 1 or 2 with malignant hypertension, K>7mmol/L, Nephrotic Syndrome, proteinuria +/− haematuria, diabetic proteinuria, macroscopic haematuria, rapid fall in eGFR or recurrent pulmonary oedema.

If stage 3 with above plus microscopic haematuria, proteinuria, anaemia, abnormal electrolytes, other disease

(SLE, vasculitis, Myeloma) severe hypertension.
If stage 4 or 5 without terminal illness.

Management: All stages: Do: BP eGFR, Prot/creat ratio, annually. Give cardiovascular prophylaxis (aspirin, statins). Ensure meticulous BP management and Rx, (especially ACEI, ARB if DM or proteinuria). Check for renal artery stenosis, stop NSAIDS, reduce salt, K retaining diuretics, ACEIs and ARBs if raised K.

Stage 3: Do Hb, K, Ca, phosphate six monthly. Refer for IV iron if Hb low. Renal USS. Review drugs, check Parathormone.

Stages 4 and 5: Check HCO3 and PTH three monthly. Advise on diet, check Hep B immunity, referral regarding Parathyroid, acidosis, treatment options, ??Dialysis etc.

Alternative algorithm CKD stages 3-5:

Bloods: Hb, U and Es, Inorg P, Gluc,.......If eGFR <20 or <30 in a diabetic............Refer
Lipids and PTH if stage 4 or 5..........

                                        :
                                        :
                            :.....If Hb<10.5, K>6, Ca<2.1, PO4 1.5,
                                        PTH>11.....Refer*

All patients:	Stage 3	Stage 4
Blood Pressure: Treat >140/90,	6 monthly eGFR annual Hb	Can Discuss with nephrologist
Aim for 130/80	Annual K Ca PO4 PTH	3 monthly eGFR to start
125/75 if Prot'uria>100mg/mmol	Renal USS if persistent raised BP	6 monthly when stable
ACEI or ARB if microalb/proteinuria	or lower urinary tract sympts.	6 monthly Hb, K, Ca, PO4, PTH
/heart failure. But in DM with	Half dose Metformin if eGFR <45	Renal tract USS
microalb use ACEI/ARB whatever the BP	Refer if progressive, eGFR incr>4	Consider stopping Metformin in
Refer if 3 drugs and still >150/90	/yr, or <50 in a patient <50 yrs or *	DM
Treat hyperlipidaemia and give aspirin		Refer if Diabetic, eGFR<20,
(>20% 10 yr risk) as appropriate		progressive (>4 incr in GFR/yr)
Flu and pneumo vaccinations		Bloods as *
Review meds, avoid NSAIDS		

Notes: If eGFR<30, stop diuretic before starting ACEI/ARB: Check U and Es 2 weeks after changing dose, starting or increasing diuretics. Any increase >20% of creatinine, D/W the Nephrologist and recheck in 2 weeks to make sure it isn't continuing to rise. If K>6 stop ACEI, and give low K diet.

Proteinuria: Significance (ie in Diabetes Mellitus)

	Spot Albumin mg/l	Albumin excretion mg/24hrs	Albumin creatinine ratio ACR mg/mmol
Normal	<30	<30	<2.5 (M) <3.5 (F)
Microalbuminuria	30-300	30-300	2.5-30 (M) 3.5-30 (F)
Clinical proteinuria (macroalbuminuria)	>300	>300	>30

Kidney Stones:

"Red flag" features which warrant further investigation:
First episode <25 yrs,

Recurrent stones,

Bilateral, multiple stones or nephrocalcinosis.

Family history,

eGFR<60,

Non-calcium oxalate stones,

Radiolucent stones (urate or cystine?)

Stones associated with medical condition such as IBD*, Gastric Bypass Surgery, Metabolic Syndrome.

*Inflammatory bowel disease.

Investigations:

U and Es, Ca++, PO4, Mg, 25OHVitD, uric acid, Parathormone, urine pH, 24 Hr urinary calcium, oxalate, citrate, sodium, (and creatinine to assess completeness when comparing repeated 24hr collections).

It is said that calcium supplementation for osteoporosis will uncover approximately 5% of your patient population who have idiopathic hypercalciuria via the formation of renal stones.

Most patients who form recurrent stones should be advised to drink more water, eat more fruit and vegetables to increase citrate excretion and this dissolves calcium stones.

Reduced animal protein plus adequate calcium reduces urine oxalate.

Thiazides reduce stone formation in hypercalciuric patients, Potassium Citrate and added bicarbonate alkalinise the urine and help dissolve uric acid, cystine and calcium oxalate stones. Too alkaline and the urine can precipitate out calcium phosphate stones though.

Renal colic:

Is said to be the worst pain there is and requires powerful and regular analgesia. Commonly used pain relief includes Diclofenac injection and suppositories and Pethidine tablets and injection.

It can also be treated with Desmopressin intranasally given acutely which reduces the need for pethidine by half. This is thought to be by reducing diuresis but it does seem slightly counter intuitive given the intermediate and longer term need to "flush" the stone out.

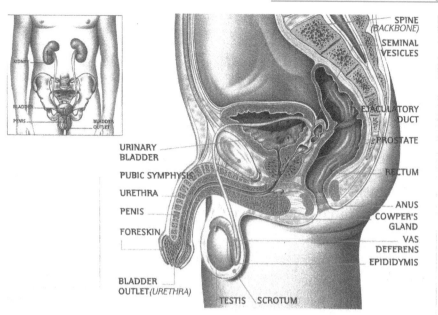

Useful Diagrams: Usual Male Anatomy and the Testicle, Anatomy for patients

(MG1, 2 and 3)

40: WORK:

Some basic work regulations:

1993 New Regulations on General Health and Safety Management, Work Equipment Safety, Manual Handling of Loads, Workplace Conditions, Personal Protective Equipment (PPE), Display Screen Equipment, -E.E. Directive "Six Pack."

Employers had to analyse workstations and reduce risks, ensure workstations reached minimum requirement (brightness and contrast controls had to upgrade). Work to be planned with appropriate breaks and changes. On request to arrange eye tests and provide special glasses where appropriate. Provide basic health and safety training related to the workstation (chair adjustment etc).

COSHH (2002)

Control of substances harmful to health. These regulations cover anything harmful from liquids and solids to dusts and vapours, gases and infectious agents. The regulations do not cover lead, asbestos or radioactivity – which have their own regulations.

The Health and Safety Executive have a selection of free publications on all COSHH matters.

Surveillance of work related occupational respiratory diseases (SWORD.)

Air intake for an average person is assumed to be 10 cu M during an 8 hr day.

Allergic alveolitis,

Asthma eg Di-isocyanates etc.

Bronchitis,

Building related disease, (Including Sick Building Syndrome).

Byssinosis,

Infectious disease,

Inhalation accidents,

Lung cancer,

Mesothelioma, (see Respiratory for asbestos related disease).

Non malignant pleural disease,

Pneumoconiosis etc.

Occupational Disease Reporting:

Asthma,

Pneumoconiosis,

Other non cancer respiratory disease,

Noise induced hearing loss,

Upper limb disorder, (WRULD – Work Related Upper Limb Disorder which used to be called RSI – Repetitive Strain Injury). WRULD is said to be commoner in patients who are depressed or who are unfulfilled at work. It is certainly rarer in self employed gardeners and musicians than you would expect. My worst two cases were a lab technician whose job was repeated pipetting with her hands above shoulder level. She was being investigated for infertility at the time she presented. Also a successful bass guitarist in a Thin Lizzie cover band who had absolutely intractable tennis elbow.

Dermatitis.

Back problems.

Stress/Depression.
Circulatory, including Vibration White Finger.
Headache, migraine, eye strain.
Cancer.

Health and Safety legislation is enforced by inspectors from the Health and Safety Executive, (The H.S.E.) or by Environmental Health Officers, (E.H.O.s) from Local Authority Environmental Health Departments.

Patients who suffer serious injury at work or who develop certain occupational diseases can claim industrial injury benefit under The Social Security Act 1975.

The Health and Safety Executive have an Employment Medical Advisory Service, (E.M.A.S.) staffed by doctors, to advise employers, employees and G.P.s and is confidential.

The Access to Medical reports act 1988 applies to GP-to-employer reports but not to reports to EMAS or to the specialist disability service of the employment service.

Hearing regulations: Noise at Work:

Noise at work Regulations 2005:
(A is average noise exposure, C is peak noise exposure):

	Average level of exposure	Peak sound pressure
Lower exposure limit	80db (A)	135db(C)
Upper exposure limit	85db (A)	137db(C)
Exposure limit value	87db(A)	140db(C)

More than 80 db average and the employer must provide a risk assessment, information and training. Over 85db (A) and there must be hearing protection and "hearing zones". 87db is the average level to which workers should not be exposed.

Reporting of Injuries Diseases and Dangerous Occurrences Regulations 1995, RIDDOR

This obliges employers, managers and responsible persons to report all the above occurrences that take place *in relation to work*. Interestingly, doctors' own patients, (accidents during medical or dental treatment or accidents during any examination carried out or supervised by a doctor or dentist) are exempt. Therefore I assume we don't have to report our own patients who happen to die during or because of treatment. RTAs (road accidents) and the armed forces are exempt though I assume we would be expected to report a colleague's death in an industrial accident at the surgery or folliculitis from contact with tar containing compounds on the skin of psoriatic patients? Other areas such as Nuclear Installations, Merchant Shipping, Radiation Accidents, Civil Aviation and some Electrical Accidents have other reporting mechanisms.

Occupational Asthma:

Very many causes including:
Isocyanates,
Flour,
Grain,
Wood dust,
Glutaraldehyde,
Solder,
Colophony,

Laboratory Animals,
Resins,
Glues,
Latex.

Pilots at work:

Must have a BP<160/95,
and are grounded with hypertension if started on centrally acting agents, adrenergic blocking drugs, alpha blockers, loop diuretics.

There must be no evidence of coronary Ischaemia, epilepsy, primary or secondary malignant disease likely to interfere with the safe performance of their duties etc etc.

I won't give the whole list but it is longer than the DVLA medical list – and so it should be, if you think of the dangers consequent to losing control of and crashing a plane.

Look it up on the C.A.A, website under "Medical" and the banned conditions are listed with all the relevant guidance. I have had many pilot patients. I have had problems with depressed pilots who were unwilling to take antidepressants as this would ("Establish their mood disorder") and disqualify them from flying during treatment despite the fact that they would thus improve much quicker. We all heard with shock and disbelief about the German Wings suicide-mass murder of pilot Andreas Lubitz. He flew his full plane into a mountain having locked the co pilot out of the cock pit. He was known to be depressed and to have "suicidal tendencies". He was declared unfit for work by a doctor but did not tell his employer. I have had pilots who deferred admitting episodes of faintness, palpitations and chest tightness as they knew they would instantly be grounded and so continued flying 300 customers across the Atlantic and back for months rather than address their own potentially serious health issues. Even though they were probably unfit to fly, they were unwilling to undertake effective investigation, treatment and admit it to their employers – a bit of a dangerous Catch 22.

Contact Dermatitis:

From Plants: Phytophotodermatitis-due to Psoralens (Just like those used in Psoriasis) which photosensitise the skin to UVA radiation. Sunblock and topical steroids help and absolute avoidance in the future. Present in many plants including:

Hogweed,
Cow Parsnip,
Celery,
Rue,
Various weeds,
Parsley,
Daisy,
Chrysanthemums,
Dandelion,
Lettuce,
Colophony in Pine,
Cypressus Leylandii,
Angelica,
Fennel, Dill, Anise, Lime, Lemon, Bergamot (as in Earl Grey Tea), Fig, Mustard, Wild Carrot etc.

Occupational causes of skin disease (80% of occupational skin disease is dermatitis) are legion but include:
Cobalt,
Nickel,
Formaldehyde,
Epoxy Resins,
Engineering oils and greases,
Cutting fluid,
Plant psoralens,
Latex,
Epoxies,
Resins,
Chromium and chromates (Cement),
Aromatic amines,
Coal tar distillation products (creosote, pitch etc),
Chloronaphthalenes, chlorodi-phenyls, chlorotriphenyls, hexachlorodibenzo-p-dioxin, tetrachloroazoxybenzene and tetrachlorodibenzodioxin, (TCDD), (Acne).
Any occupation that causes sweating etc.

Work related chest disease:

Again there are multiple causes,
Asthma and respiratory diseases may be caused by dusts, mould spores, fumes, resins, colophony, soldering, exhaust, isocyanates, laboratory animals, the dust and dander of a variety of farm and other animals, insects, flour, grain, latex, wood and MDF dust, aldehydes, (Glutaraldehyde), glues, resins, paints, solvents, perfumes, drugs, almost any breathable dust, fume or solvent in inhaled air.

Returning to work after surgery:

Vasectomy	)Usually no time off if uncomplicated
Varicose vein injections	)
PNS (provided patient can be released for regular dressings) (pilonidal sinus)	)If uninfected and wound "manageable".
Unilateral inguinal hernia or femoral hernia, appendicectomy	Two weeks for sedentary workers, four weeks for heavy workers. – Review if the appendix perforated or there were complications. Some may

	return earlier to a light job after a laparoscopic procedure.
Bilateral inguinal hernias, umbilical hernias (other than large ones),	) Four weeks sedentary workers
Incisional hernias (other than large ones)	) Six weeks heavy workers.
Gastric and duodenal surgery, femoro-popliteal grafts	) Four weeks sedentary workers) Twelve weeks heavy workers.
Open cholecystectomy, abdominal or vaginal hysterectomy large incisional or umbilical hernias, redo of inguinal hernia repair open colectomy, aortoiliac and aortic grafts, CABG, heart valve surgery, nephrectomy,	) six weeks)sedentary workers) twelve weeks) heavy workers.
Simple mastectomy	When the wound has healed
Varicose vein ligation, anal fistula	Two weeks
Haemorrhoidectomy, TURP	Four weeks.
Retinal detachment surgery	Avoid heavy manual labour forever.
Arthroscopic partial meniscectomy (etc)	May need no time off if sedentary, up to a couple of weeks if heavy manual work.

There is a superb web site resource for all things in General Practice that are work related: **www.Working fit.co.uk**

With their permission here is some of their advice to use in negotiating time off (-you can always suggest less) or when the patient should aim to get back to work. This of course depends as much on mood, mental state, enjoyment of the job, team support, family and home circumstances as it does the medical or surgical condition. The self employed will tend to go back sooner anyway.

Condition	Recommended return to non-manual	Recommended return to manual	Factors affecting return to work
Inguinal, small umbilical or incisional hernia laparoscopic repair	3-5 days[1] [2]	1-2 weeks[3]	
	1 week		
Inguinal, small umbilical or incisional hernia open repair	2 weeks	2-3 weeks[3]	
Inguinal hernia open repair	3-7 days[5]	14 days[5]	
Bilateral inguinal hernia repair laparoscopic repair	1 week	1-2 weeks	
Bilateral inguinal hernia repair open repair		3-5 weeks[2]	
Recurrent inguinal hernia laparoscopic repair	1-2 weeks	1-6 weeks	
Recurrent inguinal hernia open repair	1-3 weeks	3-12 weeks	
Large umbilical or incisional hernia laparoscopic repair	2-3 weeks[4]		
Large umbilical or incisional hernia open repair	3-5 weeks[4]		
Epigastric hernia	3-5 days[4]	10-14 days[4]	
	2 weeks	4 weeks	
Femoral hernia	2 weeks	3 weeks	
Umbilical hernia	2 weeks	6 weeks	
Cholecystectomy – laparoscopic	1-2 weeks[4]	2-3 weeks[3]	
		4 weeks	
	2 weeks[5]	2-4 weeks[5]	
Cholecystectomy – open	3 weeks	3-5 weeks[3]	
		8-12 weeks	
Laparoscopic fundoplication	10-14 days[4]	3-4 weeks[4]	providing solid foods are tolerated

Laparoscopic bowel resection	2 weeks	6 weeks	
Major laparotomy		6-8 weeks[4]	
Gastrectomy, fit before surgery	6-8 weeks[4]		
Gastrectomy or oesophagogastrectomy for malignancy	8-12 weeks[4]	unlikely[4]	Dumping from early filling of duodenum and short peak of glucose absorption
Duodenotomy for ulceration	4-6 weeks[4]	6-8 weeks[4]	
Appendicectomy – laparoscopic	7 days[4]	1-2 weeks[3]	
Appendicectomy – open	2 weeks[4]	2-3 weeks[3]	
Right hemicolectomy with end-to-end anastomosis	3-6 weeks[4]	4-8 weeks[4]	
Left hemicolectomy or anterior resection of rectum	4-6 weeks[4]	6-10 weeks[4]	stoma may delay returning to work, stoma normally closed after 3-6 months
Defunctioning stoma closure	3-4 weeks[4]		
Abdominoperineal excision of rectum with permanent colostomy	8-12 weeks[4]		General fitness and ability to cope with stoma
Anal verge haematoma	2-3 days[4]	2-3 days[4]	
Thrombosed internal haemorrhoids	Up to 2 weeks[4]	Up to 2 weeks[4]	
Haemorrhoidectomy	2-3 weeks[4]	2-3 weeks[4]	Full healing may take 5-6 weeks but should usually still be able to work
		4 weeks	
Anal fissure – lateral internal sphincterotomy	1-2 days[4]	1-2 days[4]	
Pilonidal sinus primary suture	2-4 weeks[4]	3-6 weeks[4]	
	1-3 weeks		
Pilonidal sinus secondary intention	3 weeks	6-8 weeks[4]	Earlier return if arrangements for dressing wound at work
		3-6 weeks	

Anal fistula – small, little dressing required	1 week[4]	1 week[4]	
Anal fistula – large, dressing changed by district nurse	variable[4]	variable[4]	
Abdominoplasty	2-3 weeks[6]	8 weeks[6]	

[1] Shulman AG, Amid PK, Lichtenstein IL. Returning to work after herniorrhaphy BMJ 1994;309:216-217.

[2] Wellwood J, Sculpher MJ, Stoker D, Nicholls GJ, Geddes C, Whitehead A, Singh R, Spiegelhalter D. Randomised controlled trial of laparoscopic versus open mesh repair for inguinal hernia. BMJ 1998;317:103-10.

[3] Department for Work and Pensions. Return to work following elective surgical procedures.

[4] Samuel AM, Wellwood JMcK. Fitness for work after surgery. In Palmer KT, Cox RAF and Brown I. (Eds) Fitness for Work 4th edn. Oxford University Press, Oxford 2007 pp 467-486.

[5] Royal College of Surgeons of England.

[6] Newcastle upon Tyne NHS Foundation Trust

Condition	Recommended return to non-manual	Recommended return to manual	Factors affecting return to work
Abdominal laparoscopy	2-3 days[1]	within a week[1]	If more complex procedure such as removal of ovarian cyst, return to light work after 1 week, manual work after 2-3 weeks
Endometrial ablation	1-2 days[1]	2-5 days[1]	
Hysterectomy – abdominal	2-4 weeks[1]	6-8 weeks[1]	Reduced hours recommended if early return
Hysterectomy – laparoscopic	2-4 weeks[1]	4-6 weeks[1]	Reduced hours recommended if early return
Hysterectomy – vaginal	2-4 weeks[1]	4-6 weeks[1]	Reduced hours recommended if early return
Mid-urethral sling	3-4 days[1]	2-3 weeks[1]	
Miscarriage D&C	1-2 days[1]	1-2 days[1]	Psychological issues can have a significant effect on return, but the importance of positive support from colleagues should be considered

			Avoid very heavy lifting (more than 20kg) until 6 weeks.
Pelvic floor repair	2-3 weeks[1]	3-4 weeks[1]	
[1] Royal College of Obstetricians and Gynaecologists. http://www.rcog.org.uk/recovering-well			

Recommendations based on formal analysis of evidence are in red. Where only some evidence is available, the figures are in blue, and the relevant references are provided. Consensus-based guidelines are in black.

The workingfit website has pages of recommendations and advice about all aspects of work and I haven't found a better general GP or OH resource for employment advice. My thanks to them for their help and permission to reproduce this.

Risk of suicide by occupation: (See Depression)

From data collated by the National Institute for Occupational Safety and Health. 1984-1998.

Marine engineers are 1.9X more likely than the average person to kill themselves.

Physicians are 1.87X. But surgeons have the highest risk, with access to the means of self destruction, a recent major error or complaint being factors and marriage and children being protective (Arch Surg Jan 2011). But suicides amongst doctors in general do seem to have increased since the profession has become feminised. This is something I allude to elsewhere vis a vis the GMC and "Emotional Resilience". – The suicide rate in female doctors is higher than the general population, in male doctors it is lower than the general population. This difference is statistically significant. A diagnosed psychiatric illness is present, not surprisingly, in the majority. The specialities at most risk in the UK are (surgeons) anaesthetists, community health doctors, GPs and psychiatrists. All these having increased rates compared with "general hospital doctors". Female Physicians however are increasingly retiring earlier than their male colleagues "Due to stress" (RCP Census 2015/6.)

Dentists are 1.67X

Vets are 1.54X

Finance workers 1.51X

Chiropracters 1.5X

Heavy construction worker supervisors are 1.46X

Urban planners 1.43X

Hand moulders 1.4X (No, I don't know either).

Estate Agents 1.38X

Electrical equipment assemblers 1.36X

Lawyers and Lathe operators are 1.33X

Farm managers 1.32X

It is well known that Farmers suffer high rates of suicide. This is multifactorial: Isolation, health problems, long hours alone in the cab of a tractor on deserted fields or hillsides, the poor weather and having to be outside in it, getting up in the dark and back home in the dark – the long hours, poor pay, endless legislation and unpredictable income, as well as the cold heartedness of slaughtering the animals you have worked hard to preserve. Seasonal (Spring), violent suicide is something particularly associated with male farmers.

Heat treating equipment operators 1.32X

Electricians 1.31X
Precision woodworkers 1.3X
Pharmacists 1.29X
Natural Scientists 1.28X

Between 2001 and 2005 the suicide pattern stated changing. Construction workers and plant and machine operatives had greater numbers of suicides. The highest PMRs however were for health professionals (PMR=164) and agricultural workers (PMR=133) (-**Proportional Mortality Rates**, taking into account the number of people in the profession). Among women, administrative and secretarial workers had the greatest number of suicides yet the highest PMRs were found for health (PMR=232), and sport and fitness (PMR=244) occupations.

Suicide seems more common in certain defined working groups. It has been long associated with the loneliness of farming and the stress of the psychiatric professions. It is also associated with dentistry, vets, librarians and construction workers but not with teaching or being a British police officer which are supposed to be stressful occupations.

When I researched work stress for a lecture I was asked to give to a regional meeting of head teachers a few years ago, I discovered that the main stress for teachers wasn't obnoxious or ill disciplined students but a lack of clear leadership from their own Headmaster, poor cohesion amongst the staff, absent colleague support and a lack of teamwork. In fact I realised that it was very similar to much of the stress of Medicine and General Practice in particular. You can deal with almost endless severe patient sickness, emotion, terminal illnesses, even rudeness, nastiness and personal unreasonableness from patients but only as long as you feel properly supported by a like minded, good set of partners.

Female doctors it appears are more likely to kill themselves than almost any other female group of workers. Yet another reason to rethink the current stealth feminisation of British medicine?

Actually in terms of true numbers, occupation is not a *particularly good* predictor of suicide risk when compared with, say, alcohol abuse, divorce, social isolation, previous suicide attempts.

References, Thanks and Acknowledgements:

Special thanks to my daughter Anna Woodbine who did the cover and the few better internal diagrams. She illustrates book covers for a living and wins national prizes for her work. (Annawoodbine.co.uk and thewoodbineworkshop.co.uk)
Throughout the book I have done my best to give appropriate and accurate treatment regimes and doses. Most are traditional and conventional. I would urge you however, before prescribing to consider and check each course of medication and confirm it is appropriate and safe for the patient you are treating. I take no responsibility for erroneous doses or inappropriate treatment as every prescriber is individually responsible for his or her actions and any text is but a guide. This duty of care is of course what defines a profession.
Most references are quoted in the text, those that aren't include contributions from:
Omar Ali prescribing specialist at SASH for help with prescribing information

I understand that you are interested in gaining permission to reuse some PHE material. Our materials are Crown copyright. This means you may reuse this information (excluding logos) free of charge in any format or medium, under the terms of the Open Government Licence v3.0. To view this licence, visit OGL or email psi@nationalarchives.gsi.gov.uk. Where we have identified any third party copyright information you will need to obtain permission from the copyright holders concerned.
Thanks
Phil
Philip Hemmings
Head of publications
Public Health England
philip.hemmings@phe.gov.uk

The GMC to look into higher number of complaints against overseas trained doctors. This information has been published in the BMJ and Lancet.
Peter Moszynski BMJ. 2007 August 18; 335(7615): 320.
Author: The Health and Social Care Information Centre – Workforce Directorate
The Health and Social Care Information Centre (HSCIC) was previously known as The NHS Information Centre (The NHS IC)
Responsible statistician: Kate Anderson
Version: 1.0
Date of Publication: 21 March 2012
Tramadol Prescribers Journal 1999 39/2
Diamorphine Its pharmacology and clinical use Ed Dr Bruce Scott
BCG Vaccination in England since 2005 A survey of policy and practice BMJ 10/9/12
Drug Levels Half Lives. David F McAuley Global RPh Inc
Anaphylaxis: Wikipedia
Paracetamol overdose www.healthoma.com
PPI and interactions BJCP Brit Journal Clin Pharmacology Nov 2006 62(5) 582-590
Paediatric Respiratory Rates www.healthny.gov/nysdoh/ems/pdfassmttools.pdf
P Wells PE and DVT asst tools, E Mailed pwells@ohri.ca on 20/10/12
Basic Biology: The Mitochondrial DNA Family Tree Marie-Claire King Scientific American.

Paragraph on Commissioning Simon Dean, Horsham and Chanctonbury CCG
CHADS VASC from StopAFib.org
Table 4: 2009 Birmingham Schema, CHA2DS2-VASc Scoring System
Source: adapted from Table 1(b), Refining clinical risk stratification for predicting stroke
and thromboembolism in atrial fibrillation using a novel risk factor based approach: The
Euro Heart Survey on Atrial Fibrillation, *Chest*

Safety of Soya feeds Enquiry Reference: 1-560463965
SMA.Information@pfizer.com

Enquiry Reference: 1-560463965 Pfizer information regarding infant feeding and
Wysoy
Regarding Soya feeds
Half lives of antidepressants: Harvard Health Publications Nov 2010 "Going off
Antidepressants"
My Thanks to Patricia Barby medical researcher and font of knowledge (Action
Research) for her expertise in accessing details of obscure research and factual data in
various areas for this book.
Type 2 DM and Magnesium:
The results of a meta-analysis published online on January 23, 2013 in the Journal of
Nutrition reveal an association between diets that include higher amounts of magnesium
and lower levels of fasting glucose and insulin.
An article published online on November 7, 2012 in the journal *BMJ Open* reveals an
association between black tea drinking and a lower incidence of diabetes around the world.
Chemotherapy Regimes modified from Wikipedia 2013
Particulate sizes from "Particulate article" Wikipedia 2013
Inpatient psychiatry The Guardian 29/7/2009
HIV and pregnancy: NHS Choices "Antenatal checks and tests"
Meningococcal meningitis: Meningitis Research Foundation, East Kent Hospital
University NHS Foundation Trust Staff Zone web sites
Appraisal information culled from a number of sources including various meetings and
talks one of which was given by Dr Lisa Argent.
Hepatitis in pregnancy from "Hepatitis Central" Web site
Herpes infection in pregnancy Baby Center website.
Listeria in pregnancy: The American Pregnancy Association web site, NHS Choices,
Fifth Disease: Fifth Disease.Org, CDC and *What to expect* web sites.
Swine flu in pregnancy: Mail on line
Toxoplasmosis CDC and Web MD websites etc
Head to Head Are there too many female medical graduates? Yes
*BMJ 2008; 336 doi: http://dx.doi.org/10.1136/bmj.39505.491065.94 (Published 3 April
2008)*
Cite this as: BMJ 2008;336:748
Viagra and serious visual side effects, FDA etc Bad Pharma, Ben Goldacre.
Questions@phqscreeners.com (Request for PHQ9)
The PHQ is now held in public domain and is freely available for use. No additional
permissions are needed for its inclusion in the guide you mentioned in your email. There

is an instruction manual available at the website phqscreeners.com that you may find helpful. At the end of the document there is a description for acknowledgements.

QUESTIONS REGARDING DEVELOPMENT, ACKNOWLEDGMENTS AND USE

The PHQ family of measures (see Table 1, page 3), including abbreviated and alternative versions as well as the GAD-7, were developed by Drs. Robert L. Spitzer, Janet B.W. Williams, Kurt Kroenke and colleagues, with an educational grant from Pfizer Inc.

All of the measures included in Table 1 are in the public domain. No permission is required to reproduce, translate, display or distribute.

Kind regards
Donna Burgett
Administrative Assistant to Kurt Kroenke, MD
Mediterranean Diet Benefits: Mayo Clinic retrospective study of 1.5m patients March 13.

Reported in (c) 2013 the St. Cloud Times (St. Cloud, Minn.)

Thoracic Aneurysms, size at rupture/dissection: The Annals of Thoracic Surgery, 1999. 67. 1922-1926

Infectious disease: Isolation, screening etc Mid Downs Protocol Aug 92

Weight reduction surgery and diets Atul Gawande "Complications"

Varicella in pregnancy: Crawley Hospital Dept Microbiology Memorandum March 2005

HRT Information (some) From a lecture given by Dr Malcolm Whitehead Feb 2005

Cancer screening guidelines: Sussex Cancer Network April 2007

Parenteral Drug Doses: DATB 2000, 38: 65-8

Clopidogrel duration and dose: South East London Cardiac Network Dec 2008

Splenectomy immunisation and antibiotics: advice from the Oxford public health department.

HIV statistics Clinical Medicine 12. 5 Oct 2012

Renal stones Clinical Medicine 12. 5 Oct 2012

Cystic Fibrosis Survival/Pancreatic cancer: The Practitioner 255/1742

Community Acquired Pneumonia Clinical Medicine Vol 12 No3 June 2012

Dabigatran metabolism: Personal communication Medical Information Dept Boehringer Ingelheim.

Prescribing in pregnancy The Prescriber Dec 2009

Down's Syndrome and the pill: Rothman KJ NEJM 1978 299:522

Multiple Sclerosis Clinical Medicine Vol 11 Aug 2011 p361

2 WR outcomes Clinical Medicine Vol 11 Aug 2011 p412

Gestational Diabetes: The Practitioner Jan 2012 256 pp12

Renal colic and Desmopressin The Practitioner April 2010 254 issue 1728 pp 10

Hyponatraemia Clinical Medicine Vol 11, No 5 pp 448

Inaccurate path results, sodium, calcium and the parathyroids Clinical vol 13 No 3

Frequent Attenders (etc) PL Heywood et al Family Practice, Vol 15 No 3

Chronic multiple functional somatic symptoms BMJ 325 Aug 2002 pp 323

The Drug treatment of STDs Prescriber 19/9/2011 pp 35

Cognitive decline, The Whitehall II prospective study BMJ2011 5/1/2012

Consent: Medical Law, Charles Foster. Oxford. pp50

Listeria Dept Health Circular to all Gps 16/Feb/1989

Migration and public health. Editorial Clinical Medicine Vol 13 Apr 2013

Cluster Headache: Various papers including a summary by Matharu and Goadsby.

Pertussis contacts: Who to treat: PHLS Guidelines July 2000 WSHA, Dodhia, Miller. Epidemiol infect 1998 120 143-149

Accessing primary care BMJ 4 OCT 2008 Vol337 pp768

Infected children Guidelines in Practice Feb 2008, Vol11, GD Update May 2008 pp51 etc

Septic Hips and Limps in children BMJ Aug 2010 Vol 341 pp 444

Paediatric Hip Problems Update 16 May 2002 pp654-657

Childhood infections: (Exanthems) Dermatology in Practice Vol 11 No 5 pp10 etc

Family History of Ovarian Cancer: Current Obstetrics and Gynaecology 2005 15, 54-59

Infertility: NICE, Parenting website, 10.1093 Humrep/deh 304 PMID 15205397

Iron (Pathology) Multiple sources, Incl Guidelines for Clinical Laboratory Practice June 1995 Ontario association of medical laboratories

X Rays in Cong heart disease, Radiographics Sept 2007, 27, 1323-1334

Congenital Heart Disease Dr George Sutherland Article GP June 29. 1979

Methotrimeprazine and other drug details: Clin Pharmacol Ther 1966 7(4) 436-46

Acta Med Scanda 205 191-194 1979

Canadian Anaesthetic Soc Journal 1962, 9, 153-160

Annals of Emergency Medicine 11/11/1991 1201/57

Capillary Refill Time: Pediatrics, Larry Baraff May 1993. Ann Emerg Med1988 Sep 17(9) 932-5

Emergency Medicine Journal:2008. 25: 325-326 doi:10.1136/emj.2007. 055244

Prostate cancer: Prostate Cancer Risk Management Publication (Cancer Research UK/NHS 2009)

Suicide and Occupation: Business Insider Oct 18 2011, Br J Psych. July 2008 193 (1) 73-6

Hot Children: American Family Physician Nov 15 1999

BMJ 9/4/1983 Editorial

Statin side effects: Mayo Clinic Web site: High Cholesterol, "Statin Side Effects: Weigh the benefits and risks."

Lateral Epicondylitis Christopher Greenfield and Valerie Webster Physiotherapy 88 10, 578-594

The Evolution of the NHS diagram. My thanks to the Royal College of Physicians.

Thanks to Arthritis Research UK for permission to reproduce their Exercises for Back, Knee and Neck Pain. They are from the Information and Exercise Sheet series published by the Arthritis Research Council. www.arthritisreasearchuk.org which is **uniformly excellent.**

They also do a core skills musculoskeletal online learning program for GPs with free online learning modules.

Anti convulsant guidelines with permission of Dr Oliver Charles Cockerell (Personal communication Nov 2013) and Prescriber magazine.

My thanks to Professor Paul Durrington of Manchester University for his permission to use the universal cardiovascular 10 year risk charts.

Prostate and hormones: Lee John R Hormone Balance for Men www.johnleemd.com2003 pp15 etc
Dress code/Cross infection OBG Management Editorial Nov 2008Vol 20 11
Warfarin and Bleeding: Australian Prescriber August 2004 27, 88-92
Cystic Fibrosis: New Treatments etc Clinical Medicine 14, 1, 76-78
Most of the other facts and opinions are gleaned from 40 years of clinical experience as an NHS doctor, from thousands of talks and lectures and from what all doctors do: build up a basis of knowledge, bias and opinion from our own first hand and from learnt second hand experience. This latter has to be from experienced colleagues who we (usually have worked with and) respect and not from politically, organisationally or financially motivated individuals some of whom happen to be medically qualified.

Thank you to The Royal College of Physicians for permission to use part of various publications including Atrial Fibrillation guidelines etc.

BUPA for their permission to use their diabetes risk score questionnaire

AUB Algorithms:

Dr Heath

I am happy for you to use my algorithm, (Management of acute abnormal uterine bleeding in non pregnant reproductive-aged women. Committee Opinion No. 557. American College of Obstetricians and Gynecologists. Obstet Gynecol 2013; 121:891–6.)

Thanks

Jenni

Jen Tickal Keehbauch, MD, FAAFP Director Women's Health Fellowship Assistant Director, Family Medicine Residency 133 Benmore Drive, Suite 201 Winter Park, Florida 32792

Thank you to Tony Williams Occupational Physicians at the Brilliant "Working Fit" Ltd for help and advice

Diabetes UK for permission to reproduce "Meds and kit"

Christine McDermott for all her help and permission to reproduce the various Paediatric Emergency Guidelines (NHS Coastal W Sussex CCG)

NICE for their various consents to use a number of their adapted guidelines for many conditions.

The Royal College of Physicians (again) for various permissions over the last three years to use extracts, Guidelines and Algorithms published by them.

The Resuscitation Council of Great Britain for permission to use their "Industry Standard" "Resus Guidelines" which are **superb and available to all,** regularly updated.

Professor Garrow at Bart's for permission to use his BMI charts and data.

Keith Hopcroft, David Copperfield, and many others for their encouragement and many for saying "You can't say that – but then again I don't know why, that is what we all think"

The physiotherapy department at the Nuffield Haywards Heath, for their exercise sheets.

Public Health England for permission to reproduce up to date immunisation schedules

The various admissions staff at the medical schools who replied to my E Mails and phone calls about selection processes. But not to the many who didn't.

My long suffering wife, family and friends who let me spend more than over five years of all my spare time researching and putting all the saved information together and let me bend their ears about what soft politics is doing to our once admirable NHS.

NICE Enquiry Ref EH41901

permis-
sions   x

| NICE Mail <nice@nice.org.uk> | 10/01/2014 | |
| to me | | |

Dear Chris

Thank you for contacting the National Institute for Health and Care Excellence (NICE).

I have forwarded your request to my colleagues in the publishing team. They will be in touch to discuss this shortly.

If you have any further queries then please contact the NICE Enquiry Handling team again.

Kind regards

Andrew

Andrew McGuinness

Communications Administrator (Enquiry Handling)

National   Institute   for   Health   and   Care   Excellence Level 1A | City Tower | Piccadilly Plaza | Manchester M1 4BT | United Kingdom Tel: 0845 003 7781 | Fax: 44 (0) 845 003 7785

Web: http://nice.org.uk

Dear Sir,

I am a GP of nearly 40 years experience and am writing a handbook of General Practice. I would like to include a number of NICE's Guidance protocols and algorithms – for instance on the management of Atrial Fibrillation and TB etc. May I simply include straight copies of these as they exist in the public domain, as long as I give NICE credit for them? Many Thanks,

http://www.nice.org.uk

| Iain Moir <Iain.Moir@nice.org.uk> | 13/01/2014 | |
| to me | | |

Dear Dr Health

Thank you for your recent email.

I am sure that this will not be a problem but before I can process your request and issue a licence I will need a little more information:

- The exact content you wish to include with page references
- The title/'working title' of your forthcoming publication
- The name and address of your publisher

- The rights you require – print, electronic or both

NICE has copyright in in its own publications and it is our policy to charge commercial organisations a small fee for the use of our content as most publishers do themselves.

Depending on the detail you are able to provide I will see what I can do to either reduce or waive this – I am conscious that many authors are now asked to pay their own permissions fees. If you have contributed to the development of any NICE guidance, for instance, there would be no fee involved.

I look forward to hearing from you.

Best wishes

Iain

Iain Moir

Publishing Manager

National Institute for Health and Care Excellence

10 Spring Gardens | London SW1A 2BU

Tel: 44 (0) 20 7045 2208 | Fax: 44 (0) 845 003 7784

Web: http://nice.org.uk

From: NICE Mail

Sent: 10 January 2014 15:06

To: Chris Heath

Subject: NICE Enquiry Ref EH41901

to Iain

Thank you very much Iain.

I am a GP of nearly 40 years' experience and am writing a brief Handbook of General Practice entitled "Good Practice". I intend it to be in both print and electronic formats, also possibly an "App". I will start to look for a publisher via an agent as soon as I have completed the final draft of the book and to do this I need to arrange for the reproduction of approximately 100 diagrams and charts, -and some of which I am currently negotiating permission from various sources. Thus far no clinician or organisation has refused. The NICE Charts are all from publications that NICE has already sent to every GP and I presume hospital doctor in the NHS. I need to know if I can reproduce (probably) half a dozen of NICE's clinical algorithms from their clinical guidance booklets, – on Atrial Fibrillation management and Chronic Kidney Disease certainly but for various other acute and chronic clinical situations. Do you need to know precisely which ones now? The right would be print and electronic and if you need the exact charts and algorithms I will have them for you once I have decided the final content of the book in a month or two. May I have a preliminary understanding that properly credited and accurately reproduced, NICE normally has no objection to the dissemination of its own guidance?

Best Wishes,

Dr Chris Heath

Iain Moir <Iain.Moir@nice.org.uk>	15/01/2014
to me	

Dear Dr Heath

Thanks for your email clarifying one or two points.

NICE will be quite happy to give you permission to use our content in your forth-coming book which we do on a regular basis for many authors and publishers. Nearer the time of publication, when you have a publisher and a contract with them, I will need to firm up the exact NICE content you wish to include so that we can issue you with a short electronic licence. If you intent to use material from the full clinical guidelines, I will need to direct you to the relevant National Collaborating Centre which have copyright in these outputs – NICE owns the copyright in all the derivative outputs.

I look forward to hearing from you again nearer publication.

Best wishes

Iain

From: Chris Heath Sent: 13 January 2014 12:28
To: Iain Moir
Subject: Re: FW: NICE Enquiry Ref EH41901

to Iain

Dear Iain,

The charts I would like to reproduce are these:

Emergency Treatment for people with Acute Stroke, (Nice c g 68)

Testing and Treating asymptomatic household and other close contacts of all cases with active TB (Nice c g 33)

People with TIA – assessment, early management and imaging (Nice cg 68)

The Atrial Fibrillation Algorithms Cardioversion treatment

Rhythm control in persistent AF

Rate control in permanent AF

Rhythm control in paroxysmal AF

Stroke risk stratification

and the Traffic Light System for identifying likelihood of serious illness in feverish children (Nice c g 47)

May I have you outline permission to do this and would you be kind enough to send me new copies of these nine algorithms?

Thank You very much

Dr Chris Heath

```
                    to Iain
```

Dear Ian,

I am now on the point of publishing. May I have your Final permission to go ahead with using about four or five NICE proforma in "Good Practice. These will be unchanged and NICE will, of course be fully credited.

Many Thanks

Dr Chris Heath

FRAX: IOF grants permission to use the FRAX Screenshot for the stated purpose, only if Licensee complies with the following requirements:

1. Licensee shall use the following text to describe FRAX®.

FRAX® is a sophisticated risk assessment instrument, developed by the University of Sheffield in association with the World Health Organization. It uses risk factors in addition to DXA measurements for improved fracture risk estimation. It is a useful tool to aid clinical decision making about the use of pharmacologic therapies in patients with low bone mass. The International Osteoporosis Foundation supports the maintenance and development of FRAX®. © International Osteoporosis Foundation, Reprinted with permission from the IOF. All rights reserved.

2. No mention of drug or patient information

Iain Moir <Iain.Moir@nice.org.uk>

7 Sep 2017

```
                    to me
```

Dear Dr Health

Thank you for your email and my apologies for the delay in coming back to you.

NICE UK Open Content Licence (https://www.nice.org.uk/re-using-our-content/uk-open-content-licence)

NICE has recently made all its content available for reuse free of charge to individuals and commercial/non-commercial organisations under this self-assessment licence provided the use is restricted to a UK audience. We do encourage users to complete the short online questionnaire on the web page. Use of our content outside of the UK is subject to a separate licensing arrangement and a fee – https://www.nice.org.uk/re-using-our-content#international Please let me know if you intend to use the content overseas.

Please also check the NICE guidance pages to ensure you are using the most current content in you publication.

Good luck with the book.

Best wishes

Iain

Iain Moir
Programme Manager: syndication, content and licensing
Evidence Resources
National Institute for Health and Care Excellence
10 Spring Gardens
London
SW1A 2BU

Tel: 020 7045 2208
Email: iain.moir@nice.org.uk

Lightning Source UK Ltd.
Milton Keynes UK
UKHW021842111119
353340UK00002B/19/P